KU-505-748

CROFTON AND DOUGLAS'S RESPIRATORY DISEASES

EDITED BY

ANTHONY SEATON CBE, BA, MD, FRCP, FRCPE, FFOM, FMedSci
Professor of Environmental & Occupational Medicine, University of Aberdeen, Scotland
Honorary Consultant Physician, Aberdeen Royal Hospital NHS Trust

DOUGLAS SEATON MD, FRCP
Consultant Physician, Department of Respiratory Medicine, The Ipswich Hospital NHS Trust, Suffolk, England

The late A. GORDON LEITCH BSc, MB, PhD, FRCPE, FCCP

FIFTH EDITION

IN TWO VOLUMES
VOLUME 2

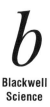

Blackwell Science

© 2000 by
Blackwell Science Ltd
Editorial Offices:
Osney Mead, Oxford OX2 0EL
25 John Street, London WC1N 2BL
23 Ainslie Place, Edinburgh EH3 6AJ
350 Main Street, Malden
   MA 02148 5018, USA
54 University Street, Carlton
   Victoria 3053, Australia
10, rue Casimir Delavigne
   75006 Paris, France

Other Editorial Offices:
Blackwell Wissenschafts-Verlag GmbH
Kurfürstendamm 57
10707 Berlin, Germany

Blackwell Science KK
MG Kodenmacho Building
7–10 Kodenmacho Nihombashi
Chuo-ku, Tokyo 104, Japan

First published 2000

Set by Excel Typesetters Co., Hong Kong
Printed and bound in Great Britain by
MPG Books Ltd, Bodmin, Cornwall

The Blackwell Science logo is a
trade mark of Blackwell Science Ltd,
registered at the United Kingdom
Trade Marks Registry

The right of the Authors to be
identified as the Authors of this Work
has been asserted in accordance
with the Copyright, Designs and
Patents Act 1988.

All rights reserved. No part of
this publication may be reproduced,
stored in a retrieval system, or
transmitted, in any form or by any
means, electronic, mechanical,
photocopying, recording or otherwise,
except as permitted by the UK
Copyright, Designs and Patents Act
1988, without the prior permission
of the copyright owner.

A catalogue record for this title
is available from the British Library

ISBN 0-86542-857-3

Library of Congress
Cataloging-in-publication Data

Crofton and Douglas's respiratory
diseases.—5th ed./edited by
   Anthony Seaton, Douglas Seaton, A.
   Gordon Leitch.
         p.   cm.
      Includes bibliographical references.
      1. Respiratory organs—Diseases.
   I. Seaton, Anthony.   II. Seaton,
   Douglas.   III. Leitch, A. Gordon
   (Andrew Gordon)   IV. Crofton, John,
   Sir, 1912–   Respiratory diseases.
   V. Title: Respiratory diseases.
      [DNLM: 1. Respiratory Tract
   Diseases.   WF 140 C9413 2000]
   RC731.C7   2000
   616.2—dc21
   DNLM/DLC
   for Library of Congress
99-15579
      CIP

DISTRIBUTORS
Marston Book Services Ltd
PO Box 269
Abingdon, Oxon OX14 4YN
(Orders: Tel: 01235 465500
          Fax: 01235 465555)

USA
Blackwell Science, Inc.
Commerce Place
350 Main Street
Malden, MA 02148 5018
(Orders: Tel: 800 759 6102
              781 388 8250
         Fax: 781 388 8255)

Canada
Login Brothers Book Company
324 Saulteaux Crescent
Winnipeg, Manitoba R3J 3T2
(Orders: Tel: 204 837 2987)

Australia
Blackwell Science Pty Ltd
54 University Street
Carlton, Victoria 3053
(Orders: Tel: 3 9347 0300
          Fax: 3 9347 5001)

For further information on
Blackwell Science, visit our website:
www.blackwell-science.com

CONTENTS

Colour plate section falls between pages 630 and 631, Vol. 1.

CONTRIBUTORS

PETER G.J. BURNEY MA, MD, FRCP, FFPHM, *Department of Public Health Sciences, King's College London, Capital House, 42 Weston Street, London SE1 3QD*

IAN A. CAMPBELL BSc, MD (Lond.), FRCP, *Consultant Chest Physician, Llandough Hospital, Cardiff CF64 2XX*

GRAHAM CROMPTON MBCHB, FRCPE, *Consultant Physician, Department of Respiratory Medicine, Western General Hospital, Crewe Road, Edinburgh EH4 2XU*

NEIL J. DOUGLAS MD, FRCPE, *Department of Respiratory Medicine, Royal Infirmary of Edinburgh, Lauriston Place, Edinburgh EH3 9YW*

RONALD J. FERGUSSON MD, FRCPE, *Consultant Physician, Respiratory Medicine Unit, Western General Hospital, Edinburgh EH4 2XU*

ANDREW P. GREENING FRCPE, *Consultant Physician and Senior Lecturer Department of Respiratory Medicine, Western General Hospital, Crewe Road, Edinburgh EH4 2XU*

CHRISTOPHER HASLETT BSc (Hons), MbchB (Hons) FRCP, FRCPE, FMedSci, *Head of Department of Respiratory Medicine Unit, University of Edinburgh, Royal Infirmary Edinburgh, Lauriston Place, Edinburgh EH3 9YW*

TIMOTHY W. HIGGENBOTTAM BSc, MA, MD, FRCP, *Consultant Physician, Section of Respiratory and Molecular Medicine, Department of Medicine and Pharmacology, University of Sheffield, Royal Hallamshire Hospital, Sheffield S10 2JF*

JULIAN M. HOPKIN MD, MSc, MA, FRCP, FRCPE, *Professor of Experimental Medicine, Experimental Medicine Unit, University of Wales, Swansea SA2 8PP*

A. GORDON LEITCH [Deceased] *RVCC, Chalmers Hospital, Lauriston Place, Edinburgh EH3 9HA*

WILLIAM MACNEE MD, FRCPE, *Department of Respiratory Medicine, Royal Infirmary of Edinburgh, Lauriston Place, Edinburgh EH3 9YW*

GEORGE RUSSELL MB, FRCP, FRCPE, FRCPCH, *Department of Child Health, Royal Aberdeen Children's Hospital, University of Aberdeen, Cornhill Road, Aberdeen AB25 2ZD*

R. ANDREW SEATON MD, MRCP, DTM & H, *Directorate of Medicine, Tayside University Hospitals NHS Trust, Ninewells Hospital, Dundee DD1 9SY*

ANTHONY SEATON CBE, BA, MD, FRCP, FRCPE, FFOM, FMedSci, *Professor of Environmental and Occupational Medicine, Aberdeen Royal Infirmary, Foresterhill, Aberdeen AB25 2ZD*

DOUGLAS SEATON MD, FRCP, *Consultant Physician, Department of Respiratory Medicine, The Ipswich Hospital NHS Trust, Heath Road, Ipswich IP4 5PD*

JOHN M. SHNEERSON MA, DM, FRCP, *Director, Respiratory Support and Sleep Centre, Papworth Hospital, Papworth Everard, Cambridge CB3 8RE*

STEPHEN J. WATT BSc, FRCPEd, AFOM, *Department of Environmental & Occupational Health, University of Aberdeen, Foresterhill, Aberdeen AB25 2ZD*

ARTHUR J.A. WIGHTMAN MBBS, DMRD, FRCR, *Consultant Radiologist, Royal Infirmary Edinburgh, Lauriston Place, Edinburgh EH3 9YW*

PREFACE

A decade has passed since we wrote the previous edition of Crofton and Douglas, in conjunction with our late colleague Gordon Leitch. Gordon's untimely death, giving his life while saving those of others, was a very sad blow not only to his family but also to his many friends and colleagues in Scotland and over the world. His work in the control and management of tuberculosis continued in the footsteps of Sir Robert Philip and Sir John Crofton, and he would undoubtedly have made a most important contribution to the international battle against the disease had he survived. He was also a splendid all-round physician; something of the flavour of this comes across in the chapters he contributed to this book and which he delivered to us just the day before he left on his tragic holiday.

The first edition of this book was published in 1969, at the end of an era in which medical research had made the most notable contributions to the direct care of patients and to the prevention of disease, marked by the discovery of antibiotics and antituberculous chemotherapy, the demonstration of the harmful effects of smoking, and the elucidation of the structure of DNA. The original volume was a relatively slim one, written by our distinguished predecessors, John Crofton and Andrew Douglas, who had themselves played a major role in the battle against tuberculosis. At that time, respiratory medicine was looking towards an uncertain future, as tuberculosis declined and other respiratory diseases remained firmly in the realm of the generalist. *Crofton and Douglas's Respiratory Diseases* was perhaps the major factor in helping chest physicians of that era find their new role, allowing us to assert the importance of respiratory disease as a cause of morbidity and mortality in both the developed and poor worlds.

The intervening three decades have seen great changes in the practice and basic science of respiratory medicine, which is now recognized as a main-line acute specialty responsible for the care of a high proportion of the sick in all countries. That our patients are often from the least privileged sections of society has meant that funds for research and clinical care have not always been so easy to obtain as in more glamorous disciplines, but we can look back with some satisfaction to the control of tuberculosis in Britain and the improved outlook for young victims of cystic fibrosis. We have, however, made little impact on the prognosis of lung cancer, have not had as much success as we would have liked in the battle against the amoral tobacco industry, and have watched in dismay as poor medical practice in other countries has encouraged the development of multi-drug resistant tuberculosis. And, in spite of all the research in the subject, we have seen asthma become progressively more prevalent in children. In our day-to-day care of sick patients, we must not take our eyes off the public health aspects of our specialty.

The previous edition of this book was well-received, and its translation into Greek and Italian, together with its production in a low-cost Asian edition, served as a reminder to us of the need to write for a world-wide readership. In this edition, we have reflected the increase in understanding of disease processes that has accrued from basic research, but we have also endeavoured to maintain the tradition of writing for the practising physician, who sees a multitude of patients with diseases common and rare, and who needs guidance on diagnosis and management. We are grateful to a number of friends and colleagues for agreeing to contribute to this edition and believe that their chapters, emphasizing the common and important, will contribute greatly to the value of the book.

One of the benefits of writing a book such as this is the amount one learns or re-learns by reading the references necessary to check up on one's statements. We have maintained a substantial bibliography, and this includes a number of older references that give graphic original accounts of diseases. It is not uncommon for old lessons to be forgotten and omitted from modern databases; while no textbook can hope to be as up-to-date as these databases, we hope we will help readers to avoid missing important earlier work while still keeping abreast of recent advances. We see this as a book to be used on the ward and in the office, where clinical problems arise and questions are asked and need clear answers.

Anthony Seaton
Douglas Seaton

ix

ACKNOWLEDGEMENTS

The observant reader will have noticed the similar names of the two editors. We should like to acknowledge certain aspects of our genetic and environmental heritage. Our late father, Dr Ronald Seaton FRCP, was a pioneer in anti-malarial chemotherapy. He inspired us to become doctors and passed on to us a broad, lively and sometimes slightly cynical interest in medicine. From our mother, Julia, a nurse who worked with Lord Moynihan in Leeds and is still busy looking after others as she approaches her tenth decade, we have inherited an aversion to a moment's idleness. We have been fortunate in our teachers, notably the late Harold Edwards who introduced us to biology and evolutionary theory at school, Dr Colin Ogilvie of Liverpool who first interested us in respiratory medicine, and Professor Keith Morgan who introduced us to the scientific basis of clinical and preventive medicine in the wilds of West Virginia, USA. Many other teachers and colleagues have of course influenced us and continue to do so, not least our juniors who impose a constant challenge to keep up-to-date.

With respect to the production of this book, we acknowledge with gratitude the tolerance of Blackwell's over our problems with deadlines and, especially, the courtesy and efficiency of Anna Woodford and the production staff. Our thanks also to the copy editor Jo Phillips for his attention to detail and his patience. We should also like to acknowledge the help of Dr Keith Kerr in providing pathological photomicrographs, Dr Lesley Gomersall for help in providing radiographs, and the Medical Illustration Department of Aberdeen University Medical School.

Most importantly, we record our gratitude to our wives, Jill and Anja, for putting up with our prolonged absence at our computers and for nevertheless helping and supporting us throughout this protracted endeavour. We promise to spend more time with them in future.

29

BRONCHIOLAR DISEASE

ANTHONY SEATON

The bronchioles have been regarded aptly as a silent part of the lung, unassociated with well-recognized diseases, invisible on radiography and the function of which is difficult to measure physiologically. Older readers may recall the interest engendered in the 1960s when it was suggested by Hogg and his Montreal colleagues [1] that the bronchioles were the site of the lesion that leads to chronic airflow obstruction in smokers, and the subsequent search for a simple test of small airways function that could be used for screening purposes. Paediatricians also have long been aware of the infective bronchiolitis syndrome in infants, most usually associated with respiratory syncytial virus. More recently, however, it has become apparent that there are a number of relatively unusual but important bronchiolitic syndromes in adults apart from that associated with smoking.

The bronchioles are airways without cartilage, lined by bronchial epithelium and leading into air sacs. They comprise three to four orders of conducting or membranous bronchioles, the terminal ones in turn bifurcating into the first of two to three orders of respiratory bronchioles. These last give rise directly to some alveoli before ending in air sacs. There are approximately 25 000 terminal bronchioles. Therefore it is not unreasonable to suppose that they may be affected not only directly but also indirectly, either by disease arising primarily in alveoli or by extension of disease occurring in the cartilagenous airways. The former situation is recognized for example in extrinsic allergic alveolitis, which were it not so difficult to pronounce might more accurately be called allergic bronchioloalveolitis; the latter situation is found in cigarette-induced lung disease.

Three factors have contributed to an increased recognition of the importance of bronchiolar disease. The first was the work on the physiology of small airways as part of a search for a means of early detection of those who would become disabled by airflow obstruction [2]. The second was the recognition of a wide spectrum of pulmonary syndromes that caused breathlessness but which did not fit easily into traditional classifications of lung disease [3,4],

and the third was the increasing availability of relatively safe and more acceptable methods of lung biopsy.

Physiological considerations

Because there are so many bronchioles, each with a diameter of about 1 mm, it would clearly require a considerable number to be obstructed before this would have a result comparable to the effect that obstruction of the larger-diameter major conducting airways has on crude overall measurements of airflow obstruction, such as forced expiratory volume in 1 s (FEV_1). Thus substantial obliteration may occur before symptoms and evidence of airflow limitation become apparent. However, other functional impairment may be detected earlier. For example, air may be trapped distal to partly occluded airways leading to a rise in residual volume and closing volume. Similarly, the presence of some narrowed small airways may produce different time constants in different parts of the lung and this may cause reductions in dynamic compliance when measured at increasing respiratory rates. These tests have provided useful information but have, perhaps undeservedly in the case of closing volume, fallen into disuse. Flow rates measured at low lung volumes may also indicate small airway obstruction, although this test proves too variable in practice to be of diagnostic value. Diffusing capacity for carbon monoxide may also be reduced, either if alveoli are involved in the pathological process or if access of the gas to the alveoli is reduced in the 10 s available during the single-breath test.

It should be apparent from this discussion that there is no one test or even combination of tests that provides diagnostic information in patients with bronchiolar disease. The patterns of abnormality described in the literature are quite variable, and need to be considered with other evidence in coming to a diagnosis.

Syndromes of bronchiolitis

There is no generally agreed clinical classification of

829

bronchiolar diseases, and many of the described syndromes are relatively unfamiliar to chest physicians. Review of the literature suggests that the 'splitters' have had a field-day, many syndromes being described on the basis of a search through pathological and clinical archives in order to describe a few cases with apparently similar features under a new name. Sometimes the same condition appears at different dates described by different names. It is important for the clinician to remember that there are in fact relatively few pathological manifestations of bronchiolar disease and that these represent inflammatory reactions to a wide range of possible causes. Clinical classifications have tended to depend on cause, known or unknown, while pathological classifications have relied on distinctive histological features. A relatively simple clinical classification suggested by the author is given in Table 29.1.

The obliterative type of bronchiolitis may be separated pathologically into two subtypes: one in which there are intrabronchiolar plugs of organizing connective tissue (proliferative bronchiolitis obliterans) and one in which the bronchiolar walls are inflamed and fibrosed with marked narrowing or complete obliteration of the lumen (constrictive bronchiolitis). The former is often accompanied by extension of the proliferative changes into alveolar ducts and alveoli, a lesion referred to as bronchiolitis obliterans with organizing pneumonia (BOOP) or, confusingly, cryptogenic organizing pneumonia.

Non-obliterative bronchiolitis

Infective bronchiolitis

Viral infections may cause direct inflammation of the airway mucosa at any point, sometimes leading to desquamation and increased airway reactivity. In children the most common syndrome is bronchiolitis due to respiratory syncytial virus occurring before the age of 1 year

Table 29.1 Aetiological classification of bronchiolar diseases.

Non-obliterative bronchiolitis
  Infective
  Toxic
  Cigarette-induced (including respiratory
    bronchiolitis–interstitial lung disease)
  Mineral dust bronchiolitis
Diffuse panbronchiolitis
Obliterative bronchiolitis
  Idiopathic
  Toxic inhalation or ingestion
  Infective
  Associated with connective tissue and bowel diseases
  Drug-related
  Transplantation-related
  Carcinoid tumour-associated

[5]. Almost all infants are infected by this virus and a proportion develop cough, wheeze, a hyperinflated chest and inspiratory crackles. The predominance of bronchiolitic symptoms in this age group is probably explained by the relatively larger contribution of the not fully developed bronchiolar airways to overall airflow resistance in such infants. Some 2–3% are sufficiently ill to require admission to hospital. While some children continue to suffer recurrent wheezy attacks afterwards, it seems likely that these represent those already predisposed to asthma and that the infection itself does not lead to this disease [6–8].

In adults it is commonplace to see patients with persistent cough after viral infections. These patients often have increased airway reactivity and respond poorly to bronchodilators and corticosteroids. It may be suspected that bronchiolitis is present in some, but histological evidence is not available. The usual course is towards slow recovery.

Toxic bronchiolitis

Persistent cough without airflow obstruction is a frequent sequel to inhalation of a very wide range of irritant gases or fumes. In more severe cases airflow obstruction is present and this is often sufficiently variable for the diagnosis of asthma to be made. In these cases airway hyperreactivity is present and the syndrome is usually called reactive airways dysfunction syndrome. Some patients respond in a different manner, with fixed airflow obstruction, and in these subjects bronchiolitis obliterans is probably present (see below). It is likely that inflammation of bronchioles is a feature of all patients with persisting symptoms after irritant gas inhalation but that relatively few develop the full-blown obliterative features.

Smokers' bronchiolitis

It has long been recognized that cigarette smokers develop inflammation in the bronchioles (Fig. 29.1) as well as in the major airways and alveoli [9,10]; morphometric studies have shown that smokers with airflow obstruction have increased thickness of bronchiolar walls with decreased luminal diameter [11]. At one time it was thought that this lesion might be the primary one leading to the development of airflow obstruction in a proportion of smokers and that early detection by lung function testing might allow targeted treatment. This hope has not been fulfilled, partly because the lung function tests have proved unable to predict reliably the future fall in airway conductance [12,13] and partly because small airway disease is but one aspect of the inflammatory damage wrought by cigarette smoke.

Correlation between CT findings and pathology in heavy smokers undergoing lung resection for peripheral

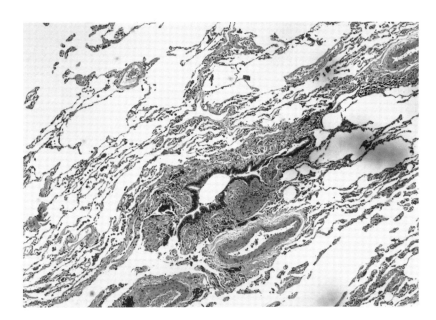

Fig. 29.1 Section from lung resected for bronchial carcinoma in a smoker showing typical peribronchiolar fibrosis (haematoxylin & eosin × 100).

tumours has shown that alveolitis and accumulation of pigmented macrophages in alveoli relate to areas of ground-glass attenuation and that bronchiolitis or bronchiolectasis relates to micronodules [14]. What may be an extreme varient of this pathological condition has been reported as 'respiratory bronchiolitis causing interstitial lung disease', in which heavy smokers develop cough, shortness of breath and diffuse infiltrates on their chest radiographs [15]. Lung function has been reported as showing a primarily restrictive pattern, with only minimal airflow obstruction. Pathologically, the few subjects described have shown pigmented macrophages throughout the acinus, some non-specific alveolar wall thickening and a mild chronic inflammatory cell infiltrate in bronchiolar walls and alveoli with alveolar cell hyperplasia. The condition appears to have had a relatively benign prognosis even when the patient continued smoking.

Mineral dust bronchiolitis

As with cigarette smoke, so also chronic inhalation of a wide variety of toxic substances is likely to cause inflammation, *inter alia*, of small airways. Pathologically, the membranous and respiratory bronchioles are the primary site of reaction to inhaled mineral dusts such as coal, quartz and asbestos [16–18] (Fig. 29.2). Physiological evidence of small airways disease has been demonstrated in coal-miners, silica-exposed workers and asbestos workers [19–21], and there has been much argument as to the significance of these lesions in terms of future development of disabling airflow obstruction. An important difficulty in assessing this has been the fact that most such workers smoke as well, while a more academic argument surrounds the attribution of the obstruction to emphysema or small airways narrowing. To the practising chest physi-

cian these matters are of little importance, although they are of relevance for the prevention of occupational disease and become extremely contentious when dust-exposed workers sue their employers for industrial injury compensation. From a preventative point of view, the evidence suggests quite strongly that mineral dust exposure contributes (with cigarette smoking) to the development of this type of physiological impairment, and account should be taken of this in setting dust standards.

Diffuse panbronchiolitis

Diffuse panbronchiolitis is a well-defined clinicopathological syndrome occurring not uncommonly among people of Japanese, Chinese and Korean descent, with a possible association with HLA-Bw54 [22,23]. It has been described infrequently in the West [24–26]. The condition occurs predominantly in males over the age of 30, who present with cough, wheeze and sputum production. Chronic sinus infection is a usual accompaniment. The chest radiograph shows diffuse small nodular shadows and high-resolution CT (HRCT) shows small rounded centrilobular lesions with linear shadows extending from them, thickened dilated peripheral airways and evidence of peripheral air trapping [27]. The pathological features are of a diffuse chronic inflammatory reaction in respiratory bronchioles, with lymphocytes, histiocytes and plasma cells extending to peribronchiolar tissues but not to alveoli. There is often ectasia of the terminal membranous bronchiole [22].

The natural history of the disease resembles that of cystic fibrosis, in that recurrent infection with *Haemophilus influenzae* becomes persistent and is succeeded by super-infection with *Pseudomonas aeruginosa*. While rapidly fatal cases occur, the usual course is chronic with gradually

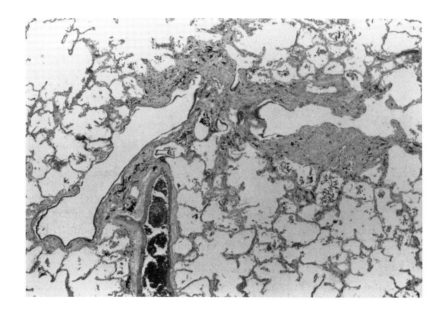

Fig. 29.2 Lung of rat showing early peribronchiolar fibrotic reaction in response to experimental inhalation of asbestos.

worsening cough, sputum production and increasing breathlessness, leading to death in cardiorespiratory failure. Lung function shows an obstructive pattern with overinflation, leading to reduction in vital capacity and diffusing capacity in the later stages. Untreated, the survival rates at 10 years have been reported as 12% in patients infected with *Pseudomonas* and 73% in those not so infected [28]. The cause of the disease is not known but is presumably related to a genetic impairment of lung defences to the infecting organisms which, once established, cause the pathological lesions [29].

The airflow obstruction in these patients is poorly if at all reversible, and bronchial reactivity is little increased [30]. Nevertheless, 8 weeks of treatment with oxitropium bromide has been shown to decrease airflow obstruction and reduce sputum production in some patients [31]. More importantly, Japanese workers have demonstrated that the prognosis can be substantially improved and symptoms relieved by long-term treatment with low-dose erythromycin (600 mg daily), which improves the 10-year survival to better than 90% [28,32]. Other new macrolide antibiotics have also been shown to be of help. It appears that these benefits may accrue, at least in part, from other than direct antibacterial properties of the drugs as a result of interference with both the ability of neutrophils to respond to chemotaxis and the capacity of *Pseudomonas* to produce the biofilm that makes it ineradicable [33–35].

Obliterative bronchiolitis

Aetiological factors

Obliterative bronchiolitis occasionally occurs without known cause, when it most usually takes the form of the proliferative type known as BOOP. However, the syndrome does occur rather more frequently, although still rarely, as a reponse to known causes, the most important of which are shown in Table 29.1. The idiopathic type sometimes follows an influenza-like illness and one suspects that it may sometimes be due to an undetected viral infection [36]. Occasional cases in adults have been described following mycoplasmal or viral infections [5,37–39] and it has been recognized as a complication of human immunodeficiency virus infection [40,41]. A dramatic outbreak in Taiwan in 1996 was caused by consumption of a salad vegetable, *Sauropus androgynus*, either eaten or drunk as a juice. It caused severe impairment in most of the 115 subjects studied and death in seven [42,43]. In infants and children, whose lungs are not fully developed, the condition is usually transient, although permanent damage to bronchioles may occur [44,45]. The development of obliterative bronchiolitis after infection in these circumstances may lead to the maldevelopment of acinar structures with a small avascular and transradiant lung and expiratory air trapping, a condition known as Macleod's or the Swyer–James syndrome [46–48]. This condition is often also associated with bronchiectasis.

Obliterative bronchiolitis may occur after inhalation of a wide range of toxic gases or fumes [49–55]. The classic episode is nitrogen dioxide exposure, although the author has seen it also after acute exposure to chlorine, dimethyl disulphide, hydrochloric acid and several other accidental gassings, as well as (on two occasions) after inhalation of a fine powder of a chlorine-liberating disinfectant. It may therefore be regarded as a possible consequence of exposure to any gas, fume or fine soluble dust with the potential to injure airways either on account of its strongly acidic or alkaline pH or because of its ability to release toxic free radicals. This latter mechanism may explain the one episode reported following inhalation of fly ash [54], which contains high concentrations of transition metals such as vanadium that are capable of releasing hydroxyl radical by a redox mechanism. It appears to be a relatively rare consequence of such exposures [55], most people recovering with simply transient symptoms or after a period of several months of bronchial hyperreactivity. The episode that leads to it usually appears to be a high-dose exposure associated with symptoms, but this is not always the case and symptoms may develop after what seems to have been a much less severe episode, sometimes unassociated with symptoms.

Bronchiolitis obliterans has been described in all connective tissue disorders, although it is a very infrequent complication in any of them. Rheumatoid disease is the one in which it is most likely to be seen, especially in women [3,56], although it has also been described in Sjögren's syndrome, scleroderma, polymyositis, lupus erythematosus, cryoglobulinaemia and various vasculitic conditions [57–61]. In some cases suspicion has been cast on drugs used to treat the condition, especially penicillamine and gold [58,62]. However, there is no doubt that bronchiolitis can occur in the absence of such treatment. Other drugs that have been associated rarely with development of the syndrome include several cytotoxics, amiodarone, acebutolol, sulfasalazine (sulphasalazine) and overdose of L-tryptophan [63–66]. A spectrum of pulmonary diseases may also be associated with inflammatory bowel disorders, both ulcerative colitis and Crohn's disease, including suppurative bronchitis, bronchiectasis and obliterative bronchiolitis [67] (see Chapter 53).

Bronchiolitis obliterans is now well described in recipients of marrow or lung transplants. In recipients of bone marrow, usually allogeneic but sometimes autologous transplants may lead to graft-versus-host disease in which some 10% develop bronchiolitis [68,69]. In heart–lung transplantation, some 10–70% of recipients develop obliterative bronchiolitis, and a similar risk applies also in single or double lung transplantation [70–72]. The risk relates more to the development of a prolonged rejection reaction, posssibly made worse by associated infection, than to the type of transplant [73–75].

In patients with peripheral lung carcinoid tumours, obliterative bronchiolitis has been found in a surprisingly high proportion, 8 of 25 in one study, suggesting that the fibrotic reaction in the small airways was a direct consequence of the tumour [76]. A similar association has been described in one patient with the very rare condition of multiple carcinoid tumourlets [77].

As a footnote to the aetiology, clinicians need to beware of too readily accepting a pathology report of bronchiolitis obliterans as meaning that there is generalized lung disease, since local inflammation and obliteration of small airways as a consequence of, for example, infection or aspiration is not uncommonly seen in biopsy specimens. As always, biopsy evidence has to be interpreted in the light of the entire clinical picture. Bronchiolitis obliterans is essentially a description of a pathological appearance that has many causes.

Presenting features

The patient usually presents with dry cough and increasing breathlessness over several weeks or months, and the diagnosis is most easily made in those cases where a predisposing condition such as collagen disease, inflammatory bowel disease or transplantation is present [78]. In idiopathic cases, the condition is most likely after the age of 40. There may be a history of a recent viral type of illness. There may be evidence of a generalized illness in patients with BOOP, with fever, malaise and loss of weight [79–81]. An exposure to inhalation of a toxic substance usually occurs some days or weeks previously; indeed it is usual for any acute symptoms to have settled and for there to have been a period of apparent recovery prior to the development of cough and breathlessness, in contrast to the reactive airways dysfunction syndrome where symptoms usually follow the episode immediately. This period relates to the time taken for obliteration of the small airways to become severe enough to cause noticeable obstruction to overall airflow, as a consequence of their very large total cross-sectional diameter.

The reason bronchiolitis goes unrecognized so often is that there is no distinctive pattern of physical signs [82]. Despite clear evidence of exertional dyspnoea, there may be no signs on auscultation. On the other hand, there may be diffuse gravity-dependent inspiratory crackles, wheezes or both. In idiopathic BOOP, crackles are the most consistent sign, being present in up to 75% of patients. Digital clubbing is not a feature.

The radiographic appearances are also quite variable. It is not uncommon for the chest film to be essentially normal and this should not be regarded as evidence against the diagnosis. Diffuse nodular or ground-glass opacities are common in idiopathic BOOP (Figs 29.3 & 29.4) and a fine interstitial nodularity may be seen in toxic gas exposure. There may be evidence of overinflation. CT may be helpful in showing subtle abnormalities even when the plain film appears normal [83]. For example, in obliterative bronchiolitis without the pneumonitis a mosaic pattern of reduced attenuation on HRCT may indicate air trapping, and expiratory CT has been used to demonstrate this in localized areas [84–86]. In the BOOP syndrome it would be expected that more obvious abnormalities might be seen on CT, reflecting the interstitial component of the disease (Fig. 29.5). Even so, CT studies of histologically diagnosed BOOP have shown a bewildering range of different appearances, including

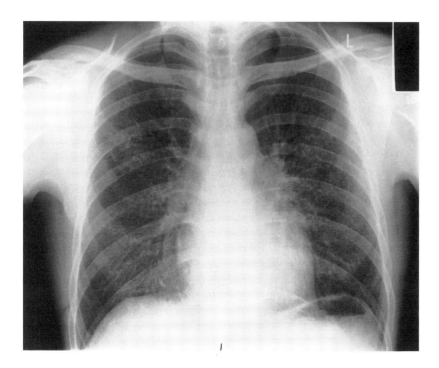

Fig. 29.3 Chest radiograph of patient with idiopathic biopsy-proven bronchiolitis obliterans with organizing pneumonia showing diffuse nodular shadows. (Courtesy of Dr Lesley Gomersal.)

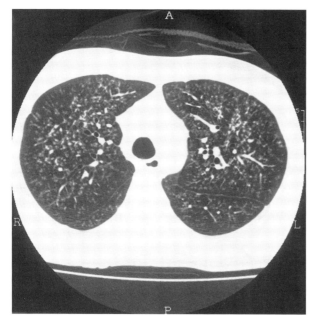

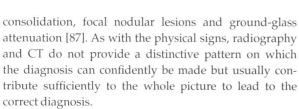

Fig. 29.4 High resolution CT of patient in Fig. 29.3 showing diffuse small centriacinar nodularity. (Courtesy of Dr Lesley Gomersal.)

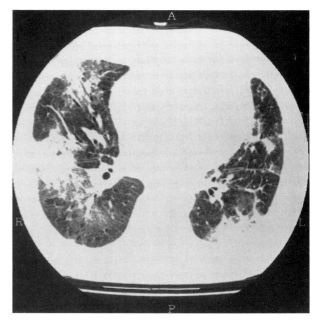

Fig. 29.5 High resolution CT of patient with biopsy-proven bronchiolitis obliterans with organizing pneumonia showing patchy irregular consolidation. (Courtesy of Dr Lesley Gomersal.)

consolidation, focal nodular lesions and ground-glass attenuation [87]. As with the physical signs, radiography and CT do not provide a distinctive pattern on which the diagnosis can confidently be made but usually contribute sufficiently to the whole picture to lead to the correct diagnosis.

Lung function tests are usually abnormal in people with symptomatic obstructive bronchiolitis, although again the findings vary. Impaired exercise tolerance and arterial desaturation are important indicators of severity. In the idiopathic type a restrictive pattern with impaired gas transfer is most common, whereas in those types that follow transplantation or toxic gas inhalation and in collagen diseases severe irreversible airflow obstruction is more frequent. However, either of these, or a mixed pattern, can occur in any of the aetiological types of bronchiolitis.

It can therefore be seen that no one distinctive clinical picture leads to the diagnosis of obliterative bronchiolitis, yet paradoxically the clinical diagnosis is not difficult if one considers the possibility. In the case of someone with predisposing disease, the onset of a persistent dry cough and increasing breathlessness in the absence of other obvious cause such as infection or heart failure should always arouse the suspicion of bronchiolitis. In otherwise previously well people, similar symptoms are usually first thought to be due to asthma or, if the chest film is abnormal, sarcoidosis or a pulmonary arteritis. The clinical features of these diseases differ quite markedly, although in cases of doubt it is usually necessary to test one's suspicion with a lung biopsy.

Pathology

Two distinct histopathological appearances may contribute to obliterative bronchiolitis [88]. In one, there is constriction of many membranous bronchioles by fibrous tissue in the adventitia and submucosa, a chronic inflammatory cell infiltrate and bronchiolar ectasia distal to the constriction with mucous plugging (Fig. 29.6). The changes are often patchy, and more proximal bronchial inflammation and fibrosis may be associated. This type is called constrictive bronchiolitis obliterans and is the one most characteristically seen in collagen diseases, inflammatory bowel disease and after transplantation, although it may occur as a consequence of all the other aetiological factors. Physiologically it is associated with an irreversible obstructive syndrome. The second type, usually known as proliferative bronchiolitis obliterans, is characterized by organizing connective tissue forming polyps that partially or completely obstruct the lumen of the bronchioles. These polyps contain fibroblasts, foamy macrophages and lymphocytes in loose connective tissue (Fig. 29.7). This type

tends to be more peripheral, sometimes involving respiratory bronchioles and alveoli; in the latter case the extension of the plugs of granulation tissue into the acinus, with some chronic inflammatory cell infiltrate in alveolar walls, allows the pathological diagnosis of BOOP or cryptogenic organizing pneumonitis [4,79]. The former term is preferable, since the condition is primarily a bronchiolar disease and may not be cryptogenic. Alveolar wall fibrosis and honeycombing are not significant features of this condition, in contrast to cryptogenic fibrosing alveolitis. Idiopathic bronchiolitis obliterans is most commonly of the proliferative type, although identical pathological features may be found after viral infections, toxic fume exposure, systemic diseases and transplantation. The physiological abnormality tends towards a more restrictive pattern of lung function.

From the foregoing, it is apparent that the pathological features do not usually help in determining the aetiology of the bronchiolitis, which is established on clinical grounds. However, lung biopsy is helpful in identifying the cause of the functional disorder, in excluding other causes of peripheral lung disease and in pointing towards prognosis, since the proliferative type is far more likely to respond to treatment than the constrictive type.

Clinical course and management

Idiopathic bronchiolitis obliterans with organizing pneumonia

Bronchiolitis obliterans with patchy or diffuse infiltrative lesions (BOOP) appears to be the most common adult presentation of bronchiolitis obliterans, being found in 57 of 67 cases of bronchiolitis analysed in Boston, USA [4]. The patients often presented with a history of cough or an

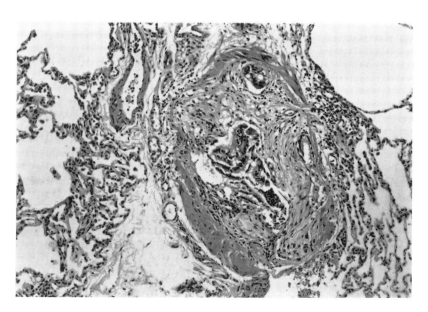

Fig. 29.6 Section of lung of patient with constrictive bronchiolitis obliterans after heart–lung transplantation showing chronic inflammatory cells and fibrous tissue occluding the bronchiolar lumen (haematoxylin & eosin ×240).

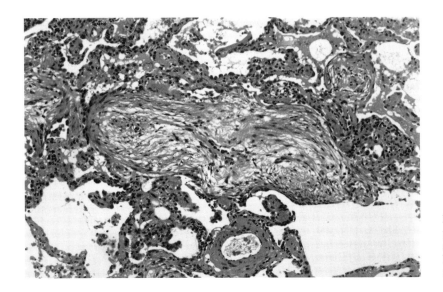

Fig. 29.7 Section of lung in patient with proliferative type of bronchiolitis obliterans showing obliteration of a respiratory bronchiole by proliferating fibrous tissue (haematoxylin & eosin × 100).

influenza-like illness 4–10 weeks previously. Age at presentation was 40–60 years with an equal sex incidence. Crepitations were audible on auscultation in the majority. The chest radiograph showed a pattern of patchy, often irregular, densities with a ground-glass background appearance in 81%. Unlike patients with bronchiolitis associated with connective tissue diseases, these patients showed evidence of restrictive lung disease in 72%, with a decreased diffusing capacity in 86%. An obstructive pattern was only seen in smokers. The pathology showed plugs of granulation tissue involving bronchiolar and alveolar ducts, with extension of the organization from distal alveolar ducts into alveoli and variable degrees of interstitial infiltration by mononuclear cells, i.e. the pattern of an organizing pneumonia.

The course of the disease is usually (though not always) progressive and may occasionally be fulminant [89,90]. Nevertheless it frequently responds to therapy with corticosteroids in an initial dose of 60–80mg daily. This dose is continued for 1–3 months, with a graduated reduction thereafter over 6–12 months to a low maintenance dose or to zero. In the Boston series 65% recovered and other authors have reported a good prognosis [91,92].

Toxic gas bronchiolitis

The characteristic feature of bronchiolitis following exposure to toxic gas or fume is a latent period between exposure and development of symptoms of a few days to several weeks. Thereafter there is progressive increase in shortness of breath over several months followed by stabilization of irreversible airflow obstruction. The condition may be, indeed usually is, preceded by acute symptoms of irritative bronchial disease and is often accompanied by persistent but slowly improving reactive airways dysfunction syndrome. Thus the clinical picture may seem complicated until one realizes that acute airway irritation may cause several effects at all levels of the airways simultaneously. Since these patients present sporadically with an acute illness it is not surprising that controlled trials of therapy have not been reported. However, based on anecdotal clinical evidence it remains sensible to treat patients with apparently progressing symptoms early with high-dose steroids and to follow their response with lung function tests [49,93–95].

Other aetiological types

Several aetiological types have rather characteristic clinical courses, although any course may occasionally occur in any type. In those of viral aetiology, the course corresponds to the histopathological type and it seems likely that in some cases the proliferative type may heal by fibrosis and become the constrictive. High-dose steroid therapy is therefore indicated in apparently progressive cases [96]. However, some less severely affected patients show spontaneous resolution without treatment. In the collagen diseases, the constrictive type is more frequent, the course more indolent with a poor prognosis and progression less likely to be arrested by steroids [3]. In contrast, in inflammatory bowel disease steroid responsiveness is more likely. An interesting feature of this condition is the occasional occurrence of lung disease after total colectomy for ulcerative colitis. Transplant-associated bronchiolitis occurs as a consequence of repeated episodes of rejection, and may be prevented by treating patients who have suffered three such episodes by daily nebulized budesonide at a dose of 500µg [97].

In progressive bronchiolitis obliterans, whatever the aetiology, a fatal outcome is possible and in these circumstances there is a case for considering lung transplantation in suitable patients. Paradoxically, this technique has been used most frequently in the management of post-transplant bronchiolitis [98,99].

References

1 Hogg JC, Macklem PT, Thurlbeck WM. Site and nature of airway obstruction in chronic obstructive lung disease. *N Engl J Med* 1968; 278: 1355.

2 Cosio M, Ghezzo H, Hogg JC *et al.* The relations between structural changes in small airways and pulmonary function tests. *N Engl J Med* 1977; 298: 1277.

3 Geddes DM, Corrin B, Brewerton DA *et al.* Progressive airway obliteration in adults and its association with rheumatoid disease. *Q J Med* 1977; 46: 427.

4 Epler GR, Colby TV, McCloud TC *et al.* Bronchiolitis obliterans organising pneumonia. *N Engl J Med* 1985; 312: 152.

5 Penn CC, Liu C. Bronchiolitis following infection in adults and children. *Clin Chest Med* 1993; 14: 645.

6 Mok JYQ, Simpson H. Outcome for acute bronchitis, bronchiolitis, and pneumonia in infancy. *Arch Dis Child* 1984; 59: 306.

7 Mok JYQ, Simpson H. Symptoms, atopy, and bronchial reactivity after lower respiratory infection in infants. *Arch Dis Child* 1984; 59: 299.

8 Landau LI. Bronchiolitis and asthma: are they related? *Thorax* 1994; 49: 293.

9 Niewoehner DE, Kleinerman J, Rice DB. Pathologic changes in the peripheral airways of young cigarette smokers. *N Engl J Med* 1974; 291: 755.

10 Leopold JG, Gough J. The centrilobular form of hypertrophic emphysema and its relation to chronic bronchitis. *Thorax* 1957; 12: 219.

11 Bosken CH, Wiggs BR, Pare PD, Hogg JC. Small airway dimensions in smokers with obstruction to airflow. *Am Rev Respir Dis* 1990; 142: 563.

12 Buist AS, Vollmer WM, Johnson LR, McCamant LE. Does the single breath N_2 test identify the smoker who will develop chronic airflow limitation? *Am Rev Respir Dis* 1988; 137: 293.

13 Stanescu DC, Rodenstein DO, Hoeven C, Robert A. 'Sensitive tests' are poor predictors of the decline in forced expiratory volume in one second in middle aged smokers. *Am Rev Respir Dis* 1987; 135: 584.

14 Remy-Jardin M, Remy J, Gosselin B, Becette V, Edme JL. Lung parenchymal changes secondary to cigarette smoking: pathologic–CT correlations. *Radiology* 1993; 186: 643.

15 Myers JL, Veal CF, Shin MS, Katzenstein A-LA. Respiratory bronchiolitis causing interstitial lung disease: a clinico-pathological study of six cases. *Am Rev Respir Dis* 1987; 135: 880.

16 Churg A, Wright JL. Small airways disease and mineral dust exposure. *Pathol Annu* 1983; 18: 233.

17 Churg A, Wright JL, Wiggs B, Paré PD, Lazar N. Small airways disease and mineral dust exposure. *Am Rev Respir Dis* 1985; 131: 139.

18 Wright JL, Cagle P, Churg A, Colby TV, Myers J. Diseases of the small airways. *Am Rev Respir Dis* 1992; 146: 240.

19 Seaton A, Lapp NL, Morgan WKC. Lung mechanics and frequency dependence of compliance in coalminers. *J Clin Invest* 1972; 51: 1203.

20 Jodoin G, Gibbs GW, Macklem PT, McDonald JC, Becklake MR. Early effects of asbestos exposure on lung function. *Am Rev Respir Dis* 1971; 104: 525.

21 Begin R, Cantin A, Berthiaume Y *et al.* Airway function in lifetime non-smoking older asbestos workers. *Am J Med* 1983; 75: 631.

22 Homma H, Yamanaka A, Tanimoto S *et al.* Diffuse panbronchiolitis. A disease of the transitional zone of the lung. *Chest* 1983; 83: 63.

23 Sugayame Y, Kudoh S, Maeda H, Suzaki H, Takaku F. Analysis of HLA antigens in patients with diffuse panbronchiolitis. *Am Rev Respir Dis* 1990; 141: 1459.

24 Poletti V, Patelli M, Poletti G, Bertanti T, Spiga L. Diffuse panbronchiolitis observed in an Italian. *Chest* 1990; 98: 515.

25 Randhawa P, Hoagland MH, Yousem SA. Diffuse panbronchiolitis in North America: report of three cases and review of the literature. *Am J Surg Pathol* 1991; 15: 43.

26 Tredaniel J, Zalcman G, Gerber F *et al.* Diffuse panbronchiolitis: efficacy of low dose erythromycin. *Respir Med* 1993; 87: 229 (see also *Respir Med* 88: 479).

27 Nishimura K, Kitaichi M, Izumi T, Itoh H. Diffuse panbronchiolitis: correlation of high resolution CT and pathologic findings. *Radiology* 1992; 184: 779.

28 Tanimoto H. A review of the recent progress in treatment of patients with diffuse panbronchiolitis associated with *Pseudomonas aeruginosa* infection in Japan. *Antibiot Chemother* 1991; 44: 94.

29 Høiby N. Diffuse bronchiolitis and cystic fibrosis: East meets West. *Thorax* 1994; 49: 531.

30 Koyama H, Nishimura K, Mio T *et al.* Bronchial responsiveness and acute bronchodilator response in chronic obstructive pulmonary disease and diffuse panbronchiolitis. *Thorax* 1994; 49: 540.

31 Tamaoki J, Chiyotani A, Tagaya E, Sakai N, Konno K. Effect of long term treatment with oxitropium bromide on airway secretion in chronic bronchitis and diffuse panbronchiolitis. *Thorax* 1994; 49: 545.

32 Nagai H, Shishido H, Yoneda R *et al.* Long-term low-dose administration of erythromycin to patients with diffuse panbronchiolitis. *Respiration* 1991; 58: 145.

33 Kadoto J-I, Sakito O, Kohno S *et al.* A mechanism of erythromycin treatment in patients with diffuse panbronchiolitis. *Am Rev Respir Dis* 1993; 147: 153.

34 Oda H, Kadota J, Kohno S, Hara K. Erythromycin inhibits neutrophil chemotaxis in bronchoalveoli of diffuse panbronchiolitis. *Chest* 1994; 106: 1116.

35 Sakata K, Yajima H, Tanaka K *et al.* Erythromycin inhibits the production of elastase by *Pseudomonas aeruginosa* without affecting its proliferation *in vivo*. *Am Rev Respir Dis* 1993; 148: 1061.

36 Laroche CM, Stewart S, Flower CDR, Stark JE. Acute resiratory failure due to bronchiolitis of unknown aetiology. *Respir Med* 1994; 88: 705.

37 Ham JC. Acute infectious obstructing bronchiolitis: a potentially fatal disease in adults. *Ann Intern Med* 1964; 60: 47.

38 Chan ED, Welsh CH. Fulminant *Mycoplasma pneumoniae* pneumonia. *West J Med* 1995; 162: 133.

39 Yeldandi AV, Colby TV. Pathologic features of lung biopsy specimens from influenza pneumonia cases. *Hum Pathol* 1994; 25: 47.

40 Leo YS, Pitchon HE, Messler G, Meyer RD. Bronchiolitis obliterans organising pneumonia in patients with AIDS. *Clin Infect Dis* 1994; 18: 921.

41 Allen JN, Wewers MD. HIV-associated bronchiolitis obliterans-organising pneumonia. *Chest* 1989; 96: 197.

42 Lai R-S, Chiang AA, Wu M-T *et al.* Outbreak of bronchiolitis obliterans associated with consumption of *Sauropus androgynus* in Taiwan. *Lancet* 1996; 348: 83.

43 Lai R-S, Wang J-S, Wu M-T, Hsu H-K. Lung transplantation in bronchiolitis obliterans associated with vegetable consumption. *Lancet* 1998; 352: 117.

44 Laraya-Cuasay LR, Deforest A, Huff D *et al.* Chronic pulmonary complications of early influenza virus infection in children. *Am Rev Respir Dis* 1977; 116: 617.

45 Becroft DM. Bronchiolitis obliterans, bronchiectasis and other sequelae of adenovirus type 21 infection in young children. *J Clin Pathol* 1971; 24: 72.

46 Macleod WM. Abnormal transradiancy of one lung. *Thorax* 1954; 9: 147.

47 Reid L, Simon G. Unilateral lung transradiancy. *Thorax* 1962; 17: 230.

48 Miravitlles M, Alvares-Castells A, Vidal R *et al.* Scintigraphy, angiography and computed tomography in unilateral hyperlucent lung due to obliterative bronchiolitis. *Respiration* 1994; 61: 324.

49 Yockey CC, Eden BM, Byrd RB. The McConnell missile accident. Clinical spectrum of nitrogen dioxide exposure. *JAMA* 1980; 244: 1221.

50 Charan NB, Myers CG, Lakshminarayan S, Spencer TM. Pulmonary injuries associated with acute sulphur dioxide inhalation. *Am Rev Respir Dis* 1979; 119: 555.

51 Tasaka S, Kanazawa M, Mori M *et al.* Long-term course of bronchiectasis and bronchiolitis obliterans as a late complication of smoke inhalation. *Respiration* 1995; 62: 40.

52 Konichezky S, Schattner A, Ezri T, Bokenboim P, Geva D. Thionyl chloride-induced lung injury and bronchiolitis obliterans. *Chest* 1993; 104: 971.

53 Ramirez RJ, Dowell AR. Silo-filler's disease. Nitrogen dioxide induced lung injury: long-term follow-up and review of literature. *Ann Intern Med* 1971; 74: 569.

54 Boswell RT, McCunney RJ. Bronchiolitis obliterans from exposure to incinerator fly ash. *J Occup Environ Med* 1995; 37: 850.

55 Zwemer FL, Pratt DS, May JJ. Silo-filler's disease in New York State. *Am Rev Respir Dis* 1992; 146: 650.

56 Murphy KC, Atkins CJ, Offer RC *et al.* Obliterative bronchiolitis in two rheumatoid arthritis patients treated with penicillamine. *Arthritis Rheum* 1981; 24: 557.

57 Newball HH, Brahim SA. Chronic airway disease in patients with Sjögren syndrome. *Am Rev Respir Dis* 1977; 115: 295.

58 Epler GR, Snider GL, Gaensler EA *et al.* Bronchiolitis and bronchitis in connective tissue disease. A possible relationship to the use of penicillamine. *JAMA* 1979; 242: 528.

59 Robinson BW, Sterrett G. Bronchiolitis obliterans associated with polyarteritis nodosa. *Chest* 1992; 102: 309.

60 Godeau B, Cormier C, Menkes CJ. Bronchiolitis obliterans in SLE: beneficial effect of intravenous cyclophosphamide. *Ann Rheum Dis* 1991; 50: 956.

61 Schwartz MI, Matthay RA, Sahn SA *et al.*

Interstitial lung disease in polymyositis and dermatomyositis: analysis of six cases and review of the literature. *Medicine* 1976; 55: 89.

62 Holness L, Tenenbaum J, Cooter NBE, Grossman RF. Fatal bronchiolitis obliterans associated with chrysotherapy. *Ann Rheum Dis* 1983; 42: 593.

63 Rosenow EC, Myers JL, Swensen SJ, Pisani RJ. Drug-induced pulmonary disease. An update. *Chest* 1992; 102: 239.

64 Camus P, Lombard JN, Perrichon M *et al.* Bronchiolitis obliterans in patients taking acebutol or amiodarone. *Thorax* 1989; 44: 711.

65 Williams T, Eidus L, Thomas P. Fibrosing alveolitis, bronchiolitis obliterans and sulfasalazine therapy. *Chest* 1982; 81: 766.

66 Mar KE, Sen P, Tan K, Krishnan R, Ratkalkar K. Bronchiolitis obliterans organising pneumonia associated with massive L-tryptophan ingestion. *Chest* 1993; 104: 1924.

67 Camus P, Piard F, Ashcroft T, Gal AA, Colby TV. The lung in inflammatory bowel disease. *Medicine* 1993; 72: 151.

68 Rosenberg ME, Vercellotti GM, Snover DC, Herd D, McGlave P. Bronchiolitis obliterans after bone marrow transplatation. *Am J Hematol* 1985; 18: 325.

69 Par HL, Crilley P, Patchefsky A, Schiffman RL, Brodsky I. Bronchiolitis obliterans after autologous bone marrow transplantation. *Chest* 1992; 101: 775.

70 Bando K, Paradis IL, Similo S *et al.* Cardiac and pulmonary replacement: obliterative bronchiolitis after lung and heart–lung transplantation. *J Thorac Cardiovasc Surg* 1995; 110: 4.

71 Keller CA, Cagle PG, Brown RW, Noon G, Frost AE. Bronchiolitis obliterans in recipients of single, double, and heart–lung transplantation. *Chest* 1995; 107: 973.

72 Burke CM, Theodore J, Dawkins KD *et al.* Post-transplant obliterative bronchiolitis and other late lung sequelae in human heart–lung transplantation. *Chest* 1984; 86: 824.

73 Burke CM, Glanville AR, Theodore J, Robin ED. Lung immunogenicity, rejection and obliterative bronchiolitis. *Chest* 1987; 92: 578.

74 Reinsmoen NL, Bolman RM, Savik K *et al.* Improved long-term graft outcome in lung transplant recipients who have donor antigen-specific hyporeactivity. *J Heart Lung Transplant* 1994; 13: 30.

75 Yousem SA, MartinT, Paradis IL, Keenan R, Griffith BP. Can immunohistological analysis of transbronchial biopsy specimens predict responder status in early acute rejection of lung allografts? *Hum Pathol* 1994; 25: 525.

76 Miller NL, Muller RR. Neuroendocrine cell hyperplasia and obliterative bronchiolitis in patients with peripheral carcinoid tumors. *Am J Surg Pathol* 1995; 19: 653.

77 Sheerin N, Harrison NK, Sheppard MN *et al.* Obliterative bronchiolitis caused by multiple tumourlets and microcarcinoids successfully treated by single lung transplantation. *Thorax* 1995; 50: 207.

78 Ezri T, Kunichezky S, Eliraz A *et al.* Bronchiolitis obliterans: current concepts. *Q J Med* 1994; 87: 1.

79 Davison AG, Heard BE, McAllister WAC, Turner-Warwick MEH. Cryptogenic organising pneumonitis. *Q J Med* 1983; 52: 382.

80 King TE, Mortenson RL. Cryptogenic organising pneumonia. The North American experience. *Chest* 1992; 102 (Suppl): 8S.

81 Cordier JF, Loire R, Brune J. Idiopathic bronchiolitis organising pneumonia: definition of characteristic clinical profiles in a series of 16 patients. *Chest* 1989; 86: 999.

82 King TE. Bronchiolitis obliterans. *Lung* 1989; 167: 69.

83 Muller NL, Miller RR. Diseases of the bronchioles: CT and histopathologic findings. *Radiology* 1995; 196: 3.

84 Eber CD, Stark P, Bertozzi P. Bronchiolitis obliterans on high resolution CT: a pattern of mosaic oligemia. *J Comput Assist Tomogr* 1993; 17: 853.

85 Padley SP, Adler BD, Hansell DM, Muller NL. Bronchiolitis obliterans: high resolution CT findings and correlation with pulmonary function tests. *Clin Radiol* 1993; 47: 236.

86 Stern EJ, Frank MS. Small airways diseases of the lungs: findings at expiratory CT. *Am J Roentgenol* 1994; 163: 37.

87 Bouchardy LM, Kuhlman JE, Ball WC *et al.* CT findings in bronchiolitis obliterans organising pneumonia (BOOP) with radiographic, clinical, and histologic correlation. *J Comput Assist Tomogr* 1993; 17: 352.

88 Colby TV, Myers JL. The clinical and histologic spectrum of bronchiolitis obliterans including bronchiolitis obliterans organising pneumonia (BOOP). *Semin Respir Med* 1992; 13: 119.

89 Nizami IY, Kissner DG, Visscher DW, Dubaybo BA. Idiopathic bronchiolitis obliterans with organising pneumonia: an acute and life-threatening syndrome. *Chest* 1995; 108: 271.

90 Cohen AJ, King TE, Downey GP. Rapidly progressive bronchiolitis obliterans with organising pneumonia. *Am J Respir Crit Care Med* 1994; 149: 1670.

91 Guerry-Force ML, Muller NL, Wright JL *et al.* A comparison of bronchiolitis obliterans with organising pneumonia, usual interstitial pneumonia and small airways disease. *Am Rev Respir Dis* 1987; 135: 705.

92 Nagai S, Kitaichi M, Nishimua K, Izumi T. Idiopathic BOOP. the prognosis of 16 Japanese patients at 5 years after onset. *Am J Respir Crit Care Med* 1996; 153: A271.

93 Wood BR, Colombo JL, Benson BE. Chlorine inhalation toxicity from vapors generated by swimming pool chlorinator tablets. *Pediatrics* 1997; 79: 427.

94 Charan NB, Meyers CG, Lackshminarayan S, Spencer TM. Pulmonary injuries associated with acute sulfur dioxide inhalation. *Am Rev Respir Dis* 1979; 119: 555.

95 Horvath EP, Dolico DGA, Barbee RA, Dickie HA. Nitrogen dioxide-induced pulmonary disease: five new cases and a review of the literature. *J Occup Med* 1978; 20: 103.

96 Hardy KA, Schidlow DV, Zaeri N. Obliterative bronchiolitis in children. *Chest* 1988; 93: 460.

97 Takao M, Higenbottam TW, Audley T *et al.* Effects of inhaled nebulised steroids on acute and chronic lung fuction in heart–lung transplant patients. *Transplant Proc* 1995; 27: 1284.

98 Burke CM, Baldwin JC, Morris AJ *et al.* Twenty-eight cases of human heart–lung transplantation. *Lancet* 1986; i: 517.

99 Novick RJ, Schäfers HJ, Sitt L *et al.* Seventy-two pulmonary retransplantations for obliterative bronchiolitis: predictors of survival. *Ann Thorac Surg* 1995; 60: 111.

30

CYSTIC FIBROSIS

ANDREW P. GREENING

Cystic fibrosis (CF) is the most common fatal inherited disease in Caucasian populations of European origin. A carrier rate of about 1 in 25 and an autosomal recessive inheritance gives rise to approximately 1 in 2500 children being affected in the UK. The consequent physiological abnormality results in faulty ion transport and water movement across epithelial cells.

Despite the disease being the result of a defect in a single gene that codes for an ion channel, there are many differences in clinical expression. Abnormality of transport of chloride and sodium ions across some epithelia is an essential feature. The respiratory tract and the pancreas are the organs that bear the predominant burden of disease, with some 80% of patients having both recurrent pulmonary infections and pancreatic insufficiency. About 15% of patients have apparently normal pancreatic function but have lung disease and some 5% have gastrointestinal problems but no overt respiratory manifestation. Clinical presentation is usually at birth, with meconium ileus, or early childhood, with recurrent respiratory infections and/or failure to thrive. However, some patients with milder variants of the disorder may present later in life, when the diagnosis may be much less obvious.

Historical review

The disease may have been recognized in folklore [1]. In old European cleansing ceremonies it was customary to lick the forehead of newborn infants. The child was feared 'bewitched' and soon to die if it tasted salty. In 1938, Dorothy Andersen in New York is credited with the first formal description of CF as a separate pancreatic pathological and clinical entity, differentiating it from coeliac disease [2]. Blackfan and May [3] reported similar findings from Boston in the same year and Blackfan and Wolbach [4] had published analogous cases in 1933 without specifically naming a 'new' disorder. In 1936, Fanconi and colleagues [5] had also identified a consistent relationship between congenital pancreatic cystic fibromatosis and bronchiectasis, which proved later to be compatible with

CF. Farber [6] introduced the term 'mucoviscidosis' in 1943 following studies which suggested that all exocrine glands had evidence of pathological changes. A high incidence of heat prostration was observed among CF patients during a New York heatwave in 1948, attracting di Sant'Agnese and colleagues [7] to study patients' sweat. They showed the sodium and chloride levels to be elevated and this formed the basis of the subsequent sweat test as the diagnostic procedure for CF; indeed it has remained the cornerstone of diagnosis to the present day. Initially this was carried out by warming the patient to produce sweating but in 1959 a test was introduced whereby sweat was induced by the iontophoresis of pilocarpine [8], which is reproducible and avoids the possible risks of heat prostration.

The autosomal recessive nature of inheritance was first suggested by Andersen and Hodges in 1946 [9] and established in the 1960s [10]. The gene was localized to the long arm of chromosome 7 in 1985 [11,12] and isolated in 1989 [13–15]. Such is the pace of current applied molecular biology that the first trial of gene therapy for CF in humans was published only 4 years later [16]. Studies of the gene product, the cystic fibrosis transmembrane conductance regulator (CFTR), have advanced the understanding of the pathogenetic processes and revealed potential new therapies. Molecular analyses of CF genotypes have taken the history of the disease full circle and helped trace its evolutionary path. Haplotype analysis of chromosomes carrying the CF mutation from different geographical regions has suggested that the most common mutation probably first occurred over 52 000 years ago during the palaeolithic era [17] in a population that migrated into Europe. It has been estimated that no lethal recessive disorder could reach the high frequency that CF has in Europe just by genetic drift. Heterozygous advantage (sickle cell disease [18], cholera [19], gastroenteritis and tuberculosis [20]) or increased fertility among CF carriers [21] have therefore been postulated. Protection against gastrointestinal disorders is an empirically attractive hypothesis and supported by recent work. A thermostable enterotoxin from *Escherichia coli* induces chloride secretion only in cells with normal CFTR, which could give a CF heterozygous person advantage for *E. coli* diarrhoea [22]. In addition, CF heterozygous mice may show resistance to cholera toxin [23].

Genetics

CF gene and CFTR

The CF gene is large, comprising 27 exons [24] and encompassing approximately 250 kb of genomic DNA. This encodes a mature mRNA of 6.5 kb [13] that codes for a protein, CFTR, with a molecular mass of approximately 168 kDa [14]. There are two hydrophobic membrane-spanning domains, two regions that bind ATP and a regulatory domain containing multiple sites for phosphorylation by protein kinases A and C [14] (Fig. 30.1). This overall structure is similar to a large family of proteins

that transports molecules into or out of cells in an ATP-dependent fashion [25]. One of these is the human multiple-drug resistance protein, which confers resistance to cancer chemotherapy by exporting drugs from cells. However, despite the similarities, CFTR does not appear to function as an ATP-dependent transporter but as a cyclic AMP-activated chloride channel [26–30]. Cross-species analyses show marked structural conservation between the human CFTR and its bovine, mouse, rat and dogshark homologues [31–34] (90% human to cow; 76% human to mouse), with 95–100% homology in some regions. These cross-species studies suggest that the function of CFTR may be similar in evolutionarily very diverse organisms.

CFTR promoter

The sequence of the CFTR promoter region has been determined. The structure has led to the proposition that the

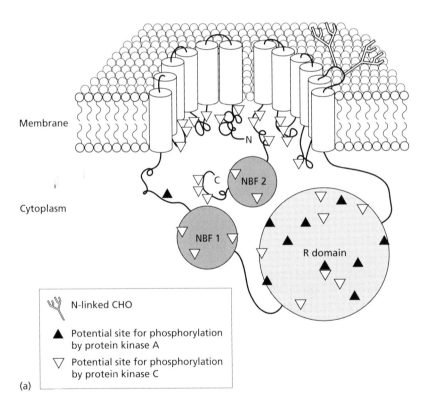

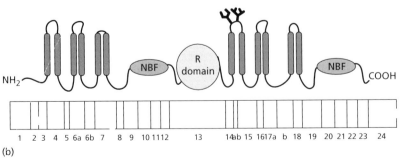

Fig. 30.1 (a) Diagrammatic representation of the structure of the cystic fibrosis transmembrane conductance regulator (CFTR) showing two transmembrane regions, two domains that bind with ATP (nucleotide-binding domains) and a regulatory domain that has multiple sites for phosphorylation by protein kinases A and C. (Adapted from Riordan *et al.* [14].) (b) Schematic representation of CFTR and the corresponding exons of the gene.

CFTR gene may belong to a group of genes that have been characterized as 'housekeeping' genes that in addition have tissue-specific functions [35]. For example, like housekeeping genes the CFTR gene contains no TATA or CAAT box element. However, there are sequences that suggest it could be under transcriptional regulation. Potential AP-1 and AP-2 binding sites have been identified, as well as candidate sequences for cyclic AMP and glucocorticoid response elements [36].

CFTR function

CFTR appears to have additional functions to those of a chloride channel in the apical membrane of epithelial cells. Endocytosis and exocytosis are defective in a CF pancreatic cell line, although this is corrected by the expression of wild-type CFTR [37]. It has also been proposed that in CF there is a defect in the acidification of the trans-Golgi network, of prelysosomes and of endosomes because of diminished chloride conductance in the membrane of these intracellular organelles [38].

In addition, there is a considerable amount of evidence that expression, and probably activity, of CFTR is capable of modulating the function of other ion channels in epithelial cells [39]. A separate chloride channel, the outward rectifying chloride channel (ORCC), has been shown to have a regulatory relationship with CFTR [40,41]. It is uncertain whether this involves direct protein–protein interactions [42], interaction through cytoskeletal elements [43] or activation of ORCC via a purinergic receptor [44] involving CFTR-mediated release of ATP from cells [45,46]. Early work had shown a consistently elevated and abnormally regulated sodium absorption in CF airway epithelia [47]. It is now recognized that these observations reflect an absence in CF cells of negative regulation of sodium channels by CFTR [48,49]. The nature of the interaction between CFTR and this epithelial sodium channel is unclear. However, the epithelial sodium channel has a two to three fold higher probability of being open in the CF cell and hence the increased sodium absorption.

CFTR expression

CFTR RNA is expressed in epithelial tissues classically affected in CF, such as the lung, pancreas, liver and sweat glands [14] but also large intestine, testis [50,51] and kidney (Table 30.1). RNA studies indicate a low level of CFTR transcripts in respiratory epithelium and much higher levels in the pancreas and intestine [50,52] and in the airway submucosal glands [53].

CF gene mutations and effects on CFTR

More than 600 mutations of the gene have now been rec-

Table 30.1 Tissue and cellular localization of CFTR.

Organ localization	Cells	Cellular
Airways	Ciliated epithelium	Apical membrane
	Submucous glands	Intracytoplasmic
Pancreas	Ductal epithelium	Apical membrane
Liver	Bile duct epithelium	Apical membrane
Sweat glands	Reabsorptive duct epithelium	Apical and basolateral membranes
Intestine	Basal cells of crypts	Apical membrane
Kidneys	Collecting tubules	Apical membrane

ognized, although the frequency of the different abnormalities is very unevenly distributed and varies between geographical regions [54–56]. The most common mutation, a deletion of three nucleotides in exon 10 resulting in the omission of a single amino acid, phenylalanine, at residue 508 (termed ΔF508), accounts for 68% of CF alleles worldwide, reported to the CF Genetic Analysis Consortium [54], and just over 70% in the UK and other parts of northern Europe. Only 13 mutations reported to the Consortium have a frequency of greater than 1% (Table 30.2) but these account for approximately 85% of all CF alleles. The majority of the rest occur infrequently, although again with significant geographical variation [57] and many in single families.

Mutations that alter CFTR mRNA

About half the mutations reported to the Consortium are predicted to affect RNA processing. These can be divided into two groups: those that introduce a premature signal for the termination of translation and those that alter the mRNA but leave the reading frame intact. The former group includes changes in a single nucleotide that substitute an amino acid with a termination signal (nonsense mutation), deletion or insertion of one, two or more nucleotides that are not multiples of three (frameshift mutation), or abnormal exon splicing (splice-site mutation).

Nonsense mutations

The most common outcome of these mutations is a severe reduction of mRNA levels from the gene containing the alteration. The RNA is produced in normal amounts but is not transported out of the nucleus into the rough endoplasmic reticulum for translation [58]. Examples of this type of mutation include G542X, R553X and W1282X [59–61]. Severe reduction in mRNA transcripts should cause reduction or absence of CFTR protein and this appears to be the case [62] (Fig. 30.2).

Table 30.2 CFTR gene mutations reported to the Cystic Fibrosis Genetic Analysis Consortium [54] with a relative frequency of >1%.

	Relative frequency	Mutation	Consequence
ΔF508	67.2	Deletion of 3 bp between nt 1652 and 1655 in exon 10	Deletion of Phe at codon 508
G542X	3.4	G→T at nt 1756 in exon 11	Gly→Stop at codon 542
G551D	2.4	G→A at nt 1784 in exon 11	Gly→Asp at codon 552
W1282X	2.1	G→A at nt 3987 in exon 20	Trp→Stop at codon 1282
3905insT	2.1	Insertion of T after nt 3905 in exon 20	Frameshift
N1303K	1.8	C→G at nt 4041 in exon 21	Asn→Lys at codon 1303
3849+10 kbC→C	1.4	C→T in a 6.2 kb EcoRI fragment 10 kb from 5′ junction on intron 19	Aberrant splicing
R553X	1.3	C→T at nt 1789 in exon 11	Arg→Stop at codon 553
621+G→T	1.3	G→T at nt 1 from 5′ junction of intron 4	Splice mutation
1717−1G→A	1.1	G→A at nt 1 from 3′ junction of intron 10	Splice mutation
1078delT	1.1	Deletion of T at nt 1078 in exon 7	Frameshift
2789+5G→A	1.1	G→A at 5 nt from 5′ end of intron 14b	Splice mutation
3849+4A→G	1.0	A→G at 4 nt from 5′ end of intron 19	Splice mutation

nt, nucleotide.

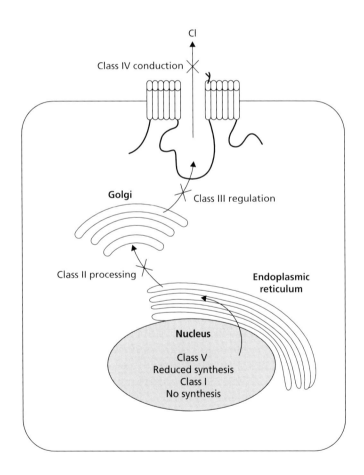

Fig. 30.2 Effects of the five classes of mutation of the cystic fibrosis transmembrane conductance regulator (CFTR) and the sites influencing CFTR synthesis, processing and function.

Splice-site mutations

The effects of splice-site mutations are more difficult to predict. Two examples, 621+1G→T and 711+1G→T, account for 1.3% and 0.9% of mutant CF alleles respectively [56]. The former mutation alters the splice site immediately following exon 4 and produces two aberrantly spliced RNAs, both of which retain an open reading frame [63,64]. The latter mutation changes the splice site following exon 5, causing skipping of the entire exon, but since the number of nucleotides here is a multiple of three the reading frame is left intact [40]. It can be predicted that these aberrant transcripts will be translated into protein products that may be unstable, non-functional or partially functional. Determining which of these possibilities occurs usually requires protein expression and analysis.

A putative disease-associated mutation was discovered that should lead to a CFTR mRNA transcript missing exon 9 [65]. This would be expected to produce non-functional protein because exon 9 encodes a critical region of the first ATP-binding domain. However, exon 9 is missing from a significant fraction of CFTR mRNA transcripts in most normal individuals [66]. The length of a polypyrimidine tract upstream of the 3′ splice acceptor site within intron 8 appears critical [67] for the splicing efficiency of exon 9 (Fig. 30.3). An optimal splice acceptor site lies downstream of 11 consecutive cytosines or thymidines [68]. In intron 8 of the CFTR gene this tract exists in three polymorphisms, consisting of five, seven or nine thymidines [69]. Consequently, the longest tract length, 9T, results in the most efficient splice acceptor, producing over 95% of CFTR transcripts with exon 9 intact. The 7T tract results in 50–90% intact transcript, but the 5T tract is inefficient and produces as little as 5% per allele [68,69]. This allows for some individuals to display variant clinical CF if they have a mutant CF allele and their 'normal' allele carries

the inefficient 5T variant or if they are homozygous for the 5T allele. Under such circumstances very little functional CFTR protein may be produced, possibly under 10% [60,61,67].

Mutations and abnormal CFTR processing and trafficking or chloride channel function

Early investigations showed that CFTR bearing the common ΔF508 mutation was incompletely glycosylated, suggesting that it was incompletely processed and not transferred to the cell membrane [70] (see Fig. 30.2). Also it appears to be temperature sensitive [71], and at lower temperatures can traffic to the cell membrane [72,73] where it has reasonable function as a cyclic AMP-dependent chloride channel [74]. Other mutations traffic to the cell membrane under normal circumstances, for example the relatively common (3% worldwide) allele G551D [75], where they display impaired function. Welsh and Smith [76] have reviewed these. At least two categories appear to exist (see Fig. 30.2). Mutations may impair the activation of CFTR; these occur in the ATP-binding domains and may respond to high levels of stimulation [77]. Other mutations alter the conduction properties of the CFTR chloride channel. Three such mutations (R117H, R334W, R347P) have been reported to be associated with milder disease and the CFTR channel appears partially functional [78–80].

CF gene mutations and patient phenotype

CFTR mutations can be grouped into five classes, as indicated above, on the basis of CFTR protein alterations (see Fig. 30.2): class I, no synthesis; class II, block in processing; class III, block in regulation; class IV, altered conductance; class V, reduced synthesis. CF shows markedly variable clinical features. Although some of these may be explained by differences in CFTR mutation, the majority show no clear relationship. On examining the common ΔF508 mutation, while there appears almost complete association with pancreatic status and sweat chloride concentrations, the pulmonary disease varies from extremely mild to very severe [81,82]. Pancreatic function does appear more closely related to the specific mutation carried, and mutations associated with exocrine pancreatic sufficiency (PS) are dominant to those associated with pancreatic insufficiency (PI) [83]. An early report linked mild disease and PS [78] and, by and large, this observation holds. A more extensive assessment of over 500 patients attending a single clinic identified five mutations (R117H, A455E, R334W, R347P and P574H) found exclusively in pancreatic sufficient patients [83]. However, the PS phenotype and genotype relationship is not absolute. In the large genotype–phenotype Consortium analysis [82], 10 of 396 ΔF508 homozygotes were pancreatic

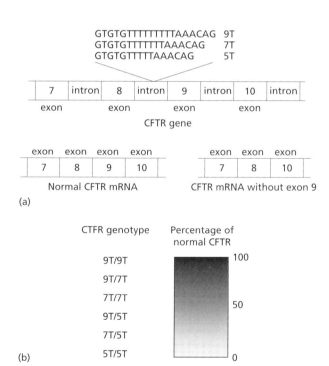

(a)

(b)

Fig. 30.3 (a) A section of the cystic fibrosis transmembrane conductance regulator (CFTR) gene. During processing, introns (sequences not involved with protein synthesis) are eliminated and the remaining sequences, exons, are spliced to form mature mRNA. DNA variations in intron 8 affect splicing efficiency and lead to different proportions of mRNA missing exon 9. (b) The relative percentage of normal CFTR depends on the number of thymines in the polyT sequence in intron 8, and the pairing of 9T, 7T and 5T alleles.

sufficient and 3 of 23 R117H/ΔF508 compound heterozygotes were pancreatic insufficient.

In CF, more than 95% of men are azoospermic because of congenital bilateral absence of vas deferens. ΔF508 mutation in men with this lesion is about 0.5 as opposed to the 0.03 in the general population [84]. A number of these men carry a second CF mutation and many who appear to have only one detectable CF mutation are also carriers of the 5T exon 9 splice variant on the other chromosome [85]. The association of specific organ involvement with specific CFTR mutations allows speculation that there exists a hierarchy of organ sensitivity to deficits in functional CFTR.

Ion transport

The evolving knowledge of CFTR function in ion transport provides a physiological basis for the more long-standing recognition of chloride, sodium and water abnormalities involving the sweat glands, airways, intestine and the pancreatic and biliary ducts. The disordered ion transport and water movement in these tissues is the basic abnormality leading to the pathophysiological consequences.

Sweat glands

While the abnormal sweat is only of clinical consequence in a hot environment, it has provided the basis of the 'gold standard' diagnostic test for CF for over 30 years. Sweat is formed from an electrolyte solution secreted into the secretory coil and is isotonic with plasma. It is modified as it passes through the duct by absorption of chloride and sodium. In CF the volume and rate of sweat production are normal [86], as is the composition of the primary secretion, but the reabsorption of ions is reduced because the ductal cells are impermeable to chloride and sodium ions are secondarily retained by the negative charge of the chloride ions. The sweat reaching the skin has a high sodium (~80 mmol/L) and chloride (~100 mmol/L) content and the duct lumen has a high negative charge [86].

However, other abnormalities of CF sweat glands are not so readily explained. Vasoactive intestinal peptide innervation is markedly reduced in comparison to normal tissues [87] and the role of prolactin in sweat formation may be altered in CF glands [88].

Airways epithelium

Cilia on airway cells beat within an aqueous environment, the 'sol'. This fluid is thought to be generated predominantly in the periphery of the lung and moved cranially by ciliary beating [89]. The alveolar surface volume is vastly greater than the airway surface volume, and if the hypoth-

esis is correct the airway epithelial cells must be predominant reabsorbers of the fluid. As in the sweat duct cells, sodium is absorbed through sodium channels in the apical membrane and transported out through the basolateral membrane by the sodium–potassium ATPase [90]. Water follows by osmosis. This sodium and water absorption is probably important for limiting the volume of the periciliary fluid layer.

Obversely, ion transport mechanisms also exist to rehydrate the airway surface. The relatively low intracellular concentration of sodium allows sodium to enter the cell from the basolateral surface via a sodium–potassium–chloride cotransporter (Fig. 30.4). Chloride is thus able to enter the cell and exits, down a gradient, via chloride channels in the apical surface. Water follows the movement of chloride, allowing hydration of the cell surface. Under basal conditions, sodium and water absorption predominate but at times of potential airway dehydration, such as exercise, chloride secretion can be activated to maintain the periciliary fluid volume.

As discussed above, CFTR is a cyclic AMP-dependent chloride channel and modulates the epithelial sodium channel and the ORCC. The consequence of an abnormal CFTR in the airway epithelium is therefore excessive inward sodium and water movement and impaired outward chloride and water movement. This gives rise to a relative dehydration of the pericellular environment, which is believed to contribute to bacterial adherence and colonization. It also leads to an increased (more negative)

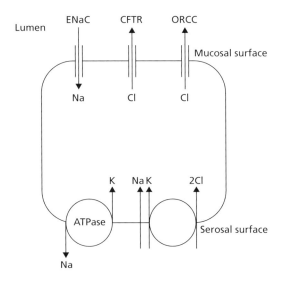

Fig. 30.4 Hydration of the mucosal cell surface depends upon interrelationships between the cystic fibrosis transmembrane conductance regulator (CFTR), the outward rectifying chloride channel (ORCC) and the epithelial sodium channel (ENaC) on the mucosal surface of the epithelial cell and the sodium–potassium ATPase cotransporter and the sodium–potassium–chloride cotransporter on the serosal surface of the cell (see text).

transepithelial potential difference. This change is also seen in the upper respiratory tract, where it is easier to make a measure of potential difference. This valuable observation was first made in 1981 [91], with subsequent research and proposal that nasal potential difference could be used as a diagnostic test [92–97]. As with the sweat test, however, patients with milder clinical disease, presumably with some preservation of CFTR function or alternative channel function, may yield equivocal rather than abnormal results [98].

Submucosal glands

CFTR is present in the submucosal glands, probably in greater amounts than in the airway epithelium [99]. Cyclic AMP-stimulated chloride secretion is defective [100,101] but there are conflicting data on calcium-stimulated chloride transport [101,102] and no data on sodium transport. The likelihood is that there is reduced mucin output and altered composition of mucus. It is unclear how important such abnormalities may be in the pathophysiological processes.

Gastrointestinal tract

There are conflicting data on basal chloride conductance [103–105] and amiloride effects on sodium transport [104–107]. However, cyclic AMP-induced chloride secretion has been reported abnormal in the jejunum [108,109], small intestine and colon [110], and rectum [105,106,111]. The combined effect of the abnormalities of ion transport appears to contribute to the development of meconium ileus and the distal intestinal obstruction syndrome. Gastric juices appear to have decreased volume, and increased viscosity and sodium levels [112]. Whether this is related to the increased frequency of gastro-oesophageal reflux is not clear.

Pancreas

Less is known about pancreatic abnormalities. *In vivo*, in response to infusion with secretin and cholecystokinin, the CF pancreas produces lower than normal chloride, sodium, potassium and bicarbonate [113–115]. The fluid secretion is lower but in proportion to the chloride and bicarbonate levels, suggesting that this is a secondary event [114]. CFTR appears localized principally to the proximal pancreatic ducts, with little at acinar level [116]. This supports the proposition that the pancreatic defect is principally of electrolyte and water secretion rather than pancreatic enzyme production.

Other tissues

B and T lymphocytes express CFTR and have abnormal

chloride transport [117]. However, this does not appear to yield a functional defect. CFTR is also expressed in the kidney but similarly renal function appears normal.

Epidemiology

Incidence

CF is found in all racial groups, although the frequency varies markedly. Reported frequencies in different populations are an underestimate. Neonatal screening does not occur widely and any molecular screening of necessity only examines a limited number of genotypes. As an increasing number of genotypes are recognized, patients with much milder variant disease are identified but will have been 'missed' from population screens.

Large population studies have been reported from Sweden [118], the former Czechoslovakia [119], The Netherlands [120], the USA [121], Ireland [122] and the UK [123], and other smaller reports provide additional information. The data are summarized in Table 30.3. These large population studies have been based on case finding rather than screening. The Swedish study of births from 1950 to 1957 found an incidence of 1 in 7700 [118], the Czechoslovakian study 1 in 5200 [119] and the Dutch study 1 in 3600 [120]. The more recent data from the American CF Registry estimates an incidence of 1 in 3500 live births for whites [121], although much lower incidences for other racial groupings (1 in 10 500 for American Indians, 1 in 14 000 for Blacks and 1 in 25 500 for Asians). The Irish and recent UK surveys give commoner frequencies, 1 in 1461 [122] and 1 in 2415 [123] births respectively.

Survival

In the 1930s most affected children died in the first few years of life. The prognosis has improved spectacularly since then, with a continuing worldwide increase in

Table 30.3 Estimated frequency of cystic fibrosis, at birth, in different populations.

National group	Birth incidence	Reference
UK	1/2500	Dodge *et al.* [123]
USA (white)	1/3500	Fitzsimmons [121]
USA (Black)	1/14 000	Fitzsimmons [121]
USA (Asian)	1/25 500	Fitzsimmons [121]
Sweden	1/7700	Selander [118]
Former Czechoslovakia	1/5200	Brunechy [119]
The Netherlands	1/3600	Ten Kate [120]
Ireland	1/1500	Cashman *et al.* [122]
Finland	1/25 000	Kere *et al.* [124]
Israel (Ashkenazi Jews)	1/3300	Kerem *et al.* [125]
Japan	1/323 000	Imaizumi [126]
Faroe Islands	1/1800	Schwartz *et al.* [127]

survival rates. In the USA, the median survival in 1969 was only 14 years but rose to 21 years in 1978 and 28 years in 1990 [121]. In the UK, the median survival was 31 years in 1994 [123] (Fig. 30.5), although estimates taking into account rates of improvement have suggested that patients born in the 1990s will survive beyond 40 years [128]. The survival of 3-year cohorts for males and females is shown in Fig. 30.6. It is clear that the reduction of mortality in the first year of life, caused principally by meconium ileus, has made a major contribution to the improved survival rates. Other factors, almost certainly antibiotic therapy and probably better nutrition, have effected the improvements beyond the first year, revealed by the progressive change in slopes of the cohort curves.

There are wide ranges in clinical severity of CF, which are reflected in the mortality rates. Genetic and environmental factors probably contribute. Although some genotypes appear to have a better prognosis, the relationship between genotype and phenotype is obtuse, with only a weak but favourable effect of pancreatic sufficiency.

Clinical decision-making may require a reasonable estimate of likely short-term to medium-term survival. Some studies have shown that a range of clinical variables may have such a predictive value [129–134], including infection with *Burkholderia (Pseudomonas) cepacia*, low weight [129–131], poor lung function [132], short stature and chronic liver disease [134], all of which may be associated with poorer prognosis.

Clinical presentation and morbidity

The majority of patients present in the first year of life (70% in the 1990 USA registry), although some patients are diagnosed later in life. The same registry indicated that 10% had not been diagnosed by 12 years. Some of the patients with much milder, variant disease escape diagnosis until their thirties or forties, although at times this is because the diagnosis had not previously been consid-

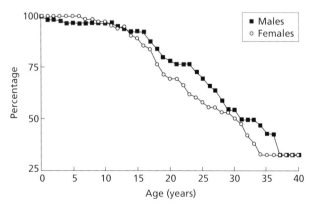

Fig. 30.5 Survival of UK residents with cystic fibrosis for both sexes for 1994. Median survival is 31 years. (Adapted from Dodge *et al.* [123].)

ered. Most patients present with the symptoms one would anticipate: the USA registry reported that meconium ileus was present at birth in 16%, and that 45% had acute or persistent respiratory problems, 36% failure to thrive and malnutrition, and 21% steatorrhoea and malabsorption at presentation.

Morbidity is a more difficult parameter to assess readily on a population basis. However, the height and weight of CF patients are simple indicators of the effectiveness of treatment. Recent data of over 3000 patients from 31 CF centres in the UK show improvement over earlier published observations [135]. Thus, during the first decade of life the height and weight of patients are now maintained at about 0.5 standard deviations below those of the general population, although they then show a progressive decline (Fig. 30.7).

Childhood presentations

Meconium ileus

Meconium ileus presents as intestinal obstruction in the neonatal period in up to 16% of children [121], although it may be diagnosed *in utero* at routine ultrasound scanning during the first trimester. The neonatal clinical features are abdominal distension, failure to pass meconium and bile-stained vomiting. Opacification of the right lower abdomen and distended loops of small bowel in the left hypochondrium are seen on radiographs. Calcification may also be seen as small specks or more extensive curvilinear areas. In one study, calcification was seen radiologically in 26% of cases of meconium ileus but identified histologically in 37% of the resected specimens, with the majority being intramural rather than serosal or luminal [138].

The obstruction is due to impaction of inspissated fetal meconium, usually occurring at the ileocaecal junction and extending proximally but sometimes found also in the ascending colon. It is associated with volvulus, ileal atresia or perforation in over 50% of cases. Rarely, a Gastrografin enema may relieve the obstruction [139] but surgery is required in the vast majority of cases. This often includes resection of a non-viable segment of ileum, usually with primary anastomosis. Improvements in the management of this complication of CF have made a major contribution to the improved survival rates.

The pathogenesis of meconium ileus is not fully elucidated. The bowel electrolyte and water transport abnormalities appear to provide the basic mechanisms. The G551D genotype, which is associated with greater apical membrane expression of CFTR than ΔF508, has a lower frequency of meconium ileus [140,141]. Pancreatic function has a less clear influence, with the severity of pancreatic insufficiency being no greater in affected individuals than in many other CF neonates. Indeed, meconium

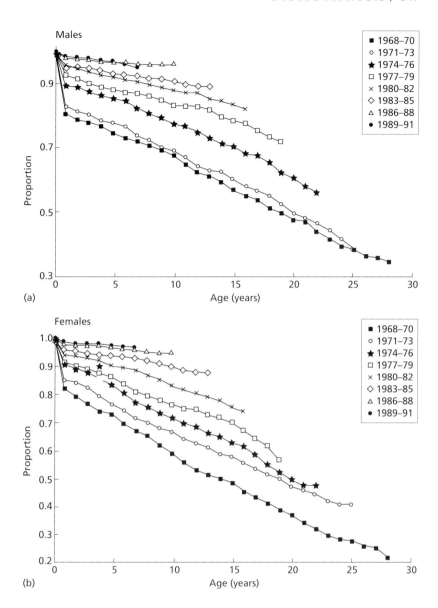

Fig. 30.6 Survival in successive 3-year cohorts of UK residents with cystic fibrosis: (a) males; (b) females. (Adapted from Dodge *et al.* [123].)

ileus can occur in infants who are pancreatic sufficient [142].

Prolonged neonatal jaundice

Prolonged cholestatic jaundice in the neonate may suggest a diagnosis of CF [143]. It is present in about 50% of patients presenting with meconium ileus.

Failure to thrive

Pancreatic insufficiency should be obvious by age 6 months in 75–80% of individuals [144]. In the absence of respiratory infections the affected infants usually have a voracious appetite but gain weight poorly. Usually the child is underweight and has obvious gaseous distension of the abdomen [145]. The stool may be frequent, bulky and offensive. In about 20% there is associated rectal

prolapse, which may be the presenting clinical problem and can be recurrent [146–149]. Rarer associated presentations include anaemia, hypoproteinaemic oedema and hypochloraemic alkalosis [150].

Recurrent infections

Respiratory symptoms have a variable age of onset and there is no clear marker for those who present early or late. A persistent cough is usually the first symptom. This is often exacerbated by viral infections and sputum appears loose. However, sputum production is uncommon in infants and young children, who tend to swallow the excessive mucus. A historical assessment from Australia (1955–78) showed that 37% of children presented with respiratory infections [151]. More recent data from the USA give a figure of 45% [121]. Wheezing is common, with up to 50% of cases being affected in some centres [152], and

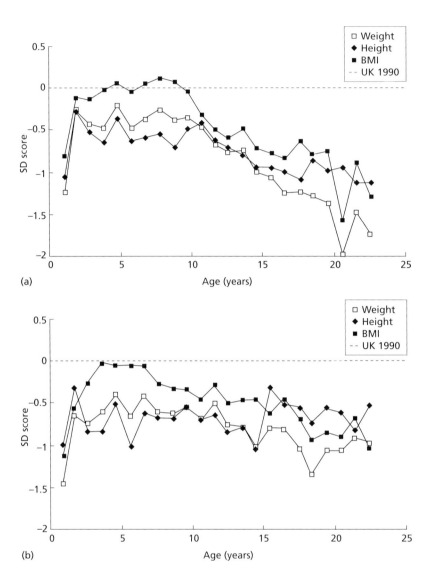

Fig. 30.7 (a) Mean weight, height and body mass index by age in patients with cystic fibrosis expressed as SD scores relative to the British 1990 growth reference [136,137]: (a) males; (b) females. (Adapted from Morison *et al.* [135].)

there is a risk that the infant may be misdiagnosed as asthmatic.

Nasal polyps and sinusitis

Nasal polyps are rare in the infant but increasingly common in preschool and school-age children. Presentation is most common between 5 and 14 years [153]. Polyps recur frequently and rapid growth may be a feature. Occasionally, they may be the only presenting feature of CF. There is a common association between sinusitis and nasal polyposis. Although the sinuses are rarely tender to palpation, over 90% are opacified radiographically [154].

Neonatal screening

Neonatal screening programmes have allowed the early recognition of CF, before any symptoms may have devel-

oped. Screening programmes and benefits of earlier diagnosis are discussed separately.

Diagnosis

Sweat test

The sweat test remains the gold standard for diagnosis, although all methods are uncertain at times. The Gibson and Cooke test of 1959 [8] has stood the test of time well and been examined in detail [155,156]. Sweat is stimulated by pilocarpine iontophoresis (a weak electric current aids the penetration of pilocarpine into the skin) and collected on preweighed filters. At least 100 mg of sweat should be analysed for sodium and chloride. Chloride is more discriminative than sodium and sodium values alone should not be used to diagnose CF [157,158]. It is probably correct to regard ion concentrations of greater than 70 mmol/L for both ions as definitely abnormal and indicative of CF, concentrations of less than 50 mmol/L as normal, and values of 50–70 mmol/L as equivocal requiring further consideration [158]. Sweat potassium concentrations are also raised in CF but there is some overlap with normal children. The data reported by Shwachman and colleagues [159] from 252 CF children and controls demonstrate these points (Table 30.4).

The sweat test is a complex procedure and there is room for misdiagnosis [160,161]. A single positive test should always be confirmed by a repeat test or with genotyping. The test should be performed by staff and a laboratory that carry out sweat tests on a frequent basis, not just occasionally. Infants under 4 weeks of age or 3 kg tend to produce too little sweat, and dry skin at any age is a problem. Thus eczema, with a small sweat volume, is a relatively common reason for raised electrolyte values. There are a number of rare conditions that may also cause raised sweat electrolytes: adrenal insufficiency, ectodermal dysplasia, hypothyroidism, familial hypoparathyroidism, nephrogenic diabetes insipidus, glucose 6-phosphatase deficiency, mucopolysaccharidoses, glycogen storage disease type I, anorexia nervosa and severe malnutrition.

Sweat sodium and chloride do show some variation with age; normal teenagers and young adults may have sweat test values, especially for sodium, that are just within the CF range. The effect of pretreatment with fludrocortisone increases the discriminating power of the sweat test in adults [162], since CF patients are relatively more resistant to its suppression of sweat electrolytes.

Nasal potential difference

If patients have an equivocal sweat test and the full genotype cannot be defined readily, it is worth while measuring the nasal potential difference [95–97], although the technique is difficult to apply in small infants and equivocal sweat tests often mean equivocal nasal potential difference.

Tests of pancreatic function

A variety of tests of pancreatic function have been described for patients with CF [163]. A simple screening test has been to look for fat globules in a stool preparation using a microscope. However, this is not specific for CF and false negatives occur. The gold standard is estimation of total faecal fat in stool collected over 3–5 days, a test designed to endear itself to patients, parents and laboratory staff! The daily dietary fat intake over the period must be adequate: 3 g/kg for infants and 30–100 g for older children and adults. Laboratory methods depend on whether medium-chain triglycerides are included in the diet [164,165]. Normal values for daily faecal fat excretion are usually less than 5 g and often less than 3 g [166].

Searches have been made for more pleasant tests. Faecal chymotrypsin concentrations have been suggested as an indicator of pancreatic exocrine insufficiency in neonates and older children [167,168]. The investigators have recommended testing three random specimens and calculating the mean value. Another alternative, the steatocrit test, examines small amounts of homogenized stool sealed into capillary tubes and centrifuged. The fat content is assessed in the resultant layers (basal solid layer, intermediate liquid layer, upper fatty layer) as the ratio of fatty layer to solid plus fatty layers, expressed as a percentage. However, there have been conflicting views of the reliability of this test [169,170].

Two urinary tests have been devised. They are based on the ability of pancreatic enzymes to cleave a compound administered orally, releasing a product that is absorbed from the gut, conjugated in the liver and excreted in the urine. *N*-benzoyl-1-tyrosyl *p*-aminobenzoic acid (NBT-PABA) releases PABA when acted upon by pancreatic chymotrypsin. PABA is then measured in the urine. However, PABA may not be fully absorbed and so a second collection is made after administration of free PABA, allowing a correction to be applied. This test gives incomplete separation between subjects with pancreatic insufficiency and normal function [171]. The pancreolauryl test is similar. On day 1 fluorescein dilaurate is given and hydrolysed to a variable degree by pancreatic arylesterases, with release of fluorescein. Fluorescein alone is given on day 3 and the overall result expressed as a ratio of the two. The test was reported as 97.6% specific for pancreatic insufficiency, and superior to an estimation of faecal chymotrypsin, in a

Table 30.4 Sweat sodium, chloride and potassium concentrations (mmol/L) for 252 patients with cystic fibrosis (CF) and 252 controls. (Adapted from Shwachman & Mahmoodian [159].)

	CF patients			Control subjects		
	Sodium	Chloride	Potassium	Sodium	Chloride	Potassium
Mean	111.2	115.3	22.9	28.2	28.0	10.3
SD	12.0	12.1	2.5	6.1	6.0	2.4
Minimum	75.4	78.6	13.8	15.9	7.7	6.0
Maximum	144.6	148.2	29.6	45.9	43.4	16.9

variety of patients not including those with CF [172]. It has distinguished between CF children with 'severe' insufficiency and controls [173]. The newest test measures pancreatic elastase in a 'spot' sample of stool. If it proves to give a true quantitative assessment of pancreatic insufficiency, it will be a welcome advance.

Genetic tests

The use of the polymerase chain reaction allows genotyping on blood spots or mouth rinses. This can be an useful adjunct to other diagnostic tests and to screening programmes. The large number of variants (>600) means that not all genotypes can be tested, although screening for approximately 20 genotypes would encompass 90–95% of all CF genes within discrete geographical populations. Nevertheless, the costs and the logistical effort involved in screening for more than a very small number of genotypes means that at present genetic tests for a diagnosis of CF are complementary to the other methods described.

Screening

The potential for neonatal screening was realized following the description of increased immunoreactive trypsin (IRT) levels in dried blood spots from infants with CF [174,175]. Possible benefits from screening were deemed to be (i) a favourable alteration in the natural history of the disorder; (ii) availability of genetic counselling to avoid the birth of a second child with CF in a family where the first child remained undiagnosed; (iii) eliminating the period of prediagnosis; and (iv) the prospect of being able to conduct critical studies of new treatments. Disadvantages were thought to include adverse effects on developing family relationships with the new baby, the trauma of false-positive tests and the stigmatization of children who might only have mild disease [176–178].

Immunoreactive trypsin

Early data that IRT is elevated in CF neonates suggested that the finding was almost always true, irrespective of pancreatic status [179,180]. However, a review of more extensive studies shows relatively high false-positive (up to 1% on the first sample) and significant false-negative rates [181]; the false-negative rate is not dependent on pancreatic function [182]. One problem with the IRT assay is that the level falls variably with age and method of assay [183,184]. Levels are raised two to five fold in the first 4 weeks of life but a negative test after 8 weeks of age is no longer informative. The value of IRT in screening was greatly enhanced by the additional ability to use the blood spots for CF gene screening.

IRT and DNA analyses

Bowling and colleagues [185] outlined a two-tiered approach of initial IRT assessment and then DNA mutation analysis on those samples with a defined elevated IRT. Similar IRT/DNA protocols have been adopted by most screening programmes and assessments are good [186–191]. The advantage of the combined IRT/DNA method compared with IRT alone is that the number of infants receiving a false-positive screening result is reduced dramatically.

Is early detection beneficial?

Short-term benefit has been shown for infants with CF who are diagnosed early by neonatal screening. Any evidence of altered long-term outcome is less clear-cut. The earlier reports on the benefits of neonatal screening were flawed in study design, since the outcomes for screened infants were compared with historical controls recognized in previous years [144,192–194]. However, these suggested that screened children at 2 years had spent less time in hospital [192] or gained weight better and had fewer chest infections [194]. Studies by Dankert-Roelse and colleagues [193,195,196] are of longer duration, although again the screened and unscreened populations are not entirely comparable since more of the screened patients were followed in a CF centre. The screened children had better clinical scores and survival and less decline in lung function [195,196]. In Wisconsin also, comparator groups have not been absolutely identical, although there has been evidence of some nutritional advantage (thus far up to the age of 10 years) in the group identified by screening [197]. A better-designed study for true comparison was carried out in Wales and the West Midlands of England between 1985 and 1990, in which screening was carried out only on alternate weeks and where screened and unscreened patients were followed in the same centres and therefore received identical management strategies [198,199]. Data have been recorded annually. Analysis to 4 years of age showed only shorter hospital admission time for the screened children in their first year [199]. By assessment at 8–10 years of age there was evidence that the screened group had (modestly) better lung function and nutrition (Weller, personal communication).

Antenatal screening

Different approaches have been used in the screening of pregnant women, such antenatal diagnosis being used in hospital and primary care settings. Stepwise screening tests the pregnant woman, and her partner is only tested if she is found to be a carrier of one of the small number of CF genes tested [200,201]. Couple screening requires mouthwash samples from both parents but only one is tested, unless that is positive, in which case the other is also tested [202,203]. A direct comparison of the two methods [204] found that couple screening allowed carriers to avoid the transient high levels of anxiety caused by stepwise screening, which occurs after the tested woman is found to be a carrier and the result from her partner is awaited. However, couple screening was associated with more anxiety and false reassurance among most screenees, who will test negative. Stepwise screening gave carriers and their relatives informative genetic facts. Population screening has also been tested in general practice [205]. Carrier testing was offered to patients of reproductive age, with an uptake of 66%. However, the cost-effectiveness of this approach is doubtful.

In one large trial when antenatal screening was offered to 8536 couples, the participation rate was 76% [203]. However, with the expected survival times of CF subjects constantly improving and the prospects of newer therapies in the future, the take-up rate is less certain. In 1998, Lothian was the only area in the UK where antenatal screening was routinely offered; neonatal screening is the preferred option of the Cystic Fibrosis Trust and others.

Childhood management

CF affects several organ systems. Many of the problems pertaining to individual systems apply to children and adults and are considered together. Similarly, the organization of care can be applied to both age groups, although the historical predominance of CF as a paediatric disease means that paediatric centres may be better established. The evidence has been convincing that CF children fare better if their care is coordinated from a specialist centre. Indeed the recommendation of the US Cystic Fibrosis Foundation is that all patients be evaluated at least quarterly at a regional CF centre [206]. In the UK the Cystic Fibrosis Trust, British Paediatric Association and the British Thoracic Society have jointly advocated care in specialist centres. The key factor is to provide care with an experienced team. The core team should include doctor(s), clinical nurse specialists, dietitian, physiotherapist, social worker and psychologist. The addition of a pharmacist is most useful. Access to other specialists and support teams is required and is considered with the specific complications.

Physical examination

The physical signs depend on the severity of disease. Often there may be no abnormal signs at all. With disease progression the lungs become hyperinflated and if this occurs in infancy thoracic cage deformity appears, revealed as bowing of the sternum (pectus carinatum),

Harrison's sulci and kyphosis. Digital clubbing develops. On auscultation, end-inspiratory and expiratory crackles appear, usually in the upper zones in the first instance. There may be polyphonic wheezes. In the abdomen there may be signs of hepatomegaly, splenomegaly or faecal 'masses'.

Other assessments

Scoring systems have been established, including clinical and radiographic evidence. Investigations at each visit include lung function, weight and height. Haematological, biochemical and microbiological assessments vary in frequency depending on the patient's condition.

Scoring systems

Clinical scoring systems in CF became pertinent once survival started to increase. The first, the Shwachman–Kulczycki score, was developed to evaluate a therapeutic programme, determine disease severity and compare one patient with the next [207]. The score is based on history, examination and chest radiograph. Respiratory function tests are not included, since at the time of the original paper these were not universally available. A maximum of 25 points and a minimum of 1 are awarded on a 5-point scale to each of four domains (Table 30.5). The 'Shwachman score' is so entrenched in CF clinical work that it is still applied even though it has been substantially outdated by the advances in CF care and patient well-being over the past 40 years and this should have confined it to historical interest; even so, there have been attempts to update it [208–210].

Other scoring systems have been suggested but also have faults. The Cooperman system [211] is rather too simple and was not really evaluated adequately. The NIH score, reported initially by Taussig and colleagues in 1973 [212], does take into account lung function tests and disease complications that were thought to influence survival (cor pulmonale, haemoptysis, pneumothorax), is reproducible and found to be useful prognostically. Stockrider and colleagues [213] have modified the NIH score in an attempt to refine it as a research tool. They found that five components accounted for 85% of the reliable consistency of the score (general pulmonary, nutrition, disability, psychosocial, acute pulmonary changes), although these had very little correlation with each other. Thus patients with the same total score could have very different component scores. Such differences limit its use as a research tool.

Chest radiographic scoring systems

Chest radiographic scores are included in the major

Table 30.5 Shwachman–Kulczycki score: a clinical evaluation score of patients with cystic fibrosis. (From Shwachman & Kulczycki [207].)

Grading	Points	General activity	Physical examination	Nutrition	Radiographic findings
Excellent (86–100)	25	Full normal activity; plays ball; goes to school regularly	Normal; no cough; pulse and respirations normal; clear lungs; good posture	Maintains weight and height above 25th centile; well-formed stools almost normal; good muscle mass and tone	Clear lung fields
Good (71–85)	20	Lacks endurance and tires at the end of the day; good school attendance	Resting pulse and respirations normal; rare coughing or clearing of the throat; no clubbing; clear lungs; minimal emphysema	Weight and height about 15th to 20th centile; stools slightly abnormal; fair muscle tone and mass	Minimal accentuation of bronchovascular markings; early emphysema
Mild (56–70)	15	May rest voluntarily during the day; tires easily after exertion; fair school attendance	Occasional cough, perhaps in the morning on rising; respirations slightly elevated; mild emphysema; coarse breath sounds; rarely localized râles; early clubbing	Weight and height above 3rd centile; stools usually abnormal, large and poorly formed; very little if any abdominal distension; poor muscle tone with reduced muscle mass	Mild emphysema with patchy atelectasis and increased bronchovascular markings
Moderate (41–55)	10	Home teacher; dyspnoeic after a short walk; rests a great deal	Frequent cough, usually productive; chest retraction; moderate emphysema; may have chest deformity; râles usually present; clubbing 2 to 3+	Weight and height below 3rd centile; poorly formed bulky fatty offensive stools; flabby muscles and reduced mass; abdominal distension mild to moderate	Moderate emphysema; widespread areas of atelectasis with superimposed areas of infection; minimal bronchial ectasia
Severe (40 or below)	5	Orthopnoeic; confined to bed or chair	Severe coughing spells; tachypnoea with tachycardia and extensive pulmonary changes; may show signs of right-sided cardiac failure; clubbing 3 to 4+	Malnutrition marked; large protuberant abdomen; rectal prolapse; large, foul, frequent, fatty movements	Extensive changes with pulmonary obstructive phenomena and infective lobular atelectasis and bronchiectasis

clinical scoring systems, although several independent radiographic scores have been developed since and have been used widely in staging disease severity. The most widely quoted was published by Chrispin and Norman in 1974 [214], which was usefully modified, standardized and validated by Brasfield and colleagues [209,215]. Independent assessments of the Shwachman, Chrispin–Norman and Brasfield scores reveal similar interobserver and intraobserver variations [216,217]. However, the rather simpler to apply Northern Score has the advantage of rapid and reproducible scoring by a single observer [218] (Table 30.6).

Pathophysiology of respiratory disease

The pulmonary disease, by far the principal cause of morbidity and mortality, is suppurative and progressive. Chronic endobronchial infection leads to bronchiectasis and eventually to respiratory failure. The abnormalities of CFTR function result in relative dehydration in the pericellular layer above the epithelial cells. This appears to facilitate bacterial adherence and inhibit mucociliary clearance. This progresses to chronic bacterial colonization with intermittent acute inflammatory responses, and a vicious cycle of further airway damage, further reduc-

Table 30.6 Northern score: a radiographic scoring system for cystic fibrosis.

Scale	Radiological changes
0	Normal: no cystic fibrosis lung disease evident
1	Mild: minimal increase in linear marking and/or nodular cystic lesions up to 0.5 cm diameter
2	Moderate: more pronounced linear marking and/or more widespread nodular cystic lesions
3	Severe: prominent increase in linear markings, profuse nodular cystic lesions, large areas of collapse/consolidation
4	Very severe: little or no area of normal lung seen, dense infiltration

Notes: The lungs are divided into four quadrants by a line drawn outwards from each hilum and each quadrant scored on a 0–4 scale based on increasing severity of chest radiographic changes. A further 0–4 points are allocated according to the observer's perception of overall severity.

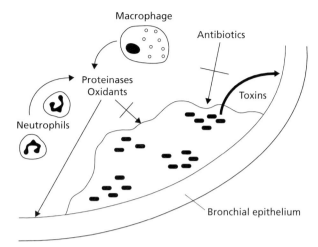

Fig. 30.8 Diagrammatic representation of *Pseudomonas aeruginosa* having undergone mucoid change and residing as microcolonies within an alginate gel. The alginate provides protection from phagocyte proteinases and oxidants and inhibits antibiotic penetrance. The bronchial epithelium is subject to damage from host defence mechanisms as well as pseudomonal toxins.

tion in mucociliary clearance and further bacterial colonization. While this rather superficial explanation for a progressive, suppurative airways disease may summarize events, it does not really address the underlying mechanisms and CF generally behaves more aggressively than other forms of bronchiectasis. Some genotypes of CF display a much milder form of airways disease. These facts suggest that there are specific biochemical events in CF that determine the inflammatory and infective responses.

Mucins are important for the viscoelastic properties of respiratory mucus. These large glycoproteins, consisting of a protein core that is extensively glycosylated, are in a highly condensed state inside secretory granules of respiratory epithelial cells. During secretion into the airway lumen they undergo rapid rehydration, with a several hundred-fold expansion in volume [219]. The pericellular relative dehydration in CF may affect this process. In addition, the mucins in CF are biochemically abnormal by being oversulphated [220,221], which may result from a defect in acidification of intracellular organelles in CF cells [38] that favours the activity of sulphotransferases over other processing enzymes in the Golgi.

Bacterial colonization

There appear to be no defects in traditional airway defences in CF. Clearly, however, bacterial colonization does take place and infective exacerbations ensue. Recent data suggest that subtle alterations in the sodium and chloride concentrations of the airway microenvironment may limit bacterial killing [222]. Further, reactive nitrogen species may be important microbicidal agents [223,224] and there is some evidence that inducible nitric oxide syn-

thase in the airway epithelium fails to upregulate [225], which could result in relative local deficiency of nitric oxide and its reactive product peroxynitrate. Also, there is new insight into CFTR function and mechanisms relating to bacterial colonization. CFTR functions as a receptor for the binding, endocytosis and clearance of *Pseudomonas aeruginosa* in the normal lung [226], and *in vitro* gene transfer of normal CFTR to CF epithelial cells reduces the binding of *Ps. aeruginosa* to the cells [227]. There is also evidence that the same organism binds to asialo-GM1, which appears to be expressed specifically by regenerating respiratory epithelial cells [228].

Bacterial adaptation can favour persistence even in the face of an active host response. After colonization, *Ps. aeruginosa* tends to undergo mucoid change. Mucoid strains appear among organisms grown *in vitro* under suboptimal conditions [229], and in CF airways *in vivo* the bacteria appear to be subject to similar nutritional limitations [230,231]. The mucoid change is due to marked production of alginate, which in the presence of calcium forms a firm gel. Microcolonies of organisms then exist in the alginate gel [232], protected from phagocytosis by host defence cells [233] and from antibiotics [234] (Fig. 30.8). The mucoid strains of *Ps. aeruginosa* express a different form of lipopolysaccharide [235] that makes the organism more sensitive to complement-mediated killing [236] and thus limits its ability to cause systemic infection. Indeed, despite the number of endobronchial bacteria, systemic sepsis is very unusual in these patients.

Infection and inflammation: a vicious circle

Bacterial colonization occurs early in CF patients and is

found even in those who apparently have clinically mild disease [237,238]. The supposition has been that the presence of bacteria stimulates and maintains a host inflammatory response that is unable to eradicate the organisms and therefore persists as a 'chronic' acute inflammatory response. Whilst this is undoubtedly of major importance, bronchoscopies in very young children have revealed the presence of an acute inflammatory response driven by interleukin (IL)-8 in the absence of bacteria [239]. In addition, laboratory-based tests have suggested an intrinsic deficiency of CF epithelial cells and cloned T cells to release IL-10 [240,241]. CF may therefore exhibit an 'intrinsic' alteration of IL-8 and IL-10 responses that would favour the persistence of inflammation.

The persistence of bacteria in the airways generates a continuous antigenic load. Coupled with an exuberant antibody response, this facilitates immune complex formation and amplification of tissue damage [242]. However, most tissue damage is mediated by neutrophils, predominantly via proteolytic mechanisms and oxidants. Neutrophil proteinases are present in substantial excess compared with their inhibitors [243], with elastase occupying a position of importance. Neutrophil elastase not only causes tissue damage but also has proinflammatory activity, activating chemotactic complement components and inducing IL-8 release from bronchial epithelial cells [244]. This aids the establishment of the 'vicious circle' of inflammation, bacterial colonization and progressive bronchiectasis.

Microbiology

A surprising feature of pulmonary infection in CF is the limited spectrum of pathogens involved, although this is increasing as patients are living longer, presumably related to the more aggressive use of antibiotics helping to 'select' organisms. Another surprising feature is that the organisms involved, which frequently are uncommon respiratory pathogens, do not cause the devastating *acute* illness that they may in other patients.

Staphylococcus aureus

In the earliest microbiological study of postmortem cultures of lung tissue from CF infants, *Staph. aureus* was the predominant organism [245]. Subsequently *Staph. aureus* and *Haemophilus influenzae* were recognized as important CF pathogens, often with repeated exacerbations [246–248]. *Staph. aureus* may cause severe infective exacerbations, although the potential for therapy is greater at present than in earlier times. However, there is an emerging problem with methicillin-resistant *Staph. aureus* (MRSA). This organism does not cause more serious infections but its presence is a major problem for patients with advanced disease, since some transplant centres do not

accept such patients on to their programmes. In some clinics the frequency of patient colonization with MRSA is greater than 10% and a number are employing segregation policies, as with *Burkholderia cepacia* (see below).

Pseudomonas aeruginosa

Ps. aeruginosa is generally regarded as the major CF pathogen but usually occurs after repeated infections with other pathogens. The incidence increases with age [249], with about 80% of patients over 26 years in the USA colonized [121], although the same survey showed an incidence of 21% under the age of 1 year. The emergence of colonization by *Ps. aeruginosa* is regarded seriously since it is often associated with an increased rate of decline in lung function. Certainly the organism has a wide range of virulence factors, including pyocyanin, elastase, exotoxin A and exoenzyme S [250–252]. Current practice is to attempt eradication procedures immediately on recognition of colonization. Different approaches include initial oral ciprofloxacin, with or without intravenous antibiotic therapy, followed by a more protracted period of nebulized antibiotics and/or intermittent ciprofloxacin [253].

An alternative, but as yet unproven, strategy to counter chronic pseudomonal infection is immunotherapy. Early attempts at using a *Pseudomonas* vaccine had proved very disappointing. A more recent polyvalent vaccine appears safe [254], and non-colonized patients who maintained high levels of antibodies in response to the vaccine have had a lower rate of infection than non-immunized patients or immunized patients who did not maintain a high-affinity response [255].

Stenotrophomonas (Xanthomonas) maltophilia

Other Gram-negative organisms, such as *E. coli* and *Klebsiella* spp., cause occasional colonization. Yet others are being seen with increasing frequency and may have serious implications for the patient. *Stenotrophomonas maltophilia* [256,257] colonization may follow *Ps. aeruginosa* infections or even occur as the first major Gram-negative problem after *Staph. aureus* and *H. influenzae* colonization. This organism usually displays multiple antibiotic resistances but its effect on the longitudinal health of the patient has to be established.

Burkholderia cepacia

B. cepacia has had a major impact in CF clinics. This organism, first identified as causing onion rot [258], was seen from the early 1970s [259] as an occasional colonizer of patients, although the frequency may have been underestimated because of inadequate laboratory culture techniques. During the 1980s and the early 1990s, the frequency of patient colonization [260–263] increased substantially and it was recognized that certain strains were being transmitted from patient to patient [262–272]. The problems with this organism are its innate resistance to very many antibiotics and the poorer clinical outcomes for many (but not all) patients colonized [273]. A number of patients succumb rapidly to 'cepacia syndrome', where severe worsening of pulmonary infection is associated with septicaemia [261,274,275]. These very serious considerations, linked with the transmissibility, have led to segregation policies between colonized and non-colonized patients and bans on summer camps and similar social events for CF patients. The psychological, social and financial implications of these infection control measures have been considerable. Recent work has identified a novel genomic marker that may help differentiate transmissible and non-transmissible lineages [276]. If so, it may prove helpful in the segregation of patients.

Opportunistic mycobacteria

The frequency of isolation of mycobacteria in the sputum of CF patients probably depends on the diligence with which these organisms are sought. Regular sputum testing and rigorous culture techniques to avoid 'contamination' by the organisms discussed above [277] appear to yield isolation rates of 10–20% of patients, with higher or lower rates in some clinics [278–283]. However, the true prevalence and effects of these mycobacteria are poorly understood. *Mycobacterium chelonei* and *M. avium* complex are the organisms reported most frequently to cause true infection (rather than colonization) and the criteria for 'infection' are not firm. Anecdotally, it has been difficult to be convinced of overt clinical deterioration in all but one of the Edinburgh Adult Clinic patients (frequency >10%), despite lack of treatment. In some the sputum becomes negative quite quickly and in others the organism persists or rarely the species changes. The one exception has been a patient colonized by *M. fortuitum*, an organism not usually viewed as pathogenic, and a fatality with this has been reported [284]. Occasional cases of *M. tuberculosis* are seen and it is important to maintain regular sputum vigilance, since the presence of such infection may be difficult to recognize clinically or radiologically, particularly in patients with more advanced disease.

Aspergillus

Aspergillus spp. are recovered quite frequently from the sputum of CF patients. The clinical relevance of this is unclear. The presence of a positive sputum culture, high IgE levels, a positive skin-prick test and precipitins are sometimes taken as evidence of allergic bronchopulmonary aspergillosis. In conjunction with new radiological shadowing and a clinical response to steroids, this

may indeed be the case. Allergic bronchopulmonary aspergillosis in CF patients has been reported [285]. One report suggests that the presence of *Aspergillus* spp. in the sputum does not contribute independently to a more rapid deterioration in pulmonary status [286]. At present the best advice is that if a patient is suspected of having clinically relevant lung disease associated with *Aspergillus* spp., treatment with steroids and itraconazole should be considered.

Viral infections

The precise role of viral infections in initiating respiratory problems or, in particular, promoting lower respiratory exacerbations is uncertain. The balance of data implies that infections with influenza A and B, rhinovirus, adenovirus and respiratory syncytial virus may be important [287–291] and affect mucociliary clearance. It is standard practice to immunize against influenza in the autumn.

Respiratory complications

Nasal polyps and sinus disease

The upper respiratory tract holds significant problems for the CF patient. The incidence of nasal polyposis is reported to vary from 10 to 32% [153,292–294]. There are differences between CF and non-CF nasal polyps, including the presence of acidic sulphated mucins in the CF patients [295], fewer eosinophils [296] and more mast cells and lymphocytes. The mast cells may show evidence of degranulation [297]. Approximately 50% of the CF patients appear to be atopic [292], although the relevance of this is uncertain [153,298]. Up to 40% of adults develop polyps [299]. The polyps may be multiple and large enough to cause visible nasal deformity. The presence of nasal polyps bears no relation to the severity of the lung disease.

The sinuses are affected in more than 90% of patients [292,300], involving predominantly the maxillary and ethmoid sinuses. The radiograph may show anything from mucosal thickening to complete opacification. While many patients are asymptomatic, others experience recurrent problems and the sinuses are colonized with the organisms found in the lower respiratory tract. Surgery and parenteral antibiotics may be required.

Progressive pulmonary pathology

The initial infections favour the development of bronchitis and bronchiolitis. Repeated infection causes ulcerative bronchitis leading to dilatation of the bronchial wall with resultant bronchiectasis. This affects the proximal airways and is usually most marked in the upper zones. The process favours progressive bacterial colonization and damage to the airways as outlined above. Bronchioles become filled with pus and there is consolidation of the surrounding lung parenchyma. Pneumonia can be seen at all stages of the evolution of the disease. Cysts occur in the lungs, particularly the upper lobes. The progressive lung damage results in deteriorating lung function, the development of pulmonary hypertension and respiratory failure.

Atelectasis and collapse

Segmental atelectasis and even lobar collapse can occur. These are usually associated with thick, retained secretions, often as a consequence of an infective exacerbation. While physiotherapy and antibiotics (see below) would be standard treatment, the importance of re-expanding the lung has led some physicians to have a low threshold for bronchoscopy with suction and even lavage of the involved segment. In the patient with more advanced disease, lavage has greater potential for causing problems and may even promote a worsening inflammatory response.

Haemoptysis

Small haemoptyses are common in CF, particularly in the patient with advanced disease. They are more frequent in the presence of an infective exacerbation and antibiotic treatment may be the appropriate course of action. However, isolated haemoptyses can occur in the stable patient and may simply require reassurance. Massive haemoptysis (>250 mL) is much less common but very disturbing for patient and clinician alike. It almost certainly reflects bronchial artery bleeding. In severe or persistent cases, interventional radiology with bronchial artery embolization may be a necessity [301–303].

Pneumothorax

Spontaneous pneumothorax (Fig. 30.9) is not very common in childhood but the risk increases in adolescence and adulthood. It is commoner in males, in whom an incidence of just under 20% has been reported [304]. Pneumothorax may be associated with a poor prognosis [305] and in our unit has been an event leading ultimately to the death of two patients. While small, asymptomatic pneumothoraces can be treated conservatively, larger pneumothoraces require aspiration or, more commonly, intercostal tube drainage. Lack of resolution results in surgical intervention. The more limited the procedure, the better. A limited abrasion surgical pleurodesis is the preferred option. More extensive pleurodesis or talc or kaolin slurry pleurodesis are less desirable because of increased risk of bleeding at any future transplant. Pleurectomy should be avoided for this reason. The problems associated with surgical interventions have encouraged us to pursue conservative intercostal tube drainage for significantly longer periods than would be the case for non-CF patients.

Pregnancy

The respiratory complications of pregnancy are considered in the section on fertility (see p. 863).

Respiratory failure

In the later stages of illness patients develop hypoxic respiratory failure, leading to pulmonary hypertension and cor pulmonale. There is usually a progressive rise in carbon dioxide, and early morning headaches are common. Oxygen therapy and nocturnal ventilatory support are valuable aids to symptom control and are described below. These strategies should not be used simply to prolong survival, unless lung transplantation is actively awaited.

Management: lung transplantation
(see Chapter 59)

Respiratory failure, lung infection and other pulmonary complications account for about 95% of CF deaths. Lung transplantation is the therapeutic option to prolong survival and return physical function and quality of life to satisfactory levels. The shortage of organ donors and the consequent wait for transplantation usually result in the referral for transplant assessment being made when the physician estimates a probable life expectancy of about 2 years. The first successful heart–lung transplant for CF was in 1983 (1985 in Europe) [306,307]. Single lung transplantation is not feasible in CF because of the chronic infection in the native lung, which could lead to fatal infections under immunosuppression. Heart–lung transplantation thus remained the treatment of choice [308] until the successful introduction of bilateral lung transplantation [309–311]. With this technique cardiopulmonary bypass can often be avoided, making it the procedure of choice. To date nearly 400 CF patients in the USA and more than 300 in Canada and Europe have undergone heart–lung or lung transplantation. In 1990 the first living-donor lobar lung transplantation took place and over 50 have now been performed. For patients with marked liver disease in addition to lung disease, heart, lung and liver transplantation may be undertaken, although numbers of such operations are few.

Referral and waiting

In general it is helpful if the referring and transplant centres have a close working relationship. This aids patients in their anticipation of what to expect at assess-

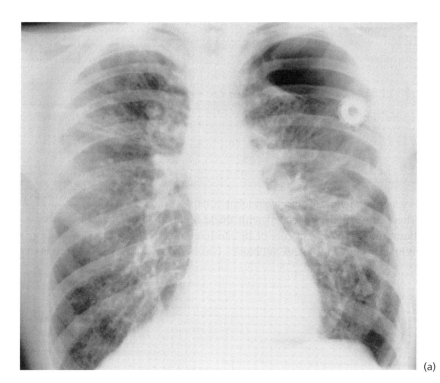

(a)

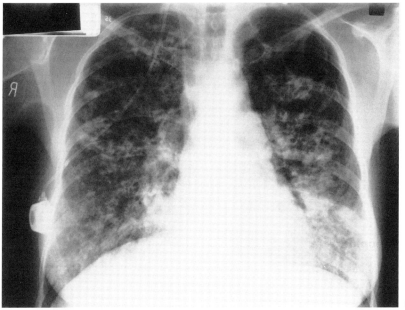

(b)

Fig. 30.9 (a) Chest film of a male patient with advanced cystic fibrosis. There are extensive bronchiectatic changes with a complicating pneumothorax on the left side. The film also shows a totally implanted venous access device in the upper left anterior chest wall accessed by a 'gripper' needle and standard connector for administration of intravenous antibiotics. (b) Chest film of a female patient with advanced cystic fibrosis. There are extensive bronchiectatic changes with a complicating pneumothorax on the left side. The film also shows a totally implanted venous access device in the right mid-axillary chest wall. The device is not being used so there is no external access needle. The tubing connecting the reservoir chamber and the central veins can be seen. It runs in the subcutaneous tissues upwards across the lateral and anterior chest wall to enter the subclavian vein above the clavicle and downwards within the veins to the superior vena cava.

ment, and may limit inappropriate referral of individuals. The whole process is very stressful for patients. Most do not believe they are unwell enough for transplantation when the subject is first broached, although once they have accepted the idea the time spent waiting for assessment and placement on the programme seems far too long to them. Once on a programme the usual wait for suitable donor lungs averages well over a year and a substantial proportion of patients die on the waiting list. Many receive 'false alarms', and may even be at the transplant centre awaiting the donor organs only to find them too

damaged for transplantation on arrival. These stresses mean that the support of family and CF unit carers may be invaluable.

Preparations

CF patients require particular attention in the waiting period. Their general health is, by definition, poor and frequent infective exacerbations are to be anticipated. Indeed many become so unwell that they receive intravenous antibiotics more often than not and undergo multiple hospital admissions. Nutrition is difficult, since most have no appetite and may become extremely breathless during eating. Nasogastric or gastrostomy tube feeding is usually essential. Supplemental oxygen therapy at night, or usually night and day, is necessary for most patients, and some benefit from nocturnal ventilatory support using BiPAP. Attention should also be paid to the bones, since a significant number of CF patients have reduced bone mineral density or overt osteoporosis. This is probably the result of low vitamin D levels through some or all of childhood combined with low exercise levels because of their respiratory disabilities. The high doses of steroid used in the immediate post-transplant period put the patients at risk of fractures. Assessment of bone mineral density before or at time of transplant referral, followed by therapeutic intervention as necessary, is important. Our policy is to use calcitriol rather than bisphosphonates, but there are no comparative studies.

Early complications

Early mortality (within 30 days) was as low as 12% even in the earlier days of transplantation and has improved since. The 1-year survival in two large series of heart–lung transplants has been about 70% [307,308], and there are similar figures for bilateral lung transplants [312,313]. Rejection episodes are the most common early complication, with almost all patients experiencing an episode within the first month. Infection is also quite common and it is difficult to distinguish between rejection and infection on clinical grounds; fever, cough, breathlessness and chest radiographic infiltrates are typical of both. In acute rejection radiographic abnormalities are less common after 1 month [314]. Cytomegalovirus (CMV) infections, especially pneumonitis, are common in lung transplantation; ideally, CMV-negative recipients should receive organs from CMV-negative donors. Ganciclovir provides important therapy for such problems. *Pneumocystis carinii* infection is common in patients not receiving prophylactic treatment [315]. The most convenient prophylaxis is with co-trimoxazole on Fridays to Sundays.

Late results and complications

Survival rates are improving. At present the 3-year survival is in the order of 56%, in contrast to 46% for transplants prior to 1992, and the 5-year survival is 48%. Survival rates are higher at centres that perform more transplants. There do not appear to be significant differences in survival attributable to differences in gender, age group or blood group.

Obliterative bronchiolitis is the most serious late pulmonary complication. Its development appears linked to repeated (perhaps unrecognized) episodes of rejection. Close assessment and treatment of rejection should limit the frequency of this complication. On the other hand, immunosuppression may allow the development of lymphoproliferative disorders caused by Epstein–Barr virus. The recognition of this requires modulation of the immunosuppressive regimen and treatment with ganciclovir. A careful watch for bacterial infections is required since CF patients have bacterial colonization of their sinuses, a ready source of *Pseudomonas* and other organisms for infection of the lower respiratory tract. The non-CF phenotype of the transplanted lungs seems to help limit permanent colonization in the lower airways.

The immunosuppressive drugs have their own problems. The steroids affect glucose handling, and thus patients already on insulin need their doses modified and other patients not previously on insulin may have to start therapy. In many patients cyclosporin causes hypertension that necessitates treatment. In the long term, cyclosporin-induced renal impairment is important and there should be careful monitoring. Some patients develop a chronic anaemia unrelated to renal impairment that presumably is drug-induced. Azathioprine may be the principal culprit, although the cause is not clear-cut.

Despite the unwanted effects of the immunosuppression, particularly the high doses of steroids in the early days, patients soon observe a dramatic improvement in exercise capacity and loss of the severe problems of chronic sputum production. Despite the very marked improvement in exercise abilities the maximum tolerable exercise capacity in transplanted patients is significantly diminished compared with healthy control subjects. Heart–lung and bilateral lung transplant patients achieve a mean maximum oxygen uptake of 50–60% predicted [316–318].

Gastrointestinal complications

Pancreatic insufficiency

Pancreatic disease was recognized before the respiratory component of CF (see above). Pancreatic function declines during the first year of life; 92% of infants diagnosed by neonatal screening were found to have steatorrhoea by age 1 year [319], while 20% of patients found to be pancreatic sufficient at birth became insufficient within 2–12 months of evaluation [320]. Various tests have been used to test pancreatic status (see above). Clinical steatorrhoea is a florid expression of pancreatic insufficiency, occurring only after patients lose greater than 97% of pancreatic lipase and colipase secretory activity [321].

Exocrine pancreatic dysfunction is treated by giving oral pancreatic enzyme supplements. These are extracts of pig pancreas. Initially, powdered extracts were used but these were inactivated by gastric acid and pepsin. In the 1970s, enteric-coated microspheres were developed, the coating not dissolving unless the pH is greater than 5.5, enabling the enclosed enzymes to escape the acid–pepsin gastric environment. Although pancreatic-insufficient patients have impaired secretion of all pancreatic enzymes, fat malabsorption presents the greatest difficulty. It leads to malodorous bulky stools and flatulence and, because of the calorie content of fat, weight loss. Pancreatic supplements are therefore ranked according to lipase content. The dose of enzyme supplements should be adjusted to the estimated fat content of a meal or snack. In reality most patients are poor at such estimations, and the number of enzyme capsules they use for the average meal is usually achieved by judging the clinical response. If a good clinical response is difficult to obtain or there remains doubt about the patient's level of absorption, a faecal fat balance is the most useful study to optimize enzyme dose [322,323].

With pancreatic insufficiency, the high-volume bicarbonate-rich fluid is not secreted and intraduodenal pH may remain low, since gastric acid is inadequately buffered [324]. When duodenal pH is less than 4, pancreatic lipase is irreversibly inactivated and most bile acids precipitate thus preventing micelle formation; this combination contributes to fat malabsorption. H_2 antagonists and proton pump inhibitors can reduce gastric acid output and enhance the alkalinity of the duodenum [325–327]. This can be a useful adjunct for patients requiring large numbers or increasing doses of pancreatic enzymes in order to control malabsorption.

Fibrosing colonopathy

In 1994 a 'new entity' for CF, fibrosing colonopathy, was reported [328]. This first report highlighted a possible association between colonic strictures and patients' intake of high-strength pancreatic enzyme preparations. It led to a UK survey, which identified 14 cases whose lipase intake was substantially higher than that of controls (46 200 units/kg daily vs. 21 500 units/kg daily) [329]. Similar cases have been identified in other countries. Although not all such cases had used high-strength enzyme preparations, the more recent USA case–control study has confirmed the association with high intake of enzyme supplements [330]; 29 patients had a mean lipase intake of 50 046 units/kg daily compared with 18 985 units/kg daily for the 105 controls. This provided a relative risk of 10.9 for patients taking 24 000–50 000 units/kg daily compared to those taking 0–24 000 units/kg daily. In the UK the Committee on Safety of Medicines has recommended a maximum lipase intake of 10 000 units/kg daily, even for adults among whom no cases have been described.

The pathology associated with the colonic strictures is that of extensive submucosal fibrosis. Some cases show evidence of mucosal injury and repair, while others show a normal mucosa. Mild infiltration with inflammatory cells is occasionally seen, and in some there is an eosinophilic infiltrate. The condition comes to clinical attention when the colonic lumen is narrowed to the point where it causes obstruction. At operation the colon wall is thickened and firm. One report has suggested that increased thickness of the colonic wall can be detected by ultrasound [331]. This has not been confirmed by other investigators and barium enema appears a more informative investigation. However, radiological appearances of a featureless and stiffened colon were reported more than 20 years ago as features of CF [145]. This was long before high-dose or even standard-strength enteric-coated microspheres were introduced. It may be unsafe therefore to assume that radiological or ultrasound evidence of a thickened colon is sufficient in itself to suggest early fibrosing colonopathy.

Pancreatitis

Pancreatitis occurs in pancreatic-sufficient patients. Pancreatic-insufficient patients usually have fatty replacement of the pancreas and too little tissue to become inflamed. Pancreatitis is seen in less than 0.5% of CF children but with greater frequency in adults (1.6–2.4% over 30 years) [121]. The diagnosis is easy to miss since pancreatic-sufficient patients are thought to be 'too healthy' or 'too old' to have CF. A sweat test should be performed in any person with unexplained recurrent pancreatitis [332,333]. Perversely, recurrent pancreatitis in pancreatic-sufficient patients may ultimately lead to pancreatic insufficiency.

Gastro-oesophageal reflux

Gastro-oesophageal reflux is common in CF. It appears to be commoner than in the general population, an 'anecdotal' observation supported by a comparative study finding increased frequency in CF patients compared with their siblings [334]. The cause is not clear, although there are probably contributions from the increased abdominal–thoracic pressure gradients associated with coughing and forced expiration during chest physiotherapy and from the postural drainage positions during physiotherapy. This would provide an explanation for the reported association with severer respiratory disease [335]. A significant proportion of patients require therapy with an H_2 antagonist or proton pump inhibitor.

Distal intestinal obstruction syndrome

Distal intestinal obstruction syndrome is an intestinal obstruction in the ileocaecal region unique to CF that occurs after the neonatal period. The true incidence is uncertain. Retrospective case reviews have reported incidences of 12–41% [336,337], with males and females equally affected. The syndrome almost always occurs in the pancreatic-insufficient patient. Relative dehydration, dietary changes and, in particular, inadequate enzyme supplementation may contribute. Distal intestinal obstruction syndrome occurs with sludging of intestinal contents in the ileocaecal region, with the process extending distally.

Clinically, there is crampy abdominal pain and distension, usually with a palpable mass in the lower right quadrant. Partial obstruction can extend to complete obstruction, with increasing pain and distension plus vomiting. The uneducated patient and the unaware surgeon have conspired occasionally to allow inappropriate surgery and resection of bowel. Successful medical treatment is almost always possible, particularly in the early stages, with repeated oral doses of Gastrografin, a contrast medium that exerts a strong osmotic effect. The consequent movement of fluid into the bowel moves the obstructing ileal contents. Success has also been reported using bowel irrigation with balanced polyethylene-glycol solutions [338]. Contrast enemas may be therapeutic for patients with complete obstruction [339].

Hepatobiliary complications

The primary liver abnormality of CF affects the cells of the bile ductules, with consequent reduced bile production and altered bile acid composition [340,341]. There is resultant biliary obstruction, portal tract inflammation and eventually portal tract fibrosis and focal biliary cirrhosis [342]. The quoted prevalence of cirrhosis in CF varies from as little as 2% to as much as 25% [121,343,344]. It is extremely difficult to obtain an accurate estimate of bile ductule function and associated focal damage. Plasma hepatocellular enzymes (alanine aminotransferase and aspartate aminotransferase) and biliary enzymes (alkaline phosphatase and γ-glutamyltransferase) are readily measured but give very poor indication of hepatobiliary status. Nevertheless, in the absence of a better measure these are generally used as the monitors of CF liver disease.

There appears to be no relationship to CF genotype, an observation confirmed by formal studies. In one, patients identified with severe liver disease had genotypes that reflected the spectrum of mutations seen in the local population [345]. In another, 29 of 111 children and young adults had severe liver disease with portal hypertension, 19 had biochemical or clinical evidence of liver disease and 63 had no evidence of liver disease. There was no correlation between hepatic disease and CF mutation [346].

Not all liver disease is as severe. In several studies over many years, fatty change has been reported to have a high incidence in CF [2,347,348]. Since CFTR is found only in the bile duct epithelium, the fatty change presumably represents a secondary effect, for example of malabsorption.

Also, there are many case reports of prolonged neonatal jaundice in CF infants. Most appear also to have had meconium ileus, although the mechanism of the jaundice is uncertain. Cholestasis may persist for months but ultimately resolves. It is not clear whether these patients are at increased risk of developing biliary fibrosis and cirrhosis later in life.

Assessment

Since conventional liver biochemistry appears to underestimate biliary and liver disease, additional assessments should be considered as part of routine monitoring, for example at the annual review. Upper abdominal ultrasound is easy, non-invasive and may be informative. Abnormal liver architecture and splenomegaly are indicators for repeated or additional investigations. In more advanced disease Doppler may reveal reversed portal blood flow. Ultrasound does not always reveal the presence of varices, and in our unit the presence of significant splenomegaly leads to CT contrast scanning to try to identify these.

Biliary scintigraphy often shows delayed excretion in the absence of extrahepatic obstruction, presumably reflecting biliary hypomotility or bile stasis [349]. In one study using endoscopic retrograde cholangiography-pancreatography, all patients had abnormalities of the intrahepatic bile ducts [350].

Treatment

Medical treatments are distinctly limited. The use of ursodeoxycholic acid has become widespread during the past 5 years, although the evidence for its benefits is, as yet, unclear. Ursodeoxycholic acid is a hydrophilic bile acid that tends to replace the more toxic hydrophobic bile acids [351]. Also, it is able to stimulate bicarbonate secretion directly and thus improves bile flow [352]. The early clinical studies reported improvement in liver function when patients with CF liver disease were given high-dose ursodeoxycholic acid [353–355]. There are no studies to show whether use of this drug prevents the development or progression of cirrhosis, or indeed to identify which patients should be treated.

For established cirrhosis with portal hypertension and varices, traditional treatments such as portosystemic shunting [356] and sclerotherapy [357] have been used. Currently, major operative portosystemic shunts have been superseded by TIPSS (transjugular, intrahepatic, portal systemic shunt) procedures [358]. Patients with severe liver disease are candidates for liver transplantation. A balanced assessment has to be taken with respect to the pulmonary status. Accompanying severe lung disease may indicate the need for heart–lung–liver transplantation. Alternatively, severe liver disease may have secondary effects on the lungs (e.g. intrapulmonary shunting; diaphragmatic splinting), which would reverse on liver transplantation. Medium-term survival for liver transplantation is good; the Cambridge group reports nine children all alive at 4–55 months (median 30 months) [359].

Extrahepatic biliary disease

Many CF patients have small shrunken gallbladders or bile sludging [360]. Gallstones and symptomatic gallbladder disease are seen frequently, usually in adults, with CF [121,361]. It is thought that the large faecal bile acid losses and decreased bile acid pool cause the bile to become supersaturated with cholesterol, which leads to stone formation [362]. The management for most patients is laparoscopic cholecystectomy.

Nutritional consequences of, and implications for, cystic fibrosis

Clinicians have long recognized that patients who are underweight have a worse prognosis than well-nourished patients, but does poor nutrition cause the decline or is it merely a marker of disease progression? Mortality patterns over a 20-year period obtained from the Canadian Patient Data Registry suggest that being underweight is, at least partly, an independent predictor of mortality [363]. Body cell mass (BCM) is the portion of metabolically active fat-free mass. Assessment of anthropometric parameters, lung function and BCM in 61 patients aged 5–17 years with moderate disease showed that change in BCM was the best predictor of change in forced vital capacity (FVC), and those patients with normal growth in BCM had less decline in FVC than those with retarded growth of BCM [364]. Generally, BCM increases with increasing calorie intake. However, the use of nutrients is controlled hormonally, particularly by insulin. In CF there may be relative insulinopenia (see below), which may contribute to reduced anabolic activity.

The association of poor nutritional status and poor lung function is presumed to be the result of increased energy expenditure from lung infection and inflammation and increased work of breathing. While these have a major effects, it has also been speculated that the CF gene defect itself may elevate energy expenditure, as a result of both abnormal ion channel kinetics and increased activity of mitochondrial electron transport.

The other aspect to consider is the dietary intake. Recommendations for daily intake are between 120 and 150% of normal recommended intake. In practical terms this is not always easy when the patients are relatively fit and well. When they are unwell, the consequent anorexia makes it even more difficult. When patients have moderate to severe disease, they have to contend with a degree of constant anorexia. At this stage also, poor nutrition has a deleterious effect on the individual's ability to resolve infection and inflammation.

Dietetic support

The dietitian has an important role in the management of CF patients by monitoring body mass index and lean body mass as well as reviewing the average daily calorie intake and pancreatic enzyme use. Dietary advice is important since it is difficult to achieve a high calorie intake without adequate use of fats, and this requires guidance with respect to pancreatic enzymes. In addition, malabsorption results in low levels of fat-soluble vitamins and it is standard practice to advise supplementation with vitamins A, D and E. When patients have difficulty keeping their body mass index in the range 19–20 or better (normal range 20–25), they should receive high energy-containing oral supplements. The newer preparations appear more palatable than some of their predecessors. In the patient with more advanced disease additional measures are often needed. Overnight enteral feeding via a nasogastric tube (passed by the patient every night) or a gastrostomy tube is a very effective way of maintaining reasonable nutrition.

Diabetes mellitus and cystic fibrosis

Changes in glucose metabolism were observed in the very early descriptions of CF [2,365] and the association between CF and diabetes mellitus was first recognized in 1955 [366]. Subsequently, different studies have reported varying prevalences of impaired glucose tolerance and diabetes mellitus, although methodologies have varied [367–373].

The Copenhagen centre has provided some of the more comprehensive data. For a planned longitudinal study over 5 years all 226 patients over 2 years of age were entered; 191 patients completed the 5 years. During the study the prevalence of diabetes increased from 11 to 24%, with an average annual incidence of 3.8%. For those aged 10 years or more the respective figures were 16%, 34% and 5.0% [374]. The median age of diagnosis for diabetes was 21 years (range 3–40); 22% of oral glucose tolerance tests showed impaired glucose tolerance, although the overall picture was complex. Nearly 60% of subjects with impaired glucose tolerance showed normal glucose tolerance at their next annual test. Overall only 37% of patients had a normal test on all five occasions and impaired glucose tolerance gave a higher risk of developing diabetes (odds ratio 5.6). This study highlighted that an oral glucose tolerance test is the gold standard for assessment. Routine assessments of hyperglycaemic symptoms, fasting hyperglycaemia and glycated haemoglobin did not identify diabetes mellitus reliably.

Pathogenesis

In patients with CF who have diabetes, there are reports of a 30–50% reduction in the number of islets and β cells [375–377]. With the additional observations of fibrotic bands, a shrunken fibrotic pancreas and presumptive distorted blood supply, the prevailing view has been that diabetes develops in CF as a secondary effect of progressive damage to the pancreas as a result of CF-related abnormalities in the exocrine pancreas. However, more recent data have shown that diabetes in CF appears to be type II diabetes [378,379] and that patients often have non-CF relatives with type II diabetes. This has led to the suggestion that CF is a risk factor that interacts with the genetic predisposition for type II diabetes, resulting in clinical disease.

Management

There is some suggestion that insulin treatment of diabetic patients improves lung function and reduces infective exacerbations [380]. In our own unit we have observed evidence of improved nutrition and body mass index after introduction of insulin treatment. In addition, diabetic patients with CF are probably no less prone to developing late diabetic complications than are other patients with diabetes of similar duration and glycaemic control. An ideal approach appears to be to run a combined clinic with an interested diabetes service. However, the dietetic input is different from that in conventional diabetes management. Since CF patients have such difficult nutritional demands, their diet should be directed accordingly and insulin therapy adjusted to the dietary intake.

Arthropathy and vasculitis in cystic fibrosis

Acute or subacute arthritis is seen in patients with CF and has been well reported [381–384]. In our own adult unit about 5% of patients have intermittent problems of arthritis, occasionally with the associated symptoms being their principal clinical concern. Usually, there is an adequate response to non-steroidal anti-inflammatory drugs (NSAIDs). However, there are reports of individuals developing persistent sinovitis and progressive erosive arthritis [383], and also isolated reports of concurrent arthritis, psoriasis and CF [385] and sarcoidosis, arthropathy and CF [386]. As an additional anecdote, one of our patients with intermittent arthropathy also has biopsy-proven sarcoidosis.

Sometimes episodic arthritis is associated with erythema nodosum or other nodular skin lesions. More commonly, purpura may be seen, particularly on the legs [387–389]. In a report of 12 patients with dermal vasculitis two had evidence of systemic vasculitis [389]. There was

no evidence of autoimmune disease but 40% had antineutrophil cytoplasmic antibodies. Purpuric vasculitis is probably associated with severer lung disease. It is a matter for conjecture as to whether lung-derived immune complexes are part of the underlying mechanism. Anecdotally, some severely ill patients awaiting transplantation experience fevers and arthralgia that are suppressed by systemic steroids.

Fertility and pregnancy in cystic fibrosis

With the marked improvements over the past 30 years in patients' well-being and survival, 'new' CF-related problems have arisen. Many now have the expectation and wish to have children. Two problems therefore have to be addressed: infertility, especially in the male, and the risks of pregnancy.

Male fertility

Infertility is almost universal among males (approximately 2% appear fertile [390,391]) as a consequence of a developmental defect of structures derived from the embryonic wolffian duct. This leads to absence, atrophy or various forms of obstruction of the vas deferens, the body and tail of the epididymis, and the seminal vesicles [392–396]. However, testicular histology appears normal and active spermatogenesis occurs, although some abnormal and immature sperm may be seen on testicular biopsy [392,397]. As discussed above, during fetal growth CFTR function appears critical for the normal development of the wolffian duct structures, and congenital absence of the vasa deferentia may be the only manifestation of CF.

The potential for fertility can be readily assessed by checking for azoospermia. It is important to introduce the likelihood of male infertility gently, during adolescence, when the concept is less threatening. However, new techniques of sperm aspiration from the epididymis or vasa efferentia and *in vitro* fertilization [398] are now being introduced in the management of male infertility in CF.

Female fertility

As a group, females with CF have reduced fertility compared with healthy subjects. The extent of the reduced fertility is unclear, and individual patients have normal fertility, subfertility or absolute infertlity. One frequently quoted study, which gives a group estimate of about 20% normal fertility [399], appears flawed in design and details. Primary and secondary amenorrhoea are common [400], often reflecting poor lung health and nutrition [401]. These contribute to overall reduced fertility. Anatomically the female reproductive tract appears normal, although relative dehydration of the cervical mucus may result in a physical barrier to sperm penetration [399].

In the absence of a simple screening test to assess fertility in women with CF, all patients of child-bearing age should be presumed to be potentially fertile and those wishing to avoid pregnancy for personal or health reasons should be counselled on appropriate forms of contraception. Oral contraceptives generally are effective and in limited-size studies have not shown problems [400,402], although there are potential difficulties. Chronic use of oral contraceptives has been associated with intrahepatic cholestasis and cholelithiasis; some of the progestogens used impair glucose tolerance; and oral contraceptives may deplete vitamin D and E levels. Finally, concern has been expressed over possible antagonistic effects of antibiotics on the intestinal absorption and bioavailability of oral contraceptives. If pregnancy is definitely contraindicated, a more definitive contraceptive measure should be given serious consideration.

Pregnancy

The first documented successful pregnancy in CF was in 1960 [403]. However, the patient died 6 months postpartum. The next report, in 1966, of a survey of 13 pregnancies in 10 patients from 34 CF centres revealed that five women experienced significant pulmonary decline during pregnancy and two died in the immediate postpartum period [404]. A further large survey of 119 CF centres in the USA and Canada, published in 1980, reviewed 129 pregnancies in 100 patients [405]; 75% of the pregnancies were completed, 89% of which resulted in viable infants; 12% of the women died within 6 months of delivery. The women who died were noted to have severe pulmonary disease before pregnancy. A similar association was observed in a smaller report published in 1983 [406]. Supporting this concept, a survey of 38 pregnancies in 25 women, predominantly with mild disease (half were pancreatic sufficient), indicated that pregnancy was well tolerated [407]. In contrast to the preceding studies, a recent UK report of 22 pregnancies in 20 patients recorded lung function before pregnancy, immediately after delivery and after pregnancy [408]; four mothers died up to 3.2 years following delivery. The previous observations were supported but with firmer data. The women with moderate to severe lung disease (forced expiratory volume in 1 s, FEV_1, <60% predicted) before pregnancy fared worse, producing preterm infants and suffering increased loss of lung function and mortality compared with mildly affected mothers.

Pregnancy is therefore not to be undertaken lightly. There should be very careful assessment of an individual's health and sound counselling provided. Patients whose FEV_1 is less than 60% predicted should be cautioned about the risks. Pregnant mothers, even those with mild CF, should be monitored closely during pregnancy. Maternal weight gain and uterine fundal height may help assess fetal growth retardation [409]. Antibiotic therapy should be given if needed. However, aminoglycosides and quinolones are potentially teratogenic and are best avoided, although they have been used by pregnant patients without consequences for the fetus [407]. From our own and others' observations, the immediate postpartum period may have its own hazards. We have seen severe respiratory exacerbations occur at this time. The reasons are unclear, although there must have been a release of the upward displacement of the diaphragm and associated possible closure of small basal airways. More importantly, the immunological changes of pregnancy, which are predominantly 'immunosuppressive' and anti-inflammatory, revert to 'normal'.

Management of respiratory aspects of cystic fibrosis

There are several well-established areas of management of the various respiratory aspects of CF. These can be viewed in respect to the pathogenetic processes involved, as outlined above and as illustrated in Fig. 30.10. Also, there is much active research in CF and new and novel approaches to management are in constant development. In this section, the standard and new management techniques are reviewed.

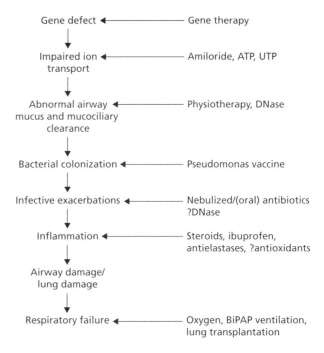

Fig. 30.10 A flow diagram outlining the pathogenetic sequence of events causing airways and lung disease in cystic fibrosis. The points of therapeutic interventions, both established and in development, are indicated.

Physiotherapy

For over 40 years chest physiotherapy has been the principal technique for attempting to remove viscid secretions from the airways and thus interrupt the cycle of infection, inflammation, tissue damage and decreased clearance. First introduced in the 1950s, the combination of postural drainage, percussion, vibration, deep breathing and coughing constitutes 'conventional' chest physiotherapy and for many years has been the gold standard [410]. When introduced, virtually all patients were children and their parents could assume responsibility for performance of the treatment. As survival has improved, more and more adolescents and adults have had to assume responsibility for carrying out their own physiotherapy. Adherence to treatment is often poor among adolescents and adults. Newer techniques have been developed to try to make physiotherapy more patient-centred and to aid compliance. The active cycle breathing technique has been shown to be as effective as conventional physiotherapy in mobilizing secretions [411–413] and is less likely to cause oxygen desaturation [414]. It undoubtedly allows patients more independence. No added benefit to this technique has been provided by a positive expiratory pressure mask or a Flutter VRP1 system [415,416], although both have had their advocates. Autogenic drainage has been reported favourably with respect to both mobilizing secretions and avoidance of oxygen desaturation [417–419]. However, since adherence to treatment is such a problem it is important to select the technique that the patient prefers. There are many likely benefits of regular exercise, including improved cardiorespiratory efficiency, respiratory muscle function, muscle strength and exercise tolerance, as well as improved self-image and well-being. Exercise alone does not appear as efficient as physiotherapy in mobilizing sputum but is a valuable adjunct [413] and to be encouraged.

Antibiotic treatment

Aggressive antibiotic therapy has probably been the major contributor to the improved survival of CF patients. Use falls principally into two categories: acute treatment for an infective exacerbation and chronic administration as maintenance therapy intended to decrease the bacterial load in the lung and to maintain lung function. Intravenous administration and nebulized antibiotics have their own intrinsic problems. In addition, pharmacokinetics are different in CF patients, who appear to have a larger volume of distribution and increased clearance of aminoglycosides and β-lactams, with a shorter elimination half-time and lower peak plasma antibiotic concentrations [420]. A larger dose and possibly more frequent dosing intervals are necessary to compensate for these differences. Children with CF appear to eliminate ciprofloxacin more rapidly than older patients and may require higher dosing of fluoroquinolones [421].

Combination therapy and aminoglycosides

Repeated courses of antibiotics lead to increased bacterial resistance patterns, and this may be an important reason for the emergence of bacterial colonization by organisms with multiple innate antibiotic resistances. Certain principles appear useful. Treatment with combinations of antibiotics appears to combine the additive benefit of two or more drugs, while in one clinic the use of monotherapy has resulted in widespread resistance to the antibiotic by *Ps. aeruginosa* [422]. Aminoglycosides in particular seem to be useful drugs to combine with other agents such as ceftazidime, aztreonam and meropenem. The ototoxicity of aminoglycosides is an important consideration, since a patient is likely to have multiple courses. Despite rigorous monitoring of blood levels and no record of 'toxic' levels, two patients in the Edinburgh adult clinic have experienced tobramycin-related vestibular problems. Once-daily aminoglycoside dosing has been used increasingly for non-CF-related disease, but in CF there are extremely limited, almost anecdotal, reports. In the Edinburgh clinic, a 6-month period of once-daily tobramycin (5 mg/kg at night) appeared to be associated with a more rapid 'relapse' rate of exacerbation, although the treatment approach has not been assessed in a prospective double-blind fashion.

Chronic antibiotic therapy

A number of centres treat children with regular anti-staphylococcal drugs, especially flucloxacillin, from the first isolation of *Staph. aureus*. Other centres prefer to treat infections aggressively as they occur, often maintaining treatment for 4 weeks. This has the advantage of including *H. influenzae* in the treatment spectrum. This regular flucloxacillin therapy has had an element of 'tradition' about it. Nevertheless, recent data from a study of infants diagnosed at neonatal screening showed that those who received continuous flucloxacillin had less frequent cough and fewer and shorter hospitalizations compared with infants treated with episodic courses of antibiotics. There was no difference in pulmonary function between the two groups at 1 year [423,424].

The use of regular antibiotics has been applied in older patients colonized by *Ps. aeruginosa*. In this instance, the route of administration has been by nebulizer. There have been differences in frequency of such treatment between the USA and Europe. Regular nebulized colistin is employed frequently in the UK, nebulized gentamicin or tobramycin less often. There are issues of drug-induced bronchoconstriction in patients (sometimes quite a high frequency) and adherence among adolescent and adult patients to a twice-daily regimen is probably even less good than to physiotherapy. There are numerous published studies with nebulized antibiotics [425] but very few address long-term use and very few are placebo-controlled [426–428]. On balance, treated patients have positive benefits including better lung function and/or fewer hospital admissions. Recent, well-controlled, multicentre studies have been performed in the USA. The first, although short term, showed benefit to lung function [429]. The second, also led by Ramsey, has been in progress for a year and has shown definite benefit [430].

Intravenous antibiotics

Recurrent infections, particularly after colonization with *Ps. aeruginosa*, require repeated courses of intravenous antibiotics. Traditionally, peripheral intravenous cannulae or long lines have been used for this purpose. However, frequent replacements are often required in a single treatment period and resulting damage to veins makes venous access difficult in the long term. The introduction of the totally implantable venous access device (TIVAD), also known as 'ports', has provided a solution to this problem. A TIVAD usually consists of a silicone septum mounted in a titanium chamber, which is inserted subcutaneously on the chest wall (see Fig. 30.9) or in the arm. The chamber is connected to a catheter, which is tunnelled into a central vein. These devices have proved successful clinically [431–435] and have greatly aided home intravenous antibiotic management. Home treatment is appreciated by patients, who avoid prolonged hospital admissions, but is dependent on adequate support. Clinical nurse specialists can provide that support and train the patients in the aseptic techniques necessary for self-administration of drugs. An important safety proviso is that the initial dose of any course of intravenous drugs is given under supervision in case of an anaphylactic response, which occasionally occurs even if the patient has received the same drugs on numerous previous occasions.

Therapy with DNase

CF sputum is remarkably tenacious and the physical effort of expectoration, particularly in patients with poor lung function, is substantial. Much of the viscosity is attributable to DNA in the sputum, the source of which appears to be dead neutrophils. In the late 1950s, use of DNase to cleave the DNA was found to be effective at reducing sputum viscosity and aided sputum clearance. Unfortunately, marked allergic reactions occurred after a short while, since the DNase was of bovine origin, and the treatment fell into disuse. More recently, human DNase has been cloned, mass produced and was licensed for use in 1994. It is markedly effective in reducing sputum

viscoelasticity *in vitro* [436] and *in vivo* early trials showed encouraging improvements in spirometry [437,438]. The large, multicentre trial (968 patients) used to support licensing [439] showed that once-daily treatment gave a relatively modest (5.8%) improvement in FEV_1 at 24 weeks, with a small reduction in exacerbations requiring parenteral antibiotics. However, there was wide variability of individual responses to treatment, with a significant proportion appearing to have no benefit. Further studies have shown no significant benefit of short-term use during exacerbations [440], improvements in spirometry but not in antibiotic use in sicker patients [441], and a wide scatter of spirometric responses with a reduction in historical antibiotic use in children [442]. One longer-term study has suggested no benefit for lung function, nutrition or hospitalization rates [443]. However, group mean data may be misleading if 'non-responders' are included in the study group. Anecdotally, in our centre there appears to be a reduction in requirement for antibiotics over about a 2-year period if the drug is targeted to patients who show a definite response to short-term testing [444]. The initial persuasive reason for testing patients' responses to DNase, i.e. to target therapy, was its great expense. The cost of therapy cannot be ignored; at more than £7000 per patient per year for once-daily dosage, it equates broadly to the per capita cost of caring for CF patients in a specialist centre [445] and thus prescription to all patients would nearly double the cost of CF care in the UK. A Scottish protocol has been developed to target the use of DNase [444], and this protocol or similar should be applied before commencing patients on long-term DNase.

Treatment of the excessive inflammatory responses

Following the recognition that host inflammatory responses are major contributors to the progressive lung damage (see above), therapeutic strategies have been directed towards control of these responses.

Corticosteroids

An initial trial reported benefit in children aged 1–12 years when given high doses of prednisone (2 mg/kg on alternate days) [446]. The steroid-treated children were said to have had better lung function and growth, and fewer hospitalizations, with no adverse effects. This trial prompted a larger, multicentre study. Two alternate-day dosing regimens (2 mg/kg and 1 mg/kg) were compared with placebo over a 4-year period in 285 children aged 6–14 years. There were benefits to lung function but growth retardation, glucose abnormalities and cataracts occurred even at the lower dose of prednisone, and the treatment limb at the higher dose had to be discontinued early because of unacceptable side-effects [447,448]. Although long-term steroid therapy is inappropriate because of this, there may be a place for short courses or inhaled treatment. A 12-week course of prednisolone produced improvements in lung function and serum IgG and cytokine concentrations [449]. Early results from trials of inhaled steroids are equivocal but suggest the approach is worth pursuing [450–452].

Non-steroidal anti-inflammatory drugs

NSAIDs have anti-inflammatory effects, for example ibuprofen can inhibit neutrophil migration and release of lysosomal enzymes. In a rat model of chronic endobronchial infection with *Ps. aeruginosa*, ibuprofen decreased inflammation without increasing the lung burden of organisms, probably in part by interfering with the production of leukotriene B_4 [453,454]. In patients it proved possible to achieve the necessary blood levels without overt side-effects [455]. A 4-year trial of ibuprofen was then conducted in 85 patients with mild lung disease aged 5–39 years. Treated patients had less decline in lung function and chest radiographic scores, preserved body weight and tended to have fewer hospital admissions than placebo-treated patients [456]. However, the effects were most pronounced in the youngest patients (5–13 years), while the data for adults were not impressive. Given that NSAIDs may cause serious problems at times, the case for treatment of adults has yet to be made.

Antiproteases

Elastase, predominantly from neutrophils, is found in the active state, often in high concentrations, in CF sputum. This implies that the natural inhibitors of neutrophil elastase in the airways, α_1-antitrypsin, secretory leukocyte protease inhibitor (SLPi) and elafin, have been 'overwhelmed' by the total elastase burden. Elastase has proinflammatory effects as well as tissue-destructive actions. It cleaves complement components to active chemotactic products and induces release of IL-8 from epithelial cells. Antielastases should therefore exert anti-inflammatory as well as tissue-protective effects. The definitive studies have yet to be done but the principles of treatment have been addressed. A preliminary study in 12 patients showed that nebulized α_1-antitrypsin twice daily for 1 week suppressed elastase activity [457]. Aerosolized recombinant SLPi 100 mg twice daily to 16 patients decreased active elastase and IL-8 in the airways [458], although a lower dose failed to decrease elastase [459]. This area of management requires further study. Empirically, an antielastase delivered via the circulation appears to have greater likelihood of action at relevant sites than nebulized drug.

Newer therapies in development and trials

Therapies based on CFTR defects

CFTR mutations that involve premature stop codons lead to early termination of CFTR mRNA (class I mutations) (see Fig. 30.2). Some aminoglycoside antibiotics can suppress these nonsense mutations and restore full-length CFTR mRNA protein to the cell [460]. There are a number of current trials of intranasal gentamicin in patients who carry two such mutant alleles (e.g. G542X, R553X, R1162X or W1282X).

Class II trafficking mutations, such as ΔF508, are defective with respect to structural assembly in the endoplasmic reticulum and are not efficiently glycosylated or transported to the cell surface. The ΔF508 protein retains some chloride channel function and may be more readily transported to the cell surface by treatment with 'chemical chaperones' such as glycerol. These are thought to facilitate protein folding and stabilize protein structure, thus promoting processing and trafficking to the cell surface [461]. A number of chaperones are being investigated *in vitro* in order to identify candidates for *in vivo* study. An alternative agent is phenylbutyrate, an oral analogue of butyrate, which was developed to treat urea cycle disorders. Phenylbutyrate regulates the expression of many genes, including CFTR, and promotes trafficking of the ΔF508 protein *in vitro* and *in vivo*. Encouraging phase I trials have been conducted at Johns Hopkins, Baltimore and been reported at the North American CF Meeting [462].

Class IV mutations have partial responses to cyclic AMP stimulation. A number of agents that may increase CFTR activation are being investigated. Milrinone is a phosphodiesterase inhibitor that improves chloride conductance by ΔF508 in a mouse model of CF [463]. Genistein is a tyrosine kinase inhibitor that augments chloride channel activity in CFTR via inhibition of protein phosphatase and possibly by a direct effect on CFTR itself [464,465]. The xanthine A_1 adenosine receptor antagonist 8-cyclophenyl-1,3-dipropylxanthine specifically activates the ΔF508 chloride channel [466] and a phase I trial is in progress. Any of these compounds, or their successors, might be used alone or in combination with other agents.

Gene therapy

The goal in gene therapy of CF is the replacement of CFTR function at a level that will prevent the progressive damage to the airways. Ideally, this would be targeted at children before the onset of pulmonary disease. The success or failure of gene therapy depends to a great extent on how much transgene expression is needed to correct the phenotype. Some individuals who are phenotypically normal have up to 92% abnormally spliced mRNA, which results in a defective protein [69]. This suggests that less than 10% of normal mRNA expressed in airway cells may be sufficient. However, since the majority of cells of the respiratory epithelium are terminally differentiated, vectors for CF gene therapy must be able to infect non-dividing cells. Both viral and non-viral strategies have been considered and numerous studies have demonstrated the principles of *in vivo* gene transfer in a variety of animal species.

Adenoviral vectors have been based on adenovirus serotypes 2 or 5, which exhibit tropism for the respiratory epithelium. Potential advantages of adenovirus vectors include this natural tropism for airway epithelium, the ability to transduce non-dividing cells and the capacity to be produced in high titre. Initial animal studies [467] demonstrated that adenoviral vectors could deliver transgene to all major cell types of the respiratory epithelium. However, these preclinical studies also made clear that adenovirus administration is associated with a dose-dependent inflammatory response and a (consequent) loss of transgene expression [468–470].

Adeno-associated virus vectors have also been considered for CF gene therapy. Like adenovirus, they exhibit tropism for the respiratory epithelium and are able to infect non-dividing cells. In contrast, they are naturally replication deficient and are not associated with any known human disease. However, they are small and CFTR cDNA is at the upper limit of packaging size, which places constraints on which promoter and enhancer can be incorporated. *In vivo* studies in rabbits [471] and monkeys [472] have demonstrated that safe and efficient delivery of transgene can be achieved following endobronchial administration, with expression persisting up to 6 months and no evidence of inflammation or other toxicity. On this basis phase I clinical trials have been initiated.

Cationic liposome-mediated gene delivery was first described in 1987 [473] and has been widely used to transfer DNA to a variety of cell types *in vitro* and *in vivo* [474]. Unlike adenoviral vectors, liposomes are non-immunogenic and offer advantages in terms of bulk production and quality control. Cationic liposome-mediated gene delivery to the airway was first demonstrated in mice in 1989 [475], and delivery and expression of CFTR in the airways of normal mice in 1992 [476]. Correction of the cyclic AMP-dependent chloride transport defect in CF mutant mice followed [477,478] and, subsequently, phase I clinical trials.

To date, nine clinical trials involving 78 CF patients have been published [16,479–486] and at least four others are in progress. These clinical trials have progressed from an open, uncontrolled study using the nasal epithelium of three patients to nebulized administration of the vector to the whole airways. They have clearly demonstrated that

the principle of transfer and expression of normal CFTR cDNA to airway epithelium can be achieved by both viral and non-viral approaches. However, in all of these trials there was low efficiency of gene transfer and no ideal method of judging the adequacy of correction of the physiological defect. Furthermore the expression of transgene was transient, lasting less than 2 weeks in most cases, confirming the need for repeated administration. Studies with current adenoviral vectors suggest that the presence of neutralizing antibodies raised against an initial administration severely limits the efficiency of subsequent doses. Clearly, improvements in delivery and persistence of expression are required for any realistic prospect of therapeutic benefit. Attempts have been made to reduce the immune response by modifications of the adenoviral genome, which reduces expression of adenovirus proteins [487], or by interfering with MHC class I expression on the cell surface of infected cells, thus suppressing viral antigen presentation [488,489]. For non-viral delivery systems the most important issue is to improve the efficiency of transfection. Cationic liposome-based gene therapy has the further drawback of being non-specific. Attempts have been made to circumvent this problem by incorporating ligands for cell surface molecules into the DNA–liposome complexes. However, despite initial successes *in vitro* [474], this approach has yet to be proved *in vivo*. Effort has gone into the development of novel cationic liposome formulations and to optimizing formulations of currently available liposomes by mixing with neutral colipids [490]. Some of these novel cationic liposomes appear more inflammatory than the original formulations, raising concerns for clinical safety. The first reports of a phase I clinical trial involving application of the cationic lipid GL67 to the lung supports such concerns.

Thus, after 5 years of clinical gene therapy trials (and only 9 years after identification of the CF gene), trial results hold promise of effective therapy but, realistically, the delivery of that promise appears a further decade away.

Holistic care for adults and adolescents with cystic fibrosis

The idea that the management of CF can be neatly packaged into therapeutic areas (exciting and new though they are) avoids the realities of care. Patients' problems are psychosocial as well as physical and require holistic care provided by a team of experienced people. Adolescents with CF have all the problems of healthy adolescents but compounded by physical limitations and additional requirements. The extra nutritional needs and the time for self-treatment (physiotherapy, nebulized therapies) test patient adherence to the limits. Educational pressures, limitations on close contact with friends with CF (*B. cepacia* transmission), parental difficulties in 'letting go', and the move from paediatric to adult clinic care all severely test patients' emotional strengths. Transition clinics, with adult clinic team members meeting the patients in their familiar paediatric clinic surroundings, and contact with patients and families in their home surroundings may smooth the passage of patients into adult clinics. Adults too have many psychosocial problems that have to be addressed. These include independent living, establishment of permanent relationships and further education and employment, usually in the face of declining physical health. Generally, carers in CF centres are experienced in the support of patients with regard to employment and education [491].

It remains a little unclear how the health problems of CF patients influence their quality of life. Often psychological studies find similar quality-of-life scores to people with minor health problems and even healthy controls [492–494]. However, this may reflect the limitations of the tools used to measure quality of life and patients' reduced expectations. Certainly their health perceptions impact on their therapies. One study has suggested that patients who cope well with their disease may be less adherent to their various management regimens than those who worry about their disease and who perceive that they have little personal control over it [495].

All these issues emphasize the need for 'art' as well as 'science' in providing care for CF and the need to be involved in the 'whole' patient contributes to the rewarding nature of CF management.

References

1 Busch R. The history of cystic fibrosis. *Acta Univ Carol Med* 1990; 36: 13.

2 Andersen DH. Cystic fibrosis of the pancreas and its relation to celiac disease: a clinical and pathologic study. *Am J Dis Child* 1938; 56: 344.

3 Blackfan KD, May CD. Inspissation of secretion and dilatation of ducts and acini. Atrophy and fibrosis of the pancreas in infants. *J Pediatr* 1938; 13: 627.

4 Blackfan KD, Wolbach SB. Vitamin A deficiency in infants. *J Pediatr* 1933; 3: 679.

5 Fanconi G, Uehlinger E, Knaver C. Das Coeliaksyndrom bei Angeborener zystischer Pankreas fibromatose und Bronchiektasein. *Wien Med Wochenschr* 1936; 86: 753.

6 Farber S. Pancreatic insufficiency and the celiac syndrome. *N Engl J Med* 1943; 229: 653, 682.

7 di Sant'Agnese PA, Darling RC, Perera GA, Shea E. Abnormal composition of the sweat in cystic fibrosis of the pancreas. Clinical significance and relationship to the disease. *Pediatrics* 1953; 12: 549.

8 Gibson LE, Cooke RE. A test for concentration of electrolytes in sweat in cystic fibrosis of the pancreas utilizing pilocarpine by iontophoresis. *Pediatrics* 1959; 23: 545.

9 Andersen DH, Hodges RG. Celiac syndrome. V. Genetics of cystic fibrosis of the pancreas with a consideration of etiology. *Am J Dis Child* 1946; 72: 62.

10 Danks DM, Allan J, Anderson CM. A genetic study of fibrocystic disease of the pancreas. *Ann Hum Genet* 1965; 28: 323.

11 Wainwright BJ, Scambler PJ, Schmidtke J *et al.* Localization of cystic fibrosis locus to human chromosome 7cen-q22. *Nature* 1985; 318: 384.

12 Eiberg H, Mohr J, Schmiegelow K, Nielsen LS, Williamson R. Linkage relationships of paraoxonase (PON) with other markers: indication of PON-cystic fibrosis synteny. *Clin Genet* 1985; 28: 265.

13 Rommens JM, Iannuzzi MC, Kerem B-S *et al.* Identification of the cystic fibrosis gene: chromosome walking and jumping. *Science* 1989; 245: 1059.

14 Riordan JR, Rommens JM, Kerem B-S *et al.* Identification of the cystic fibrosis gene: cloning and characterization of complementary DNA. *Science* 1989; 245: 1066.

15 Kerem B-S, Rommens JM, Buchanan JA *et al.* Identification of the cystic fibrosis gene: gene analysis. *Science* 1989; 245: 1073.

16 Zabner J, Couture LA, Gregory. RJ, Granham SM, Smith AE, Welsh MJ. Adenovirus-mediated gene transfer transiently corrects the chloride transport defect in nasal epithelia of patients with cystic fibrosis. *Cell* 1993; 75: 207.

17 Morral N, Bertanpetit J, Estivill X *et al.* Tracing the origin of the major CF mutation (ΔF508) in European populations. *Nature Genet* 1994; 7: 169.

18 Super M, van Schalkwyk DJ. Heterozygote advantage in cystic fibrosis: mosquito tests. *Clin Genet* 1979; 16: 65.

19 Quinton PM. Chloride impermeability in cystic fibrosis. *Nature* 1983; 301: 421.

20 Meindl RS. Hypothesis: a selective advantage for cystic fibrosis heterozygotes. *Am J Phys Anthropol* 1987; 74: 39.

21 Pritchard DJ. Cystic fibrosis allele frequency, sex ratio anomalies and fertility: a new theory for the dissemination of mutant alleles. *Human Genet* 1991; 87: 671.

22 Chao AC, de Sauvage FJ, Dong Y-J, Wagner JA, Goeddel DV, Gardner P. Activation of intestinal CFTR Cl- channel by heat-stable enterotoxin and guanylin via cAMP-dependent protein kinase. *EMBO J* 1994; 13: 1065.

23 Gabriel SE, Brigman KN, Koller BH, Boucher RC, Stutts MJ. Cystic fibrosis heterozygote resistance to cholera toxin in the cystic fibrosis mouse model. *Science* 1994; 266: 107.

24 Zielenski J, Rozmahe! R, Bozon D *et al.* Genomic DNA sequence of the cystic fibrosis transmembrane conductance regulator (CFTR) gene. *Genomics* 1991; 10: 214.

25 Hyde SC, Emsley P, Hartshorn MJ *et al.* Structural model of ATP-binding proteins associated with cystic fibrosis, multidrug resistance and bacterial transport. *Nature* 1990; 346: 362.

26 Rich DP, Anderson MP, Gregory RI *et al.* Expression of the cystic fibrosis transmembrane conductance regulator corrects defective chloride channel regulation in cystic fibrosis airway epithelial cells. *Nature* 1990; 347: 358.

27 Anderson MP, Rich DP, Gregory RJ *et al.* Generation of cAMP-activated chloride currents by expression of CFTR. *Science* 1991; 251: 679.

28 Kartner N, Hanrahan JW, Jenson TJ *et al.* Expression of the cystic fibrosis gene in non-epithelial invertebrate cells produces a regulated anion conductance. *Cell* 1991; 64: 681.

29 Anderson MP, Gregory RJ, Thompson S *et al.* Demonstration that CFTR is a chloride channel by alteration of its anion selectivity. *Science* 1991; 253: 202.

30 Bear CE, Canhui L, Kartner N *et al.* Purification and functional reconstitution of cystic fibrosis transmembrane conductance regulator (CFTR). *Cell* 1992; 68: 809.

31 Diamond G, Scanlin TF, Zasloff MA, Bevins CL. A cross-species analysis of the cystic fibrosis transmembrane conductance regulator. *J Biol Chem* 1991; 266: 22761.

32 Tata F, Stanier P, Wicking C *et al.* The mouse homologue of the cystic fibrosis gene. *Genomics* 1991; 10: 298.

33 Fiedler MA, Nemecz ZN, Shull GE. Cloning and sequence analysis of the rat cystic fibrosis transmembrane conductance regulator. *Am J Physiol* 1992; 262: L779.

34 Riordan JR, Forbush B, Hanrahan JW. The molecular basis of chloride transport in shark rectal gland. *J Exp Biol* 1994; 196: 405.

35 Yoshimura K, Nakamura H, Trapnell BC *et al.* The cystic fibrosis gene has a 'housekeeping'-type promoter and is expressed at low levels in cells of epithelial origin. *J Biol Chem* 1991; 266: 9140.

36 Trapnell BC, Zeitlin PL, Chu C-S *et al.* Down-regulation of cystic fibrosis gene mRNA transcript levels and induction of the cystic fibrosis chloride secretory phenotype in epithelial cells by phorbol ester. *J Biol Chem* 1991; 266: 10319.

37 Bradbury NA, Jilling T, Berta G, Sorscher EJ, Bridges RJ, Kirk KL. Regulation of plasma membrane recycling by CFTR. *Science* 1992; 256: 530.

38 Barasch J, Kiss B, Prince A, Saimon L, Gruenert D, Al-Awqati Q. Defective acidification of intracellular organelles in cystic fibrosis. *Nature* 1991; 352: 70.

39 Al-Awqati Q. Regulation of ion channels by ABC transporters that secrete ATP. *Science* 1995; 269: 805.

40 Egan M, Flotte T, Afione S *et al.* Defective regulation of outwardly rectifying Cl- chan-

nels by protein kinase A corrected by insertion of CFTR. *Nature* 1992; 358: 581.

41 Gabriel SE, Clarke LL, Boucher RC, Stutts MJ. CFTR and outward rectifying chloride channels are distinct proteins with a regulatory relationship. *Nature* 1993; 363: 263.

42 Jovov B, Ismailov II, Benos DJ. Cystic fibrosis transmembrane conductance regulator is required for protein kinase A activation of an outwardly rectified anion channel purified from bovine tracheal epithelia. *J Biol Chem* 1995; 270: 1521.

43 Morris AP, Frizzell RA. Vesicle targeting and ion secretion in epithelial cells: implications for cystic fibrosis. *Annu Rev Physiol* 1994; 56: 371.

44 Stutts MJ, Chinet TC, Mason SJ *et al.* Regulation of chloride channels in normal and cystic fibrosis airway epithelial cells by extracellular ATP. *Proc Natl Acad Sci USA* 1992; 89: 1621.

45 Reisen IL, Prat AG, Abraham EH *et al.* The cystic fibrosis transmembrane conductance regulator is a dual ATP and chloride channel. *J Biol Chem* 1994; 269: 20584.

46 Schwiebert EM, Egan ME, Hwang T *et al.* CFTR regulates outwardly rectifying chloride channels through an autocrine mechanism involving ATP. *Cell* 1995; 81: 1063.

47 Boucher RC, Stutts MJ, Knowles MR *et al.* Na+ transport in cystic fibrosis respiratory epithelia. Abnormal base rate and response to adenylate cyclase activation. *J Clin Invest* 1986; 78: 1245.

48 Chinet TC, Fulton JM, Yankaskas JR *et al.* Mechanism of hyperabsorption in cultured cystic fibrosis nasal epithelium: a patch clamp study. *Am J Physiol* 1994; 266: C1061.

49 Stutts MJ, Canessa CM, Olsen JC *et al.* CFTR as a cAMP-dependent regulator of sodium channels. *Science* 1995; 269: 847.

50 Trezise AEO, Buchwald M. *In vivo* cell-specific expression of the cystic fibrosis transmembrane conductance regulator. *Nature* 1991; 353: 434.

51 Crawford I, Maloney P, Zeitlin PL *et al.* Immunocytochemical localization of the cystic fibrosis gene product CFTR. *Proc Natl Acad Sci USA* 1991; 88: 9262.

52 Trapnell BC, Chu C-S, Paakko PK *et al.* Expression of the cystic fibrosis transmembrane conductance regulator gene in the respiratory tract of normal individuals with cystic fibrosis. *Proc Natl Acad Sci USA* 1991; 88: 6565.

53 Engelhardt JF, Yankaskas JR, Ernst SA *et al.* Submucosal glands are the predominant site of CFTR expression in the human bronchus. *Nature Genet* 1992; 2: 240.

54 Cystic Fibrosis Genetic Analysis Consortium. Worldwide survey of the ΔF508 mutation: report from the Cystic Fibrosis Genetic Analysis Consortium. *Am J Hum Genet* 1990; 50: 222.

55 Tsui L-C, Buchwald M. Biochemical and molecular genetics of cystic fibrosis. *Adv Hum Genet* 1991; 20: 153.

56 Tsui L-C. The spectrum of cystic fibrosis mutations. *Trends Genet* 1992; 8: 392.

57 Gilfillan A, Warner JP, Kirk JM *et al.* P67L: a cystic fibrosis allele with mild effects found at high frequency in the Scottish population. *J Med Genet* 1998; 35: 122.

58 Urlaub G, Mitchell PJ, Ciudad CJ, Chasin LA. Nonsense mutations in the dihydrofolate reductase gene affect RNA processing. *Mol Cell Biol* 1989; 9: 2868.

59 Hamosh A, Trapnell BC, Zeitlin PL *et al.* Severe deficiency of CFTR mRNA carrying nonsense mutations R553X and W1316X in respiratory epithelial cells of patients with cystic fibrosis. *J Clin Invest* 1991; 88: 1880.

60 Hamosh A, Rosenstein BJ, Cutting GR. CFTR nonsense mutations G542X and W1282X associated with severe reduction of CFTR mRNA in nasal epithelial cells. *Hum Mol Genet* 1282; 1: 542.

61 Jones CT, McIntosh I, Keston M *et al.* Three novel mutations in the cystic fibrosis gene detected by chemical cleavage: analysis of variant splicing and nonsense mutation. *Hum Mol Genet* 1992; 1: 11.

62 Zeitlin PL, Crawford I, Lu L *et al.* CFTR protein expression in primary and cultured epithelia. *Proc Natl Acad Sci USA* 1992; 89: 344.

63 Zielenski J, Bozon D, Markiewicz D *et al.* Analysis of CFTR transcripts in nasal epithelial cells and lymphoblasts of a cystic fibrosis patient with 621 + 1G→T and 711 + 1G→T mutations. *Hum Mol Genet* 1993; 2: 683.

64 Hull J, Shackleton S, Harris A. Abnormal mRNA splicing resulting from three different mutations in the CFTR gene. *Hum Mol Genet* 1993; 2: 689.

65 Cutting GR, Curristin SM, Nash E *et al.* Analysis of four diverse population groups indicates that a subset of cystic fibrosis mutations occur in common among Caucasians. *Am J Hum Genet* 1992; 50: 1185.

66 Chu C-S, Trapnell BC, Murtagh JJ *et al.* Variable deletion of exon 9 coding sequences in cystic fibrosis transmembrane conductance regulator gene mRNA transcripts in normal bronchial epithelium. *EMBO J* 1991; 10: 1355.

67 Chu C-S, Trapnell BC, Curristin SM *et al.* Genetic basis of variable exon 9 skipping in cystic fibrosis transmembrane conductance regulator mRNA. *Nature Genet* 1993; 3: 151.

68 Krainer AR, Maniatis T. RNA splicing. In: Hames BD, Glover DM, eds. *Transcription and Translation*. Oxford: IRL Press, 1988: 131.

69 Chu C-S, Trapnell BC, Curristin SM, Cutting GR, Crystal RG. Extensive posttranscriptional deletion of the coding sequences for part of nucleotide-binding fold 1 in respiratory epithelial cell mRNA transcripts of the cystic fibrosis transmembrane conductance regulator gene is not associated with the clinical manifestations of cystic fibrosis. *J Clin Invest* 1992; 90: 785.

70 Cheng SH, Gregory RJ, Marshall J *et al.* Defective intracellular transport and processing of CFTR is the molecular basis of most cystic fibrosis. *Cell* 1990; 63: 827.

71 Denning GM, Anderson MP, Amara JF *et al.* Processing of mutant cystic fibrosis transmembrane conductance regulator is temperature-sensitive. *Nature* 1992; 358: 761.

72 Kartner N, Hanrahan JW, Jenson TJ *et al.* Expression of the cystic fibrosis gene in nonepithelial invertebrate cells produces a regulated anion conductance. *Cell* 1991; 64: 681.

73 Bear CE, Duguay F, Naismith AL *et al.* Cl- channel activity in *Xenopus* oocytes expressing the cystic fibrosis gene. *J Biol Chem* 1991; 266: 19142.

74 Li C, Ramjeesingh M, Reyes E *et al.* The cystic fibrosis mutation (deltaF508) does not influence the chloride channel activity of CFTR. *Nature Genet* 1993; 3: 311.

75 Kartner N, Augustinas O, Jensen TJ, Naismith AL, Riordan JR. Mislocalization of deltaF508 CFTR in cystic fibrosis sweat gland. *Nature Genet* 1992; 1: 321.

76 Welsh MJ, Smith AE. Molecular mechanisms of CFTR chloride channel dysfunction in cystic fibrosis. *Cell* 73: 1251.

77 Drumm ML, Wilkinson DJ, Smit LS *et al.* Chloride conductance expressed by deltaF508 and other mutant CFTRs in *Xenopus* oocytes. *Science* 1991; 254: 1797.

78 Dean M, White MB, Amos J *et al.* Multiple mutations in highly conserved residues are found in mildly affected cystic fibrosis patients. *Cell* 1990; 61: 863.

79 Carroll TP, McIntosh I, Egan ME *et al.* Transmembrane mutations alter the channel characteristics of the cystic fibrosis transmembrane conductance regulator expressed in *Xenopus* oocytes. *Cell Physiol Biochem* 1994; 4: 10.

80 Sheppard DN, Rich DP, Ostedgaard LS *et al.* Mutations in CFTR associated with mild disease form Cl- channels with altered pore properties. *Nature* 1993; 362: 160.

81 Kerem E, Corey M, Kerem B-S *et al.* The relationship between genotype and phenotype in cystic fibrosis: analysis of the most common mutation (F508). *N Engl J Med* 1990; 323: 1517.

82 Hamosh A, Rosenstein BJ, Nash E *et al.* Cystic fibrosis genotype/phenotype consortium: correlation between genotype and phenotype in cystic fibrosis. *N Engl J Med* 1994; 329: 1308.

83 Kristidis P, Bozon D, Corey M, Markiewicz D, Rommens J, Tsui L-C, Durie P. Genetic determination of exocrine pancreatic function in cystic fibrosis. *Am J Hum Genet* 1992; 50: 1178.

84 Anguiano A, Oates RD, Amos JA *et al.* A primarily genital form of cystic fibrosis. *JAMA* 1992; 267: 1794.

85 Chillon M, Casals T, Mercier B *et al.* Mutations in the cystic fibrosis gene in patients with congenital absence of the vas deferens. *N Engl J Med* 1995; 332: 1475.

86 Quinton PM, Bijman J. Higher bioelectric potentials due to decreased chloride absorption in the sweat glands of patients with cystic fibrosis. *N Engl J Med* 1983; 308: 1185.

87 Heinz-Erian P, Dey RD, Flux M, Said SI. Deficient vasoactive intestinal peptide innervation in the sweat glands of cystic fibrosis patients. *Science* 1985; 229: 1407.

88 Kulczycki LL, Robertson MT. The sweat chloride concentration and prolactin activity in cystic fibrosis. *Scand J Gastroenterol* 1988; Suppl 143: 28.

89 Kilburn KH. A hypothesis for pulmonary clearance and its implications. *Am Rev Respir Dis* 1967; 98: 449.

90 Welsh MJ. Electrolyte transport by airway epithelia. *Physiol Rev* 1987; 67: 1143.

91 Knowles M, Gatzy J, Boucher R. Increased bioelectric potential difference across respiratory epithelia in cystic fibrosis. *N Engl J Med* 1981; 305: 1489.

92 Knowles M, Gatzy J, Boucher R. Relative ion permeability of normal and cystic fibrosis nasal epithelium. *J Clin Invest* 1983; 71: 1410.

93 Hay JG, Geddes DM. Transepithelial potential difference in cystic fibrosis. *Thorax* 1985; 40: 493.

94 Gowen CW, Lawson EE, Gingras-Leatherman J *et al.* Increased nasal potential difference and amiloride sensitivity in neonates with cystic fibrosis. *J Pediatr* 1986; 108: 517.

95 Sauder RA, Chesrown SE, Loughlin GM. Clinical application of transepithelial potential difference measurements in cystic fibrosis. *J Pediatr* 1987; 111: 353.

96 Alton EW, Hay JG, Munro C, Geddes DM. Measurement of nasal potential difference in adult cystic fibrosis, Young's syndrome, and bronchiectasis. *Thorax* 1987; 42: 815.

97 Alton EWFW, Currie D, Logan-Sinclair R *et al*. Nasal potential difference: a clinical diagnostic test for cystic fibrosis. *Eur Respir J* 1990; 3: 922.

98 Ho LP, Sammways JM, Porteous DJ *et al*. Correlation between nasal potential difference measurements, genotype and clinical condition in patients with cystic fibrosis. *Eur Respir J* 1997; 10: 2018.

99 Engelhardt JF, Yankaskas JR, Ernst SA *et al*. Submucosal glands are the predominant site of CFTR expression in the human bronchus. *Nature Genet* 1992; 2: 240.

100 Dwyer TM, Farley JM. Intracellular chloride in submucosal gland cells. *Life Sci* 1991; 48: 2119.

101 Yamaya M, Finkbeiner WE, Widdicombe JH. Altered ion transport by tracheal glands in cystic fibrosis. *Am J Physiol* 1991; 261: L491.

102 Cozens AL, Yezzi MJ, Chin L *et al*. Characterization of immortal cystic fibrosis tracheobronchial gland epithelial cells. *Proc Natl Acad Sci USA* 1992; 89: 5171.

103 Patton CJ, Jenkins MQ, Briggman JV, Spicer SS. Effect of amiloride on potential difference across rectal mucosa in cystic fibrosis patients. *Pediatr Res* 1982; 16: 1035.

104 Goldstein JL, Nash NT, al-Bazzaz F *et al*. Rectum has abnormal ion transport but normal cAMP-binding proteins in cystic fibrosis. *Am J Physiol* 1988; 254: C719.

105 Orlando RC, Powell DW, Croom RD *et al*. Colonic and esophageal transepithelial potential difference in cystic fibrosis. *Gastroenterology* 1989; 96: 1041.

106 Veeze HJ, Sinaasappel M, Bijman J *et al*. Ion transport abnormalities in rectal suction biopsies from children with cystic fibrosis. *Gastroenterology* 1991; 101: 398.

107 Hardcastle J, Hardcastle PT, Taylor CJ, Goldhill J. Failure of cholinergic stimulation to induce a secretory response from the rectal mucosa in cystic fibrosis. *Gut* 1991; 32: 1035.

108 Taylor CJ, Baxter PS, Hardcastle J, Hardcastle PT. Failure to induce secretion in jejunal biopsies from children with cystic fibrosis. *Gut* 1988; 29: 957.

109 O'Loughlin EV, Hunt DM, Gaskin KJ *et al*. Abnormal epithelial transport in cystic fibrosis jejunum. *Am J Physiol* 1991; 260: G758.

110 Berschneider HM, Knowles MR, Azizkhan RG *et al*. Altered intestinal chloride transport in cystic fibrosis. *FASEB J* 1988; 2: 2625.

111 Goldstein JL, Shapiro AB, Rao MC, Layden TJ. *In vivo* evidence of altered chloride but not potassium secretion in cystic fibrosis rectal mucosa. *Gastroenterology* 1991; 101: 1012.

112 Schmidt KD, Abiodun P, Tolckmitt W. Viscocity and electrolyte concentrations in gastric juice from cystic fibrosis children compared to healthy children. *Eur J Pediatr* 1981; 136: 193.

113 Davidson GP, Kirubakaran CP, Ratcliffe G *et al*. Abnormal pancreatic electrolyte secretion in cystic fibrosis. Reliability as a diagnostic marker. *Acta Paediatr Scand* 1986; 75: 145.

114 Kopelman H, Corey M, Gaskin K *et al*.

115 Kopelman H, Forstner G, Durie P, Corey M. Origins of chloride and bicarbonate secretory defects in the cystic fibrosis pancreas, as suggested by pancreatic function studies on control and CF subjects with preserved pancreatic function. *Clin Invest Med* 1989; 12: 207.

116 Marino CR, Matovcik LM, Gorelick FS, Cohn JA. Localization of the cystic fibrosis transmembrane conductance regulator in pancreas. *J Clin Invest* 1991; 88: 712.

117 Chen JH, Schulman H, Gardner P *et al*. A cAMP-regulated chloride channel in lymphocytes that is affected in cystic fibrosis. *Science* 1989; 243: 657.

118 Selander P. The frequency of cystic fibrosis of the pancreas in Sweden. *Acta Paediatr Scand* 1962; 51: 65.

119 Brunechy Z. The incidence and genetics of cystic fibrosis. *J Med Genet* 1972; 9: 33.

120 Ten Kate LP. Cystic fibrosis in the Netherlands. *Int J Epidemiol* 1977; 6: 23.

121 Fitzsimmons SC. The changing epidemiology of cystic fibrosis. *J Pediatr* 1993; 122: 1.

122 Cashman SM, Patino A, Delgado MG, Byrne L, Denham B, De Arce M. The Irish cystic fibrosis database. *J Med Genet* 1995; 32: 972.

123 Dodge JA, Morison S, Lewis PA *et al*. Incidence, population, and survival of cystic fibrosis in the UK 1968–95. *Arch Dis Child* 1997; 77: 493.

124 Kere J, Estivill X, Chillon M *et al*. Cystic fibrosis in a low-incidence population: two major mutations in Finland. *Hum Genet* 1994; 93: 162.

125 Kerem E, Kalman YM, Yahav Y *et al*. Highly variable incidence of cystic fibrosis and different mutation distribution among different Jewish ethnic groups in Israel. *Hum Genet* 1995; 96: 193.

126 Imaizumi Y. Incidence and mortality rates of cystic fibrosis in Japan 1969–1992. *Am J Med Genet* 1995; 58: 161.

127 Schwartz M, Sorensen N, Brandt NJ, Hogdall E, Holm T. High incidence of cystic fibrosis on the Faroe Islands: a molecular and genealogical study. *Hum Genet* 1995; 95: 703.

128 Elborn JS, Shale DJ, Britton JR. Cystic fibrosis: current survival and population estimates to the year 2000. *Thorax* 1991; 46: 881.

129 Kraemer R, Rudeberg A, Hadorn B, Rossi E. Relative underweight in cystic fibrosis and its prognostic value. *Acta Paediatr Scand* 67: 33.

130 Huang NN, Schidlow DV, Szatrowski TH *et al*. Clinical features, survival rate and prognostic factors in young adults with cystic fibrosis. *Am J Med* 1987; 82: 871.

131 Corey M, McLaughlin FJ, Williams M, Levison H. A comparison of survival, growth and pulmonary function in patients with cystic fibrosis in Boston and Toronto. *J Clin Epidemiol* 1988; 41: 583.

132 Kerem E, Reisman J, Corey M, Canny GJ, Levison H. Prediction of mortality in patients with cystic fibrosis. *N Engl J Med* 1992; 326: 1187.

133 Nixon PA, Orenstein DM, Kelsey SF, Doershuk CF. The prognostic value of exercise testing in patients with cystic fibrosis. *N Engl J Med* 1992; 327: 1785.

134 Hayllar KM, Williams SGJ, Wise AE *et al*. A prognostic model for the prediction of survival in cystic fibrosis. *Thorax* 1997; 52: 313.

135 Morison S, Dodge JA, Cole TJ *et al*. Height and weight in cystic fibrosis: a cross sectional study. *Arch Dis Child* 1997; 77: 497.

136 Freeman JV, Cole TJ, Chinn S, Jones PRM, White EM, Preece MA. Cross-sectional stature and weight reference curves for the UK 1990. *Arch Dis Child* 1995; 73: 17.

137 Cole TJ, Freeman JV, Preece MA. Body mass index reference curves for the UK. *Arch Dis Child* 1995; 73: 25.

138 Daneman A, Cutz E, Hagen P, Shandling B. Abdominal calcification in cystic fibrosis with meconium ileus: radiologic–pathologic correlation. *Pediatr Radiol* 1997; 27: 523.

139 Wagget J, Johnson DG, Borns P, Bishop HC. The non-operative treatment of meconium ileus by Gastrografin enema. *J Pediatr* 1970; 77: 407.

140 Hamosh A, King TM, Rosenstein BJ *et al*. Cystic fibrosis patients bearing both the common missense mutation Gly→Asp at codon 551 and the delta F508 mutation are clinically indistinguishable from delta F508 homozygotes, except for decreased risk of meconium ileus. *Am J Hum Genet* 1992; 51: 245.

141 Eggermont E. Gastrointestinal manifestations in cystic fibrosis. *Eur J Gastroenterol Hepatol* 1996; 8: 731.

142 Lands L, Zinman R, Wise M, Kopelman H. Pancreatic function testing in meconium disease in CF: two case reports. *J Pediatr Gastroenterol Nutr* 1988; 7: 276.

143 Valman HB, France NE, Wallis BG. Prolonged neonatal jaundice in cystic fibrosis. *Arch Dis Child* 1971; 46: 805.

144 Wilcken B, Towns SJ, Mellis CM. Diagnostic delay in cystic fibrosis: lessons from newborn screening. *Arch Dis Child* 1983; 58: 863.

145 Shwachman H. Gastrointestinal manifestations of cystic fibrosis. *Pediatr Clin North Am* 1975; 22: 787.

146 Kulczycki LL, Shwachman H. Studies in cystic fibrosis of the pancreas. Occurrence of rectal prolapse. *N Engl J Med* 1958; 259: 409.

147 Stern RC, Izant RJ, Boat TF, Wood RE, Matthews LW, Doershuk CF. Treatment and prognosis of rectal prolapse in cystic fibrosis. *Gastroenterology* 1982; 82: 707.

148 Zemsky WT, Rosenstein BJ. The cause of rectal prolapse in children. *Am J Dis Child* 1988; 142: 338.

149 Kopelman H. Cystic fibrosis. Gastrointestinal and nutritional aspects. *Thorax* 1991; 46: 261.

150 Lee PA, Roloff DW, Howatt WF. Hypoproteinemia and anemia in infants with cystic fibrosis. A presenting sympom complex often misdiagnosed. *JAMA* 1974; 228: 585.

151 Allan JL, Robbie M, Phelan PD, Dorks DM. The incidence and presentation of cystic fibrosis in Victoria 1955–1978. *Austr Paediatr J* 1980; 6: 270.

152 Hiatt P, Eigen H, Yu P, Tepper RS. Bronchodilator responsiveness in infants and young children with cystic fibrosis. *Am Rev Respir Dis* 1988; 137: 119.

153 Stern RC, Boat TF, Wood RE *et al*. Treatment and prognosis of nasal polyps in cystic fibrosis. *Am J Dis Child* 1982; 136: 1067.

154 Ledesma-Medina J, Osman MZ, Girdany BR. Abnormal paranasal sinuses in patients with cystic fibrosis of the pancreas. *Pediatr Radiol* 1980; 9: 61.

Impaired chloride secretion, as well as bicarbonate secretion, underlies the fluid secretory defect in the cystic fibrosis pancreas. *Gastroenterology* 1988; 95: 349.

155 Denning CR, Huang NN, Cuasay LR et al. Cooperative study comparing three methods of performing sweat tests to diagnose cystic fibrosis. *Pediatrics* 1980; 66: 752.

156 Littlewood JM. The sweat test. *Arch Dis Child* 1986; 61: 1041.

157 Gleeson M, Henry RL. Sweat sodium or chloride? *Clin Chem* 1991; 37: 112.

158 Kirk J, Keston M, McIntosh I, Essa SA. The variation of sweat sodium and chloride with age in cystic fibrosis and normal populations: further investigations in equivocal cases. *Ann Clin Biochem* 1992; 29: 145.

159 Shwachman H, Mahmoodian A, Neff RK. The sweat test: sodium and chloride values. *J Pediatr* 1981; 98: 576.

160 David TJ, Phillips BM. Overdiagnosis of cystic fibrosis. *Lancet* 1982; ii: 1204.

161 Shaw NJ, Littlewood JM. Misdiagnosis of cystic fibrosis. *Arch Dis Child* 1987; 62: 1271.

162 Hodson ME, Beldon I, Power R et al. Sweat test to diagnose cystic fibrosis in adults. *Br Med J* 1983; 286: 1381.

163 Durie PR, Gaskin KJ, Corey M et al. Pancreatic function testing in cystic fibrosis. *J Pediatr Gastroenterol Nutr* 1984; 3 (Suppl 1): S89.

164 van de Kamer JH, ten Bokkel Huinick H, Weyers HA. Rapid method for the determination of fat in feces. *J Biol Chem* 1949; 177: 347.

165 Jeejeebhoy KN, Ahmed S, Kozak G. Determination of faecal fats containing both medium and long-chain triglycerides and fatty acids. *Clin Biochem* 1970; 3: 157.

166 Goldstein R, Blondheim O, Levy H et al. The fatty meal test: an alternative to stool fat analysis. *Am J Clin Nutr* 1983; 38: 763.

167 Brown GA, Halliday RB, Turner PJ, Smalley CA. Faecal chymotrypsin concentrations in neonates with cystic fibrosis. *Arch Dis Child* 1988; 63: 1229.

168 Brown GA, Sule D, Williams J et al. Faecal chymotrypsin: a reliable index of exocrine pancreatic function. *Arch Dis Child* 1988; 63: 785.

169 Colombo C, Maiavacca R, Ronchi M et al. The Steatocrit: a simple method for monitoring fat malabsorption in patients with cystic fibrosis. *J Pediatr Gastroenterol Nutr* 1987; 6: 926.

170 Walters MP, Kelleher J, Gilbert J, Littlewood JM. Clinical monitoring of steatorrhoea in cystic fibrosis. *Arch Dis Child* 1990; 65: 99.

171 Puntis JWL, Berg JD, Buckley BM et al. Simplified oral pancreatic function test. *Arch Dis Child* 1988; 63: 780.

172 Lankisch PG, Schreiber A, Otto J. Pancreolauryl test. Evaluation of a tubeless pancreatic function test in comparison with other indirect tests for exocrine pancreatic function. *Dig Dis Sci* 1983; 28: 490.

173 Dalzell AM, Heaf DP. Fluoroscein dilaurate test on exocrine pancreatic function in cystic fibrosis. *Arch Dis Child* 1990; 65: 788.

174 Crossley JR, Elliot RB, Smith PA. Dried blood spot screening for cystic fibrosis in the newborn. *Lancet* 1979; i: 472.

175 Crossley JR, Smith PA, Edgar BW et al. Neonatal screening for cystic fibrosis using immunoreactive trypsin assay in dried blood spots. *Clin Chim Acta* 1981; 113: 111.

176 Gibson LE. Screening of newborns for cystic fibrosis. *Am J Dis Child* 1980; 134: 925.

177 Dodge JA, Riley HC. Screening for cystic fibrosis. *Arch Dis Child* 1982; 57: 774.

178 Farrell PM. Early diagnosis of cystic fibrosis:

to screen or not to screen – an important question. *Pediatrics* 1984; 73: 115.

179 Heeley AF, Heeley ME, King DN et al. Screening for cystic fibrosis by dried blood spot trypsin assay. *Arch Dis Child* 1982; 57: 18.

180 Wilcken B, Brown ARD, Urwin R, Brown DA. Cystic fibrosis screening by dried blood spot trypsin assay: results for 75,000 newborn infants. *J Pediatr* 1983; 102: 383.

181 Ryley HC, Goodchild MC, Dodge JA. Screening for cystic fibrosis. *Br Med Bull* 1992; 48: 805.

182 Waters DL, Dorney SF, Gaskin KJ et al. Pancreatic function in infants identified as having cystic fibrosis in a neonatal screening programme. *N Engl J Med* 1990; 322: 303.

183 Rock MJ, Mischler EH, Farrell PM et al. Newborn screening for cystic fibrosis is complicated by age-related decline in immunoreactive trypsinogen levels. *Pediatrics* 1990; 85: 1001.

184 Hammond KB, Abman SH, Sokol RJ, Accurso FJ. Efficacy of state wide screening for cystic fibrosis bioassay of trypsinogen concentrations. *N Engl J Med* 1991; 325: 769.

185 Bowling FG, McGill JJ, Shepherd RW, Danks DM. Screening for cystic fibrosis: use of ΔF508 mutation. *Lancet* 1990; 335: 925.

186 Ranieri E, Ryall RG, Morris CP et al. Neonatal screening strategy for cystic fibrosis using immunoreactive trypsinogen and direct gene analysis. *Br Med J* 1991; 302: 1237.

187 Ranieri E, Lewis BD, Gerace RL et al. Neonatal screening for cystic fibrosis using immunoreactive trypsinogen and direct gene analysis: four years experience. *Br Med J* 1994; 308: 1469.

188 Wilken B, Wiley V, Sherry G, Bayliss U. Neonatal screening for cystic fibrosis: a comparison of two strategies for case detection in 1.2 million babies. *J Pediatr* 1995; 127: 965.

189 Larsen J, Campbell S, Faragher EB et al. Cystic fibrosis screening in neonates: measurment of immunoreactive trypsin and direct genotype analysis for ΔF508 mutation. *Eur J Pediatr* 1994; 153: 569.

190 Ferec C, Verlingue C, Parent P et al. Neonatal screening for cystic fibrosis: result of a pilot study using both immunoreactive trypsinogen and cystic fibrosis gene mutation analyses. *Hum Genet* 1995; 96: 542.

191 Gregg RG, Simantel A, Farrell PM et al. Newborn screening for cystic fibrosis in Wiscons: comparison of biochemical and molecular methods. *Pediatrics* 1997; 99: 819.

192 Wilcken B, Chalmers G. Reduced morbidity in patients with cystic fibrosis detected by neonatal screening. *Lancet* 1985; ii: 1319.

193 Dankert-Roelse JE, te Meerman GJ, Knol K, ten Kate LP. Effect of screening for cystic fibrosis on the influence of genetic counselling. *Clin Genet* 1987; 32: 271.

194 Bowling F, Cleghorn G, Chester A et al. Neonatal screening for cystic fibrosis. *Arch Dis Child* 1988; 63: 196.

195 Dankert-Roelse JE, te Meerman GJ, Martijn A et al. Survival and clinical outcome in patients with cystic fibrosis, with and without neonatal screening. *J Pediatr* 1989; 114: 362.

196 Dankert-Roelse JE, te Meerman GJ. Long term prognosis of patients with cystic fibrosis in relation to early detection by neonatal screening and treatment in a cystic fibrosis centre. *Thorax* 1995; 50: 712.

197 Farrell PM, Kosorok MR, Laxova A. Nutritional benefits of neonatal screening for cystic fibrosis. Wisconsin Cystic Fibrosis Neonatal Screening Study Group. *N Engl J Med* 1997; 337: 963.

198 Ryley HC, Deam SM, Williams J et al. Neonatal screening for cystic fibrosis in Wales and the West Midlands: 1. Evaluation of immunoreactive trypsin test. *J Clin Pathol* 1988; 41: 726.

199 Chatfield S, Owen G, Ryley HC et al. Neonatal screening for cystic fibrosis in Wales and the West Midlands: clinical assessment after five years of screening. *Arch Dis Child* 1991; 66: 29.

200 Mennie ME, Gilfillan A, Compton M et al. Prenatal screening for cystic fibrosis. *Lancet* 1992; 340: 214.

201 Cuckle H, Quirke P, Sehmi I et al. Antenatal screening for cystic fibrosis. *Br J Obstet Gynaecol* 1996; 103: 795.

202 Wald NJ. Couple screening for cystic fibrosis. *Lancet* 1991; 338: 1318.

203 Livingstone J, Axton RA, Gilfillan A. Antenatal screening for cystic fibrosis: a trial of the couple model. *Br Med J* 1994; 308: 1459.

204 Miedzybrodzka ZH, Hall MH, Mollison J. Antenatal screening for carriers of cystic fibrosis: randomised trial of stepwise v couple screening. *Br Med J* 1995; 310: 353.

205 Watson EK, Mayall E, Chapple J. Screening for carriers of cystic fibrosis through primary health care services. *Br Med J* 1991; 303: 504.

206 Schidlow DV, Ramsey BW, Chesrovon S et al. Guidelines for CF care centers. *Am J Dis Child* 1990; 144: 1311.

207 Shwachman H, Kulczycki LL. Long-term study of one hundred and five patients with cystic fibrosis: studies made over a five to fourteen year period. *Am J Dis Child* 1958; 96: 6.

208 Doershuk CF, Matthews LW, Tucker AS et al. A five year clinical evaluation of a therapeutic program for patients with cystic fibrosis. *J Pediatr* 1964; 65: 677.

209 Brasfield D, Hicks G, Soong S, Tiller RE. The chest roentgenogram in cystic fibrosis: a new scoring system. *Pediatrics* 1979; 63: 24.

210 Lewiston N, Moss R, Hindi R, Rubinstein S, Sullivan M. Interobserver variance in clinical scoring for cystic fibrosis. *Chest* 1987; 91: 878.

211 Cooperman EM, Park M, McKee J, Assad JP. A simplified scoring system (a preliminary report). *Can Med Assoc J* 1971; 105: 580.

212 Taussig LM, Kattwinkel J, Friedewald WT, di Sant'Agnese PA. A new prognostic score and clinical evaluation system for cystic fibrosis. *J Pediatr* 1973; 82: 380.

213 Stockrider MM, Swank PR, Seilheimer DK, Schidlow DV. Measuring clinical status in cystic fibrosis: internal validity and reliability of a modified NIH score. *Pediatr Pulmonol* 1994; 17: 86.

214 Chrispin AR, Norman AP. The systematic evaluation of the chest radiograph in cystic fibrosis. *Pediatr Radiol* 1974; 2: 101.

215 Brasfield D, Hicks G, Soong S et al. Evaluation of a scoring system of the chest radiograph in cystic fibrosis: a collaborative study. *Am J Roentgenol* 1980; 134: 1195.

216 Meerman GJ, Dankert-Roelse J, Martijn A, van Woerden HH. Comparison of the Shwachman, Chrispin–Norman and Brasfield methods for scoring of chest radiographs for patients with cystic fibrosis: a

collaborative study. *Pediatr Radiol* 1985; 15: 98.

217 Wong EB, Regnis J, Shnier RC, Bye PT, Stewart ME. The relationship between tests of lung function and three chest radiological scoring systems in patients with cystic fibrosis. *Australas Radiol* 1993; 37: 265.

218 Conway SP, Pond MN, Bowler I *et al*. The chest radiograph in cystic fibrosis: a new scoring system compared with the Chrispin–Norman and Brasfield scores. *Thorax* 1994; 49: 860.

219 Verdugo P. Mucin exocytosis. *Am Rev Respir Dis* 1991; 144: S33–S37.

220 Gupta R, Jentoft N. The structure of tracheo-bronchial mucins from cystic fibrosis and control patients. *J Biol Chem* 1992; 267: 3160.

221 Cheng PW, Boat TF, Cranfill K *et al*. Increased sulfation of glycoconjugates by cultured nasal epithelial cells from patients with cystic fibrosis. *J Clin Invest* 1989; 84: 68.

222 Smith JJ, Travis SM, Greenberg EP, Welsh MJ. Cystic fibrosis airway epithelia fail to kill bacteria because of abnormal airway surface fluid. *Cell* 1996; 85: 229.

223 Malawista SE, Montgomery RR, van Blaricom G. Evidence for RNI in killing of staphylococci by human neutrophil cytoplasts. *J Clin Invest* 1992; 90: 631.

224 Evan TJ, Buttery LDK, Carpenter A, Springall DR, Polak JM, Cohen J. Cytokine treated human neutrophils contain iNOS that produces nitration of ingested bacteria. *Proc Natl Acad Sci USA* 1992; 93: 9553.

225 Meng Q-H, Springall DR, Bishop AE *et al*. Lack of inducible nitric oxide synthase in bronchial epithelium: a possible mechanism of susceptibility to infection in CF. *J Pathol* 1998; 184: 323.

226 Pier GB, Grout M, Zaidi TS. Cystic fibrosis transmembrane conductance regulator is an epithelial cell receptor for clearance of *Pseudomonas aeruginosa* from the lung. *Proc Natl Acad Sci USA* 1997; 94: 12088.

227 Davies JC, Stern M, Dewar A *et al*. CFTR gene transfer reduces the binding of *Pseudomonas aeruginosa* to cystic fibrosis respiratory epithelium. *Am J Respir Cell Mol Biol* 1997; 16: 657.

228 de Bentzmann S, Roger P, Dupuit F *et al*. Asialo GM1 is a receptor for *Pseudomonas aeruginosa* adherence to regenerating respiratory epithelial cells. *Infect Immun* 1996; 64: 1582.

229 Speert DP, Farmer SW, Campbell ME *et al*. Conversion of *Pseudomonas aeruginosa* to the phenotype characteristic of strains from patients with cystic fibrosis. *J Clin Microbiol* 1990; 28: 188.

230 Anwar H, Brown MRW, Day A, Weller PH. Outer membrane antigens of mucoid *Pseudomonas aeruginosa* isolated directly from the sputum of a cystic fibrosis patient. *FEMS Microbiol Lett* 1984; 24: 235.

231 Haas B, Kraut J, Marks J *et al*. Siderophore presence in sputa of cystic fibrosis patients. *Infect Immun* 1991; 59: 3997.

232 Lam J, Chan R, Lam K, Costerton JW. Production of mucoid microcolonies by *Pseudomonas aeruginosa* within infected lungs in cystic fibrosis. *Infect Immun* 1980; 28: 546.

233 Schwarzman S, Boring JR. 1. Antiphagocytic effect of slime from a mucoid strain of *Pseudomonas aeruginosa*. *Infect Immun* 1971; 3: 762.

234 Anwar H, Dasgupta M, Lam K, Costerton JW. Tobramycin resistance of mucoid *Pseudomonas aeruginosa* biofilm grown under iron limitation. *J Antimicrob Chemother* 1989; 24: 647.

235 Hancock RE, Mutharia LM, Chan L *et al*. *Pseudomonas aeruginosa* isolates from patients with cystic fibrosis: a class of serum-sensitive, non-typable strains deficient in lipopolysaccharide O side chains. *Infect Immun* 1983; 42: 170.

236 Pitt TL. Lipopolysaccharide and virulence of *Pseudomonas aeruginosa*. *Antibiot Chemother* 1989; 42: 1.

237 Konstan MW, Hilliard KA, Norvell TM, Berger M. Bronchoalveolar lavage findings in cystic fibrosis patients with stable, clinically mild lung disease suggest ongoing infection and inflammation. *Am J Respir Crit Care Med* 1994; 150: 448.

238 Birrer P, McElvaney NG, Rudeberg A *et al*. Protease–antiprotease imbalance in the lungs of children with cystic fibrosis. *Am J Respir Crit Care Med* 1994; 150: 207.

239 Khan TZ, Wagener JS, Bost T, Martinez J, Accurso FJ, Riches DWH. Early pulmonary inflammation in infants with cystic fibrosis. *Am J Respir Crit Care Med* 1995; 151: 1075.

240 Bonfield TL, Konstan MW, Burfiend P, Panuska JR, Hilliard JB, Berger M. Normal bronchial epithelial cells constitutively produce the anti-inflammatory cytokine interleukin-10, which is downregulated in CF. *Am J Respir Cell Mol Biol* 1995; 13: 257.

241 Moss RB, Bocian RC, Hsu YP *et al*. Reduced IL-10 secretion by CD4+ T lymphocytes expressing mutant cystic fibrosis transmembrane conductance regulator (CFTR). *Clin Exp Immunol* 1996; 106: 374.

242 Høiby N, Döring G, Schiøtz PO. Role of immune complexes in the pathogenesis of bacterial infections. *Ann Rev Microbiol* 1986; 40: 29.

243 Suter S. Imbalance between granulocyte neutral proteases and anti-proteases in bronchial secretions from patients with cystic fibrosis. *Antibiot Chemother* 1989; 42: 158.

244 Nakamura H, Yoshimura K, McElvaney NG, Crystal RG. Neutrophil elastase in respiratory epithelial lining fluid of individuals with cystic fibrosis induces interleukin-8 gene expression in a human bronchial epithelial cell line. *J Clin Invest* 1992; 89: 1478.

245 Di Sant'Agnese PA, Andersen DH. Celiac syndrome: chemotherapy in infections of the respiratory tract associated with cystic fibrosis of the pancreas: observations with penicillin and drugs of the sulphonamide groups, with special reference to penicillin aerosol. *Am J Dis Child* 1946; 72: 17.

246 Andersen DH. Therapy and prognosis in fibrocystic disease of the pancreas. *Pediatrics* 1949; 3: 406.

247 Høiby N. Microbiology of lung infections in cystic fibrosis patients. *Acta Paediatr Scand* 1974; 301 (Suppl): 33.

248 Watson KC, Kerr EJC, Baillie M. Temporal changes in biotypes of *Haemophilus influenzae* isolated from patients with cystic fibrosis. *J Med Microbiol* 1988; 26: 129.

249 Pedersen SS, Espersen F, Pressler T, Høiby N, Rosendal K. Does centralized treatment of cystic fibrosis increase the risk of *P. aeruginosa* infection? *Acta Paediatr Scand* 1986; 75: 840.

250 Kharazmi A. Mechanisms involved in the evasion of the host defence by *Pseudomonas aeruginosa*. *Immunol Lett* 1991; 30: 201.

251 Döring G, Buhl V, Høiby N *et al*. Detection of proteases of *Pseudomonas aeruginosa* in immune complexes isolated from sputum of cystic fibrosis patients. *Acta Pathol Microbiol Scand C* 1984; 92: 307.

252 Baker NR, Minor V, Deal C *et al*. *Pseudomonas aeruginosa* exoenzyme-S is an adhesin. *Infect Immun* 1991; 59: 2859.

253 Valerius NH, Koch C, Høiby N. Prevention of chronic *Pseudomonas aeruginosa* colonisation in cystic fibrosis by early treatment. *Lancet* 1991; 338: 725.

254 Cryz SJ, Wedgwood J, Lang AB *et al*. Immunization of noncolonized cystic fibrosis patients against *Pseudomonas aeruginosa*. *J Infect Dis* 1994; 169: 1159.

255 Lang AB, Schaad UB, Rudeberg A *et al*. Effect of high-affinity anti-*Pseudomonas aeruginosa* lipopolysaccharide antibodies induced by immunization on the rate of *Pseudomonas aeruginosa* infection in patients with cystic fibrosis. *J Pediatr* 1995; 127: 711.

256 Karpati F, Malmborg AS, Alfredsson H, Hjelte L, Strandvik B. Bacterial colonisation with *Xanthomonas maltophilia*: a retrospective study in a cystic fibrosis patient population. *Infection* 1994; 22: 258.

257 Spencer RC. The emergence of epidemic, multiple-antibiotic-resistant *Stenotrophomonas (Xanthomonas) maltophilia* and *Burkholderia (Pseudomonas) cepacia*. *J Hosp Infect* 1995; 30 (Suppl): 453.

258 Burkholder WH. Sour skin, a bacterial rot of onion bulbs. *Phytopathology* 1950; 40: 115.

259 Ederer GM, Matsen JM. Colonization and infection with *Pseudomonas cepacia*. *J Infect Dis* 1972; 125: 613.

260 Isles A, Maclusky I, Corey M *et al*. *Pseudomonas cepacia* infection in cystic fibrosis: an emerging problem. *J Pediatr* 1984; 104: 206.

261 Thomassen MJ, Demko CA, Klinger JD, Stern RC. *Pseudomonas cepacia* colonization among patients with cystic fibrosis: a new opportunist. *Am Rev Respir Dis* 1985; 131: 791.

262 Govan JRW, Brown PH, Maddison J *et al*. Evidence for transmission of *Pseudomonas cepacia* by social contact in cystic fibrosis. *Lancet* 1993; 342: 15.

263 Smith DL, Gumery LB, Smith EG, Stableforth DE, Kaufmann ME, Pitt TL. Epidemic of *Pseudomonas cepacia* in an adult cystic fibrosis unit: evidence of person-to-person transmission. *J Clin Microbiol* 1993; 31: 3017.

264 LiPuma JJ, Dasen SE, Nielson DW, Stern RC, Stull TL. Person-to-person transmission of *Pseudomonas cepacia* between patients with cystic fibrosis. *Lancet* 1990; 336: 1094.

265 Millar-Jones L, Paull A, Saunders Z, Goodchild MC. Transmission of *Pseudomonas cepacia* among cystic fibrosis patients. *Lancet* 1992; 340: 491.

266 Corkill JE, Sisson PR, Smyth A *et al*. Application of pyrolysis mass spectroscopy and SDS-PAGE in the study of the epidemiology of *Pseudomonas cepacia* in cystic fibrosis. *J Med Microbiol* 1994; 41: 106.

267 Pegues DA, Carson LA, Tablan OC *et al*. Acquisition of *Pseudomonas cepacia* at summer camps for patients with cystic fibrosis. *J Pediatr* 1994; 124: 694.

268 Johnson WM, Tyler SD, Rozee KR. Linkage analysis of geographic and clinical clusters

in *Pseudomonas cepacia* infections by multilocus enzyme electrophoresis and ribotyping. *J Clin Microbiol* 1994; 32: 924.

269 LiPuma JJ, Marks-Austin KA, Holsclaw DS, Winnie GB, Gilligan PH, Stull PL. Inapparent transmission of *Pseudomonas (Burkholderia) cepacia* among patients with cystic fibrosis. *Pediatr Infect Dis J* 1994; 13: 716.

270 Ryley HC, Millar-Jones L, Paull A, Weeks J. Characterisation of *Burkholderia cepacia* from cystic fibrosis patients living in Wales by PCR ribotyping. *J Med Microbiol* 1995; 43: 436.

271 Whiteford ML, Wilkinson JD, McColl JH *et al*. Outcome of *Burkholderia (Pseudomonas) cepacia* colonisation in children with cystic fibrosis following a hospital outbreak. *Thorax* 1995; 50: 1194.

272 Pitt TL, Kaufmann ME, Patel PS, Benge LCA, Gaskin S, Livermore DM. Type characterisation and antibiotic susceptibility of *Burkholderia (Pseudomonas) cepacia* isolates from patients with cystic fibrosis in the United Kingdom and the Republic of Ireland. *J Med Microbiol* 1996; 44: 203.

273 Govan JRW, Nelson JW. Microbiology of lung infections: themes and issues. *J R Soc Med* 1996; 86 (Suppl 20): 11.

274 Rosenstein BJ, Hall DE. Pneumonia and septicaemia due to *Pseudomonas cepacia* in a patient with cystic fibrosis. *Johns Hopkins Med J* 1980; 147: 188.

275 Govan JRW, Glass S. The microbiology and therapy of cystic fibrosis lung infections. *Rev Med Microbiol* 1990; 1: 19.

276 Mahenthiralingam E, Simpson DA, Speert DP. Identification and characterization of a novel DNA marker associated with epidemic *Burkholderia cepacia* strains recovered from patients with cystic fibrosis. *J Clin Microbiol* 1997; 35: 808.

277 Whittier S, Hopfer RL, Knowles MR, Gilligan PH. Improved recovery of mycobacteria from respiratory secretions of patients with cystic fibrosis. *J Clin Microbiol* 1993; 31: 861.

278 Hjelte L, Petrini B, Kallenius G, Strandvik B. Prospective study of mycobacterial infections in patients with cystic fibrosis. *Thorax* 1990; 45: 397.

279 Kilby JM, Gilligan PH, Yankaskas JR, Highsmith WE, Edwards LJ, Knowles MR. Nontuberculous mycobacteria in adult patients with cystic fibrosis. *Chest* 1992; 102: 70.

280 Aitken ML, Burke W, McDonald G *et al*. Non-tuberculous mycobacterial disease in adult cystic fibrosis patients. *Chest* 1993; 103: 1096.

281 Hjelt K, Hojlyng N, Howitz P *et al*. The role of mycobacteria other than tuberculosis (MOTT) in patients with cystic fibrosis. *Scand J Infect Dis* 1994; 26: 569.

282 Fauroux B, Delaisi B, Clement A *et al*. Mycobacterial lung disease in cystic fibrosis: a prospective study. *Pediatr Infect Dis J* 1997; 16: 354.

283 Torrens JK, Dawkins P, Conway SP, Moya E. Non-tuberculous mycobacteria in cystic fibrosis. *Thorax* 1998; 53: 182.

284 Efthimiou J, Smith MJ, Hodson ME *et al*. Fatal pulmonary infection with *Mycobacterium fortuitum* in cystic fibrosis. *Br J Dis Chest* 1984; 78: 299.

285 Brueton MJ, Omerod LP, Shah KJ, Anderson CM. Allergic bronchopulmonary aspergillosis complicating cystic fibrosis. *Arch Dis Child* 1980; 55: 348.

286 Milla CE, Wielenski CL, Regelmann WE. Clinical significance of the recovery of

Aspergillus species from the respiratory secretions of cystic fibrosis patients. *Pediatr Pulmonol* 1996; 21: 6.

287 Ramsey BW, Gore EJ, Smith AL *et al*. The effect of respiratory viral infections on patients with cystic fibrosis. *Am J Dis Child* 1989; 43: 662.

288 Hordvik NL, König P, Hamory B *et al*. Effects of acute viral respiratory infections in patients with cystic fibrosis. *Pediatr Pulmonol* 1989; 7: 217.

289 Shale DJ. Viral infections: a role in the lung disease of cystic fibrosis. *Thorax* 1992; 47: 69.

290 Johansen HK, Høiby N. Seasonal onset of initial colonisation and chronic infection with *Pseudomonas aeruginosa* in patients with cystic fibrosis in Denmark. *Thorax* 1992; 47: 109.

291 Conway SP, Simmonds EJ, Littlewood JM. Acute severe deterioration in cystic fibrosis associated with influenza-A virus infection. *Thorax* 1992; 47: 112.

292 Shwachman H, Kulczycki LL, Mueller HL, Flake CG. Nasal polyposis in patients with cystic fibrosis. *Pediatrics* 1962; 30: 389.

293 Taylor B, Evans JNG, Hope GA. Upper respiratory tract in cystic fibrosis. *Arch Dis Child* 1982; 49: 133.

294 Bak-Pedersen K, Kildegaard Larsen P. Inflammatory middle ear diseases in patients with cystic fibrosis. *Acta Otolaryngol* 1979; 360: 138.

295 Puchelle E. Airway secretions: new concepts and functions. *Eur Respir J* 1992; 5: 3.

296 Tos M, Morgensen C, Thomsen J. Nasal polyps in cystic fibrosis. *J Laryngol Otol* 1977; 91: 827.

297 Henderson WR, Chi EY. Degranulation of cystic fibrosis nasal polyp mast cells. *J Pathol* 1992; 166: 395.

298 Drake-Lee AB, Morgan DW. Nasal polyps and sinusitis in children with cystic fibrosis. *J Laryngol Otol* 1989; 103: 753.

299 Kerrebijn JDF, Poublon RML, Overbeek SE. Nasal and paranasal disease in adult cystic fibrosis patients. *Eur Respir J* 1992; 5: 1239.

300 Neely J, Harrison GM, Jerger JF *et al*. The otolaryngologic aspects of cystic fibrosis. *Am Acad Ophthalmol Oto Trans* 1972; 76: 313.

301 Fairfax AJ, Ball J, Batten JC, Heard BE. A pathological study following bronchial artery embolisation for haemoptysis in cystic fibrosis. *Br J Dis Chest* 1980; 74: 345.

302 Sweezey NB, Fellows KE. Bronchial artery embolization for severe hemoptysis in cystic fibrosis. *Chest* 1990; 97: 1322.

303 Stern RC, Wood RE, Boat TF *et al*. Treatment and prognosis of massive hemoptysis in cystic fibrosis. *Am Rev Respir Dis* 1978; 177: 825.

304 Penketh AR, Knight RK, Hodson ME, Batten JC. Management of pneumothorax in adults. *Thorax* 1982; 37: 850.

305 Spector ML, Stern RC. Pneumothorax in cystic fibrosis: a 26 year experience. *Ann Thorac Surg* 1989; 47: 204.

306 Scott JP, Higenbottam TW, Hutter J *et al*. Heart–lung transplantation for cystic fibrosis. *Lancet* 1988; ii: 192.

307 Madden BP, Hodsen ME, Tsang V *et al*. Intermediate-term results of heart–lung transplantation for cystic fibrosis. *Lancet* 1992; i: 1583.

308 De Leval MR, Smyth RL, Whithead B *et al*. Heart and lung transplantation for terminal cystic fibrosis: a $4\frac{1}{2}$-year experience. *J Thorac Cardiovasc Surg* 1991; 101: 633.

309 Cooper JD, Patterson GA, Grossmann R *et al*. Double-lung transplant for advanced chronic obstructive lung disease. *Am Rev Respir Dis* 1989; 139: 303.

310 Noirclerc M, Chazalette JP, Metras D *et al*. Les transplantations Bi pulmonies. Rapport de la première observation francaise et commentaire des cinq suivantes. *Ann Chir Thorac Cardiovasc* 1989; 43: 597.

311 Pasque MK, Cooper JD, Kaiser LR *et al*. Improved technique for bilateral lung transplantation: rationale and initial experience. *Ann Thorac Surg* 1990; 49: 785.

312 Shennib H, Noirclerc N, Ernst P *et al*. Double lung transplantation for cystic fibrosis. *Ann Thorac Surg* 1992; 54: 27.

313 Snell GI, de Hoyos A, Krajden M *et al*. *Pseudomonas cepacia* in lung transplant recipients with cystic fibrosis. *Chest* 1993; 103: 466.

314 Millet B, Higenbottam TW, Flower CD *et al*. The radiographic appearances of infection and acute rejection of the lung after heart–lung transplantation. *Am Rev Respir Dis* 1989; 140: 62.

315 Kramer MR, Stoehr C, Lewiston NJ *et al*. Trimethoprim–sulfamethoxazole prophylaxis for *Pneumocystis carinii* infections in heart–lung and lung transplantation. *Transplantation* 1992; 53: 586.

316 Theodore J, Morris AJ, Burke CM *et al*. Cardiopulmonary function at maximum tolerable constant work rate exercise following human heart–lung transplantation. *Chest* 1987; 92: 433.

317 Sciurla FC, Owens GR, Sanders MH *et al*. Evidence of an altered pattern of breathing during exercise in recipients of heart–lung transplants. *N Engl J Med* 1988; 319: 1186.

318 Williams TJ, Patterson GA, McClean PA *et al*. Maximal exercise testing in single and double lung transplant recipients. *Am Rev Respir Dis* 1992; 145: 101.

319 Bronstein MN, Sokol RJ, Abman SH *et al*. Pancreatic insufficiency, growth, and nutrition in infants identified by newborn screening as having cystic fibrosis. *J Pediatr* 1992; 120: 533.

320 Walters DL, Dorney SFA, Gaskin KJ *et al*. Pancreatic function in infants identified as having cystic fibrosis in a neonatal screening program. *N Engl J Med* 1990; 322: 303.

321 Gaskin KJ, Durie PR, Lee L *et al*. Colipase and lipase secretion in childhood-onset pancreatic insufficiency. *Gastroenterology* 1984; 86: 1.

322 Robinson PJ, Sly PD. High dose pancreatic enzymes in cystic fibrosis. *Arch Dis Child* 1990; 65: 311.

323 Brady MS, Rickard K, Yu PL, Eigen H. Effectiveness and safety of small vs. large doses of enteric coated pancreatic enzymes in reducing steatorrhea in children with cystic fibrosis: a prospective randomized study. *Pediatr Pulmonol* 1991; 10: 79.

324 Weber AM, Roy CC. Intraduodenal events in cystic fibrosis. *J Pediatr Gastroenterol Nutr* 1984; 3 (Suppl 1): S113.

325 Boyle BJ, Long WB, Balistreri WF *et al*. Effect of cimetidine and pancreatic enzymes on serum and fecal bile acids and fat absorption in cystic fibrosis. *Gastroenterology* 1980; 78: 950.

326 Durie PR, Bell L, Linton W *et al*. Effect of cimetidine and sodium bicarbonate on pancreatic replacement therapy in cystic fibrosis. *Gut* 1980; 21: 778.

327 Heijerman HG, Lamers CB, Bakker W. Omeprazole enhances the efficacy of pancreatin (pancrease) in cystic fibrosis. *Ann Intern Med* 1991; 114: 200.

328 Smyth RL, van Velzen D, Smyth AR, Lloyd DA, Heaf DP. Strictures of ascending colon in cystic fibrosis and high-strength pancreatic enzymes. *Lancet* 1994; 343: 85.

329 Smyth RL, Ashby D, O'Hea U *et al.* Fibrosing colonopathy in cystic fibrosis. Results of a case-control study. *Lancet* 1995; 346: 1247.

330 FitzSimmons SC, Burkhart GA, Borowitz D *et al.* High-dose pancreatic-enzyme supplements and fibrosing colonopathy in children with cystic fibrosis. *N Engl J Med* 1997; 336: 1283.

331 MacSweeney EJ, Oades PJ, Buchdahl R, Rosenthal N, Bush A. Relation of thickening of colon wall to pancreatic enzyme treatment in cystic fibrosis. *Lancet* 1995; 345: 752.

332 Masaryk TJ, Achkar E. Pancreatitis as initial presentation of cystic fibrosis in young adults. A report of two cases. *Dig Dis Sci* 1983; 28: 874.

333 Gross V, Schoelmerich J, Denzel K, Gerok W. Relapsing pancreatitis as initial manifestation of cystic fibrosis in a young man without pulmonary disease. *Int J Pancreatol* 1989; 4: 221.

334 Scott RB, O'Loughlin EV, Gall DG. Gastroesophageal reflux in patients with cystic fibrosis. *J Pediatr* 1985; 106: 223.

335 Feigelson J, Girault F, Pecau Y. Gastro-oesophageal reflux and oesophagitis in cystic fibrosis. *Acta Paediatr Scand* 1987; 76: 989.

336 Rubenstein S, Moss R, Lewiston N. Constipation and meconium ileus equivalent in patients with cystic fibrosis. *Pediatrics* 1986; 78: 473.

337 Rosenstein BJ, Langbaum TS. Incidence of distal intestinal obstruction syndrome in cystic fibrosis. *J Pediatr Gastroenterol Nutr* 1983; 2: 299.

338 Koletzko S, Stringer DA, Cleghorn GJ, Durie PR. Lavage treatment of distal intestinal obstruction syndrome in children with cystic fibrosis. *Pediatrics* 1989; 83: 727.

339 Consensus Conferences. Gastroesophageal reflux. *Cystic Fibrosis Foundation*, II, section II 1991.

340 Cohn JA, Strong TV, Picciotto MR, Nairn AC, Collins FS, Fitz JG. Localization of the cystic fibrosis transmembrane conductance regulator in human bile duct epithelial cells. *Gastroenterology* 1993; 105: 1857.

341 Weizman Z, Drie PR, Kopelman HR, Vesely SM, Forstner GG. Bile acid secretion in cystic fibrosis: evidence for a defect unrelated to fat malabsorption. *Gut* 1986; 27: 1043.

342 Tanner MS. Liver and biliary problems in cystic fibrosis. *J R Soc Med* 1992; 85 (Suppl 19): 20.

343 Scott-Jupp R, Lama M, Tanner MS. Prevalence of liver disease in cystic fibrosis. *Arch Dis Child* 1991; 66: 698.

344 Feigelson J, Anagnostopoulos C, Poquet M, Munck A, Navarro J. Liver cirrhosis in cystic fibrosis: therapeutic implications and long term follow up. *Arch Dis Child* 1993; 68: 653.

345 Kovesi T, Corey M, Tsui L-C *et al.* The association between liver disease and mutations of the cystic fibrosis gene (abstract). *Pediatr Pulmonol* 1992; Suppl. 8: 244.

346 Duthie A, Doherty DG, Williams C *et al.* Analysis of ΔF508, G551D and R553X mutations in children and young adults

347 Craig JM, Haddad H, Shwachman H. The pathological changes in the liver in cystic fibrosis of the pancreas. *Am J Dis Child* 1957; 93: 357.

348 Hultcrantz R, Mengarelli S, Strandvik B. Morphological findings in the liver of children with cystic fibrosis: a light and electron microscopical study. *Hepatology* 1986; 6: 881.

349 O'Brien S, Keogan M, Casey M *et al.* Biliary complications of cystic fibrosis. *Gut* 1992; 33: 387.

350 Nagel RA, Javaid A, Meire HB *et al.* Liver disease and bile duct abnormalities in adults with cystic fibrosis. *Lancet* 1989; ii: 1422.

351 Nakagawa M, Colombo C, Setchell KDR. Comprehensive study of the biliary bile acid composition of patients with cystic fibrosis and associated liver disease before and after ursodeoxycholic acid administration. *Hepatology* 1990; 12: 322.

352 Scharschmidt BF. Bile formation and gallbladder acid bile duct function. In: Sleisenger MH, Fordtran JS, eds. *Gastrointestinal Disease: Pathophysiology, Diagnosis and Management.* Philadelphia: WB Saunders, 1989: 1656.

353 Colombo C, Castellani MR, Balistreri WF *et al.* Scintigraphic documentation of an improvement in hepatobiliary excretory function after treatment with ursodeoxycholic acid in patients with cystic fibrosis and associated liver disease. *Hepatology* 1992; 15: 667.

354 Galabert C, Montet JC, Legrand D *et al.* Effects of ursodeoxycholic acid on liver function in patients with cystic fibrosis and chronic cholestasis. *J Pediatr* 1992; 121: 138.

355 Colombo C, Setchell KDR, Podda M *et al.* Effects of ursodeoxycholic acid therapy for liver disease associated with cystic fibrosis. *J Pediatr* 1990; 117: 482.

356 Stern RC, Stevens DP, Boat TF *et al.* Symptomatic hepatic disease in cystic fibrosis: incidence, course, and outcome of portal systemic shunting. *Gastroenterology* 1976; 70: 645.

357 Donovan TJ, Ward M, Shepherd RW. Evaluation of endoscopic sclerotherapy of esophageal varices in children. *J Pediatr Gastroenterol Nutr* 1986; 5: 696.

358 Conn HO. Transjugular intrahepatic portal systemic shunts: the state of the art. *Hepatology* 1993; 17: 148.

359 Noble-Jamieson G, Barnes N, Jamieson N, Friend P, Calne R. Liver transplantation for hepatic cirrhosis in cystic fibrosis. *J R Soc Med* 1996; 89 (Suppl 27): 31.

360 Wilson-Sharp RC, Irving HC, Brown RC *et al.* Ultrasonography of the pancreas. liver, and biliary system in cystic fibrosis. *Arch Dis Child* 1984; 59: 923.

361 Stern RC, Rothstein FC, Doershuk CF. Treatment and prognosis of symptomatic gallbladder disease in patients with cystic fibrosis. *J Pediatr Gastroenterol Nutr* 1986; 5: 35.

362 Weber AM, Roy CC. Bile acid metabolism in children with cystic fibrosis. *Acta Paediatr Scand* 1985; 317 (Suppl): 9.

363 Corey M, Farewell V. Determinants of mortality from cystic fibrosis in Canada. *Am J Epidemiol* 1996; 143: 1007.

364 Thomson MA, Quirk P, Swanson CE *et al.* Nutritional growth retardation is associated with defective lung growth in cystic fibrosis:

with cystic fibrosis with and without chronic liver disease. *Hepatology* 1992; 15: 660.

a preventable determinant of progressive pulmonary dysfunction. *Nutrition* 1995; 11: 350.

365 Lowe CU, May CD, Reed SC. Fibrosis of the pancreas in infants and children. *Am J Dis Child* 1949; 78: 349.

366 Shwachman H, Leubner H, Catzel P. Mucoviscidosis. *Adv Pediatr* 1955; 7: 249.

367 Handwerker S, Roth J, Gorden P *et al.* Glucose intolerance in cystic fibrosis. *N Engl J Med* 1969; 281: 451.

368 Mitchell-Heggs P, Mearns M, Batten JC. Cystic fibrosis in adolescents and adults. *Q J Med* 1976; 45: 479.

369 Lippe BM, Sperling MA, Dooley RR. Pancreatic alpha and beta cell functions in cystic fibrosis. *J Pediatr* 1977; 90: 751.

370 Di Sant'Agnese PA, Davis PB. Cystic fibrosis in adults: 75 cases and a review of 232 cases in the literature. *Am J Med* 1979; 66: 121.

371 Stutchfield PR, O'Halloran S, Teale JD *et al.* Glycosylated haemoglobin and glucose intolerance in cystic fibrosis. *Arch Dis Child* 1987; 62: 805.

372 Hartling SG, Garne S, Binder C *et al.* Proinsulin, insulin, and C-peptide in cystic fibrosis after an oral glucose tolerance test. *Diabetes Res* 1988; 7: 165.

373 Lanng S, Thorsteinsson B, Erichsen G, Nerup J, Koch C. Glucose tolerance in cystic fibrosis. *Arch Dis Child* 1991; 66: 612.

374 Lanng S, Hansen A, Thorsteinsson B, Nerup J, Koch C. Glucose tolerance in patients with cystic fibrosis: five year prospective study. *Br Med J* 1995; 311: 655.

375 Abdul-Karim FW, Dahms BB, Velasco ME, Rodman HM. Islets of Langerhans in adolescents and adults with cystic fibrosis. *Arch Pathol Lab Med* 1986; 110: 602.

376 Iannucci A, Mukai K, Johnson D, Burke B. Endocrine pancreas in cystic fibrosis: an immunohistochemical study. *Hum Pathol* 1984; 15: 278.

377 Soijima K, Landing BH. Pancreatic islets in older patients with cystic fibrosis with and without diabetes mellitus: morphometric and immunocytologic studies. *Pediatr Pathol* 1986; 6: 25.

378 Couce M, O'Brien TD, Moran A, Roche PC, Butler PC. Diabetes mellitus in cystic fibrosis is characterized by islet amyloidosis. *J Clin Endocrinol Metab* 1996; 81: 1267.

379 Moran A, Doherty L, Wang X, Thomas W. Abnormal glucose metabolism in cystic fibrosis. *J Pediatr* 1998; 133: 10.

380 Lanng S, Thorsteinsson B, Nerup J, Koch C. Diabetes mellitus in cystic fibrosis: effect of insulin therapy on lung function and infections. *Acta Paediatr Scand* 1994; 83: 849.

381 Newman AJ, Ansell BM. Episodic arthritis in children with cystic fibrosis. *J Pediatr* 1979; 94: 594.

382 Schidlow DV, Goldsmith DP, Palmer J, Huang NN. Arthritis in cystic fibrosis. *Arch Dis Child* 1984; 59: 377.

383 Rush PJ, Shore A, Coblentz C *et al.* The musculoskeletal manifestations of cystic fibrosis. *Semin Arthritis Rheum* 1986; 15: 213.

384 Dixey J, Redington AN, Butler RC *et al.* The arthropathy of cystic fibrosis. *Ann Rheum Dis* 1988; 47: 218.

385 Benjamin CM, Clague RB. Psoriatic or cystic fibrosis arthropathy? Difficulty with diagnosis and management. *Br J Rheumatol* 1990; 29: 301.

386 Soden M, Tempany E, Bresnihan B. Sarcoid

arthropathy in cystic fibrosis. *Br J Rheumatol* 1989; 28: 341.

387 Nielsen HE, Lundh S, Jacobsen SV, Høiby N. Hypergammaglobulinemic purpura in cystic fibrosis. *Acta Paediatr Scand* 1978; 67: 443.

388 Fradin MS, Kalb RE, Grossman ME. Recurrent cutaneous vasculitis in cystic fibrosis. *Pediatr Dermatol* 1987; 4: 108.

389 Finnegan MJ, Hinchcliffe J, Russell-Jones D *et al.* Vasculitis complicating cystic fibrosis. *Q J Med* 1989; 72: 609.

390 Taussig LM, Lobeck CC, di Sant'Agnese PA *et al.* Fertility in males with cystic fibrosis. *N Engl J Med* 1972; 287: 586.

391 Barreto C, Marques Pinto L, Duarte A *et al.* A fertile male with cystic fibrosis. *J Med Genet* 1991; 28: 420.

392 Kaplan E, Shwachman H, Perlmutter AD *et al.* Genital abnormalities in males with CF. *N Engl J Med* 1968; 279: 65.

393 Valman HB, France NE. The vas deferens in CF. *Lancet* 1969; ii: 566.

394 Olson JR, Weaner DK. Congenital mesonephric defects in male infants with mucoviscidosis. *J Clin Pathol* 1969; 22: 725.

395 Oppenheimer EH, Esterly JR. Observations on CF of the pancreas. V. Developmental changes in the male genital system. *J Pediatr* 1969; 75: 808.

396 Holsclaw DS, Perlmutter AD, Jocklin H. Genital abnormalities in male patients with CF. *J Urol* 1971; 106: 568.

397 Gottlieb C, Ploen L, Kvist U, Strandvik B. The fertility potential of male cystic fibrosis patients. *Int J Androl* 1991; 14: 437.

398 Silber SJ, Ord T, Balmaceda J *et al.* Congenital absence of the vas deferens. The fertilizing capacity of human epididymal sperm. *N Engl J Med* 1990; 323: 1788.

399 Kopito LE, Kosasky HJ, Shwachman H. Water and electrolytes in cervical mucus from patients with cystic fibrosis. *Fertil Steril* 1973; 24: 512.

400 Penketh ARL, Wise A, Mearns MB *et al.* Cystic fibrosis in adolescents and adults. *Thorax* 1987; 42: 526.

401 Stead RJ, Hodson ME, Batten JC *et al.* Amenorrhoea in cystic fibrosis. *Clin Endocrinol* 1987; 26: 187.

402 Fitzpatrick SB, Stokes DC, Rosenstein BJ *et al.* Use of oral contraceptives in women with cystic fibrosis. *Chest* 1984; 86: 863.

403 Siegel B, Siegel S. Pregnancy and delivery in a patient with CF of the pancreas. *Obstet Gynecol* 1960; 16: 439.

404 Grand RJ, Talamo RC, di Sant'Agnese PA, Schwartz RH. Pregnancy in cystic fibrosis of the pancreas. *JAMA* 1966; 195: 117.

405 Cohen LF, di Sant'Agnese PA, Friedlander J. Cystic fibrosis and pregnancy: a national survey. *Lancet* 1980; ii: 842.

406 Palmer J, Dillon-Baker C, Tecklin JS *et al.* Pregnancy in patients with cystic fibrosis. *Ann Intern Med* 1983; 99: 596.

407 Canny GJ, Corey M, Livingstone RA *et al.* Pregnancy and cystic fibrosis. *Obstet Gynecol* 1991; 77: 850.

408 Edenborough FP, Stableforth DE, Webb AK, MacKenzie WE, Smith DL. Outcome of pregnancy in women with cystic fibrosis. *Thorax* 1995; 50: 170.

409 Hilman BC, Aitken ML, Constantinescu M. Pregnancy in patients with cystic fibrosis. *Clin Obstet Gynecol* 1996; 39: 70.

410 Reisman JJ, Rivington-Law B, Corey M *et al.* Role of conventional physiotherapy in cystic fibrosis. *J Pediatrics* 1988; 113: 632.

411 Pryor JA, Webber BA. An evaluation of the forced expiratory technique as an adjunct to postural drainage. *Physiotherapy* 1979; 65: 304.

412 Webber BA, Hofmeyr JL, Morgan MDL, Hodson ME. Effects of postural drainage incorporating the forced expiration technique on pulmonary function in cystic fibrosis. *Br J Dis Chest* 1986; 80: 353.

413 Thomas J, Cook DJ, Brooks D. Chest physical therapy management of patients with cystic fibrosis. *Am J Respir Crit Care Med* 1995; 151: 846.

414 Webber BA, Hodson ME. Effect of chest physiotherapy on oxygen saturation in patients with cystic fibrosis. *Thorax* 1990; 45: 77.

415 Hofmeyr JL, Webber BA, Hodson ME. Evaluation of positive expiratory pressure as an adjunct to chest physiotherapy in the treatment of cystic fibrosis. *Thorax* 1986; 41: 951.

416 Pryor JA, Webber BA, Hodson ME, Warner JO. The Flutter VRP1 as an adjunct to chest physiotherapy in cystic fibrosis. *Respir Med* 1994; 88: 677.

417 Schoni MH. Autogenic drainage: a modern approach to physiotherapy in cystic fibrosis. *J R Soc Med* 1989; 82 (Suppl 16): 32.

418 Miller S, Hall DO, Clayton CB, Nelson R. Chest physiotherapy in cystic fibrosis: a comparative study of autogenic drainage and the active cycle breathing techniques with postural drainage. *Thorax* 1995; 50: 165.

419 Giles DR, Wagener JS, Accurso FJ, Butlersimon N. Short-term effects of postural drainage on oxygen saturation and sputum recovery in patients with cystic fibrosis. *Chest* 1995; 108: 952.

420 Lindsay CA, Bosso JA. Optimisation of antibiotic therapy in cystic fibrosis patients: pharmacokinetic considerations. *Clin Pharmacokinet* 1993; 24: 496.

421 Rubio TT, Miles MV, Church DA, Echols RM, Pickering LK. Pharmacokinetic studies of ciprofloxacin in children with cystic fibrosis. *Pediatr Pulmonol* 1994; Suppl 10: 251.

422 Cheng K, Smyth RL, Govan JRW *et al.* Spread of β-lactam-resistant *Pseudomonas aeruginosa* in cystic fibrosis clinic. *Lancet* 1996; 348: 639.

423 Weaver LT, Green MR, Nicholson K *et al.* Prognosis in cystic fibrosis treated with continuous flucloxacillin from the neonatal period. *Arch Dis Child* 1994; 70: 84.

424 Beardsmore CS, Thompson JR, Williams A *et al.* Pulmonary function in infants with cystic fibrosis: the effect of antibiotic treatment. *Arch Dis Child* 1994; 71: 133.

425 Touw DJ, Brimicombe RW, Hodson ME, Heijerman HGM, Bakker W. Inhalation of antibiotics in cystic fibrosis. *Eur Respir J* 1996; 8: 1594.

426 Nolan G, McIvor P, Levison H, Fleming PC, Corey M, Gold R. Antibiotic prophylaxis in cystic fibrosis: inhaled cephaloridine as an adjunct to oral cloxacillin. *J Pediatr* 1982; 4: 626.

427 Kun P, Landau LI, Phelan P. Nebulized gentamicin in children and adolescents with cystic fibrosis. *Aust Paediatr J* 1984; 20: 43.

428 MacLusky I, Gold R, Corey M, Levison H. Long-term effects of inhaled tobramycin in patients with cystic fibrosis colonized with *Pseudomonas aeruginosa*. *Pediatr Pulmonol* 1989; 7: 42.

429 Ramsey B, Dorkin HL, Eisenberg JD, Gibson RL, Harwood IR, Kravitz RM. Efficacy of aerosolized tobramycin in patients with cystic fibrosis. *N Engl J Med* 1993; 328: 1740.

430 Ramsey B. *N Engl J Med* 1999.

431 Cassey J, Ford WDA, O'Brien L, Martin AJ. Totally implantable system for venous access in children with cystic fibrosis. *Clin Pediatr* 1988; 27: 91.

432 Morris JB, Occhionreo ME, Gauderer MWL, Stern RC, Doershuk CF. Totally implantable vascular access devices in cystic fibrosis: a four year experience with fifty-eight patients. *J Pediatr* 1990; 117: 82.

433 Ball ABS, Duncan FR, Foster FJ, Davidson TI, Watkins RM, Hodson ME. Long term venous access using a totally implantable drug delivery system in patients with cystic fibrosis and bronchiectasis. *Respir Med* 1989; 83: 429.

434 Yung B, Campbell IA, Elborn JS, Harvey JS, Shale DJ. Totally implantable venous access devices in adult patients with cystic fibrosis. *Respir Med* 1996; 90: 353.

435 Rodgers HC, Liddle K, Nixon SJ, Innes JA, Greening AP. Totally implantable venous access devices in cystic fibrosis: complications and patients' opinions. *Eur Respir J* 1998; 12: 217.

436 Shak S, Capon DJ, Hellmiss R, Marsters SA, Baker CL. Recombinant human DNase I reduces the viscosity of cystic fibrosis sputum. *Proc Natl Acad Sci USA* 1990; 87: 9188.

437 Ramsey BW, Astley SJ, Aitken ML *et al.* Efficacy and safety of short-term administration of aerosolized recombinant human deoxyribonuclease in patients with cystic fibrosis (CF). *Am Rev Respir Dis* 1993; 148: 145.

438 Ranasinha C, Assoufi B, Christiansen D *et al.* Efficacy and safety of short-term administration of aerosolised recombinant human DNase I in adults with stable stage cystic fibrosis. *Lancet* 1993; 342: 199.

439 Fuchs HJ, Borowitz DS, Christiansen DH *et al.* Effect of aerosolized recombinant human DNase on exacerbations of respiratory symptoms and pulmonary function in patients with cystic fibrosis. *N Engl J Med* 1994; 331: 637.

440 Wilmott RW, Amin RS, Colin AA *et al.* Aerosolized recombinant human DNase in hospitalized cystic fibrosis patients with acute pulmonary exacerbations. *Am J Respir Crit Care Med* 1996; 153: 1914.

441 McCoy K, Hamilton S, Johnson C. Effects of 12-week administration of dornase alfa in patients with advanced cystic fibrosis lung disease. *Chest* 1996; 110: 889.

442 Davies J, Trindade M-T, Wallis C, Rosenthal M, Crawford O, Bush A. Retrospective review of the effects of DNase in children with cystic fibrosis. *Pediatr Pulmonol* 1997; 23: 243.

443 Milla CE. Long term effects of aerosolised rhDNase on pulmonary disease progression in patients with cystic fibrosis patients. *Thorax* 1998; 53: 1014.

444 Böllert FGE, Paton JY, Marshall TG, Calvert J, Greening AP, Innes JA. (on behalf of the Scottish Cystic Fibrosis Group). Recombinant DNase in cystic fibrosis: a protocol for targeted introduction through n-of-1 trials. *Eur Respir J* 1999; 13: 107.

445 Robson M, Abbott J, Webb K *et al.* A cost description of an adult CF unit and cost

analyses of different categories of patients. *Thorax* 1992; 47: 684.

446 Auerbach HS, Williams M, Kirkpatrick JA, Colten HR. Alternate day prednisone reduces morbidity and improves pulmonary function in cystic fibrosis. *Lancet* 1985; ii: 686.

447 Rosenstein BJ, Eigen H. Risks of alternate day prednisone in patients with cystic fibrosis. *Pediatrics* 1991; 87: 245.

448 Eigen H, Rosenstein BJ, Fitzsimmons S, Schidlow DV. A multicenter study of alternate-day prednisone therapy in patients with cystic fibrosis. *J Pediatr* 1995; 126: 515.

449 Greally P, Hussain MJ, Vergani D, Price JF. Interleukin-1α, soluble interleukin-2 receptor, and IgG concentrations in cystic fibrosis treated with prednisolone. *Arch Dis Child* 1994; 71: 35.

450 van Haren EHJ, Lammers JWJ, Festen J, Heijerman HGM, Groot CAR, van Herwaarden CLA. The effects of the inhaled corticosteroid budesonide on lung function and bronchial hyperresponsiveness in adult patients with cystic fibrosis. *Respir Med* 1995; 89: 209.

451 Nikolaizik WH, Schoni MH. Pilot study to assess the effect of inhaled corticosteroids on lung function in patients with cystic fibrosis. *J Pediatr* 1996; 128: 271.

452 Balfour-Lynn IM, Klein NJ, Dinwiddie R. Randomised controlled trial of inhaled corticosteroids (fluticasone propionate) in cystic fibrosis. *Arch Dis Child* 1997; 77: 124.

453 Konstan MW, Vargo KM, Davis PB. Ibuprofen attenuates the inflammatory response to *Pseudomonas aeruginosa* in a rat model of chronic pulmonary infection: implications for anti-inflammatory therapy in cystic fibrosis. *Am Rev Respir Dis* 1990; 141: 186.

454 Konstan MW, Walenga RW, Hilliard KA, Hilliard JB. Leukotriene B₄ markedly elevated in the epithelial lining fluid of patients with cystic fibrosis. *Am Rev Respir Dis* 1993; 143: 896.

455 Konstan MW, Hoppel CL, Chai B, Davis PB. Ibuprofen in children with cystic fibrosis: pharmacokinetics and adverse effects. *J Pediatr* 1991; 118: 956.

456 Konstan MW, Byard PJ, Hoppel CL, Davis PB. Effect of high-dose ibuprofen in patients with cystic fibrosis. *N Engl J Med* 1995; 332: 848.

457 McElvaney NG, Hubbard RC, Birrer P *et al.* Aerosol α₁-antitrypsin treatment for cystic fibrosis. *Lancet* 1991; 337: 392.

458 McElvaney NG, Nakamura H, Birrer P *et al.* Modulation of airway inflammation in cystic fibrosis: *in vivo* suppression of interleukin-8 levels on the respiratory epithelial surface by aerosolization of recombinant secretory leukoprotease inhibitor. *J Clin Invest* 1992; 90: 1296.

459 McElvaney NG, Doujaiji B, Moan MJ, Burnham MR, Wu MC, Crystal RG. Pharmacokinetics of recombinant secretory leukoprotease inhibitor aerosolized to normals and individuals with cystic fibrosis. *Am Rev Respir Dis* 1993; 148: 1056.

460 Howard M, Frizzell RA, Bedwell DM. Aminoglycoside antibiotics restore CFTR function by overcoming premature stop mutations. *Nature Med* 1996; 2: 467.

461 Brown CR, Hong-Brown LQ, Welch WJ. Correcting temperature-sensitive protein folding defects. *J Clin Invest* 1997; 99: 1432.

462 Zeitlin PL, Rubenstein RC. Phenylbutyrate therapy for cystic fibrosis. *Pediatr Pulmonol* 1997; Suppl 14: 132.

463 Kelly TJ, Thomas K, Milgram LJ, Drumm ML. *In vivo* activation of the cystic fibrosis transmembrane conductance regulator mutant deltaF508 in murine nasal epithelium. *Proc Natl Acad Sci USA* 1997; 94: 2604.

464 Illek B, Fischer H, Santos G, Widdicombe JH, Machen TE, Reenstra WW. cAMP-independent activation of CFTR Cl channels by the tyrosine kinase inhibitor genistein. *Am J Physiol* 1995; 268: C886.

465 Yang IC, Cheng TH, Wang F, Price EM, Hwang TC. Modulation of CFTR chloride channels by calyculin A and genistein. *Am J Physiol* 1997; 272: C142.

466 Guay-Broder C, Jacobson KA, Barnoy S *et al.* A1 receptor antagonist 8-cyclopentyl-1,3-dipropylxanthine selectively activates chloride efflux from human epithelial and mouse fibroblast cell lines expressing the cystic fibrosis transmembrane regulator delta F508 mutation. *Biochemistry* 1995; 34: 9079.

467 Wilson JM. Gene therapy for cystic fibrosis: challenges and future directions. *J Clin Invest* 1995; 96: 2547.

468 St George JA, Pennington SE, Kaplan JM *et al.* Biological response of nonhuman primates to long-term repeated lung exposure to Ad2/CFTR-2. *Gene Ther* 1996; 3: 103.

469 Yang Y, Qin L, Ertl HCJ, Wilson JM. Cellular and humoral immune responses to viral antigens create barriers to lung-directed gene therapy with recombinant adenoviruses. *J Virol* 1995; 69: 2004.

470 Yei S, Mittereder N, Tang K, O'Sullivan C, Trapnell B. Adenovirus-mediated gene transfer for cystic fibrosis: quantitative evaluation of repeated *in vivo* vector administration to the lung. *Gene Ther* 1994; 1: 192.

471 Flotte TR, Afione SA, Conrad C *et al.* Stable *in vivo* expression of the cystic fibrosis transmembrane conductance regulator with an adeno-associated virus vector. *Proc Natl Acad Sci USA* 1993; 90: 10613.

472 Conrad CK, Allen SS, Afione SA *et al.* Safety of single-dose administration of an adeno-associated virus (AAV)-CFTR vector in the primate lung. *Gene Ther* 1996; 3: 658.

473 Felgner PL, Gadek TR, Holm M *et al.* Lipofection: a highly efficient, lipid-mediated DNA-transfection procedure. *Proc Natl Acad Sci USA* 1987; 84: 7413.

474 Gao X, Huang L. Cationic liposome-mediated gene transfer. *Gene Ther* 1995; 2: 710.

475 Brigham KL, Meyrick B, Christman B, Magnuson M, King G, Barry LC. *In vivo* transfection of murine lungs with a functioning prokaryotic gene using a liposome vehicle. *Am J Med Sci* 1989; 298: 278.

476 Yoshimura K, Rosenfeld MA, Nakanura H *et al.* Expression of the human cystic fibrosis transmembrane conductance regulator gene in the mouse lung after *in vivo* intratracheal plasmid-mediated gene transfer. *Nucleic Acids Res* 1992; 20: 3233.

477 Alton EWFW, Middleton PG, Caplen NJ *et al.* Non-invasive liposome-mediated gene delivery can correct the ion transport defect in cystic fibrosis mutant mice. *Nature Genet* 1993; 5: 135.

478 Hyde SC, Gill DR, Higgins CF *et al.* Correction of the ion-transport defect in cystic-fibrosis transgenic mice by gene-therapy. *Nature* 1993; 362: 250.

479 Crystal RG, McElvaney NG, Rosenfeld MA *et al.* Administration of an adenovirus containing human CFTR cDNA to the respiratory tract of individuals with cystic fibrosis. *Nature Genet* 1994; 8: 42.

480 Knowles MR, Hohneker KW, Zhaoqing Z *et al.* A controlled study of adenovirus-vector-mediated gene transfer in the nasal epithelium of patients with cystic fibrosis. *N Engl J Med* 1995; 333: 823.

481 Zabner J, Ramsey BW, Meeker DP *et al.* Repeat administration of an adenovirus vector encoding cystic fibrosis transmembrane conductance regulator to the nasal epithelium of patients with cystic fibrosis. *J Clin Invest* 1996; 97: 1504.

482 Bellon G, Michel-Calemard L, Thouvenot D *et al.* Aerosol administration of a recombinant adenovirus expressing CFTR to cystic fibrosis patients: a phase I clinical trial. *Hum Gene Ther* 1997; 8: 15.

483 Caplen NJ, Alton EWFW, Middleton PG *et al.* Liposome-mediated *CFTR* gene transfer to the nasal epithelium of patients with cystic fibrosis. *Nature Med* 1995; 1: 39.

484 Gill DR, Southern KW, Mofford KA *et al.* A placebo-controlled study of liposome-mediated gene transfer to the nasal epithelium of patients with cystic fibrosis. *Gene Ther* 1997; 4: 199.

485 Porteous DJ, Dorin JR, McLachlan G *et al.* Evidence for the safety and efficacy of DOTAP cationic liposome mediated *CFTR* gene transfer to the nasal epithelium of patients with cystic fibrosis. *Gene Ther* 1997; 4: 210.

486 Wagner JA, Reynolds T, Moran ML *et al.* Efficient and persistent gene transfer of AAV-CFTR in maxillary sinus. *Lancet* 1998; 351: 1702.

487 Yang Y, Nunes FA, Berencsi K, Gonczol E, Engelhardt JF, Wilson JM. Inactivation of *E2a* in recombinant adenoviruses improves the prospect for gene therapy in cystic fibrosis. *Nature Genet* 1994; 7: 362.

488 Zabner J, Petersen DM, Puga AP *et al.* Safety and efficacy of repetitive adenovirus-mediated transfer of CFTR cDNA to airway epithelia of primates and cotton rats. *Nature Genet* 1994; 6: 75.

489 Kaplan JM, St George JA, Pennington SE *et al.* Humoral and cellular immune responses of nonhuman primates to long-term repeated lung exposure to Ad2/CFTR-2. *Gene Ther* 1996; 3: 117.

490 Lee ER, Marshall J, Siegel CS *et al.* Detailed analysis of structures and formulations of cationic lipids for efficient gene transfer to the lung. *Hum Gene Ther* 1996; 7: 1701.

491 Davis PB. Saturday's children. *Am J Respir Crit Care Med* 1995; 152: 1.

492 Shepherd SL, Hovell MF, Harwood IR *et al.* A comparative study of the psychosocial assets of adults with cystic fibrosis and their healthy peers.

493 Blair C, Cull A, Freeman CP. Psychosocial functioning of young adults with cystic fibrosis and their families. *Thorax* 1994; 49: 798.

494 Congleton J, Hodson ME, Duncan-Skingle F. Quality of life in adults with cystic fibrosis. *Thorax* 1996; 51: 936.

495 Abbott J, Dodd M, Webb AK. Health perceptions and treatment adherence in adults with cystic fibrosis. *Thorax* 1996; 51: 1233.

31

PULMONARY FIBROSIS

ANTHONY SEATON

Pulmonary fibrosis is the end-result of a multiplicity of pathological processes, from infections to autoimmune diseases. Many of these are of unknown aetiology but have characteristic features that allow them to be classified as distinct disease entities. Among them is one that typically occurs in older males, is slowly progressive, poorly responsive to therapy and has well-defined clinical, radiological, pathological and functional characteristics, known as idiopathic pulmonary fibrosis or cryptogenic fibrosing alveolitis. The latter term, coined by Scadding [1], is probably to be preferred as it emphasizes the inflammatory reaction in the alveoli that precedes the fibrosis. The danger implicit in either term is that all patients with pulmonary fibrosis are labelled 'of unknown aetiology' and the doctor forgets that all diseases must have a cause that is worth seeking. As with cardiac failure, the term 'pulmonary fibrosis' describes a clinical end-point of many different pathological processes, and the adjective 'idiopathic' or 'cryptogenic' should only be applied after appropriate thought.

In fact, the first description of the idiopathic condition concerned a rather atypical and acutely progressive variant, which still sometimes goes by the names of the original authors, the Hamman–Rich syndrome. They described five patients with progressive dyspnoea, following a fulminant course and leading to death with cor pulmonale or respiratory failure within 6 months [2,3]. It subsequently became apparent that this form of the disease was uncommon and that the majority of patients pursue a more chronic course lasting for several years [4–6].

Cryptogenic fibrosing alveolitis is a progressive fibrosing inflammatory disease of the lung of unknown aetiology. Most patients present with dyspnoea, although some are detected at an asymptomatic stage by the coincidental finding of clubbing, crepitations or radiological changes. Bilateral pulmonary crepitations are almost always audible and finger clubbing is often present. In the author's experience, very marked clubbing denotes a more chronic process. Lung function testing shows a restrictive defect with diminished gas transfer, and inflammation and fibrosis are evident distal to the terminal bronchioles on lung biopsy. Similar clinical, radiological and pathological findings may occur in pulmonary fibrosis associated with connective tissue diseases (see Chapter 53), asbestosis (see Chapter 54) and certain drugs (see Chapter 55).

Aetiology

By definition, cryptogenic fibrosing alveolitis is of unknown aetiology. However, this should not close the clinician's mind, since the disease must have some cause or causes, be they genetic or environmental. As with most diseases it is likely that there will eventually prove to be several contributing environmental causes operating in someone who is genetically susceptible. There are now some clues relevant to both factors.

The evidence for a genetic cause is not strong, most cases occurring quite sporadically. However, many familial cases have been described [7–11], including the finding of subclinical disease in relatives of patients [12]. Occasionally the occurrence of the condition in monozygotic twins separated from birth has suggested a genetic influence [10,13]. When the condition occurs in families it is probably transmitted as an autosomal dominant with incomplete penetrance. No consistent association with human leucocyte antigen (HLA)-A or HLA-B foci has been found [14–16], although one study has recorded an increased frequency of the B-cell alloantigen HLA-DR2 in patients (65%) compared with controls (26%) [17]. Studies of gene loci in patients with familial disease have also been confusing, in some subjects pointing to loci on chromosome 14 and in others to chromosome 6 [11,18]. Evidence from animal studies and from studies of human responses to fibrogenic stimuli due to drugs suggests that individuals differ on a genetic basis in their lung fibrogenic responses, although it is likely that these differences are mediated by complex mechanisms that probably differ from person to person. They presumably involve the genotypic control of HLA type or of any one or more of the large number of cytokines and receptors involved in the processes between the environmental stimulus and the deposition of collagen [19,20].

The more likely primary causes in most cases are environmental. This is supported by the considerable similarities between the cryptogenic disease and pulmonary fibrosis caused by asbestos and cytotoxic drugs, by the increasing evidence that the condition is becoming more prevalent and by the differences in trends in different countries, evidence not wholly explained by changes in diagnostic preferences [21–23]. It has been suggested that there is an association with infection by Epstein–Barr virus, although studies of viral genes have shown markedly different frequencies [24,25]. Nevertheless, patients not infrequently give a history suggestive of viral infection prior to the development of the disease [26]. Diffuse fibrosis has also followed infection by *Mycoplasma* [27], and a study in rats has suggested that adenovirus gene products in type II alveolar cells may be capable of promoting type I collagen formation [28].

Infectious causes aside, a case–control study has suggested that in up to about 20% of patients with the disease, exposure to wood or metal dust at work may have been an aetiological factor [29]; a recent British study of 588 patients has shown 47% to have had a history of a dusty occupation [30]. Recent work suggesting that the toxic effects of the ultra-fine fraction of particulate air pollution may lie in the transition metals on the particle surface (see Chapter 11) points towards what may be an interesting line of future research in this area [31]. Further evidence for an environmental factor comes from another case–control study in which it has been shown that cigarette smoking is a risk factor [32]. Another important clue to the aetiology is the occurrence of pulmonary fibrosis in rheumatoid and other collagen diseases. In the absence of the clinical manifestations of these diseases, rheumatoid factor and antinuclear factor are found in a proportion of patients with cryptogenic fibrosing alveolitis, suggesting a spectrum of response to whatever it is that causes these diseases. Again, the association of collagen diseases with quartz exposure [33] (see Chapter 54) serves as a reminder that these may also have environmental causes.

Epidemiology

Cryptogenic fibrosing alveolitis is a disease affecting males rather more frequently than females, the median age at diagnosis being in the seventh decade. However it may occur in either sex at any age. The prevalence has been estimated, using somewhat different methods, to be about 6 per 100000 in England and Wales and 20 per 100000 in the USA [34,35]. It is the cause of some 2000 deaths annually in the UK and 10000 annually in the USA. It appears to be becoming a more frequent cause of death in the UK, Australia and Canada, and this may reflect a real rise in incidence as well as greater diagnostic awareness [21,23]. It seems to show no racial preference and is diagnosed in developing as well as developed countries [36].

Pathology

In many patients with features suggesting a diagnosis of cryptogenic fibrosing alveolitis, a lung biopsy is carried out to provide both diagnostic and prognostic information prior to the initiation of therapy. Transbronchial lung biopsy is not suitable for establishing this diagnosis and open, trephine or, most frequently nowadays, thoracoscopic lung biopsy should be employed to obtain satisfactory tissue specimens [37–41]. There are two principal features of the disease identifiable on the biopsy: (i) cellular thickening of the alveolar walls with a tendency to fibrosis and (ii) the presence of large mononuclear cells within the alveolar spaces. The more prominent the second feature and the thinner the alveolar walls, the better the response to corticosteroid drugs [5,39,42]. In early disease, proliferation of type II alveolar epithelial cells and loss of type I cells may be seen [43]. The intra-alveolar mononuclear cells, once thought to be type II alveolar cells, are now known on the basis of ultrastructural and cytochemical studies to be predominantly alveolar macrophages [44–48]. Other cells, including lymphocytes, eosinophils, neutrophils and plasma cells, may be seen both in the interstitium and the alveoli. At an early phase, there may be fibrinous exudate in the alveoli with hyaline membrane formation. In the later stages, the lung architecture is distorted by fibrosis and there may be hyperplasia of the bronchiolar epithelium to line the residual airspaces. Interestingly, the collagen content of the lung does not differ from that found in controls but the ratio of type I to type III collagen is increased from 2:1 in controls to 4:1 in fibrosing alveolitis, reflecting increased production of type I collagen by the fibroblasts [49,50]. Release of fibronectin and alveolar macrophage-derived growth factor is not suppressed by corticosteroid therapy in these patients, which may explain the relatively poor response to such therapy [51]. Haemosiderosis and squamous metaplasia of bronchiolar and alveolar epithelium may occur [52,53], and occasionally deposits of bone may be found [54,55]. B-lymphocyte follicles with occasional germinal centres and containing helper T cells may be seen and indicate a local B-lymphoid immune response [56]. Occasionally when a particular cell type predominates, for example the lymphocyte, giant cell or plasma cell, the terms lymphocytic, giant cell or plasma cell interstitial pneumonia are used, although this differentiation is probably not clinically useful since all are likely to progress to end-stage fibrosis.

Livingstone and colleagues [57] divided their cases

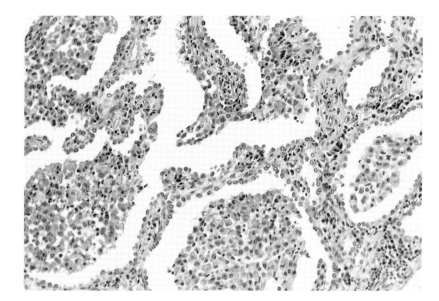

Fig. 31.1 Open lung biopsy from patient with a diffuse pneumonitis on radiography showing thickened alveolar walls lined by hyperplastic type II cells. The alveoli are filled with a mixture of macrophages and desquamated type II cells. This is the pattern of 'desquamative interstitial pneumonitis' (haematoxylin & eosin × 150).

pathologically into five grades according to the amount of disruption of lung architecture. Grade I is the mildest stage, in which change is confined to the alveolar walls, the alveolar spaces being empty. In grade II, the architecture of the lung is still intact, although the alveolar space is now filled with fluid or cellular exudate. In grade III, the alveolar architecture is becoming blurred and perhaps lost altogether, though bronchioles may still be recognized. Elastic fibre staining shows that the alveolar pattern is no longer intact. In grade IV, the normal lung structure is distorted by fibrosis, although remnants of bronchiolar epithelium and muscle may still be recognized. In grade V, the lung is converted to cystic spaces varying in diameter up to 1 cm or more. Grades IV and V commonly coexist and correlate with the presence of honeycombing on the chest radiograph, whereas grades I and II more often show

fine and coarse mottling on the chest film and a ground-glass appearance on high-resolution CT (HRCT).

The terms 'usual' and 'desquamative' interstitial pneumonitis have been used by pathologists to describe discrete pathological and clinical entities [6,58,59]. Most workers now consider 'desquamative' change to indicate the early stage of the disease with active alveolitis and minimal fibrosis (Fig. 31.1) and 'usual' change to indicate the late stage of the disease when fibrosis is established and alveolitis is minimal (Fig. 31.2) [1,60,61].

Injection studies have shown a dramatic increase in bronchial arteries with numerous precapillary bronchopulmonary anastomoses. In contrast, pulmonary angiograms show the peripheral pruning characteristic of pulmonary hypertension [62]. Pulmonary muscular hyperplasia may occur in some patients, resulting in

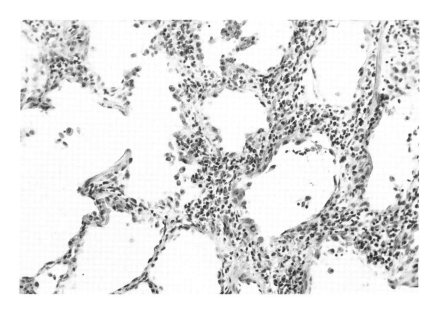

Fig. 31.2 Open lung biopsy from patient with a familial type of interstitial lung disease showing expanded alveolar walls containing an interstitial infiltrate of chronic inflammatory cells and some fibrosis. A few hyperplastic alveolar lining cells are visible. This is the pattern of 'usual interstitial pneumonitis' (haematoxylin & eosin × 150).

pathological descriptions of 'bronchiolar emphysema' or 'muscular cirrhosis of the lung' [63–65]. Most such examples are probably variants of fibrosing alveolitis and radiologically honeycombing is common.

Pathogenesis

The pathogenesis of cryptogenic fibrosing alveolitis is not understood. This statement is intended to prevent the reader feeling discouraged when confronted by all the trees and wondering where the wood is. After a promising start, most reviews of the subject finish as an enumeration of cytokines that may or may not be important, leaving the reader somewhat bewildered, as one might perhaps feel from trying to appreciate a symphony by studying small collections of notes played by individual instruments.

It may be helpful to think of the condition as an aberrant defensive reaction at the alveolar level, these defences having evolved specifically to deal with invading airborne microorganisms. The unknown initial stimulus, candidates for which have been discussed above, appears to initiate an uncontrolled inflammatory reaction that involves recruitment of macrophages, neutrophils and smaller numbers of other cells including lymphocytes, eosinophils and mast cells. This inflammatory reaction leads in turn to 'healing' by inappropriate alveolar wall fibrosis and destruction of the normal alveolar wall of type I and endothelial cells, with proliferation of type II cells, the normal progenitors of the type I cell. It is noteworthy that emphysema, which often accompanies fibrosis in sarcoidosis, allergic alveolitis and mineral pneumoconioses, is not a common feature of the cryptogenic disease but that late development of carcinoma is—this is the wood.

Whatever triggers the process, mystery number one, seems to be responsible for attracting the greatly increased numbers of alveolar macrophages, which in turn attract other inflammatory cells, leading to the alveolar wall damage. Mystery number two is why this process continues and is not checked, as it is in almost all infective alveolar inflammatory conditions. The answer to this is likely to be that the triggering stimulus remains *in situ*, perhaps as a consequence of virus-induced genetic change in epithelial or endothelial cells. This would be analogous to the pathogenesis of asbestosis, where the fibres remain embedded at alveolar level and continue to stimulate macrophage ingress, and consistent with bleomycin-induced fibrosis that generally arrests when the drug is stopped. However, another possibility is that the lungs in some people lose their ability to downregulate the inflammatory response, making them unable to control the process once initiated. This would be consistent with the studies of familial fibrosis and with the observation that the disease occurs only in relatively few of those people treated with bleomycin. It is possible, indeed likely, that

both mechanisms may operate together in those unfortunate enough to develop the disease.

Research intended to elucidate the pathogenetic mechanisms has studied both these possibilities. Less effort has been expended on what at first sight might appear more fundamental, the initial triggering factors and possible alterations in alveolar cells. The majority of the effort seems to have been devoted, perhaps understandably, to a search for cytokines that may be present to excess and therefore possibly amenable to drug therapy [66,67]. With respect to the former, the most promising research relates to alteration of cultured rat alveolar cells by adenovirus infection, leading to increased type I collagen production [28]. Viral alteration of the genetic material of alveolar cells could lead not only to uncontrolled fibrosis but also to the development of carcinoma, which is a feature of the condition.

The aspect of pathogenesis that has attracted most attention is the link between inflammatory cells, once recruited, and the deposition of fibrosis. Studies have concentrated on the demonstration of the actions of an increasingly large number of cytokines and cell receptors able to stimulate fibrogenesis, in the hope that an understanding of these mechanisms may lead to the development of drugs able to block them. Of the cytokines, those currently attracting most interest are transforming growth factor (TGF)-β_1 and tumour necrosis factor (TNF)-α [68]. TGF-β_1 has been shown to be able to cause expression of the gene for procollagen in fibroblasts, increase protein synthesis and inhibit breakdown of collagen. TNF-α has also been shown to cause increased collagen formation and is released in increased amounts from macrophages of patients with fibrosing alveolitis. In the case of both cytokines, there is experimental evidence that their fibrogenic action may be inhibited by antibodies, thus raising hopes of possible future therapeutic options [69,70]. Other cytokines that may play a part in fibrogenesis include platelet-derived growth factor and insulin growth factor 1. Endothelin 1, derived from capillary endothelial cells, may have a similar effect [71]. Finally, there is increasing interest in the presence of coagulation activity in the lung, based on the production by alveolar macrophages of thromboplastin and factor VII [72,73]. The very number of substances thought to be of interest in the genesis of lung fibrosis, and the fact that all are inflammatory cell products normally available and controlled by homeostatic mechanisms, indicate the difficulties that still lie ahead of those who hope to discover a curative treatment.

To pursue the symphonic analogy, the cytokines are the notes while the instruments are the inflammatory cells. Typically, in active cryptogenic fibrosing alveolitis, the total number of cells obtained at lavage is increased, with significant increases in percentages of neutrophils and eosinophils and occasionally a small increase in percentage of lymphocytes. Although the macrophage percent-

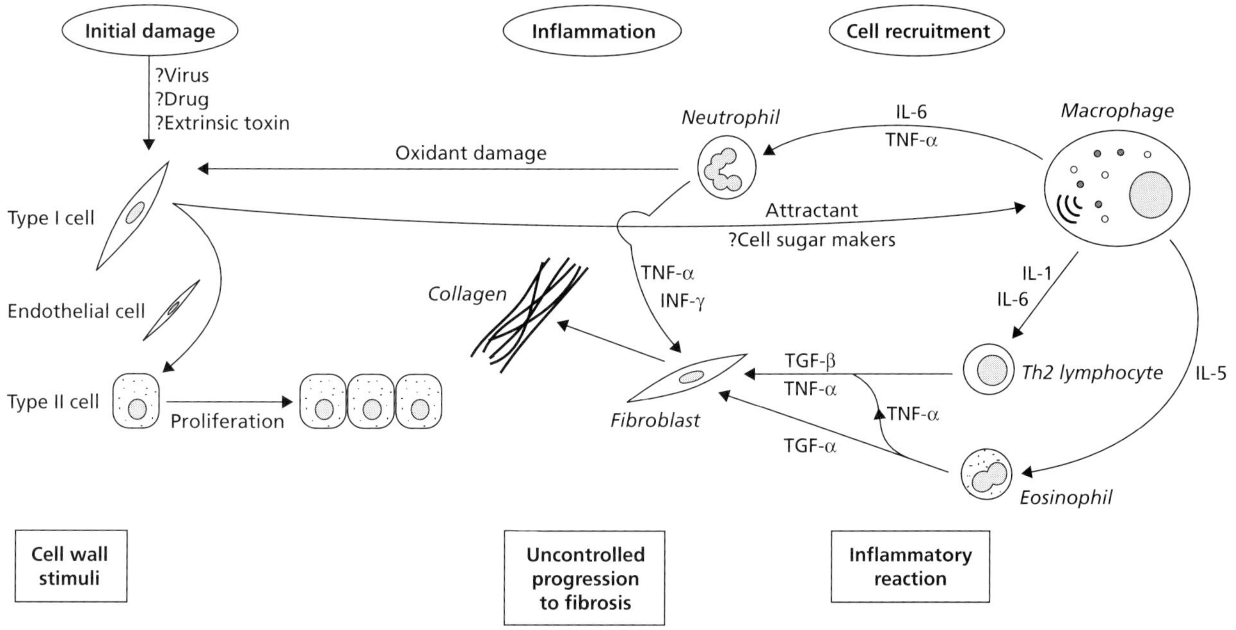

Fig. 31.3 An outline scheme for the pathogenesis of cryptogenic fibrosing alveolitis. The initial stimulus to inflammation, acting through macrophage recruitment, and the reasons for uncontrolled progression to fibrosis are unknown.

age is usually decreased, the absolute numbers of macrophages are much increased [74–76]. A scheme, necessarily simplified, of some of the roles of each cell type in the pathogenesis of the disease is discussed below (Fig. 31.3).

Alveolar macrophages

Not only are the alveolar macrophages increased in numbers in cryptogenic fibrosing alveolitis but the macrophages are activated, as demonstrated by increased surface expression of markers [77,78]. They have been shown to secrete a large number of cytokines, including interleukin (IL)-1, IL-6 and IL-12, interferon (IFN)-γ, granulocyte–macrophage colony-stimulating factor (GM-CSF), TGF-β and TNF. Mechanisms promoted by these substances are able between them to explain attraction and activation of further macrophages, neutrophils and lymphocytes [79–83]. However these mechanisms are all designed for anti-infection purposes and why they go awry in pulmonary fibrosis remains unknown.

B lymphocytes

Although the percentage of lung B lymphocytes is not usually increased in cryptogenic fibrosing alveolitis, the absolute number is increased because the total number of lymphocytes is increased several-fold. B-lymphocytic fol-

licles with germinal centres have been identified in lung tissue from patients with cryptogenic fibrosing alveolitis [56] and the number of B lymphocytes producing immunoglobulin, particularly IgG, is increased [84]. In keeping with these observations, IgG levels in bronchoalveolar lavage (BAL) fluid of fibrosing alveolitis patients are increased, suggesting that there is active local production of immunoglobulins [85,86]. Coupled with the finding of immune complexes in BAL fluid, this suggests that immunoglobulins are produced locally in the lung and combine with antigens to form complexes that may subsequently be demonstrated both in the lung and in circulating blood. The antigen or antigens against which the antibodies are directed have not been identified but the observation that blood lymphocytes from patients with fibrosing alveolitis release lymphokines on exposure to type I collagen suggests one possible antigenic site in the alveolar wall [87].

T lymphocytes

The percentage of T lymphocytes is not increased in BAL fluid of patients with cryptogenic fibrosing alveolitis but the absolute numbers are, under the control of macrophage-derived cytokines including IL-6 and IL-12. There is a suggestion that a shift from the Th1 subtype (which produces IFN-γ, a cytokine that suppresses fibroblast proliferation and collagen synthesis) towards the Th2 subtype (which produces IL-4 and IL-5, both of which have been implicated in fibrogenesis) may be relevant to the production of fibrous tissue [88]. IL-5 is an eosinophil chemoattractant, and the presence of eosinophils in pulmonary fibrosis is an indicator of poor prognosis.

Neutrophils

As already noted, the percentage and total number of neutrophils have been shown to be increased in BAL fluid of patients with fibrosing alveolitis, though not all studies are consistent in this respect [74–76]. However, tissue concentrations of these cells and evidence of their elastase activity are considerably increased from normal [89]. Their presence is probably a response to macrophage-derived attractants, including IL-6, IL-8, GM-CSF and TNF-α. When activated, they can perpetuate the inflammatory response by producing IL-1, IL-8, IFN-γ and TNF-α themselves. These neutrophils are cytotoxic to normal lung parenchymal cells and their cytotoxic properties are related to the release of reactive oxidant species [90,91]. This is consistent with the demonstration of myeloperoxidase in BAL fluid of patients with the disease [92]. In addition, one neutrophil protease, a collagenase, has been found in lavage fluids from patients with the disease and shown to be cytolytic to normal lung explants [93,94]. The damage to alveolar walls may therefore be secondary to release of reactive oxidant species and proteases from neutrophils. The identification of fibronectin fragments in lavage fluid from patients with cryptogenic fibrosing alveolitis suggests that fibronectin degradation may also be occurring *in vivo* [95].

Eosinophils

Eosinophils are often increased in percentage and total numbers in BAL fluid of patients with cryptogenic fibrosing alveolitis, attracted by macrophage-derived cytokines particularly IL-6. They may damage normal lung parenchymal cells by release of cytokines, including TGF-α and TNF-α, and also release a collagenase capable of cleaving types I and III collagen [94,96,97]. Their presence is generally taken to indicate a poor response to treatment.

Conclusion

The pathogenesis of cryptogenic fibrosing alveolitis appears to hinge around activation of alveolar macrophages. The triggers of this reaction are unknown but could be infections, environmental pollutants or both. The activated macrophages produce chemotactic factors leading to accumulation of increased numbers of neutrophils and eosinophils which, by the generation of reactive oxidant species and proteases, produce local lung damage. The generation of cytokines promoting fibrosis by these cells and by lymphocytes promotes the collagenous scarring found in association with the lung tissue destruction characteristic of this disease. The condition is characterized by a failure of control mechanisms that would normally be expected to halt the repair process, and this may have a partly genetic aetiology.

Clinical features

Cryptogenic fibrosing alveolitis [1,3,30,53,57,98] is approximately twice as common in males and most commonly presents in older patients, the mean age in the largest survey reported being 67 years [30]. It commences in some 90% of patients with progressive dyspnoea on exertion. A non-productive cough is present in 75% at presentation. About 5% of patients are discovered at an asymptomatic stage by an incidental chest film or by a doctor hearing crepitations at the bases. The subacute, rapidly progressive type of the disease originally described by Hamman and Rich is much less common than the more slowly progressive chronic form of the disease, and may declare itself as an illness with systemic symptoms such as fever, weight loss, fatigue, myalgia and arthralgia

Finger clubbing is found in about half the patients, while auscultation of the chest reveals bilateral, gravity-dependent, inspiratory crepitations. With progression of disease, cyanosis becomes a feature and evidence of pulmonary hypertension may be found. In some patients, signs of connective tissue disease, such as rheumatoid arthritis, systemic lupus erythematosus or scleroderma, may coexist (see Chapter 53). Subgroups of patients with associated digital vasculitis or peripheral neuropathy have also been described [99,100], and rare associations with chronic active hepatitis and autoimmune haemolytic anaemia have been reported [101]. Hypertrophic pulmonary osteoarthropathy and spontaneous pneumothorax may occasionally occur [102,103]. Bronchogenic carcinoma is 14 times more common in patients with cryptogenic fibrosing alveolitis than in a control population [104]. In one series, carcinoma showed the usual distribution of histological types and was found in 13% of 155 patients followed to death [104].

The course of the disease is very variable. It ranges from an acute, rapidly progressive condition that may progress to death within months to a very slowly progressive or even apparently arrested pulmonary fibrosis. Most patients fall between these extremes and show gradual deterioration over 3 or 4 years. It is not uncommon in such circumstances to find that chest films taken several years before symptoms developed show early changes of fibrosis. In general, the younger the patient and the more acute the history, the more likely is the condition to respond to treatment. However, in an initial report of the large UK study 47% of patients had died within 2–4 years of enrolment, indicating a poor overall prognosis with or without treatment [30].

Radiology

Chest radiography

In the early stages the chest film can be normal despite the presence of dyspnoea. In one study of lung biopsies in breathless patients, 26% of 47 with a 'desquamative' histological picture had normal films compared with only 7% of 68 with the 'usual' type of alveolitis [105]. In the subacute type of disease, the initial chest radiograph may resemble bronchopneumonia with extensive patchy shadows, confluent in places, and more extensive in the lower zones (Fig. 31.4). In the commoner chronic type, mottling may give rise to a ground-glass appearance, although more often individual shadows up to 2mm in diameter may be identified and these may later increase in size (Fig. 31.5). In the majority of patients the shadowing is predominantly in the lower zones. As the shadowing coarsens, translucencies up to 3mm in diameter may appear, and this may finally develop into classical honeycomb lung (Fig. 31.6). Larger translucencies may also

occur and, in the later stages of the disease, emphysematous bullae and irregular streaky fibrosis may be seen [106]. Shrinkage of the lungs occurs, with progressive elevation of the diaphragms. In the presence of cor pulmonale the proximal pulmonary artery shadows increase in diameter.

When the disease is advanced, bronchograms may show shrinkage of the lung and bronchial dilatation. In the late stages, the distortion of lung architecture is reflected in bronchiolectasis and bronchial distortion [57]. In one reported case, diffuse dense mottled opacities seen on the chest film proved to be deposits of bone, some containing marrow cavities [55].

Computed tomography

Because of the risks associated with lung biopsy and the generally poor response to treatment, non-invasive diagnostic methods find favour with most clinicians, especially in older patients. The dilemma regarding the decision to investigate has been made less taxing by the

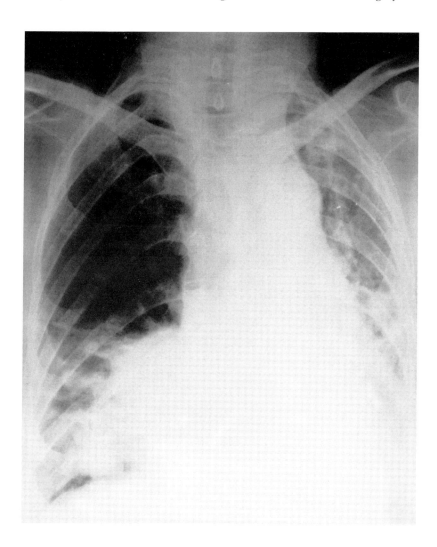

Fig. 31.4 Chest film of a female with a relatively rapid onset of pulmonary fibrosis. The patient presented with increasing breathlessness over 9 months. After 2 months of treatment with corticosteroids, the left lung remained unchanged but much clearing had occurred in the right lower zone.

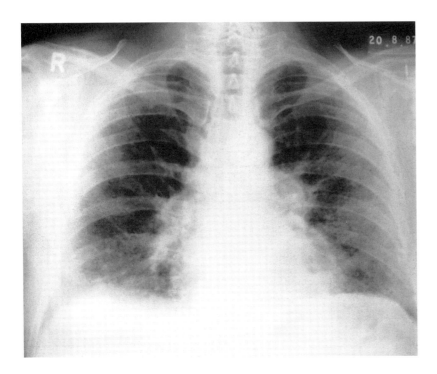

Fig. 31.5 Chest film of a patient with early fibrosing alveolitis showing diffuse, predominantly lower zone, micronodular infiltrates. This patient made a good response to corticosteroids.

advent of HRCT [107,108]. The features found on HRCT reflect histopathology quite well [109] and three types of shadow may be recognized. Early, active inflammatory disease is characterized by a ground-glass appearance,

Fig. 31.6 Extensive honeycomb change in a patient with slowly progressing, irreversible fibrosis.

with hazy attenuation of the normal lung parenchyma but preservation of vascular shadows (Fig. 31.7). Usually such appearances coexist with areas of more mature fibrosis in the same film, and if biopsy is to be carried out it should be directed at an area of ground-glass opacity. As fibrous tissue is laid down, the appearances are of thickened inter-lobular and intralobular septa, giving a reticular pattern

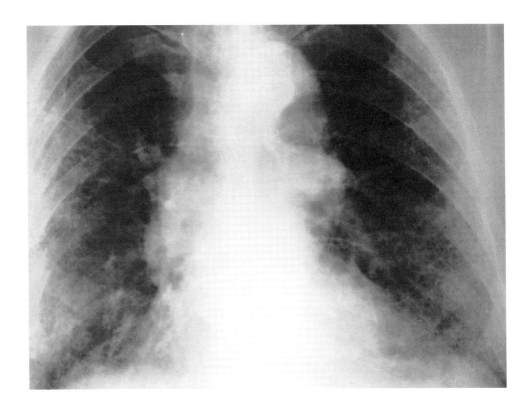

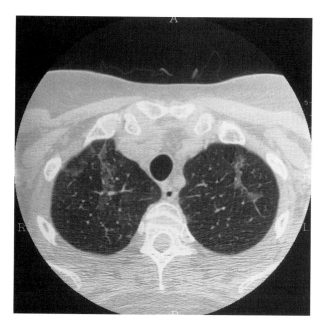

Fig. 31.7 High-resolution CT of patient with predominantly 'desquamative' alveolitis, in this case associated with rheumatoid disease, showing patchy ground-glass appearances. (Courtesy of Dr Lesley Gomersal.)

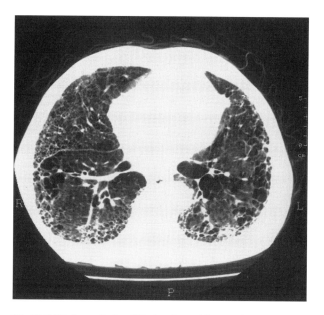

Fig. 31.8 High-resolution CT of patient with 'usual' type of fibrosing alveolitis showing reticular pattern of interlobular and intralobular fibrosis. (Courtesy of Dr Lesley Gomersal.)

(Fig. 31.8); the distribution of shadows is predominantly lower zone and subpleural initially, though as the disease progresses it becomes more generalized. Finally, mature fibrosis with bronchial ectasia and destruction of lung architecture is represented by thick-walled cystic changes 5–10 mm in diameter, so-called honeycombing (Fig. 31.9). In smokers, emphysematous changes in the upper zones often coexist with the fibrosis [110].

These appearances are reasonably characteristic and, taken with the clinical features, allow a confident diagnosis to be made in most cases. They do not differ in any important respects from the changes seen in systemic sclerosis or asbestosis, although the differentiation from these diseases is made on other clinical grounds and, in the case of asbestosis, by the frequent presence of associated pleural lesions. In younger patients, differentiation from the rare diseases, Langerhans' cell histiocytosis and lymphangioleiomyomatosis, is aided by the more generalized appearances, nodular change and thinner-walled cysts in these conditions.

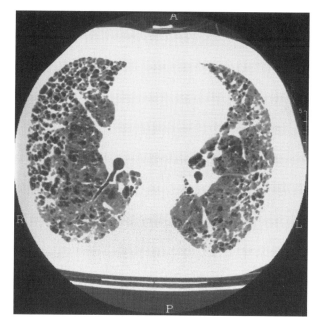

Fig. 31.9 High-resolution CT of patient with advanced disease showing honeycomb pattern of fibrosis with destruction of normal lung architecture. (Courtesy of Dr Lesley Gomersal.)

Gallium-67 lung scanning

Pulmonary uptake of gallium occurs in many diffuse interstitial lung diseases, including cryptogenic fibrosing alveolitis [76]. The pattern of uptake is usually diffuse and confined to the lung parenchyma. Such scans are positive in about 70% of all patients with cryptogenic fibrosing alveolitis [76,98], and the intensity of gallium uptake correlates well with the degree of alveolitis on open lung biopsy and the percentage of polymorphonuclear leucocytes present in BAL fluid [111]. However, this technique does not make a major contribution to the clinical assessment of patients with cryptogenic fibrosing alveolitis.

Pulmonary function

The lung volumes may be normal in early cryptogenic fibrosing alveolitis but as the disease progresses all the compartments of lung volume decrease, with a relatively greater reduction in vital capacity [98,112,113]. In the absence of extensive emphysema the forced expiratory volume in 1s (FEV_1)/forced vital capacity (FVC) ratio is normal, although abnormalities in sophisticated tests of small airways function (e.g. frequency dependence of compliance, the terminal portion of the maximum expiratory flow–volume curve and the maximum flow–static recoil curve) correlate with morphological evidence of small airways disease [114,115].

The single-breath diffusing capacity for carbon monoxide is reduced early in cryptogenic fibrosing alveolitis [76,112]. In the early stages of the disease, Pao_2 may be normal at rest but falls during exercise when the alveolar–arterial Po_2 gradient is increased [76,116–119]. With progression of disease, resting hypoxaemia develops. The major part of this hypoxaemia can be explained by mismatching of ventilation and perfusion [120–122]. During exercise, because of the reduced transit time of erythrocytes in the pulmonary capillaries, up to 20% of the exercise-induced widening of the alveolar–arterial Po_2 difference may be due to impaired oxygen diffusion [123]. Hypoxaemia in fibrosing alveolitis worsens during sleep, particularly in the rapid eye movement stage [119,124].

Lung compliance is reduced in fibrosing alveolitis, with greater transpulmonary pressure changes on breathing and consequent increase in the work of breathing, which may be responsible for the sensation of dyspnoea. Exercise tolerance is reduced and there is an increased heart rate and ventilatory response to exercise compared with normal individuals [125]. The maximal achievable exercise ventilation correlates with lung volumes. The tidal volume is reduced in proportion to the reduction in vital capacity and increased ventilation during exercise is achieved by increases in respiratory rate rather than by the predominant increase in tidal volume seen in normal subjects [125,126]. The 12-min walking test provides a useful measure of limitation of exercise tolerance in these patients [127].

Bronchoalveolar lavage

BAL fluid usually shows an excess of neutrophils and eosinophils compared with normal non-smokers. There is considerable overlap, making this little use as a diagnostic test; it is more informative in a prognostic sense, in that high proportions of neutophils (>4%) or eosinophils (>3%) are indicative of a poor response to steroids. A relative lymphocytosis (>11%) may also be an indicator of active alveolar inflammation and a better response to steroid treatment [128,129].

Other investigations

The erythrocyte sedimentation rate is usually elevated in this disease, but apart from the occasional detection of antinuclear antibodies, rheumatoid factor, cryoglobulins or other autoimmune phenomena, no other abnormalities are found in the peripheral blood [98,130,131].

Diagnosis

The diagnosis is suggested by the clinical features of dyspnoea, cough and bilateral basal crepitations in an elderly or middle-aged individual, the presence of reticulonodular shadowing predominantly at the lung bases on the chest film in the absence of a known cause, the typical findings on HRCT, and appropriate pulmonary function findings. In most cases these investigations are sufficient to make a confident clinical diagnosis, although differential cell counting of BAL fluid may assist in indicating likely response to treatment. The main decision required is whether to proceed to lung biopsy, which provides definitive proof of the diagnosis and somewhat better prognostic evidence. It has been established that the small specimens obtained by transbronchial biopsy through the fibreoptic bronchoscope are not suitable [37] and open or thoracoscopic lung biopsy, guided by HRCT to areas of active alveolitis if present, is preferred [37–41]. This therefore subjects the patient to some risk and discomfort and should be undertaken only if it is considered that knowledge of the histological appearances would influence the physician's treatment regimen. Thus the serious possibility of some other disease, more acute presentations or a relatively young patient in whom a very persistent trial of treatment, often including consideration of transplantation, is likely to be considered are usually influential factors in coming to a decision to proceed to biopsy. With appropriate ethical safeguards, biopsy would also usually be advised if the patient has agreed to participate in a trial of new therapy. Physicians differ in their practices but ultimately rather fewer than half of all patients are biopsied in the UK. In the majority of patients the clinical findings, including HRCT, give sufficient diagnostic information to justify a therapeutic trial monitored by response in terms of change in lung function. However, patients with an acute or rapidly progressive presentation in whom HRCT suggests active disease should almost always have early biopsy if considered fit enough, since the differential diagnosis of such patients is wide and treatment may well be influenced by the histological findings.

Treatment

It is disappointing to record that the prognosis of this condition appears not to have altered appreciably nor has any important advance in treatment occurred since the first edition of this book in 1969. The mainstay of therapy in cryptogenic fibrosing alveolitis remains corticosteroids, prednisolone being the drug of choice. Since occasionally the disease is very slowly progressive, or has even arrested, it is wise in patients suspected of such a course to allow a period of several months to elapse, monitoring the patient's lung function and exercise performance carefully in order to assess whether treatment is likely to be necessary. In fact, the major recent UK study showed that the option not to treat was taken in over 50% of cases [30]. After the diagnosis has been established and baseline measurements of pulmonary function (i.e. lung volumes, D_{LCO} and exercise tolerance) have been obtained, treatment is usually initiated with prednisolone in a dose of 40–60 mg daily for at least 4 weeks. This is followed by a graduated reduction in dosage over 2–3 months to the lowest maintenance dose capable of sustaining any objective improvement in chest radiograph, lung volumes, exercise tolerance or D_{LCO} that has been achieved. Objective improvement is most likely to be found in those with histological evidence of early disease with marked cellularity and little fibrosis on the lung biopsy [6,39], in younger patients and in those with recent onset of disease [39,132], and in those with less severe radiographic and functional abnormality [132].

Although it is common (almost 60% in one series [133]) for patients to report some subjective improvement with corticosteroid therapy, objective evidence of improvement is found relatively rarely (17% in the same study). Clearly, many patients with established fibrotic disease do not respond, although a trial of therapy is often warranted. BAL studies suggest that high eosinophil or neutrophil counts or low lymphocyte counts predict a poor clinical response to corticosteroids, whereas a lymphocyte count of greater than 11% appears to be related to improvement [128,134–136]. Serial lavage studies suggest that objective improvement is associated in general with return of elevated cell counts towards normality; however, there is no indication at present that such studies, although interesting from the research point of view, influence the clinical management of patients [136]. Indeed, striking decreases in neutrophil counts in BAL fluid occasioned by high-dose parenteral steroid therapy have resulted in no greater changes radiologically and functionally than occurred in a conventionally treated group [137]. Also, confusingly, corticosteroid therapy may lead to an increase in lavage neutrophils in smokers with fibrosing alveolitis [138].

In patients who do not respond to corticosteroids or for whom steroid therapy is contraindicated, immunosuppressant drugs such as azathioprine 150 mg daily or cyclophosphamide 100–120 mg daily may be tried. There have been reports of successful treatment with these agents, which may also be employed for their steroid-sparing effect [136,139,140]. Patients treated with a combination of cyclophosphamide or aziathioprine and prednisolone fare little if any better than those treated with prednisolone alone [141,142], although there is a case for considering such a combination for its steroid-sparing properties. No other drugs have proved of clinical value, but it is to be hoped that the new understanding of pathogenetic mechanisms discussed above will lead to therapeutic trials of specific cytokine antibodies or receptor antagonists that may eventually prove of more promise. Possible new therapeutic options have been discussed in detail [67,68].

The author's approach is to make an initial assessment of likelihood of response, based mainly on HRCT and either biopsy or BAL findings. In the presence of evidence of active alveolitis, combined steroids and cyclophosphamide are started immediately and continued until it becomes apparent that no physiological response is occurring or side-effects become intolerable. In the absence of such evidence, a judgement is made as to whether treatment is justified after several months of follow-up with repeated lung function and exercise tolerance tests. Old radiographs are particularly helpful in assessing progression if they are available. The patient's age and general condition are also taken into consideration; most important are the views of the patients themselves, after explanation of the chances of response, the likely prognosis and the side-effects of treatment. Many older patients prefer to wait and see when presented with this information.

In younger non-smoking patients without systemic disease, there is now the option of lung transplantation [143,144] (see Chapter 59) and pulmonary fibrosis is responsible for 20% of transplants done currently [145]. The results indicate a 50% survival at 3 years [146].

Since only a small minority of patients with chronic disease respond in any worthwhile way to steroids or immunosuppressants and many find the side-effects of the former intolerable, the drugs are usually discontinued after a trial of several months and (except in younger patients intended for transplantation) efforts should be made to relieve the symptoms as far as possible. In some cases, small doses of benzodiazepine may help relieve the intractable breathlessness. In the later stages of the disease, oxygen therapy and treatment for right heart failure may be required. Appropriate sedation with opiates should be given in the terminal stages of the disease to relieve the intense distress occasioned by dyspnoea.

Prognosis

The duration of the illness is variable but may range from a few months in patients whose disease follows a fulminant course to over 20 years. In several large series the average duration of survival from diagnosis has been 4–5 years [39,57,133]. Carrington and colleagues [6] found

5-year mortality in the 'desquamative' type of disease to be 27.5% with a mean survival of 12.2 years compared with 66% and 5.6 years in the 'usual' type. Only the 'desquamative' type improved spontaneously (22%). With corticosteroid drugs, 61.5% of the 'desquamative' but only 11.5% of the 'usual' type improved. In Stack's series the 5-year survival was 43% in those responding to corticosteroids compared with only 20% for those who did not respond [147]. As already mentioned, survival is longest in those with the most cellular and least fibrotic lung biopsies. Wright and colleagues [39] showed that patients with little fibrosis on lung biopsy had a 5-year survival of 90% compared with a 25% 5-year survival in those with severe fibrosis on biopsy. Most patients die from respiratory or cardiac failure, although there is a significant excess of lung cancer in patients with cryptogenic fibrosing alveolitis [104].

Differential diagnosis of diffuse interstitial lung disease

Contrary to the impression conveyed by accounts of the differential diagnosis of diffuse interstitial lung disease (Table 31.1), the diagnosis of the usual type of cryptogenic fibrosing alveolitis is quite straightforward. A good history and examination, coupled with some experience of the more usual radiographic and HRCT appearances of given diseases makes the task of differential diagnosis easy. The most important aspect of diagnosis is to exclude both more readily treatable causes of the radiological appearances and also conditions with different prognoses. Thus, in practice, sarcoidosis, pneumoconioses (especially asbestosis), extrinsic allergic alveolitis and, most importantly, adverse reactions to drugs need to be considered. The more acute form of the disease, with ground-glass HRCT appearances, has a wider differential diagnosis that is usually only resolved by lung biopsy, a procedure that should not be delayed in such cases.

Clinical features

History

Cough productive of sputum is suggestive of airway involvement, and diffuse shadowing on the chest film with associated cough and purulent sputum would suggest pneumonia in relation to underlying airway disease, such as might be found in chronic bronchitis, bronchiectasis and cystic fibrosis. Cough with purulent sputum may also be features of allergic bronchopulmonary aspergillosis, tuberculosis and chronic eosinophilic pneumonia.

Wheeze is a usual accompaniment of acute allergic bronchopulmonary aspergillosis and chronic eosinophilic

Table 31.1 Some causes of interstitial lung disease.

Occupational and environmental (Chapter 54)
Asbestos
Quartz, cristobolite, silicates
Beryllium
Bauxite
Coal, graphite
Cobalt, antimony

Organic dusts (Chapter 37)
Microorganisms
    Fungal spores
    Actinomycetes
Animal protein
    Bird bloom
    Small mammal protein

Collagen diseases (Chapter 53)
Rheumatoid
Systemic sclerosis
Lupus erythematosus
Sjögren's syndrome

Inherited disorders (Chapter 53)
Tuberous sclerosis
Neurofibromatosis
Ankylosing spondylitis
Familial pulmonary fibrosis
Weber–Christian disease
Hermansky–Pudlak syndrome

Vasculitis/granulomas (Chapter 40)
Churg–Strauss syndrome
Polyarteritis nodosa
Wegener's granulomatosis

Toxic fumes and vapours (Chapters 54, 55)
Oxygen
Chlorine, fluorine and other gases
Nitrogen dioxide
Lipids

Drugs (Chapter 55)
Cytotoxics
Nitrofurantoin
Sulfasalazine, salicylates
Gold
Penicillamine
Amiodarone

Poisons (Chapter 55)
Paraquat
Toxic oil syndrome
Radiation

Infections (Chapter 13)
Viral pneumonias
Mycoplasma pneumonia
HIV-associated disease (Chapter 52)

Unknown aetiology
Cryptogenic fibrosing alveolitis
Sarcoidosis (Chapter 39)
Langerhans' cell histiocytosis (Chapter 42)
Haemosiderosis (Chapter 51)
Amyloidosis (Chapter 51)
Lymphangioleiomyomatosis (Chapter 42)

pneumonia and is also found in the pulmonary vasculitides and pulmonary oedema. Dyspnoea is a common presenting symptom in diffuse interstitial lung disease. When acute in onset and associated with fever, infection should be suspected although in some instances a connective tissue disorder such as disseminated lupus erythematosus is responsible. Acute dyspnoea is of course commonly due to left ventricular failure. Episodic acute dyspnoea is a feature of extrinsic allergic alveolitis, when a history of exposure to the relevant antigen will be obtained and influenza-type symptoms may be associated. Slowly progressive rather than acute dyspnoea suggests a chronic progressive disease. The rate of progression of dyspnoea varies widely between different processes. Slow progression over a decade or more is usual in asbestosis and some other pneumoconioses and is also found in pulmonary sarcoidosis evolving to fibrosis. In contrast, in some of the complications of human immunodeficiency virus (HIV) infection, including *Pneumocystis* pneumonia, or the more acute cryptogenic fibrosing alveolitis, dyspnoea may progress more rapidly, often over a few months. The relative severity of dyspnoea in relation to the radiographic extent of disease is also important, for example sarcoidosis may cause minimal dyspnoea despite substantial radiographic extent of disease, whereas in cryptogenic fibrosing alveolitis dyspnoea may be disproportionately severe.

Chest pain of a pleuritic nature may suggest a diagnosis of connective tissue disease or pleural involvement in, for example, rheumatoid arthritis or sarcoidosis. Acute pleuritic pain due to pneumothorax may be consequent on rupture of bullae or blebs in chronic fibrotic processes, such as cryptogenic fibrosing alveolitis, or be a manifestation of less common diseases, such as Langerhans' cell histiocytosis or lymphangioleiomyomatosis.

Haemoptysis may occur in left ventricular failure and is a feature of less common conditions such as idiopathic pulmonary haemosiderosis and Goodpasture's syndrome.

As is apparent from Table 31.1, an occupational and environmental history is of cardinal importance. Not only the present occupation but previous occupations should be documented and explored for possible exposure to inhaled agents. If necessary, the workplace should be visited and possible agents obtained for challenge tests if indicated. A domiciliary visit may be required in some cases. The author has seen extrinsic allergic alveolitis in a patient who persistently denied keeping birds until a home visit revealed the offending budgerigars, which an astute ward sister had overheard twittering during a telephone call from the patient's husband. In a similar case, bird fanciers' lung was diagnosed in a patient who eventually revealed that he was keeping doves in his kitchen.

A drug history should be vigorously pursued. Many cytotoxic drugs cause pulmonary fibrosis. Nitrofurantoin, still frequently prescribed for recurrent urinary tract infections, and sulfasalazine (sulphasalazine) for ulcerative colitis are not uncommon causes of pulmonary eosinophilia or chronic progressive fibrosis. The problems of differential diagnosis of diffuse pulmonary shadowing in the immunosuppressed host are discussed in Chapter 52.

Extrapulmonary symptoms may suggest systemic disease. Arthralgia and skin lesions are found in sarcoidosis, connective tissue disease and Wegener's granulomatosis. Eye and skin symptoms are common in sarcoidosis and upper respiratory tract symptoms in Wegener's granulomatosis. Bone lesions may be found in Langerhans' cell histiocytosis and chronic sarcoidosis. Increasingly in the UK, and to a much greater extent in Africa and parts of Asia and the USA, it is necessary to consider HIV infection as a cause of interstitial lung disease, either infective or infiltrative, and some of these manifestations, such as *Pneumocystis* infection or lymphocytic interstitial pneumonitis, cause diagnostic difficulties. A history designed to elicit risk factors and HIV testing should now be considered in all patients with diffuse lung disease of obscure aetiology.

Examination

Finger clubbing is a feature of cryptogenic fibrosing alveolitis and asbestosis and may also be found in bronchiectasis and cystic fibrosis. Bilateral crepitations on auscultation are a feature of pulmonary oedema, cryptogenic fibrosing alveolitis, extrinsic allergic alveolitis and asbestosis. Crepitations are not a feature of the other pneumoconioses or sarcoidosis (except in the late fibrotic stages). A full examination of all systems should be undertaken in a search for relevant signs, with particular attention being paid to bones and joints, the skin and the eyes.

Other investigations

The routine full blood count may be diagnostically useful. A neutrophil leucocytosis suggests bacterial infection, while eosinophilia is found in pulmonary eosinophilia of whatever cause (see Chapter 38). A very high erythrocyte sedimentation rate may be found in connective tissue diseases, Wegener's granulomatosis, Goodpasture's syndrome and in chronic eosinophilic pneumonia. Sputum examination may reveal bacterial or fungal infection or malignant cells. Iron-laden macrophages are found in the sputum in idiopathic pulmonary haemosiderosis and PAS-positive material in alveolar proteinosis. Sputum eosinophilia may suggest pulmonary eosinophilia and bronchial casts may be found in allergic bronchopulmonary aspergillosis.

Precipitins to the causative antigen may be detected in extrinsic allergic alveolitis. Antinuclear antibodies and anti-DNA antibodies are found in disseminated lupus erythematosus; antinuclear and rheumatoid factors may also be found in cryptogenic fibrosing alveolitis and antineutrophil cytoplasmic antibodies in Wegener's granulomatosis. Serological evidence of HIV infection should be sought where relevant and after appropriate discussion with the patient.

BAL may be of value in diagnosing infection and differential cell counting may suggest diagnoses of fibrosing alveolitis, extrinsic allergic alveolitis or sarcoidosis. Birkbeck (or X) bodies may be found in Langerhans' cell histiocytosis, and evidence of HIV-related infection may be found with appropriate stains. Transbronchial biopsy is of value in diagnosing infection, malignancy, alveolar proteinosis, haemosiderosis and sarcoidosis but open lung biopsy may be necessary to establish a firm diagnosis particularly in cryptogenic fibrosing alveolitis.

Chest radiograph

The radiographic appearances of specific conditions are described in detail in the relevant chapters. In many conditions the distribution of pulmonary opacities is characteristic and examples of generalized, upper, middle and lower zone opacities are listed in Table 31.2.

Table 31.2 Patterns of distributions of pulmonary opacities on the chest radiograph.

Upper zones
Tuberculosis
Chronic sarcoidosis
Extrinsic allergic alveolitis
Langerhans' cell histiocytosis
Subacute silicosis
Progressive massive fibrosis

Middle zones
Pulmonary oedema
Alveolar proteinosis
Pneumocystis carinii infection

Lower zones
Cryptogenic fibrosing alveolitis
Asbestosis
Bronchopneumonia
Collagen diseases
Tropical eosinophilia

Generalized
Pneumoconioses
Miliary tuberculosis
Sarcoidosis
Cystic fibrosis
Complications of human immunodeficiency virus infection
Metastases
Lymphangitic carcinomatosis
Adult respiratory distress syndrome
Drug reactions
Haemosiderosis
Microlithiasis

References

1 Scadding JG, Hinson KF. Diffuse fibrosing alveolitis (diffuse interstitial fibrosis of the lungs). Correlation of histology at biopsy with prognosis. *Thorax* 1967; 22: 291.
2 Hamman L, Rich AR. Fulminating diffuse interstitial fibrosis of the lungs. *Trans Am Clin Climatol Assoc* 1935; 51: 154.
3 Hamman L, Rich AR. Acute diffuse interstitial fibrosis of the lungs. *Bull Johns Hopkins Hosp* 1944; 74: 177.
4 Rubin EH, Lubliner R. The Hamman–Rich syndrome: review of the literature and analysis of 15 cases. *Medicine* 1957; 36: 397.
5 Turner-Warwick M, Burrows B, Johnson A. Cryptogenic fibrosing alveolitis: clinical features and their influence on survival. *Thorax* 1980; 35: 171.
6 Carrington CB, Gaensler EA, Coutu RE, Fitzgerald MX, Gupta RG. Natural history and treated course of usual and desquamative interstitial pneumonia. *N Engl J Med* 1978; 298: 801.
7 Peabody JW, Peabody JW Jr, Hayes EW, Hayes EW Jr. Idiopathic pulmonary fibrosis: its occurrence in identical twin sisters. *Dis Chest* 1950; 18: 330.
8 MacMillan JM. Familial pulmonary fibrosis. *Dis Chest* 1951; 20: 426.
9 Donohue WL, Laski B, Uchida F, Munn JD. Familial fibrocystic pulmonary dysplasia and its relation to Hamman–Rich syndrome. *Pediatrics* 1959; 24: 786.

10 Bitterman PB, Crystal RG. Is there a fibrotic gene? *Chest* 1980; 78: 549.
11 Musk AW, Zilco PJ, Manners P, Kay PH, Kamboh MI. Genetic studies in familial fibrosing alveolitis: possible linkage with immunoglobulin allotypes (Gm). *Chest* 1986; 89: 206.
12 Bitterman PB, Rennard SI, Keogh BA, Wewers MD, Adelberg S, Crystal RG. Familial idiopathic pulmonary fibrosis: evidence of lung inflammation in unaffected family members. *N Engl J Med* 1986; 314: 1343.
13 Javaheri S, Lederer DH, Pella JA *et al.* Idiopathic pulmonary fibrosis in monozygotic twins. *Chest* 1980; 78: 591.
14 Fulmer JD, Sposovska MS, von Gal ER *et al.* Distribution of HLA antigens in idiopathic pulmonary fibrosis. *Am Rev Respir Dis* 1978; 118: 141.
15 Strimlan CV, Taswell HF, DeRemee RA, Kueppers F. HL-A antigens and fibrosing alveolitis. *Am Rev Respir Dis* 1977; 116: 1120.
16 Evans CC. HLA antigens in diffuse fibrosing alveolitis. *Thorax* 1976; 31: 483.
17 Libby DM, Gibofsky A, Fotino M *et al.* Immunogenetic and clinical findings in idiopathic pulmonary fibrosis. *Am Rev Respir Dis* 1983; 127: 618.
18 McDevitt HO. Current concepts in immunology: regulation of the immune response by the major histocompatibility system. *N Engl J Med* 1980; 303: 1514.

19 Marshall RP, McAnulty RJ, Laurent GJ. The pathogenesis of pulmonary fibrosis: is there a fibrosis gene? *Int J Biochem Cell Biol* 1997; 29: 107.
20 Lympany PA, duBois RM. Diffuse lung disease: product of genetic susceptibility and environmental encounters. *Thorax* 1997; 52: 92.
21 Hubbard R, Johnston I, Coultas DB, Britton J. Mortality rates from cryptogenic fibrosing alveolitis in seven countries. *Thorax* 1996; 51: 711.
22 Mannino DM, Etzel RA, Parrish RG. Pulmonary fibrosis deaths in the United States, 1979–1991. An analysis of multiple cause mortality data. *Am J Respir Crit Care Med* 1996; 153: 1548.
23 Johnston I, Britton J, Kinnear W, Logan R. Rising mortality from cryptogenic fibrosing alveolitis. *Br Med J* 1990; 301: 1017.
24 Egan JJ, Stewart JP, Haselton PS, Arrand JR, Carroll KB, Woodcock AB. Epstein–Barr virus replication within pulmonary epithelial cells in cryptogenic fibrosing alveolitis. *Thorax* 1995; 50: 1234.
25 Barbara JA, Hayashi S, Hegele RG, Hogg JC. Detection of Epstein–Barr virus in lymphocytic interstitial pneumonia by *in situ* hybridisation. *Am Rev Respir Dis* 1992; 145: 940.
26 Vergnon JM, Vincent M, de The G, Mornex JF, Weynets P, Brune J. Cryptogenic fibrosing

alveolitis and Epstein-Barr virus: an association? *Lancet* 1984; ii: 768.

27 Kaufman JM, Cuvelier CA, van der Straeten M. *Mycoplasma* pneumonia with fulminant evolution into diffuse interstitial fibrosis. *Thorax* 1980; 35: 140.

28 Matsui R, Goldstein RH, Mihal K, Brody JS, Steele MP, Fine A. Type I collagen formation on rat type II alveolar cells immortalised by viral gene products. *Thorax* 1994; 49: 201.

29 Hubbard R, Lewis S, Richards K, Johnston I, Britton J. Occupational exposure to metal or wood dust and aetiology of cryptogenic fibrosing alveolitis. *Lancet* 1996; 347: 284.

30 Johnston IDA, Prescott RJ, Chalmers JC, Rudd RM. British Thoracic Society study of cryptogenic fibrosing alveolitis: current presentation and initial management. *Thorax* 1997; 52: 38.

31 Donaldson K, Brown DM, Mitchell C *et al.* Free radical activity of PM_{10}: iron-mediated generation of hydroxyl radical. *Environ Health Perspect* 1997; 105 (Suppl 5): S1285.

32 Baumgartner KB, Samet JM, Stidley CA, Colby TV, Waldron JA. Cigarette smoking: a risk factor for idiopathic pulmonary fibrosis. *Am J Respir Crit Care Med* 1997; 155: 242.

33 Koeger AC, Lang T, Alcaix D *et al.* Silica-associated connective tissue disease. A study of 24 cases. *Medicine* 1995; 74: 221.

34 Scott J, Johnston I, Britton J. What causes cryptogenic fibrosing alveolitis? A case-control study of environmental exposure to dust. *Br Med J* 1990; 301: 1015.

35 Coultas DB, Zumwalt RE, Black WC, Sobonya RE. The epidemiology of interstitial lung diseases. *Am J Respir Crit Care Med* 1994; 150: 967.

36 Jindal SK, Gupta D. Incidence and recognition of interstitial pulmonary fibrosis in developing countries. *Curr Opin Pulm Med* 1997; 3: 378.

37 Wall CP, Gaensler EA, Carrington CB, Hayes JA. Comparison of transbronchial and open biopsies in chronic infiltrative lung disease. *Am Rev Respir Dis* 1981; 123: 280.

38 Gaensler EA, Moister MVB, Hamm J. Open lung biopsy in diffuse pulmonary disease. *N Engl J Med* 1964; 270: 1319.

39 Wright PH, Heard BE, Steel SJ, Turner-Warwick M. Cryptogenic fibrosing alveolitis: assessment by graded trephine lung biopsy histology compared with clinical, radiographic and physiological features. *Br J Dis Chest* 1981; 75: 61.

40 Krasner MJ, White CS, Aisner SC, Templeton PA, McLaughlin JS. The role of thoracoscopy in the diagnosis of interstitial lung disease. *Ann Thorac Surg* 1995; 59: 348.

41 Mouroux J, Clary-Meinesz C, Padovani B *et al.* Efficacy and safety of videothoracoscopic lung biopsy in the diagnosis of interstitial lung disease. *Eur J Cardiothorac Surg* 1997; 11: 22.

42 Bjoraker JA, Ryu JH, Edwin MK *et al.* Prognostic significance of histopathologic subsets in idiopathic pulmonary fibrosis. *Am J Respir Crit Care Med* 1998; 157: 199.

43 Spencer H. Interstitial pneumonia. *Annu Rev Med* 1967; 18: 423.

44 Shortland JR, Darke CS, Crane WAJ. Electron microscopy of desquamative interstitial pneumonia. *Thorax* 1969; 24: 192.

45 Fromm GB, Dunn LJ, Harris JO. Desquamative interstitial pneumonitis: characterization of free intra-alveolar cells. *Chest* 1980; 77: 552.

46 Stachura I, Singh G, Whiteside TL. Mechanisms of tissue injury in desquamative interstitial pneumonitis. *Am J Med* 1980; 68: 733.

47 Tubbs RR, Benjamin SP, Osborne DG, Barenberg S. Surface and transmission ultrastructural characteristics of desquamative interstitial pneumonitis. *Hum Pathol* 1978; 9: 693.

48 Tuder RM. A pathologist's approach to interstitial lung disease. *Curr Opin Pulm Med* 1996; 2: 357.

49 Fulmer JD, Bienkowsk RS, Cowan MJ *et al.* Collagen concentration and rates of synthesis in idiopathic pulmonary fibrosis *Am Rev Respir Dis* 1980; 122: 289.

50 Hance AJ, Crystal RG. The connective tissue of lung. *Am Rev Respir Dis* 1975; 112: 657.

51 Lachronique JG, Rennard SL, Bitterrnan PB *et al.* Alveolar macrophages in idiopathic pulmonary fibrosis have glucocorticoid receptors, but glucocorticoid therapy does not suppress alveolar macrophage release of fibronectin and alveolar macrophage derived growth factor. *Am Rev Respir Dis* 1984; 130: 450.

52 Herbert FA, Nahmias BB, Gaensler EA, McMahon HE. Pathophysiology of interstitial pulmonary fibrosis. Report of 19 cases and follow up with corticosteroids. *Arch Intern Med* 1962; 110: 628.

53 Stack BHR, Grant IWB, Irvine WJ, Moffat MAJ. Idiopathic diffuse interstitial lung disease. A review of 42 cases. *Am Rev Respir Dis* 1965; 92: 939.

54 Douglas AC. Diffuse interstitial pulmonary fibrosis. Report of a case. *Br J Dis Chest* 1960; 54: 86.

55 Mendeloff J. Disseminated nodular pulmonary ossification in the Hamman–Rich lung. *Am Rev Respir Dis* 1971; 103: 269.

56 Campbell DA, Poulter LW, Janossy G, duBois RM. Immunohistological analysis of lung tissue from patients with cryptogenic fibrosing alveolitis suggesting local expression of immune hypersensitivity. *Thorax* 1985; 40: 405.

57 Livingstone JL, Lewis JG, Reid L, Jefferson KE. Diffuse interstitial pulmonary fibrosis. A clinical, radiological and pathological study based on 45 patients. *Q J Med* 1964; 33: 71.

58 Gaensler EA, Goff AM, Prowse CM. Desquamative interstitial pneumonia. *N Engl J Med* 1964; 274: 113.

59 Liebow AA, Steer A, Billingsley JG. Desquamative interstitial pneumonia. *Am J Med* 1965; 39: 369.

60 Patchefsky AS, Israel HL, Hoch WS, Gordon G. Desquamative interstitial pneumonia: relationship to interstitial fibrosis. *Thorax* 1973; 28: 680.

61 Tubbs RR, Benjamin SP, Reich NE *et al.* Desquamative interstitial pneumonitis: cellular phase of fibrosing alveolitis. *Chest* 1977; 72: 159.

62 Turner-Warwick M. Cryptogenic fibrosing alveolitis. *Br J Hosp Med* 1972; 7: 697.

63 Davies D, MacFarlane A, Darke CS, Dodge OG. Muscular hyperplasia ('cirrhosis') of the lung and bronchial dilatations as features of chronic diffuse fibrosing alveolitis. *Thorax* 1966; 21: 272.

64 Fraimow W, Cathcart RT. Clinical and physiological considerations in pulmonary muscular hyperplasia. *Ann Intern Med* 1962; 56: 752.

65 Ziskind MM, Weill H, George RB. Diffuse pulmonary diseases. *Am J Med Sci* 1967; 254: 117.

66 Goldstein RH, Fine A. Potential therapeutic initiatives for fibrogenic lung diseases. *Chest* 1995; 108: 848.

67 Phan SH. New strategies for treatment of pulmonary fibrosis. *Thorax* 1995; 50: 415.

68 Coker RK, Laurent GJ. Anticytokine approaches in pulmonary fibrosis: bringing factors into focus. *Thorax* 1997; 52: 294.

69 Zang K, Gharaee-Kermani M, McGarry B, Remick D, Phan SH. TNF-alpha mediated lung cytokine networking and eosinophil recruitment in pulmonary fibrosis. *J Immunol* 1997; 158: 954.

70 Giri S, Hyde D, Hollinger M. Effect of antibody to transforming growth factor β on bleomycin-induced accumulation of lung collagen in mice. *Thorax* 1993; 48: 959.

71 Cambrey A, Harrison NK, Dawes KE *et al.* Increased levels of endothelin-1 in bronchoalveolar lavage fluid from patients with systemic sclerosis contribute to fibroblast mitogenic activity *in vitro*. *Am J Respir Cell Mol Biol* 1994; 11: 439.

72 Hernandez-Rodriguez NA, Cambrey AD, Harrison NK *et al.* Role of thrombin in pulmonary fibrosis. *Lancet* 1995; 346: 1071.

73 Lyberg T, Nakstad B, Hetland O, Boye NP. Procoagulant (thromboplastin) activity in human bronchoalveolar lavage fluids is derived from alveolar macrophages. *Eur Respir J* 1990; 3: 61.

74 Crystal RG, Bitterman PB, Rennard Sl *et al.* Interstitial lung diseases of unknown cause. *N Engl J Med* 1984; 310: 154.

75 Hunninghake GW, Kawanami O, Ferrans VJ *et al.* Characterisation of the inflammatory and immune effector cells in the lung parenchyma of patients with interstitial lung disease. *Am Rev Respir Dis* 1981; 123: 407.

76 Crystal RG, Gadek JE, Ferrans VJ *et al.* Interstitial lung disease: current concepts of pathogenesis, staging and therapy. *Am J Med* 1981; 70: 542.

77 Campbell DA, Poulter LW, duBois RM. Phenotypic analysis of alveolar macrophages in normal subjects and patients with interstitial lung disease. *Thorax* 1986; 41: 429.

78 Noble B, duBois RM, Poulter LW. The distribution of phenotypically distinct macrophage subsets in the lungs of patients with cryptogenic fibrosing alveolitis. *Clin Exp Immunol* 1989; 76: 41.

79 Hunninghake GW, Gadek JE, Lawley TJ, Crystal RG. Mechanisms of neutrophil accumulation in the lungs of patients with idiopathic pulmonary fibrosis. *J Clin Invest* 1981; 68: 259.

80 Martin WJ, Davis WB, Gadek JE *et al.* Alveolar macrophages from patients with idiopathic pulmonary fibrosis contribute to lung cell injury. *Am Rev Respir Dis* 1982; 125: 91.

81 Bittenan PB, Adelberg S, Crystal RG. Mechanisms of pulmonary fibrosis. Spontaneous release of the alveolar macrophage-derived growth factor in the interstitial lung disorders. *J Clin Invest* 1983; 72: 1801.

82 Rennard SI, Hunninghake GW, Bitterman PB, Crystal RG. Production of fibronectin by the human alveolar macrophage: mechanism for the recruitment of fibroblasts to sites of tissue injury in interstitial lung diseases. *Proc Natl Acad Sci USA* 1981; 78: 7147.

83 Hunninghake GW, Hemken C, Brady M, Monick M. Immune interferon is a growth factor for human lung fibroblasts. *Am Rev Respir Dis* 1986; 134: 1025.

84 Lawrence EC, Martin RR, Blaese RM *et al.* Increased bronchoalveolar IgG-secreting cells in interstitial lung diseases. *N Engl J Med* 1980; 302: 1186.

85 Reynolds HY, Fulmer JD, Kazmierowski JA *et al.* Analysis of cellular and protein content of bronchoalveolar lavage fluid from patients with idiopathic pulmonary fibrosis and chronic hypersensitivity pneumonitis. *J Clin Invest* 1977; 59: 165.

86 Weinberger SE, Kelman JA, Elson NA *et al.* Bronchoalveolar lavage in interstitial lung disease. *Ann Intern Med* 1978; 89: 459.

87 Kravis TC, Ahmed A, Brown TE *et al.* Pathogenic mechanisms in pulmonary fibrosis: collagen induced migration inhibition factor production and cytotoxicity mediated by lymphocytes. *J Clin Invest* 1976; 58: 1223.

88 Huninghake GW, Kalica AR. Approaches to the treatment of pulmonary fibrosis. *Am J Respir Crit Care Med* 1995; 151: 915.

89 Obayashi Y, Yamadori I, Fujita J, Yoshinouchi T, Ueda N, Takahara J. The role of neutrophils in the pathogenesis of idiopathic pulmonary fibrosis. *Chest* 1997; 112: 1338.

90 Martin WJ, Gadek JE, Hunninghake GW, Crystal RG. Neutrophil mediated lung injury: a lung explant system of cytotoxicity. *Am Rev Respir Dis* 1980; 121: 82.

91 Martin WJ, Davis WB, Gadek JE *et al.* Alveolar macrophages from patients with pulmonary fibrosis contribute to lung cell injury. *Am Rev Respir Dis* 1982; 125: 91.

92 Gadek JE, Fells GA, Zimmerman RT *et al.* Role of proteolytic and oxidative products of the neutrophil in determining the specificity of the pulmonary lesions in fibrotic and destructive lung disease. *Chest* 1983; 83 (Suppl 5): 595.

93 Gadek JE, Kelman JA, Fells G *et al.* Collagenase in the lower respiratory tract of patients with idiopathic pulmonary fibrosis. *N Engl J Med* 1979; 301: 737.

94 Davis WB, Sun XH, Gadek JE *et al.* Cytotoxicity of eosinophils for lung parenchymal cells. *Am Rev Respir Dis* 1982; 125: 178.

95 Rennard SI, Crystal RG. Fibronectin in human bronchopulmonary lavage fluid. Elevation in patients with interstitial lung diseases. *J Clin Invest* 1981; 69: 113.

96 Davis WB, Gadek JE, Fells GA, Crystal RG. Role of eosinophils in connective tissue destruction. *Am Rev Respir Dis* 1981; 123: 55.

97 Libby DM. The eosinophil in idiopathic pulmonary fibrosis. *Chest* 1987; 92: 7.

98 Crystal RG, Fulmer JD, Roberts WC *et al.* Idiopathic pulmonary fibrosis: clinical, histologic, radiographic, physiologic, scintigraphic, cytologic and biochemical aspects. *Ann Intern Med* 1976; 85: 769.

99 Hodson ME, Haslam PL, Spiro SG, Turner-Warwick M. Digital vasculitis in patients with cryptogenic fibrosing alveolitis. *Br J Dis Chest* 1984; 78: 140.

100 Turton C, Jacobs JM. Cryptogenic fibrosing alveolitis associated with peripheral neuropathy. *Q J Med* 1983; 52: 417.

101 Williams AJ, Marsh J, Stableforth DE. Cryptogenic fibrosing alveolitis, chronic active hepatitis and autoimmune haemolytic anaemia in the same patient. *Br J Dis Chest* 1985; 79: 200.

102 Galko B, Grossman RF, Day A *et al.* Hypertrophic pulmonary osteoarthropathy in four patients with interstitial lung disease. *Chest* 1985; 88: 94.

103 Picado C, Gomez De Almeida R, Xaubet A *et al.* Spontaneous pneumothorax in cryptogenic fibrosing alveolitis. *Respiration* 1985; 48: 77.

104 Turner-Warwick M, Lebowitz M, Burrows B, Johnson A. Cryptogenic fibrosing alveolitis and lung cancer. *Thorax* 1980; 35: 496.

105 Epler GR, McCloud TC, Gaensler EA *et al.* Normal chest roentgenograms in chronic diffuse infiltrative lung disease. *N Engl J Med* 1978; 798: 934.

106 Wright PH, Buxton-Thomas M, Kreel L, Steel SJ. Cryptogenic fibrosing alveolitis: pattern of disease in the lung. *Thorax* 1984; 39: 857.

107 DuBois RM. Diffuse lung disease: an approach to management. *Br Med J* 1994; 309: 175.

108 Hansell DM, Wells AU. CT evaluation of fibrosing alveolitis: applications and insights. *J Thorac Imag* 1996; 11: 231.

109 Wells AU, Hansell DM, Rubens MB, Cullinan P, Black CM, duBois RM. The predictive value of appearances on thin section computed tomography in fibrosing alveolitis. *Am Rev Respir Dis* 1993; 148: 1076.

110 Wiggins J, Strickland B, Turner-Warwick M. Combined cryptogenic fibrosing alveolitis and emphysema: the value of high resolution computed tomography in assessment. *Respir Med* 1990; 84: 365.

111 Line BR, Fulmer JD, Reynolds HY *et al.* Gallium-67 citrate scanning in the staging of idiopathic pulmonary fibrosis: correlation with physiologic and morphologic features and bronchoalveolar lavage. *Am Rev Respir Dis* 1978; 118: 355.

112 Boushy SF, North LB. Pulmonary function in infiltrative lung disease. *Chest* 1973; 64: 448.

113 Herbert FA, Nahmias BB, Gaensler EA *et al.* Pathophysiology of interstitial pulmonary fibrosis. *Arch Intern Med* 1962; 110: 628.

114 Fulmer ID, Roberts WC, von Gal ER, Crystal RG. Small airways in idiopathic pulmonary fibrosis: comparison of morphologic and physiologic observations. *J Clin Invest* 1977; 60: 595.

115 Ostrow D, Cherniack RM. Resistance to airflow in patients with diffuse interstitial lung disease. *Am Rev Respir Dis* 1973; 108: 205.

116 Gaensler EA, Carrington CB. Open biopsy for chronic diffuse infiltrative lung disease: clinical, roentgenographic and physiological correlations in 502 patients. *Ann Thorac Surg* 1980; 30: 411.

117 Stanek V, Widimsky J, Kasalicky J *et al.* The pulmonary gas exchange during exercise in patients with pulmonary fibrosis. *Scand J Respir Dis* 1967; 48: 11.

118 Bye PTP, Anderson SD, Woolcock AJ *et al.* Bicycle endurance performance of patients with interstitial lung disease breathing air and oxygen. *Am Rev Respir Dis* 1982; 126: 1005.

119 Midgren B, Hansson L, Eriksson L. Oxygen desaturation during sleep and exercise in patients with interstitial lung disease. *Thorax* 1987; 42: 353.

120 Finley TN, Swenson EW, Comroe JH. The cause of arterial hypoxaemia at rest in patients with 'alveolar–capillary block syndrome'. *J Clin Invest* 1962; 41: 618.

121 Hamer J. Cause of low arterial oxygen saturation in pulmonary fibrosis. *Thorax* 1964; 19: 507.

122 McCarthy D, Cherniack RM. Regional ventilation–perfusion and hypoxia in cryptogenic fibrosing alveolitis. *Am Rev Respir Dis* 1973; 107: 200.

123 Wagner PD, Dantzker DR, Dueck R *et al.* Distribution of ventilation-perfusion ratios in patients with interstitial lung diseases. *Chest* 1976; 69: 256.

124 Perez-Padilla R, West P, Lertzman M, Kryger MH. Breathing during sleep in patients with interstitial lung disease. *Am Rev Respir Dis* 1985; 132: 224.

125 Spiro SG, Dowdeswell IRG, Clark TJH. An analysis of submaximal exercise responses in patients with sarcoidosis and fibrosing alveolitis. *Br J Dis Chest* 1981; 75: 169.

126 Jones NL, Rebuck AS. Tidal, during exercise in patients with diffuse fibrosing alveolitis. *Bull Eur Physiopathol Respir* 1979; 15: 321.

127 McGavin CR, Artvinli M, Naoe H, McHardy GJR. Dyspnoea, disability and distance walked: comparison of estimates of exercise performance in respiratory disease. *Br Med J* 1978; ii: 241.

128 Haslam P, Turton CWG, Lukoszek A *et al.* Bronchoalveolar lavage fluid cell counts in cryptogenic fibrosing alveolitis and their relation to therapy. *Thorax* 1980; 35: 328.

129 Rudd RM, Haslam P, Turner-Warwick M. Cryptogenic fibrosing alveolitis: relationships of pulmonary physiology and bronchoalveolar lavage to response to treatment and prognosis. *Am Rev Respir Dis* 1981; 124: 1.

130 Turner-Warwick M, Doniach D. Autoantibody studies in interstitial pulmonary fibrosis. *Br Med J* 1965; i: 886.

131 Haslam P, Turner-Warwick M, Lukoszek A. Antinuclear antibody and lymphocyte responses to nuclear antigens in patients with lung disease. *Clin Exp Immunol* 1975; 20: 379.

132 Tukiainen P, Taskinen E, Holsti P *et al.* Prognosis of cryptogenic fibrosing alveolitis. *Thorax* 1983; 38: 349.

133 Turner-Warwick M, Burrows B, Johnson A. Cryptogenic fibrosing alveolitis: response to corticosteroid treatment and its effect on survival. *Thorax* 1980; 35: 593.

134 Rudd RM, Haslam PL, Turner-Warwick M. Cryptogenic fibrosing alveolitis. Relationship of pulmonary physiology and bronchoalveolar lavage to response to treatment and prognosis. *Am Rev Respir Dis* 1981; 124: 1.

135 Peterson MW, Monick M, Hunninghake GW. Prognostic role of eosinophils in pulmonary fibrosis. *Chest* 1987; 92: 51.

136 Turner-Warwick M, Haslam PL. The value of serial bronchoalveolar lavages in assessing the clinical progress of patients with cryptogenic fibrosing alveolitis. *Am Rev Respir Dis* 1987; 135: 26.

137 Keogh BA, Bernardo J, Hunninghake GW *et al.* Effect of intermittent high dose parenteral corticosteroids on the alveolitis of idiopathic pulmonary fibrosis. *Am Rev Respir Dis* 1983; 127: 18.

138 Watters LC, King TE, Cherniack RM *et al.* Bronchoalveolar lavage neutrophils increase after corticosteroid therapy in smokers with

idiopathic pulmonary fibrosis. *Am Rev Respir Dis* 1986; 133: 104.

139 Brown CH, Turner-Warwick M. The treatment of cryptogenic fibrosing alveolitis with immunosuppressant drugs. *Q J Med* 1971; 40: 289.

140 Weese WC, Levine BW, Kazemi H. Interstitial lung disease resistant to corticosteroid therapy: report of three cases treated with azathioprine or cyclophosphamide. *Chest* 1975; 67: 57.

141 Johnson MA, Kwan S, Snell NJC, Nunn AJ, Darbyshire JH, Turner-Warwick M. Randomised controlled trial comparing prednisolone alone with cyclophosphamide and low dose prednisolone in combination in cryptogenic fibrosing alveolitis. *Thorax* 1989; 44: 280.

142 Raghu G, Depaso WJ, Cain K *et al.* Azathioprine combined with prednisolone in the treatment of idiopathic pulmonary fibrosis: a prospective, double blind, randomized, placebo controlled trial. *Am Rev Respir Dis* 1991; 144: 291.

143 Toronto Lung Transplant Group. Unilateral lung transplantation for pulmonary fibrosis. *N Engl J Med* 1986; 314: 1140.

144 Anon. Lung transplantation in perspective. *N Engl J Med* 1986; 314: 1186.

145 Hosenpud JD, Novick RJ, Bennett LE, Keck BM, Fiol B, Dail OP. The registry of the International Society for Heart and Lung Transplantation: thirteenth official report – 1996. *J Heart Lung Transplant* 1996; 15: 655.

146 Trulock EP. Lung transplantation: state of the art. *Am J Respir Crit Care Med* 1997; 155: 789.

147 Stack BHR, Choo-Kang YFJ, Heard BE. The prognosis of cryptogenic fibrosing alveolitis. *Thorax* 1972; 27: 535.

32

ASTHMA: EPIDEMIOLOGY

PETER G. J. BURNEY

Asthma is an important condition with a very variable prevalence that has become an increasing burden on health in both developing and market economies. The condition is associated with atopy, although its causes are otherwise poorly understood. Most people with asthma have mild disease with occasional exacerbations but some develop chronic airflow obstruction and patients with diagnosed asthma have a reduced expectation of life.

Definition and presentation

Asthma remains undefined. In 1958 a CIBA guest symposium set out to define chronic lung diseases and provided a definition of asthma as 'the condition of subjects with widespread narrowing of the bronchial airways which changes its severity over short periods of time either spontaneously or under treatment' [1]. This remains the benchmark definition, and several groups have refined or altered it to suit current hypotheses from time to time. However, it was pointed out soon after the publication of the symposium that this was less a definition than a description of the condition [2]. A true definition provides unambiguous criteria for deciding whether an individual has asthma or not. Despite this we are no nearer a definition and one recent attempt is perhaps even vaguer than the original on which it is based:

> a chronic inflammatory disorder of the airway in which many cells play a role, including mast cells and eosinophils. In susceptible individuals this inflammation causes symptoms which are usually associated with widespread but variable airflow obstruction that is often reversible either spontaneously or with treatment, and causes an associated increase in airway responsiveness to a variety of stimuli [3].

Because asthma is used to convey a complex idea, a simple definition is probably not possible and clarification has generally come through restricting the use of the term. For instance, 'renal asthma', a term used at the beginning of the century, is now not recognized and it is increasingly archaic to talk of 'cardiac asthma'. The utility of discussing all obstructive lung disease as a spectrum of disease with common aetiology (the Dutch hypothesis) is still debated [4]. Against the hypothesis, smoking and atopy are independent risk factors for bronchial hyperresponsiveness and appear to have their effects through different mechanisms [5,6]. The hyperresponsiveness associated with cigarette smoking only emerges in middle life and is more strongly associated with low lung function, whereas the hyperresponsiveness associated with atopy is seen much earlier in life. A number of people develop a condition very similar to atopic asthma, although they are not atopic in the conventional sense of having specific IgE to common inhalant allergen. Nevertheless these 'intrinsic asthmatics' have a histology similar to that of atopic asthmatics and it is speculated that the mechanisms are also similar [7].

In studying asthma, working definitions are required and a number of inconsistent methods have been used; the most common are given in Table 32.1. A clinical diagnosis of asthma is often used in clinical research. However, there is evidence for important differences, at least between countries, in the way that doctors identify patients with asthma [8], and the implicit lack of standardization in this method is unacceptable in epidemiological studies even when the study is small enough for the method to be feasible.

Patients' own reports of whether they have asthma are closely related to their reports on taking treatment for asthma and are largely determined by a doctor's diagnosis. This therefore has the same problem of poor standardization. In addition patients may not always know the doctor's diagnosis [9], and the diagnosis depends on the accessibility and quality of the local health services. This is a particularly severe restriction where surveys are being used in part to assess the quality of healthcare.

Questions concerning symptoms are less prone to these problems and as such are preferable, though they also have their limitations. There is no clear-cut symptom or symptom complex that is pathognomonic of asthma [10] and perception and reporting of symptoms

Table 32.1 Common methods for identifying asthma in surveys.

Clinical
    Doctor's assessment
    Patient's report of asthma
Symptomatic
    Wheeze
Physiological
    Peak flow variability
    Bronchial response to stimulus
        Direct: histamine, methacholine
        Indirect: cold air, exercise, adenosine
    Bronchial response to bronchodilators
    Bronchial response to steroids

may be affected by a number of psychological and cultural factors. Nevertheless there are now some well-standardized, symptom-based questionnaires that can be used [10–12].

Where questionnaires are potentially cheap and quick, physiological measures tend to be expensive to undertake in large surveys. Nevertheless they are less open to cultural influences and are a useful adjunct in epidemiological surveys. Once again, however, there is no physiological measure that is pathognomonic of asthma as it is generally understood and the different tests do not give closely related answers [13].

Improved lung function following administration of a bronchodilator is a useful clinical test but is probably less useful in surveys where 'asthmatic' subjects may have good lung function prior to the medication and therefore may not respond.

Bronchial challenge tests using bronchoconstrictor agents are now commonly used in surveys and simplified dosage schedules have been introduced [14]. Indirect challenge with cold air, non-isotonic saline, exercise or adenosine may be more specific for asthma, although there is less experience with adenosine in large surveys and standardization of the other methods is even more difficult. Extensive use has been made of histamine and methacholine challenge in surveys and there is now a great deal of experience with these. However, patients with cigarette-induced airway damage also respond to these tests. Challenge tests also tend to be relatively poorly standardized, as the effective dose delivered depends on the nature of the aerosol and this may vary considerably from one machine to another. Using the slope of the dose–response curve as the measure of responsiveness mitigates this problem and has the additional advantage that it provides a continuous measure of responsiveness [15].

In reality, the distinction between the normal and the abnormal is somewhat arbitrary and the level of abnormality selected as being significant is as important as the method of detection. In general it can be shown that specific tests give less misclassification, while the best test depends on the circumstances in which it is being used

and on the prevalence of disease in the population under study.

Distribution

Geography

Asthma is widely distributed but very variable in its prevalence. The use of standardized methods ensures that even though the absolute prevalence of the disease is unknowable, because the disease is undefined, the relative prevalence of the condition can be studied. It appears from surveys of children [16,17] and young adults [18] that the disease is more common in the English-speaking world and in some other areas such as France, of relatively lower prevalence in Scandinavia and in most of southern and eastern Europe, and very low in prevalence in some parts of rural Africa and other areas with markedly undeveloped ways of life [19–22]. There is some broad correlation between the prevalence of asthma and the prevalence of IgE antibodies to common inhaled allergens [23].

Age and sex

The incidence of diagnosed asthma as recorded in the USA is highest in the first year of life. In childhood the incidence is higher in boys than girls but reverses in the age group 15–50 years and reverses again in the older age group when the incidence among men increases once more [24]. The prevalence of bronchial responsiveness has been shown to follow a similar pattern, with boys having greater responsiveness than girls but adult women having higher levels than men and older men having similar levels of hyperresponsiveness as older women [25].

Women have lower levels of total and specific IgE than men and cross-sectional surveys show an increase in prevalence of sensitization during childhood and a marked decline with age in adult life [26,27]. However, cohort studies suggest that at least part of this later decline is due not to ageing but to the year of birth, implying that people who were born longer ago were less likely to become sensitized in the first place [28].

Ethnicity

Differences in atopy and asthma have been reported between different ethnic groups but whether these are due to genetic, environmental or cultural differences is unclear.

In the UK, there is greater respiratory morbidity in inner city areas, particularly among Afro-Caribbean and white children, although Afro-Caribbean children report slightly less asthma [29–31]. Black British and Caribbean children have also been found to have more atopic dermatitis [32,33], though in one of the surveys this was not true of black children from Africa [33]. In the USA, both serum IgE levels [34] and the prevalence of skin sensitivity [26] are slightly higher in African-Americans. Schwartz and colleagues [35] also found a significantly increased prevalence of diagnosed asthma (and to a lesser extent wheeze) in black children in the NHANES II study.

By contrast, in Southern Africa there was no difference in the prevalence of exercise-induced bronchoconstriction between black and white children living in the affluent northern suburbs of Harare [22].

In the UK, children from the Indian subcontinent tend to report fewer symptoms [36–38] but have been estimated to have either a greater prevalence of exercise-induced responsiveness [37] or equal prevalence of methacholine-induced responsiveness and a greater prevalence of atopy [38]. They have also been reported to have an increased tendency to respond to food additives, particularly fizzy drinks [39].

In New Zealand [40], European children have a higher prevalence of bronchial responsiveness than the Maoris, who in turn have a higher prevalence of responsiveness than the Pacific Islanders. However the Maoris report more symptoms than either the Europeans or Pacific Islanders. In young adults the Maoris also report more symptoms, though this is largely due to higher prevalence rates in those aged 30–44 years and the Maoris have lower rates of hay fever and are heavier smokers than the Europeans, suggesting that their increased symptoms may not be due to asthma.

Poverty/social status

The relation between poverty and wheezing is strongly confounded by exposure to cigarette smoke. Children from the 1958 birth cohort whose fathers were of higher social class were more likely to have hay fever and atopic dermatitis [41] and were more likely to be sensitive to common allergens at 33 years old [42], though there was no association with wheezy illness at that age when other factors had been taken into account [43]. The children of fathers of higher social class studied in the 1970 birth cohort were more likely to have persistent wheeze at the age of 16, though they had had less wheeze at the age of 5 [44]. Much of the excess risk of asthma in Baltimore could be explained better by poverty than by ethnicity alone [45]. In England and Wales more severe asthma has also been reported among adults from lower social classes [46].

Time

There is good evidence that the prevalence of wheezy illness has been increasing over the last couple of decades at least. Indirect evidence suggests that this may have been happening in some places from the early part of the

century, at least in those countries with high prevalence rates. It appears that this has been accompanied for the most part by changes in the prevalence of other atopic conditions [47,48] and in the prevalence of sensitivity to common aeroallergens [49,50]. It would be natural to conclude that much of the increase was secondary to this change in the prevalence of atopy. However it is likely that other factors are also involved and these would have to explain the changes in Australia, where there is evidence for an increasing prevalence of asthma but for a constant prevalence of atopy as measured by skin tests [51].

Admissions to hospitals with asthma have been increasing at approximately the same rate as the increase in the prevalence of disease. There is good reason to believe that hospital admission rates are affected by both health service factors and local prevalence rates [52,53], and the recent slowing down in the increase of admission rates in several countries may be due to health service pressure on costs and, in particular, financial pressure to reduce the use of inpatient facilities [54,55].

The major changes in mortality during the latter half of the twentieth century probably have little to do with changes in prevalence, although it is likely that mortality rates have been affected by changes in prevalence and this may be what is implied by the weak cohort effects found in mortality trends [56]. The changes in prevalence that have almost certainly occurred make it difficult to assess any long-term changes in the case fatality of the disease. Although evidence from life assurance companies, mostly in the USA, suggests that these have been relatively constant over the century, their interpretation is difficult [57].

Although the changes reported here are widespread, it should not be assumed that they have been universal. Trends are more likely to be studied where there is a prior belief that the rates are rising. Only a more systematic estimate of trends would allow generalizations to be made about such changes. The question of whether the same upward trends in prevalence are continuing is difficult to answer.

Early life

There are several characteristics of early life that predict atopy and asthma later in life. However, it is possible that these are, at least in some cases, predictors of continuing exposures that also persist into adult life. In the case of asthma at least, there is evidence for continuing plasticity as evidenced, for instance, in the effect of migration. In the UK, where there is regional variation in the prevalences of wheezy illness, children at the age of 5 or 7 years have prevalences of wheezy illness closer to those of the regions to which they have migrated than to those in the regions where they were born [58].

There are consistent reports that children from larger

families have less hay fever and atopy than those from smaller families. There is more debate as to whether this is an effect of large families or whether it is more specifically related to the number of older siblings. This finding has not generally been replicated when looking at the prevalence of asthma [59], although Seidman and colleagues [60] have described a similar relationship for asthma in Israeli military recruits.

Younger mothers have been noted to have infants with more wheezy lower respiratory tract infections [61] and 3–4 year olds with more asthma [62]. In the 1970 British birth cohort, children at the age of 16 were more likely to have persistent wheeze if their mothers were younger, but this was not the case at the age of 5 nor was it the case in the 1958 birth cohort. On the other hand, adolescents in Sheffield were found to have rather less hay fever if their mothers were younger [63].

Children who are born prematurely have a greater prevalence of sensitization to allergens [64]. They are also more likely to have wheezy illness [35,65,66] and asthma [67] at primary school age. However, prematurity was not associated with wheezy illness in either the 1958 [43] or 1970 [44] birth cohorts and Olesen and colleagues [68] concluded that atopic dermatitis was more common in postmature children. Bertrand and colleagues [69] hypothesized that both children who were born prematurely and their mothers might be more likely to have airway hyperresponsiveness, though others [70], while confirming the association between low birthweight and later airway responsiveness, were unable to link this with maternal airway responsiveness.

Low birthweight children have been reported to have a greater risk of having asthma and wheeze in childhood [35,70], asthma or wheeze at 16 [71] and asthma as young adults [60] and a lower lung function as primary school children [65] and adults [72]. However, others have reported no greater risk of asthma in childhood [65,67,73] and a reduced risk of atopic dermatitis in low birthweight babies [68].

Exposure to allergens

Exposure to allergen is necessary for sensitization and for subsequent expression of disease, although as allergens are widespread other factors may well be more important in determining whether sensitization takes place. Some studies have shown that sensitivity to house-dust mite is rare among children where antigen levels are less than 2 pg/g of dust but is increasingly likely as levels rise above this value [74,75]; areas with low levels of dust mite antigens have low prevalence of sensitivity to the allergen [76,77]. Studies have also suggested that cat ownership is associated with sensitization to cats in children [64,78]. However, others have shown very little relation between domestic levels of allergen and sensitivity to mites [79,80]

or cat [79] and Rugtveit [81] was unable to find an association between pet ownership and sensitization to cat or dog.

There is considerable interest in the possibility that early exposure to allergen may be particularly important. The evidence for this is based largely on the association between sensitization to particular allergens and month of birth. A number of studies have shown a strong association between mite allergen sensitivity and birth in the latter part of the year [82–85]. However, in the UK at least, mite is not a strongly seasonal allergen, and there is only very inconsistent evidence that pollen allergen is related to month of birth.

It is unlikely that increased exposure to allergen has led to the increase in sensitization mentioned earlier. Although insulation of housing has increased and it has been shown that reduced ventilation leads to increases in levels of both cat [86] and mite [87] allergens in the home, the two studies that have documented increases in sensitivity to allergens [49,50] have shown that the increase is not due to increases in indoor allergens alone and there is little evidence for an increase in other allergens [88].

Exposure of sensitized subjects to allergen increases bronchial reactivity and this increase is associated with the late asthmatic response [89]. In the USA the increase in emergency room visits with asthma that occurs in the spring has been associated with raised IgE to grass pollen allergen [90] and several studies have shown an association between indoor mite allergen levels and clinical disease [80,91]. There is further evidence that acute severe asthma may be associated with exposure to high ambient levels of indoor allergen [92].

Epidemics of asthma are rare but those that have been recorded have mostly been associated with allergen. The best documented of these were the epidemics of asthma in Barcelona associated with the release of soybean allergen [93]. Other epidemics have been associated with castor bean allergen [94,95] and possibly grass allergen released from pollen during thunderstorms [96,97].

Mortality among young asthmatics also shows a seasonal variation and this is particularly marked in those who die suddenly [98,99]. Increases in acute severe asthma and asthma deaths have been reported following exposure to moulds [100–102] and to soybean dust [93]. The role of indoor allergen in asthma deaths is poorly understood.

Smoking

Smoking has frequently been associated with higher levels of total serum IgE [103–106]. Although adjustment for age and gender, which are important confounders, reduces the size of this association, the association is not entirely explained by these [107,108].

Allergy to occupational allergens has been found to be

increased in smokers compared with non-smokers [109–111], though the same studies often showed no increase in the sensitivity to common inhaled allergens among smokers. In contrast, a number of studies have shown that the sensitivity to common allergens is reduced among smokers [42,104,107,108]. In two of these studies [107,108], the response to mite allergens was apparently dissimilar to that of the other common inhaled allergens including grass and cat. All these studies are cross-sectional and might be biased by the tendency of those who are sensitized to avoid smoking. However, evidence from the Tucson study suggests that this is not the explanation [28].

The effect of maternal smoking on sensitization is disputed. Magnusson reported an increase in cord IgE and subsequent infant allergy in the children of mothers who smoked during pregnancy. However subsequent investigators have generally not been able to replicate this [112].

Smoking causes a temporary increase in airway responsiveness [113], although smokers also develop a more persistent airway hyperresponsiveness [5,114,115]. This is associated with a fall in baseline airway function and does not reverse on quitting smoking [6], suggesting that it is secondary to structural damage to the lung. Patients with asthma who give up smoking experience a reduction of airway responsiveness [116], but there is little evidence that smokers are at any increased risk of developing asthma [117].

Since Colley [118] first drew attention to the effects of 'passive' smoking on the respiratory health of infants, a large body of literature has grown up to support his conclusions [119], although this effect is generally less marked after the first year of life [120]. Some studies have shown an increase in airway responsiveness in the children of mothers who smoke [121,122] but others have found either inconsistent [123,124] or negative [125–127] results. In Saskatchewan, non-allergic children and adolescents exposed to smoking had an increased prevalence of 'asthma' that was not found in the allergic children [128]. Evans and colleagues [129] found that asthmatic children from families that smoked were more likely to use emergency rooms, though this may have been due to unresolved confounding by other social factors. In contrast, Ehrlich and colleagues [127] found an increased prevalence of asthma in the children of mothers who smoked but were unable to show an increased risk of acute attacks of asthma.

Air pollution

Air pollution is frequently cited as an important cause of asthma and its exacerbation. There is no good evidence that air pollution in general causes asthma, though it has been hypothesized that traffic pollution may be a cause of the increased prevalence noted recently in the market economies. The pollution traditionally associated with cities, where coal burning was a major source of sulphur dioxide and particulates, has largely disappeared from the countries that have experienced the major increase in asthma prevalence.

Changes in symptoms and lung function have been noted in both normal and asthmatic populations in relation to increases in air pollution, although these have been for the most part relatively mild changes. Studies of mortality and admissions for asthma in relation to air pollution episodes have generally shown equally small and inconsistent effects. Several investigators have been surprised by such findings. During the famous London smog of December 1952 John Fry, a general practitioner in south London, reported that there was almost no effect of the smog on his young asthmatic patients [130]. In the air pollution episode that affected a large part of central Europe in 1985, admissions rose in affected areas compared with unaffected areas for stroke, ischaemic heart disease and chronic obstructive pulmonary disease but, if anything, fell for asthma [131]. These findings seem to bear out the observations of Henry Hyde Salter that 'it is, one may almost say, a *law* of asthma for it to be better in the air of great cities' [132].

On the other hand, there have been major [133] and some less extensive [134] episodes in which asthma has been reported to have been a problem, and the APHEA studies in Europe showed a modest increase in asthma admissions related to increases in nitrogen dioxide and, in children, with increases in sulphur dioxide levels [135].

One complicating factor in all of this is the role that might be played by allergen. The dramatic effects of exposure to allergen have already been described and the question arises whether allergen may play a role also in more normal circumstances. It is notable that the epidemics in Barcelona that were eventually shown to be due to the release of soybean allergen were at first attributed to oxides of nitrogen [136]. The reason for this is that the same weather conditions that lead to the build-up of one type of pollution may also lead to the build-up of another. The problem has been that there is no way of monitoring allergen, only a limited range of allergenic particles, such as pollens and molds, or specific allergens that have been identified and are under suspicion. However, the data from Barcelona suggest that low levels of allergen can contribute to asthma admissions without producing epidemics [137] and other allergens such as latex have been demonstrated in respirable particles from ambient air [138]. Such confounding could explain the relatively weak and inconsistent effects of air pollution on asthma.

Infection and infestation

Frick [139,140] suggested that viruses could potentiate

sensitization to aeroallergens. Some bacterial antigens can act in the same way and pertussis vaccine can enhance IgE responses in animals [141], though natural pertussis infection does not lead to persistent respiratory disease [142,143].

As many as 70% of children respond to respiratory syncytial virus (RSV) with specific IgE, although those that have persistent anti-RSV IgE tend to have a family history or a personal history of wheeze [144]. This suggests that response with IgE may be normal but that persistence of the response is dependent on some other personal characteristic, possibly a genetic susceptibility. While it is true that children who develop RSV bronchiolitis are more likely to go on to develop episodic airways obstruction [145], it is not clear that this is cause and effect; it may simply be that those who are going to develop asthma and who become infected with RSV are more likely to have a severe episode of bronchiolitis. It has been shown, for instance, that children who are born with small airways are more likely to develop wheezing when they contract a lower respiratory tract infection [146]. The principal evidence against this interpretation in the case of RSV is the coincidence between the month of birth of those who develop asthma severe enough to be admitted to hospital and the month of birth of those who develop bronchiolitis [147]. It has also been suggested that persistent steroid-resistant asthma may be induced by chronic adenoviral infection [148].

On the other hand, there are alternative theories that suggest that early infection may suppress allergic responses and even the development of the atopic phenotype. In West Africa, a history of severe infection with measles was shown to be associated with a reduced prevalence of atopy, particularly sensitivity to mite allergen [149]. A strong response to tuberculin in Japanese schoolchildren who had received bacille Calmette–Guérin (BCG) vaccine was also inversely related to atopy [150]. Serological evidence of infection by hepatitis A has also been shown to be inversely related to the prevalence of atopy in Italian military recruits [151]. All of these studies have been used to argue the case that early infection may affect the development of the immune response from one characterized by T lymphocytes producing interleukin (IL)-2, interferon γ and tumour necrosis factor to one characterized by T lymphocytes producing IL-4, IL-5, IL-6 and IL-10. At least in the second of these studies it is likely that those who respond to BCG with a tuberculin response are less likely to respond to allergen with an atopic response, rather than that BCG infection itself alters the immune response [150].

The simple view that any early infection reduces the risk of atopy is not well substantiated. Although Martinez and colleagues [152] have found that children experiencing non-wheezing lower respiratory tract infections in early life have a lower prevalence of atopy, Strachan and colleagues [63] found no association between early infection and subsequent atopy. Nor is there evidence of an inverse relationship between atopy and the common childhood infections [153].

There is much better evidence that acute viral infections of the respiratory tract, particularly rhinovirus and parainfluenza virus infections, cause acute exacerbations of asthma. Viruses cause exacerbations of asthma in both children [154] and adults [155] and infections are the commonest reported cause of exacerbations of asthma at all ages [27]. It seems likely that there is an interactive effect of viral infections and allergy in causing severe episodes of respiratory disease in children [156].

Diet

Until the introduction of effective treatments for managing asthma, there was considerable interest in the effects of diet on the condition, and early in the twentieth century there were already hypotheses that food might induce asthma by anaphylaxis or by pharmacological means. The resulting fashion for restrictive diets was reversed in the middle of the century following increasing concern over the effects of these diets on nutrition and the introduction of double-blind food challenge as the criterion for assessing hypersensitivity to food. Although food sensitivity is common in children, and as many as 13% of adults complain of food-associated symptoms, current estimates of true food sensitivity in adults lie between 1 per 10000 and 2.3 per 1000 [157].

Infant feeding

There is some evidence that allergy in early life may be reduced by breast-feeding and allergen avoidance. A randomized controlled trial of breast milk in premature neonates found less allergy in the treated children, but only among those who had a family history [158]. Zeiger and colleagues [159] also found a reduction of atopic disease in breast-fed babies where both mother and baby avoided allergen in the diet, but were unable to show a reduction in either rhinitis or asthma or in sensitization to inhalant allergens. Although Burr and colleagues [160] were able to show a reduction in wheezy illness early in life in those babies who had been breast-fed on any occasion, most studies show little difference in the incidence of asthma in those who were breast-fed and those who were not [161]. This is the conclusion from the two large British birth cohorts [162,163] and the Melbourne cohort in which the subjects with the longest history of breast-feeding had the worst asthma [164].

Overall nutrition

There is little evidence on the effects of overall nutrition on asthma, although there is some evidence that children with protein-calorie malnutrition are less likely to show skin sensitivity to common allergens [165]. At an ecological level, Keeley showed that the response to exercise in African children was related to body size, with the communities with smaller and lighter children having the least response to exercise. Such ecological data are hard to interpret, but Sommerville and colleagues [166] have also shown that children who are heavy for their height are more likely to have wheezy illnesses and in the Second National Health and Nutritional Examination Survey in the USA a two standard deviation increase in triceps skin-fold thickness increased the prevalence of frequent wheeze by 60% [167].

Lipid

The Victorians believed in the efficacy of cod liver oil for asthma [168] and interest in this was revived by a corresponding interest in the role of lipid mediators in asthma. Clinical studies showed that fish oil in the diet could reduce the production of lipid mediators and blunt the late allergic response [169] but this had little influence on clinical asthma and aspirin-sensitive asthmatic patients deteriorated [170]. More recently interest has returned to this mechanism, with some epidemiological evidence that those who eat a diet rich in fish are less likely to have asthma [171]. However, others have been unable to demonstrate any difference in the ω-3 fatty acid content of the diet of women who became asthmatic in middle life [172].

Antioxidants

The lung has elaborate defences against oxidant damage and these are likely to be stressed in patients with asthma. Some of these defences are dietary in origin and Seaton has suggested that the increase in asthma may be due in part to a change in the diet with, in particular, a decline in the consumption of vitamin C. Trials of vitamin C in patients with asthma were first undertaken in the 1930s, with little success [173,174], and trials since that time have had mixed results. While neither Kreisman and colleagues [175] nor Malo and colleagues [176] were able to demonstrate any effect on either symptoms or hyperresponsiveness, others have reported reductions in the number and severity of attacks, the response to exercise and the response to methacholine. There are moreover several studies that have demonstrated lower levels of vitamin C in asthmatic patients [177–180] and those with hyperresponsiveness [181]. Low levels of vitamin C have also been associated with low lung function in men [182] and symptoms of chronic bronchitis [167].

In addition to the effects of vitamin C, there is suggestive evidence that vitamin E may also protect against the onset of asthma in mid-life [172]. Selenium is a further micronutrient that has an important role in antioxidant activity in the lung. A number of studies have demonstrated a low level of selenium in patients with asthma [183–186]. One small randomized controlled trial has shown a clinical improvement in those taking selenium supplements but no change in lung function or airway reactivity [187].

Electrolytes

Two electrolytes have received most attention with regard to their effects on asthma. Magnesium has been used for a long time as a bronchodilator [188], although it has disappointing results in acute severe asthma. A number of studies have shown that dietary magnesium is associated with lower prevalence of airway hyperresponsiveness in population surveys [181,189], though experimental studies have not suggested a strong effect on airway responsiveness [190]. Dietary sodium has been associated with increased bronchial responsiveness in one study [191], while other cross-sectional studies have shown weak or negative effects [192,193]. Experimental studies have suggested that a high sodium load does increase airway responsiveness in men [194,195] but not in women, and this is consistent with a finding that regions of England with high sales of table salt had an increased mortality from asthma for men and children but not for women [196]. The mechanism is unknown but it has been shown that serum from men with asthma increased sodium influx into donor cells and that this influx and dietary sodium were independently related to the airway responsiveness [197].

Prognosis

Symptoms and lung function

A high proportion of children wheeze, though relatively few persist with severe respiratory problems. In the 1958 birth cohort, of all the children whose parents had reported wheeze in the first 7 years of life, only 50% were still wheezing at 7 years, 18% at 11 years and 10% at 16 years. At 23 years, this figure was still only 10% but by 33 the figure had risen again to 27% [43]. During childhood the reduction in symptoms with age is paralleled by a fall in airway responsiveness [198]. A relatively poor prognosis is associated with the presence of atopy and severity of disease, which is itself associated with atopy. Of those with persistent symptoms in childhood, relatively few are symptom-free in adult life [199].

A low lung function and bronchial responsiveness in childhood are predictive of low lung function and bronchial responsiveness in adult life [200]. Furthermore, those who have persistent wheeze during childhood and are still wheezing in adulthood have low lung function that is not fully reversed by salbutamol. However, although symptomatic children have low lung function, the growth of their lung function with age is normal [201]. It seems likely therefore that asthma does not have an adverse effect on lung growth in childhood. In adulthood the effects of asthma on decline in lung function are unclear. Poor lung function is clearly associated with severe asthma [202] and is also associated with an increased mortality both in those with asthma [203] and others [204]. However, although two studies have reported a more rapid decline in lung function in patients with asthma [205,206], others have not [207] and Burrows and colleagues [208] found a normal rate of decline in lung function in those who had an unequivocal diagnosis of asthma with evidence of atopy and no history of smoking.

Mortality

Follow-up of representative populations in the UK [209] and the USA [210] has shown an excess of mortality in those with diagnosed asthma. This excess increases with age and is negligible under the age of 45 years. Evidence from the life assurance companies also suggests that there is a small excess of mortality in those with a diagnosis of asthma, but this source also identifies a reduced mortality in those with other allergic diseases. This latter observation may explain why there is no excess of mortality in younger age groups although deaths from asthma do occur.

Recording

Most studies of the validity of mortality statistics in asthma have studied the certificates and circumstances of death of those who have been certified as dying of asthma. These have generally concluded that, at least in younger subjects, the certificates are fairly accurate [211,212] though others have suggested that the certificates overestimate the number of deaths due to asthma [213]. For a clear view of accuracy, a study needs to assess both false-positive and false-negative rates. Where this has been done it has been found that the false-positive certificates are likely to balance or outweigh the false-negative certificates [214–216].

Vagueness in the definition of asthma and the presence of multiple pathology in older subjects inevitably leads to some uncertainty in ascribing any death to asthma in this age group. However, it also seems likely that there are more systematic biases in the variation in certification from country to country. Kelson and Heller [217] sent case histories to samples of doctors who had signed death certificates in eight European countries and asked them to complete death certificates for each of the cases. There was

considerable variation between countries and these differences related to the recorded mortality rates from asthma for the countries in the study [8].

Trends

Overall mortality rates from asthma in England and Wales have not changed greatly over the course of the century. However this has not been consistent in all age groups. While mortality from asthma in the older age groups has declined throughout the century, that in adolescents and young adults has tended to rise [99]. In addition, there have been increases in mortality in the 1960s [218] and the 1980s [219].

Overtreatment

Possibly because the early writers on asthma assumed that it was a largely benign condition that did not kill patients, much of what has been written on the subject since has related to iatrogenic causes of death. Early case reports concentrated on the dangers associated with respiratory depressants [220,221], while in more recent times the dangers of aspirin and other non-steroidal anti-inflammatory drugs have been emphasized. Of greater concern, however, has been the possibility that the drugs used to treat asthma might themselves be responsible for the deaths.

The first to suggest this were Benson and Perlman [222] who noticed that patients using epinephrine (adrenaline) sprays, mostly sold by door-to-door salesmen, had a seven-fold risk of death from asthma. The problem that was unresolved by this study was whether those taking the sprays had more severe disease. The hypothesis was revived in the 1960s when there was an increase in mortality from asthma in a number of countries that had licensed high-dose isoproterenol inhalers for the management of asthma. Early enquiries showed that a high proportion of the asthmatics who died were using these [223], while other studies showed a close association between the time course of the deaths and the use of these medications [218,224].

A further epidemic of deaths from asthma in New Zealand in the 1980s led to renewed interest in this hypothesis, in this case implicating the drug fenoterol. This was another potent bronchodilator prescribed in high doses and widely used in New Zealand. Case–control studies identified patients treated with fenoterol as being at increased risk, and the time course of the epidemic of deaths was interpreted as being compatible with fenoterol having been responsible. Despite this, a prospective study in Canada was unable to confirm the finding, though it showed that both salbutamol and fenoterol were prescribed in increasing amounts prior to the death of an asthmatic patient. The question of how far fenoterol was to blame for the increase in asthma deaths in New Zealand in the 1970s and 1980s is still controversial. However, it is clear that there were less spectacular increases in deaths in other countries such as the USA at the same time where fenoterol was not licensed.

Undertreatment

Another line of inquiry into asthma deaths has focused on undertreatment. Historically, much of the evidence for undertreatment being associated with death has come from uncontrolled enquiries into asthma deaths [225–229]. More recently, however, there has emerged more specific evidence that treatment with steroids may reduce mortality substantially [230,231]. Those treated with regular inhaled steroids appear to have approximately one-third the risk of death of those who are not.

Summary

Asthma is a disease that has become increasingly common over the last century. Although it is very variable in its severity, it is now a common cause of disability. The causes are still unknown. It has a genetic component although this cannot explain the increase in the disease or much of the variation in prevalence. It is associated with atopy but only a minority of atopic individuals are asthmatic. The major questions remain what circumstances lead to an increase in the disease and what factors lead to a deterioration in the condition.

References

1 Anon. Terminology, definitions, and classification of chronic pulmonary emphysema and related conditions: a report of the conclusions of a CIBA guest symposium. *Thorax* 1959; 14: 286.

2 Scadding JG. Meaning of diagnostic terms in broncho-pulmonary disease. *Br Med J* 1963; 7: 1425.

3 National Institutes of Health, National Heart, Lung and Blood Institute. International consensus report on diagnosis and treatment of asthma. *Eur Respir J* 1992; 5: 601.

4 Pride N. Smoking, allergy and airways obstruction: revival of the 'Dutch hypothesis'. *Clin Allergy* 1986; 16: 3.

5 Burney PGJ, Britton JR, Chinn S et al. Descriptive epidemiology of bronchial reactivity in an adult population: results from a community study. *Thorax* 1987; 42: 38.

6 Lim TK, Taylor RG, Watson A, Joyce H, Pride NB. Changes in bronchial responsiveness to inhaled histamine over four years in middle aged male smokers and ex-smokers. *Thorax* 1988; 43: 599.

7 Bentley AM, Menz G, Storz C et al. Identification of T lymphocytes, macrophages, and activated eosinophils in the bronchial mucosa in intrinsic asthma. Relationship to symptoms and bronchial responsiveness. *Am Rev Respir Dis* 1992; 146: 500.

8 Burney PGJ. The effect of death certification practice on recorded national asthma mortality rates. *Rev Epidemiol Sante Publique* 1989; 37: 385.

9 Burney PGJ, Laitinen LA, Perdrizet S et al. Validity and repeatability of the IUATLD (1984) Bronchial Symptoms Questionnaire: an international comparison. *Eur Respir J* 1989; 2: 940.

10 Burney PGJ, Chinn S, Tattersfield AE, Papacosta AO. What symptoms predict the bronchial response to histamine? *Int J Epidemiol* 1989; 18: 165.

11 Abramson MJ, Hensley MJ, Saunders NA, Wlodarczyk JH. Evaluation of a new asthma questionnaire. *J Asthma* 1991; 28: 129.

12 Shaw R, Woodman K, Ayson M et al. Measuring the prevalence of bronchial hyperresponsiveness in children. *Int J Epidemiol* 1995; 24: 597.

13 Sierstedt HC, Mostgaard G, Hyldebrandt N, Hansen HS, Boldsen J, Oxhoj H. Interrelationships between diagnosed asthma, asthma like symptoms and abnormal airway behaviour in adolescence: the Odense schoolchild study. *Thorax* 1996; 51: 503.

14 Yan K, Salome C, Woolcock AJ. Rapid method for measurement of bronchial responsiveness. *Thorax* 1983; 38: 760.

15 Chinn S, Arossa WA, Jarvis DL, Luczynska CM, Burney PG. Variation in nebulizer aerosol output and weight output from the Mefar dosimeter: implications for multicentre studies. *Eur Respir J* 1997; 10: 452.

16 Burr ML, Limb ES, Andrae S, Barry DMJ, Nagel F. Childhood asthma in four countries: a comparative study. *Int J Epidemiol* 1994; 23: 341.

17 Pearce N, Weiland S, Keil U et al. Self-reported prevalence of asthma symptoms in children in Australia, England, Germany and New Zealand: an international comparison using the ISAAC protocol. *Eur Respir J* 1993; 6: 1455.

18 Burney P, Chinn S, Jarvis D, Luczynska C, Lai E. Variations in the prevalence of respiratory symptoms, self-reported asthma attacks, and use of asthma medication in the European Community Respiratory Health Survey (ECRHS). *Eur Respir J* 1996; 9: 687.

19 Anderson HR. The epidemiological and allergic features of asthma in the New Guinea Highlands. *Clin Allergy* 1974; 4: 171.

20 Godfrey RC. Asthma and IgE levels in rural and urban communities of The Gambia. *Clin Allergy* 1975; 5: 201.

21 Van Niekerk CH, Weinberg EG, Shore SC, Heese H, Van Schalkwyk J. Prevalence of asthma: a comparative study of urban and rural Xhosa children. *Clin Allergy* 1979; 9: 319.

22 Keeley DJ, Gallivan S. Comparison of the prevalence of reversible airways obstruction in rural and urban Zimbabwean children. *Thorax* 1991; 46: 549.

23 Burney P, Malmberg E, Chinn S, Jarvis D, Luczynska C, Lai E. The distribution of total and specific IgE in the European Community Respiratory Health Survey. *J Allergy Clin Immunol* 1997; 99: 314.

24 Yunginger JW, Reed CE, O'Connell EJ, Melton LJ, O'Fallon WM, Silverstein MD. A community-based study of the epidemiology of asthma. *Am Rev Respir Dis* 1992; 146: 888.

25 Paoletti P, Carrozzi L, Viegi G et al. Distribution of bronchial hyperresponsiveness in a general population: effect of sex, age, smoking and level of pulmonary function. *Am J Respir Crit Care Med* 1995; 151: 1770.

26 Anon. Percutaneous immediate hypersensitivity to eight allergens: United States 1976. *Vital Health Stat* 1998; 235: 1.

27 Prescott-Clarke P, Primatesta P. Health survey for England 1995. 1997.

28 Barbee RA, Kaltenborn W, Lebowitz MD, Burrows B. Longitudinal changes in allergen skin test reativity in a community population sample. *J Allergy Clin Immunol* 1987; 79: 16.

29 Melia RJW, Chinn S, Rona RJ. Respiratory illness and home environment of ethnic groups. *Br Med J* 1988; 296: 1438.

30 Johnston IDA, Bland JM, Anderson HR. Ethnic variation in respiratory morbidity and lung function in childhood. *Thorax* 1987; 42: 542.

31 Duran-Tauleria E, Rona RJ, Chinn S, Burney P. Influence of ethnic group on asthma treatment in children in 1990–1: national cross sectional study. *Br Med J* 1996; 313: 148.

32 Golding J, Peters TJ. The epidemiology of childhood eczema: I. A population based study of associations. *Paediatr Perinat Epidemiol* 1987; 1: 67.

33 Williams HC, Pembroke AC, Forsdyke H, Boodoo G, Hay RJ, Burney PGJ. London-born black Caribbean children are at increased risk of atopic dermatitis. *J Am Acad Dermatol* 1995; 32: 212.

34 Grundbacher FJ, Massie FS. Levels of immunoglobulin F, M, A, and E at various ages in allergic and non allergic black and white individuals. *J Allergy Clin Immunol* 1985; 75: 651.

35 Schwartz J, Gold D, Dockery DW, Weiss ST, Speizer FE. Predictors of asthma and persistent wheeze in a national sample of children in the United States. *Am Rev Respir Dis* 1990; 142: 555.

36 Pararajasingam CD, Sittampalam L, Damani

P, Pattemore K, Holgate S. Comparison of the prevalence of asthma among Asian and European children in Southampton. *Thorax* 1992; 47: 529.

37 Jones CO, Qureshi S, Rona RJ, Chinn S. Exercise-induced bronchoconstriction by ethnicity and presence of asthma in British nine year olds. *Thorax* 1996; 51: 1134.

38 Carey OJ, Cookson JB, Britton J, Tattersfield AE. The efrect of lifestyle on wheeze, atopy, and bronchial hyperreactivity in Asian and white children. *Am J Respir Crit Care Med* 1996; 154: 537.

39 Wilson MN. Food related asthma: a differ-ence between two ethnic groups. *Arch Dis Child* 1985; 60: 861.

40 Mitchell EA. Racial inequalities in childhood asthma. *Soc Sci Med* 1991; 32: 831.

41 Williams HC, Strachan DP, Hay RJ. Child-hood eczema: disease of the advantaged? *Br Med J* 1994; 308: 1132.

42 Strachan DP, Harkins LS, Johnston IDA, Anderson HR. Childhood antecedents of allergic sensitization in young British adults. *J Allergy Clin Immunol* 1997; 99: 6.

43 Strachan DP, Butland BK, Anderson HR. Incidence and prognosis of asthma and wheezing illness from early childhood to age 33 in a national British cohort. *Br Med J* 1996; 312: 1195.

44 Lewis S, Richards D, Bynner J, Butler N, Britton J. Prospective study of risk factors for early and persistent wheezing in child-hood. *Eur Respir J* 1995; 8: 349.

45 Mak H, Johnston P, Abbey H, Talamo R. Prevalence of asthma and health service utilization of asthmatic children in an inner city. *J Allergy Clin Immunol* 1982; 70: 367.

46 Littlejohns P, Macdonald LD. The relation-ship between severe asthma and social class. *Respir Med* 1993; 87: 139.

47 Burr ML, Butland BK, King S, Vaughan-Williams E. Changes in asthma prevalence: two surveys 15 years apart. *Arch Dis Child* 1989; 64: 1452.

48 Taylor B, Wadsworth M, Wadsworth J, Peckham C. Changes in the reported preva-lence of childhood eczema since the 1939–45 war. *Lancet* 1984; i: 1255.

49 Gassner M. Immunologische-allergologische reactionen unter veran-derten umweltbedudngingen. *Schweiz Rundsch Med Prax* 1992; 81: 426.

50 Nakagomi T, Itaya H, Tominaga T, Yamaki M, Hisamatsu N, Nakagomi O. Is atopy increasing? *Lancet* 1994; 343: 121.

51 Peat JK, van den Berg. RH, Green WF, Mellis CM, Leeder SR. Changing prevalence of asthma in Australian children. *Br Med J* 1994; 308: 1591.

52 Burney PGJ, Papacosta AO, Withey CH, Colley JRT, Holland WW. Hospital admis-sion rates and the prevalence of asthma symptoms in 20 local authority districts. *Thorax* 1991; 46: 574.

53 Connett GJ, Warde C, Wooler E, Lenney W. Audit strategies to reduce hospital admis-sions for acute asthma. *Arch Dis Child* 1993; 69: 202.

54 Vollmer WM, Osborne ML, Buist S. Tempo-ral trends in hospital-based episodes of asthma care in a health maintenance organi-sation. *Am Rev Respir Dis* 1993; 147: 347.

55 Hyndman SJ, Williams DRR, Merill SL, Lipscombe JM, Palmer CR. Rates of admis-sion to hospital for asthma. *Br Med J* 1994; 308: 1596.

56 Burney P. Asthma deaths in England and Wales 1931–85: evidence for a true increase in asthma mortality. *J Epidemiol Community Health* 1988; 42: 316.

57 Brackenridge RDC. Respiratory system disease. In: Lew EA, Gajewski J, eds. *Medical Risks: Trends in Mortality by Age and Time Elapsed*. New York: Praeger, 1990: 8-1.

58 Strachan DP, Golding J, Anderson HR. Regional variations in wheezing illness in British children: effect of migration during early childhood. *J Epidemiol Community Health* 1990; 44: 231.

59 Jarvis D, Chinn S, Luczynska C, Burney P. The association of family size with atopy and atopic disease. *Clin Exp Allergy* 1997; 27: 240.

60 Seidman DS, Laor A, Gale R, Stevenson DK, Danon YL. Is low birth weight a risk factor for asthma during adolescence? *Arch Dis Child* 1991; 66: 584.

61 Martinez FD, Wright AL, Holberg CJ, Morgan WJ, Taussig LM. Maternal age as a risk factor for wheezing lower respiratory illnesses in the first year of life. *Am J Epi-demiol* 1992; 136: 1258.

62 Infante-Rivard C. Young maternal age: a risk factor of childhood asthma? *Epidemiology* 1995; 6: 178.

63 Strachan DP, Taylor EM, Carpenter RG. Family structure, neonatal infection, and hay fever in adolescence. *Arch Dis Child* 1996; 74: 422.

64 Kuehr J, Frischer T, Karmaus T et al. Early childhood risk factors for sensitization at school age. *J Allergy Clin Immunol* 1992; 90: 358.

65 Rona RJ, Gulliford MC, Chinn S. Effects of prematurity and interuterine growth on res-piratory health and lung function in child-hood. *Br Med J* 1993; 306: 817.

66 Frischer T, Kuehr J, Meinert R, Karmaus W, Urbanek R. Risk factors for childhood asthma and recurrent wheezy bronchitis. *Eur J Pediatr* 1993; 152: 771.

67 Kelly YJ, Brabin BJ, Millgan P, Heaf DP, Reid J, Pearson MG. *Thorax* 1995; 50: 525.

68 Olesen AB, Ellingsen AR, Olesen H, Juul S, Thestrup-Pedersen K. Atopic dermatitis and birth factors: historical follow up by record linkage. *Br Med J* 1997; 314: 1003.

69 Bertrand J-M, Riley SP, Popkin J, Coates AL. The long-term pulmonary sequelae of pre-maturity: the role of familial airway hyper-reactivity and the respiratory distress syndrome. *N Engl J Med* 1985; 312: 742.

70 Chan KN, Noble-Jamieson CM, Elliman A, Bryan EM, Silverman M. Lung function in children of low birth weight. *Arch Dis Child* 1989; 64: 1284.

71 Lewis S, Butland B, Strachan D et al. Study of the aetiiology of wheezing illness at age 16 in two national British birth cohorts. *Thorax* 1996; 51: 670.

72 Barker DJP, Godfrey KM, Fall C, Osmond C, Winter PD, Shaheen SO. Relation of birth weight and childhood respiratory infection to adult lung function and death from chronic obstructive airways disease. *Br Med J* 1991; 303: 671.

73 Sears MR, Holdaway MD, Flannery EM, Herbison GP, Silva PA. Parental and neona-tal risk factors for atopy, airway hyper-responsiveness, and asthma. *Arch Dis Child* 1996; 75: 392.

74 Lau S, Falkenhorst G, Weber A et al. High mite-allergen exposure increases the risk of

sensitization in atopic children and young adults. *J Allergy Clin Immunol* 1989; 84: 718.

75 Sporik R, Holgate T, Platts-Mills TAE, Cogswell JJ. Exposure to house-dust mite allergen (*Der p I*) and the development of asthma in childhood. *N Engl J Med* 1990; 323: 502.

76 Charpin D, Kleisbauer JP, Lanteaume A et al. Asthma and allergy to house-dust mites in populations living in high altitudes. *Chest* 1988; 93: 758.

77 Britton WJ, Woolcock AJ, Peat JK, Sedgewick CJ, Lloyd DM, Leeder SR. Preva-lence of bronchial hyperresponsiveness in children: the relationship between asthma and skin reactivity to allergens in two com-munities. *Int J Epidemiol* 1986; 15: 202.

78 Suoniemi I, Bjorksten F, Haahtela T. Depen-dence of immediate hypersensitivity in the adolescent period on factors encountered in infancy. *Allergy* 1981; 36: 263.

79 Burr ML, Limb ES, Maguire MJ et al. Infant feeding, wheezing, and allergy: a prospec-tive study. *Arch Dis Child* 1993; 68: 724.

80 Hart B, Whithead L. Ecology of house dust mites in Oxfordshire. *Clin Exp Allergy* 1990; 20: 203.

81 Rugtveit J. Environmental factors in the first months of life and the possible relationship to later development of hypersensitivity. *Allergy* 1990; 45: 154.

82 Warner JO, Price JF. House dust mite sensi-tivity in childhood asthma. *Arch Dis Child* 1978; 53: 710.

83 Morrison Smith J, Springett H. Atopic disease and month of birth. *Clin Allergy* 1979; 9: 153.

84 Korsgaard J, Dahl R. Sensitivity to house dust mite and grass pollen in adults. *Clin Allergy* 1983; 13: 529.

85 Businco L, Cantani A, Farinella F, Businco E. Month of birth and grass pollen or mite sen-sitization in children with respiratory allergy: a significant relationship. *Clin Allergy* 1988; 18: 269.

86 Luczynska CM, Li Y, Chapman MD, Platts-Mills TAE. Airborne concentrations and par-ticle size distribution of allergen derived from domestic cats (*Felis domesticus*). *Am Rev Respir Dis* 1990; 141: 361.

87 Harving H, Korsgaard J, Dahl R. House-dust mite exposure reduction in specially designed, mechanically ventilated 'healthy' homes. *Allergy* 1994; 49: 713.

88 Emberlin J, Savage M, Jones S. Annual varia-tions in grass pollen seasons in London 1961–90: trends and forecast models. *Clin Exp Allergy* 1993; 23: 911.

89 Cockcroft DW, Ruffin RE, Dolovich J, Hargreave FE. Allergen-induced increase in non-allergic bronchial reactivity. *Clin Allergy* 1977; 7: 503.

90 Pollart SM, Reid MJ, Fling JA, Chapman MD, Platss-Mills TAE. Epidemiology of emergency room asthma in northern Cali-fornia: association with IgE antibody to rye-grass pollen. *J Allergy Clin Immunol* 1988; 82: 224.

91 Korsgaard J. Mite asthma and residency. *Am Rev Respir Dis* 1983; 128: 231.

92 Rosenstreich DL, Eggleston P, Kattan M et al. The role of cockroach allergy and exposure to cockroach allergen in causing morbidity among inner-city children with asthma. *N Engl J Med* 1997; 336: 1356.

93 Anto JM, Sunyer J, Rodriguez-Roisin R, Suarez-Cervera M, Vazquez L. Community

outbreaks of asthma associated with inhalation of soybean dust. *N Engl J Med* 1989; 320: 1097.

94 Figley KD, Elrod RH. Endemic asthma due to castor bean dust. *JAMA* 1928; 90: 79.

95 Ordman D. An outbreak of bronchial asthma in South Africa affecting more than 200 persons caused by castor bean dust from an oil processing factory. *Int Arch Allergy Appl Immunol* 1955; 7: 10.

96 Bellomo R, Gigliotti P, Treloar A *et al*. Two consecutive thunderstorm associated epidemics of asthma in the city of Melbourne. The possible role of rye grass pollen. *Med J Aust* 1992; 156: 834.

97 Suphioglu C, Singh MB, Taylor P *et al*. Mechanism of grass-pollen-induced asthma. *Lancet* 1992; 339: 569.

98 Weiss KB. Seasonal trends in US asthma hospitalizations and mortality. *JAMA* 1990; 263: 2323.

99 Marks G, Burney P. Diseases of the respiratory system. In: Charlton J, Murphy M, eds. *The Health of Adult Britain 1841–1991*. London: HMSO, 1998.

100 Jenkins PF, Mullins J, Davies BH, Williams DA. The possible role of aero-allergens in the epidemic of asthma deaths. *Clin Allergy* 1981; 11: 611.

101 O'Hollaren MT, Yunginger JW, Offord KP *et al*. Exposure to an aeroallergen as a possible precipitating factor in respiratory arrest in young patients with asthma. *N Engl J Med* 1991; 324: 359.

102 Targonski PV, Persky VW, Ramekrishnan V. Respiratory pathophysiologic responses: effect of environmental molds on risk of death from asthma during the pollen season. *J Allergy Clin Immunol* 1995; 95: 955.

103 Gerrard JW, Heiner DC, Mink J, Meyers A, Dosman JA. Immunoglobulin levels in smokers and non-smokers. *Ann Allergy* 1980; 44: 261.

104 Burrows B, Halonen M, Barbee RA, Lebowitz MD. The relationship of serum immunoglobulin E to cigarette smoking. *Am Rev Respir Dis* 1981; 124: 523.

105 Warren CPW, Holford-Strevens V, Wong C, Manfreda J. The relationship between smoking and total immunoglobulin E levels. *J Allergy Clin Immunol* 1982; 69: 370.

106 Bahna SL, Heiner DC, Myhre BA. Immunoglobulin E pattern in cigarette smokers. *Allergy* 1983; 38: 57.

107 Omenaas E, Bakke P, Elsayed S, Hanoa R, Gulsvik A. Total and specific serum IgE levels in adults: relationship to sex, age and enviromental factors. *Clin Exp Allergy* 1994; 24: 530.

108 Jarvis D, Luczynska C, Chinn S, Burney P. The association of age, gender and smoking with total IgE and specific IgE. *Clin Exp Allergy* 1995; 25: 1083.

109 Zetterström O, Osterman K, Machado L, Johansson SGO. Another smoking hazard: raised serum IgE concentration and increased risk of occupational allergy. *Br Med J* 1981; 283: 1215.

110 Venables KM, Topping MD, Howe W, Luczynska CM, Hawkins R, Newman-Taylor AJ. Interaction of smoking and atopy in producing specific IgE antibody against a hapten protein conjugate. *Br Med J* 1985; 290: 201.

111 McSharry C, Wilkinson P. Cigarette smoking and the antibody response to inhaled antigens. *Immunol Today* 1986; 7: 98.

112 Strachan D, Cook DG. Parental smoking and allergic sensitisation in children. *Thorax* 1998; 53: 117.

113 Nadel JA, Comroe JH. Acute effects of inhalation of cigarette smoke on airway conductance. *J Appl Physiol* 1961; 16: 713.

114 Woolcock AJ, Peat JK, Salome CM *et al*. Prevalence of bronchial hyperresponsiveness and asthma in a rural adult population. *Thorax* 1987; 42: 361.

115 Cerveri I, Bruschi C, Zoia MC *et al*. Distribution of bronchial nonspecific reactivity in the general population. *Chest* 1988; 92: 26.

116 Fennerty AG, Banks J, Ebden P, Bevan C. The effect of cigarrette withdrawal on asthmatics who smoke. *Eur J Respir Dis* 1987; 71: 395.

117 Vesterinen E, Kaprio J, Koskenvuo M. Prospective study of asthma in relation to smoking habits among 14,729 adults. *Thorax* 1988; 43: 534.

118 Colley JRT. Influence of passive smoking and parental phlegm on pneumonia and bronchitis in early childhood. *Lancet* 1974; ii: 1031.

119 Strachan DP, Cook DG. Parental smoking and lower respiratory illness in infancy and early childhood. *Thorax* 1997; 52: 905.

120 Fergusson DM, Horwood LJ, Shannon FT, Taylor B. Parental smoking and lower respiratory illness in the first three years of life. *J Epidemiol Community Health* 1981; 35: 180.

121 Murray AB, Morrison BJ. The effect of cigarette smoke from the mother on bronchial responsiveness and severity of symptoms in children with asthma. *J Allergy Clin Immunol* 1986; 77: 575.

122 Young S, Le Souef PN, Geelhoed GC *et al*. The influence of family history of asthma and parental smoking on airway responsiveness in early infancy. *N Engl J Med* 1991; 324: 1168.

123 O'Connor G, Weiss ST, Tager IB, Speizer FE. The effect of passive smoking on pulmonary function and non-specific bronchial responsiveness in a population based sample of children and young adults. *Am Rev Respir Dis* 1985; 135: 800.

124 Martinez FD, Antognoni G, Macri F *et al*. Parental smoking enhances bronchial responsiveness in nine-year old children. *Am Rev Respir Dis* 1988; 138: 518.

125 Weiss ST, Tager IB, Munoz A, Speizer FE. The relationship of respiratory infections in early childhood to the occurrence of increased levels of bronchial responsiveness and atopy. *Am Rev Respir Dis* 1985; 131: 573.

126 Strachan DP, Jarvis MJ, Feyerabend C. The relationship of salivary cotinine to respiratory symptoms, spirometry, and exercise-induced bronchospasm in seven-year-old children. *Am Rev Respir Dis* 1990; 142: 147.

127 Ehrlich R, Kattan M, Godbold J *et al*. Childhood asthma and passive smoking. *Am Rev Respir Dis* 1992; 145: 594.

128 Chen Y, Rennie DC, Dosman J. Influence of environmental tobacco smoke on asthma in allergic and non-allergic children. *Epidemiology* 1996; 7: 536.

129 Evans D, Levison MJ, Feldman CH *et al*. The impact of passive smoking on emergency room visits of urban children with asthma. *Am Rev Respir Dis* 1987; 135: 567.

130 Fry J. Effects of a severe fog on a general practice. *Lancet* 1953; i: 235.

131 Wichmann HE, Mueller W, Allhof P *et al*. Health effects during a smog episode in West Germany in 1985. *Environ Health Perspect* 1989; 79: 89.

132 Salter HH. Diseases of the chest. *Lancet* 1870; i: 183.

133 Firket J. Sur les causes des accidents survenus dans la vallee de la Meuse, lors des brouillards de Decembre 1930. *Bull Mem Acad R Med Belg* 1931; 11: 683.

134 Hoek G, Brunekreef B, Hofschrueder P, Lumens M. Effect of air pollution episodes on pulmonary function and respiratory symptoms. *Toxicol Ind Health* 1990; 6: 189.

135 Sunyer J, Spix C, Quenel P *et al*. Urban air pollution and emergency admissions for asthma in four European cities: the APHEA Project. *Thorax* 1997; 52: 760.

136 Ussetti P, Roca J, Agusti AGN, Montserrat JM, Rodriguez-Roisin R, Agusti-Vidal A. Asthma outbreak in Barcelona. *Lancet* 1983; ii: 280.

137 Soriano JB, Anto JM, Plasencia A and the Barcelona Soybean-Asthma Group. Repeaters count: a sentinel method for asthma outbreaks. *Thorax* 1995; 50: 1101.

138 Williams PB, Buhr MP, Weber RW, Volz MA, Koepke JW, Selner JC. Latex allergen in respirable particulate air pollution. *J Allergy Clin Immunol* 1995; 95: 88.

139 Frick OL, German DF, Mills J. Development of allergy in children. *J Allergy Clin Immunol* 1979; 63: 228.

140 Frick OL. Effect of respiratory and other virus infections on IgE immunoregulation. *J Allergy Clin Immunol* 1986; 78: 1013.

141 Pauwels R, Van Der Straeten M, Platteau B, Bazin H. The non-specific enhancement of allergy. *Allergy* 1983; 38: 239.

142 Johnston EDA, Anderson HR, Lambert HP, Patel S. Respiratory morbidity and lung function after whooping-cough. *Lancet* 1983; 2: 1104.

143 Teculescu DB, Aubry C, Pham QT, Locuty J, Deschamps JP, Manciaux M. Lung function in adolescents after uncomplicated whooping cough in childhood. *Eur Respir J* 1989; 2: 733.

144 Welliver RC, Kaul T, Ogra PL. The appearance of cell-bound IgE in respiratory epithelium after respiratory-syncytial-virus infection. *N Engl J Med* 1980; 303: 1198.

145 Sigurs N, Bjarnason R, Sigurbergsson F, Kjellman B, Bjorksten B. Asthma and immunoglobulin E antibodies after respiratory synctial virus bronchiolitis: a prospective cohort study with matched controls. *Pediatrics* 1995; 95: 500.

146 Martinez FD, Morgan WJ, Wright AL, Holberg CJ, Taussig LM. Diminished lung function as a predisposing factor for wheezing respiratory illness in infants. *N Engl J Med* 1988; 319: 1112.

147 Strachan DP, Seagroatt V, Cook DG. Chest illness in infancy and chronic respiratory disease in later life: an analysis by month of birth. *Int J Epidemiol* 1994; 23: 1060.

148 Macek V, Sorli J, Kopriva S, Marin J. Persistent adenoviral infection and chronic airway obstruction in children. *Am J Respir Crit Care Med* 1994; 150: 7.

149 Shaheen SO, Aaby P, Hall AJ *et al*. Measles and atopy in Guinea-Bissau. *Lancet* 1996; 347: 1792.

150 Shirakawa T, Enomoto T, Shimazu S, Hopkin JM. The inverse association between tuberculin responses and atopic disorder. *Science* 1997; 275: 77.

151 Matricardi PM, Rosmini F, Ferrigno L *et al*.

Cross sectional retrospective study of prevalence of atopy among Italian military students with antibodies against hepatitis A virus. *Br Med J* 1997; 314: 999.

152 Martinez FD, Stern DA, Wright AL, Taussig LM, Halonen M, Group Health Medical Associates. Association of non-wheezing lower respiratory tract illness in early life with persistently diminished serum IgE levels. *Thorax* 1995; 50: 1067.

153 Bodner C, Godden D, Seaton A. Family size, childhood infections and atopic disease. *Thorax*, 1998; 53: 28.

154 Johnston SL, Pattemore PK, Sanderson G *et al.* Community study of role of viral infections in exacerbations of asthma in 9–11 year old children. *Br Med J* 1995; 310: 1225.

155 Nicholson KG, Kent J, Ireland DC. Respiratory viruses and exacerbations of asthma in adults. *Br Med J* 1993; 307: 982.

156 Duff AL, Pomeranz ES, Gelber LE *et al.* Risk factors for acute wheezing in infants and children: viruses, passive smoke, and IgE antibodies to inhalant allergens. *Pediatrics* 1993; 92: 535.

157 Young E, Patel S, Stoneham M, Rona R, Wilkinson JD. The prevalence of reaction to food additives in a survey population. *J R Coll Physicians Lond* 1987; 21: 241.

158 Lucas A, Brooke OG, Morley R, Cole TJ, Bamford MF. Early diet of preterm infants and development of allergic or atopic disease: randomised prospective study. *Br Med J* 1990; 300: 837.

159 Zeiger RS, Heller S, Mellon MH *et al.* Effect of combined maternal and infant food-allergen avoidance on development of atopy in early infancy: a randomized study. *J Allergy Clin Immunol* 1989; 84: 72.

160 Burr M, Miskelly FG, Butland BK, Merrett TG, Vaughan-Williams E. Environmental factors and symptoms in infants at high risk of allergy. *J Epidemiol Community Health* 1989; 43: 125.

161 Wjst M, Dold S, Reitmeier P, Wulff A, Nicolai T, von Mutius E. Does breast feeding protect against asthma and allergies? Results of the Munich survey on asthma and allergies. *Monatsschr Kinderheilkd* 1992; 140: 769.

162 Taylor B, Wadsworth J, Golding J, Butler N. Breast feeding, eczema, asthma, and hayfever. *J Epidemiol Community Health* 1983; 37: 95.

163 Omar AH. Respiratory symptoms and asthma in primary school children in Kuala Lumpur. *Acta Paediatr Jpn* 1990; 32: 183.

164 Martin AJ, Landau LI, Phelan PD. Natural history of allergy in asthmatic children followed to adult life. *Med J Aust* 1981; 2: 470.

165 Abbassy AS, Badr E, Hassan AI, Aref GH, Hammad SA. Studies of cell mediated immunity and allergy in protein energy malnutrition. II. Immediate hypersensitivity. *J Trop Med Hyg* 1974; 77: 18.

166 Somerville SM, Rona RJ, Chinn S. Obesity and respiratory symptoms in primary school. *Arch Dis Child* 1984; 59: 940.

167 Schwartz J, Weiss ST. Dietary factors and their relation to respiratory symptoms. *Am J Epidemiol* 1990; 132: 67.

168 Martin S. Asthma and its treatment. *Br Med J* 1898; 2: 1861.

169 Arm JP, Horton CE, Spur BW, Mencia-Huerta J, Lee TH. The effects of dietary supplementation with fish oil lipids on the airways response in inhaled allergen in

bronchial asthma. *Am Rev Respir Dis* 1989; 139: 1395.

170 Picado C, Castillo JA, Schinca N *et al.* Effects of fish oil enriched diet on aspirin intolerant asthmatic patients: a pilot study. *Thorax* 1988; 43: 93.

171 Hodge L, Salome CM, Peat JK, Haby MM, Xuan W, Woolcock AJ. Consumption of oily fish and childhood asthma risk. *Med J Aust* 1996; 164: 137.

172 Troisi RJ, Willett WC, Weiss ST, Trichopoulos D, Rosner B, Speizer FE. A prospective study of diet and adult-onset asthma. *Am J Respir Crit Care Med* 1995; 151: 1401.

173 Epstein A. De l'emploi de la vitamine C dans le traitement de l'asthme bronchique. *Schweiz Med Wochenschr* 1936; 7: 1087.

174 Hunt HB. Ascorbic acid in bronchial asthma: report of a therapeutic trial on twenty-five cases. *Br Med J* 1938; i: 726.

175 Kreisman H, Mitchell C, Bouhuys A. Inhibition of histamine-induced airway constriction negative results with oxtriphylline and ascorbic acid. *Lung* 1977; 154: 223.

176 Malo J, Cartier A, Pineau L, L'Archeveque J, Ghezzo H, Martin RR. Lack of acute effects of ascorbic acid on spirometry and airway responsiveness to histamine in subjects with asthma. *J Allergy Clin Immunol* 1986; 78: 1153.

177 Goldsmith GA, Ogaard AT, Gowe DF. Vitamin C (ascorbic acid) nutrition in bronchial asthma. *Arch Intern Med* 1941; 67: 597.

178 Olusi SO, Ojutiku OO, Jessop WJE, Iboko MI. Plasma and white blood cell ascorbic acid concentrations in patients with bronchial asthma. *Clin Chim Acta* 1979; 92: 161.

179 Aderele WI, Ette SI, Oduwole O, Ikpeme SJ. Plasma vitamin C (ascorbic acid) levels in asthmatic children. *Afr J Med Sci* 1985; 14: 115.

180 Akinkugbe FM, Ette SI. Role of zinc, copper, and ascorbic acid in some common clinical paediatric problems. *J Trop Pediatr* 1987; 33: 337.

181 Soutar A, Seaton A, Brown K. Bronchial reactivity and dietary antioxidants. *Thorax* 1997; 52: 166.

182 Ness AR, Khaw KT, Bingham S, Day NE. Vitamin C status and respiratory function. *Eur J Clin Nutr* 1996; 50: 573.

183 Stone J, Hinks LJ, Beasley R, Holgate ST, Clayton BA. Reduced selenium status of patients with asthma. *Clin Sci* 1989; 77: 495.

184 Flatt A, Pearce N, Thomson CD, Sears MR, Robinson MF, Beasley R. Reduced selenium in asthmatic subjects in New Zealand. *Thorax* 1990; 45: 95.

185 Shaw R, Woodman K, Crane J, Moyes C, Kennedy J, Pearce N. Risk factors for asthma symptoms in Kawerau children. *N Z Med J* 1994; 107: 387.

186 Misso NLA, Powers KA, Gillon RL, Stewart, GA, Thompson PJ. Reduced platelet glutathione peroxidase activity and serum selenium concentration in atopic asthmatic patients. *Clin Exp Allergy* 1996; 26: 838.

187 Hasselmark L, Malmgren R, Zetterstrom O, Unge G. Selenium supplementation in intrinsic asthma. *Allergy* 1993; 48: 30.

188 Rosello HJ, Pla JC. *La Prensa Med Argentina* 1936; 1677.

189 Britton J, Pavord I, Richards K *et al.* Dietary magnesium, lung function, wheezing, and airway hyperreactivity in a random adult population sample. *Lancet* 1994; 344: 357.

190 Hill J, Micklewright A, Lewis S, Britton J. Investigation of the effect of short-term change in dietary magnesium intake in asthma. *Eur Respir J* 1997; 10: 2225.

191 Burney PGJ, Britton JR, Chinn S *et al.* Response to inhaled histamine and 24 hour sodium excretion. *Br Med J* 1986; 292: 1483.

192 Britton JR, Pavord I, Richards K *et al.* Dietary sodium intake and the risk of airway hyperreactivity in a random adult population. *Thorax* 1994; 49: 875.

193 Devereux G, Beach JR, Bromly C *et al.* Effect of dietery sodium on airways responsiveness and its importance in the epidemiology of asthma: an evaluation in three areas of northern England. *Thorax* 1995; 50: 941.

194 Burney PGJ, Neild JE, Twort CHC *et al.* Effects of changing dietary sodium on the airway response to histamine. *Thorax* 1989; 44: 36.

195 Carey OJ, Lock CR, Cookson JB. The effect of alterations of dietary sodium on the severity of asthma in men. *Thorax* 1993; S23: 714.

196 Burney P. A diet rich in sodium may potentiate asthma. *Chest* 1987; 91: 143S.

197 Tribe RM, Barton JR, Poston L, Burney PGJ. Dietary sodium intake, airway responsiveness and cellular sodium transport. *Am J Respir Crit Care Med* 1994; 149: 1426.

198 Peat JK, Salome CM, Sedgwick CS, Kerrebjn J, Woolcock AJ. A prospective study of bronchial hyperresponsiveness and respiratory symptoms in a population of Australian schoolchildren. *Clin Exp Allergy* 1989; 19: 299.

199 Giles GG, Gibson HB, Lickiss N, Shaw K. Respiratory symptoms in Tasmanian adolescents: a follow up of the 1961 birth cohort. *Aust N Z J Med* 1984; 14: 631.

200 Gerritsen J, Koeter GH, Postma DS, Schouten FP, Knol K. Prognosis of asthma from childhood to adulthood. *Am Rev Respir Dis,* 1989; 140: 1325.

201 Borsboom GJJM, Van Pelt W, Quanjer PH. Pubertal growth curves of ventilatory function: relationship with childhood respiratory symptoms. *Am Rev Respir Dis* 1993; 147: 372.

202 Martin AJ, McLennan LA, Landau LI, Phelan PD. The natural history of childhood asthma to adult life. *Br Med J* 1980; 280: 1397.

203 Lange P, Suppli Ulrik C, Vestbo J. Mortality in adults with self-reported asthma. *Lancet*, 1996; 347: 1285.

204 Beaty, Cohen BH, Newill CA, Menkes HA, Diamond EL, Chen CJ. Impaired pulmonary fuction as a risk factor for mortality. *Am J Epidemiol* 1982; 116: 102.

205 Schachter EN, Doyle CA, Beck GJ. A prospective study of asthma in a rural community. *Chest* 1984; 85:

206 Peat JK, Woolcock AJ, Cullen K. Rate of decline of lung function in subjects with asthma. *Eur J Respir Dis* 1987; 70: 171.

207 Suppli Ulrik C, Lange P. Decline of lung function in adults with bronchial asthma. *Am J Respir Crit Care Med* 1994; 150: 629.

208 Burrows B, Bloom JW, Traver GA, Cline MG. The course and prognosis of different forms of chronic airways obstruction in a sample from the general population. *N Engl J Med* 1987; 317: 1309.

209 Markowe HLJ, Bulpitt CJ, Shipley MJ, Crombie DL, Fleming DM. Prognosis in adult asthma: a national study. *Br Med J* 1987; 295: 949.

210 McWhorter WP, Polis MA, Kaslow RA. Occurrence, predictors and consequences of adult asthma in NHANESI and follow-up survey. *Am Rev Respir Dis* 1989; 139: 721.

211 Beaty TH, Menkes HA, Cohen BH, Newill CA. Risk factors associated with longitudinal change in pulmonary function. *Am Rev Respir Dis* 1984; 129: 660.

212 Sutherland DC, Beaglehole R, Jackson RT, Rea HH. Death from asthma in Auckland: circumstances and validation of causes. *N Z Med J* 1984; 97: 845.

213 Berrill WT. Is the death rate from asthma exaggerated? Evidence from west Cumbria. *Br Med J* 1993; 306: 193.

214 Hunt LWJ, Silverstein MD, Reed CE, O'Connell EJ, O'Fallon WM, Yunginger JW. Accuracy of the death certificate in a population-based study of asthmatic patients. *JAMA* 1993; 269: 1947.

215 Goldacre MJ. Cause-specific mortality: understanding uncertain tips of the disease iceberg. *J Epidemiol Community Health* 1993; 47: 491.

216 Guite HF, Burney PG. Accuracy of recording of deaths from asthma in the UK: the false negative rate. *Thorax* 1996; 51: 924.

217 Kelson MC, Heller RF. The effects of death certification and coding practices on observed differences in respiratory disease mortality in 8 EEC countries. *Rev Epidemiol Sante Publique* 1983; 31: 423.

218 Inman WH, Adelstein AM. Rise and fall of asthma mortality in England and Wales in relation to use of pressurised aerosols. *Lancet* 1969; 279.

219 Burney PGJ. Asthma mortality in England and Wales: evidence for a further increase, 1974. *Lancet* 1986; 323.

220 Clarke JA. Pulmonary atalectasis as a complication of bronchial asthma. *Arch Intern Med* 1930; 45: 624.

221 Wright CB. Death from bronchial asthma. *JAMA* 1930; 94: 1218.

222 Benson RL, Perlman F. Clinical effects of epinephrine by inhalation. *J Allergy Clin Immunol* 1948; 19: 129.

223 Speizer FE, Doll R, Heaf P, Strang LB. Investigation into use of drugs preceding death from asthma. *Br Med J* 1968; 1: 339.

224 Stolley PD, Schinnar R. Association between asthma mortality and isoproterenol aerosols: a review. *Prev Med* 1978; 7: 519.

225 British Thoracic Association. Death from asthma in two regions of England. *Br Med J* 1982; 285: 1251.

226 Macdonald JB, Seaton A, Williams DA. Asthma deaths in Cardiff 1963–74: 90 deaths outside hospital. *Br Med J* 1976; 1: 1493.

227 Macdonald JB, Macdonald ET, Seaton A, Williams DA. Asthma deaths in Cardiff 1963–74: 53 deaths in hospital. *Br Med J* 1976; 721: 723.

228 Johnson AJ, Nunn AJ, Somner AR, Stableforth DE, Stewart CJ. Circumstances of death from asthma. *Br Med J* 1984; 288: 1870.

229 Ormerod LP, Stableforth DE. Asthma mortality in Birmingham 1975–7: 53 deaths. *Br Med J* 1980; 687.

230 Ernst P, Spitzer WO, Suissa S *et al.* Risk of fatal and near-fatal asthma in relation to inhaled corticosteroid use. *JAMA* 1992; 268: 3462.

231 Suissa S, Ernst P. Optical illusions from visual data analysis: example of the New Zealand asthma mortality epidemic. *J Clin Epidemiol* 1997; 50: 1079.

33

ASTHMA: CELLULAR AND HUMORAL MECHANISMS

CHRISTOPHER HASLETT

The cellular and mediator mechanisms of asthma must be considered in relation to the clinical definition and classification. The widespread acknowledgement that asthma is caused by a chronic inflammatory response in the airways has been arrived at as a result of information gained from histological studies in autopsy specimens (and more recently bronchoscopic bronchial biopsies in patients), the study of mediator and cellular interactions in allergen-challenged atopic patients and, to a lesser extent, the study of experimental animal models. In this chapter, the cellular and mediator mechanisms likely to underlie the asthmatic state and the effector mechanisms that may explain the pathological features are described.

Clinical definition and classification

A full understanding of basic mechanisms must ultimately explain the clinical picture of airways obstruction that is variable (or reversible) as a result of therapy or spontaneously. It should also account for the propensity of asthmatic patients to show markedly heightened responses to direct bronchoconstrictor agents, or indirectly to triggers such as exercise and cold air. It is now widely considered that in many or most cases, the syndrome of asthma or the asthmatic state arises from a number of poorly understood inducing stimuli, such as allergens and chemicals, in a group of patients who are in some way genetically predisposed. The patient with asthma is 'primed' or at risk of severe bronchospasm if exposed to trigger factors, which may be specific allergens or non-specific trigger factors such as viruses or exposure to cold air (Fig. 33.1).

Pathology

The macroscopic and histological appearances of the airways of patients dying from status asthmaticus show quite clearly that severe asthma involves much more than simple bronchoconstriction. Naked eye examination shows that many airways are blocked with thick, tena-

cious mucus [1]. Histological analysis reveals that airway narrowing is not just brought about by shortening of the airway musculature but also by inflammatory oedema of the whole airway, particularly the submucosal layer [2]. There is often marked thickening of the epithelial basement membrane and in many patients, particularly those with severe asthma, the bronchial epithelial lining is damaged, with evidence of epithelial injury, desquamation and even large areas of complete epithelial denudation and exposure of the epithelial basement membrane (see Fig. 34.6) [3,4]. In keeping with the excessive mucus production, there is marked hypertrophy and hyperplasia of submucous glands and goblet cell hyperplasia [5]. There is also evidence of smooth muscle cell hypertrophy and hyperplasia in the muscularis layer, and microvascular vasodilatation in the adventitia layer of the airway. Throughout the layers of the airway there is an intense inflammatory and immunological cellular infiltration, with large numbers of granulocytes (particularly eosinophils) in the submucosa and within the epithelial layer and mucous plugs [5,6], together with evidence of eosinophil degranulation and disgorgement of highly histotoxic products, e.g. major basic protein (MBP), on histochemical staining [7]. Elsewhere in the airway there are heavy infiltrations of chronic inflammatory mononuclear cells, including large numbers of T lymphocytes, particularly CD4+ cells [8].

Although it may have been thought that these features were predominant only in the catastrophic forms of asthma, early studies of sputum, necropsy studies on patients dying from unrelated causes (e.g. road traffic accidents) and the application of bronchoscopic biopsy techniques in asthmatic patients have clearly demonstrated that many are also found in the background histological picture of asthma [9–14] and in atopic patients challenged experimentally with relevant antigens [15–17].

Atopic asthma and allergen provocation

Atopic asthmatics constitute the larger subgroup of

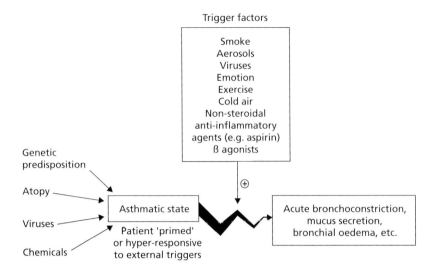

Fig. 33.1 The asthmatic state.

patients, and the study of their bronchial secretions (by bronchoalveolar lavage) and histology (by bronchial biopsy) at various times after deliberate antigen challenge has led to important insights into the mechanisms of asthma. While this experimental approach does not compare exactly with natural exposure to allergens, it has been extremely useful as a human model of asthma, providing much valuable information on the likely pathogenesis of allergic asthma and in the design and testing of new therapeutic agents. When the airways of most atopic asthmatic patients are challenged with specific allergen, the bronchial responses occur in two phases. The first rapid phase of bronchoconstriction (the early asthmatic response) reaches a peak within 20 min of challenge and recovers spontaneously within 60 min or so [18]. This response is thought to resemble a type I anaphylactic response, occurring as a result of IgE-triggered mast cell secretion of histamine and other rapidly acting bronchoconstrictor agents [19,20]. It can be prevented by prior treatment with the mast cell-stabilizing agent sodium cromoglicate (cromoglycate) and abrogated by β agonists [21]. This response is not significantly influenced by a single treatment with corticosteroids. The late asthmatic response occurs in around 50% of atopic individuals. It begins 4–6 h after challenge and persists for 12 h or more [18]. The mast cell is again likely to play an important role in this phase of bronchoconstriction since it is also attenuated by sodium cromoglycate. However, cytological and histological studies also show submucosal oedema, vascular dilatation and a complex cellular infiltration of granulocytes (especially eosinophils) and CD4+ T lymphocytes, which are linked to a Th2-type cytokine secretion profile including interleukin (IL)-3, IL-4 and IL-5 [22].

The distinction between the early and late phases, which is a useful simplification in research, is of little value in the clinical context as most cases of severe asthma are likely to involve a multiplicity of mechanisms combining elements of both the acute and chronic inflammatory responses.

The cells

In this section the role of important cell types in asthma is considered. Although it is a somewhat artificial separation they can be segregated into the following groups.

1 Constitutive or resident cells of the airway, including tissue macrophages, dendritic cells and mast cells. These resident airway cells generally function to initiate the inflammatory and immune responses, although the mast cell clearly has many important effector functions in asthma.

2 Inflammatory/immune blood-borne cells, including the granulocytes and lymphocytes recruited to the inflamed asthmatic airway and which are likely to play additional important pathogenetic roles.

Resident cells

Cells of the monocyte/macrophage series and dendritic cells

By far the most numerous cell in the airway is the resident tissue macrophage. Under homeostatic conditions in healthy airways this population of cells is continuously replenished by bone marrow-derived, blood-borne monocytes. The resident macrophage expresses the low-affinity IgE receptor and can secrete a wide range of proinflammatory cytokines and chemokines [23]. These cells perform a key sensing and regulatory function in the inflammatory response, particularly in its initiation phase, although their precise contribution to the pathogenesis of asthma is uncertain. They rapidly secrete cytokines (Table 33.1) such as IL-1 and tumour necrosis factor (TNF)-α that act on microvascular endothelial cells [24,25], causing them to express

Table 33.1 Some important cytokines: their source and major function.

Cytokine	Source	Functions
IL-1	Macrophages and other cell types	Activation of endothelial cells and macrophages, fever, T cell co-stimulation
IL-2	T cells	T-cell growth factor, NK cell activation
IL-3	Bone marrow stromal cells, T cells	Growth factor for neutrophils, eosinophils, mast cells
IL-4	T cells (Th2) and mast cells	B-cell IgE isotype switching, growth factor for B cells and T cells
IL-5	T cells (Th2) and mast cells	Eosinophil differentiation, recruitment activation and inhibition of apoptosis. Growth factor for B cells
IL-6	Macrophages, T cells and other cells	Acute-phase protein production, B and T cell growth and differentiation
IL-7	Bone marrow stromal cells	Growth factor for pre-B and T cells
IL-8	Reclassified as C-X-C chemokine	
IL-9	T cells	Mast cell activation
IL-10	B cells and macrophages	Inhibits macrophage function
IL-11	Bone marrow stromal cells	Growth factor for haematopoietic stem cells
IL-12	Macrophages and B cells	Promotes differentiation of Th1 cells, activates NK cells
IL-13	T cells (Th2)	B-cell IgE isotype switch, B-cell growth factor
IL-14	T cells	Development of memory B cells
IL-15	Macrophages and other cell types	Growth factor for T cells
IL-16	T cells (CD8+)	Chemoattractant for CD4+ T cells and macrophages
TNF-α	Macrophages, monocytes and T cells	Activates endothelial cells, stimulates release of IL-8 and other chemokines from resident cells
TNF-β	T and B cells	Activates endothelial cells, CD8+-mediated cytotoxicity
IFN-α	Macrophages, T and B cells	Antiviral activity, increased MHC class I expression
IFN-β	Fibroblasts and other cells	Antiviral activity, increased MHC class I expression
IFN-γ	Macrophages, T cells and other cells	Activates macrophages and CD+ T cells, antiviral activity
TGF-β	Macrophages, monocytes and T cells	Inhibits macrophage function, promotes fibrosis and wound repair
GM-CSF	Monocytes, macrophages and T cells	Growth factor for myeloid cells, primes macrophages, primes and inhibits apoptosis in neutrophils and eosinophils
PDGF	Macrophages and platelets	Growth factor for fibroblasts, repair, fibrosis
FGF	Macrophages	Growth factor for fibroblasts, repair, fibrosis

FGF, fibroblast growth factor; GM-CSF, granulocyte–macrophage colony-stimulating factor; IFN, interferon; IL, interleukin; NK, natural killer; PDGF, platelet-derived growth factor; TGF, transforming growth factor; TNF, tumour necrosis factor.

the adhesion molecules (Table 33.2) required for leucocyte trapping and emigration. They also secrete certain chemokines such as IL-8 and gro-α that are specifically chemotactic for neutrophil granulocytes [26,27], whereas others such as RANTES and monocyte chemotachi protein-1 (MCP-1) attract eosinophils and monocytes [28,29]. Macrophage-derived IL-1 and TNF-α can also act on other resident tissue cells, for example fibroblasts and epithelial cells, inducing them to secrete IL-8 and other chemokines [30,31] and thus amplifying the inflammatory response.

In the development of an acute inflammatory response, the initial emigration of granulocytes from blood into tissues is followed by a wave of monocyte emigration. These cells rapidly mature into inflammatory macrophages, which can also secrete cytokines and chemokines and amplify the inflammatory response. However, these cells possess much more effective mechanisms for the secretion of enzymes and reactive oxygen species than do resident macrophages and may thus play an important role in the effector limb of asthma. Macrophages also secrete the cyclooxygenase products thromboxane (TX)B_2 and prostaglandin (PG)E_2, the 5-lipoxygenase product leukotriene (LT)D_4 and platelet-activating factor (PAF), which are capable of inducing many of the features of

asthma [9,32,33]. Cells of the monocyte/macrophage series are also able to influence T-lymphocyte function through the secretion of cytokines, and while resident macrophages are poor presenters of antigen, monocytes and immature inflammatory macrophages are more effective. Although there is little direct evidence for the macrophage in the pathogenesis of asthma *in vivo*, the circumstantial evidence is impressive and it is hard to believe that it does not play an important role.

The lung dendritic cell is likely to play the major role in antigen presentation to T lymphocytes. These cells are prominent in the submucosal layer of the airway, particularly beneath the epithelial lining.

Mast cells

These highly granular tissue cells have long been implicated in the pathogenesis of allergic conditions, particularly asthma. Ultrastructural examination (Fig. 33.2) reveals large numbers of cytoplasmic granules with a characteristic morphology. Reports vary as to whether there are increased numbers of mast cells in the asthmatic airway, although most ultrastructural studies show that those present display an activated, degranulated

Table 33.2 Some surface adhesion molecules controlling leukocyte–endothelial interactions.

Family	Receptor	Distribution	Ligand/counter-receptor	Promotes adhesion to
Integrin family	LFA-1 (CD11a/CD18)	All leucocytes	ICAM-1, ICAM-2, ICAM-3	Endothelial cells
	Mac-1/CR3 (CD11b/CD18)	Granulocytes Monocytes Lymphocytes	ICAM-1, C3bi, factor X	Endothelial cells Opsonized particles
	P150.95 (CD11c/CD18)	Granulocytes Monocytes	Endothelial ligand?	Endothelial cells
Selectin family	L-selectin (CD)	Neutrophils Monocytes Lymphocytes	?E selectin ?P selectin CD15 C5(ex)	Endothelial cells
	P-selectin (CD62)	Endothelium	Sialyl Lewis X (CD15)	Neutrophils
	ICAM-1 (CD54)	Endothelium Epithelium	LFA-1 (CD11a/CD18) MAC-1 (CD11b/CD18)	All leucocytes
Immunoglobulin superfamily	ICAM-2	Monocytes Lymphocytes Endothelium	LFA-1 (CD11a/CD18)	All leucocytes
	VCAM-1	Activated endothelium	VLA-4	Monocytes Eosinophils

ICAM, intercellular adhesion molecule; VCAM, vascular cell adhesion molecule; VLA, very late antigen.

appearance. Being the most important cellular source of histamine, it has been clear for some time that the mast cell plays a key role in the effector limb of asthma. In addition to secreting preformed mediators such as histamine, mast cells can also synthesize other mediators in the cyclooxygenase pathway, especially PGD_2, and 5-lipoxygenase arachidonic acid pathways that exert rapid effects on the airway [34–37]. Another important granule component is tryptase, which besides exerting a number of effects on the airway also activates the kinin cascade. Mast cells may be triggered by direct binding of IgE via their high-affinity surface receptors or by cross-linking of these receptors but can also be triggered indirectly by cold air or by changes in tonicity of the fluids in the airways [38,39]. Recent studies suggest that the mast cell, like the resident macrophage, is an important regulatory cell: when atopic airways are challenged with specific allergen, airway mast cells rapidly generate mRNA for IL-3, IL-4 and IL-5, the Th2-type cytokines [40,41]. This cell is clearly a major player in the pathogenesis of asthma (Figs 33.2 and 33.4).

Basophils

The role of these cells in asthma has been difficult to establish, partly because they lack specific surface markers that would aid histological identification and purification for detailed *in vitro* study. While there is uncertainty about whether increased numbers are present in asthmatic airways, they can be found in the blood during the asthmatic response [42,43]. Like mast cells, basophils possess

the high-affinity IgE receptor and when triggered can secrete histamine and a wide range of other mediators relevant to the pathogenesis of asthma [44–48]. Unlike mast cells they can also be stimulated by the cytokines IL-1 and IL-3 and by the chemokines IL-8 and RANTES.

Circulating leucocytes

Eosinophils

Eosinophils are bone marrow-derived, blood-borne polymorphonuclear leucocytes, the cytoplasmic granules of which stain a deep pink with haematoxylin/eosin; hence the name and their distinction from the neutrophil granulocyte. Ultrastructural examination (see Fig. 33.2) reveals large angular granules possessing the dark, crystalline core that characterizes this cell type. Eosinophil granules contain not only many of the potentially histotoxic agents found in the neutrophil but also a number of eosinophil-specific agents, including major basic protein (MBP) and eosinophil cationic protein (ECP) that help identify the cell and provide evidence of its secretory activity *in situ* [7,49,50]. Atopic asthmatics have long been recognized to display high circulating levels of eosinophils in the blood and large numbers of eosinophils and Charcot–Leyden crystals (lysolecithin from degraded eosinophils) in their sputum [51,52]. Histological studies of severe asthmatics reveal heavy infiltrations of the airways with eosinophils [6,53,54], many of which show evidence of degranulation on electron microscopy, together with evidence of dis-

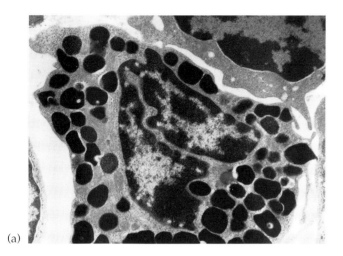

(a)

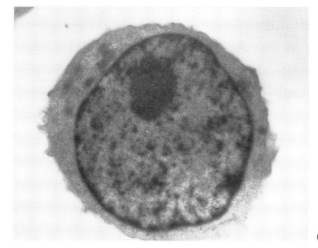

(b)

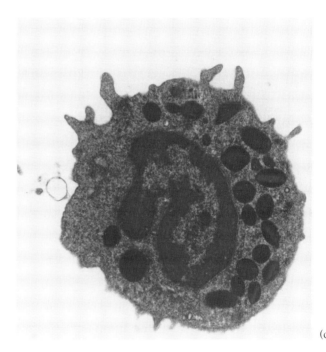

(c)

Fig. 33.2 Key cellular players in asthma (see text). (a) Tissue mast cell (×13 000, courtesy of Professor H. Miller). A key cell in the early pharmacological mechanisms of asthma. (b) T. Lymphocyte (×7000) controller of the allergic immune response. It secretes mediators that attract eosinophils. (c) Eosinophilic granulocyte (×7000, courtesy of Dr Tom Henson). Important in the effector limb causing bronchial epithelial injury.

gorged MBP and eosinophil peroxididase (EPO) in tissues [7]. These cationic products are highly toxic to epithelial cells *in vitro*, and eosinophils are widely considered to be responsible for much of the epithelial damage described in cases of severe asthma. Eosinophils possess functional low-affinity IgE receptors and can synthesize PAF and other important lipid mediators [55–65]. They can also secrete a variety of cytokines, including IL-4 that is so important in IgE secretion [66,67], and their reputation as a centrally important cell in the pathogenesis of asthma seems fully justified. Airway challenge of atopic patients with specific allergen results in eosinophil accumulation in the airways and bronchoalveolar lavage fluid, together with evidence of extracellular secretion of ECP and MBP. The characteristic eosinophil accumulation in the tissues in an allergic response is probably brought about by the local

secretion of specific chemokines (MCP-1 and RANTES) and cytokines (IL-5) that attract eosinophils, together with the expression of specific components of the adhesive molecule repertoire that trap them in local microvessels prior to their directed emigration. CD4+ T cells and mast cells are probably responsible for most of the IL-5, granulocyte–macrophage colony-stimulating factor (GM-CSF) and IL-3 necessary for eosinophil production, recruitment and activation. Extravasated eosinophils are much longer-lived in tissues than are neutrophils, and cytokines such as IL-5 and GM-CSF that are important in the 'supply side' of eosinophils also have major effects in prolonging the functional longevity of these cells in tissues by exerting major inhibitory effects on eosinophil apoptosis, the process of natural cell death that controls the ultimate removal of extravasated granulocytes [68].

Neutrophils (neutrophilic polymorphonuclear leucocytes)

The importance of these cells in human asthma is uncertain at present. In a number of experimental animal models of asthma there is a relationship between neutrophil influx and airway hyperresponsiveness, and the *Alternaria*–rabbit model appears to be neutrophil-dependent [69]. In equine 'heaves', a syndrome very like asthma that is due to exposure to allergens in mouldy hay, the disease is associated with neutrophil, not eosinophil, accumulation in the airways. However, in established human asthma, eosinophils rather than neutrophils are usually the dominant granulocyte in histological sections of the airway, although neutrophils are certainly present in significant numbers in most cases. In dynamic studies of allergen-challenged atopic patients, a wave of neutrophil migration precedes eosinophil migration. The neutrophil contains an enormous armamentarium of preformed agents in its granules (see Chapter 27) and is able to rapidly synthesize a range of agents, including PAF and cyclooxygenase products that are important in the effector limb of asthma pathogenesis. It is perhaps also worth considering that because the neutrophil lives for a much shorter time in tissues than do the eosinophil, lymphocyte and macrophage, the comparative paucity of neutrophils on histological sections could in fact represent a major tissue throughput and the neutrophil may play a more important role than has hitherto been thought.

Lymphocytes

Lymphocytes are blood-borne leucocytes responsible for the classical immune response. They can also be regarded as tissue cells since, in the process of lymphocyte recirculation, they pass through the high endothelial venules of organs including the lung, transit the tissues and return to the bloodstream via the lymphatics. The expression of clonally distributed specific receptors for antigen is characteristic of both B and T lymphocytes, although the function of B lymphocytes is generally restricted to immunoglobulin synthesis and, in the lymph nodes, antigen presentation. T cells can be separated broadly into helper or regulatory (CD4+) cells and effector/cytotoxic (CD8+) cells based on their surface expression of CD4 or CD8 coreceptors. The important role of allergen-specific B lymphocytes in synthesizing IgE has long been recognized as a key mechanism in allergic asthma, although it is now clear that the T cell also plays a vital role in this response by acting as a helper cell and by secreting IL-4, which is responsible for switching B-cell immunoglobulin secretion from IgG to IgE.

However, it is now becoming apparent that CD4+ T cells may play a number of other important roles: they are the only cells that can recognize and directly respond to processed antigen on the surface of antigen-presenting cells (APC) and they are likely to represent the major airway tissue source of IL-5, GM-CSF and IL-3, which promote eosinophil recruitment, activation and longevity. In mice, antigen-activated CD4+ T-cell clones can be divided broadly into two functional phenotypes [70,71]:
1 Th1: secretes IL-2, interferon (IFN)-γ and TNF-α (*not* IL-4, IL-5, IL-6);
2 Th2: secretes IL-4, IL-5 and IL-6 (*not* IL-2, IFN-γ, TNF-α). However, both types of cell secrete IL-3 and GM-CSF. It is not yet certain how directly applicable this subdivision is to humans, but it is clear that Th1 and Th2 patterns of cytokines may be dominant in different circumstances. A Th2 type of response would favour IgE synthesis (which is also inhibited by IFN-γ) and activation of mast cells and eosinophils, and there is preliminary evidence for this pattern of response in human asthma [72–75]. Bronchoalveolar lavage fluid from asthmatics contains increased concentrations of Th2 cytokines and the mononuclear cells from bronchoalveolar lavage fluid contain mRNA for IL-4, IL-5 and GM-CSF [76–78]. However the exact role of CD4+ cells and possible regulatory role of CD8+ cells require further clarification.

Mediators

Hundreds of mediators have been implicated in the inflammatory and immunological processes that contribute to the pathogenesis of asthma, and it is difficult to know how best to categorize them, whether as biochemical groupings or under headings relating to their biological effects. One of the problems with the latter approach is that single mediators may possess a number of very different actions. Furthermore, for a single key function there are usually many different mediators, often from different biochemical cascades, that exert the same action. For example, there are a large number of agents that are chemotactic for neutrophil granulocytes, such as C5a in the complement cascade, LTB_4 in the prostanoid cascade and a variety of chemokines from the C-X-C subclass including IL-8, ENA-78 and gro-α (see Table 33.3). There are numerous examples of this type of redundancy, which probably evolved as an important part of the inflammatory and immune responses against microorganisms, for example should a bacterium develop an escape mechanism against a particular mediator, then there are a number of different back-up mediators to perform that action. Thus the mediators to be described should perhaps be considered as a network or web rather than as a series of pathways. Rather like a spider's web, if one strand is lacking this does not necessarily impair its overall integrity. This remarkable redundancy is undoubtedly of enormous value in antimicrobial host defence. However, when this same concept is considered from the perspective of designing effective mechanism-based therapy in inflammatory and immuno-

Table 33.3 Some members of the chemokine family of small peptides. ENA, epithelial neutrophil-activating protein; MCP, monocyte chemotactic protein; MIP, macrophage inflammatory protein; NAP, neutrophil-activating peptide.

C-X-C subgroup
IL-8 (NAP-1)
NAP-2
ENA-78
gro-α1
Platelet factor 4

C-C subgroup
MIP-1α
MIP-1β
RANTES
MCP-1
MCP-2
MCP-3

logical diseases such as asthma, where these complex networks are part of the disease pathogenesis, the prospects are indeed daunting. Although, intuitively, it would seem futile in established inflammatory/immunological diseases to adopt a single mediator stategy, there have indeed been attempts to do just this. To exemplify this problem, PAF can provoke virtually all the features of asthma (see below), yet when an extremely effective PAF antagonist (WEB2086), which blocks almost all its effects in model systems, was assessed in human asthma it was found to have no beneficial effects [79]. Glucocorticoids are likely to be effective in most cases of asthma because they have multiple actions at different points in the cellular and mediator events, yet unfortunately they also cause adverse effects. It seems likely that unless we are fortunate to identify key anchor strands of the spider's web of mediators, therapeutic stategies will need to be directed at more than one mediator or mechanism.

In this section the important mediators are described under the headings histamine, kinins, lipid mediators, cytokines and chemokines. The mechanisms whereby these agents might cooperate in the integrated cellular and mediator responses that characterize the asthmatic state are then considered.

Histamine

The main source of histamine is the mucosal mast cell, although eosinophils may also contribute. Via the airway H_1 receptors, histamine causes rapid bronchoconstriction and induces dilatation and leakage of microvessels, which results in airway oedema and further narrowing of the bronchial lumen [80,81]. Histamine is thought to stimulate secretion of mucus in human airways via the H_2 receptor [82]. While it is likely to be an important mediator in all stages of asthma and particularly the early response, antihistamines have proved disappointing in the treatment of human asthma, perhaps because of the redundancy factor

since prostanoids, leukotrienes and PAF can mimic most of its actions.

Kinins

Bradykinin is detected in the bronchoalveolar lavage fluid of atopic patients after allergen challenge of the airways [83]. It acts as a potent constrictor of human airways *in vivo* [84], perhaps acting by indirect mechanisms such as the release of sensory neuropeptides and lipid mediators. Bradykinin is probably generated from preformed kininogens in plasma as a result of the action of kallikrein and mast cell tryptase. In addition to its action on smooth muscle and airway sensory nerves, it is a potent vasodilator and inducer of microvascular leakage and airway mucous secretion [85,86].

Lipid mediators (Fig. 33.3)

Cyclooxygenase products

A wide range of inflammatory cells are able to synthesize the cyclooxygenase products (or prostanoids, i.e. prostaglandins and thromboxane) from membrane phospholipids; certainly macrophages and granulocytes are potent in this regard. Recent research has identified two forms of cyclooxygenase: COX1, a constitutive form present in unstimulated cells; and COX2, a form induced by TNF-α and other proinflammatory cytokines [87]. Unlike COX1, COX2 is inhibited by corticosteroids [87] and is likely to be responsible for the increased level of prostanoids found in the airways of asthmatic patients and atopic patients challenged with allergens [88,89]. PGD_2 and PGE_2 cause constriction of the airways by activating thromboxane TP_1 receptors, as do TXA_2 and its more stable metabolite TXB_2. PGD_2 also primes or enhances the airway bronchoconstrictor response to histamine in asthmatic patients. Other prostanoids, including PGE_2 and PGI_2 (prostacyclin), may exert bronchodilator effects. The prostanoid family is likely to contribute to the bronchoconstrictor effect *in vivo*, as do many other redundant mediators, although potent cyclooxygenase inhibitors alone do not exert major benefical effects on asthma *in vivo* [90].

Leukotrienes

Activation of 5-lipoxygenase, particularly in macrophages, mast cells and granulocytes, results in the synthesis of LTB_4, LTC_4, LTD_4 and LTE_4. Raised levels of these agents are found in bronchoalveolar lavage fluid after allergen challenge of atopic subjects [89,91]. LTB_4 is a potent neutrophil chemoattractant that has little effect on eosinophils and its role in asthma is uncertain. The sulphidopeptide leukotrienes (LTC_4, LTD_4 and LTE_4) are potent

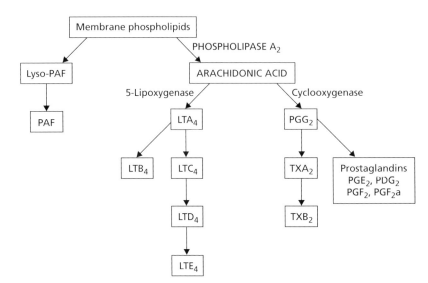

Fig. 33.3 Lipid mediators derived from membrane phospholipids that have a role in the inflammatory processes involved in asthma.

bronchoconstrictors and can induce bronchial hyperresponsiveness [92,93]. They can also exert potent effects on airway microvascular leakage and airway mucous secretion. It is possible that these agents may play a centrally important role in asthma and new 5-lipoxygenase inhibitors are being developed commercially, particularly directed against 5-lipoxygenase-activating protein (FLAP) [94]. Preliminary studies with LTD_4 antagonists show effectiveness against exercise- and aspirin-induced asthma.

Platelet-activating factor

This lipid mediator is synthesized by inflammatory macrophages and granulocytes. It was originally discovered through its action on platelets [95], although it has now become clear that it can mimic many of the features of asthma, including; bronchoconstriction and mucous secretion [93,96,97], and is a potent inducer of microvascular leakage [98]. It has also been found to exert important influences on inflammatory cells, including eosinophil recruitment, endothelial activation and eosinophil degranulation [99–102]. While it is likely that PAF makes important contributions to the mediator network in asthma, it does not seem to have a unique role because the powerful PAF antagonists (e.g. WEB2086) that block the effects of PAF *in vitro* and *in vivo* [103,104] are of little benefit in human asthma [79].

Cytokines and growth factors

The cytokines are a family of peptides secreted by inflammatory cells (and also some resident tissue cells) that cooperate to orchestrate the initiation, amplification and, finally, cessation of the inflammatory and immune responses, plus the regulation of repair responses required to restore tissue integrity. The family now exceeds 50 members (see Table 33.1 for some of the more important ones), which are involved in a complex interplay with each other and with a variety of cells types in the regulation of these important tissue responses. Full understanding of the roles of the cytokine network has been hindered not only by the discovery of new family members almost weekly but also by the facts that (i) there is marked redundancy in many of the mechanisms (a variety of cytokines may exert the same action), (ii) the same cytokine may have multiple effects including different effects on different cells and (iii) some cytokines may require prior interaction with other cytokines before their own effects are revealed.

Interleukin 1

IL-1 has important direct actions on microvascular endothelial cells, activating them and upregulating their expression of adhesion molecules necessary for leucocyte trapping and emigration. It exerts important secondary effects by stimulating resident cells, such as fibroblasts and airway epithelial cells, to secrete IL-8 and GM-CSF [105,106]. Thus it is considered to be a key mediator in the control of the early-release mediators involved in the initiation of the inflammatory response, although it is not specific to the allergic response seen in asthma.

Tumour necrosis factor α

There is much evidence for the release of this peptide and expression of the TNF-α gene in asthmatic tissues and in allergen-provoked atopic patients [107,108]. It is secreted by macrophages and other inflammatory cells and also by bronchial epithelial cells. Like IL-1, it is likely to play an important role in the initiation of inflammation because it is a potent inducer of GM-CSF and IL-8 secretion by epithelial cells and fibroblasts and it activates microvascular endothelial cells to express intercellular adhesion molecule (ICAM)-1 and vascular cell adhesion molecule (VCAM)-1 [105,106,109,110].

Interleukin 3

IL-3 is centrally important in haematopoiesis, particularly the growth and differentiation of neutrophil and eosinophil granulocytes, mast cells and basophils. At the inflamed site it is likely to promote eosinophil survival.

Interleukin 4

Like IL-3, IL-4 is one of the Th2 group of cytokines produced by a subpopulation of CD4+ T lymphocytes, although it can also be produced by mast cells in asthmatic patients [40]. Together with CD40L it is likely to play a critical role in switching B-lymphocyte immunoglobulin secretion from IgG to IgE [111]. It may also be important in inducing the expression of endothelial adhesion molecules (e.g. VCAM-1) that are important in monocyte and eosinophil emigration [112].

Interleukin 5

IL-5 is produced by the Th2 subpopulation of CD4+ lymphocytes and can also be secreted by mast cells. This cytokine is likely to be centrally important in asthma because of its major effects on various aspects of eosinophil function. It is necessary for the final differentiation of eosinophils in the bone marrow, their recruitment to the inflamed site, their activation [113] and, by inhibiting their inherent rate of apoptosis, is likely to exert important inflammatory amplification effects by prolonging their tissue longevity [68]. Raised levels of IL-5 have been found in the bronchoalveolar lavage fluid of asthmatic patients and atopic patients who have been challenged with allergens [114,115].

Granulocyte–macrophage colony-stimulating factor

GM-CSF is produced by macrophages, granulocytes, lymphocytes and airway epithelial cells. It is important in the haematopoiesis of inflammatory cells, in priming macrophages, neutrophils and eosinophils for subsequent secretory responses and, by inhibiting apoptosis, in prolonging the functional lifespan of neutrophils and eosinophils. Once again, there is evidence for the expression and secretion of this important cytokine in asthma

and in allergen-induced bronchoconstriction in atopic patients.

Growth factors

Attention has recently been drawn to the possible importance of thickening of the subepithelial basement membrane and the subepithelial fibrosis that has been observed in necropsy studies of asthmatic patients. Platelet-derived growth factor (PDGF), which in spite of its name is mostly derived from macrophages, exerts potent effects on fibroblast functions, including proliferation and collagen synthesis. Transforming growth factor β (TGF-β) and fibroblast growth factor (FGF) also stimulate fibroblast replication and collagen secretion. These cytokine growth factors may also promote smooth muscle proliferation and vascular remodelling in the chronic asthmatic airway.

Most cytokines so far discovered exert proinflammatory or profibrotic effects, yet in the healthy individual the beneficial inflammatory response to injury or infection is exquisitely controlled, with minimal damage to host tissues, prompt resolution and a fibroproliferative response (see Chapter 27) just sufficient to complete the minor repairs necessary to restore tissue integrity. It is possible that this tight regulation is achieved at the level of synthesis and secretion, although analogies in other cascades such as blood coagulation suggest that there are likely to be numerous inhibitory cytokines or partner molecules that keep cytokine responses in check. IL-12 exerts a number of inhibitory influences, particularly on macrophages, and the soluble form of the IL-1 receptor inhibits several early events in the initiation of inflammation; there are probably many more inhibitory cytokines to be discovered, some of which may yet be of therapeutic value.

Chemokines

The comparatively recent discovery of this family of small peptides, many of which exert powerful and specific chemoattractant influences, has generated much interest. Until now there has been no really plausible explanation for the attraction of specific cell types at different stages of the inflammatory response and in different types of inflammation. Furthermore, the molecular characterization of specific chemokine receptors may lead to incisive therapeutic approaches in allergic inflammation. This family of mediators has been broadly divided into the C-X-C subgroup, in which the cysteine residues of the peptide are separated by an interposed amino acid, and the C-C subgroup where this is not the case (Table 33.3). In humans, the genes encoding the C-X-C group are located on chromosome 4 and those encoding the C-C group on chromosome 17. The C-X-C group contains the neutrophil chemoattractants IL-8, neutrophil attractant protein (NAP)-2, gro-α and ENA-78. Platelet factor 4 is closely related molecularly but is not a chemoattractant. Lung macrophages are extremely potent producers of IL-8, which was originally classified as a cytokine but molecular characterization resulted in its reclassification as a chemokine. It is specifically chemotactic for neutrophils, although it is thought that in the presence of IL-4 it may also attract eosinophils. It also has important but poorly understood roles in neovascularization. In contrast, the C-C chemokine RANTES is a potent and specific chemoattractant for eosinophils [116,117], whereas its close relative macrophage-inhibitory protein-1α (MIP-1α) is involved in monocyte and eosinophil chemoattraction.

Orchestration of cellular and mediator events in the pathogenesis of asthma

As mentioned above, most asthma attacks in human disease probably involve elements of both the early and late responses observed when atopic individuals are exposed to airway-delivered specific allergens. Nevertheless, as a simplification of the very complex events *in vivo* it is helpful to consider each separately.

Early asthmatic response

In the sensitized individual, mast cells and perhaps also basophils are triggered by IgE, which binds via the high-affinity IgE receptor (FcεR1), causing prompt degranulation and secretion of preformed granule contents including histamine and tryptase (Fig. 33.4). Histamine causes rapid airway responses, including bronchoconstriction, vasodilatation/oedema and mucous section. Mast cell tryptase exerts direct actions on the airway but also activates the kinin system to generate bradykinin, a

Fig. 33.4 Summary of the acute asthmatic response.

powerful bronchoconstrictor. Activated mast cells also synthesize potent vasoactive and bronchoconstrictor agents, including PGD_2 and $LTC_4/LTD_4/LDE_4$. The IgE that triggers mast cells is generated by T lymphocytes that have been activated by processed antigen on the surface of antigen presenting cells (APCs). Mast cells can also be triggered by cold air or by changes in the osmolality of the local tissue fluids. In the complex inflammatory picture of the chronic asthmatic airway, other cells including macrophages and granulocytes that display the low-affinity IgE receptor may also contribute to the synthesis and secretion of important vasoactive and bronchoconstrictor agents, including leukotrienes, prostanoids and PAF.

Late asthmatic response

Most asthmatic attacks in patients probably include elements of the mechanisms involved in the early asthmatic response but also involve major contributions from inflammatory cells (macrophages, neutrophils, eosinophils) and immune cells (lymphocytes), which have more complex, more prolonged and perhaps more damaging effects. The likely cellular events that follow the acute events described above when a sensitized individual is exposed to specific antigens are considered now. The discussion is divided into the cell recruitment phase and the effector mechanism phase, where products of inflammatory cells are likely to cause the histological features seen in severe asthma. However, while useful as a framework for understanding, the distinction is again somewhat artificial because in asthmatic patients acute and chronic inflammatory cells are often already present in airway tissues and because some damaging mechanisms are likely to have been initiated before cellular recruitment is complete.

Cell recruitment

Neutrophils are the first cells to arrive in the challenged

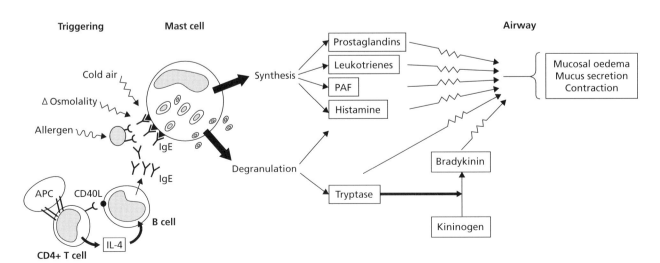

airways, followed by eosinophils and monocytes, which mature into inflammatory macrophages. The attraction of specific inflammatory cells is mediated by chemotactic factors. For the neutrophil, these would include the complement product C5a, LTB_4 and a number of chemotactic chemokines in the C-X-C group. IL-8 is perhaps the most relevant and powerful neutrophil chemokine in the lung. Eosinophils are attracted by a number of mechanisms, perhaps by the specifically eosinophilic chemoattractant peptide RANTES and a new member of the family the eosinophil-specific eotaxin [116–118]. Monocytes can be attracted by a number of chemokines in the C-C group. The selective emigration of neutrophils, eosinophils and monocytes is mediated initially by a trapping phase in the local microvessels followed by transmigration of the endothelial cell layer in the microvessels within the airway. This is a multistep process, the adhesion component occurring in at least two phases that utilize different components of the adhesion molecule repertoire (see Table 33.2). The early arrest phase of transient adhesion in microvessels requires adhesion molecules of the selectin family, whereas the tight adhesion that is a necessary prelude to capillary transmigration (Fig. 33.5) depends upon activation of molecules of the integrin family. Although current reports are a little confusing, it seems that under some circumstances eosinophils and monocytes may use components of the adhesion molecule repertoire (such as VCAM-1) that differ from those used by neutrophil granulocytes. This selective use of the adhesion molecule repertoire, together with the generation of chemokines with specificity for the different inflammatory cells, probably accounts for the selective accumulation of eosinophils in allergic responses and also for the differential timing of arrival of inflammatory cells at the inflamed site (neutrophils followed by monocytes and eosinophils). These selective mechanisms may also provide potential targets for the development of new therapies in asthma and other allergic conditions.

There is *in vivo* evidence that these early recruitment mechanisms are operating in human asthma and its models. During the late response to inhaled allergen, a number of poorly characterized chemotactic factors for neutrophils and eosinophils can be detected in circulating blood [50,119,120]. Bronchial biopsies taken after allergen challenge show increased numbers of neutrophils, eosinophils and T cells [121,122]. Immunocytochemistry shows increased expression of ICAM-1, which correlates with the accumulation of leucocytes, and other molecules (see Table 33.2) involved in leucocyte adhesion to vascular endothelium [123,124]. Experimental studies in non-human primates have shown that monoclonal antibodies directed against ICAM-1 and E-selectin are able to attenuate the allergen-induced late reaction. The increased expression of ICAM-1 and other adhesion molecules on the surface of activated endothelial cells is likely to be mediated by cytokines such as IL-1, TNF-α and IL-5, which are probably derived from macrophages and T lymphocytes in the asthmatic airway [125]. However, these cells take several hours to synthesize these agents, whereas mucosal mast cells store preformed TNF-α, IL-5, IL-6 and other cytokines and chemokines in their granules and which can be released rapidly by cross-linking of the IgE receptor. Thus mast cells may make a variety of important contributions to early pathogenetic events in asthma.

Effector mechanisms (Fig. 33.6)

Once recruited to the airways, extravasated neutrophils and eosinophils are able to secrete a large number of histotoxic granule contents (see Chapter 27), including elastase, collagenase, MBP and EPO, many of which have been implicated in endothelial injury but which also contribute

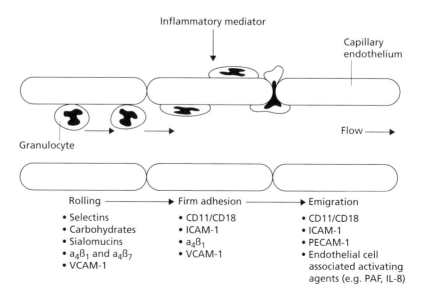

Fig. 33.5 Stages of granulocyte adhesion and emigration in microvessels.

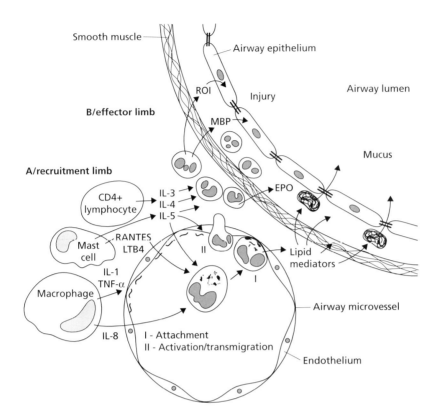

Fig. 33.6 Inflammatory response and asthma effector mechanisms. ROI, reactive oxygen intermediate.

to vascular responses and mucous secretion. They can also release a wide range of highly histotoxic reactive oxygen intermediates, including superoxide anion, hydrogen peroxide and hydroxyl radicals, and synthesize a range of important leukotrienes and prostanoids that cause airway narrowing, mucosal oedema and increased mucous secretion.

Vascular responses

The inflammatory response stimulates increased blood flow in the local airway microvessels which, in concert with increased vascular permeability, causes mucosal oedema and extravasation of plasma proteins. Mucosal oedema probably plays a major role in the airway narrowing and increased airflow resistance that characterizes severe asthma. Plasma-derived mediators like bradykinin cause bronchoconstriction, mucosal oedema, increased mucous secretion and, by inhibiting mucociliary clearance, contribute to mucous plugging of the airways. In chronic severe asthma, angiogenesis is probably involved in the process of airway remodelling. A number of inflammatory cytokines, including IL-1, FGF and PDGF, and the chemokine IL-8 have been implicated in angiogenesis.

Airway smooth muscle

There may well be no inherent change in smooth muscle contractility in asthma [126], although clearly many mediators cause bronchoconstriction both directly and indirectly via release of neuropeptides and by influencing local nerve axon responses. There is also evidence of increased smooth muscle thickness, which may be the result of both hypertrophy and hyperplasia. Like vascular remodelling these changes are probably brought about by the action of growth factor cytokines such as PDGF.

Epithelial injury and shedding

Epithelial changes range from epithelial stimulation and minor injury to epithelial shedding and even extensive areas of denudation [4,122]. Many inflammatory cell products, including reactive oxygen intermediates and granule enzymes, are capable of injuring the airway epithelium, but the highly cationic eosinophil products MBP and EPO are particularly implicated. The fact that a diverse range of agents, such as viruses, allergies, chemicals and toxic gases, may lead to airway hyperresponsiveness may in part be explained by their common property of causing epithelial damage. Depending on the degree of epithelial injury, there may be a variety of consequences of relevance to the pathogenesis of asthma.

1 Injured and stimulated epithelial cells may themselves secrete a variety of important mediators, cytokines and chemokines, for example GM-CSF, IL-1, IL-8, RANTES. In responding to macrophage-derived IL-1 and TNF-α by secreting a range of chemokines, it is believed that the epithelium, a rich source of IL-8 for example, may exert important amplification effects in the evolution of the inflammatory response.

2 Significant denudation of the epithelium may itself result in a variety of important secondary effects:

(a) loss of the epithelial barrier function may permit direct access and influence of allergens and other proinflammatory factors (e.g. pollutants) on tissue cells including mast cells;

(b) loss of airway epithelial cells reduces the ability to degrade peptide and kinin mediators and to secrete

epithelial-derived relaxant factor, which may help to maintain airway dilatation;

(c) sensory nerve exposure may promote inflammation and bronchoconstriction by local nerve axon reflex mechanisms [127].

(d) epithelial denudation may provoke proliferation of myofibroblasts normally located beneath the epithelial membrane, and proliferation of these cells and their secretion of extracellular matrix protein including collagen may contribute to the thickened basement membrane described in chronic asthma [128].

References

1 Messer JW, Peters GA, Bennett WA. Causes of death and pathologic findings in 304 cases of bronchial asthma. *Dis Chest* 1960; 38: 616.

2 Lungren R, Soderberg M, Horstedt P, Stenling R. Morphological studies on bronchial mucosal biopsies from asthmatics before and after ten years treatment with inhaled steroids. *Eur Respir J* 1988; 1: 883.

3 Naylor B. The shedding of the mucosa of the bronchial tree in asthma. *Thorax* 1962; 17: 69.

4 Laitinen LA, Heino M, Laitinen A, Kava T, Haahtela T. Damage of the airway epithelium and bronchial respiratory tract in patients with asthma. *Am Rev Respir Dis* 1985; 131: 599.

5 Dunnill MS. The pathology of asthma, with special reference to the changes in the bronchial mucosa. *J Clin Pathol* 1960; 13: 27.

6 Huber HL, Koessler KK. The pathology of bronchial asthma. *Arch Intern Med* 1992; 30: 689.

7 Filley WV, Holley KE, Kephart GM, Gleich GJ. Identification by immunofluorescence of eosinophil granule major basic protein in lung tissue of patients with bronchial asthma. *Lancet* 1982; ii: 11.

8 Azzawi M, Bradley B, Jeffrey PK *et al.* Identification of activated T lymphocytes and eosinophils in bronchial biopsies in stable atopic asthma. *Am Rev Respir Dis* 1990; 142: 1407.

9 Godard P, Chaintreuil J, Damon M *et al.* Functional assessment of alveolar macrophages: comparison of cells from asthmatic and normal subjects. *J Allergy Clin Immunol* 1982; 70: 88.

10 Flint KC, Leung KB, Hudspith BN, Brostoff J, Pearce FL, Johnson NM. Bronchoalveolar mast cells in extrinsic asthma: a mechanism for the initiation of antigen specific bronchoconstriction. *Br Med J* 1985; 291: 923.

11 Kelly C, Ward C, Stenton CS, Bird G, Hendricks DJ, Walters EH. Number and activity of inflammatory cells in bronchoalveolar lavage fluid in asthma and their relation to airway hyperresponsiveness. *Thorax* 1988; 43: 684.

12 Wardlaw AJ, Cromwell O, Celestino D *et al.* Morphological and secretory properties of bronchoalveolar lavage mast cells in respiratory diseases. *Clin Allergy* 1986; 16: 163.

13 Wardlaw AJ, Dunnette S, Gleich GJ, Collins JV, Kay AB. Eosinophils and mast cells in bronchoalveolar lavage fluid and mild asthma: relationship to bronchial hyperreactivity. *Am Rev Respir Dis* 1988; 137: 62.

14 Djukanovic R, Roche WR, Wilson JW *et al.* Mucosal inflammation in asthma. *Am Rev Respir Dis* 1990; 142: 434.

15 Metzger WJ, Zavala D, Richerson HB *et al.* Local allergen challenge and bronchoalveolar lavage of allergic asthmatic lungs: description of the model and local airway inflammation. *Am Rev Respir Dis* 1987; 135: 433.

16 Lam S, LeRichie J, Phillips D *et al.* Cellular and protein changes in bronchial lavage fluid after late asthmatic reaction in patients with red cedar wood asthma. *J Allergy Clin Immunol* 1987; 80: 44.

17 Frew AJ, Kay AB. The relationship between infiltrating CD4+ lymphocytes, activated eosinophils and the magnitude of the allergen induced late-phase response in man. *J Immunol* 1988; 141: 4158.

18 Pepys J, Hutchcroft BJ. Bronchial provocation tests in etiologic diagnosis and analysis of asthma. *Am Rev Respir Dis* 1978; 112: 829.

19 Gell PGH, Coombs RRA. *Clinical Aspects of Immunology*, 2nd edn. Oxford: Blackwell, 1968.

20 Ishizaka T, Soto S, Ishizaka K. Mechanisms of passive sensitization. III. Number of IgE molecules and their receptor sites in human basophil granulocytes. *J Immunol* 1973; 111: 500.

21 Booij-Noord H, Orie NGM, de Bries K. Immediate and late bronchial obstructive reactions to house dust mite and protective effects of disodium cromoglycate and prednisolone. *J Allergy Clin Immunol* 1971; 48: 344.

22 Bradley BL, Azzawi M, Jacobson M *et al.* Eosinophils, T-lymphocytes, mast cells, neutrophils, and macrophages in bronchial biopsy specimens from atopic subjects with asthma: comparison with biopsy specimens from atopic subjects without asthma and normal control subjects and relationships to bronchial hyperresponsiveness. *J Allergy Clin Immunol* 1991; 88: 661.

23 Spielberg HL. Structure and function of Fc receptors for IgE on lymphocytes, monocytes and macrophages. *Adv Immunol* 1984; 35: 51.

24 Larick JW, Kunkel SL. The role of tumor necrosis factor and interleukin-1 in the immunoinflammatory response. *Pharmacol Res* 1988; 5: 129.

25 Dinarello CA. Interleukin-1 and its biologically related cytokines. *Adv Immunol* 1989; 44: 153.

26 Baggiolini M, Walz A, Kunkel SL. Neutrophil-activating peptide-1/interleukin 8, a novel cytokine that activates neutrophils. *J Clin Invest* 1989; 84: 1045.

27 Walz A, Burgener R, Car B *et al.* Structure and neutrophil-activating properties of a novel inflammatory peptide (ENA-78) with homology to interleukin-8. *J Exp Med* 1991; 174: 1355.

28 Wolpe SD, Davatelis G, Sherry B *et al.* Macrophages secrete a novel heparin-binding protein with inflammatory and neutrophil chemokinetic properties. *J Exp Med* 1988; 167: 570.

29 Schall TJ, Jangstra J, Dyer BJ *et al.* A human T cell-specific molecule is a member of a new glue family. *J Immunol* 1988; 141: 1018.

30 Sherry B, Cerami A. Cachectin/tumor necrosis factor exerts endocrine, paracrine and autocrine control of inflammatory responses. *J Cell Biol* 1988; 107: 1269.

31 Le J, Vilcek J. TNF and IL-1: cytokines with multiple overlapping biological activities. *Lab Invest* 1987; 56: 234.

32 Damon M, Chavis C, Godard P, Michel EB, Crastes de Paulet A. Purification and mass spectrometry identification of LTD4, synthesized by human alveolar macrophages. *Biochem Biophys Res Commun* 1983; 111: 518.

33 Amoux B, Simeos-Caerio MH, Landes A, Mathieu M, Daroux P, Benveniste J. Alveolar macrophages from asthmatic patients release platelet activating factor (PAF-acether) and lyso-PAF-acether when stimulated with specific allergens. *Am Rev Respir Dis* 1982; 125: 70.

34 Campbell AM, Robinson C. Further studies on IgE-mediated eicosanoid release by dispersed lung cells. *Br J Pharmacol* 1988; 95 (Suppl): 674.

35 Schulman ES, Newball HH, Demers LM, Fitzpatrick FA, Adkinson NF. Anaphylactic release of thromboxane A2, prostaglandin D2 and prostacyclin from human lung parenchyma. *Am Rev Respir Dis* 1981; 124: 402.

36 Robinson C. Mast cells and newly-generated lipid mediators. In: Holgate ST, ed. *Mast Cells, Mediators and Disease.* Dordrecht: Kluwer Academic, 1988: 149.

37 Holgate ST, Robinson C, Church MK. Mediators of immediate hypersensitivity. In: Middleton E, Reed CE, Ellis EF, Adkinson NF, Yuninger JW, eds. *Allergy: Principles and Practice.* St Louis: Mosby, 1988: 135.

38 Lee TH, Nagakura T, Papageogiou N, Cromwell O, Ikura Y, Kay AB. Mediators in

exercise-induced asthma. *J Allergy Clin Immunol* 1984; 73: 634.

39 Flint KC. Hyperosmolar histamine release from human lung mast cells: its relevance to exercise-induced asthma. In: Flint KC, Hudspith BN, eds. London: Springer Verlag, 1987: 43.

40 Bradding P, Feather IH, Howarth PH *et al.* Interleukin 4 is localised to and released by human mast cells. *J Exp Med* 1992; 176: 1381.

41 Bradding P, Feather IH, Wilson S *et al.* Immunolocalisation of cytokines in the nasal mucosa of normal and perennial rhinitic subjects. *J Immunol* 1993; 151: 3853.

42 Akagi K, Townley RG. Spontaneous histamine release and histamine content in normal subjects with asthma. *J Allergy Clin Immunol* 1989; 83: 742.

43 Gaddy JH, Busse WW. Enhanced IgE-dependent basophil histamine release and airway reactivity in asthma. *Am Rev Respir Dis* 1986; 134: 969.

44 Sampson D, Archer GT. Release of histamine from human basophils. *Blood* 1967; 29: 722.

45 Ishizaka TR, De Bernardo R, Tomioka H, Lichtenstein LM, Ishizaka K. Identification of basophil granulocyte as a site of allergic histamine release. *J Immunol* 1972; 108: 1000.

46 Kaplan AP, Haak-Frendscho M, Fauci A, Dinarello C, Halbert E. A histamine-releasing factor from activated human mononuclear cells. *J Immunol* 1985; 135: 2027.

47 MacDonald SM, Lichtenstein LM, Proud D *et al.* Studies of IgE-dependent histamine releasing factors: heterogeneity of IgE. *J Immunol* 1987; 139: 506.

48 Columbo M, Casolaro V, Warner JA, McGlashan DW Jr, Kagey-Sabotka A, Lichtenstein LM. The mechanism of mediator release from human basophils induced by platelet-activating factor. *J Immunol* 1990; 145: 3855.

49 Frigas E, Loegering DA, Solley GO, Farrow GM, Gleich GJ. Elevated levels of the eosinophil granule major basic protein in the sputum of patients with bronchial asthma. *Mayo Clin Proc* 1981; 56: 345.

50 de Monchy JGR, Kauffman HF, Venge P *et al.* Bronchoalveolar eosinophilia during allergen-induced late asthmatic reactions. *Am Rev Respir Dis* 1985; 131: 373.

51 Horn BR, Robin ED, Theodore J, Van Kessel A. Total eosinophil counts in the management of bronchial asthma. *N Engl J Med* 1975; 292: 1152.

52 Durham SR, Kay AB. Eosinophils, bronchial hyperreactivity and late-phase asthmatic reactions. *Clin Allergy* 1985; 15: 411.

53 Ellis AG. The pathological anatomy of bronchial asthma. *Am J Med Sci* 1908; 136: 407.

54 Dunnill MS. *Pulmonary Pathology.* Edinburgh: Churchill Livingstone, 1982: Chapter 6.

55 Capron M, Capron A, Dessaint JP, Torpier G, Johansson GS, Prin A. Fc receptors for IgE on human and rat eosinophils. *J Immunol* 1981; 126: 2087.

56 Khalife J, Capron M, Cesbron JY *et al.* Role of specific IgE antibodies in peroxidase (EPO) release from human eosinophils. *J Immunol* 1986; 137: 1659.

57 Burke LA, Crea REG, Wilkinson JRW, Arm JP, Spur BW, Lee TH. Comparison of the generation of platelet activating factor and leukotriene C4 in human eosinophils stimulated by unopsonized zymosan and the

calcoum inophore A23187: the effects of nedocromil sodium. *J Allergy Clin Immunol* 1990; 85: 26.

58 Cromwell O, Wardlaw AJ, Champion A, Moqbel R, Osei D, Kay AB. IgG-dependent generation of platelet activating factor by normal and low density human eosinophils. *J Immunol* 1990; 145: 3862.

59 Hubscher T. Role of the eosinophil in allergic reactions. II. Release of prostaglandins from human eosinophilic leukocytes. *J Immunol* 1975; 114: 1389.

60 Parsons WG, Roberts LJ. Transformation of prostaglandin D$_2$ to isomeric prostaglandin F$_2$ compounds by human eosinophils. A potential mast cell–eosinophil interaction. *J Immunol* 1988; 141: 2413.

61 Shaw RJ, Walsh GM, Cromwell O, Moqbel R, Spry CJF, Kay AB. Activated human eosinophils generate SRS-A leukotrienes following physiological (IgG-dependent) stimulations. *Nature* 1985; 316: 150.

62 Cromwell O, Moqbel R, Fitzharris P *et al.* Leukotriene C4 generation from human eosinophils stimulated with IgG–*Aspergillus fumigatus* antigen immune complexes. *J Allergy Clin Immunol* 1988; 82: 535.

63 Jorg A, Henderson WR, Murphy RC, Klebanoff SJ. Leukotriene generation by eosinophils. *J Exp Med* 1982; 155: 390.

64 Weller PF, Lee CN, Foster DW, Corey EJ, Susten KF, Lewis RA. Generation and metabolism of 5-lipoxygenase pathway leukotrienes by human eosinophils; predominant production of leukotriene C4. *Proc Natl Acad Sci USA* 1983; 80: 7625.

65 Turk J, Maas RL, Brash AR, Roberts L, Oates JA. Arachidonic acid and 5-lipoxygenase products from human eosinophils. *J Biol Chem* 1982; 257: 7068.

66 Moqbel R, Lacy P, Levi-Schaffer F *et al.* Interleukin-6 is a granule-associated preformed mediator in eosinophils from asthmatic subjects. *Am J Respir Crit Care Med* 1994; 149: A836.

67 Wardlaw AJ, Moqbel RM, Kay AB. Eosinophils and the allergic inflammatory response. In: Kay AB, ed. *Allergy and Allergic Diseases.* Oxford: Blackwell Science, 1997: Chapter 10.

68 Stern M, Meagher L, Savill J, Haslett C. Apoptosis in human eosinophils: programmed cell death in the eosinophil leads to phagocytosis by macrophages and is modulated by IL-5. *J Immunol* 1992; 148: 3543.

69 Murphy KR, Wilson MC, Irvin CG *et al.* The requirement for polymorphonuclear leukocytes in the late asthmatic response and heightened airways reactivity in an animal model. *Am Rev Respir Dis* 1986; 134: 62.

70 Gajewski TF, Joyce J, Fitch FW. Antiproliferative effect of interferon-γ in immune regulation. III. Differential selection of Th1 and Th2 murine helper T lymphocyte clones using recombinant IL-2 and recombinant IFN-γ. *J Immunol* 1989; 143: 15.

71 Fiorentino D, Bond HW, Mossmann TR. Two types of mouse T helper cells. IV. Th2 clones secrete a factor that inhibits cytokine production by Th1 clones. *J Exp Med* 1989; 170: 65.

72 Robinson DR, Hamid Q, Ying S *et al.* Evidence for a predominant 'Th2 type' bronchoalveolar lavage T-lymphocyte population in atopic asthma. *N Engl J Med* 1992; 326: 298.

73 Corrigan CJ, Hamid Q, North J *et al.* Peripheral blood CD4, but not CD8 T lymphocytes in patients with exacerbation of asthma transcribe and translate messenger RNA encoding cytokines which prolong eosinophil survival in the context of a Th2-type pattern: effect of glucocorticoid therapy. *Am J Respir Cell Mol Biol* 1995; 12: 567.

74 Kamei T, Ozaki T, Kawaji K *et al.* Production of interleukin-5 and granulocyte/macrophage colony-stimulating factor by T cells of patients with bronchial asthma in response to *Dermatophagoides farinae* and its relation to eosinophil colony-stimulating factor. *Am J Respir Crit Care Med* 1993; 9: 378.

75 Del Prete GF, De Carli M, D'Elios MM *et al.* Allergens exposure induces the activation of allergen-specific Th2 cells in the airway mucosa of patients with allergic respiratory disorders. *Eur J Immunol* 1993; 23: 1445.

76 Robinson DS, Ying S, Bentley AM *et al.* Relationships among numbers of bronchoalveolar lavage cells expressing messenger ribonucleic acid for cytokines, asthma symptoms, and airway methacholine responsiveness in atopic asthma. *J Allergy Clin Immunol* 1993; 92: 397.

77 Ying S, Durham SR, Corrigan CJ, Hamid Q, Kay AB. Phenotype of cells expressing mRNA for Th2-type (interleukin-4 and interleukin-5) and Th1-type (interleukin-2 and interferon-γ) cytokines in bronchoalveolar lavage and bronchial biopsies from atopic asthmatics and normal control subjects. *Am J Respir Cell Mol Biol* 1995; 12: 477.

78 Virchow JC, Walker C, Hafner D *et al.* T cells and cytokines in bronchoalveolar lavage fluid after segmental allergen provocation in atopic asthma. *Am J Respir Crit Care Med* 1995; 151: 960.

79 Wilkens M, Wilkens JH, Busse S *et al.* Effects of an inhaled PAF antagonist (WEB 2086BS) on allergen-induced early and late asthmatic responses and increased bronchial responsiveness to methacholine. *Am Rev Respir Dis* 1991; 143: A812.

80 Finney MJB, Karlson JA, Persson CGA. Effects of bronchoconstriction and bronchodilation on a novel human small airway preparation. *Br J Pharmacol* 1985; 85: 29.

81 Evans TW, Rogers DF, Aursudjij B, Chung KF, Barnes PJ. Inflammatory mediators involved in antigen-induced airway microvascular leakage in guinea pigs. *Am Rev Respir Dis* 1988; 138: 395.

82 Shelhamer J, Marom Z, Kaliner M. Immunologic and neuropharmacologic stimulation of mucous glycoprotein release from human airways in vitro. *J Clin Invest* 1980; 66: 1400.

83 Christiansen SC, Proud D, Sarnoff RB, Juergens U, Cochrane CG, Zuran BL. Elevation of tissue kallikrein and kinin in the airways of asthmatic subjects after endobronchial allergen challenge. *Am Rev Respir Dis* 1992; 145: 900.

84 Fuller RW, Dixon CMS, Cuss FMC, Barnes PJ. Bradykinin-induced bronchoconstriction in man: mode of action. *Am Rev Respir Dis* 1987; 135: 176.

85 Ichinose M, Nakajima N, Takahashi T, Yamauchi H, Inoue H, Takishima T. Protection against bradykinin-induced bronchoconstriction in asthmatic patients by a neurokinin receptor antagonist. *Lancet* 1992; 340: 1248.

86 Barnes PJ. Bradykinin and asthma. *Thorax* 1992; 47: 979.

87 O'Banion MK, Winn VD, Young DA. cDNA cloning and functional activity of a glucocorticoid-regulated inflammatory cyclooxygenase. *Proc Natl Acad Sci USA* 1992; 89: 4888.

88 Liu MC, Hubbard WC, Proud D *et al*. Immediate and late inflammatory responses to ragweed antigen challenge of the peripheral airways in allergic asthmatics: cellular, mediator and permeability changes. *Am Rev Respir Dis* 1991; 144: 51.

89 Smith HR, Larsen GL, Cherniak RM *et al*. Inflammatory cells and eicosanoid mediators in subjects with late asthmatic responses and increased airway responsiveness. *J Allergy Clin Immunol* 1992; 89: 1076.

90 O'Byrne PM, Fuller RW. The role of thromboxane A_2 in the pathogenesis of airway hyperresponsiveness. *Eur Respir J* 1989; 2: 782.

91 Wenzel SE, Larsen GL, Johnston K, Voelkel NP, Wescott JY. Elevated levels of leukotriene C_4 in bronchoalveolar lavage fluid from atopic asthmatics after allergen challenge. *Am Rev Respir Dis* 1990; 142: 112.

92 Arm JP, Spur BW, Lee TH. The effects of inhaled leukotriene E_4 on the airway responsiveness to histamine in subjects with asthma and normal subjects. *J Allergy Clin Immunol* 1988; 82: 654.

93 Kaye MG, Smith LJ. Effects of inhaled leukotriene D_4 and platelet activating factor on airway reactivity in normal subjects. *Am Rev Respir Dis* 1990; 141: 993.

94 Ford-Hutchison AW. FLAP: a novel drug target for inhibiting the synthesis of leukotrienes. *Trends Pharmacol Sci* 1991; 21: 68.

95 Benveniste J, Henson PM, Cochrane CG. Leukocyte-dependent histamine release from rabbit platelets: the role of IgE, basophils and a platelet-activating factor. *J Exp Med* 1972; 136: 1356.

96 Cuss FM, Dixon CMS, Barnes PJ. Effects of inhaled platelet activating factor on pulmonary function and bronchial responsiveness in man. *Lancet* 1986; ii: 189.

97 Evans TW, Chung KF, Rogers DF, Barnes PJ. Effect of platelet activating factor on airway vascular permeability: possible mechanisms. *J Appl Physiol* 1987; 63: 479.

98 Rogers DF, Alton EWFW, Aursudkij B, Boschetto P, Dewar A, Barnes PJ. Effect of platelet activating factor on formation and composition of airway fluid in the guinea pig trachea. *J Physiol* 1991; 43: 643.

99 Sanjar S, Smith D, Kings MA, Morley J. Pre-treatment with rh-GMCSF, but not rh-IL3, enhances PAF-induced eosinophil accumulation in guinea pig airways. *Br J Pharmacol* 1990; 100: 399.

100 Kimani G, Tonnesen MG, Henson PG. Stimulation of eosinophil adherence to human vascular endothelial cells *in vitro* by platelet activating factor. *J Immunol* 1988; 140: 3161.

101 Kroegel C, Yukawa T, Dent G, Chanez P, Chung KF, Barnes PJ. Platelet activating factor induces eosinophil peroxidase release from human eosinophils. *Immunology* 1988; 64: 559.

102 Kroegel C, Yukawa T, Dent G, Venge P, Chung KF, Barnes PJ. Stimulation of degranulation from human eosoinophils by platelet activating factor. *J Immunol* 1989; 142: 3518.

103 Adamus WS, Heuer H, Meade CJ, Kempe ER, Brecht HM. Inhibitory effect of oral WEB 2086, a novel selective PAF-acether antagonist, on *ex vivo* platelet aggregation. *Eur J Clin Pharmacol* 1988; 35: 237.

104 Hayes J, Ridge SM, Griffiths S, Barnes PJ, Chung KF. Inhibition of cutaneous and platelet responses to platelet activating factor by oral WEB 2086 in man. *J Allergy Clin Immunol* 1991; 88: 83.

105 Cromwell O, Hamid Q, Corrigan CJ *et al*. Expression and generation of interleukin-8, IL-6 and granulocyte colony-stimulating factor by bronchial epithelial cells and enhancement by IL-1β and tumour necrosis factor-α. *Immunology* 1992; 77: 330.

106 Kwon OJ, Collins PD, Au B *et al*. Glucocorticoid inhibition of TNFα-induced IL-8 gene expression in human primary cultured epithelial cells. *Am Rev Respir Dis* 1993; 147: A752.

107 Ohno I, Ohkawara Y, Yamauchi K, Tanno Y, Takisima T. Production of tumor necrosis factor with IgE receptor triggering from sensitized lung tissue. *Am J Respir Cell Mol Biol* 1990; 3: 285.

108 Ohkawara Y, Yamauchi K, Tanno Y *et al*. Identification of TNF producing cells in sensitized human lung after IgE receptor triggering. *Am Rev Respir Dis* 1991; 143: 201.

109 Tosi MF, Stark JM, Smith CW, Hamedani A, Gruenert DC, Infeld MD. Induction of ICAM-1 expression on human airway epithelial cells by inflammatory cytokines: effects on neutrophil–epithelial cell adhesion. *Am J Respir Cell Mol Biol* 1992; 7: 214.

110 Thornhill MH, Wellicome SM, Mahiouz DL, Lanchbury JSS, Kyan-Aung V, Haskard DO. Tumor necrosis factor combines with IL-4 or IFN-γ to selectively enhance endothelial cell adhesiveness for T cells. The contribution of vascular adhesion molecule-1-dependent and -independent binding mechanisms. *J Immunol* 1991; 146: 592.

111 Gauchat J-F, Henchoz S, Mazzei G *et al*. Induction of human IgE synthesis in B cells by mast cells and basophils. *Nature* 1993; 365: 340.

112 Schleimer RP, Sterbinsky CA, Kaiser CA *et al*. Interleukin-4 induces adherence of human eosinophils and basophils but not neutrophils to endothelium: association with expression of VCAM-1. *J Immunol* 1992; 148: 1086.

113 Sanderson CJ. Interleukin-5, eosinophils and disease. *Blood* 1992; 79: 3101.

114 Broide D, Paine MM, Firestein GS. Eosinophils express interleukin 5 and granulocyte-macrophage colony-stimulating factor mRNA at sites of allergic inflammation in asthmatics. *J Clin Invest* 1992; 90: 1414.

115 Ohnishi T, Sur S, Collins DS, Fish JE, Gleich GJ, Peters SP. Eosinophil survival activity identified as interleukin-5 is associated with eosinophil recruitment and degranulation and lung injury 24 hours after segmental antigen lung challenge. *J Allergy Clin Immunol* 1993; 92: 607.

116 Rot A, Krieger M, Brunner T, Bischoff SC, Schall TJ, Dahinden CA. RANTES and macrophage inhibitory protein 1α induce the migration and activation of normal human eosinophil granulocytes. *J Exp Med* 1992; 176: 1489

117 Kameyoshi Y, Dorschner A, Mallet AI, Christophers E, Schroder JM. Cytokine RANTES released from thrombin-stimulated platelets is a potent attractant for human eosinophils. *J Exp Med* 1992; 176: 587.

118 Jose PH, Griffiths-Johnson DA *et al*. Eotaxin: a potent eosinophil chemoattractant cytokine detected in a guinea pig model of allergic airways inflammation. *J Exp Med* 1994; 179: 881.

119 Fabbri LM, Boschetto P, Zocca E. Bronchoalveolar neutrophilia during late asthmatic reactions induced by toluene diisocyanate. *Am Rev Respir Dis* 1987; 136: 36.

120 Aalbers R, Kauffman HF, Vrugt B *et al*. Bronchial lavage and bronchoalveolar lavage in allergen-induced single early and dual asthmatic responders. *Am Rev Respir Dis* 1993; 147: 76.

121 Gonzalez MC, Diaz P, Galleguilos FR, Ancic P, Cromwell O, Kay AB. Allergen-induced recruitment of bronchoalveolar helper (OKT4) and suppressor (OKT8) T cells in asthma: relative increases in OKT8 cells in single early responders compared with those in late-phase responders. *Am Rev Respir Dis* 1987; 136: 600.

122 Beasley R, Roche WR, Roberts AJ, Holgate ST. Cellular events in the bronchi in mild asthma and after bronchial provocation. *Am Rev Respir Dis* 1989; 139: 806.

123 Wegner CD, Gundel RH, Reilly N, Haynes L, Letts G, Rothlein R. Intercellular adhesion molecule-1 (ICAM-1) in the pathogenesis of asthma. *Science* 1990; 247: 456.

124 Bentley AM, Durham SR, Robinson DS *et al*. Expression of endothelial and leukocyte adhesion molecules intercellular adhesion molecule-1, E-selectin, and vascular cell adhesion molecule-1 in the bronchial mucosa in steady state and allergen-induced asthma. *J Allergy Clin Immunol* 1993; 92: 857.

125 Bentley AM, Qui Meng, Robinson DS *et al*. Increases in activated T lymphocytes, eosinophils, and cytokine mRNA expression for IL-5 and GM-CSF in bronchial biopsies after allergen inhalation challenge in atopic asthmatics. *Am J Respir Cell Mol Biol* 1993; 8: 35.

126 Thomson NC. *In vivo* versus *in vitro* human airway responsiveness to different pharmacologic stimuli. *Am Rev Respir Dis* 1987; 136: S58.

127 Barnes PJ. Asthma as an axon reflex. *Lancet* 1986; i: 242.

128 Roche WR, Beasley R, Williams JH, Holgate ST. Subepithelial fibrosis in the bronchi of asthmatics. *Lancet* 1989; i: 520.

34

ASTHMA: CLINICAL FEATURES

ANTHONY SEATON AND GRAHAM CROMPTON

What is asthma?

The word 'asthma' is Greek, meaning 'breathless' or 'to breathe with open mouth'. Originally applied to shortness of breath of any cause, as in the description of the mode of death of metal miners ('from the disease the Greeks call asthma') by Agricola in 1556 [1], it has come to be applied particularly to episodic breathlessness due to bronchial disease. Sir John Floyer in his *Treatize of the Asthma* (1698) used the term in its general sense but confined himself largely to discussing the episodic type from which he himself suffered [2]. By the last century, as in another famous book by an asthma sufferer, Henry Hyde Salter's *On Asthma, its Pathology and Treatment* (1860), it was used specifically to describe this type of breathlessness [3]. Nevertheless, its application, as cardiac asthma, to left ventricular failure has only recently fallen into disuse.

The condition from which Floyer and Salter suffered is so distinctive that it may readily be diagnosed by non-medical people and its name is used in common parlance. It might therefore surprise the layman that there is so much debate about the definition of asthma, but such debate continues and is likely to do so unresolved. This is because, as far as can be seen, asthma results from the interaction of many genetic and environmental influences on the tone or reactivity of the airways, usually by causing inflammation; the response varies from individual to individual and from time to time. No single definition will ever cover all these variables in a way that is likely to be useful, particularly when one considers that asthmatic responses are not likely to be all-or-nothing phenomena but rather gradations of change on a continuum. As with other common diseases, the concept of what asthma is has been modified as knowledge of the disease increases. Originally it was acceptable to think of it in terms of a complex of symptoms and signs, then in terms of distinctive physiological and pathological features. Recently it has been popular to define it in terms of bronchial reactivity, although this leads to the uncomfortable recognition that some quite typically asthmatic subjects have normally

reactive airways between attacks. Of course, any definition in physiopathological terms requires arbitrary decisions about cut-off points between normality and asthma that make artificial distinctions between health and illness on that continuum.

It might therefore be appropriate to consider first why it is necessary to define asthma. From the point of view of the patient and the doctor, the name is unimportant; what matters is the management. Diagnosis leads to treatment and prognosis. For the former, it is necessary to demonstrate a response of the airflow obstruction to various drugs or to exclude exposure to a provoking agent, but for the latter it is desirable to fit the patient's disease into some broad category about which there is a body of medical knowledge on which attempts at prognosis may be based. Thus clinicians have tended to prefer definitions based on variability of symptoms and expiratory flow rates [4]. In contrast, pathologists, based on their experience particularly of fatal asthma, have inclined towards histopathological definitions, for example the presence of characteristic patterns in the sputum or of inflammation on bronchial biopsies or lavage [5,6]. Others, pursuing an interest in clinical pharmacology, have required tighter definitions based on physiological criteria; these definitions have often selected specific subgroups, for example in terms of exercise response [7] or the presence of evidence of cardiac stress in acute severe asthma [8]. Finally, epidemiologists have also needed to devise their own definitions for studies of asthma in populations; these range from positive answers to certain questions in a questionnaire to predefined responses to exercise or bronchial challenge [9,10].

Ultimately, it is conceivable that the propensity to develop asthma given appropriate environmental stimuli may be definable in terms of several chromosomal mutations. It is likely that there are separately inherited components of asthma, some genes leading to the development of atopy and others responsible for the many factors leading to bronchial inflammation and clinical asthma [11]. It has been suggested that the tendency for IgE responses to occur is conferred by an 'atopy locus' on chromosome 11q [12], although there is dispute about this and other loci have been described [13,14]. However, studies of bronchial hyperresponsiveness in twins that have been adjusted for atopic status have suggested that environmental factors are at least as important as genetic [15,16]. Until we have more knowledge about the inheritance of atopy and asthma we will have to make do with more or less unsatisfactory definitions influenced by clinical, physiological and pathological factors that are inevitably imprecise. No harm will be done by this if physicians are aware of their reasons for using a particular definition or description of the disease, and the uncertainties surrounding it. A useful description of chronic asthma, based on the clinical, physiological and pathological findings, is

> A common and chronic inflammatory condition of the airways. As a result of the airway inflammation the bronchi are hyperreactive and narrow readily in response to a wide range of stimuli. Whilst initially reversible, the inflammation may lead to irreversible obstruction to airflow.

This may then be qualified by a more quantitative definition in terms of, for example, sputum cytology, airway pathology, spontaneous change in flow rates, or responses to bronchodilators, steroids, exercise or bronchoconstrictors.

Natural history

What happens to asthmatic children in adult life remains somewhat unpredictable [17]. It is a common observation that children with mild asthma tend to improve about the time of adolescence. Clinical and epidemiological studies indicate that 30–80% of asthmatics become asymptomatic during puberty [18–22]. In the UK the prevalence of asthma or wheeze at the age of 7 has been assessed as 8.3% compared with 4.7% at the age of 11 and 3.5% at the age of 16 [23]. In a study of a 1958 birth cohort of over 18 000 British children, Strachan and colleagues [24] showed a cumulative incidence of wheezy illness of 18% by age 7, rising to 43% by age 33. The prognosis in this cohort is shown in Fig. 34.1. Roughly one-quarter of those wheezing at age 7 were still wheezing at 33, and within this overall pattern there was a tendency for remission and later recurrence of symptoms in adult life. Furthermore, new wheezers added to the overall incidence throughout the study. Similarly, in a 25-year follow-up of 2500 primary school children in Scotland, Godden and colleagues [25,26] showed the incidence of new wheezy illness over this period to be 11% of those who had not wheezed in childhood and that these new incidences occurred steadily throughout the period. In a cohort study of Australian schoolchildren tested initially at the age of 8–10 years and then again at 12–14 years of age, the persistence of bronchial hyperresponsiveness at age 12–14 was found to be related to severity of disease at age 8–10, atopic status and parental asthma [27]. It has been suggested that improvement in asthma during adolescence may result from diminished clinical and immunological responsiveness directly related to hormonal changes [28], and that the effect of age on the prevalence of asthma in each sex may relate to differences in hormonal status, influencing airway size, inflammation and smooth muscle and vascular functions [29]. Factors found to predict persistence of asthma appear to be early age of onset of disease (younger than 3 years), infantile eczema (atopic status) and severe disease [30–32], as well as parental asthma [27]. When a cohort of children was assessed at the age of 20, about one-quarter were free from symptoms and had

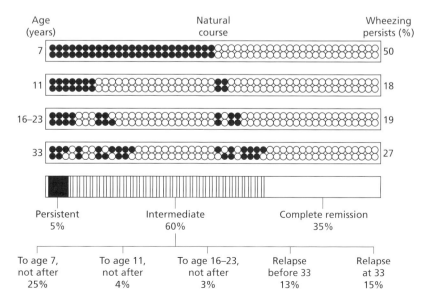

Fig. 34.1 Prognosis of children who developed asthma or wheezy bronchitis by age 7, each symbol representing 1% of such children. Solid circles represent children reporting asthma or wheeze in the previous year at ages 7 and 11, since their 16th birthday at age 23, and in the previous year at age 33. (From Strachan *et al.* [24] with permission.)

normal pulmonary function tests, half had occasional mild wheezing and some 20% had persistent or frequent wheeze or subnormal pulmonary function tests [33,34]. At the age of 28, 30% of those who were free from symptoms at the age of 21 had relapsed and had recurrent wheeze [35]. This supports the clinical experience that patients who appear to develop asthma in adult life often remember chest symptoms during childhood.

There has been much speculation about the genetic and environmental determinants of childhood asthma. Some of the factors related to the development of atopic sensitization that have been discussed include exposure to allergens, infectious diseases, or tobacco smoke early in life. The dietary habits of the mother may also be important but the effects of outdoor air pollution are likely to be unimportant [36]. This and other potential risk factors for asthma are discussed below. One cross-sectional study of elderly people with a history of asthma, detected in a random survey of a town's population, attempted to trace back the natural history of the disease by clinical questioning [37]. Even allowing for problems with memory and diagnosis, this illustrated the liability of asthma both to start and to remit at any age (Fig. 34.2).

Prospective population-based studies of the natural history of asthma in adults are few and, like the studies in children, are limited by difficulties in defining the disease. Most of the patients whose asthma persists from childhood have allergy to various aeroallergens, although the genuine new-onset adult asthmatics have allergic symptoms less commonly unless they have developed occupational asthma (see below). The term 'intrinsic' asthma was introduced in 1940 to emphasize that this type is distinct from allergic 'extrinsic' asthma with respect to the absence of an obvious precipitating exogenous cause [38]. The debate about whether intrinsic asthma is a distinct immunopathological entity persists [39]. Of a group of 85 children consecutively referred to an allergy clinic in Copenhagen when aged 5–15, 70 were seen 10 years later [40]; 24 originally had intrinsic asthma, i.e. normal serum IgE and no evidence of allergy from history, skin tests, radioallergosorbent test (RAST) and, in some, specific bronchial provocation tests; the remaining 46 were labelled extrinsic asthmatics. At the 10-year follow-up, 60 (24 intrinsic and 46 extrinsic) had current symptoms and 54 were receiving maintenance therapy. In the patients with intrinsic asthma, outcome appeared to be predicted by a combination of initial frequency of symptoms, initial forced expiratory volume in 1s (FEV_1), active smoking and age at onset of symptoms. In the extrinsic group, initial FEV_1 was the strongest predictor for outcome and it was suggested that these differences pointed to different pathogenic mechanisms in the two types of asthma. However, a careful follow-up study of a cohort of wheezy children in Australia, to the age of 28, concluded that there is no difference in outcome between asthma and 'wheezy

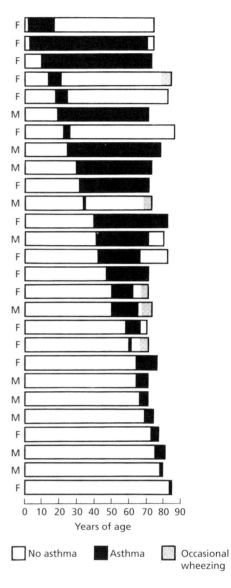

Fig. 34.2 History of asthma symptoms in 27 subjects found in a random sample of people aged 70 or more from a South Wales town. (From Burr *et al.* [37].)

bronchitis' in childhood [33,35]. In the view of the authors, asthma is best thought of as an inflammatory disease of the airways with multiple precipitating causes acting throughout life. In those most strongly predisposed genetically, atopy is a dominant factor and such individuals tend to present early in life. Those presenting in adult life are somewhat less frequently atopic, and factors such as smoking, poor diet, occupational exposures and infections appear to be more relevant to the aetiology than in childhood.

Several studies have investigated mortality from asthma. Interest in this subject was aroused by a sharp rise in mortality in the UK, New Zealand and other westernized countries (but not the USA) in the mid-1960s [41]. Among young people, death rates attributed to asthma rose to about 2 per 100 000 population per annum, subsequently falling to the more usual levels of about half that (Fig. 34.3). In New Zealand there was a second rise in mortality in the 1970s to about 4 per 100 000 [43]. These changes stimulated a number of clinical and case–control investigations of possible causative factors; excess use of bronchodilators and inadequate use of corticosteroids have been suggested as likely ones [44–50]. The possible role of β-agonist bronchodilators and the increase in mortality, particularly in New Zealand, has caused most concern and has stimulated much debate. The New Zealand 'epidemic' was originally attributed to fenoterol [51]. However, the explanation is not straightforward; although the drug was also available in The Netherlands and the UK, the asthma mortality rates in these countries had returned to the levels observed before 1940 and remained there. Taken together, the time trends suggest a causal relationship between death from asthma and inhalation therapy with β agonists. However, others have rejected the view that the use of β agonists, one of the cornerstones of asthma treatment, is potentially dangerous [52], the argument being that β agonists merely served as a marker of patients with a poor prognosis. There are two main questions that remain unanswered with regard to β agonists: does regular inhaled treatment with these drugs make asthma worse or increase bronchial hyperreactivity either during therapy or after withdrawal and is this form of treatment dangerous when given to, or taken in excess by, the hypoxaemic asthmatic? Of course, β-agonist therapy cannot be an explanation of the increased prevalence of asthma, and whether it has had any role in the fluctuation in severity of patients with severe disease over

the years remains to be answered. There is evidence from experiments with animals that β agonists are much more toxic in the presence of hypoxaemia [53], and this has tended to be forgotten. It has been reported that similar findings resulted when human volunteers were studied in a hypoxaemic state [54]. In general the message from all studies is the slightly depressing one that death commonly occurs as a result of failure by patient or doctor to appreciate the severity of the condition or to take appropriate therapeutic action until too late. The pros and cons of β-agonist therapy are discussed in more detail in Chapter 35.

The actual risk of an asthmatic patient dying of the disease clearly depends on such factors as age, severity of disease, and availability and quality of medical care. Asthma deaths are rare in children, accounting for just over 1% of total deaths [55]. Thereafter, the risk increases exponentially with age (Fig. 34.4). Interpretation of geographical variations and time trends in mortality usually concentrates on deaths among children and adults up to age 35 where there is more confidence in the accuracy of diagnosis. However, only 10% of deaths occur in this age group and the rates for all countries where reliable data are available were similar in the 1990s at 1 per 100 000 or fewer [56].

Pathology

Gross pathology

The greatest amount of information on the pathology of the lungs in asthma originally came from necropsy studies of patients who had died from acute attacks [57–61]. However, some information has also been obtained from lungs of asthmatic patients dying of other causes while in remission and from the study of bronchial biopsies, bronchoalveolar lavage (BAL) fluid and sputum from asthmatics. Recently, developments in bronchoscopic techniques and methods to enable patients to produce sputum, together with electron microscopy, have allowed a much more detailed knowledge of pathological airway morphology to be obtained from living patients with mild, moderate and severe disease.

The lungs of asthmatic patients who have died of incidental disease may show the features seen in those who have died of asthma but in a less advanced form. There is usually some overdistension and plugging of airways. In contrast, patients with chronic asthma may die with lungs that look grossly quite normal, despite having had intractable symptoms in life [62]. The lungs of patients who have died of acute asthma are voluminous and do not collapse when the chest is opened at autopsy. When cut, thick and tenacious mucus is seen to be occluding almost all small- and medium-sized airways, but this can extend into the large bronchi. There may be small focal areas of

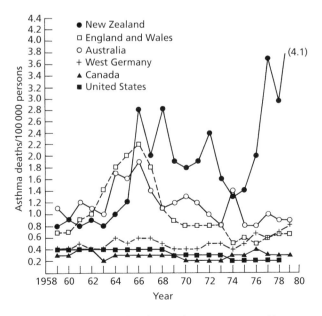

Fig. 34.3 Trends in mortality from asthma in 5–34 year olds in six countries, 1959–79. (From Jackson *et al.* [42].)

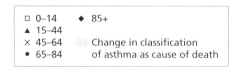

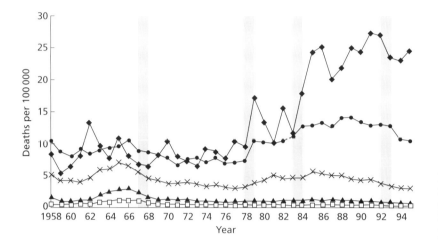

Fig. 34.4 Age-specific asthma mortality rates, males and females combined, England and Wales 1958–95. (From Lung and Asthma Information Agency factsheet 97/3, with permission of Professor Ross Anderson.)

pulmonary collapse. Occasionally, when death has been sudden, widespread airway plugging is absent. Although the lungs are hyperinflated, there is usually no macroscopic evidence of emphysema.

Bronchial biopsies

Much has been learned about the pathological processes in asthma by examination of bronchial biopsies and BAL fluid. These investigations are safe providing that they are performed by an experienced bronchoscopist and that published recommendations are followed [63,64]. The airway mucosa sampled by biopsy comprises surface epithelium and its supportive subepithelial tissue, often referred to as the lamina propria.

Data obtained by biopsy have shown beyond doubt that asthma is an inflammatory condition, and have provided the basis for the validation of less invasive techniques, such as airway lavage, bronchial brush biopsy and the examination of sputum, either produced spontaneously or induced. Pioneering studies of relatively large biopsy samples obtained using the rigid bronchoscope revealed the mucosal inflammation of asthma, contrasted the pathological appearances in asthma and chronic bronchitis and demonstrated the efficacy of inhaled corticosteroid therapy [65–68]. These studies also revealed the marked airway epithelial disruption in asthma, now accepted as a characteristic pathological feature of the disease even though described as early as 1962 [69]. With the advent of flexible fibreoptic bronchoscopy as a research tool there has been an explosion of interest in the pathological changes in the bronchial epithelium of the asthmatic patient [70]. Initial electron microscopic studies of biopsies

in mild chronic asthma reported the involvement and degranulation of mast cells [71], highlighted a controlling role for the lymphocyte in the inflammatory response, and demonstrated an association between loss of surface epithelium and airways hyperresponsiveness [72]. Most, if not all, of these pathological changes had previously been described in autopsy studies of patients dying from asthma [57,59–61]. These features of inflammation were shown to be present even in patients with newly diagnosed asthma or asthma of apparently recent onset [73].

Studies of bronchial biopsies together with clinical observations have led to the conclusion that early intervention with anti-inflammatory therapy is the most rational approach to treatment of asthma [74]. Homogeneous thickening of the basement membrane, also referred to as the lamina reticularis, is a constant pathological finding and has been shown to occur early in the disease process [72,75], in contrast to the lack of this change in chronic obstructive airways disease [76,77]. Basement membrane thickening in asthma is assumed to represent subepithelial fibrosis and is associated with close proximity of myofibroblasts [75,78]. Studies of bronchial biopsies from large numbers of patients have revealed activation of the CD4+ subset of T lymphocytes and also eosinophils [79,80]. There appears to be a negative correlation between eosinophil activation and bronchial reactivity [80]. Observation of upregulation of gene expression for the proinflammatory cytokine interleukin (IL)-5, in association with the CD4+ T lymphocyte, particularly in symptomatic patients [81], has led to the concept of a prevailing Th2 allergic inflammatory profile in asthma in which IL-4, IL-5 and IL-10 predominate [82,83]. Verification of these findings has been achieved by using reverse transcriptase–polymerase chain reaction techniques. The profile of inflammatory cell and cytokine gene expression appears to be similar in different types of disease, such as atopic (extrinsic), non-atopic (intrinsic) and occupational asthma, although there is some debate about the role of IL-4 in intrinsic asthma [84–87].

Bronchial and nasal biopsies have been studied after exposure to allergens. The use of immunohistological and molecular (*in situ* hybridization) techniques has supported the involvement of CD4+ T cells, mast cells and eosinophils, together with IL-4, IL-5 and IL-10 [82,88–90]. There is also great interest in the role of cell-surface adhesion molecules in the epithelial inflammatory events of asthma and allergy [91–93]. Myofibroblast numbers increase in response to allergen and transitional ultrastructural forms between fibroblasts and bronchial smooth muscle cells are found [94]. This suggests a possible mechanism to explain the increase in bronchial smooth muscle that is a characteristic feature of the airway wall remodelling found in severe asthma [95]. Exposure to toluene diisocyanate (TDI) in workers who develop occupational asthma resembles allergen exposure in many aspects, although in addition there is a marked recruitment of neutrophils [86,96,97].

Bronchial biopsies have been used to assess the effects of various treatments on the asthmatic bronchial epithelial inflammation. Inhaled corticosteroid therapy has been shown to improve these pathological changes [98–100] and the changes in bronchial biopy appearances have been asssociated with symptomatic improvement. Similar improvements in symptoms and bronchial epithelial pathology have been reported in non-allergic asthma [101]. The anti-inflammatory properties of some other drugs have been assessed by bronchial biopsies, and oral theophylline has been shown to have some activity after 6 weeks of treatment compared with placebo in that it decreased cell numbers and the expression of IL-4 [102].

Bronchial biopsies sample mainly the proximal airways and it is somewhat surprising that so much inflammation and remodelling has been found in the large airways in asthma. There is some evidence that the changes in large airways reflect more peripheral pathology in the small airways, and perhaps also in the alveoli [103]. Since biopsies sample such a small fragment of epithelium, one would expect considerable variation between specimens, such that very large numbers of patients would have to be studied to obtain any meaningful data. However, it is reassuring that there seems to be larger intersubject than interbiopsy site variation, and it has been estimated that study of groups numbering 15 patients should provide sufficient statistical power to detect most of the changes of interest in biopsies from inflamed airways [104].

The inflammatory cell that predominates within the surface epithelium may be different to that in the tissue beneath it, and cells harvested from the bronchial lumen by BAL may not reflect the cell populations in any section of the bronchial mucosa. This may partly explain differences between biopsy and BAL findings. The correlations between cellular findings of lavage and biopsy specimens are poor and bronchial biopsy remains the gold standard [70]. Bronchial brush biopsies are being used to harvest cells from the bronchial mucosa and may in the future be of value in the assessment of the degree of pathological change in asthma and its response to treatment, if there proves to be a good correlation between these and bronchial biopsies.

Sputum

Sputum is characteristically viscous. When held up to the light, pale green or white streaks can often be seen in the mucus and, when teased out, these can be shown to be bronchial casts (Fig. 34.5). Recently there has been considerable interest in the cell content and immunobiochemical characteristics of sputum from asthmatics [105]. Sputum is defined as expectorated lower respiratory tract secretions and is composed of fluid and cellular components, including macrophages, bronchial epithelial cells and inflammatory cells. As well as containing water and inorganic ions, it also contains non-dialysable components such as albumin, lysozyme, glycoproteins (including immunoglobulins, macroglobulin, complement and proteases), proteoglycan and lipids, perhaps in part derived from surfactant. Proteins and glycoproteins appear to occur in considerably higher concentration in asthmatic than in bronchitic sputum [106]. IgE is also increased, even in

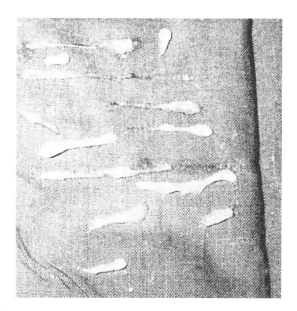

Fig. 34.5 Bronchial casts teased out from the sputum of a patient with asthma.

non-atopic asthma [107]. When expectorated, sputum is always mixed with saliva, composed mainly of fluid, squamous epithelial cells and oropharyngeal bacteria. Sputum contaminated with saliva may be examined for evidence of bronchial inflammation [108], although it is apparent that examination of sputum *selected* from the expectorate is preferable [109–111]. In asthmatic subjects, sputum may be induced by the inhalation of an aerosol of hypertonic saline after pretreatment with inhaled salbutamol [105,112].

Sputum eosinophils

Sputum eosinophilia is a hallmark of asthma and was shown to be associated with the disease almost 100 years ago. The eosinophil is probably the major effector cell in asthma [113]. Eosinophils arise from a bone marrow-derived progenitor cell and circulate via the bloodstream to the airways [114]. Under the influence of cellular adhesion molecules and cytokines the eosinophils migrate across the endothelium to the airway lumen. Sputum eosinophils in asthma are in an activated state, expressing cleaved eosinophil cationic protein (ECP) and CD11b [115]. Cell adhesion molecules ICAM-1 and HLA-DR are present in sputum eosinophils but not blood eosinophils, and these may allow migration across the endothelium and facilitate interaction with other immunocompetent cells such as T lymphocytes [116]. The eosinophil plays an important role in the pathogenesis of asthma, and sputum eosinophil counts reflect disease severity [112]. Eosinophils occur spontaneously and after allergen challenge in asthma [108,113–118]. Thus eosinophil counts and measurement of their products in sputum have a potentially important role in acting as objective markers of bronchial inflammation in asthma. Sputum eosinophils, and the biochemical markers ECP, albumin and fibrinogen, correlate with the diagnosis of asthma [108,112,117] but not with airway hyperresponsiveness in the absence of symptoms [119]. There is also correlation with disease activity and the magnitude of response following allergen challenge [112,114,120]. Patients with sputum eosinophilia tend to respond well to corticosteroid therapy [118,121,122].

Sputum mast cells

There is in the region of a 10-fold increase in the number of mast cells in spontaneously produced and induced sputum from asthmatic patients compared with normal subjects or patients with chronic bronchitis [112,117]. Mast cell counts are highest during exacerbations of asthma and increase after allergen challenge [120]. There is no correlation between sputum mast cell numbers and markers of disease severity such as FEV_1 and bronchial provocation tests, whereas in BAL and bronchial brushings mast cells appear to correlate with airway responsiveness [123,124]. Mast cell mediators such as tryptase and histamine can be detected in induced sputum, although there are no major differences between normal and asthmatic subjects [108].

Bronchoalveolar lavage

BAL is a useful research technique but its role in the investigation and assessment of asthma has yet to be established. Together with other research techniques it has contributed to the understanding of disease mechanisms and treatment effects [125]. Interlobar variability of BAL findings has been assessed. Eosinophil and neutrophil counts are consistent between two lobes from the same individual, indicating that a single-site lavage yields fluid representative of the whole lung; however, there is poor agreement between soluble markers such as the neutrophil product myeloperoxidase and the eosinophil marker ECP [126]. In stable asthma there are increased numbers of eosinophils and mast cells in BAL fluid compared with normals [123], and the same pattern of BAL cell increases has been found in allergic and non-allergic asthma [124]. BAL eosinophils correlate with asthma symptoms, airflow obstruction and airway responsiveness [123,127]. Allergen challenge causes an increase in BAL eosinophils [128] and in eosinophil activation. This is accompanied by increased gene transcription for those cytokines that control eosinophilic function, IL-5 and granulocyte–macrophage colony-stimulating factor (GM-CSF) [127]. Treatment with prednisolone reduces BAL eosinophils and IL-5 gene transcription at the same time as symptoms are improved [129]. In general there is a correlation between the severity of airways responsiveness in asthma and the numbers of eosinophils, mast cells and their mediators in BAL [130]. In a comparison of induced sputum, bronchial washings and BAL in 16 patients, it was concluded that induced sputum is rich in neutrophils and eosinophils and poor in lymphocytes, suggesting an origin in the larger airways. It was also concluded that induced sputum adequately reflects the findings in fluid collected by BAL [131].

Histological features

Many of the microscopic features of the asthmatic airway are mirrored in the sputum. The airways of patients who have died from asthma characteristically show smooth muscle hypertrophy and thickening of the basement membrane (Fig. 34.6). The mucous glands are often considerably enlarged. The submucosa is oedematous, infiltrated with eosinophils and lymphocytes, and contains dilated capillaries with swollen endothelial cells. Mast cells may be found in the submucosa, especially in association with small vessels. Internal to the basement

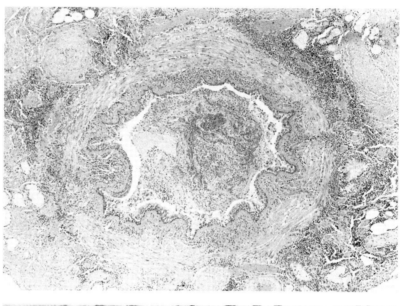

(a)

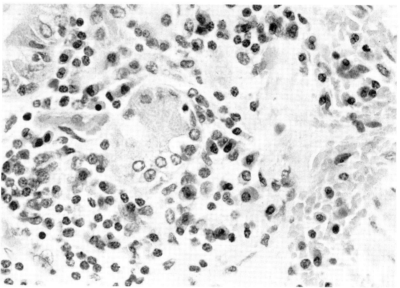

(b)

Fig. 34.6 (a) Cross-section of bronchus from patient who died of acute severe asthma showing plugging of the lumen by mucus. Note also irregular loss of epithelium, thick basement membrane and hyperplastic smooth muscle. A conspicuous inflammatory cell infiltrate involves the full thickness of the wall (haematoxylin & eosin ×35). (b) Detail of the inflammatory infiltrate showing mixture of lymphocytes, plasma cells, macrophages and eosinophils (haematoxylin & eosin ×335). (Courtesy of Dr Peter Johnston, Department of Pathology, University of Aberdeen.)

membrane, the mucosa may have been almost totally destroyed. It is often very oedematous, the oedema being associated with a denudation of the internal surface cells leaving only basal cells. Remaining epithelium is often metaplastic, showing a stratified non-ciliated structure with prominent goblet cells. Eosinophils are a conspicuous feature of the inflammatory exudate. Within the airway lumen lies thick tenacious mucus that under the microscope is seen to contain strips of desquamated epithelial cells (Curschmann's spirals), eosinophils, isolated metaplastic epithelial cells or clumps of cells (Creola bodies) and crystalline material consisting largely of major basic protein derived from eosinophils (Charcot–Leyden crystals) [5,60,132–134]. These plugs may occur throughout airways of all sizes, sometimes reaching the smallest respiratory bronchioles, possibly by aspiration.

The consequences of these histological abnormalities may be found in the sputum of patients with symptomatic asthma, and are not confined to patients with severe disease (Fig. 34.7).

In contrast to the dramatic evidence of disease in patients dying of asthma, much less marked yet nevertheless similar changes are found in patients who have suffered from chronic asthma but have died from another cause [61]. There may be no plugging and little or no smooth muscle hypertrophy, and relatively few eosinophils in patients who have been treated with corticosteroids. Basement membrane thickening is the only characteristic feature, although mucosal and submucosal infiltration with lymphocytes and plasma cells, mucous gland hyperplasia and some peribronchiolar fibrosis may be seen.

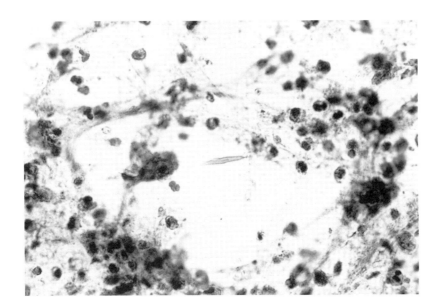

Fig. 34.7 Photomicrograph of asthmatic sputum showing strands of mucus containing eosinophils, some macrophages and one Charcot–Leyden crystal (×340).

Pathogenesis

An understanding of the pathogenesis of asthma requires answers to two questions: what predisposes an individual to show the characteristic pathophysiological airway changes, and how do the known provoking stimuli cause these changes? With respect to the first question, it is a matter of common observation that genetic factors must be important, particularly when the asthma is accompanied by the manifestations of atopy. This is discussed later. However, it is now clear that environmental factors may initiate the asthmatic process, rather than simply provoke attacks in someone already predisposed. The differences in prevalence of asthma in populations transferred to westernized from more primitive societies, between people living different lifestyles in the same country, and the secular changes in prevalence noted in developed countries over the past three decades all suggest an important environmental factor, as does the evidence that certain chemicals may act as initiators of asthma (which persists after exposure has ceased) in some workforces. Similarly, it is also a matter of common observation that adult asthma may be initiated by upper respiratory tract infections, sometimes for a short time but not infrequently permanently. Studies of bronchial reactivity and of responses to inhalation of irritant substances suggest that the liability of airways to constrict in response to such stimuli is distributed normally in the population, and is variable over time, indicating perhaps that all of us may be liable to develop some of the features of asthma in response to stimuli of appropriate severity.

The answers to the second question, namely the mechanisms whereby a stimulus provokes the airway reaction, lie in the study of the cellular, immunological and biochemical control of airway function. Any hypothesis must explain why similar reactions occur in response to infection, allergic challenge, chemical challenge, exercise, sleep, emotion, ingestion of certain drugs and, indeed, for no obvious reason at all. It must also explain the presence of the characteristic histological and biochemical changes in the airways and their exudate, and must take account of the recognized patterns of response (and, in some cases, failure to respond) to therapy. Not surprisingly, understanding of the mechanisms of asthma remains incomplete; nevertheless, much research effort has been devoted towards this end and much interesting, if somewhat confusing, information has been obtained. In the following discussion, this evidence is considered under the headings of cellular mechanisms, mediators, neural mechanisms and bronchial smooth muscle function. There is evidence that all these factors, which interrelate with each other, play a part in producing the pathophysiological changes of asthma. Before embarking on this discussion, some relatively simple models of asthma are described.

Simple models of asthmatic mechanisms

Exercise and hyperventilation

The simplest model of asthma, and one that has been much used in research, is the induction of airflow obstruction by exercise or breathing cold air [135,136]. In most but not all patients with clinical asthma, either of these manoeuvres causes an increase in airways resistance that lasts for some 30 min. This gave rise to the hypothesis that hyperventilation, with its associated drying and cooling of the airways, leads to the release of bronchoconstrictor substances or to a neural bronchoconstriction reflex, or to both [137,138]. Only rarely has exercise been shown to provoke a delayed and more prolonged reaction [139,140], suggesting that in most cases if release of mediators occurs these are likely to be short-acting bronchial muscle constrictors rather than agents that lead to bronchial wall inflammation and oedema. This concept is supported by studies which have shown that once an attack has been provoked by exercise and the subject has recovered, further exercise does not provoke increasingly severe attacks [141]. On the contrary, subjects may be able to continue exercise and find that the asthma improves.

Thus exercise provocation provides an opportunity to study the mechanisms of the immediate component of the asthmatic reaction. Two approaches have been used: search for release of mediators and attempts to block the reaction with drugs. Studies of arterial total and plasma histamine have shown raised baseline levels (compared with controls) that increase during exercise [142–144]; however, similar rises have been described in exercising control subjects [143]. Rises in the levels of neutrophil chemotactic factor during exercise have also been observed [139,145]. Since asthmatic airways show increased sensitivity to histamine, it is likely that histamine release during exercise contributes to the production of airflow obstruction; this concept has been supported by demonstration of a protective effect of selective H_1-receptor antihistamine inhalation prior to exercise [146]. The exercise response can be blocked by inhaled β-sympathomimetic drugs and, in a proportion of cases, by sodium cromoglicate (cromoglycate) and high-dose inhaled antiparasympathetic drugs [147–149]. The former observation is explicable on the basis of bronchodilatation, although it is interesting that studies of cyclic AMP levels show that subjects developing exercise-induced asthma do not show the marked rise seen in the non-asthmatic exercise response, indicating a reduced sympathetic response to exercise in such subjects [150–152]. Furthermore, the blocking effect of antiparasympathetic drugs suggests that vagal reflex mechanisms may be involved in some cases.

Thus, what appears superficially to be a simple model of part of the asthmatic reaction can be seen to involve release of histamine and other mediators, reduced sympathetic response and sometimes parasympathetic reflexes. This leaves unexplained both the mechanisms whereby the response is triggered and also the increased susceptibility of airway muscle to histamine stimulation. Perhaps the clue to the latter lies in the failure of the cyclic AMP response, an area of research that has lately been neglected in favour of search for mediators. The mechanism of the trigger seems to be related to hyperventilation and associated drying and cooling of airways, although this is a feature of exercise common to asthmatics and non-asthmatics; the reason that one responds and the other does not may lie in differences in the reactions of mast cells or neural receptors in airway mucosa to these stimuli.

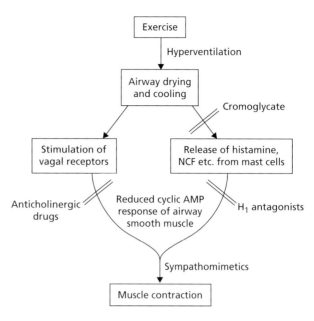

Fig. 34.8 Mechanisms of exercise-induced asthma showing the three possible pathways: mediator release, vagal stimulation and reduced sympathetic drive in smooth muscle. The most effective preventive drugs are sympathomimetics, although H_1 antagonists and anticholinergics are also moderately effective in adequate doses. Steroids have only a rather weak long-term preventive effect. (NCF, neutrophil chemotactic factor.)

Here, again, the reduced cyclic AMP response may be an important clue. A suggested scheme for the mechanisms of exercise-induced asthma is shown in Fig. 34.8.

Antigen challenge

Another model of the asthmatic reaction that has been much studied is the response to inhalation of antigen. This differs from the response to exercise in one important particular: it commonly comprises an immediate and a delayed reaction (Fig. 34.9). The immediate reaction is similar to that occurring after exercise and is blocked by sympathomimetics and cromoglicate but not by corticosteroids. The delayed reaction usually starts during recovery from the immediate (which is shown by the fact that flow rates rarely rise to baseline levels between the two), is prolonged up to 24 or 48 h, and may be followed by a period of increased bronchial reactivity or even by recurrent asthma attacks for several days [153]. It is usually blocked by corticosteroids and cromoglicate but not by sympathomimetics [154–156]. An identical dual reaction may occur in response to inhalation of low molecular weight chemicals such as isocyanates or colophony that are known to cause workplace asthma, probably by combining as haptens with plasma proteins.

This dual reaction and its modification by drugs are clearly suggestive of immediate bronchial muscle constriction followed by a progressive bronchial wall inflammation and mucosal swelling. Moreover, the persistence of the late reaction and the fact that it is only partly responsive to sympathomimetic drugs suggest that it is a more realistic model of the situation in most patients with attacks of asthma. It is reasonable to hypothesize that the initial antigenic stimulus results in the release of both short-acting and long-acting mediators, which initiate both reactions; it is known that the combination of antigen molecules with pairs of IgE antibody molecules on the surface of mast cells leads to release of such substances [157]. Studies of blood and urine levels of histamine and its metabolites and of neutrophil chemotactic activity after bronchial challenge with antigen have shown an initial rise, consistent with the hypothesis [158,159]. Furthermore, bronchial lavage studies during the late reaction have shown evidence of an influx of eosinophils and ECP

at that time, indirect evidence for the release of eosinophil chemotactic factor during the earlier part of the reaction [160]. The cellular and humoral mechanisms of the late response are discussed further in Chapter 33.

Thus, as far as the evidence goes at present, antigen challenge may be regarded as a means of releasing short-acting and delayed-acting mediators, almost certainly from mast cells, which produce immediate broncho-constriction and later bronchial wall, predominantly eosinophilic, inflammation. In most subjects, the basic requirement is atopic sensitization, with the ability to react to antigen with an IgE antibody response. These reactions are illustrated in Fig. 34.10.

Challenge with mediators

In concept, the simplest model of asthma results from the identification of mediators of the reaction and their use in a challenge test. Histamine is the one most studied; its inhalation provokes an immediate increase in airflow obstruction that can be blocked by prior administration of inhaled H_1-receptor but not H_2-receptor antagonists [161,162]. The response to inhaled histamine varies in the population, most people showing very little reaction, some showing a moderate reaction and a few being very sensitive [163,164]. There is no clear distinction between reactors and non-reactors, rather a gradation. Moreover, some people show reactivity at one time and much less or none at others [165]. The test may therefore be used as an index of bronchial reactivity but does not in itself shed much light on the mechanisms of asthma.

Methacholine, a parasympathomimetic agent, affects airflow similarly to histamine and is also used as a non-specific indicator of bronchial reactivity [166]. Similar effects have been demonstrated by inhaled prostaglandin $(PG)D_2$ and $PGF_{2\alpha}$ and leukotriene $(LT)C_4$ and LTD_4, which are more potent than histamine on the asthmatic

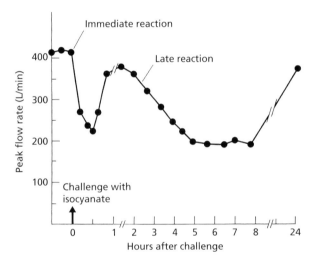

Fig. 34.9 Response of peak flow rate to challenge with toluene diisocyanate vapour from varnish showing immediate and late reactions.

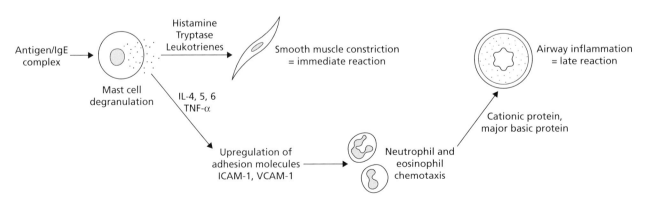

Fig. 34.10 Mechanisms of response to inhaled antigen. Mast cell degranulation provoked by surface binding of IgE–allergen complex releases both short-term mediators, which cause immediate smooth muscle constriction, and also interleukins and

tumour necrosis factor α, which upregulate adhesion molecules. These in turn cause chemotaxis of neutrophils and eosinophils, leading to airway inflammmation and the later more prolonged reaction.

airway [167–171]. The leukotrienes exert a rather slower and more prolonged effect than does histamine.

All these studies indicate that such chemicals are able to provoke airflow obstruction much more readily in people with hyperreactive airways than in those without. They thus suggest that at least part of the mechanism of asthma is related to reactivity of airways rather than excessive release of mediators. However, it is possible that prolonged exposure to these or other mediators may in some way sensitize the airways. This subject remains an area of active research.

Immunological mechanisms

While it is clear that what would be regarded as classical immunological reactions are not responsible for all the manifestations of asthma, there is little doubt that they are among the important factors in the genesis of the disease in atopic individuals. Such people have the inherited ability to produce IgE antibody in response to allergenic stimulation (see p. 939). The reaginic antibody described as the important factor in allergy by Prausnitz and Kustner in 1921 [172] was characterized as IgE in 1966 [173]. It is a glycoprotein of molecular mass 190 kDa, with two heavy (ε) chains bound by disulphide bridges to two light (κ) chains. It is synthesized and secreted by B lymphocytes and plasma cells in response to specific antigen challenge, the response being under the control of T helper and suppressor lymphocytes [174]. In common with other immunoglobulins, IgE has two functional components, an Fc (crystallizable) part responsible for eliciting the biological response and two identical Fab (antigen-binding) parts responsible for attachment to the allergen.

The simplest concept of allergic asthma is that an antigenic response to allergen provocation results in the binding of an antigen with multiple binding sites to the Fab part of the IgE molecule. At least two of these IgE molecules bound to a common antigenic particle then link to Fc-binding sites on a basophil or mast cell, leading to a sequence of events in the cell resulting in the release of mediators [174]. It is now known that this is only part of the story and that other cells, including macrophages, eosinophils, lymphocytes and platelets, also have IgE Fc receptors and may well play a part in the pathogenesis of the disease. Much is known of the changes occurring in the mast cell membrane in response to antigen–antibody binding [175]. The bridging of two Fc receptors by the IgE–antigen complex leads to two parallel biochemical events, the influx of calcium into the cell and the conversion of ATP to cyclic AMP. Cyclic AMP, in the presence of an appropriate calcium concentration, activates protein kinases that phosphorylate the specific enzymes concerned with histamine release. The conversion of ATP to cyclic AMP is promoted by augmentation of the activity of adenylate cyclase by the bridging event, this enzyme in turn cleaving the ATP molecule. The influx of calcium is governed by the methylation, again in response to the bridging event, of phosphatidylethanolamine to phosphatidylcholine. This phospholipid migrates to the cell surface and the consequent change in the structure of the cell membrane allows the influx of calcium. The same biochemical reactions probably result in the release of other preformed mediators, including the low molecular weight eosinophil chemotactic factor [176].

Antigen–antibody binding to the surface of mast cells or basophils can also lead to the release of mediators derived from arachidonic acid [177]. This substance is stored in the phospholipids of the cell membrane and is released by activation of phospholipase during influx of calcium following the bridging event described above. Platelet-activating factor (PAF) may also be derived by similar mechanisms from basophils and other cells [178–180].

The basophil and mast cell are not the only cells involved in the release of mediators of asthmatic inflammation [181,182]. Macrophages, eosinophils, lymphocytes and platelets also have receptors for the Fc portion of IgE. Macrophages have been shown to release reactive oxygen intermediates, lysosomal enzymes and derivatives of arachidonic acid in response to surface binding of multiple IgE molecules bound to antigen. Eosinophils are attracted by the binding of IgE–antigen complexes to mast cells and this may lead to release of the major basic protein, which is very toxic to airway epithelium [183,184]. T-lymphocyte IgE receptors may play a role in the control of IgE production by B lymphocytes via a process of negative or positive feedback [181,185]. Platelet receptors may facilitate the secretion of serotonin.

Thus the events related to the immunological induction of asthma may be summarized as follows. In an individual with a predisposition to react to antigen challenge by production of IgE from B lymphocytes, such challenge leads to the formation of IgE–antigen complexes that bind to the surface of basophils, mast cells and macrophages in particular. Release of preformed mediators, such as histamine and eosinophil chemotactic factor, leads to bronchoconstriction and an influx of eosinophils. Release of other inflammatory mediators leads to progressive oedema and infiltration of the bronchial wall, while toxic substances such as major basic protein and PAF cause epithelial cellular disruption. Enzymes released from macrophages may be responsible for the characteristic separation of the epithelium from the basement membrane.

Immunopathogenic mechanisms

It is, of course, of some interest to speculate why the human organism should have evolved such a sophisticated mechanism of self-injury; the answer must lie in a biological advantage obtained by those with the ability to produce IgE in these amounts [186,187]. One simple and perhaps partial explanation is that this may be related to the role of IgE in defence against parasitic organisms, by facilitating the binding of such organisms to cells such as eosinophils and macrophages able to secrete substances toxic to the invaders. More interestingly, it has been suggested that the reason may be found in the need for the fetus to protect itself from attack by the mother *in utero* [188]. This concept relates to the fact that the propensity to mount an IgE-mediated allergic reaction depends upon a predominant differentiation of T-helper lymphocytes into the Th2 subtype responsible for production of cytokines, especially IL-4, which stimulate B lymphocytes to produce IgE. It is argued that undifferentiated helper T cells may produce clones of predominantly Th1 or Th2 type. The former secrete, *inter alia*, interferon (IFN)-γ, important in defence against many infecting organisms, including viruses and intracellular bacteria, but which is also very toxic to the conceptus; the latter produce IL-4 and IL-5. These cytokines may counter the effect of IFN-γ, and it appears that the natural state of the fetus is skewed towards production of Th2 cells. This bias persists in infant life, but in the majority is displaced by a predominantly Th1 clone as the baby develops. At least one stimulus to this may be infections acquired in childhood, which promote the development of Th1 clones. Thus it has been argued that early childhood infections, perhaps particularly the intestinal infections associated with relatively poor living conditions, may switch newborn children from an atopic to a non-atopic potential. This concept fits well with evolutionary theory and provides an explanation not only for the persistence of atopy but also possibly for the increase in asthma and allergic diseases.

The interrelationships of Th1 and Th2 cells and their cytokines are complex and far from fully understood. It is thought that the initial stage of differentiation involves the dendritic cell, which is derived from CD34 lymphocytes and which is present in asthmatic airway walls [189]. Cytokines, including tumour necrosis factor α and IL-4, cause dendritic cells to express receptors for antigen; after binding with this, they migrate to local lymph nodes where they present their major histocompatibility complex (MHC) class II antigens to naive T lymphocytes, leading to Th2 differentiation. In contrast, infections leading to secretion of IL-12 from dendritic cells can influence naive T cells to differentiate into Th1 cells. In atopic disease, allergen is processed and presented by the dendritic cells to T lymphocytes, which then differentiate into the Th2 phenotype; this secretes IL-4 that further aids in the maturation of the Th2 cell and in switching B lymphocytes from production of IgM and IgG to IgE. In contrast, IFN-γ from Th1 cells, driven by IL-12, downregulates Th2 differentiation and IgE production. The Th1 phenotype is associated with cell-mediated cytotoxicity and delayed-type hypersensitivity, and it is likely that early induction of high levels of IFN-γ may reinforce T-cell differentiation in the Th1 direction, leading to unresponsiveness to allergens.

Whatever the precise relationships between T lymphocytes and their cytokines, it is apparent that there are opportunities for understanding the reasons why one person develops asthma and another does not; even more importantly, this may lead to explaining the reasons for the rise in atopic diseases as societies become wealthier and more sophisticated. This is discussed below. A simplified summary of the proposed cellular and humoral mechanisms in the allergic asthmatic reaction is shown in Fig. 34.11.

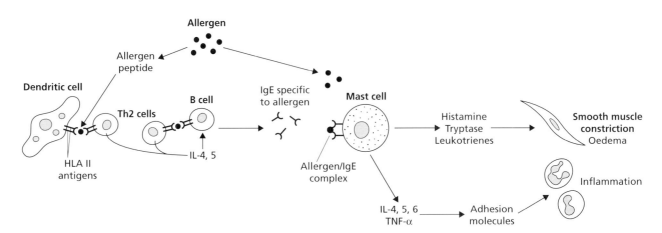

Fig. 34.11 A summary of the main proposed cellular and humoral mechanisms in the allergic asthmatic reaction. Allergen fragments are presented to T lymphocytes by the major histocompatibility complex (MHC) class II antigens on dendritic cells. They are then presented to B cells, which under the influence of interleukins from T cells produce allergen-specific IgE. This then binds to allergen on the surface of mast cells, leading to release of mediators and the pathological features of the asthmatic airway.

Mediators of the asthmatic reaction

It is generally agreed that the final common pathway to the asthmatic reaction involves the release of mediators from mast cells and other inflammatory cells and their actions on the bronchial wall. Immunological reactions involving IgE are the best understood mechanisms for triggering mediator release, although other factors such as exercise, infection and drugs may have similar effects. Moreover, the actions of mediators on the target cells in the bronchial wall may well be modified by the action of the nerves supplying that structure and, indeed, the liability of cells to produce mediators may also be under humoral, nervous or genetic control. This section discusses briefly the mediators thought to be most relevant to the asthmatic reaction.

Histamine

Histamine (Fig. 34.12) is stored in the granules of mast cells and basophils, each basophil containing about 0.01 pmol (6×10^9 molecules) of the substance [190]. It is formed in the cell from L-histidine by enzymatic decarboxylation and after release is metabolized rapidly in tissues by oxidation to *N*-methyl-imidazoleacetic acid or to imidazoleacetic acid, both of which are excreted in the urine.

Histamine exerts its pharmacological effects through two types of receptor, called H_1 and H_2, the former being blocked by the original antihistamines and the latter by cimetidine. Studies on humans have shown that blockade of H_1 receptors can prevent the bronchial response to histamine, whereas H_2-receptor blockade does not have this effect [146,161,162]. In the airways, the main effect of histamine is probably to produce smooth muscle constriction. This is likely to be effected by a direct action on the muscle and also by an indirect action via stimulation of vagal receptors.

The role of histamine in asthma has been much debated. There is evidence of raised levels in the plasma of patients with severe asthma compared with normal controls, although controls with other diseases have raised levels also [162,190]. There is also a tendency for the plasma histamine response to challenge to increase in relation to age [142]. Studies of changes in histamine level in response to exercise and antigen challenge have been mentioned above [142–144]. On balance, it seems likely that histamine is an important mediator in asthma, though its rapid metabolism, the rapid depletion of stores in attacks and

suppression of its release by corticosteroids make it difficult to find in increased amounts in the circulation [191].

Leucocyte chemotactic factors

Three chemotactic factors occur in preformed state in the mast cell and basophil granules and may be released in response to challenge. Eosinophil chemotactic factor is a low molecular mass (0.3–1 kDa) acidic polypeptide [192]. An intermediate molecular mass (1.5–3 kDa) eosinophil chemoattractant and a high molecular mass (>750 kDa) neutrophil chemoattractant have also been isolated from human lung and from mast cells [193,194].

Prostaglandins

Prostaglandins comprise one of two groups of mediators produced by the metabolism of arachidonic acid derived from cell membranes, the other group being the leukotrienes. The biochemical pathways involved are shown in Fig. 34.13. Prostaglandins are produced by the cyclooxygenase pathway. At least two prostaglandins, PGD_2 and prostacyclin, may have a role in asthma. Large amounts of PGD_2 are released on immunological challenge of human mast cells, while inhalation of this compound causes bronchoconstriction, asthmatic subjects being more responsive than controls [195,196]. $PGF_{2\alpha}$ is also a potent bronchoconstrictor in humans [196]. Prostacyclin may also be released from human mast cells following immune challenge and it has been suggested that it may antagonize the bronchoconstrictor effects of other prostaglandins [197]. PGE_2 has been shown to be a bronchodilator in humans [198].

These paradoxical effects of the prostaglandins may be mirrored in the effects of aspirin and other non-steroidal anti-inflammatory drugs in asthma. Most aspirin-sensitive subjects present with a syndrome of nasal polyposis, non-atopic asthma and aspirin-induced bronchoconstriction, the potency of this effect being related to the strength of the drug's inhibitory effects on prostaglandin synthetase. However, a small number of asthmatic subjects actually derive benefit, and show bronchodilatation, from aspirin therapy.

Leukotrienes

Leukotrienes are produced from arachidonic acid via the lipoxygenase pathway, particularly in leucocytes and macrophages (Fig. 34.14). Different cells probably have the

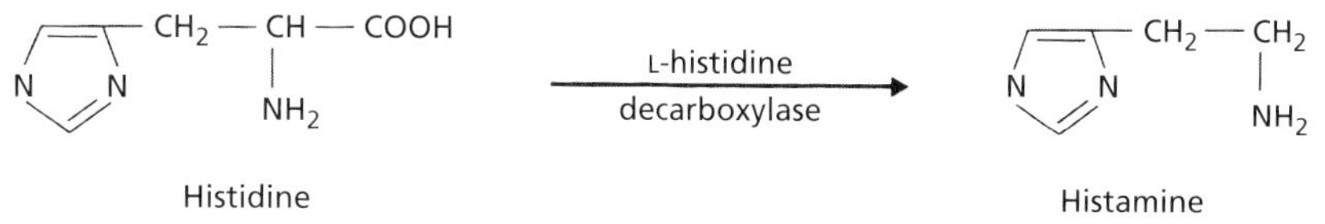

Fig. 34.12 Biosynthesis of histamine.

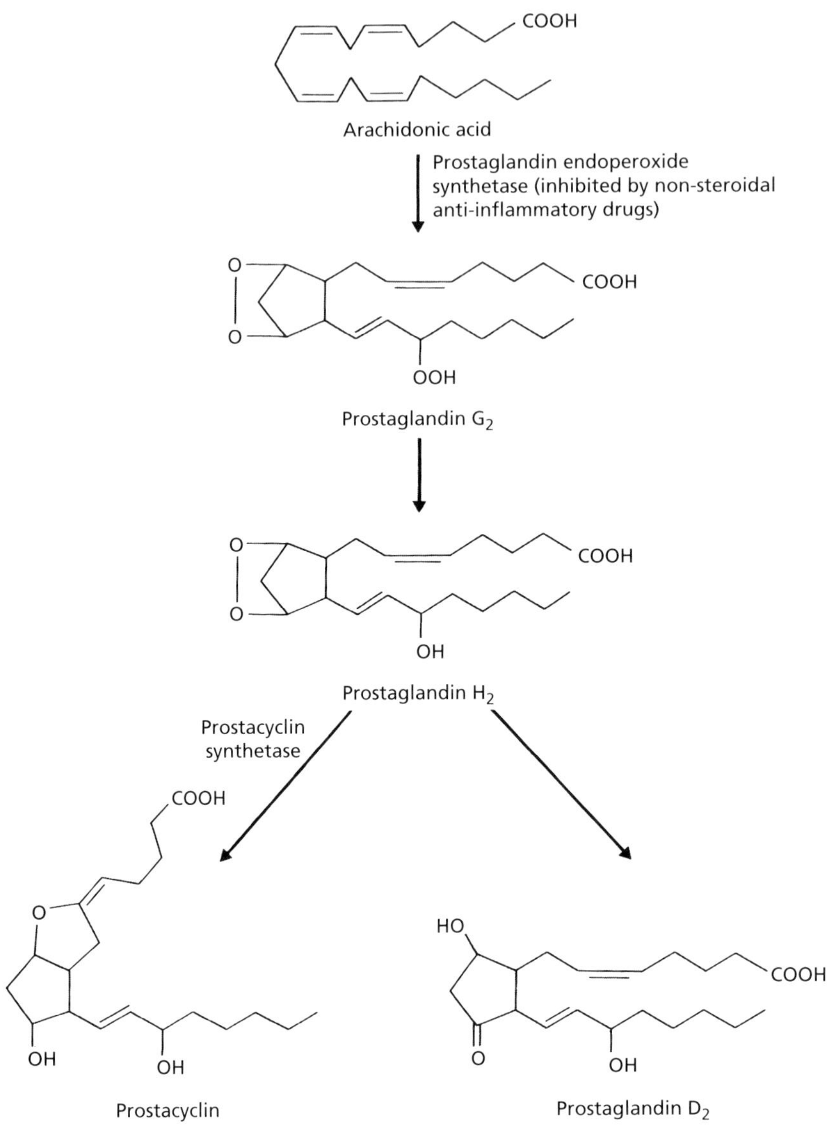

Fig. 34.13 Biosynthesis of some of the prostaglandins.

capacity to produce different metabolites. LTD_4, LTE_4 and LTC_4 (which together were originally described as slow-reacting substance of anaphylaxis, SRS-A) are most potent in terms of bronchial smooth muscle constriction and LTB_4 in terms of causing neutrophil chemotaxis and release of lysosomal enzymes [199]. Leukotrienes have been shown to be released from allergen-challenged human lung and to be present in sputum and blood from patients with asthma [200–202].

Platelet-activating factor

PAF (1-*O*-alkyl-2-acetyl-*n*-glyceryl-3-phosphorylcholine also known as PAF-acether or AGEPC) is a lipid substance derived from phospholipids in a large number of cells, including basophils, neutrophils, mast cells, eosinophils, macrophages and platelets [203]. Its actions include aggre-

gation of platelets, induction of lysosomal enzyme and oxygen free radical release from neutrophils and macrophages, and bronchoconstriction and pulmonary oedema. These latter effects may well be secondary to the release of other lipid mediators from cells stimulated by PAF. It is of interest also that it is able to produce both immediate and delayed local reactions when injected into the skin [204].

Kinins

Kinins are polypeptides generated in plasma from kinino-gen precursors with molecular masses of about 200 and 500 kDa. The enzymes responsible are called kallikreins, which in turn are derived from prekallikreins by the action of activated Hageman factor. While this process may take place wholly within the plasma, there is evidence that

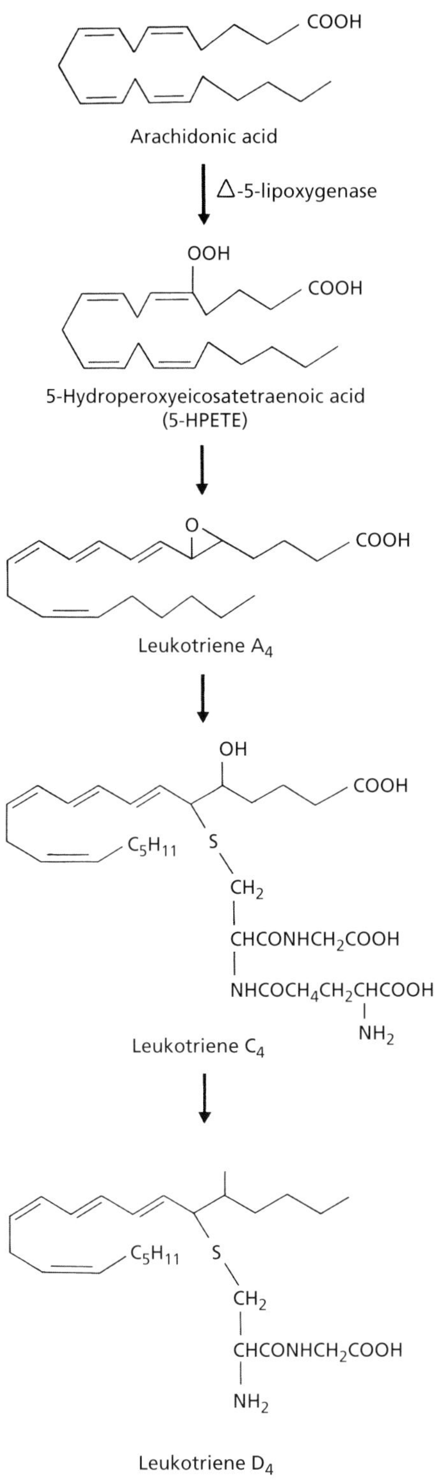

COOH

Arachidonic acid

Δ-5-lipoxygenase

OOH

COOH

5-Hydroperoxyeicosatetraenoic acid
(5-HPETE)

O

COOH

Leukotriene A_4

OH

COOH

C_5H_{11}

S

CH_2

CHCONHCH_2COOH

NHCOCH_4CH_2CHCOOH

NH_2

Leukotriene C_4

C_5H_{11}

S

CH_2

CHCONHCH_2COOH

NH_2

Leukotriene D_4

Fig. 34.14 Biosynthesis of some of the leukotrienes.

mast cells may produce a kallikrein-like substance [205]. The best-known kinin is bradykinin, a nonapeptide to which asthmatic airways are hypersensitive and which has been found in the skin reactions of atopic subjects [206]. It has no action on normal airways, and it has been

suggested that it may act via a local axon reflex, its release in airways stimulating exposed non-myelinated afferent nerve endings and causing release of sensory neuropeptides [207,208] These in turn may cause bronchoconstriction, mucosal oedema and hypersecretion of mucus.

Neural mechanisms

The allergic or immunological model of asthma discussed above provides the best-understood key to the mechanisms of the disease. However, it is plain that allergic sensitization is of little or no importance in a great number of people with asthma. Moreover, studies of mediators have so far been unable to demonstrate convincing qualitative differences between people with asthma and those without, except that patients with asthma tend to show increased susceptibility to their actions. Thus it is necessary to search elsewhere for an understanding of the disease. Two observations in particular have led to an interest being taken in neural mechanisms: first, patients with asthma usually show non-specific bronchoconstrictor responses to a wide variety of non-immunological stimuli such as infection or inhalation of irritants; and, second, psychological stress may lead to exacerbations of the disease. Even more importantly, from a practical point of view, the first-line drugs used in asthma are most frequently those that act upon autonomic nervous control of the bronchi.

Three components of the autonomic nervous system play a part in control of the airways and their secretions [209]: the parasympathetic system via the vagus; the sympathetic system via its hormonal control of cyclic AMP levels; and the peptidergic or non-adrenergic non-cholinergic (NANC) system.

Parasympathetic control

The vagus nerve includes afferent fibres from sensory receptors in the bronchial epithelium. It is thought, largely on the basis of studies on animals, that stimulation of these receptors by irritants can initiate a reflex impulse along vagal efferents that causes release of acetylcholine and bronchoconstriction [210,211]. Bronchial glands are also under parasympathetic control, and vagal stimulation can also lead to secretion of mucus [212]. The vagal efferent nerves end in ganglia close to bronchial smooth muscle in the posterior walls of the larger airways. The postsynaptic fibres are short and connect with muscle and glands. Vesicles containing norepinephrine (noradrenaline) have been found in the parasympathetic ganglia, suggesting that the sympathetic system may have a modulatory effect on the parasympathetic [213].

In terms of relevance to asthma, parasympathomimetic drugs induce bronchial constriction in patients in much the same way as histamine [214]. Antiparasympathetic drugs cause bronchodilatation in normal subjects and in patients with asthma [215,216]. In high doses they usually block the bronchoconstrictor response to exercise [149]. Finally, vagal receptors may be stimulated by a number of inflammatory mediators, including bradykinin and histamine [217–219], and this may explain in part the effects of respiratory infections in provoking asthmatic symptoms [220].

Sympathetic contro1

The lung receives sympathetic innervation mainly via the stellate ganglion [221]. The postsynaptic nerves supply bronchial vessels but not smooth muscle. Nevertheless, bronchial tone is influenced to a major degree by the sympathetic system, β-receptor agonists causing bronchial relaxation that is antagonized by β blockers. Other studies have demonstrated β receptors on smooth muscle, mast cells and bronchial glands that are presumably stimulated by circulating catecholamines [222,223].

The β receptors exist on the surface of cell membranes, though they should not be regarded as unchanging structures because their numbers may vary from time to time in response to external stimuli. The receptor receives a hormone that has a steric configuration complementary to its own, the binding of hormone to receptor initiating a chain of events that leads to the cell producing its effect. The first step is conversion, in the cell membrane, of guanine nucleotide regulatory protein into its active state, when it combines with the hormone–receptor complex. This leads to activation of adenylate cyclase that catalyses the conversion of ATP to cyclic AMP, the so-called second messenger, which in turn activates the particular cell's specific protein kinases. Cyclic AMP is metabolized by phosphodiesterase to AMP. The actions of the protein kinases depend on the cell; in smooth muscle they phosphorylate myosin light chain kinase and reduce actin–myosin coupling in order to produce relaxation. The release of preformed mediators from mast cells also appears to be under the control of cyclic AMP, reduced levels being involved in the process of degranulation. The relevance of β-receptor mechanisms to clinical asthma is clear from the effects of sympathetic agonist and antagonist drugs. However, study of these mechanisms has pointed to something more fundamental to the understanding of the disease [221]. It has been known for many years that asthmatic subjects may show diminished responsiveness to adrenergic stimulation, in terms of a rise in blood sugar, free fatty acids and levels of cyclic AMP in blood and urine. Much evidence has now accumulated to support the hypothesis that subjects with asthma have a relative reduction of β receptors and a reciprocal increase in excitatory α receptors. Such differences may be related to genetic factors or may be acquired as a result of allergic, infective or possibly autoimmune factors.

Peptidergic control

The NANC nervous system was originally described in the gut. Fibres of this system run with the vagus and supply postganglionic fibres to bronchial muscle, glands and vessels [224–226]. Two neuroendocrine peptides in particular have been demonstrated in human sensory airway nerves, substance P and neurokinin A. Activation of these nerves by such stimuli as mechanical or chemical irritation may lead to a form of neurogenic inflammation, with bronchoconstriction, extravasation of protein-rich fluid and vasodilatation in the airways. There is also evidence that release of these transmitter substances may influence the attraction of inflammatory cells to the site. Both substance P and neurokinin A administered by inhalation cause bronchoconstriction; this effect is reduced by prior inhalation of cromoglicate and amplified if the action of neutral endopeptidase, the enzyme responsible for their natural breakdown, is blocked. It seems reasonable to propose that neural mechanisms such as these play an important part in the initiation of non-immunological asthma, such as occurs after viral infection or exposure to irritant substances, the so-called reactive airways dysfunction syndrome.

Bronchial muscle

The contractile mechanism of bronchial smooth muscle is due to the ability of the proteins actin and myosin to interact and to slide over one another [227,228]. In outline, myosin is composed of a pair of filamentous heavy chains coiled around each other, ending in a globular structure to which are attached two pairs of light chains. The globular head is attached by a cross-bridging mechanism to actin, which is also a filamentous protein consisting of two intertwined polymers. These in turn are wrapped round two intertwined molecules of tropomyosin. Contraction takes place by detachment of the globular part of the myosin from the actin and reattachment further along the structure, the energy for the reaction being derived from breakdown of AMP by activated myosin ATPase. The sequence of events leading to activation of myosin ATPase is as follows [228,230]. A fundamental requirement appears to be an approximately 10-fold increase in intracellular calcium ion concentration. Normally the concentration of calcium in smooth muscle cells is about 10 000 times less than that in extracellular fluid, the differential being maintained by the cell membrane and an active energy-dependent removal mechanism whereby it is exchanged for sodium. However, the cell membrane may allow calcium to enter when channels are opened, either via the actions of drugs or hormones on receptors or by changes in the transmembrane potential difference. Influxing calcium combines with the protein calmodulin and this combination activates myosin light chain kinase. The activated enzyme then phosphorylates one of the pairs of myosin light chains on the globular part of the molecule, leading in turn to activation of myosin ATPase and contraction. Another calcium-dependent pathway has also been described in the activation of myosin ATPase; an enzyme present in the cell membrane called protein kinase C alters the sensitivities of actin and myosin to calcium. The protein kinase C is in turn activated by calcium flux across the membrane.

Thus calcium is thought to play a central role in the contraction of smooth muscle. Yet calcium channel blocking drugs have proved of little therapeutic value in asthma, in contrast to β-sympathomimetic drugs that act to increase levels of cyclic AMP in the smooth muscle cell. The part played by cyclic AMP is not clear, although rises in its concentration have a wide range of effects including activation of various protein kinases (that may inhibit calcium transfer and activation of protein kinase C) and by increasing the inward flow of sodium in exchange for calcium. The lack of efficacy of calcium-blocking drugs may be explained partly by their inability to block the receptor-dependent channels. Despite the well-recognized bronchial hyperreactivity of asthmatic airways, no clear picture has yet emerged of the biochemical correlates of this process. Although it is tempting to believe that a fundamental abnormality may be present in the regulation of intracellular calcium metabolism, the evidence seems to indicate that bronchial reactivity *in vivo* does not relate to altered mechanical properties and responses of the excised muscle *in vitro* [231]. However, there is some evidence that asthmatic airway smooth muscle does have altered mechanical properties [232].

Genetic factors

The frequent clinical observation that asthma runs in families has been supported by many more formal investigations [233–237]. There is a greater concordance for asthma in monozygotic than dizygotic twin pairs. The risk of having an asthmatic child is greater if both parents have the disease than if one does, and greater if one has it than if neither does. However, study of the genetics of asthma is made particularly complex by the absence of agreement on definition of the phenotype, which could for example include atopy, bronchial hyperresponsiveness and any number of consequences due to genetic polymorphisms involving individual cytokines and cell receptors [238]. Recent studies, in which atopy has been defined in terms of one or more positive skin tests, positive specific IgE or raised total IgE levels, have produced somewhat contradictory results. The original findings suggestive of autosomal dominant inheritance based on a gene on chromosome 11q13 have been supported by work that has shown an association between atopy and an amino acid substitution in the β subunit of the receptor for IgE, the

gene for which is also located on chromosome 11q13 [239–241]. This receptor is responsible for the changes in calcium flux leading to mediator release. However, studies of other family groups have failed to replicate these findings and it seems very likely that different genetic polymorphisms in different populations can produce what to the clinician appears to be the same phenotype [238]. Other linkages have been demonstrated between chromosome 14, the T-cell receptor and specific IgE reactions to major allergens [242], and between chromosome 5q and a cluster of cytokines including IL-3, IL-4 and IL-5 [243]. The complexity of the multiple mechanisms and network of cells, cytokines and chemokines involved in asthma, the differences in the clinical manifestations of the disease and the now very obvious increasing prevalence of atopic diseases, and thus the dominance of environmental factors in their expression, make one wonder whether the current emphasis on genetic research is likely to pay the rich dividends anticipated by some of the pharmaceutical companies investing in it. While it will surely lead to new and possibly better drugs, it may be that a greater research emphasis on factors influencing the expression of whatever genes are involved in determining atopy and bronchial reactivity may produce greater dividends in terms of prevention.

Why has asthma increased?

One of the greatest enigmas in the study of asthma arises from the repeated observation that the disease has become more common in prosperous societies. This has been demonstrated in repeated cross-sectional studies in the same place, in studies of populations that have migrated from poorer to richer societies, and in studies of people of similar racial background living traditional or more sophisticated lifestyles. The increase in asthma appears to be paralleled by increases in atopy and the other allergic diseases, hay fever and eczema. These observations provide an important challenge in understanding and reversing the environmental factors that lie behind them.

Early attempts to attribute these changes to an increasingly toxic environment, whether due to maternal smoking, increases in exposure to mites and other allergens or to air pollution, are likely to provide at best a very partial explanation [244]. The changes in prevalence of atopy seem to be occurring very early in infancy, and possible or recorded changes in these toxic factors are unlikely to be large enough to have produced the observed effects. For example in the UK, smoking prevalence in women of child-bearing age has decreased over the relevant period, pet ownership has not increased and urban particulate air pollution has decreased substantially. If the increase in asthma was due to a large increase in exposure to mites, an unlikely event given the high exposures in bedclothes almost universal 30 years ago [245], it is strange that hay fever has increased despite no change in grass pollen levels [246]. Thus it seems much more likely that the increase in prevalence is primarily a consequence of an increase in population susceptibility (Fig. 34.15).

Two hypothetical but plausible means by which population susceptibility could have increased suggest themselves. First, the diet of the population could have altered in such a way as to decrease resistance to allergens [244,247]. Secondly, falling rates of infection in infants could have removed a stimulus towards development of the anti-infection Th1 phenotype, leaving a population with an increased proportion of the atopic Th2 phenotype [248,249]. There is evidence that newborn babies destined to become atopic already show decreased concentrations of IFN-γ, a cytokine associated with the Th1 phenotype, and evidence of *in utero* sensitization to allergen in their cord blood [250], suggesting that the key determinant of atopic and therefore likely asthmatic status in childhood may occur before birth. Other evidence, from studies of populations, has suggested that early childhood infections may protect against later atopy, though not asthma. Children in Guinea-Bissau who had severe measles were less likely to become atopic, while the same was true of children in Japan who were tuberculin positive and of Italian military recruits who had serological evidence of past hepatitis A infection [251–253]. In contrast, except for measles which had a weak effect, the common childhood infections in Aberdeen schoolchildren did not protect from (but rather in general appeared to increase the risk of) later asthma [254]. All these studies have pointed to an intriguing effect of family size on risk of atopy, in that children in larger families were relatively protected, an observation not wholly explained by infection but which also may point to some subtle intrauterine effect.

It is becoming apparent that the change in asthma prevalence is associated with a rising standard of living rather than with westernization *per se*. Thus children in the same country, be it Ethiopia or Saudi Arabia, neither of which can be regarded as westernized, show a much greater prevalence of asthma and allergic symptoms among the wealthier urban than among the poorer rural children [255,256], whereas urban–rural differences do not exist in countries that are relatively uniformly wealthy. Some factor associated with increased prosperity, be it a different diet, reduced opportunity for childhood infection, increased use of immunization or a combination, must be responsible. The authors favour a dietary hypothesis, since increasing prosperity is accompanied by the consumption of less fruit and vegetables and a different pattern of fat intake. A lowered consumption of vitamins C and E, coupled with changes from ω-3 to ω-6 fatty acids in the diet of the pregnant woman, could theoretically influence T-lymphocyte differentiation in the unborn child and tip the balance towards a predominantly Th2 phenotype persisting at birth when the child first meets inhaled allergens [247,257] (Fig. 34.16). At this stage a lowered antioxidant level in the child could further reduce its resistance to substances capable of causing bronchial inflammation. As childhood progresses, it is conceivable that immunization and freedom from, say, intestinal infections reinforce rather than switch the Th2 phenotype, so that by the age of 12, the stage at which most of the epidemiological studies have been done, atopic symptoms have become commonplace. It must be stressed that this hypothesis remains unproven but forms a useful template for further research and may point the way to future prevention.

Clinical features

Taking the history

The diagnosis of asthma is usually made as a result of careful history-taking, supported by a few tests or by a trial of therapy. In most cases a properly taken history gives the diagnosis. The history should discover the presenting symptoms, their periodicity and evolution and factors related to their variability. In particular, factors provoking attacks should be sought. An assessment of the patient's level of disablement should be made, not forgetting that disturbed nights lead to impaired performance in the day. The history should also discover any associated features, such as other atopic disease and drug sensitivity.

Presentation

Asthma may present at any age, including the extremes of life. The most common presenting symptom is breathlessness usually associated with chest tightness, often coming on in attacks, although in older people it is frequently a chronic symptom. Wheeze is often not the primary complaint and is a term usually put into their mouths by their

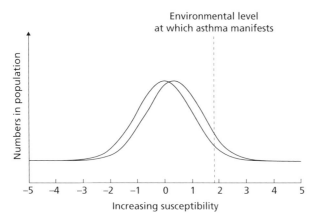

Fig. 34.15 Distribution of susceptibility to asthma in a population showing how a small overall shift can substantially increase the prevalence of overt disease.

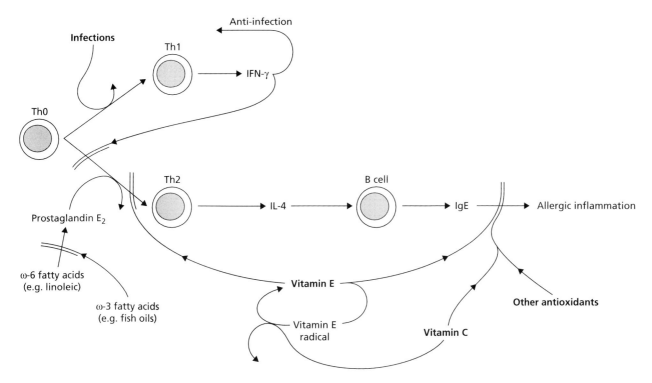

Fig. 34.16 Possible factors influencing susceptibility to asthma. The undifferentiated T lymphocyte may become either the antimicrobial Th1 cell, producing interferon γ under the stimulus of certain infections, or the Th2 cell, producing interleukin 4 and leading to allergic inflammation through the production of IgE by B cells. Antioxidants might protect directly against allergic inflammation and vitamins E and C may together downregulate Th2 differentiation. The balance of fatty acids in the diet may also affect T-cell differentiation.

doctors, patients often preferring to refer to tightness in the chest. A large minority of patients present with cough, which may be the only symptom, especially in children. When cough is troublesome, bilateral aches or pains in the chest are common. In some patients cough is productive of small amounts of sticky sputum, although it is rare for profuse or frothy sputum to be produced. Sputum is usually described as being white or clear; sometimes more solid or greenish streaks are noticed in it.

Of particular importance in making the diagnosis of asthma is the periodicity of symptoms. In children and young adults the usual complaint is of episodes of cough, wheeze and breathlessness. These characteristically occur shortly after exertion and at night. Persistent dry cough may be the only symptom. Exercise-induced symptoms occur after several minutes of usually unaccustomed exertion, increase in severity over a minute or two and wane over about half an hour, though mild attacks may last only a few minutes. The patient may or may not notice wheeze. Nocturnal symptoms typically disturb sleep in the small hours of the morning. Many patients feel the need to get up and out of bed to go to a window for air. Others make themselves a cup of tea after being awakened by symptoms, an almost pathognomonic symptom. Attacks also vary greatly in severity, from a mild episode of cough lasting a few minutes to a night repeatedly disturbed by

frightening breathlessness, wheeze, chest tightness and cough. In general, the frequency and severity of nocturnal episodes may be taken to be a useful guide to the current severity of asthma. If a patient is seen during the day and is clinically reasonably well but describes distressing nocturnal symptoms, more weight should be put on the history than on the immediate apparent good health when assessing the severity of asthma and the planning of its treatment. Moreover, the time at which the attacks occur is also a guide to severity. Most patients with mild to moderate untreated asthma wake in the morning at their normal time with a tight chest and some wheeze, or a dry cough. Measurement of peak flow rates, which are characteristically lower in the mornings in asthma, has led to this being described as the 'morning dip'. As asthma, and presumably airways hyperreactivity, becomes more severe, symptoms occur earlier and disturb sleep, until in some cases the patient barely sleeps at all or is woken repeatedly through the night by breathlessness, wheeze and cough. Nocturnal asthmatic symptoms are discussed further in the next section, but it should be pointed out that they are a feature of asthma of all types at all ages and not simply related to house-dust mite hypersensitivity.

Particular attention should be paid to factors provoking attacks. Exercise has been mentioned; almost as frequently, patients comment on attacks following 'colds'.

Care should be taken to distinguish genuine viral infections, with fever and malaise, from rhinitis. While the latter is common in asthmatics and frequently accompanies attacks, the former commonly provoke them. Often a bad upper respiratory tract infection leads to cough and wheeziness that persist, sometimes for weeks, and do not respond to the antibiotic therapy which is often unnecessarily given in repeated courses. Such patients do not have persistent bronchial infection despite their cough and sputum. Their sputum, if apparently purulent initially, rapidly becomes mucoid and sticky and they usually have troublesome nocturnal symptoms. Sputum may occasionally appear to be purulent in asthmatics; this green colour is due to peroxidase, which is released from eosinophils as well as neutrophils. Symptoms are due to bronchial hyperreactivity following the infection and respond to anti-inflammatory therapy but not antibiotics. Other common factors that may provoke asthma are exposure to allergens, cold air, chemicals in the workplace, drugs and emotional upsets. These are discussed in subsequent sections.

In terms of making a diagnosis from the history, the most difficult presentation is in middle-aged and elderly people. While most such patients present with typical symptoms, some present with progressively increasing cough and dyspnoea, without the characteristic day-to-day variability. Nevertheless, they usually admit to nocturnal symptoms and these are frequently assumed to be manifestations of cardiac disease. One important feature of the history should always be sought, namely the relationship of the start of symptoms to cigarette smoking. Anyone who starts wheezy breathlessness and cough some weeks or months after stopping smoking is likely to have asthma. It is a commonplace observation that such patients complain that their chest has never been right since they stopped, although a careful history reveals that the symptoms usually started some time after cessation. If symptoms were present when the patient stopped smoking, a diagnosis of smoking-induced chronic obstructive airways disease is more likely. In terms of management this distinction is less important than it appears, since all such patients developing airflow obstruction are treated similarly initially in order to assess their response and many initially categorized as having smoking-induced disease nevertheless respond at least partially to such treatment. This is discussed further below.

Provoking factors

Allergy

The possible mechanisms whereby allergy provokes asthma have been discussed. Over 90% of childhood asthmatics are atopic, though this proportion falls among adults to some 50% [258–260]. In most atopic subjects allergy is only one of many factors, including exercise, infection and emotional upsets, that provokes attacks. Nevertheless it is always desirable to consider possible allergic factors and to try to eliminate important ones wherever possible.

The chest physician confronted by an asthmatic patient is faced with a daunting task in investigating allergic factors. The most important guide to the relevance of these comes from the history. Allergens may be encountered in the general, the domestic and the occupational environment, and timing of the symptoms may give an important clue. Seasonal variation suggests allergy to pollens or spores in the air. Symptoms in the working week and improvement when away from work throw suspicion on occupational factors. Associated rhinitis or conjunctivitis is a useful pointer to an allergen; house dust, animals and pollen rarely cause attacks of asthma without some nasal manifestations. Allergy to food or food additives is usually very difficult to detect from the history, although many such patients find that certain foods or drinks make their symptoms worse. The following sections discuss the main allergens with the exception of those encountered in an occupational setting, which are dealt with separately.

House dust and mites

Most atopic asthmatics report symptoms on exposure to house dust, usually when making beds and when dusting. Exposure while in bed may cause perennial rhinitis and nocturnal attacks of asthma, although this is by no means the only cause of asthma during the night. The major allergen in house dust was shown in the 1960s to be due to mites [261–263], though an occasional patient shows sensitivity to house dust alone and not to the mites in it. At least in temperate climates, *Dermatophagoides pteronyssinus* (Fig. 34.17) is the most prevalent of the mites found in house dust; others such as *Euroglyphus maynei*, *Chyletus* spp., *Glycyphagus* spp. and *Tyrophagus* spp. may also be found in small numbers [245]. *Dermatophagoides farinae* is rare in the European house habitat and is a more common organism in the USA; it should be noted that different species become dominant in different environments such as holiday caravans or stored grain. *D. pteronyssinus* lives mainly on skin scales and the fungi that feed on them [264]; it prefers a dark, warm and humid environment, around 25°C and 80% relative humidity, being in temperature and fluid equilibrium with its environment. These conditions are ideally provided by a bed. It breeds rapidly, the female producing up to 300 eggs in its short life. It is easily found in the small collections of dust round buttons and piping on mattresses and in blankets, pillows and other bedclothes, as well as in dust accumulated in curtains, carpets and other household sources. The highest

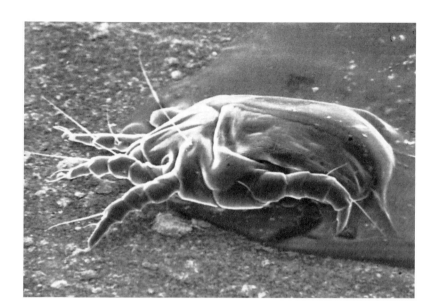

Fig. 34.17 Scanning electron micrograph of *Dermatophagoides pteronyssinus*.

concentrations, up to 13000/g of dust in one study, are found in mattresses [245], although large numbers (up to 100000/m²) may be present in a carpet. Interestingly, hospital mattresses are usually free of mites, indicating that regular disturbance of the colony by changing beds and exposing the mattresses to light makes the microenvironment unsuitable for their survival [245,265]. Conversely, low standards of domestic hygiene encourage house-dust mite colonies to thrive. The main allergen from mites seems to be excreted in the 20 or so faecal pellets each mite produces daily [266]. The faecal pellets are some 10–40 μm in diameter and thus easily become briefly airborne and inhaled into the nose and conducting airways [267,268]. Once inhaled and deposited onto a moist mucous membrane, the soluble allergens leach out of the faecal pellet. The main allergens have been characterized and are known as *Der p*I, II, III and IV indicating the order in which they were found [269]. Monoclonal antibodies to these allergens allow their quantification in air, dust and other media. *Der p*I is a cysteine protease with a molecular mass of about 25 kDa, while *Der p*III is a trypsin with a molecular mass of about 30 kDa; these are the two allergens to which almost all mite-sensitive subjects react. *Der p*II is probably unimportant as an allergen and *Der p*IV, an amylase with a molecular mass of about 60 kDa, sensitizes a minority of subjects. The fact that these allergens, derived as they are from the gut of mites, are enzymes is interesting in terms of their ability to obtain access to submucosal lymphocytes in the respiratory tract.

Other allergens in house dust include animal dander and feathers. Hair itself is not allergenic. The presence of an animal in the house ensures that it makes some contribution to the dust's antigenicity, though the main threat is usually posed by more direct contact between patient and pet (see below). Feather allergy seems to be related to a mixture of proteins from keratin, although apparent allergy to feathers in pillows or downies may rather be related to their mite content.

Pollens

Plant pollen grains are major causes of seasonal rhinitis (hay fever) and in such patients commonly provoke asthmatic symptoms as well. Allergy to pollens causes a distinctive illness in that the rhinitis is usually associated also with itchy conjunctivitis and lacrimation, and the symptoms have a distinctly seasonal pattern. Pollination of plants occurs at the same season each year but the amount of pollen that becomes airborne depends on the plant's natural method of pollination (via wind, water or insects) and the climatic conditions [270,271] Pollen allergens therefore differ considerably between different regions of the world and from time to time in the same region. In Europe, the most frequent allergens are grass pollens and these cause symptoms from about April to August; pollination is promoted by wind and sunshine and occurs earlier in more southern latitudes. Counts of grass pollen may rise as high as 1000/m³ on a hot summer's day. Symptoms typically start in the mid-morning and may persist through the next night.

Grass pollens are 30–50 μm in diameter and soluble antigens with molecular masses of 30–40 kDa are found on their surface. Osmotic rupture of the grain may cause release of starch granules bearing these antigens; this has been proposed as a mechanism whereby heavy rain during a thunderstorm may be responsible for epidemic outbreaks of asthma [272,273]. There is considerable cross-reactivity between pollens from different species of grass [274]. Certain weeds, generally of the family Compositae, may also be important sources of allergen. As with mites, the major allergens are denoted by letters and numbers indicating the source species and the order in which they were characterized. In North America in particular, especially in agricultural areas of the central and eastern regions, ragweed (*Ambrosia* sp.) is a major source of allergen [275–277]. It pollinates in August and September. Mid and late summer allergic symptoms may be due to nettle or mugwort pollen, while symptoms in the spring may be due to pollen from trees such as alder, elm, ash, birch, beech or oak, all of which pollinate between February and May in temperate climates. The seasons of some of the important pollen allergens in the UK are shown in Fig. 34.18.

Seasonal asthma always suggests an airborne biological allergen. However, it should be clear that this depends on the local flora and a knowledge of this is essential for making a diagnosis. Pollens may travel hundreds of miles in the air, although high concentrations are obviously only likely to occur close to a source. The introduction of new species of plant into a region may be followed by important epidemics of respiratory symptoms, as occurred in Kuwait when decorative trees of the species *Prosopis* were planted in previously desert areas [278]. The widespread cultivation of oilseed rape in the European Community has given rise to fears that it may be an important new cause of epidemic asthma; however, since it produces large grains and is primarily pollinated by insects, this seems not to be the case [279,280]. Nevertheless, it does occasionaly sensitize people working with it in agricultural laboratories and therefore has allergenic potential with respect to heavily exposed atopic individuals.

Fungal spores

Like plant pollens, fungal spores may also become airborne and cause sensitization. Fungal spores are usually smaller than pollen, being about 5–20 μm in diameter [270,271]. Each species has its distinctive shape, varying from roughly spherical to torpedo-like. They usually appear to cause asthmatic symptoms without rhinitis. Although the total numbers of spores in the air may be exceedingly large, because of their smaller size the antigenic load is usually much less than that from grass pollen and this probably explains why fungal allergy is generally less of a problem than pollen allergy. Nevertheless, some patients do become sensitized and also develop seasonal symptoms in relation to the sporing season of the organism [281,282] (Fig. 34.19). Most fungi are either parasites or saprophytes of plants or live on dead organic matter. Their classification and nomenclature are discussed in Chapter 21. Different fungi predominate in different macroclimates and microclimates, according to the availability of suitable substrates. In Britain and other temperate climates, *Cladosporium* spp., basidiomycetes (including smuts and rusts), ascospores, *Sporobolomyces* spp., *Alternaria* spp., *Fusarium* spp. and *Penicillium* spp. are the most common spores in the air generally. However, local factors such as fields of cereals, compost heaps or rotting wood may cause very high local concentrations of other organisms. *Aspergillus fumigatus* may sensitize people working with compost, farmers may develop asthma in relation to large numbers of spores liberated at harvest time, and people living in damp mouldy houses or exposed to dry rot may develop asthma related to organ-

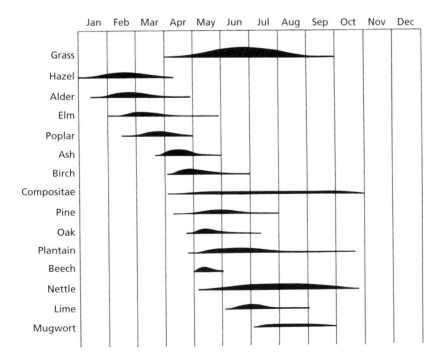

Fig. 34.18 A guide to the pollen season of common British plants. This varies somewhat according to latitude and weather.

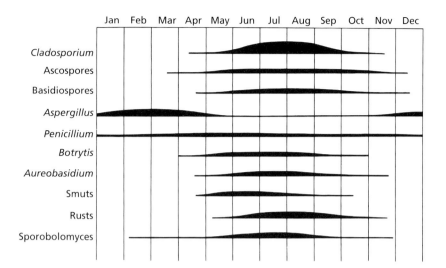

Fig. 34.19 A guide to the spore season of common British fungi. This varies according to the weather and local availability of substrates.

isms such as *Aspergillus niger, Merulius lacrimans* or *Penicillium* spp. It is of interest that *Aspergillus* spp. are not among the most frequent fungi in the air spora and yet they are probably the most troublesome species of fungus in terms of sensitization and disease; this is discussed separately in the section on bronchopulmonary aspergillosis. It has been postulated that the presence of activated epithelial cells and the exposure of basement membrane that occurs in asthma, together with oxidant stress, may facilitate the colonization of the asthmatic lung by *A. fumigatus* [283]. The incidence of positive skin reactions to *A. fumigatus* in unselected atopic asthmatics ranges from 10 to 20% [258]. A prerequisite for the development of aspergillar hypersensitivity is repeated exposure to the *Aspergillus* antigen [284]. Two distinct antigens, *Asp f*I (an 18-kDa protein) and a 48-kDa protein, have been identified as important causes of IgE antibody responses [285].

In clinical terms, fungal allergy (apart from aspergillosis) is probably not a frequent cause of troublesome symptoms [286]. However, there is increasing evidence that damp housing, which predisposes to the growth of moulds, is associated with a higher prevalence of asthma [287–290], although it is often difficult to separate this from the effects of the house-dust mite which also thrives in some damp houses [290]. Suspicion should be aroused in seasonal asthma without rhinitis [282] and when symptoms point to some specific site of asthma provocation, such as the house or workplace. The use of fungi in biotechnology is another area where sensitization may occur [291]. Fungal-induced asthmatic reactions in general have been well reviewed [292].

Animals

Up to 25% of atopic asthmatics show skin sensitivity to an animal [293]. Sensitization usually arises as a result of regular contact, and therefore is normally to a household pet or farm animals. Cats, dogs, horses and guinea-pigs are those most commonly encountered, though rabbits, white mice and even rats and ferrets are kept as house pets. Occupational sensitization to laboratory animals is a widespread problem. Birds, such as budgerigars, occasionally provoke asthma, although allergic alveolitis is a more common problem. All asthmatic patients should be asked about pets and animal contact. If sensitization is of clinical significance, the patient is likely to have noticed rhinitis and conjunctivitis as well as wheeze on contact with the animal. The sensitization is to animal proteins on particles derived from urine or saliva. In occupational cases, animal allergy may be the only cause of the asthma, which often remits when exposure ceases; occasionally this may be the case with domestic exposure. Allergy to the major cat allergen, *Fel d*I, is much more of a problem than allergies to other domestic pets. Cat-owning asthmatics with proven allergy to their pets rarely (and understandably) take medical advice about removal of the animal from their households [294], and there is evidence to suggest that asthmatics with cats require higher doses of inhaled corticosteroid therapy to control their symptoms than patients with dogs and other pets [295]. It has been suggested that in some countries, such as Sweden, cat allergy is the most important problem in childhood asthma [296].

Occasionally arthropods other than mites may cause asthma, and in some parts of the world cockroaches rather than mites are the main domestic allergen. Research workers studying locusts have been reported to develop symptoms, as have people exposed to various flies and to cockroaches [297–300]. Epidemic asthma has been reported in the Sudan due to a midge [301].

Food, drink and drugs

Atopic asthmatics may occasionally notice that their

symptoms are provoked by certain foods or drinks and it is worth asking all asthmatic patients whether they have noticed such an association. In the authors' experience it occurs in less than 10% of patients. The foods most frequently suspected are milk, eggs, fish, cereals, nuts and chocolates, but very many others have been described [302,303]. Meats containing antibiotics fed to animals or tenderized with enzymes are recognized as occasional causes. It is thought that sensitization occurs as a result of pinocytosis of antigenic protein molecules by intestinal mucosal cells (perhaps in the Peyer's patches) and induction of an IgE antibody response [304]. Subsequent entry of antigen into the bloodstream provokes an IgE-mediated reaction. Some of these patients notice gastrointestinal symptoms as well as wheeze; indeed such symptoms alone are a more frequent consequence of food allergy than is asthma. Anaphylaxis is a serious consequence of food allergy and appears to be occurring more frequently than before; peanuts, widely used in a large number of prepared foods, are most commonly to blame. Such patients need to exclude the offending substance absolutely from their diet and to be instructed in use of emergency epinephrine (adrenaline) injections.

Food may also provoke asthma via mechanisms that may not be related to IgE-mediated allergy. Preservatives such as benzoates, sodium nitrite and sodium metabisulphite, synthetic antioxidants, dyes such as tartrazine, and flavourings may be found in many foods and may provoke asthma. Red wines contain a number of congeners that give them their distinctive flavours but which also may provoke attacks of asthma, perhaps by a direct effect on mast cells causing liberation of mediators [305,306]. In general, however, alcohol itself is a mild bronchodilator [307,308]. It has been postulated that asthma associated with chewing betel-nut is chemically mediated by cholinergic stimulation [309].

An observation of some interest was that regional variations in asthma mortality in England and Wales correlated with dietary intake of sodium [310]. It has also been shown that bronchial reactivity to histamine is related to 24-h urinary sodium excretion [311], and it is possible that changes in dietary salt intake could alter the activity of the bronchial smooth muscle cellular sodium pump, which may be relevant to bronchial reactivity [312]. However, in a study of Montreal schoolchildren no association was found between asthma or exercise-induced bronchospasm and dietary salt intake, although bronchial responsiveness to methacholine did appear to increase with greater salt intake [313]. Absence of a relationship with peak flows and and peak flow variability has been reported [314], as has presence of a relationship to bronchial reactivity in some populations and not in others [315]. Yet other studies have linked increasing dietary salt intake with worsening asthma symptoms and increased bronchodilator use [316–318]. These discrepancies suggest

that the effect of salt intake is unlikely to be an important determinant of asthma [315], and it may be that it is a marker of an otherwise unsatisfactory diet [319].

Recently it has been suggested that omissions from, or changes in, the pattern of diet rather than allergenic additions may have played some part in the increase in allergic diseases in developed countries (see p. 940) [244]. Although diet may be responsible for some of the differences in the prevalence rates of asthma between countries, the extent of the effect is not known [56]. Breast-feeding is often cited as a protective factor, although the evidence is contradictory. A regular fish diet appears to reduce the risk of airway hyperresponsiveness in Australian children [257] and there are theoretical reasons why fish oils might alter the course of asthma via metabolites produced from arachidonic acid. Recently it has been postulated that dietary polyunsaturated fats, notably ω-6 fatty acids such as linoleic acid, may influence the development of allergic sensitization by increasing the formation of PGE_2, promoting Th2 lymphocyte responses and IgE generation [247]. Also dietary changes leading to a decrease in the intake of antioxidants such as vitamins C, E and β-carotene have been suggested as a possible cause of alterations in population susceptibility to atopic disorders [244], and some evidence now supports the concept that a diet high in fats and low in vitamins C and E is an important risk factor for adult-onset asthma and bronchial hyperreactivity [320,321]. Vitamin E may also be immunomodulatory and able to influence T-helper cell development in the direction of Th1, while vitamin C acts to reduce oxidized vitamin E radical and thus regenerate the active vitamin. It now seems likely that diet will prove to play a role in the development of susceptibility to allergens, although the magnitude of this effect has yet to be determined.

Drugs are an important but occasional cause of asthmatic attacks. Aspirin and other non-steroidal anti-inflammatory drugs are the most frequent offenders, followed closely by β blockers. The drugs and mechanisms are discussed in more detail in Chapter 55. It should be noted that aspirin sensitivity occurs particularly in non-atopic adult asthmatics, the combination of asthma, anti-inflammatory drug sensitivity and nasal polyposis constituting a well-defined syndrome. Tartrazine, a well-recognized chemical cause of asthma, may also be present in many drugs as well as in foods [322].

Infection

Viral infections are one of the most common and important triggers of asthma exacerbations, especially in atopic infants [323]. There is some evidence that viral infections in childhood may predispose to the development of asthma and bronchial hyperreactivity in later life [324–326]. Both respiratory syncytial virus infection and croup may be followed by persistent wheezing and hyperreactivity, and it has been suggested that such infections may also precede sensitization to common allergens in children of atopic parents [327–330]. The other view is that genetic predisposition is required to allow this to happen, and only transient damage occurs in previously normal individuals [331]. Asthma and acute viral infections are among the commonest of respiratory afflictions. There is a strong association between viral respiratory infections and both the onset and exacerbation of asthma, and the nature of the association is an important area for future research. Recent information suggests that this link may not be wholly accidental but may reflect specific interactions of viral proteins with the host immune system [332].

From the point of view of the chest physician, viral infections in adults are frequently followed by protracted cough and wheeze indistinguishable from asthma [333,334]. The viruses usually responsible are influenza, rhinovirus and respiratory syncytial virus, together with the bacterium *Mycoplasma pneumoniae*. Asthmatic patients with these infections usually suffer attacks of wheeze lasting several weeks. Even non-asthmatic subjects can be shown to have a prolonged period of hyperreactivity, probably related to the mucosal epithelial damage and irritation of vagal receptors [220,335,336]. In contrast, infection with pyogenic bacteria rarely causes acute exacerbations of asthma, though such infections may occasionally be superimposed on a previous viral infection.

Air pollution

Certain air pollutants, notably sulphur dioxide (SO_2), ozone and nitrogen dioxide (NO_2), are able to cause bronchoconstriction when inhaled at high concentrations, although the concentrations that cause this effect are rarely reached in outdoor air in the West nowadays. Nevertheless, epidemiological studies have shown an association between episodes of pollution, primarily with particles and ozone, and exacerbations of asthma [337]. Some reports from the UK indicate that currently encountered levels of air pollution may have measurable but small effects on hospital admissions for asthma and on the lung function of adult asthmatics [338,339]. Studies in the USA and Canada have also shown positive correlations between asthma admissions and ozone, SO_2 and sulphates [340,341], and fluctuations in the concentrations of SO_2 and ozone have been associated with patterns of attendance at casualty departments for acute wheezy episodes [342]. In children a small but statistically significant adverse effect on lung function has been linked with airborne respirable particulate matter, measured as PM_{10} (particles <10 μm in diameter), but not with levels of ozone or NO_2 [343,344].

Although these studies point towards an interaction of air pollution and asthma, the results are not entirely consistent, particularly when linking an individual pollutant to asthma. The main problems with these studies have been difficulty in differentiating asthma and other chronic airway disease and in controlling for confounding variables, including geographical variations in weather, other pollutant levels, occupation, lifestyle, smoking habits, infections, allergens, socioeconomic status and healthcare facilities [345]. Air pollution in general has lessened in the UK at a time when asthma and atopic disorders have increased, and there is the well-known paradox that heavily polluted countries have in general more chronic obstructive pulmonary disease (COPD) and less asthma than do less polluted countries. It is highly unlikely therefore that air pollution is responsible for the increased prevalence of childhood asthma, episodic wheezing and hay fever seen over the last two decades [346]. Functional responses of asthmatics to ozone, NO_2 and SO_2 have been extensively evaluated in controlled exposure studies [346,347] and these studies have shown that asthmatics are abnormally sensitive to SO_2 but not to NO_2 or ozone. However, the possibility of some synergistic effects of combinations of ozone, NO_2 and SO_2 cannot be excluded.

Controlled human exposure studies suggest that air pollutants can potentiate inhaled responses to aeroallergens [348–351]. The mechanisms contributing to the potentiation of responses to aeroallergens following exposure to outdoor and indoor air pollutants is not well understood, but could be the result of pollutants causing shedding of the bronchial basal epithelial cells [345], allowing access of antigen to submucosal lymphocytes and possibly exaggerating the immune response by increasing IgE synthesis [352].

There is thus good evidence that air pollution can influence asthma morbidity and mortality in those who have the disease. However, the evidence does not support the view that air pollution could account for the increasing prevalence of asthma, nor does it support the view that chronic exposure to raised levels of ambient air pollutants can trigger asthma in normal healthy individuals [345].

Smoking

The interrelations of smoking, asthma and atopy are ill understood. Smokers appear to be at greater risk of developing asthma and have a higher prevalence of hyperreactivity [353,354] but the role of smoking as an independent cause of asthma has been questioned [355]. In a long-term follow-up study of a childhood cohort, atopy and smoking were two important predictors of adult-onset wheezy illness [356]. It seems likely that smoking is an important risk factor for reversible airflow obstruction in adults, although the very fact that a patient is a smoker inclines doctors towards a diagnosis of COPD rather than asthma, causing unnecessary confusion to epidemiologists.

The role of environmental tobacco smoke as a cause of asthma remains uncertain. Asthma has been associated with tobacco smoke more strongly in young children [357–359] than in school-aged children in whom the evidence is confusing [360–365]. On the other hand, there are many reports of a significantly increased risk of wheeze in school-aged children. While wheeze is often used as a surrogate measure of asthma, different definitions of wheeze have been used in various studies, making comparisons between studies difficult. Another difficulty with these studies is the confounding effect of other factors associated with social class, and it seems to the authors that in general a relatively poor environment in the West, associated with parental smoking, poor housing and a bad diet, combine to increase the risks of wheezy illness in adolescents and adults.

To add further complexity, it has often been observed by clinicians that asthmatic symptoms commence more frequently than would be expected in individuals who have recently stopped smoking; in some of these, symptoms improve if they restart. There may be an immunosuppressant effect of smoke (which could also explain the relative resistance of smokers to the development of allergic alveolitis) and this is an area that requires further research.

Psychological factors

Most patients with asthma acknowledge that exacerbations may be provoked by psychological events, such as shock, bereavement or excitement. However, such factors are rarely the dominant cause of the disease [366,367]. Suggestion (and its extreme form, hypnosis) may have important effects in modifying asthmatic reactions to provoking factors in either direction [368,369], and good doctors make use of this in their management of such patients. In one study hypnosis abolished skin sensitivity, even though the presence of antibody in serum was still demonstrable by the Prausnitz–Kustner reaction [370].

The psychogenic effects on airways reactivity are presumably mediated by the autonomic nervous system, and the effects of suggestion in provoking bronchospasm may be blocked by atropine [371]. Hyperventilation induced by anxiety or laughter may also be responsible for asthmatic reactions.

The severe asthmatic attack may be very frightening, and such patients are understandably anxious. It is important to recognize this and to reassure the patient, while treating the asthma rather than the anxiety with drugs. The parents of an asthmatic child frequently and understandably become anxious and tend to be overprotective towards the child. This also should be recognized by the doctor, and managed by proper care of the child and reassurance of the parents. It is likely that such psychosocial factors in a family contribute to the severity of the asthma,

and they should always be sought for and dealt with as far as possible. Occasionally, psychological illness, family disputes or marital problems may be major factors in the aetiology of intractable asthma and expert psychiatric help may be necessary.

Gastro-oesophageal reflux

It is now well recognized that episodes of gastro-oesophageal reflux may provoke wheeze as well as the more familiar symptoms of heartburn [372,373]. Not all asthmatics respond in this way to reflux, but in those that do a lowered intraoesophageal pH seems to initiate a fall in FEV_1 over about 90 min [374,375]. Acidic drinks, such as colas and fruit juices, and iced water produce similar effects. In some cases where reflux symptoms are troublesome, fundal plication or treatment with an H_2 blocker has also resulted in amelioration of the asthmatic symptoms [376,377]. Gastro-oesophageal reflux is common and enquiry about it should be routine in history-taking in the asthmatic. While it plays no part in the generation of the common nocturnal symptoms in most patients [378], reflux should always be considered as a possible provocative factor in the 'difficult to control' asthmatic [379]. If an asthmatic patient has prominent reflux symptoms, a trial of treatment with an H_2 blocker or a proton pump inhibitor is justified.

Exercise

Almost all young, active asthmatic subjects may provoke attacks by exercise, although their responsiveness to this form of challenge varies according to other factors such as associated allergen challenge and baseline bronchial reactivity and the ambient temperature. The typical exercise required to provoke an attack is several minutes of running, though a quick sprint for a bus on a cold winter morning may be sufficient. The bronchoconstriction usually starts at or towards the end of the exercise and lasts 20–30 min. The mechanisms have been discussed above.

Weather

Almost all asthmatic patients notice effects of the weather on their symptoms and learn which individual patterns suite them best or least. Aside from the effects of air pollution and seasonal airborne pollen and spores, extremes of temperature seem most likely to provoke attacks in the susceptible. Notable epidemics of asthma have been described on many occasions in association with thunderstorms [380–382], although the causes of these are not understood and not all such storms are associated with epidemics. It has been suggested that in some cases they may be due to release by the associated rainfall of large numbers of fungal spores or allergenic grass pollen particles, and epidemics are most likely to occur if the storm follows a period of high pollen counts [272,383].

Occupational factors

Work-related factors are important provokers of asthma, and asthma is now the most common type of work-related respiratory disease in industrialized countries [384,385]. Occupational asthma can be defined as variable airways narrowing causally related to exposure in the working environment to airborne dusts, gases, vapours or fumes [386]. Most authorities now recognize that typical asthma may occur following exposure to high concentrations of irritant gases or fumes [387], the so-called reactive airways dysfunction syndrome discussed further in Chapter 36. This section concerns itself with asthma following exposure to a sensitizer. Symptoms usually commence within 2 years of starting the job, although this period is sometimes much longer, and may be associated with a particular place or process. Typically, the symptoms initially occur towards the end of the working day and in the evening, and are relieved at weekends and on holiday. As the condition progresses, so the symptoms become more persistent and may last over weekends and even for several weeks after work has ceased [385,388]. Indeed, there is no doubt that exposure to allergens, particularly those of low molecular weight, in the workplace can act as a trigger of persistent asthma that continues despite complete cessation of exposure; unless the patient ceases exposure relatively quickly after symptoms commence, this is the usual outcome [387,389,390]. Thus, if the patient presents for diagnosis when the condition has become well established, typical patterns of work-related peak flow rate changes may be absent. There are a number of factors that influence prognosis. Further occupational exposure in sensitized subjects leads to persistence and sometimes progressive deterioration of asthma, irrespective of any reduction of exposure to the specific sensitizer. Other determinants of an unfavourable prognosis are long duration of exposure before the development of asthma, long duration of symptoms before diagnosis, poor baseline pulmonary function, dual responses after specific challenge tests and the persistence of markers of airway inflammation in BAL and bronchial biopsies [388]. The diagnosis of occupational asthma is discussed in a later section.

Occupational asthma is considered for medicolegal purposes to be asthma provoked by some agent in the work process that was not present before the individual was so exposed. The agent (identified or not) should be specific to the workplace as well as causally related to the disease [386,389,391]. A previous history of asthma does not exclude a diagnosis of occupational asthma, but in such individuals the diagnosis is much more difficult to estab-

lish. People with pre-existing asthma are of course liable to develop exacerbations if they choose jobs in which allergen exposure is a problem. Atopic individuals are also at greater risk of developing asthma in jobs where they are exposed to one of the classical high molecular weight allergens, such as animal dander, grain dust or other organic debris. In general, however, this is not true of exposures to low molecular weight chemicals, where atopics appear to be at relatively little greater risk [392], with some exceptions such as platinum complex salts. Nor are non-atopics immune from asthma even when exposed to classical allergens, so prevention of the condition by screening out atopics is not usually a very effective means of control. More than one immunological mechanism must be involved in occupational asthma. The mechanisms of asthma due to small molecular weight substances are not known, and it is unlikely that classical IgE-mediated allergic processes are responsible in all cases. There is evidence to confirm that T-lymphocyte activation and local accumulation of activated eosinophils in the bronchial wall occurs in asthma of diverse aetiology [392]. It should be noted in passing that bronchoconstriction in response to workplace exposures may not always imply the potential of persisting hypersensitivity. For example, it may be a transient phenomenon provoked by irritant exposures, such as to smoke, chlorine, SO_2 or citric acid, or by exposure to the anticholinesterase organophosphate insecticides [393].

Causes of occupational asthma

The list of proven causes of asthma in the workplace is long and inevitably increasing. For a detailed review, the reader is referred to the article by Chan-Yeung and Malo [394]. However, it is more important always to bear in mind the possibility of occupational factors, which may not have been recognized previously, and to make appropriate investigations than to remember a long list of known causes. The list may be simplified by subdivision into categories that may prompt a question in the history, i.e. exposure to animals or animal products, plants or their derivatives, and enzymes, drugs and chemicals. The best known of these are listed in Tables 34.1–34.3.

Table 34.1 Causes of occupational asthma of animal origin.

Agent	Occupation
Cats, dogs, horses	Veterinarians
Rats, mice, guinea-pigs	Laboratory workers
Grain mites	Farmers
Locusts	Research workers
Moths, silkworms, flies	Breeding
Pigeons, chickens	Breeding, farming
Oyster, prawn, crab, salmon	Food production

Table 34.2 Causes of occupational asthma of vegetable and bacteriological origin.

Agent	Occupation
Grains and flour	Farmers, millers, bakers
Hardwood dusts	Millers, joiners, carpenters
Castor, coffee beans	Processing
Gum acacia	Pharmaceuticals
Tragacanth	Sweet manufacture
Colophony	Soldering
Enzymes	
Alcalase	Detergent production
Trypsin	
Papain	Pharmaceuticals, food technology
Amylase	
Ispaghula	Laxative manufacture

Table 34.3 Causes of occupational asthma of chemical origin.

Agent	Occupation
Isocyanates	Paints, varnishes, plastics
Epoxy resin hardeners	Adhesives, varnishes
Ethanolamines	Aluminium soldering
Formaldehyde, glutaraldehyde	Hospital workers
Azodicarbonamide	Plastics
Platinum	Refining
Nickel	Plating
Chromium	Leather tanning
Cobalt	Hard-metal work
Vanadium	Boiler cleaning
Persulphates, henna	Hair colouring
Reactive dyes	Manufacture, dyeing
Pharmaceuticals	Pharmaceutical industry
Penicillins	
Tetracyclines	
Cephalosporins	
Piperazine	
Psyllium	
Chloramine T	
Ceftazidime	

Important animal causes include small laboratory mammals, where urinary protein is usually the principal allergen [395–397], insects such as locusts [297], fruit flies [398] and honey-bee dust [399], grain mites [400], fowl mites [401], moths (including silkworms) and flies [299,402], birds such as pigeons and chickens [401,403], and molluscs such as oyster, prawn and crab [404,405]. Sensitization occurs as a result of exposure to airborne particles such as urine droplets, mite faeces or small fragments of insect parts. Prawn workers may be exposed because of the water jets used to blow the meat from the exoskeleton. Farmers and veterinarians may become sensitized to any number of animals that they handle, as may laboratory workers.

The best-known vegetable causes are wood dusts, especially from hardwoods such as western red cedar [389] and grain dusts [406–408]. The largest numbers of subjects sensitized to wood have been reported from sawmills, although joiners and carpenters not infrequently develop symptoms [409]. They can usually prevent attacks by avoiding the particular wood. It is probable that the active agent in hardwood dust is a small molecular weight chemical, plicatic acid, which can combine with serum albumin to form a sensitizing hapten [410]. In common with other types of asthma provoked by small molecules, atopic individuals do not seem to be at increased risk of western red cedar sensitization. Less is known of the immunological mechanisms of asthma caused by other wood dusts, although in view of their common characteristic of hardness it is likely that they act similarly. Grain dust contains a complex mixture of allergens and has been known to cause respiratory problems among bakers and millers since the eighteenth century. Flour itself may be allergenic, and not uncommonly sensitization to enzymes used in the process, notably α-amylase, occurs [411,412]. Occasionally the grain may be contaminated by fungi and mites. The grain mites *Tyrophagus* and *Acarus* spp. have been shown to be an important cause of asthma in farmers in Scotland handling stored grain [413]. Other vegetable causes of asthma include castor and coffee beans [414,415], in workers manufacturing their products, and gums from acacia and tragacanth used previously in printing and currently in pharmaceuticals and sweet manufacture [416,417].

Colophony (or rosin), the residue that remains when oil of turpentine has been distilled from pine resin, is known to be an important cause of asthma [418,419]. It is used as a component of multicore solders and has widespread industrial application in the manufacture of circuitry in electronics. The principal component of the fume liberated when it is heated is a small molecular weight chemical, abietic acid. The mechanism whereby this provokes asthma is not known, although there is no evidence that it causes IgE-mediated sensitization. Asthma caused by colophony is commonplace in the electronic industry and again affects atopics and non-atopics, even though atopy may be a weak predisposing factor [420,421]. Occupational asthma caused by enzymes was first described in workers making so-called biological washing powders, where proteolytic enzymes derived from *Bacillus subtilis* were introduced into the product [422–424]. This problem has now been controlled by careful attention to industrial hygiene in the process [425]. Sporadic cases may be seen of workers sensitized to other enzymes such as trypsin, papain and amylase in plastic, pharmaceutical laboratory and food technology work [426–428]. Asthma caused by drugs administered to patients is discussed in Chapter 55. Pharmaceutical products or chemical compounds involved in their synthesis may also sensitize workers. Among these are penicillins, tetracyclines, cephalosporins, piperazine, chloramine disinfectants and psyllium [429–435].

In recent years, the substances that have attracted most attention as causes of occupational asthma have been low molecular weight chemicals. Isocyanates, especially TDI but also the diphenyl methane, hexamethylene and naphthylamine compounds and prepolymers [436–444], are particularly important because of the large numbers of workers exposed in the production of polyurethanes and synthetic rubbers and in the use of foundry binding materials, varnishes and other surface coatings. Isocyanates are irritant substances and in high concentration can cause non-specific bronchial reactivity, although sensitized subjects react to extremely low concentrations. They are reactive chemicals but the method by which they cause sensitization is not known; there is no strong evidence that they cause their effect via hapten formation and an IgE-mediated reaction, though occasional subjects show a positive RAST to TDI–albumin complexes [445]. Isocyanates may occasionally also cause hypersensitivity pneumonitis (see Chapter 37).

Epoxy resins are polymers that are converted into solids by the addition of acid anhydrides or other chemicals as curing agents. Mixing of the two components in their use as adhesives, surface coatings or plastics may cause liberation of anhydride fumes that can produce asthmatic sensitization, as can heating materials containing them, as in meat-wrappers' asthma [446–448]. There are several such chemicals in use: phthalic, trimellitic, hexahydrophthalic, maleic and tetrachlorophthalic anhydrides. Trimellitic anhydride may also cause alveolitis, an influenza-like syndrome and haemolytic anaemia and haemoptysis [447,449]. These reactive chemicals do act as haptens, and both IgE and IgG antibodies have been described in exposed subjects [450,451]. Aliphatic amines are also potent causes of occupational asthma, described in shellac and lacquer handlers and also in aircraft fitters [452–454]. These compounds include ethylenediamine, dimethylethanolamine, triethylenetetramine and aminoethylethanolamine.

Several metals or their salts may cause bronchial (and skin) sensitization: complex salts of platinum in refining [455,456], nickel in polishing and plating [457], chromium in plating, printing and tanning leather [458,459], cobalt in coolants used in making and machining tungsten carbide (hard metal) and diamond polishing [460,461] and vanadium in cleaning residues from boilers which have burned oil containing the metal [462]. Exposure to cobalt in hard-metal work may also lead to an alveolitis and pulmonary fibrosis, so-called hard metal disease [463]. Asthma in aluminium refinery workers is probably due to fumes of fluoride rather than to the metal itself [464].

Many other chemicals have been described as occasional causes of asthma and no doubt many others will be in the future. Worthy of note are formaldehyde and glutaraldehyde in hospital workers [465,466], azodicarbonamide (a blowing agent in plastic manufacture) [467], paraphenylenediamine in fur dyeing [468], various dyes in hairdressing [469] and aminoethylethanolamine in aluminium soldering [470]. Reactive dyes in the textile industry, when handled in powder form, are another cause that has on occasion proved fatal [471]. More recently, a large variety of causes have been reported including latex especially in rubber gloves used in hospitals [472], fungicides [473,474], and polyethylene shrink wrapping [475]. Latex allergy is becoming an important and increasing problem in hospitals, causing both allergic dermatitis and asthma. It is caused by liberation of particles of protein from the gloves, which are now generally made of cheaper, less well-washed latex.

Some studies have shown that asthma related to chemical and vegetable agents occurs more commonly in cigarette smokers. It has been speculated that this may be due to the effect of smoke on bronchial epithelium, improving access of the sensitizer to submucosal lymphocytes and mast cells [476,477]

Several mechanisms, including immunological, pharmacological and genetic, have been suggested as causes of occupational asthma, acting in concert with airway and neurogenic inflammation [392]. It is likely that more than one mechanism is operative, and it is certain that many more causes or 'inducers' of this problem will be identified in the future. The medicolegal and compensation aspects of occupational asthma have been well reviewed [478].

Clinical course

The only certain things about the course of asthma are its variability and its unpredictability. However, some general points about the natural history can be made and are useful in discussing prognosis with patients and their relatives at the time of diagnosis. The course of asthma is usually one of periods of normality punctuated by attacks of cough, wheeze and breathlessness. Factors provoking attacks have been discussed above; however, attacks often occur without obvious provocation. They may be brief, as after exertion, or last several weeks, as after a viral illness. Between attacks, patients are usually free of symptoms though symptoms may be provoked by exercise or exposure to allergens. During symptomatic periods, patients are usually more sensitive to such stimuli than when well. In atopic asthmatics, exacerbations provoked by allergens are commonly accompanied by rhinitis, while perennial rhinitis of non-allergic but uncertain aetiology commonly accompanies non-atopic asthma. During periods of poor symptom control the characteristic features are variation of symptoms and expiratory flow rates within the 24-h cycle, usually being worst in the small hours and first thing in the morning and least troublesome in the early afternoon [479,480]. Appropriate changes in the timing of this cycle occur in shift workers [481]. There has been much discussion of the cause of diurnal variation and, particularly, nocturnal deterioration in asthma. Suggestions that it might be related to feather pillows or mites in the bed do not explain its occurrence as frequently in non-atopic as in atopic patients. Circadian corticosteroid variation does not explain its occurrence in those on regular medication with these drugs. On balance, it seems likely to be related to increased vagal tone and reduced NANC tone acting on a hyperreactive airway at night [482,483]. It has been shown that bronchial inflammation is increased at night [484] and this is likely to contribute to airway narrowing and hyperreactivity [485].

When asthma starts in childhood, there is a reasonable probability that it will remit (sometimes temporarily) at about the time of adolescence and it usually improves at that age [486–488]. In a Finnish study, 108 asthmatic children were followed up to 20–24 years of age [489]; one-quarter were symptom-free, while another quarter had symptoms at least once a week, half had increased airway responsiveness but only 18% had a below-normal FEV_1. Risk factors for persistence of asthma appear to be severe childhood asthma starting at an early age aociated with atopic eczema. Asthma starting in adult life remits less frequently, except when it occurs simply as a prolonged response to a viral infection. The disease may start at any age, from infancy to extreme old age [37], and may announce itself with an acute severe attack, with increasing wheeze and breathlessness, or with persistent cough. When it presents in middle age or later in this insidious manner, especially if cough is a prominent symptom, it is very liable to be misdiagnosed as chronic bronchitis by the unwary physician. A patient developing asthma for the first time in adult life frequently gives a family history of the disease and atopy is a major risk factor [356], although personal allergic factors are much less important than in childhood, unless the asthma is occupational in origin. It is common clinical experience that older more severe asthmatic patients frequently develop a substantial degree of fixed airway obstruction, and the rate of decline in lung function tends to be accelerated in these patients [490,491].

Acute severe attacks, previously called status asthmaticus, occur spasmodically and unpredictably. They are usually provoked by one of the factors mentioned above. Some patients suffer such episodes frequently but some never (this condition is discussed in the next section). A relatively small proportion of patients develop progressive chronic disease that becomes largely irreversible, even to large doses of corticosteroids. This syndrome, chronic severe asthma, is also discussed below.

Acute severe asthma

Acute severe attacks represent progression of airways narrowing to the point where the patient is distressed at rest and may have signs of cardiac stress. Episodes may be of extremely sudden onset, as in an anaphylactic reaction, but more commonly build up over several hours or days. Often they are initiated by a viral infection and preceded by a period of a few hours or days during which asthmatic symptoms are increasingly troublesome, especially at night.

The symptoms are of increasing breathlessness, wheeze, cough and chest tightness, culminating in difficulty in talking or inability to do anything other than concentrating on breathing, usually in an upright position but sometimes crouching on hands and knees. Anxiety to the stage of panic is a usual and understandable feature. The patient sits up in bed or chair [492], wheezing is audible without the stethoscope, unless the patient is desperately sick, and the chest is visibly overinflated. Sweating may be profuse in severe attacks, and more often than not patients are pale and sweaty. If cyanosis is present this indicates life-threatening severe acute asthma. Considerable effort is clearly being expended on inspiration, the hyperinflated thoracic cage working at a great mechanical disadvantage, even though all accessory respiratory muscles are being used in an attempt to improve breathing. Cough is usually not prominent, as it is almost impossible for the ill patient to generate sufficient expiratory flow; if it is a feature, it is rarely productive of sputum. Indeed, production of sputum can be taken as an encouraging sign of recovery or indicative of an episode that at this time is not life-threatening. Tachycardia is always present, unless the episode has caused profound hypoxaemia. A paradoxical pulse (pulsus paradoxicus) is frequently detected; the extent of the fall in systolic pressure on inspiration may be as much as 50–60 mmHg and if present is a good indicator of the severity of the condition [493–495]. However it is not always present in patients with severe acute asthma and therefore its absence may be misleading [496]. Because of this, it has been withdrawn from the most recent British Thoracic Society guidelines on the management of asthma [497].

Assessment of the severity of the attack prior to treatment includes judging the degree of breathlessness by the patient's ability to talk (e.g. complete sentences in one breath) and measurement of heart rate and pulsus paradoxicus, peak flow rate and arterial blood gases [493,498]. Of these, the ability to talk, pulse rate and arterial blood gases provide the best indicators of severity and prognosis. The degree of breathlessness can be categorized conveniently according to the scheme of Sherwood Jones, which ranges from 'able to carry out housework or job with moderate difficulty (Grade 1A)' to 'immobilized and exhausted (Grade 4)' [498]. Blood gases, as discussed later, show hypoxaemia and hypocapnia initially, hypercapnia only occurring in the preterminal stages of an attack [499].

Even before the introduction of corticosteroids, the majority of attacks resolved spontaneously after several very frightening and stressful days. Nowadays, the use of aerosol and intravenous bronchodilators usually brings some symptomatic relief within minutes, while resolution of the attack can be expected to start some 6–12 h after the commencement of high-dose corticosteroids. A few patients prove resistant to this treatment and require several days or even weeks of steroids before the attack resolves, while some patients have attacks of such suddenness (or present for treatment at such a late stage) that assisted ventilation is necessary immediately. These matters are discussed in Chapter 35. A proportion of patients die of cardiorespiratory arrest in the course of such attacks, and management of asthma patients should foresee and plan to prevent this possibility.

Chronic severe asthma

Some patients with long-standing asthma develop increasingly severe airflow obstruction progressively over several years. While this may occasionally occur in young people, it is more frequently seen in the middle-aged and elderly [500,501]. Sometimes it is due to bronchopulmonary aspergillosis but usually there is no clinically obvious cause. The characteristic feature is failure to respond, more than partially, to high doses of prednisolone [502], although sometimes change to an alternative corticosteroid in high dose (e.g. intravenous methylprednisolone or intramuscular triamcinolone acetonide) may produce some improvement [503]. Bronchodilator responsiveness in these patients is usually preserved. The frequency with which this condition develops in asthma patients is not high but, because of the therapeutic problems it presents, it is disproportionately represented in specialist respiratory medicine clinics.

The pathology of the disease does not apparently differ from that of more steroid-responsive asthma [62]. Occasional such patients show unexpectedly dramatic improvement, sometimes lasting months, following a severe febrile illness; this was recognized by the generations of physicians before the advent of steroids, who occasionally treated such patients with fever therapy induced by injections of milk or vaccines. Understanding this syndrome, which is probably due to corticosteroid resistance [504–506], is an urgent priority of asthma research in order that appropriate therapy may be found. For the present, chronic severe asthma causes untold misery to large numbers of older asthmatics, misery compounded usually by the side-effects of high-dose corticosteroids. Glucocorticosteroid responsiveness in asthma can be defined as an increase in FEV_1, or mean peak expiratory flow (PEF), of 30% or greater during a 14-day course of prednisolone 40 mg daily, and glucocorticosteroid resistance as a less than 15% improvement in FEV_1, or mean

PEF, with the same 2-week treatment with prednisolone [507]. Glucocorticosteroid resistance is not caused by altered pharmacokinetics and the defect in asthmatics is not organ-specific [507,508]. Comparison of cells from normal individuals and from patients with corticosteroid-sensitive asthma has shown peripheral blood mononuclear cells and T lymphocytes to have different *in vitro* characteristics, especially with regard to their response to corticosteroids [504,505,509,510]. All aspects of corticosteroid-resistant asthma have been comprehensively reviewed [506].

Bronchopulmonary aspergillosis

Skin sensitivity to *A. fumigatus* is commonly present in atopic individuals and occurs also in a proportion of otherwise 'non-atopic' patients with chronic asthma. The frequency with which this occurs varies between 16 and 38% in different studies which, being based on clinic populations, may be assumed to be biased towards the more severe end of the asthmatic spectrum [511–513]. In some of these patients, bronchial hypersensitivity to the fungus is also present, while in a small proportion attacks of asthma provoked by the organism are accompanied by a systemic illness with fever and malaise associated with radiographic evidence of peripheral patchy infiltrates or collapse of a lobe, segment or even a whole lung [514–516]. Sputum can be shown to contain hyphae of *A. fumigatus*, which therefore may be presumed to be growing in the airways. Characteristically, the sputum contains typical bronchial casts, with eosinophils, Curschmann's spirals, desquamated epithelial cells and hyphae (Fig. 34.20). The serum contains both IgE and IgG antibodies to *A. fumigutus*, and the total IgE is usually markedly raised. Both immediate and delayed skin sensitivity to intradermal injection of antigen are present [517–519]. Blood eosinophilia ($1–3 \times 10^9/L$) is a common finding. The full-blown picture is known as allergic bronchopulmonary aspergillosis (one of the causes of pulmonary eosinophilia; see Chapter 38). Attacks are recurrent and tend to occur at first predominantly in the winter months. Untreated, an episode may last many weeks before resolving; recurrent attacks characteristically cause a proximal form of bronchiectasis, with evidence of distal pulmonary fibrotic changes [520,521]. Occasionally, especially in patients treated with long-term corticosteroids, typical radiographic exacerbations may occur without clinical symptoms [522–524]. Usually, however, attacks are noticed by the patient; they may present with chest pain and fever, as well as worsening of asthmatic symptoms, so appropriate therapeutic action can be taken. In patients with frequent attacks, progressive disease may occur leading to extensive, mainly upper zone, bronchiectasis and fibrosis. Radiological features are described in the following section. A diagnosis of allergic bronchopulmonary aspergillosis

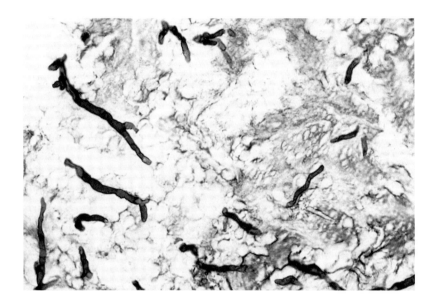

Fig. 34.20 Asthmatic sputum smear showing hyphae of *Aspergillus fumigatus* and a Charcot–Leyden crystal at bottom right (Papanicolaou ×350).

should be suspected in any patient with asthma who has an abnormal chest radiograph and a high peripheral blood eosinophil count. The diagnostic criteria include:

1 asthma (in most cases);

2 peripheral blood eosinophilia of greater than $0.5 \times 10^9/L$;

3 presence or history of chest radiograph abnormalities;

4 positive skin-prick test to an extract of *A. fumigatus*;

5 serum precipitating antibodies to *A. fumigatus*;

6 raised total serum IgE;

7 fungal hyphae of *A. fumigatus* on microscopic examination of sputum.

Patients may sometimes present with typical attacks without having previously had asthma; in these cases diagnosis is often delayed [525,526]. Bronchoscopy is sometimes necessary to make a diagnosis and is of great value therapeutically. This often reveals thick tenacious plugs, which should be removed to restore an airway and to allow cytological examination to reveal the diagnosis. Occasionally, lobes or segments are excised surgically in the mistaken belief that bronchial occlusion has been caused by tumour. The histological features in the lung infiltrates are infiltration with eosinophils, areas of collapse, typical asthmatic bronchial inflammatory changes with intraluminal hyphae and sometimes intramural granulomas [527]. The more florid features of bronchocentric granulomatosis may sometimes be present [528].

The spectrum of response of the lungs to *A. fumigatus* is wide (see Chapter 21). Typical allergic bronchopulmonary aspergillosis may occasionally occur in people with aspergilloma and vice versa, and aspergillomas may occur as a sequel to treated invasive or allergic aspergillosis [529,530]. Very occasionally, allergic bronchopulmonary aspergillosis may develop features of invasive disease [531].

The immediate cause of the clinical manifestations of allergic bronchopulmonary aspergillosis appears to be the development of both immediate and delayed hypersensitivity to *A. fumigatus*, with an important cell-mediated component [532,533]. *A. fumigatus* spores are inhaled into the lungs since they are present in the air spora, predominantly in winter, the natural habitat of the organism being dead leaves, compost heaps and other decaying organic matter [534]. Since *A. fumigatus* is not by any means the most profuse fungal organism in the air, its special propensity to cause pulmonary problems requires explanation. This is probably related partly to its small spore size, which allows inhalation to alveolar level, and partly to its optimal temperature requirement of 37°C. In addition, its spores have developed sophisticated antiphagocytic defences that allow it to survive macrophage attack [535–537], and colonization may be facilitated by the pathological changes in the asthmatic's bronchial wall that expose the basement membrane [283]. A syndrome similar to allergic bronchopulmonary aspergillosis has been described occasionally in response to other fungal spores, both other species of *Aspergillus* and unrelated organisms such as *Curvularia* spp. and *Dreschlera* spp. It would be surprising if others were not to be described in the future, as the fungal air spora varies according to local climate and vegetation. For further discussion of these matters, see Chapter 21. The natural history of the condition is for recurrent episodes of pulmonary infiltration associated almost always with symptoms of exacerbation of asthma to occur over many years [538]. Between attacks, which tend to occur in autumn or winter when spores are most prevalent in the air, the patient is usually well. If attacks are treated promptly with oral corticosteroids, the condition does not usually result in progressive lung or airway damage, though early unrecognized or untreated episodes often leave some localized bronchiectatic change [538]. The management of allergic bronchopulmonary aspergillosis is discussed in Chapter 35.

Other complications of asthma

The most common complications of asthma relate to the long-term use of corticosteroid drugs. Facial changes, skin dystrophy, bruising, osteoporosis and vertebral collapse, and adrenal suppression are all commonplace and distressing features in chronic asthmatics. In children, growth retardation may be blamed on the drugs, but was a feature of chronic childhood asthma prior to their introduction [539]. In general the literature on the effects of inhaled corticosteroids on growth is reassuring, although long-term oral corticosteroid therapy, even in low doses equivalent to prednisolone 2.5–5 mg daily, significantly stunts short-term and intermediate-term growth and can reduce final height [540]. Treatment with inhaled budesonide in doses up to 400 µg daily seems not to affect growth adversely in children with asthma [541]. Higher doses can be seen to have an effect on short-term lower leg growth as assessed by knemometry; while no firm conclusions can be made about the long-term effects of inhaled corticosteroids, studies addressing this question suggest that children with asthma treated with these drugs usually attain a normal final height [542]. The question of the possibility of individually increased sensitivity to a growth-retarding effect of inhaled corticosteroids needs further study. Structural chest cage deformities caused by uncontrolled severe chronic asthma [543], such as pigeon chest and kyphosis, are now rarely seen in countries in which modern drug therapy can be afforded.

Other complications are relatively uncommon, except for respiratory infections. These are often difficult to differentiate from acute asthmatic exacerbations, especially as purulent sputum may be mimicked by sputum containing large numbers of eosinophils. Pulmonary infiltration on chest radiographs in adult asthmatics is very suggestive of allergic bronchopulmonary aspergillosis, although other eosinophilic pneumonias or segmental collapse due to plugging may be responsible. The latter is not uncommon in children [544]. Very rarely, lung collapse unrelated to aspergillosis may occur [545]. Cough fractures of ribs may occur, especially in osteoporotic bones, and acute attacks may rarely be complicated by pneumothorax or mediastinal and subcutaneous emphysema [546,547]. Even patients with long-standing chronic severe asthma occasionally develop pulmonary hypertension and cor pulmonale, and chronic hypercapnia is also a most unusual feature. When these complications do occur, the patient usually has cigarette-induced COPD as well; nevertheless, occasional non-smoking chronic asthmatics do ultimately develop cor pulmonale and, in contrast to the clinical findings, right ventricular hypertrophy at necropsy is a not uncommon finding in chronic asthma [548].

Physical findings and functional effects

The characteristic clinical findings in a patient with asthma are wheezes (sometimes, harking back to Laënnec, called rhonchi). They are usually polyphonic, indicating their origin from many airways of different calibre. A wheeze is generated by vibration in the wall of an airway on the point of closure, in the same way as a reed in a woodwind instrument generates a note [549]. The airway narrowing is due to smooth muscle constriction, mucosal oedema and mucous plugging. From this central principle of asthma derive all the physiological abnormalities, which may be considered in terms of primary alterations in pulmonary mechanics and secondary changes in gas exchange and cardiac function. However, the cardinal feature of asthma is its variability, and the main role of lung function testing is in demonstrating change in expiratory flow rates in response to bronchodilators or various forms of challenge. It should also be noted that lung function is often completely normal when the patient is in clinical remission, or even during the day at a time when nocturnal symptoms are troublesome. During the asthma attack there is widespread narrowing of airways and this has the effect of reducing airflow rates. Measurements of this by FEV_1, PEF or flow rates at different lung volumes derived from the flow–volume curve therefore show reduction in proportion to the severity of the attack [550]. Inspiratory flow rates are also reduced, though not to the same extent as those on expiration. In partial compensation for the airway narrowing the patient breathes at a higher lung volume, which increases the (negative) pressure within the thorax acting to distend the airways. This, and the widespread closure and partial closure of small airways, results in increased residual volume and increased work of breathing. These changes are illustrated in Fig. 34.21, which shows a progressive increase in residual volume. As the attack becomes progressively more severe, tidal breathing moves up towards total lung capacity and the tidal expiratory flow rate approaches the maximal expiratory flow rate. At this point, the thoracic system is working on a part of the pressure–volume relationship that is relatively inefficient, large negative pressures being required to generate adequate tidal volumes. This inefficiency is due to the increased elastic recoil pressures in the lungs and thoracic cage, together with the shorter initial length of the intercostal and diaphragmatic muscles at high lung volumes. At the same time, the reduced vital capacity and the low flow rates available mean that adequate ventilation can be maintained only by increasing the frequency of breathing. Thus the patient in an acute attack expends a considerable amount of energy in maintaining rapid inspiratory efforts at high lung

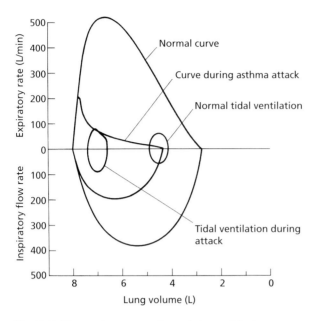

Fig. 34.21 Flow–volume curves in remission and during an asthma attack. Note that during the attack residual volume is increased and tidal breathing takes place at a high lung volume. Also during the attack, tidal expiratory flows approach maximal values.

volumes. Indeed, there is evidence that total lung capacity actually increases during an acute attack of asthma, thereby putting the patient's respiratory muscles at an even greater mechanical disadvantage [551–553]. These physiological features are easily seen in the patient with acute severe asthma, who sits upright fighting to breathe in, and are the reason for the increasing fatigue that occurs terminally in this condition.

At one time there was much discussion about the site of airway narrowing in asthma, as determined by physiological tests [554,555]. There is little purpose in such studies, and the validity of so-called tests of small airways resistance is dubious in subjects with the patchy changes one might anticipate in asthma. There is little doubt that airways at all levels, from the larynx to the bronchioles, may be narrowed in an attack; glottic and major bronchial narrowing have been seen at bronchoscopy and demonstrated physiologically [556,557], and widespread plugging of small airways seen pathologically is universal in fatal attacks, unless death has occurred within minutes of the onset of the attack. It would be expected that different patterns of obstruction would occur in different attacks. Irregular distribution of airway narrowing through the lungs has been demonstrated by studies using inert gas washout and by ventilation scanning using radioactive isotopes [558–560].

Changes in gas exchange

The irregular distribution of ventilation of lung units men-

tioned above is matched by local reduction in perfusion, resulting in patchy but similarly distributed areas of reduced activity on ventilation–perfusion scans [560]. The mechanisms of this are likely to be reflex, due to local hypoxia, together with increased local alveolar pressure from the elastic recoil of overdistended parts of the lung acting on capillaries in alveolar walls. Thus a compensatory mechanism exists that permits excessive physiological shunting and thus hypoxaemia in the stable, less severe, asthmatic. The infrequency with which segmental or subsegmental collapse occurs despite widespread hypoventilation is suspected to be due to collateral ventilation between acini, maintaining an air supply to alveoli distal to blocked bronchi. The asthmatic in remission and in the early stages of an attack may therefore have evidence of gross unevenness of ventilation, with only slight increase in alveolar–arterial oxygen gradient and mild hypoxaemia. Similarly, the diffusing capacity for carbon monoxide is rarely reduced in asthma (a useful point in differentiating the chronic asthmatic from the patient with emphysema) and indeed during remissions is often raised [561,562]. The reason for this high $D\text{LCO}$ is not clear; it is not wholly due to a raised alveolar volume and may be related to increased pulmonary capillary blood volume, perhaps as a consequence of distension of the capillary bed by the increased negative transpulmonary pressure [563]. Small reductions in $D\text{LCO}$ may be found in chronic bronchopulmonary aspergillosis [520,538], after administration of bronchodilator drugs (perhaps due to increased mismatch of ventilation and perfusion when both airways and vessels respond to the drug) [563] and when the steady-state rather than the single-breath method is used [564].

However, there is in general a direct relationship in asthma between FEV_1 and Pao_2. The lower the FEV_1, as a patient deteriorates, the lower the Pao_2, and in acute severe asthma the patient is often markedly hypoxaemic [499,565] (Fig. 34.22). This presumably relates to the inability of reflex changes in perfusion to match exactly the increasingly severe and diffuse reductions in ventilation as the attack progresses. In contrast to the case in patients with smoking-induced chronic airways disease, the asthmatic patient is able to respond to this acute episode by hyperventilation. Because of the shape of the oxygen–haemoglobin dissociation curve, this has minimal effect on hypoxaemia, only allowing a rise roughly in proportion to the reduction in Pco_2 in the alveoli. In contrast, however, hyperventilation of those units of lung still accessible to inspired air allows removal of sufficient carbon dioxide to maintain normal pressures of this gas in the arterial blood; indeed, during most of a severe asthmatic attack the $Paco_2$ is below normal, and a rise to normal levels together with increasing hypoxaemia is an ominous sign. The arterial pH usually simply reflects the ventilation and, except in prolonged attacks,

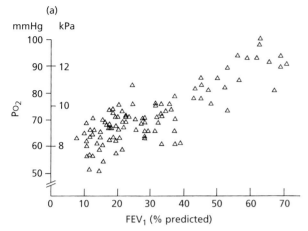

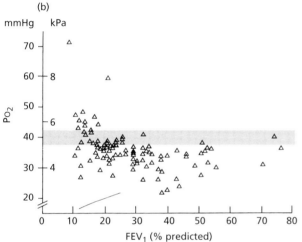

Fig. 34.22 Effects of increasing airflow obstruction on (a) Pao_2 and (b) $Paco_2$. Progressive decline in Pao_2 is accompanied by a fall in $Paco_2$ until severe airflow obstruction, when a rise to, or above, normal levels may occur. (From McFadden & Lyons [565].)

metabolic compensation for respiratory alkalosis is unusual [566].

Cardiac function

Cardiac function is not normally altered in asthma except in an acute attack and, as mentioned above, right-sided heart disease of sufficient severity to present clinical problems is rare even in patients with chronic severe asthma. Indeed, when such a patient does have evidence of cor pulmonale, other diagnoses such as smoking-induced COPD or recurrent pulmonary embolism should be considered.

In the acute severe attack, tachycardia and pulsus paradoxus are evidence of cardiac stress, and the ECG may show P pulmonale and inverted anterior chest T waves [493]. Few studies of the pulmonary circulation in such circumstances have (understandably) been carried out,

although there is little doubt that pulmonary arterial pressure would normally be raised both in response to hypoxaemia and as a consequence of the high intra-alveolar pressures [567]. These pressures are due to the high recoil pressure of the lungs when breathing towards the top of the pressure–volume curve and are, of course, transmitted directly to the pulmonary capillary bed in the alveolar walls. In very severe attacks requiring assisted ventilation, it is noteworthy that the high ventilator pressures required to inflate these already overinflated lungs commonly provoke a marked decrease in venous return that can result in cardiac arrest [45]. In patients with respiratory acidosis and high inflation pressures, attempts to normalize blood gases quickly are abandoned and 'controlled hypoventilation' is employed, providing an adequate Pao_2 can be maintained [568].

Perhaps also related to cardiac stress is the occasional occurrence of myocardial infarction during an acute severe attack [569]. Such episodes are usually painless and rarely fatal, being identified from ECG changes. Plasma free fatty acids are raised, presumably reflecting greatly increased sympathetic activity [570]; this, together with impaired coronary circulation, may be the explanation of infarction. It is reasonable to suppose that the lack of pain in such episodes may be related to raised levels of endogenous opioids, the stress of the attack being not dissimilar to that occurring during severe prolonged exercise in which painless infarction and raised β-endorphin levels may occur [571].

Variability in function

The greatest value of lung function testing in asthma is derived from measuring variability in flow rates. Fortunately this requires only the simplest of equipment, a peak flow meter or spirometer; the portability of the former makes it invaluable. Three types of testing are within the scope of every physician: measuring response to bronchodilators, examining the effect of exercise, and measuring variability over a period of days or weeks, with or without a course of steroids. A fourth type, assessing the effect of challenge testing, is usually carried out by specialists.

Many asthmatic patients when first presenting to their general practitioner do so during an attack. Measurement of FEV_1 or PEF, followed by two puffs of a fast-acting inhaled bronchodilator, a wait of a few minutes and repeat measurement help to confirm the diagnosis in most cases and give an immediate indication of the patient's likely responsiveness to further treatment. It has the added bonus of encouraging patients to believe that they have found a physician who understands their condition. However, there are a few snags to this simple test. It should be borne in mind that responsiveness to bronchodilator varies according to the degree of airflow

958 / CHAPTER 34

obstruction at the time of administration, and little or none would be expected in someone with no obstruction or in someone with very severe obstruction. In the latter case, poor access of the bronchodilator to the airways may be a partial explanation, though intravenous bronchodilator may not be much better and it is therefore probable that in this situation airway oedema and plugging are making the major contribution to the obstruction [572,573].

Exercise testing can also be carried out with ease in clinic or surgery, and finds its application in confirming a suspected diagnosis in a (usually younger) patient who is not obstructed at the time of presentation. The simplest procedure is to measure PEF or FEV$_1$ and then to ask the patient to jog at a steady pace for about 8 min. While laboratory treadmill or bicycle are perfectly satisfactory means of ensuring appropriate exercise is taken and are necessary for scientific study of the effect of different forms of exercise [574] and therapy, lack of a laboratory should not be a deterrent to the physician; a hospital corridor, the adjacent street or a nearby staircase are adequate substitutes [575]. The response to exercise, as discussed previously, varies from time to time depending on the pre-existing bronchial reactivity. A patient with typical asthma shows a period of bronchodilatation in the early stages of exercise but by the end of 8 min usually has started to bronchoconstrict. The expiratory flow rates usually continue to decline for a few minutes after exercise has ceased, then gradually recover to normal over an hour or less depending on the severity of the initial fall [576] (Fig. 34.23). The recovery can be speeded up by administration of a bronchodilator.

Another method of confirming the diagnosis of asthma is to record measurements of PEF several times daily over

a period of days or weeks. This is also of inestimable value both in the investigation of suspected provocative factors, such as occupational or environmental sensitizers, and in investigating patients in whom the history of episodic breathlessness is equivocal. For the latter purpose, it is usually sufficient to ask the patient to record PEF morning, midday and at bedtime, together with recordings during any attacks (especially if any occur at night). In patients with normal flow rates when first seen, this allows assessment of the amount and severity of variability, while in those with a persistently reduced PEF it allows a baseline to be measured for comparison with similar readings during a period of treatment. In many patients with relatively severe airways obstruction, there is doubt about whether asthma or cigarette-induced disease is the dominant condition, and monitoring of PEF during a 2-week course of high-dose prednisolone usually resolves this matter. In investigating possible occupational factors, it is desirable to ask the patient to record PEF more frequently, up to every 2h during work [577]. Unfortunately, such records are very time-consuming to analyse, and a compromise number of recordings (four or five times daily) is usually adequate. This should be combined with a diary kept by the patient, noting work activities, times away from work and symptoms. The use of lung function in challenge testing is discussed in the section on diagnosis. Again, simple and repeatable tests such as FEV$_1$ and PEF are ideal for this purpose.

Radiological features

In most patients with asthma, either in remission or during an attack, the chest radiograph looks normal. Slight overinflation, with depressed diaphragm, laterally spread ribs and enlarged retrosternal airspace, may be seen in some patients during an attack and in some with chronic severe asthma [578,579]. In contrast to emphysema, the diaphragm normally retains its upwardly convex curvature and the pulmonary vessels do not show the same degree of attenuation. The most usual abnormality seen on the asthmatic radiograph is thickening of bronchial walls, as tramline shadows and rings close to the hilum [580]. This is a non-specific finding that is seen also in chronic bronchitis.

The most important function of a chest radiograph in asthma is the exclusion of other abnormalities. In acute attacks pneumothorax may (rarely) occur and may be difficult to detect clinically. There may be evidence of mediastinal and subcutaneous emphysema, usually in the absence of pneumothorax. If consolidation is present, it is likely to be due to pneumonia but the possibility of allergic bronchopulmonary aspergillosis should always be considered.

Episodes of allergic bronchopulmonary aspergillosis are characterized by recurrent fleeting pulmonary

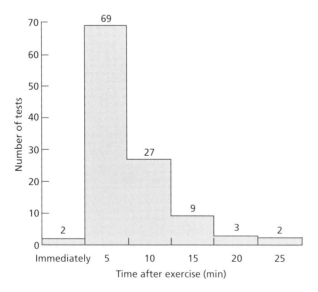

Fig. 34.23 Time of maximal fall in peak flow rate after exercise in 112 tests on asthmatic patients. (From Hartley [152].)

shadows [538], although lobar or segmental collapse, nodular or band shadows may occur (Figs 34.24 & 34.25). If untreated they resolve only slowly over several weeks, but with corticosteroid treatment they may be expected to clear within days. In some patients they recur at the same site; equally, recurrences occur apparently at random sites in the lungs. Recurrent episodes may, but do not always, lead to chronic lung damage [538]. This shows radiologically as tubular (tramline), 'gloved-finger' and ring shadows, lobar or segmental fibrosis and lung shrinkage (Fig. 34.26) and the end-result in severe cases may resemble the appearances in cystic fibrosis. CT or

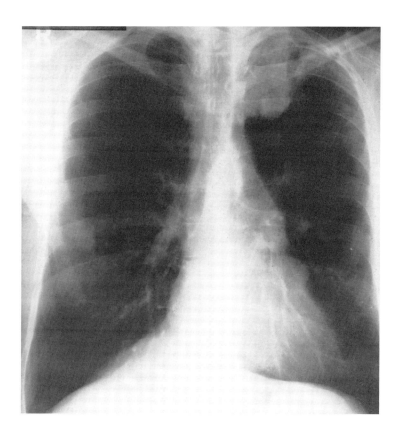

Fig. 34.24 Radiograph of patient with acute episode of allergic aspergillosis showing segmental consolidation in left upper lobe. This resolved after a 2-week course of corticosteroid.

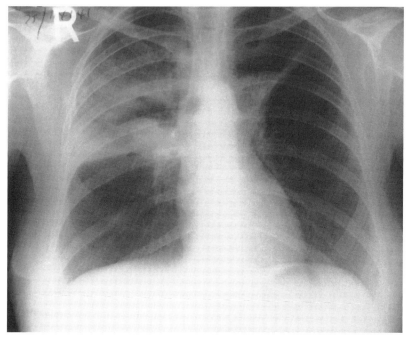

Fig. 34.25 Acute allergic aspergillosis showing segmental consolidation in both upper lobes.

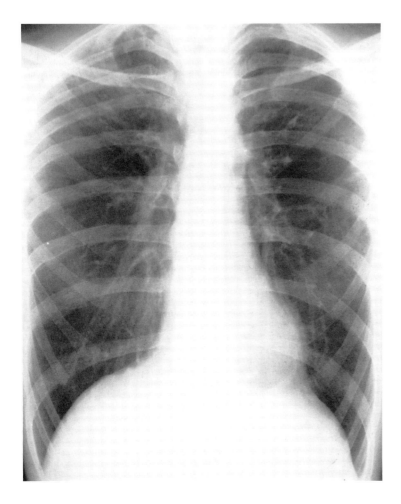

Fig. 34.26 Chronic allergic aspergillosis showing shrunken upper lobes with linear and ring shadows.

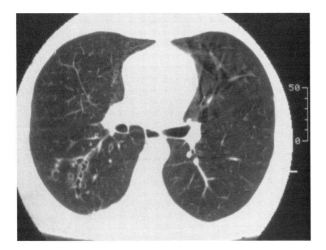

Fig. 34.27 CT of a patient who had had repeated attacks of allergic aspergillosis, the first of which had resulted in bronchiectasis in the right lower lobe.

bronchography shows bronchiectasis [538] (Fig. 34.27), commonly though not always confined to more proximal bronchi, giving a characteristic appearance of normal-looking bronchi distal to the ectatic lesions.

Diagnosis and investigation

In most cases the diagnosis of asthma is made readily from the history. An account of episodic wheezy breathlessness, interspersed with periods of normality, is sufficient evidence on which to suspect asthma. In children and younger adults almost nothing else can cause such symptoms. However, a few conditions do need to be considered in the differential diagnosis at different ages, as all can mimic asthma when the disease presents in a less typical manner. Further evidence in support of asthma comes from a history of marked diurnal variability, attacks in the small hours of the night, and provocation by strong smells, exercise, changes in ambient temperature and allergens.

In infants, acute respiratory infections and asthma are hard to differentiate, and this problem persists in early childhood. When it presents with predominantly respiratory symptoms, cystic fibrosis may also be misdiagnosed as asthma. In older children and adults, bronchiectasis may be associated with wheezy breathlessness and airflow obstruction mimicking asthma, although these patients usually have productive cough as their predominant problem. In adults there can be great difficulty in differentiating asthma from COPD due to smoking. The two conditions coexist in many patients, and it is often impossible to be sure whether an asthmatic component is present without a formal trial of treatment.

Two other conditions must be considered in older patients presenting with wheeze, namely carcinoma of the larynx and proximal bronchial or tracheal tumours not visible on the chest radiograph. Both present with persistent symptoms rather than with attacks of breathlessness, although in this age group asthma also frequently presents in a similar manner. Both may cause wheezy breathlessness on exertion and at night. Clues may come from other symptoms, such as voice changes, haemoptysis or weight loss, but the diagnosis of main airway partial obstruction should follow the physical examination, when a fixed monophonic inspiratory wheeze or stridor is heard. Confirmation is obtained by laryngoscopy or bronchoscopy. Extrathoracic airflow obstruction causes disproportionate inspiratory obstruction (hence stridor) and this may be demonstrated in the laboratory on flow–volume loops. However, this investigation is usually less readily available and less specific than laryngoscopy/bronchoscopy.

Confirmation of the diagnosis of asthma is usually achieved by serial PEF monitoring, which in the majority of cases shows a diurnal variation of more than 15%, and the response to therapy. In most cases no other investigations are necessary. General support for the diagnosis is usually obtained by showing a response in ventilatory function (FEV_1 or PEF) to an aerosol bronchodilator or, in younger subjects, the demonstration of a fall in FEV_1 or PEF following exercise. A raised eosinophil count (above 5% of the total white cell count) is common in untreated asthma [581]. Sputum eosinophilia is a useful indication of an asthmatic type of airways reaction, though it does not invariably predict a response to corticosteroids [582,583]. The demonstration of all the histopathological features of the asthmatic exudate by examining stained sections of sputum fixed in alcohol or formalin is probably a more reliable indication of asthma than a sputum eosinophil count [5]. This technique is also useful for the demonstration of hyphae of *A. fumigatus*.

Skin-prick tests may be useful in identifying suspected provocative allergens. The tests should be chosen from the history and should include a control solution, the most common allergens (house dust, *D. pteronyssinus* and grass pollen or whatever airborne allergens are most common in the locality), together with any allergens that are suspected of causing the patient's reaction in the home or work environment. There is no point in routinely performing a large battery of skin tests. In general, RAST for specific IgE levels correlates closely with the results of skin-prick testing [584]; as it is more expensive and cannot be performed in the clinic immediately, most physicians manage without it in the investigation of most of their patients. In the past, not all commercially available methods of allergy testing have been entirely reliable and care must be taken before using results of these tests in the decision about whether 'hyposensitizing' vaccines should be recommended [585]. The sensible physician relies on a good history and skin testing for the detection of suspected allergens, backed by selective use of RAST, reserving challenge testing for the few occasions when it is thought necessary.

The skin-prick test is performed by putting a drop of allergen on the skin, usually the front surface of the forearm, and lifting the skin lightly through the drop with the point of an intradermal needle. Blood should not be drawn. The test should be read about 15–20 min later. A wheal is a positive result and should be compared in size to that obtained with the control solution, as some subjects react simply to the prick. Intradermal injection of allergen can be used for showing delayed reactions. It requires a larger dose of antigen and there is a higher risk of provoking an anaphylactic reaction; this method of testing is best confined to specialized investigations of aspergillosis or allergic alveolitis and should not be used in outpatient clinics. It should be noted that a positive skin test does not prove that the subject has bronchial hypersensitivity to the allergen in question, but simply adds support to the clinical suspicion. Conversely, bronchial sensitivity may sometimes be present in the absence of skin sensitivity, and when this is suspected RAST may indeed be useful. RAST also has undoubted value in investigating food allergy and in following patients for a quantitative fall in titres after control of exposure, for example to occupational allergen or to pets.

Challenge testing

When it is necessary to investigate provocative factors, challenge testing may be desirable. Normally the first step is to demonstrate a response to a particular environment in terms of changes in PEF over a period. As the suspect environment in most such cases is the workplace, it is often necessary to record PEF four to eight times daily during periods off work, periods at work and periods again off work. The differences may be immediately obvious on looking at the record or particular patterns may be noticed [586]. Figure 34.28 illustrates one such test, where flow rates were persistently lower (and a bronchodilator was required frequently) when the patient was at work. More complex patterns may show increasing fall in flow rates as the week progresses, carry-over into the following week and intermittent falls, depending on such factors as the frequency and duration of exposure and the length of time the patient has had asthma. Sometimes in individuals in whom the asthmatic response has been over a prolonged period, recovery of flow rates may take weeks after exposure ceases (Fig. 34.29). Occasionally in these

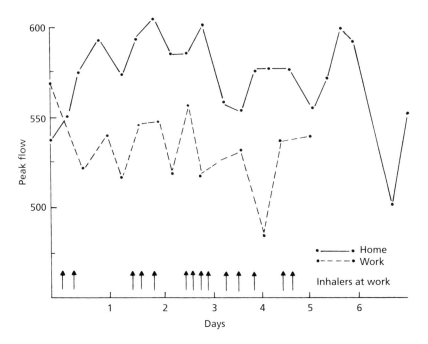

Fig. 34.28 Peak flow record of a patient with allergy to rubber gloves worn in laboratory work. Upper trace was recorded while he was on holiday, lower trace while at work. During the latter period he had frequent need of his inhaler. The one fall when at home followed a drink of red wine, to which he was also allergic.

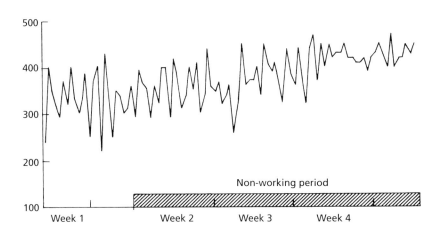

Fig. 34.29 Peak flow record of female electronic soldering supervisor. Full recovery and reduction in diurnal variability did not occur until about 2 weeks after cessation of exposure to colophony.

circumstances, where the aetiological diagnosis remains uncertain and when it is important to find out, challenge testing may be necessary.

As far as possible, all inhalation challenge tests should include exposure to an 'identical' placebo. The patient should be admitted to hospital overnight and the substance administered in a manner mimicking as closely as possible exposure at work. For example, isocyanate exposure may be produced by mixing certain two-component varnishes and applying them to a surface. Flour or sawdust exposure can be produced by pouring the dust from one bowl to another. In one study, a patient who thought he reacted to powder from his surgical gloves was challenged with placebo powder (talc), glove powder (starch), gloves of a different but apparently identical latex and gloves with which he worked [587]. He only reacted to the last, which were subsequently shown to give off

traces of carene vapour, previously known as a potent skin sensitizer.

The effects of the challenge are most conveniently monitored by peak flow rate, which the patient can carry out at home for a few days before and on the morning of challenge in order to obtain a baseline. The measurements should be carried out every 5–10 min after challenge until the immediate reaction is over (if necessary, a bronchodilator aerosol may be given if a severe attack is induced) and then every 30 min until it is certain that a late reaction will not occur. Such late reactions, starting after 3–4 h and lasting about 24 h, are common after challenge and may require treatment with corticosteroids (see Fig. 34.9).

In some cases the only convenient way of administering the challenge is by nebulized aerosol of extracts of the suspect material. It is difficult to judge the dose, and it is therefore wise to start with high dilutions given for only a few minutes. The advantage of an exposure which mimics that in the workplace is that the patient is unlikely to be given a dose higher than that received previously. Nevertheless, length of administration is a matter for judgement, based on assessment of the patient's history. Severe reactions can occur, and nebulized bronchodilators for the initial reaction together with corticosteroids and bronchodilators for the late reaction should be available. Challenge tests are, of course, affected by drugs. The initial response is blocked by bronchodilators and cromoglicate and the late response by corticosteroids. These drugs should therefore be stopped before challenge and this may lead to difficulties in control of the asthma and in interpretation of the results. In general, challenge tests should be carried out on patients whose asthma is in remission and who are managing without regular medication. The techniques and problems of aerosol challenge testing have been reviewed by Burge [588].

Two other types of challenge test may occasionally be necessary. If ingested drug-related asthma is suspected, a small dose of the drug should be given orally. The above-mentioned precautions of hospitalization, baseline investigations, placebo tests and cessation of antiasthma treatment should be taken. The dose should be estimated from the severity of previous responses but initially should not be more than one-tenth of that contained in the preparation under suspicion. The other type of challenge test is that related to investigation of food allergy. In the simple case, the suspected food can be administered in a suitably disguised form (e.g. in a capsule or down a nasogastric tube). In complex cases, it may be necessary to establish the patient on an allergen-free diet and gradually introduce other foods one by one until reactions occur [589]. A typical such exclusion diet might consist of lamb or mutton, gluten-free bread or rice, fresh fruit and vegetables (though reactions to these are not unknown), tea, coffee, sugar and water. If this diet results in disappearance of symptoms and recovery of lung function over 2 weeks, foods under suspicion may be added. Those most likely to cause reactions are ones containing artificial flavours and colours, nuts, milk, eggs and wheat. The investigation of food allergy is complex and the results of such tests are subject to some variability in most cases; therefore clinical importance should only be attached to clear-cut results from placebo-controlled challenges.

References

1 Agricola G (1556) *De re metallica* (translated by Hoover HC, Hoover LH). The Mining Magazine (London) 1912.
2 Sakula A. Sir John Floyer's 'A treatise of the asthma' (1698). *Thorax* 1984; 39: 248.
3 Sakula A. Henry Hyde Salter (1823–71): a biographical sketch. *Thorax* 1985; 40: 887.
4 Porter R, Birch J. *Identification of Asthma*. Edinburgh: Churchill Livingstone, 1971.
5 Sanerkin NG. Terminology and classification of 'bronchial asthma' and 'chronic bronchitis': a reappraisal. *Ann Allergy* 1971; 29: 187.
6 Djukanovic R, Roche WR, Wilson JW *et al*. Mucosal inflammation in asthma. *Am Rev Respir Dis* 1990; 142: 434.
7 Jones RS, Buston MH, Wharton MJ. The effect of exercise on ventilatory function in the child with asthma. *Br J Dis Chest* 1962; 56: 78.
8 Williams SJ, Parrish RW, Seaton A. Comparison of intravenous aminophylline and salbutamol in acute severe asthma. *Br Med J* 1975; iv: 685.
9 Burr ML, St Leger AS, Bevan C, Merrett TG. A community survey of asthmatic characteristics. *Thorax* 1975; 30: 663.
10 Ramsdale EH, Roberts RS, Morris MM, Hargreave FE. Differences in responsiveness to histamine and metacholine in asthma and chronic bronchitis. *Thorax* 1985; 40: 422.
11 Daniels SA, Battacharrya S, James A *et al*. A genome-wide search for quantitative trait loci underlying asthma. *Nature* 1996; 383: 247.
12 Cookson W, Sharp PA, Faux JA, Hopkin JM. Linkage between immunoglobulin E responses underlying asthma and rhinitis and chromosome 11q. *Lancet* 1989; i: 1292.
13 Lympany P, Welsh KI, Cochrane GM,

Kemeny DM, Lee TH. Genetic analysis of the linkage between chromosome 11q and atopy. *Clin Exp Allergy* 1992; 22: 1085.
14 Amelung PJ, Panhuysen CIM, Postma DS *et al*. Atopy and bronchial hyperresponsiveness: exclusion of linkage to markers on chromosomes 11q and 6p. *Clin Exp Allergy* 1992; 22: 1077.
15 Falliers CJ, de Cardoso RR, Bane HN, Coffey R, Middleton E. Discordant allergic manifestations in monozygotic twins: genetic identity versus clinical, physiologic, and biochemical differences. *J Allergy* 1971; 47: 207.
16 Zamel N, Leroux M, Vanderdoelen JL. Airway response to inhaled methacholine in healthy nonsmoking twins. *J Appl Physiol* 1984; 56: 936.
17 von Mutius E. Progression of allergy and asthma through childhood to adolescence. *Thorax* 1996; 51 (Suppl 1): S3.
18 Kraepelien S. Prognosis of asthma in childhood with special reference to pulmonary function and the value of specific hyposensitization. *Acta Paediatr Scand* 1963; Suppl 140: 92.
19 Ogilvie AG. Asthma: a study of prognosis in 1000 patients. *Thorax* 1962; 17: 183.
20 Blair H. Natural history of wheezing in childhood. *J R Soc Med* 1979; 72: 42.
21 Park ES, Golding J, Carswell F, Stewart-Brown S. Pre-school wheezing and prognosis at 10. *Arch Dis Child* 1986; 61: 642.
22 Balfour-Lynn L. Childhood asthma and puberty. *Arch Dis Child* 1985; 60: 231–5.
23 Anderson HR, Bland JM, Patel S, Peckham C. The natural history of asthma in childhood. *J Epidemiol Community Health* 1986; 40: 121.
24 Strachan DP, Butland BK, Anderson HR.

Incidence and prognosis of asthma and wheezing illness from early childhood to age 33 in a national British cohort. *Br Med J* 1996; 312: 1195.
25 Godden DJ, Ross S, McMurray D *et al*. Outcome of wheeze in childhood: symptoms and pulmonary function 25 years later. *Am J Respir Crit Care Med* 1994; 149: 106.
26 Bodner C, Ross S, Douglas G, Little J *et al*. The prevalence of adult onset wheeze: longitudinal study. *Br Med J* 1997; 314: 792.
27 Peat JK, Salome CM, Sedgwick CS, Kerrebijn J, Woolcock AJ. A prospective study of bronchial hyperresponsiveness and respiratory symptoms in a population of Australian schoolchildren. *Clin Exp Allergy* 1989; 19: 299.
28 Hill DJ, Hosking CS, Shelton MJ, Turner MW. Growing out of asthma: clinical and immunological changes over 5 years. *Lancet* 1981; ii: 1359.
29 Redline S, Gold D. Challenges in interpreting gender differences in asthma. *Am J Respir Crit Care Med* 1994; 150: 1219.
30 Williams H, McNicol KN. Prevalence, natural history and relationship of wheezy bronchitis and asthma in children. An epidemiological study. *Br Med J* 1969; iv: 321.
31 McNicol KN, Williams H. Spectrum of asthma in children. 1. Clinical and physiological components. *Br Med J* 1973; iv: 7.
32 McNicol KN, Williams H. Asthma in children. 2. Allergic components. *Br Med J* 1973; iv: 12.
33 Martin AJ, McLennan LA, Landau LI, Phelan PD. The natural history of childhood asthma to adult life. *Br Med J* 1980; 280: 1397.
34 Martin AJ, Landau LI, Phelan PD. Lung function of young adults who had asthma in childhood. *Am Rev Respir Dis* 1980; 122: 609.

35 Kelly WJW, Hudson I, Phelan PD, Pain MCF, Olinski A. Childhood asthma in adult life: a further study at 28 years of age. *Br Med J* 1987; 294: 1059.

36 Seaton A, Godden DJ, Brown K. Increase in asthma: a more toxic environment or a more susceptible population? *Thorax* 1994; 49: 171.

37 Burr ML, Charles TJ, Roy K, Seaton A. Asthma in the elderly: an epidemiological survey. *Br Med J* 1979; i: 1041.

38 Rackemann FM. Intrinsic asthma. *J Allergy* 1940; 11: 147.

39 Kroegel C, Jäger L, Walker C. Is there a place for intrinsic asthma as a distinct immunopathological entity? *Eur Respir J* 1997; 10: 513.

40 Ulrik CS, Backer V, Dirksen A, Pedersen M, Koch C. Extrinsic and intrinsic asthma from childhood to adult age: a 10-yr follow-up. *Respir Med* 1995; 89: 547.

41 Speizer FE, Doll R, Heaf P. Observations on recent increase in mortality from asthma. *Br Med J* 1968; i: 335.

42 Jackson RT, Beaglehole R, Rea HH, Sutherland DC. Martality from asthma: a new epidemic in New Zealdn. *Br Med J* 1982; 285: 771.

43 Sears MR, Rea HH, Beaglehole R *et al.* Asthma mortality in New Zealand: a two year national study. *N Z Med J* 1985; 98: 271.

44 Frazer PM, Speizer FE, Waters SDM *et al.* The circumstances preceding death from asthma in young people in 1968–69. *Br J Dis Chest* 1971; 65: 71.

45 Macdonald JB, Macdonald ET, Seaton A, Williams DA. Asthma deaths in Cardiff 1963–74: 53 deaths in hospital. *Br Med J* 1976; i: 721.

46 Macdonald JB, Seaton A, Williams DA. Asthma deaths in Cardiff 1963–74: 90 deaths outside hospital. *Br Med J* 1976; i: 1493.

47 Ormerod LP, Stableforth DE. Asthma mortality in Birmingham 1975–77: 53 deaths. *Br Med J* 1980; 280: 687.

48 British Thoracic Association. Death from asthma in two regions of England. *Br Med J* 1982; 285: 1251.

49 Rea HH, Scragg R, Jackson R *et al.* A case-control study of deaths from asthma. *Thorax* 1986; 41: 833.

50 Eason J, Markowe HLJ. Controlled investigation of deaths from asthma in hospitals in the North East Thames region. *Br Med J* 1987; 294: 1255.

51 Crane J, Pearce N, Flatt A *et al.* Prescribed fenoterol and death from asthma in New Zealand, 1981–83: case-control study. *Lancet* 1989; i: 917.

52 Sly RM. Adverse effects and complications of treatment with beta-adrenergic agonist drugs. Position statement, the American Acadamy of Allergy and Immunology. *J Allergy Clin Immunol* 1985; 75: 443.

53 Collins JM, McDevitt DG, Shanks RG, Swanton JG. The cardiotoxicity of isoprenaline during hypoxia. *Br J Pharmacol* 1969; 36: 35.

54 Blauw GJ, Westendorp RGJ. Asthma deaths in New Zealand: whodunnit? *Lancet* 1995; 345: 2.

55 Anderson HR. Epidemiology of asthma. *Br J Hosp Med* 1992; 47: 99.

56 Woolcock AJ, Peat JK. Definition, classification, epidemiology and risk factors for asthma. In: O'Byrne P, Thomson NC, eds. *Manual of Asthma Management.* London: WB Saunders, 1995.

57 Dunnill MS, Massarella GR, Anderson JA. A comparison of the quantitative anatomy of the bronchi in normal subjects, in status asthmaticus, in chronic bronchitis, and in emphysema. *Thorax* 1969; 24: 176.

58 Gough J. Correlation of radiological and pathological changes in some diseases of the lung. *Lancet* 1955; i: 161.

59 Thurlbeck WM, Henderson JA, Fraser RG, Bates DV. Chronic obstructive lung disease. A comparison between clinical, roentgenologic, functional and morphologic criteria in chronic bronchitis, emphysema, asthma and bronchietasis. *Medicine* 1970; 49: 81.

60 Dunnill MS. *Pulmonary Pathology.* Edinburgh: Churchill Livingstone, 1982: Chapter 6.

61 Messer JW, Peters GA, Bennett WA. Cause of death and pathological findings in 304 cases of bronchial asthma. *Dis Chest* 1960; 38: 616.

62 Sobonya RE. Quantitative structural alterations in long-standing allergic asthma. *Am Rev Respir Dis* 1984; 130: 289.

63 Workshop summary and guidelines. Investigative use of bronchoscopy, lavage and bronchial biopsies in asthma and other airway diseases. *J Allergy Clin Immunol* 1991; 88: 808.

64 Djukanovic R, Wilson JW, Lai CKW, Holgate ST, Howarth PH. The safety aspects of fibreoptic bronchoscopy, bronchoalveolar lavage and endobronchial biopsy in asthma. *Am Rev Respir Dis* 1991; 143: 772.

65 Glynn AA, Michaels L. Bronchial biopsy in chronic bronchitis and asthma. *Thorax* 1960; 15: 142.

66 Salvato G. Some histological studies in chronic bronchitis and asthma. *Thorax* 1968; 23: 168.

67 Lundgren R. Scanning electron microscopic studies of bronchial mucosa before and during treatment with beclomethasone dipropionate inhalations. *Scand J Respir Dis* 1977; Suppl 101: 179.

68 Laitinen LA, Heino M, Laitinen A, Kava T, Haahtela T. Damage of the airway epithelium and bronchial reactivity in patients with asthma. *Am Rev Respir Dis* 1985; 131: 599.

69 Naylor B. The shedding of mucosa of the bronchial tree in asthma. *Thorax* 1962; 17: 69.

70 Jeffery PK. Bronchial biopsies and airway inflammation. *Eur Respir J* 1996; 9: 1583.

71 Beasley R, Roche W, Roberts JA, Holgate ST. Cellular events in the bronchi in mild asthma and after bronchial provocation. *Am Rev Respir Dis* 1989; 139: 806.

72 Jeffery PK, Wardlaw A, Nelson FC, Collins JV, Kay AB. Bronchial biopsies in asthma: an ultrastructural quantification study and correlation with hyperreactivity. *Am Rev Respir Dis* 1989; 140: 1745.

73 Laitinen LA, Laitinen A, Haahtela T. Airway mucosal inflammation even in patients with newly diagnosed asthma. *Am Rev Respir Dis* 1993; 147: 697.

74 Jackson B. *Early Intervention in Asthma. The Role of Inhaled Steroid Therapy.* Clinical Vision Ltd, Harwell UK, 1994.

75 Roche WR, Beasley R, Williams JH, Holgate ST. Sub-epithelial fibrosis in the bronchi of asthmatics. *Lancet* 1989; i: 520.

76 Ollerenshaw SL, Woolcock AJ. Characteristics of the inflammation in biopsies from large airways of subjects with asthma and

subjects with chronic airflow limitation. *Am Rev Respir Dis* 1992; 145: 922.

77 O'Shaughnessy TC, Ansari TW, Barnes NC, Jeffery PK. Reticular basement membrane thickness in moderately severe asthma and smokers' chronic bronchitis with and without airflow obstruction. *Am J Respir Crit Care Med* 1996; 153: A879.

78 Brewster CEP, Howarth PH, Djukanovic R *et al.* Myofibroblasts and subepithelial fibrosis in bronchial asthma. *Am J Respir Cell Mol Biol* 1990; 3: 507.

79 Azzawi M, Bradley B, Jeffery PK *et al.* Identification of activated T-lymphocytes and eosinophils in bronchial biopsies in stable atopic asthma. *Am Rev Respir Dis* 1990; 142: 1407.

80 Bradley BL, Azzawi M, Jacobson M *et al.* Eosinophils, T-lymphocytes, mast cells, neutrophils and macrophages in bronchial biopsies from atopic asthmatics: comparison with with atopic non asthma and relationship to bronchial hyperresponsiveness. *J Allergy Clin Immunol* 1991; 88: 661.

81 Hamid Q, Azzawi M, Ying S *et al.* IL-5 mRNA in bronchial biopsies from asthmatic patients. *J Clin Invest* 1991; 87: 1541.

82 Robinson DS, Tsicopoulos A, Meng Q *et al.* Increased interleukin-10 messenger RNA expression in atopic allergy and asthma. *Am J Respir Cell Mol Biol* 1996; 14: 113.

83 Robinson DS, Durham SR, Kay AB. Cytokines. 3. Cytokines in asthma. *Thorax* 1992; 48: 845.

84 Bentley AM, Menz G, Stortz C *et al.* Identification of T-lymphocytes, macrophages and activated eosinophils in the bronchial mucosa in intrinsic asthma: relationship to symptoms and bronchial responsiveness. *Am Rev Respir Dis* 1992; 146: 500.

85 Bentley AM, Maesrelli P, Saetta M *et al.* Activated T-lymphocytes and eosinophils in the bronchial mucosa in isocyanate-induced asthma. *J Allergy Clin Immunol* 1992; 89: 821.

86 Boulet L-P, Boutet M, Laviolette M *et al.* Airway inflammation after removal from the causal agent in occupational asthma due to high and low molecular weight agents. *Eur Respir J* 1994; 7: 1567.

87 Ackerman V, Marini M, Vittori E *et al.* Detection of cytokines and their cell sources in bronchial biopsy specimens from asthmatic patients; relationship to atopic status, symptoms and level of airway hyperresponsiveness. *Chest* 1994; 105: 687.

88 Aalbers R, De Monchi JGR, Kauffman HK *et al.* Dynamics of eosinophil infiltration in the bronchial mucosa before and after the late phase reaction. *Eur Respir J* 1993; 6: 840.

89 Durham SR, Ying S, Varney V *et al.* Cytokine mRNA expression for IL-3, IL-4 and GM-CSF on nasal mucosa after local allergen provocation: relation to tissue eosinophilia. *J Immunol* 1992; 148: 2390.

90 Djukanovic F, Feather I, Gratziou C *et al.* Effect of natural allergen exposure during the grass pollen season on airways inflammatory cells and asthma symptoms. *Thorax* 1996; 51: 575.

91 Montefort S, Holgate ST, Howarth PH. Leucocyte endothelial adhesion molecules and their role in bronchial asthma and allergic rhinitis. *Eur Respir J* 1993; 6: 1044.

92 Montefort S, Gratziou C, Goulding R *et al.* Bronchial biopsy evidence for leukocyte infiltration and upregulation of leukocyte–endothelial cell adhesion mole-

cules 6 hours after local allergen challenge of sensitised asthmatic airways. *J Clin Invest* 1994; 93: 1411.

93 Bentley AM, Durham SR, Robinson DS *et al*. Expression of endothelial and leukocyte intercellular adhesion molecule-1, E-selectin and vascular cell adhesion molecule-1, in the bronchial mucosa in steady-state and allergen-induced asthma. *J Allergy Clin Immunol* 1993; 92: 857.

94 Gizycki MJ, Adelroth E, Rogers AV, O'Byrne PM, Jeffery PK. Myofibroblast involvement during the late phase reaction in the airways of mild atopic asthma. *Am J Respir Crit Care Med* 1996; 153: A250.

95 Redington AE, Howarth PH. Airway wall remodelling in asthma. *Thorax* 1997; 52: 310.

96 Fabbri LM, Boschetto P, Zocca E *et al*. Bronchoalveolar neutrophilia during late asthmatic reactions induced by toluene diisocyanate. *Am Rev Respir Dis* 1987; 136: 36.

97 Saetta M, Di Stefano A, Maestrelli P *et al*. Airway mucosal inflammation in occupational asthma induced by toluene diisocyanate. *Am Rev Respir Dis* 1992; 145: 160.

98 Laitinen LA, Laitinen A, Haahtela T. A comparative study of the effects of an inhaled corticosteroid, budesonide, and a beta$_2$-agonist, terbutaline, on airway inflammation in newly diagnosed asthma. *J Allergy Clin Immunol* 1992; 90: 32.

99 Djukanovic R, Wilson JW, Britten KM *et al*. Effect of an inhaled corticosteroid on airway inflammation and symptoms in asthma. *Am Rev Respir Dis* 1992; 145: 669.

100 Trigg CJ, Manolitas ND, Wang J *et al*. Placebo-controlled immunopathologic study of four months of inhaled corticosteroids in asthma. *Am J Respir Crit Care Med* 1994; 150: 17.

101 Hoshino M, Nakamura Y. Anti-inflammatory effects of inhaled beclomethasone dipropionate in nonatopic asthmatics. *Eur Respir J* 1996; 9: 696.

102 Finnerty JP, Lee C, Wilson S *et al*. Effects of theophylline on inflammatory cells and cytokines in asthmatic subjects: a placebo-controlled parallel group study. *Eur Respir J* 1996; 9: 1672.

103 Saetta M, Turato G, Cresci C *et al*. Inflammation of the central airways reflects that of the peripheral airways in smokers. *Am J Respir Crit Care Med* 1996; 153: A709.

104 Richmond I, Booth H, Ward C, Walters EH. Intrasubject variability in the airway inflammation in biopsies in mild-to-moderate stable asthma. *Am J Respir Crit Care Med* 1996; 53: 899.

105 Pavord ID, Pizzichini MMM, Pizzichini E, Hargreave FE. The use of induced sputum to investigate airway inflammation. *Thorax* 1997; 52: 498.

106 Brogan TD, Ryley HC, Neale L, Yassa J. Soluble proteins of bronchopulmonary secretions from patients with cystic fibrosis, asthma and bronchitis. *Thorax* 1975; 30: 72.

107 Kay AB. The sputum in bronchial asthma. In: Clark TJH, Godfrey S, eds. *Asthma*, 2nd edn. London: Chapman & Hall, 1983: Chapter 5.

108 Fahy JV, Liu J, Wong X, Boushey HA. Cellular and biochemical analysis of induced sputum from asthmatic and healthy individuals. *Am Rev Respir Dis* 1993; 147: 1126.

109 Popov T, Gottschalk R, Kolendowicz R, Dolovich J, Powers P, Hargreave FE. The evaluation of a cell dispersion method of sputum examination. *Clin Exp Allergy* 1994; 24: 778.

110 Chodosh S, Zaccheo CV, Segal MS. The cytology and histochemistry of sputum cells. *Am Rev Respir Dis* 1962; 85: 635.

111 Pizzichini E, Pizzichini MMM, Efthimiadis A, Hargreave FE, Dolovich J. Measurement of inflammatory indices in induced sputum: effects of selection of sputum to minimize salivary contamination. *Eur Respir J* 1996; 9: 1174.

112 Pin I, Gibson PG, Kolendovicz R *et al*. Use of induced sputum cell counts to investigate airway inflammation in asthma. *Thorax* 1992; 47: 25.

113 Frigas E, Gleich GJ. The eosinophil and the pathophysiology of asthma. *J Allergy Clin Immunol* 1986; 77: 527.

114 Gibson PG, Wong BJ, Hepperle MJ *et al*. A research method to induce and examine a mild exacerbation of asthma by withdrawal of inhaled corticosteroid. *Clin Exp Allergy* 1992; 22: 525.

115 Walker C, Rihs S, Braun RK, Betz S, Bruijnzeal PL. Increased expression of CD11b and functional changes in eosinophils after migration across endothelial monolayers. *J Immunol* 1993; 150: 4061.

116 Hassall TT, Braunstein JB, Walker C *et al*. Sputum eosinophils from asthmatics express ICAM-1 and HLA-DR. *Clin Exp Immunol* 1991; 86: 271.

117 Gibson PG, Girgis-Gabardo A, Morris AM *et al*. Cellular characteristics of sputum from patients with asthma and chronic bronchitis. *Thorax* 1989; 44: 693.

118 Baigelman W, Chodosh S, Pizzuto D, Cupples LA. Sputum and blood eosinophils during corticosteroid treatment of acute exacerbations of asthma. *Am J Med* 1983; 75: 929.

119 Virchow JG, Holscher U, Virchow C. Sputum ECP levels correlate with parameters of airflow obstruction. *Am Rev Respir Dis* 1992; 146: 604.

120 Pin I, Freitag AP, O'Byrne PM *et al*. Changes in the cellular profile of induced sputum after allergen-induced asthmatic responses. *Am Rev Respir Dis* 1992; 145: 1265.

121 Brown HM. Corticosteroids in asthma. *Lancet* 1958; ii: 1245.

122 Gibson PG, Dolovich J, Denburg J, Ramsdale EH, Hargreave FE. Chronic cough: eosinophilic bronchitis without asthma. *Lancet* 1989; i: 1346.

123 Kirby PG, Hargreave FE, Gleich GJ, O'Byrne PM. Bronchoalveolar cell profiles of asthmatics and non-asthmatic subjects. *Am Rev Respir Dis* 1987; 136: 379.

124 Gibson PG, Allen CJ, Yang JP *et al*. Intraepithelial mast cells in allergic and non-allergic asthma. *Am Rev Respir Dis* 1993; 148: 80.

125 Smith DL, Deshazo RD. Bronchoalveolar lavage in asthma. *Am Rev Respir Dis* 1993; 148: 523.

126 Schmekel B, Blom-Bulow B, Hornblad Y *et al*. Granulocytes and their secretory products, myeloperoxidase and eosinophilic cationic protein, in bronchoalveolar lavage fluids from two lung lobes in normal subjects. *Eur Respir J* 1991; 4: 867.

127 Bousquet J, Chanez P, Lacoste JY. Eosinophilic inflammation in asthma. *N Engl J Med* 1990; 323: 1033.

128 Wenzel SE, Fowler A, Schwartz LB. Activation of pulmonary mast cells by bronchoalveolar allergen challenge. *In vivo* release of histamine and tryptase in atopic subjects with and without asthma. *Am Rev Respir Dis* 1986; 137: 1002.

129 Robinson D, Hamid Q, Ying S *et al*. Prednisolone treatment in asthma is associated with modulation of bronchoalveolar lavage cell interleukin-4, interleukin-5 and interferon-gamma cytokine gene expression. *Am Rev Respir Dis* 1993; 148: 401.

130 Gibson P, Saltos N. In: O'Byrne P, Thomson NC, eds. *Manual of Asthma Management*. London: WB Saunders, 1995.

131 Keatings VM, Evans DJ, O'Connor BJ, Barnes PJ. Cellular profiles in asthmatic airways: a comparison of induced sputum, bronchial washings, and bronchoalveolar lavage fluid. *Thorax* 1997; 52: 372.

132 Dunnill MS. The pathology of asthma with special reference to changes in the bronchial mucosa. *J Clin Pathol* 1960; 13: 27.

133 Sanerkin NG. Causes and consequences of airways obstruction in bronchial asthma. *Ann Allergy* 1970; 28: 528.

134 Sakula A. Charcot–Leyden crystals and Curschmann spirals in asthmatic sputum. *Thorax* 1986; 41: 503.

135 Hartley JPR. Exercise-induced asthma. *Thorax* 1979; 34: 571.

136 Anderson SD. Recent advances in the understanding of exercise-induced asthma. *Eur J Respir Dis* 1983; 64 (Suppl 128): 225.

137 Strauss RH, McFadden ER, Ingram RH *et al*. Influence of heat and humidity on the airway obstruction induced by exercise in asthma. *J Clin Invest* 1978; 61: 433.

138 Lee TH, Assoufi BK, Kay AB. The link between exercise, respiratory heat exchange, and the mast cell in bronchial asthma. *Lancet* 1983; i: 520.

139 Lee TH, Nagakura T, Papageorgiou N *et al*. Exercise-induced late asthmatic reactions with neutrophil chemotactic activity. *N Engl J Med* 1983; 308: 1502.

140 Bierman CW, Spiro SG, Petheram I. Characterization of the late response in exercise-induced asthma. *J Allergy Clin Immunol* 1985; 74: 701.

141 Godfrey S, Silverman M, Anderson SD. Problems of interpreting exercise-induced asthma. *J Allergy Clin Immunol* 1973; 52: 109.

142 Hartley JPR, Charles TJ, Money RDH *et al*. Arterial plasma histamine after exercise in normal individuals and in patients with exercise-induced asthma. *Clin Sci* 1981; 61: 151.

143 Barnes PJ, Brown MJ. Venous plasma histamine in exercise and hyperventilation-induced asthma in man. *Clin Sci* 1981; 61: 159.

144 Anderson SD, Bye PTP, Schoeffel RE *et al*. Arterial plasma histamine levels at rest, during and after exercise in patients with asthma: effects of terbutaline aerosol. *Thorax* 1981; 36: 259.

145 Lee TH, Nagy L, Nakagura T *et al*. Identification and partial characterization of an exercise-induced neutrophil chemotactic factor in bronchial asthma. *J Clin Invest* 1982; 69: 889.

146 Hartley JPR, Nograd SG. Effect of an inhaled antihistamine on exercise-induced asthma. *Thorax* 1980; 35: 675.

147 Godfrey S, Konig P. Inhibition of exercise-induced asthma by different pharmacological pathways. *Thorax* 1976; 31: 137.

148 Davies SE. Effect of disodium cromoglycate on exercise-induced asthma. *Br Med J* 1968; iii: 593.

149 Hartley JPR, Davies BH. Cholinergic blockade in the prevention of exercise-induced asthma *Thorax* 1980; 35: 680.

150 Hartley JPR, Davies CJ. Plasma cyclic nucleotides in exercise-induced asthma. *Thorax* 1978; 33: 668.

151 Barnes PJ, Brown MJ, Silverman M, Dollery CT. Circulating catecholamines in exercise and hyperventilation induced asthma. *Thorax* 1981; 36: 435.

152 Hartley JPR. *Studies of exercise-induced asthma in adults*. DM thesis, University of Oxford, 1982.

153 Cockcroft DW. Mechanism of perennial allergic asthma. *Lancet* 1983; ii: 253.

154 Pepys J, Hargreave FE, Chan M, McCarthy DS. Inhibitory effects of disodium cromoglycate on allergen inhalation tests. *Lancet* 1968; ii: 134.

155 Pepys J, Hutchcroft BJ. Bronchial provocation tests in etiologic diagnosis and analysis of asthma. *Am Rev Respir Dis* 1978; 112: 829.

156 Booij-Noord H, Orie NGM, de Vries K. Immediate and late bronchial obstruction reactions to inhalation of house dust and protective effects of disodium cromoglycate and prednisolone. *J Allergy Clin Immunol* 1971; 48: 344.

157 Wasserman SI. Mediators of immediate hypersensitivity. *J Allergy Clin Immunol* 1983; 72: 101.

158 Durham SR, Lee TH, Cromwell O *et al.* Immunologic studies in allergen-induced late phase asthmatic reactions. *J Allergy Clin Immunol* 1984; 74: 49.

159 Kayzer N, Kaufmann HF, Monchy JGR *et al.* Urinary *N*-methyl histamine during early and late allergen-induced bronchial-obstructive reactions. *J Allergy Clin Immunol* 1984; 74: 240.

160 De Monchy JGR, Kaufmann HF, Venge P *et al.* Bronchoalveolar lavage and the late asthmatic reaction. In: Kay AB, ed. *Asthma: Clinical Pharmacology and Therapeutic Progress.* Oxford: Blackwell Scientific Publications, 1986: Chapter 5.

161 Nogrady SG, Bevan C. Inhaled antihistamines: bronchodilatation and effects on histamine and metacholine-induced bronchoconstriction. *Thorax* 1978; 33: 700.

162 Nogrady SG, Bevan C. H_2 receptor blockage and bronchial hyperreactivity to histamine in asthma. *Thorax* 1981; 36: 268.

163 Mortagy AK, Howell JBL, Waters WE. Respiratory symptoms and bronchial reactivity: identification of a syndrome and its relation to asthma. *Br Med J* 1986; 293: 525.

164 Scadding JG. Asthma and bronchial reactivity. *Br Med J* 1987; 294: 1115.

165 Platts-Mills TAE, Tovey ER, Mitchell EB *et al.* Reduction of bronchial hyperreactivity during prolonged allergen avoidance. *Lancet* 1982; ii: 675.

166 Juniper EF, Frith PA, Dunnett C *et al.* Reproducibility and comparison of responses to inhaled histamine and metacholine. *Thorax* 1978; 33: 705.

167 Smith LJ, Greenberger PA, Patterson R *et al.* The effect of inhaled leukotriene D_4 in humans. *Am Rev Respir Dis* 1985; 131: 368.

168 Barnes NC, Piper PJ, Costello JF. Comparative effects of inhaled leukotriene C_4, leukotriene D_4, and histamine in normal subjects. *Thorax* 1984; 39: 500.

169 Bisgaard H, Groth S, Madsen F, Taudorf E. Hyperreactive airway response to LTD_4 in exogenous asthmatics compared to non-atopics. *Prostaglandins* 1984; 28: 635.

170 Hardy CC, Robinson C, Tattersfield AE, Holgate ST. The bronchoconstrictor effect of inhaled prostaglandin D_2 in normal and asthmatic man. *N Engl J Med* 1984; 311: 209.

171 Thomson NC, Roberts R, Bandouvakis J *et al.* Comparison of bronchial response to prostaglandin $F_{2\alpha}$ and metacholine. *J Allergy Clin Immunol* 1981; 68: 392.

172 Prausnitz C, Kustner H. Studien uber die Ueberempfindlichkeit. *Zentralbl Bakteriol* 1921; 86: 160.

173 Ishizaka K, Ishizaka T, Hornbrook MM. Physicochemical properties of human reaginic antibody. *J Immunol* 1966; 97: 75.

174 Johansson SGO, Bennich HH. Advances in the biology of IgE. In: Weiss EB, Segal MS, Stein M, eds. *Bronchial Asthma: Mechanisms and Therapeutics*, 2nd edn. Boston: Little, Brown, 1985: Chapter 9.

175 Ishizaka T. Analysis of triggering events in mast cells for immunoglobulin E-mediated release. *J Allergy Clin Immunol* 1981; 67: 90.

176 Kay AB, Austen KF. The IgE-mediated release of an eosinophil leukocyte chemotactic factor from human lung. *J Immunol* 1971; !07: 899.

177 Irvine RF. How is the level of free arachidonic acid controlled in mammalian cells? *Biochem J* 1982; 204: 3.

178 Knauer KA, Lichtenstein LM, Adkinson NF, Fish JE. Platelet activation during antigen-induced airway reactions in asthmatic subjects. *N Engl J Med* 1981; 304: 1404.

179 Benveniste J, Henson PM, Cochrane CG. Leukocyte-dependent histamine release from rabbit platelets: the role of IgE, basophils and a platelet activating factor. *J Exp Med* 1972; 136: 1356.

180 Benveniste J, Chignard M, Le Couedic JP, Vargaftig BB. Biosynthesis of platelet activating factor (PAF-acether). II. Involvement of phospholipase A2 in the formation of PAF-acether and lyso-PAF-acether from rabbit platelets. *Thromb Res* 1982; 25: 375.

181 Melewicz FM, Plummer JM, Spiegelburg HL. Comparison of the Fc receptors for IgE on human lymphocytes and monocytes. *J Immunol* 1982; 129: 563.

182 Rouzer CA, Scott WA, Hamill AL, Cohn ZA. Dynamics of leukotriene C production by macrophages. *J Exp Med* 1980; 152: 1236.

183 Dessein AJ, Parker WL, James SL, David JR. IgE antibody and resistance to infection. *J Exp Med* 1981; 153: 423.

184 Gleich GJ, Frigas E, Loegering DA *et al.* Cytotoxic properties of the eosinophil major basic protein. *J Immunol* 1979; 123: 2925.

185 Spiegelburg HL, Simon RA. Increases of lymphocytes with Fc receptors for IgE in patients with allergic rhinitis during the grass pollen season. *J Clin Invest* 1981; 68: 845.

186 Holgate S. Mediators and cytokine mechanisms in asthma. *Thorax* 1993; 48: 103.

187 Holgate ST. The cellular and mediator basis of asthma in relation to natural history. *Lancet* 1997; 350 (Suppl 2): 5.

188 Holt PG, Sly PD. Allergic respiratory disease: strategic targets for primary prevention during childhood. *Thorax* 1997; 52: 1.

189 Semper AE, Hartley JA. Dendritic cells in the lung: what is their relevance to asthma? *Clin Exp Allergy* 1996; 26: 485.

190 Charles J, Williams SJ, Seaton A *et al.* Histamine, basophils and eosinophils in severe asthma. *Clin Sci* 1979; 57: 39.

191 Bruce C, Weatherstone R, Seaton A, Taylor WH. Histamine levels in plasma, blood and urine in severe asthma, and the effect of corticosteroid treatment. *Thorax* 1976; 31: 724.

192 Goetzl EJ, Austen KF. Purification and synthesis of eosinophilotactic tetrapeptides of human lung tissue: identification as eosinophil chemotactic factor of anaphylaxis. *Proc Natl Acad Sci USA* 1975; 72: 4123.

193 Lewis RA, Austen KF. Mediation of local homeostasis and inflammation by leukotrienes and other mast cell dependent compounds. *Nature* 1981; 293: 103.

194 Nagy L, Lee TH, Kay AB. Neutrophil chemotactic activity in antigen-induced late asthmatic reactions. *N Engl J Med* 1982; 306: 497.

195 Lewis RA, Soter NA, Diamond P *et al.* Prostaglandin D_2 generation after activation of rat and human mast cells with anti-IgE. *J Immunol* 1982; 129: 1627.

196 Hardy CC, Robinson C, Tattersfield AE, Holgate ST. The bronchoconstrictor effect of inhaled prostaglandin D_2 in normal and asthmatic men. *N Engl J Med* 1984; 311: 209.

197 Hardy CC, Robinson C, Bradding P, Holgate ST. Prostacyclin: a functional antagonist of prostaglandin D_2-induced bronchoconstriction. *Thorax* 1984; 39: 696.

198 Smith AP, Cuthbert MF, Dunlop LS. Effects of inhaled prostaglandins E_1, E_2, and $F_{2\alpha}$ on the airway resistance of healthy and asthmatic man. *Clin Sci Mol Med* 1975; 48: 421.

199 Lee TH. Biological properties of lipoxygenase products: an overview. In: Kay AB, ed. *Asthma: Clinical Pharmacology and Therapeutic Progress.* Oxford: Blackwell Scientific Publications, 1986: Chapter 15.

200 O'DrisColl BRC, Kay AB. Leukotrienes and lung disease. *Thorax* 1982; 37: 241.

201 Barnes NC, Costello JF. Leukotrienes and asthma. In: Kay AB, ed. *Asthma: Clinical Pharmacology and Therapeutic Progress.* Oxford: Blackwell Scientific Publications, 1986: Chapter 16.

202 Zakrzewski JT, Barnes NC, Piper PJ, Costello JF. Measurement of leukotrienes in arterial and venous blood from normal and asthmatic subjects by radioimmunossay. *Br J Clin Pharmacol* 1985; 19: 574.

203 Mencia-Huerta JM, Benhamon M. PAF-acether (platelet activating factor): an update. In: Kay AB, ed. *Asthma: Clinical Pharmacology and Therapeutic Progress.* Oxford: Blackwell Scientific Publications, 1986: Chapter 20.

204 Basran GS, Morley J, Page CP, Paul W. Platelet activating factor: a potential mediator of acute and chronic asthma. *Am Rev Respir Dis* 1982; 125 (Suppl): 52.

205 Basran GS, Morley J, Paul W, Turner-Warwick M. Evidence in man of synergistic interaction between putative mediators of acute inflammation and asthma. *Lancet* 1982; i: 935.

206 Michel B, Russell T, Winkelman RK, Gleitch GJ. Release of kinins during wheal and flare allergic reactions. *J Clin Invest* 1968; 47: 68a.

207 Barnes PJ. Asthma as an axon reflex. *Lancet* 1986; i: 242.

208 Fuller RW, Dixon CMS, Dollery CT, Barnes PJ. Bradykinin induced bronchoconstriction in man. *Clin Sci* 1985; 68: 35P.

209 Nadel JA, Barnes PJ. Autonomic regulation of the airways. *Annu Rev Med* 1984; 35: 451.

210 Widdicombe JG. Regulation of tracheo-bronchial smooth muscle. *Physiol Rev* 1963; 43: 1.

211 Roberts AM, Kaufman MP, Baker DG *et al.* Reflex tracheal contraction induced by stimulation of bronchial C-fibers in dogs. *J Appl Physiol* 1981; 51: 485.

212 Nadel JA, Davis B, Phipps RJ. Control of mucus secretion and ion transport in airways. *Annu Rev Physiol* 1979; 41: 369.

213 Nadel JA. Autonomic regulation of airway smooth muscle. In: Nadel JA, ed. *Physiology and Pharmacology of the Airways.* New York: Marcel Dekker, 1980.

214 Laitinen LA. Histamine and metacholine challenge in the testing of bronchial reactivity. *Scand J Respir Dis* 1974; Suppl 86: 1.

215 Chamberlain DA, Muir DCF, Kennedy KP. Atropine methonitrate and isoprenaline in bronchial asthma. *Lancet* 1962; ii: 1019.

216 Mann JS, George CF. Anticholinergic drugs in the management of airways disease. *Br J Dis Chest* 1985; 79: 209.

217 Fuller RW, Dixon CMS, Cuss F, Barnes PJ. Bradykinin induced bronchoconstriction in humans. *Am Rev Respir Dis* 1987; 135: 176.

218 Dekock MA, Nadel JA, Zwi S *et al.* New method for perfusing bronchial arteries: histamine bronchoconstriction and apnea. *J Appl Physiol* 1966; 21: 185.

219 White J, Eiser NM. The role of histamine and its receptors in the pathogenesis of asthma. *Br J Dis Chest* 1983; 77: 215.

220 Empey DW, Laitinen LA, Jacobs L *et al.* Mechanisms of bronchial hyperreactivity in normal subjects after upper respiratory tract infection. *Am Rev Respir Dis* 1976; 113: 131.

221 Szentivanyi A, Polson JB, Szentivanyi J. Adrenergic regulation. In: Weiss EB, Segal MS, Stein M, eds. *Bronchial Asthma: Mechanisms and Therapeutics*, 2nd edn. Boston: Little, Brown, 1985: Chapter 13.

222 Barnes PJ, Karliner JS, Dollery CT. Human lung adrenoceptors studied by radioligand binding. *Clin Sci* 1980; 58: 457.

223 Carstairs JR, Nimmo AJ, Barnes PJ. Autoradiographic localization of β-adrenoceptors in human lung. *Eur J Pharmacol* 1984; 103: 189.

224 Barnes PJ, Baraniuk JN, Belvisi MG. Neuropeptides in the respiratory tract. Part 1. *Am Rev Respir Dis* 1991; 144: 1187.

225 Barnes PJ, Baraniuk JN, Belvisi MG. Neuropeptides in the respiratory tract. Part 2. *Am Rev Respir Dis* 1991; 144: 1391.

226 Joos GF, Germonpre PR, Pauwels RA. Neurogenic inflammation in human airways: is it important? *Thorax* 1995; 50: 217.

227 Small JV, Sobieszek A. The contractile apparatus of smooth muscle. *Int Rev Cytol* 1980; 64: 241.

228 Adelstein RS, Pato MN, Conti MA. The role of phosphorylation in regulating contractile proteins. *Adv Cycl Nucleotide Res* 1981; 14: 361.

229 Bolton TB. Mechanisms of action of transmitters and other substances on smooth muscle. *Physiol Rev* 1979; 59: 606.

230 Rodger IW. Calcium ions and contraction of smooth muscle. In: Kay AB, ed. *Asthma: Clinical Pharmacology and Therapeutic Progress.* Oxford: Blackwell Scientific Publications, 1986: Chapter 10.

231 Vicenc KS, Black JL, Yam K *et al.* Comparison of *in vivo* and *in vitro* responses to histamine in human airways. *Am Rev Respir Dis* 1983; 128: 875.

232 Stephens NL. Airway smooth muscle. *Am Rev Respir Dis* 1987; 135: 960.

233 Van Arsdel PP, Motulski AG. Frequency of asthma and allergic rhinitis in college students. *Acta Genet Statis Med* 1959; 9: 104.

234 Edfors-Lubs ML. Allergy in 7000 twin pairs. *Acta Allergol* 1971; 26: 249.

235 Marsh DG, Meyers DA, Bias WB. The epidemiology and genetics of atopic allergy. *N Engl J Med* 1981; 305: 1551.

236 Sibbald B, Turner-Warwick M. Factors influencing the prevalence of asthma among first degree relatives of extrinsic and intrinsic asthmatics. *Thorax* 1979; 34: 332.

237 Sibbald B, Horn MEC, Gregg I. A family study of the genetic basis of asthma and wheezy bronchitis. *Arch Dis Child* 1980; 55: 354.

238 Wilkinson J, Holgate ST. Candidate gene loci in asthmatic and allergic inflammation. *Thorax* 1996; 51: 3.

239 Cookson WOCM, Hopkin JM. Dominant inheritance of atopic, immunoglobulin E responsiveness. *Lancet* 1988; i: 86.

240 Sandford AJ, Shirakawa T, Moffatt MF *et al.* Localisation of atopy and β subunit of high affinity IgE receptor (FcεR1) on chromosome 11q. *Lancet* 1993; 341: 332.

241 Shirakawa T, Li A, Dubowitz M *et al.* Association between atopy and variants of the β subunit of the high affinity Immunoglobulin E receptor. *Nature Genet* 1994; 7: 125.

242 Moffatt MF, Hill MR, Cornelis F *et al.* Genetic linkage of T cell receptor α/δ complex to specific IgE responses. *Lancet* 1994; 343: 1597.

243 Marsh DG, Neely JD, Breazeale DR *et al.* Linkage analysis of IL-4 and other chromosome 5q31.1 markers and total serum immunoglobulin E concentrations. *Science* 1994; 264: 1152.

244 Seaton A, Godden DG, Brown K. Increase in asthma: a more toxic environment or a more susceptible population? *Thorax* 1994; 19: 171.

245 Rao VRM, Dean B, Seaton A, Williams DA. A comparison of mite populations in mattress dust from hospital and from private houses in Cardiff, Wales. *Clin Allergy* 1975; 5: 209.

246 Seaton A, Soutar A, Mullins J. The increase in hay fever: pollen, particulate matter and SO_2 in ambient air. *Q J Med* 1996; 89: 279.

247 Black PN, Sharpe S. Dietary fat and asthma: is there a connection? *Eur Respir J* 1997; 10: 6.

248 Strachan DP. Hay fever, hygiene and household size. *Br Med J* 1989; 299: 1259.

249 Shaheen SO. Changing patterns of childhood infection and the rise in allergic disease. *Clin Exp Allergy* 1995; 25: 1034.

250 Tang MLK, Kemp AS, Thorburn J, Hill DJ. Reduced interferon-γ secretion in neonates and subsequent atopy. *Lancet* 1994; 344: 983.

251 Shaheen SO, Aaby P, Hall AJ *et al.* Measles and atopy in Guinea-Bissau. *Lancet* 1996; 347: 1792.

252 Shirakawa T, Enomoto T, Shimazu S-I, Hopkin JM. The inverse association between tuberculin responses and atopic disorder. *Science* 1997; 275: 77.

253 Matricardi PM, Rosmini F, Ferrigno L *et al.* Cross-sectional retrospective study of prevalence of atopy among Italian military students with antibodies to hepatitis A virus. *Br Med J* 1997; 314: 999.

254 Bodner C, Godden D, Seaton A. Family size, childhood infections and atopic disease. *Thorax* 1998; 53: 28.

255 Yemaneberhan H, Bekele Z, Venn A *et al.* Prevalence of wheeze and asthma and relation to atopy in urban and rural Ethiopia. *Lancet* 1997; 350: 85.

256 Hijazi N, Abalkhail B, Seaton A. Asthma and respiratory symptoms in urban and rural Saudi Arabia. *Eur Respir J* 1998; 12: 41.

257 Hodge L, Salome CM, Peat JK *et al.* Consumption of oily fish and childhood asthma risk. *Med J Aust* 1996; 64: 137.

258 Hendrick DJ, Davies RJ, D'Souza MF, Pepys J. An analysis of skin prick tests in 656 asthmatic patients. *Thorax* 1975; 30: 2.

259 McNichol KN, Williams HB. Spectrum of asthma in children. II. Allergic components. *Br Med J* 1973; iv: 12.

260 Ford RM. Aetiology of asthma: a review of 11,551 cases. *Med J Aust* 1969; i: 628.

261 Voorhorst R, Spieksma FIM, Varekamp H *et al.* The house dust mite (*Dermatophagoides pteronyssinus*) and the allergens it produces. Identity with the house dust allergen. *J Allergy* 1967; 39: 325.

262 Maunsell K, Wraith DG, Cunnington AM. Mites and house dust allergy in bronchial asthma. *Lancet* 1968; i: 1267.

263 McAllen MK, Assem ESK, Maunsell K. House dust mite asthma. Results of challenge tests on five criteria with *Dermatophagoides pteronyssinus*. *Br Med J* 1970; ii: 501.

264 Van Bronswijk JEMH, Sinha RN. Role of fungi in the survival of *Dermatophagoides* (Acarina: Pyroglyphidae) in house-dust environment. *Environ Entomol* 1973; 2: 142.

265 Sesay HR, Dobson RM. Studies on the mite fauna of house dust in Scotland, with special reference to that of bedding. *Acarologia* 1972; 14: 384.

266 Chapman MD, Platts-Mills TAE. Purification and characterization of the major allergen from *Dermatophagoides pteronyssinus*-antigen P1. *J Immunol* 1980; 125: 587.

267 Tovey ER, Chapman MD, Platts-Mills TAE. Mite faeces are a major source of house dust allergen. *Nature* 1981; 289: 592.

268 Tovey ER, Chapman MD, Wells CW, Platts-Mills TAE. The distribution of dust mite allergen in the houses of patients with asthma. *Am Rev Respir Dis* 1981; 124: 630.

269 Feather IH, Warner JA, Holgate ST, Thompson PJ, Stewart GA. Cohabiting with domestic mites. *Thorax* 1993; 48: 5.

270 Hyde HA. Atmospheric pollen grains and spores in relation to allergy I. *Clin Allergy* 1972; 2: 153.

271 Hyde HA. Atmospheric pollen grains and spores in relation to allergy II. *Clin Allergy* 1973; 3: 109.

272 Knox RB. Grass pollen, thunderstorms and asthma. *Clin Exp Allergy* 1993; 23: 354.

273 Suphioglu C, Singh MB, Taylor P *et al.* Mechanism of grass-pollen-induced asthma. *Lancet* 1992; 339: 569.

274 Weber RW. Cross reactivity among pollens. *Ann Allergy* 1981; 46: 208.

275 Hoehne JH, Reed CE. Where is the allergic reaction in ragweed asthma? *J Allergy Clin Immunol* 1971; 48: 36.

276 Busse WW, Reed CE, Hoehne JH. Where is the allergic reaction in ragweed asthma? II. Demonstration of ragweed antigen in particles smaller than pollen. *J Allergy Clin Immunol* 1972; 50: 289.

277 King TP, Norman PS. Isolation studies of allergens from ragweed pollen. *Biochem*, 1962; 1: 709.

278 Ellul-Micallef R, Al-Ali S. The spectrum of bronchial asthma in Kuwait. *Clin Allergy* 1984; 14: 509.

279 Soutar A, Harker C, Seaton A, Brooke M, Marr I. Oilseed rape and seasonal symptoms: epidemiological and environmental studies. *Thorax* 1994; 49: 352.

280 Seaton A, Soutar A. Oilseed rape and seasonal symptoms. *Clin Exp Allergy* 1994; 24: 1089.

281 Herxheimer H, Hyde HA, Williams DA. Allergic asthma caused by fungal spores. *Lancet* 1966; i: 572.

282 Herxheimer H, Hyde HA, Williams DA. Allergic asthma caused by basidiospores. *Lancet* 1969; ii: 131.

283 Bromley IMJ, Donaldson K. Binding of *Aspergillus fumigatus* spores to lung epithelial cells and basement membrane proteins: relevance to the asthmatic lung. *Thorax* 1996; 51: 1203.

284 Bateman ED. A new look at the natural history of *Aspergillus* hypersensitivity in asthmatics. *Respir Med* 1994; 88: 325.

285 Arruda LK, Platts-Mills TAE, Longbottom JL, El-Dahr Chapman MD. *Aspergillus fumigatus*: identification of 16, 18 and 45 kd antigens recognised by human IgG and IgE antibodies and murine monoclonal antibodies. *J Allergy Clin Immunol* 1992; 89: 1166.

286 Salvaggio J, Aukrust L. Mold-induced asthma. *J Allergy Clin Immunol* 1981; 68: 327.

287 Platt S, Martin C, Hunt S, Lewis C. Damp housing, mould growth, and symptomatic health state. *Br Med J* 1989; 298: 1673.

288 Dales R, Burnett R, Zwanenburg H. Respiratory health effects of home dampness and moulds among Canadian children. *Am J Epidemiol* 1991; 134: 196.

289 Brunekreef B. Damp housing and adult respiratory symptoms. *Allergy* 1992; 47: 498.

290 Williamson IJ, Martin CJ, McGill G, Monie RDH, Fennerty AG. Damp housing and asthma: a case-control study. *Thorax* 1997; 52: 229.

291 Topping MD, Scarisbrick DA, Luczynska CM *et al.* Clinical and immunological reactions to *Aspergillus niger* among workers in a biotechnology plant. *Br J Ind Med* 1985; 42: 312.

292 Kauffman HF, Tomee JFC, van der Werf TS, de Monchy JGR, Koeter GK. Review of fungus-induced asthmatic reactions. *Am J Respir Crit Care Med* 1995; 151: 2109.

293 Ohman JL, Kendall S, Lowell FC. IgE antibody to cat allergens. *J Allergy Clin Immunol* 1977; 60: 317.

294 Coren S. Allergic patients do not comply with doctors' advice to stop owning pets. *Br Med J* 1997; 314: 517.

295 Crompton GK. How I manage the difficult asthmatic. *Proc R Coll Physicians Edinb* 1997; 27: 194.

296 Munir AKM, Björkstén B, Einarsson R *et al.* Cat (*Fel d*1), dog (*Can f*1) and cockroach allergens in homes of asthmatic children from three climatic zones of Sweden. *Allergy* 1992; 49: 508.

297 Burge PS, Edge G, O'Brien IM *et al.* Occupational asthma in a research centre breeding locusts. *Clin Allergy* 1980; 10: 355.

298 Kang B, Vellody D, Homburger H, Yunginger JW. Cockroach cause of allergic asthma. *J Allergy Clin Immunol* 1979; 63: 80.

299 Figley KD. Mayfly (Ephemerida) sensitivity. *Allergy* 1940; 11: 376.

300 Gibbons HL, Dille JR, Cowley RG. Inhalant allergy to screw worm fly. *Arch Environ Health* 1965; 10: 424.

301 Kay AB, McLean CMU, Wilkinson AH, Gad EL, Rab MO. The prevalence of asthma and rhinitis in a Sudanese community seasonally exposed to a potent allergen, the green nimitti midge. *J Allergy Clin Immunol* 1983; 71: 345.

302 Lessof MH, Wraith DG, Merrett TG *et al.* Food allergy and intolerance in 100 patients, local and systemic effects. *Q J Med* 1980; 49: 259.

303 Aas K. The diagnosis of hypersensitivity to ingested food. *Clin Allergy* 1978; 8: 39.

304 Walker WA, Isselbacher KJ. Uptake of macromolecules by the intestine: possible role in clinical disorders. *Gastroenterology* 1974; 67: 531.

305 Breslin ABX, Hendrick DJ, Pepys J. Asthma and alcohol. *Clin Allergy* 1973; 3: 71.

306 Ayres J, Clark TJH. Alcohol in asthma and the bronchoconstrictor effect of chlorpropamide. *Br J Dis Chest* 1982; 76: 79.

307 Ayres J, Clark TJH. Contrasting effects of ethanol on airflow in asthma. *Br J Dis Chest* 1981; 75: 316.

308 Herxheimer H, Stresemann E. Ethanol and lung function in bronchial asthma. *Arch Int Pharmacodyn* 1963; 144: 310.

309 Taylor RFH, al-Jarad N, John LME *et al.* Betel-nut chewing and asthma. *Lancet* 1992; 339: 1134.

310 Burney PG. Asthma mortality: England and Wales. *J Allergy Clin Immunol* 1987; 80: 397.

311 Burney PGJ, Britton JR, Chinn S *et al.* Response to inhaled histamine and 24 hour sodium excretion. *Br Med J* 1986; 292: 1483.

312 Souhrada M, Souhrada JF. Immunologically induced alterations of airway smooth muscle cell membrane. *Science* 1984; 225: 723.

313 Demissie K, Ernst P, Donald KG, Joseph L. Usual dietary salt intake and asthma in children: a case-control study. *Thorax* 1996; 51: 59.

314 Lieberman D, Heimer D. Effect of dietary sodium on the severity of asthma in men. *Thorax* 1992; 47: 360.

315 Devereux G, Beach JR, Bromly C *et al.* Effect of dietary sodium on airways responsiveness and its importance in the epidemiology of asthma: an evaluation in three areas of northern England. *Thorax* 1995; 50: 941.

316 Medici TC, Schmid AZ, Häcki M, Vetter W. Are asthmatics salt-sensitive? A preliminary controlled study. *Chest* 1993; 104: 1138.

317 Carey OJ, Locke C, Cookson JB. Effect of alterations of dietary sodium on severity of asthma in men. *Thorax* 1993; 48: 714.

318 Pistelli R, Forastiere F, Corbo GM *et al.* Respiratory symptoms and bronchial responsiveness are related to dietary salt intake and urinary potassium excretion in male children. *Eur Respir J* 1993; 6: 517.

319 Demissie K, Ernst P. Is increased dietary salt intake a cause of increased airway respon-

320 Bodner C, Godden DJ, Little J, Ross S, Brown K, Seaton A. Antioxidant intake and adult-onset wheeze: a case-control study. *Eur Respir J* 1999; 13: 22.

321 Soutar A, Seaton A, Brown K. Bronchial reactivity and dietary antioxidants. *Thorax* 1997; 52: 166.

322 Settipane GA. Adverse reactions to aspirin and related drugs. *Arch Intern Med* 1981; 141: 328.

323 Johnston SL, Bardin PG, Holgate ST. Viral infections in acute exacerbations of asthma: epidemiology and mechanisms. *Eur Respir J* 1992; 5: 429s.

324 Burrows B, Knudsen RG, Lebowitz MD. The relationship of childhood respiratory illness to adult obstructive airway disease. *Am Rev Respir Dis* 1970; 115: 751.

325 Sly PD, Hibbert ME. Childhood asthma following hospitalisation with acute viral bronchiolitis in infancy. *Pediatr Pulmonol* 1989; 7: 153.

326 Murray M, Webb MSC, O'Callaghan C, Swarbrick AS, Milner AD. Respiratory status and allergy after bronchiolitis. *Arch Dis Child* 1992; 67: 482.

327 Frick DL, Gerrnan DF, Mills J. Development of allergy in children. 1. Association with virus infections. *J Allergy Clin Immunol* 1979; 63: 228.

328 Rooney JC, Williams HE. The relationship between proved viral bronchitis and subsequent wheezing. *J Pediatr* 1971; 79: 744.

329 Zach MS, Schnall RP, Landau LI. Upper and lower airway hyperreactivity in recurrent croup. *Am Rev Respir Dis* 1980; 121: 979.

330 Pattemore PK, Johnston SL, Bardin PG. Viruses as precipitants of asthma symptoms. 1. Epidemiology. *Clin Exp Allergy* 1992; 22: 325.

331 Burney PGJ. Epidemiology. *Br Med Bull* 1992; 48: 10.

332 Openshaw PJM, O'Donnell DR. Asthma and the common cold: can viruses imitate worms? *Thorax* 1994; 49: 101.

333 Hudgel DW, Langston LA, Selner JC, McIntosh K. Viral and bacterial infections in adults with chronic asthma. *Am Rev Respir Dis* 1979; 120: 393.

334 Minor TE, Dick EC, Baker JW *et al.* Rhinovirus and influenza type A infections as precipitants of asthma. *Am Rev Respir Dis* 1976; 113: 149.

335 Walsh JJ, Dietlein LF, Low FN *et al.* Tracheobronchial response in human influenza. *Arch Intern Med* 1961; 108: 376.

336 Little JW, Hall WJ, Douglas RG *et al.* Airway hyperreactivity and peripheral airway dysfunction in influenza A infection. *Am Rev Respir Dis* 1978; 118: 295.

337 Devalia JL, Rusznak C, Davies RJ. Air pollution in the 1990s: cause of increased respiratory disease? *Respir Med* 1994; 88: 241.

338 Walters S, Griffiths RK, Ayres J. Temporal association between hospital admissions for asthma in Birmingham and ambient levels of sulphur dioxide and smoke. *Thorax* 1994; 49: 133.

339 Higgins BG, Francis HC, Yates CJ *et al.* Effects of air pollution on symptoms and peak expiratory flow measurements in subjects with obstructive lung disease. *Thorax* 1995; 50: 149.

340 Bates DV, Sitzo R. The Ontario air pollution

siveness or a marker of an unhealthy life style? *Respir Med* 1994; 88: 79.

study: identification of the causal agent. *Environ Health Perspect* 1989; 79: 69.

341 Thurston GD, Ito K, Hayes CG, Bates DV, Lippmann M. Respiratory hospital admissions and summertime haze air pollution in Toronto, Ontario: consideration of role of acid aerosols. *Environ Res* 1994; 65: 271.

342 Buchdahl R, Parker A, Stebbings T, Babiker A. Association between air pollution and acute childhood wheezy episodes: prospective observational study. *Br Med J* 1996; 312: 661.

343 Scarlett JF, Abbott KJ, Peacock JL, Strachan DP, Anderson HR. Acute effects of summer air pollution on respiratory function in primary school children in southern England. *Thorax* 1996; 51: 1109.

344 Peters A, Dockery DW, Heinrich J, Wichmann HE. Short-term effects of particulate air pollution on respiratory morbidity in asthmatic children. *Eur Respir J* 1997; 10: 872.

345 Krishna MT, Chauhan AJ, Frew AJ. Air pollution and asthma: what is the association? *Clin Asthma Rev* 1997; 1: 7.

346 Committee of the Environmental and Occupational Health Assembly of the American Thoracic Society. State of the art: health effects of outdoor pollution. Part 1. *Am J Respir Crit Care Med* 1996; 153: 3.

347 Committee of the Environmental and Occupational Health Assembly of the American Thoracic Society. State of the art: health effects of outdoor air pollution. Part 2. *Am J Respir Crit Care Med* 1996; 153: 477.

348 Molfino NA, Wright SC, Katz I. Effect of low concentrations of ozone on inhaled allergen responses in asthmatic subjects. *Lancet* 1991; 338: 199.

349 Peden DB, Woodrow Setzer R, Devlin RB. Ozone exposure has both priming effect on allergen-induced responses and an intrinsic inflammatory action in the nasal airways of perennially allergic asthmatics. *Am J Respir Crit Care Med* 1995; 151: 1336.

350 Tunnicliffe WS, Burge PS, Ayres JG. Effect of domestic concentrations of nitrogen dioxide on airway responses to inhaled allergen in asthmatic patients. *Lancet* 1994; 344: 1733.

351 Rusznak C, Devalia JL, Davies RJ. Airway response of asthmatic subjects to inhaled allergen after exposure to pollutants. *Thorax* 1996; 51: 1105.

352 Osebold JW, Owens SL, Zee YC, Dotson WM, Labarre DD. Immunological alterations in the lungs of mice following ozone exposure: changes in immunological levels and antibody containing cells. *Arch Environ Health* 1979; 34: 258.

353 Dodge RR, Burrows B. The prevalence and incidence of asthma and asthma-like symptoms in a general population sample. *Am Rev Respir Dis* 1980; 122: 567.

354 Burney PGJ, Britton JR, Chinn S *et al.* Descriptive epidemiology of bronchial reactivity in an adult population: results from a community study. *Thorax* 1987; 42: 38.

355 Troisi RJ, Speizer FE, Rosner B, Trichopoulos D, Willet WC. Cigarette smoking and incidence of chronic bronchitis and asthma in women. *Chest* 1995; 108: 1557.

356 Ross S, Godden DJ, Abdalla M *et al.* Outcome of wheeze in childhood: the influence of atopy. *Eur Respir J* 1995; 8: 2081.

357 Weitzman MS, Gortmaker S, Walker DK, Sobol A. Maternal smoking and childhood

asthma. *Pediatrics* 1990; 85: 505.

358 Martinez FD, Cline M, Burrows B. Increased incidence of asthma in children of smoking mothers. *Pediatrics* 1992; 89: 21.

359 Infante-Rivard C. Childhood asthma and indoor environmental risk factors. *Am J Epidemiol* 1993; 137: 834.

360 Dekker C, Dales R, Bartlett S, Brunekreef B, Zwanenburg H. Childhood asthma and the indoor environment. *Chest* 1991; 100: 922.

361 Ehrlich R, Kattan M, Godbold J *et al.* Childhood asthma and passive smoking: urinary cotinine as a biomarker of exposure. *Am Rev Respir Dis* 1992; 145: 594.

362 Schmitzberger R, Rhomberg K, Buchele H *et al.* Effects of air pollution on the respiratory tract of children. *Pediatr Pulmonol* 1993; 15: 68.

363 McConnochie KM, Roghmann KJ. Wheezing at 8 and 13 years: changing importance of bronchiolitis and passive smoking. *Pediatr Pulmonol* 1989; 6: 138.

364 Sherman CB, Tosteson TD, Tager IB, Speizer FE, Weiss ST. Early childhood predictors of asthma. *Am J Epidemiol* 1990; 132: 83.

365 Cunningham J, O'Connor GT, Dockery DW, Speizer FE. Environmental tobacco smoke, wheezing and asthma in children in 24 communities. *Am J Respir Crit Care Med* 1996; 153: 218.

366 Rees L. Physical and emotional factors in bronchial asthma. *J Psychosom Res* 1956; 1: 98.

367 De Araujo G, Van Arsdel PP, Holmes TH, Dudley DL. Life change, coping ability and chronic intrinsic asthma. *J Psychosom Res* 1973; 17: 359.

368 Dekker E, Groen J. Reproducible psychogenic attacks of asthma. *J Psychosom Res* 1956; 1: 58.

369 Luparello TJ, Leist N, Lourie CH, Sweet P. The interaction of psychologic stimuli and pharmacologic agents on airway reactivity in asthmatic subjects. *Psychosom Med* 1970; 32: 509.

370 Mason AA, Black S. Allergic skin responses abolished under treatment of asthma and hay fever by hypnosis. *Lancet* 1958; i: 877.

371 McFadden ER, Luparello TJ, Lyons HA, Bleeker E. The mechanism of action of suggestion in the induction of acute asthma attacks. *Psychosom Med* 1969; 31: 134.

372 Babb RR, Notarangelo J, Smith VM. Wheezing: a clue to gastroesophageal reflux. *Am J Gastroenterol* 1970; 53: 230.

373 Overholt RH, Voorhees RJ. Esophageal reflux as a trigger in asthma. *Dis Chest* 1966; 49: 464.

374 Wilson NM, Charette L, Thomson AH, Silverman M. Gastro-oesophageal reflux and childhood asthma: the acid test. *Thorax* 1985; 40: 592.

375 Wilson NM, Chudry N, Silverman M. Role of the oesophagus in asthma induced by the ingestion of ice and acid. *Thorax* 1987; 42: 506.

376 Foglia RP, Fonkalsrud EW, Ament ME *et al.* Gastroesophageal fundoplication for the management of chronic pulmonary disease in children. *Am J Surg* 1980; 140: 72.

377 Goodall RJR, Earis JE, Cooper DN *et al.* Relationship between asthma and gastro-oesophageal reflux. *Thorax* 1981; 36: 116.

378 Tan WC, Martin RJ, Pandey R *et al.* Effects of spontaneous and simulated gastroesophageal reflux on sleeping asthmatics. *Am Rev Respir Dis* 1990; 141: 1394.

379 Irwin RS, Curley FJ, French CL. Difficult-to-control asthma. Contributing factors and outcome of a systematic management protocol. *Chest* 1993; 103: 1662.

380 Packe GE, Ayres JG. Asthma outbreak during a thunderstorm. *Lancet* 1985; ii: 199.

381 Bellomo R, Gigliotti P, Treloar A *et al.* Two consecutive thunderstorm associated epidemics of asthma in the city of Melbourne. *Med J Aust* 1992; 156: 834.

382 Davidson AC, Emberlin J, Cook AD, Venables KM. A major outbreak of asthma associated with a thunderstorm: experience of accident and emergency patients' characteristics. *Br Med J* 1996; 312: 601.

383 Newson R, Strachan D, Archibald E *et al.* Effect of thunderstorms and airborne grass pollen on the incidence of acute asthma in England, 1990–94. *Thorax* 1997; 52: 680.

384 Meredith S, Taylor V, McDonald J. Occupational respiratory disease in the United Kingdom 1989: a report to the British Thoracic Society and Society of Occupational Medicine by the SWORD project group. *Br J Ind Med* 1991; 48: 292.

385 Cartier A. Definition and diagnosis of occupational asthma. *Eur Respir J* 1994; 7: 153.

386 Newman Taylor AJ. Occupational asthma. *Thorax* 1980; 35: 241.

387 Chan-Yeung M, Malo J-L. Occupational asthma. *N Engl J Med* 1995; 333: 107.

388 Paggiaro PL, Vagaggini B, Boscci E *et al.* Prognosis of occupational asthma. *Eur Respir J* 1994; 7: 761.

389 Chan-Yeung M, Lam S, Koener S. Clinical features and natural history of occupational asthma due to western red cedar (*Thuja plicata*). *Am J Med* 1982; 72: 411.

390 Burge PS. Occupational asthma in electronic workers caused by colophony fumes: follow-up of affected workers. *Thorax* 1982; 37: 348.

391 Pauli G, Bessot JC, Dietemann-Molard A. Occupational asthma: investigation and aetiological factors. *Bull Eur Physiopathol Respir* 1986; 22: 339.

392 Mapp CE, Saetta M, Maestrelli P *et al.* Mechanisms and pathology of occupational asthma. *Eur Respir J* 1994; 7: 544.

393 Weiner A. Bronchial asthma due to the organic phosphate insecticides. *Ann Allergy* 1961; 19: 397.

394 Chan-Yeung M, Malo J-L. Aetiological agents in occupational asthma. *Eur Respir J* 1994; 7: 346.

395 Cockcroft A, Edwards J, McCarthy P, Andersson N. Allergy in laboratory animal workers. *Lancet* 1981; i: 827.

396 Newman Taylor AJ, Longbottom JL, Pepys J. Respiratory allergy to urine proteins of rats and mice. *Lancet* 1977; ii: 847.

397 Venables KM, Tee RD, Hawkins ER *et al.* Laboratory animal allergy in a pharmaceutical company. *Br J Ind Med* 1988; 45: 660.

398 Spieksma FTM, Vooren PH, Kramps JA, Dijkmzn JH. Respiratory allergy to laboratory fruit flies (*Drosophila melanogaster*). *J Allergy Clin Immunol* 1986; 77: 108.

399 Ostrom NK, Swanson MC, Agarwal MK, Yuninger JW. Occupational allergy to honey-bee dust in a honey processing plant. *J Allergy Clin Immunol* 1986; 77: 736.

400 Cuthbert OD, Brostoff J, Wraith DG, Brighton WD. Barn allergy. Asthma and rhinitis due to storage mites. *Clin Allergy* 1979; 9: 229.

401 Lutsky I, Bar-Sela S. Northern fowl mite (*Ornithonyssus sylvianum*) in occupational asthma of poultry workers. *Lancet* 1982; ii: 874.

402 Stevenson DD, Mathews KP. Occupational asthma following inhalation of moth particles. *J Allergy* 1967; 39: 274.

403 Bar-Sela S, Teichtahl H, Lutsky I. Occupational asthma in poultry workers. *J Allergy Clin Immunol* 1984; 73: 271.

404 Cartier A, Malo JL, Forest F *et al.* Occupational asthma in snow crab processing workers. *J Allergy Clin Immunol* 1984; 74: 261.

405 Gaddie J, Legge JS, Friend JAS, Reid TMS. Pulmonary hypersensitivity in prawn workers. *Lancet* 1980; ii: 1350.

406 Darke CS, Knowleden J, Lacey J, Ward AM. Respiratory disease of workers harvesting grain dusts. *Thorax* 1976; 31: 294.

407 Chan-Yeung M, Wong R, Maclean L. Respiratory abnormalities among grain elevator workers. *Chest* 1979; 75: 461.

408 Chan-Yeung M, Schulzer M, MacLean L, Dorken E, Grzybowski S. Epidemiologic health survey of grain elevator workers in British Columbia. *Am Rev Respir Dis* 1980; 121: 329.

409 Ishizaki T, Shida T, Miyamoto T *et al.* Occupational asthma from western red cedar dust (*Thuja plicata*) in furniture factory workers. *J Occup Med* 1973; 15: 580.

410 Chan-Yeung M, Barton GM, Maclean L, Grzybowski S. Occupational asthma and rhinitis due to western red cedar (*Thuja plicata*). *Am Rev Respir Dis* 1973; 108: 1094.

411 Cullinan P, Lowson D, Nieuwenhuijsen MJ *et al.* Work-related symptoms, sensitisation and estimated exposure in workers not previously exposed to flour. *Occup Environ Med* 1994; 51: 579.

412 Vanhanen M, Tuomi T, Hokkanen H *et al.* Enzyme exposure and enzyme sensitisation in the baking industry. *Occup Environ Med* 1996; 53: 670.

413 Ingram CG, Jeffrey IG, Symington IS, Cuthbert OD. Bronchial provocation studies in farmers allergic to storage mites. *Lancet* 1979; ii: 1330.

414 Kathren RL, Price H, Rogers JC. Airborne castor bean pomace allergy. *Arch Ind Health* 1959; 19: 487.

415 Lehrer SB, Karr RM, Salvaggio IE. Extraction and analysis of coffee bean allergens. *Clin Allergy* 1978; 8: 217.

416 Fowler PBS. Printer's asthma. *Lancet* 1952; ii: 755.

417 Gelfand HH. The allergenic properties of vegetable gums. A case of asthma due to tragacanth. *J Allergy* 1943; 14: 203.

418 Burge PS, Harries MGO, Brien IM, Pepys J. Respiratory disease in workers exposed to solder flux fumes containing colophony (pine resin). *Clin Allergy* 1978; 8: 1.

419 Burge PS, Edge G, Hawkins R, White V, Taylor AN. Occupational asthma in a factory making flux-cored solder containing colophony. *Thorax* 1981; 36: 828.

420 Burge PS, Perks WH, O'Brien M *et al.* Occupational asthma in an electronics factory. A case control study to evaluate aetiological factors. *Thorax* 1979; 34: 300.

421 Perks WH, Burge PS, Rehahn M, Green M. Work-related respiratory disease in employees leaving an electronics factory. *Thorax* 1979; 34: 19.

422 Flindt MLH. Pulmonary disease due to inhalation of derivatives of *Bacillus subtilis* containing proteolytic enzyme. *Lancet* 1969; i: 1177.

423 Newhouse ML, Tagg B, Pocock SJ, McEwan AC. An epidemiological study of workers producing enzyme washing powders. *Lancet* 1970; i: 689.

424 Franz T, McMurrain KD, Brooks S, Bernstein IL. Clinical, immunologic and physiologic observations in factory workers exposed to *B. subtilis* enzyme dust. *J Allergy* 1971; 47: 170.

425 Juniper CP, How MJ, Goodwin BFJ, Kinshott AK. *Bacillus subtilis* enzymes: a 7 year clinical, epidemiological and immunological study of an industrial allergen. *J Soc Occup Med* 1977; 27: 3.

426 Colten HR, Polakoff PL, Weinstein SF, Strieder DJ. Immediate sensitivity to hog trypsin resulting from industrial exposure. *N Engl J Med* 1975; 292: 1050.

427 Baur X, Konig G, Bencze K, Fruhmann G. Clinical symptoms and results of skin test, RAST and bronchoprovocation tests in thirty three papain workers. *Clin Allergy* 1982; 12: 9.

428 Flindt MLH. Allergy to alpha amylase and papain. *Lancet* 1979; i: 1407.

429 Davies RJ, Hendrick DJ, Pepys J. Asthma due to inhaled chemical agents: ampicillin, benzyl penicillin, 6-amino penicillanic acid and related substances. *Clin Allergy* 1974; 4: 227.

430 Fawcett IW, Pepys J. Allergy to a tetracycline preparation. *Clin Allergy* 1976; 6: 301.

431 Coutts II, Dally MB, Newman Taylor AJ *et al.* Asthma in workers manufacturing cephalosporins. *Br Med J* 1981; 283: 950.

432 Pepys J, Pickering CAC, Loudon HWG. Asthma due to inhaled chemical agents: piperazine dihydrochloride. *Clin Allergy* 1972; 2: 189.

433 Bourne MS, Flindt MLH, Walker JM. Asthma due to industrial use of chloramine. *Br Med J* 1979; ii: 10.

434 Bardy J-D, Malo J-L, Seguin P *et al.* Occupational asthma and IgE sensitization in a pharmaceutical company processing psyllium. *Am Rev Respir Dis* 1987; 135: 1033.

435 Stenton SC, Dennis JH, Hendrick DJ. Occupational asthma due to ceftazidime. *Eur Respir J* 1995; 8: 1421.

436 Butcher BT, Salvaggio JE, Weil H, Ziskind MM. Toluene diisocyanate (TDI) pulmonary disease: immunologic and inhalation challenge studies. *J Allergy Clin Immunol* 1976; 58: 59.

437 Pepys J, Pickering CAC, Breslin ABX, Terry DJ. Asthma due to inhaled chemical agents: toluene diisocyanate. *Clin Allergy* 1972; 2: 225.

438 Tanser AR, Bourke MP, Blandford AG. Isocyanate asthma; respiratory symptoms caused by diphenylmethane isocyanate. *Thorax* 1973; 28: 596.

439 Zammit-Tabana M, Sherkin M, Kijek K *et al.* Asthma caused by diphenyl methane isocyanate in foundry workers. Clinical, bronchoprovocation and immunologic studies. *Am Rev Respir Dis* 1983; 128: 226.

440 Johnson A, Chan-Yeung M, Maclean L *et al.* Respiratory abnormalities among workers in an iron and steel foundry in Vancouver. *Br J Ind Med* 1985; 42: 94.

441 Harries MG, Burge PS, Samson M *et al.* Isocyanate asthma: respiratory symptoms due

to 1,5-naphthylene diisocyanate. *Thorax* 1979; 34: 762.

442 Mapp CE, Boschetto P, Vecchio L, Maestrelli P, Fabbri LM. Occupational asthma due to isocyanates. *Eur Respir J* 1988; 1: 273.

443 Vandenplas O, Cartier A, Lesage J, Perrault G, Grammer LC, Malo JL. Occupational asthma caused by a pre-polymer but not the monomer of toluene diisocyanate (TDI). *J Allergy Clin Immunol* 1992; 89: 1183.

444 Vandenplas O, Cartier A, Lesage J *et al.* Pre-polymers of hexamethylene diisocyanate (HDI) as a cause of occupational asthma. *J Allergy Clin Immunol* 1993; 91: 850.

445 Gallagher JS, Tse CST, Brooks SM, Bernstein IL. Diverse profiles of immunoreactivity in toluene diisocyanate asthma. *J Occup Med* 1981; 23: 610.

446 Fawcett IW, Newman Taylor AJ, Pepys J. Asthma due to inhaled chemical agents. Epoxy resin systems containing phthalic acid anhydride, trimellitic anhydride and triethylene tetramine. *Clin Allergy* 1977; 7: 1.

447 Zeiss CR, Wolkonsky P, Chacon R *et al.* Syndromes in workers exposed to trimellitic anhydride: a longitudinal clinical and immunologic study. *Ann Intern Med* 1983; 99: 8.

448 Pauli G, Bessot JC, Kopferschmitt MC *et al.* Meatwrappers' asthma: identification of the causal agent. *Clin Allergy* 1980; 10: 263.

449 Zeiss CR, Patterson R, Pruzansky JJ *et al.* Trimellitic anhydride-induced airways syndromes: clinical and immunologic studies. *J Allergy Clin Immunol* 1977; 60: 96.

450 Venables KM. Low molecular weight chemicals, hypersensitivity and direct toxicity: the acid anhydrides. *Br J Ind Med* 1989; 46: 222.

451 Nielsen J, Welinder H, Horstmann V, Skerfving S. Allergy to methyltetrahydrophthalic anhydride in epoxy resin workers. *Br J Ind Med* 1992; 49: 769.

452 Gelfand HH. Respiratory allergy due to chemical compounds encountered in the rubber, lacquer, shellac, and beauty culture industries. *J Allergy* 1963; 34: 374.

453 Lam S, Chan-Yeung M. Ethylenediamine-induced asthma. *Am Rev Respir Dis* 1980; 121: 151.

454 Aleva RM, Aalbers R, Koëter GH, de Monchy JGR. Occupational asthma caused by a hardener containing an aliphatic and cycloliphatic diamine. *Am Rev Respir Dis* 1992; 145: 1217.

455 Pepys J, Pickering CAC, Hughes EG. Asthma due to inhaled chemical agents: complex salts of platinum. *Clin Allergy* 1972; 2: 391.

456 Brooks SM, Baker DB, Gannn PH *et al.* Cold air challenge and platinum skin reactivity in platinum refinery workers. *Chest* 1990; 97: 1401.

457 Block GT, Yeung M. Asthma induced by nickel. *JAMA* 1982; 247: 1600.

458 Joules H. Asthma from sensitization to chromium. *Lancet* 1932; ii: 182.

459 Novey HS, Habib M, Wells ID. Asthma and IgE antibodies induced by chromium and nickel salts. *J Allergy Clin Immunol* 1983; 72: 407.

460 Sjorgren I, Hillerdahl G, Anderson A, Zetterstrom O. Hard metal lung disease: importance of cobalt in coolants. *Thorax* 1980; 35: 653.

461 Gheysens B, Auxwerx J, van den Eeckhout A, Demedts M. Cobalt-induced bronchial asthma in diamond polishers. *Chest* 1985; 88: 740.

462 Williams N. Vanadium poisoning from cleaning oil-fired boilers. *Br J Ind Med* 1952; 9: 50.

463 Davison AG, Haslam PL, Corrin B *et al.* Interstitial lung disease and asthma in hard metal workers: bronchoalveolar lavage, ultrastructural and analytical findings, and results of bronchial challenge tests. *Thorax* 1983; 38: 119.

464 Saric M, Zuskin E, Gonzi M. Bronchoconstriction in potroom workers. *Br J Ind Med* 1979; 36: 211.

465 Hendrick DJ, Lane DJ. Occupational formalin asthma. *Br J Ind Med* 1977; 34: 11.

466 Gannon PFG, Bright P, Campbell M, O'Hickey SP, Burge PS. Occupational asthma due to glutaraldehyde and formaldehyde in endoscopy and X ray departments. *Thorax* 1995; 50: 156.

467 Slovak AJM. Occupational asthma caused by plastics blowing agent, azodicarbonamide. *Thorax* 1981; 36: 906.

468 Silberman DE, Sorrell AH. Allergy in fur workers, with special reference to paraphenylene diamine. *J Allergy* 1959; 30: 11.

469 Pepys J, Hutchcroft BJ, Breslin ABX. Asthma due to inhaled chemical agents: persulphate salts and henna in hairdressers. *Clin Allergy* 1976; 6: 399.

470 Sterling GM. Asthma due to aluminium soldering flux. *Thorax* 1967; 22: 533.

471 Docker A, Wattie JM, Topping MD *et al.* Clinical and immunological investigations of respiratory disease in workers using reactive dyes. *Br J Ind Med* 1987; 44: 534.

472 Tarlo SM, Wong L, Roos J, Booth N. Occupational asthma caused by latex in surgical glove manufacture. *J Allergy Clin Immunol* 1990; 85: 626.

473 Honda I, Kohrogi H, Andro M *et al.* Occupational asthma induced by the fungicide tetrachloroisophthalonitrile. *Thorax* 1992; 47: 760.

474 Shelton D, Urch B, Tarlo SM. Occupational asthma induced by a carpet fungicide, tributyl tin oxide. *J Allergy Clin Immunol* 1992; 90: 274.

475 Gannon PFG, Burge PS, Benfield CFA. Occupational asthma due to polyethylene shrink wrapping (paper wrapper's asthma). *Thorax* 1992; 47: 759.

476 Venables KM, Topping MD, Howe W *et al.* Interaction of smoking and atopy in producing specific IgE antibody against a hapten protein conjugate. *Br Med J* 1985; 290: 201.

477 Anon. Smoking, occupation and allergic lung disease. *Lancet* 1985; i: 965.

478 Dewitte J-D, Chan-Yeung M, Malo J-L. Medicolegal and compensation aspects of occupational asthma. *Eur Respir J* 1994; 7: 969.

479 Hetzel MR, Clark TJH. Comparison of normal and asthmatic rhythms in peak expiratory flow rate. *Thorax* 1980; 35: 732.

480 Hetzel MR. The pulmonary clock. *Thorax* 1981; 36: 481.

481 Clark TJH, Hetzel MR. Diurnal variation of asthma. *Br J Dis Chest* 1977; 71: 87.

482 Soutar CA, Carruthers M, Pickering CAC. Nocturnal asthma and urinary adrenaline and noradrenaline excretion. *Thorax* 1977; 32: 677.

483 Barnes P, Fitzgerald G, Brown M, Dollery C. Nocturnal asthma and changes in circulating epinephrine, histamine and cortisol. *N Engl J Med* 1980; 303: 263.

484 Douglas NJ. Nocturnal asthma. *Thorax* 1993; 48: 100.

485 Martin RJ. Nocturnal asthma: circadian rhythms and therapeutic interventions. *Am Rev Respir Dis* 1993; 147: 525.

486 Martin AJ, McLennan LA, Landau LI, Phelan PD. The natural history of childhood asthma to adult life. *Br Med J* 1980; 280: 1391.

487 Balfour-Lynn L, Tooley NI, Godfrey S. A study comparing the relationship of exercise induced asthma to clinical asthma in childhood. *Arch Dis Child* 1980; 56: 450.

488 Blair H. Natural history of childhood asthma: 20 year follow-up. *Arch Dis Child* 1977; 52: 613.

489 Kokkonen J, Linna O. The state of childhood asthma in young adulthood. *Eur Respir J* 1993; 6: 657.

490 Braman SS, Kaemmerlen JT, Davis SM. Asthma in the elderly: a comparison between patients with recently acquired and long standing disease. *Am Rev Respir Dis* 1991; 143: 336.

491 Peat JK, Woolcock AJ, Cullen K. Rate of decline of lung function in subjects with asthma. *Eur J Respir Dis* 1987; 70: 171.

492 Brenner BE, Abraham E, Simon RR. Position and diaphoresis in acute asthma. *Am J Med* 1983; 74: 1005.

493 Rebuck AS, Reid J. Assessment and management of severe asthma. *Am J Med* 1971; 51: 788.

494 Rebuck AS, Pengelly LD. Development of pulsus paradoxus in the presence of airways obstruction. *N Engl J Med* 1973; 288: 66.

495 Knowles GK, Clark TJH. Pulsus paradoxus as a valuable sign indicating severity of asthma. *Lancet* 1973; ii: 1356.

496 Pearson MG, Spence DP, Ryland I, Harrison BDW. Value of pulsus paradoxus in assessing acute severe asthma. *Br Med J* 1993; 307: 659.

497 British Thoracic Society. The British guidelines on asthma management: 1995 review and position statement. *Thorax* 1997; 52 (Suppl 1): S2.

498 Jones ES. The intensive therapy of asthma. *Proc R Soc Med* 1971; 64: 1151.

499 Rees HA, Millar JS, Donald KW. A study of the clinical course and arterial blood gas tensions of patients in status asthmaticus. *Q J Med* 1968; 37: 541.

500 Traver GA, Cline MG, Burrows B. Asthma in the elderly. *J Asthma* 1993; 302: 81.

501 Ulrik CS, Backer D, Dirksen A. A 10 year follow up of 180 adults with bronchial asthma: factors important for the decline in lung function. *Thorax* 1992; 47: 14.

502 Carmichael J, Paterson IC, Diaz P *et al.* Corticosteroid resistance in chronic asthma. *Br Med J* 1981; 282: 1419.

503 McLeod DT, Capewell SJ, Law J *et al.* Intramuscular triamcinolone acetonide in chronic severe asthma. *Thorax* 1985; 40: 840.

504 Poznansky MC, Gordon ACH, Douglas JG, Krajewski AS, Wyllie AH, Grant IWB. Resistance to methylprednisolone in cultures of blood mononuclear cells from glucocorticoid-resistant asthmatic patients. *Clin Sci* 1984; 67: 639.

505 Poznansky MC, Gordon ACH, Grant IWB, Wyllie AH. A cellular abnormality in glucocorticoid resistant asthma. *Clin Exp Immunol* 1985; 61: 135.

506 Barnes PJ, Greening AP, Crompton GK. Glucocorticoid resistance in asthma. *Am J Respir Crit Care Med* 1995; 152: S125.

507 Lane SJ, Palmer JBD, Skidmore IF, Lee TH. Corticosteroid pharmacokinetics in asthma. *Lancet* 1990; 336: 1265.

508 Brown PJ, Teelucksingh S, Matusiewicz SP, Greening AP, Crompton GK, Edwards CRW. Cutaneous vasoconstrictor response to glucocorticoids in asthma. *Lancet* 1991; 337: 576.

509 Corrigan CJ, Brown PJ, Barnes NC, Tsai J-J, Frew AJ, Kay AB. Peripheral blood T lymphocyte activation and comparison of the T lymphocyte inhibitory effects of glucocorticoids and cyclosporin. *Am Rev Respir Dis* 1991; 144: 1026.

510 Corrigan CJ, Bungre JK, Assoufi B, Cooper AE, Seddon H, Kay AB. Glucocorticoid resistant asthma: T-lymphocyte steroid metabolism and sensitivity to glucocorticoids and immunosuppressive agents. *Eur Respir J* 1996; 9: 2077.

511 Longbottom IL, Pepys J. Pulmonary aspergillosis: diagnostic and immunological significance of antigens and C-substance in *Aspergillus fumigatus*. *J Pathol Bacteriol* 1964; 88: 141.

512 Malo JL, Paquin R. Incidence of immediate hypersensitivity to *Aspergillus fumigatus* in a North American asthmatic population. *Clin Allergy* 1979; 9: 377.

513 Schwartz HJ, Citron KM, Chester EH *et al.* A comparison of the prevalence of sensitization to *Aspergillus* antigens among asthmatics in Cleveland and London. *J Allergy Clin Immunol* 1978; 62: 9.

514 McCarthy DS, Pepys J. Allergic bronchopulmonary aspergillosis. Clinical immunology. 1. Clinical features. *Clin Allergy* 1971; 1: 261.

515 Henderson AH. Allergic aspergillosis: review of 32 cases. *Thorax* 1968; 23: 501.

516 McCarthy DS, Simon G, Hargreave FE. The radiological appearances in allergic bronchopulmonary aspergillosis. *Clin Radiol* 1970; 21: 366.

517 Patterson R, Fink JN, Pruzansky JJ *et al.* Serum immunoglobulin levels in pulmonary allergic aspergillosis and certain other lung diseases, with special reference to immunoglobulin E. *Am J Med* 1973; 54: 16.

518 Rosenberg M, Patterson R, Mintzer R. Clinical and immunologic criteria for the diagnosis of allergic bronchopulmonary aspergillosis. *Ann Intern Med* 1977; 86: 405.

519 McCarthy DS, Pepys J. Allergic bronchopulmonary aspergillosis. Clinical immunology. 2. Skin, nasal and bronchial tests. *Clin Allergy* 1971; 1: 415.

520 Malo JL, Hawkins R, Pepys J. Studies in chronic bronchopulmonary aspergillosis. 1. Clinical and physiological findings. *Thorax* 1977; 32: 254.

521 Malo JL, Pepys J, Simon G. Studies in chronic bronchopulmonary aspergillosis 2. Radiological findings. *Thorax* 1977; 32: 262.

522 Safirstein BH, D'Souza MF, Simon G *et al.* Five year follow-up of allergic bronchopulmonary aspergillosis. *Am Rev Respir Dis* 1973; 108: 450.

523 Basich JE, Graves TS, Baz NM *et al.* Allergic bronchopulmonary aspergillosis in corticosteroid dependent asthmatics. *J Allergy Clin Immunol* 1981; 68: 98.

524 Crompton GK. Inhaled beclomethasone dipropionate in allergic bronchopulmonary aspergillosis. Report to the Research Committee of the British Thoracic Association. *Br J Dis Chest* 1979; 73: 349.

525 Glancy JJ, Elder J, McAleer R. Allergic bron-

chopulmonary fungal disease without clinical asthma. *Thorax* 1981; 36: 345.

526 Berkin KE, Vernon DRH, Kerr JW. Lung collapse caused by allergic bronchopulmonary aspergillosis in non-asthmatic patients. *Br Med J* 1982; 285: 87.

527 Sanerkin NG, Seal RME, Leopold JG. Plastic bronchitis, mucoid impaction of the bronchi and allergic bronchopulmonary aspergillosis, and their relationship to bronchial asthma. *Ann Allergy* 1966; 24: 586.

528 Clee MD, Lamb D, Clark RA. Bronchocentric granulomatosis: a review and thoughts on pathogenesis. *Br J Dis Chest* 1983; 77: 227.

529 Israel RH, Poe RH, Bomba PA, Gross RA. The rapid development of an aspergilloma secondary to allergic bronchopulmonary aspergillosis. *Am J Med Sci* 1980; 280: 41.

530 Ein ME, Wallace RJ, Williams TW. Allergic bronchopulmonary aspergillosis-like syndrome consequent to aspergilloma. *Am Rev Respir Dis* 1979; 119: 811.

531 Anderson CJ, Craig S, Bardana EJ. Allergic bronchopulmonary aspergillosis and bilateral fungal balls terminating in disseminated aspergillosis. *J Allergy Clin Immunol* 1980; 65: 140.

532 Forman SR, Fink JN, Moore VL *et al.* Humoral and cellular immune responses in *Aspergillus fumigatus* pulmonary disease. *J Allergy Clin Immunol* 1978; 62: 131.

533 Haslam P, Lukoszek A, Longbottom JL, Turner-Warner M. Lymphocyte sensitization to *Aspergillus fumigatus* antigens in pulmonary disease in man. *Clin Allergy* 1976; 6: 277.

534 Mullins J, Harvey R, Seaton A. Sources and incidence of airborne *Aspergillus fumigatus* (Fres). *Clin Allergy* 1976; 6: 209.

535 Robertson MD, Seaton A, Milne LJR, Raeburn JA. Suppression of host defences by *Aspergillus fumigatus*. *Thorax* 1987; 42: 19.

536 Robertson MD, Seaton A, Raeburn JA, Milne LJR. Resistance of spores of *Aspergillus fumigatus* to ingestion by phagocytic cells. *Thorax* 1987; 42: 466.

537 Robertson MD, Seaton A, Raeburn JA, Milne LJR. Inhibition of phagocyte migration and spreading by spore diffusates of *Aspergillus fumigatus*. *J Med Vet Mycol* 1987; 25: 389.

538 Seaton A, Seaton RA, Wightman AJA. Management of allergic bronchopulmonary aspergillosis without maintenance oral corticosteroids: a fifteen-year follow-up. *Q J Med* 1994; 87: 529.

539 Cohen MB, Abram LE. Growth patterns of allergic children. A statistical study using the grid technique. *J Allergy* 1948; 19: 165.

540 Pedersen S. Importance of early intervention in children: efficacy and safety. In: Schleimer R, Busse W, O'Byrne P, eds. *Topical Glucocorticosteroids in Asthma: Mechanisms and Clinical Actions. New York:* Marcel Dekker, 1995.

541 Pedersen S. Safety aspects of corticosteroids in children. *Eur Respir Rev* 1994; 4: 33.

542 Pedersen S. Important issues in childhood asthma. *Eur Respir Rev* 1996; 6: 192.

543 Derbes VJ, Weaver NK, Cotton AL. Complications of bronchial asthma. *Am J Med Sci* 1951; 222: 88.

544 Eggleston PA, Ward BH, Pierson WE, Bierman CW. Radiographic abnormalities in acute asthma in children. *Pediatrics* 1974; 54: 442.

545 Hopkirk JAC, Stark JE. Unilateral pul-

546 Burke GH. Pneumothorax complicating acute asthma. *S Afr Med J* 1979; 55: 508.

547 D'Assumpcao C, Smith WG. Spontaneous mediastinal and subcutaneous emphysema complicating bronchial asthma. *Med J Aust* 1967; i: 328.

548 Dunnill MS. *Pulmonary Pathology.* Edinburgh: Churchill Livingstone, 1982: 59.

549 Forgacs P. *Lung Sounds.* London: Baillière Tindall, 1978.

550 Freedman S, Tattersfield AE, Pride NB. Changes in lung mechanics during asthma induced by exercise. *J Appl Physiol* 1975; 38: 974.

551 Woolcock AJ, Read J. Lung volumes in exacerbations of asthma. *Am J Med* 1966; 41: 259.

552 Woolcock AJ, Rebuck AS, Cade JF, Read J. Lung volume changes in asthma measured concurrently by two different methods. *Am Rev Respir Dis* 1971; 104: 703.

553 Peress L, Sybrecht G, Macklem PT. The mechanism of increase in total lung capacity during acute asthma. *Am J Med* 1976; 61: 165.

554 Cade JE, Woolcock AJ, Rebuck AS, Pain MCF. Lung mechanics during provocation of asthma. *Clin Sci* 1971; 40: 381.

555 McFadden ER, Kiser R, De Groot WJ. Acute bronchial asthma: relations between clinical and physiologic manifestations. *N Engl J Med* 1973; 288: 221.

556 Lisboa C, Jardim J, Angus E, Macklem PT. Is extrathoracic airway obstruction important in asthma? *Am Rev Respir Dis* 1980; 122: 115.

557 McCarthy D, Milic-Emili J. Closing volume in asymptomatic asthma. *Am Rev Respir Dis* 1973; 107: 559.

558 Hecksher T, Bass H, Oriol A *et al.* Regional lung function in patients with bronchial asthma. *J Clin Invest* 1968; 47: 1063.

559 Fazio F, Palla A, Santolicandro A *et al.* Studies of regional ventilation in asthma using ^{81m}Kr. *Lung* 1979; 156: 185.

560 Wagner PD, Dantzker DR, Lacovoni VE *et al.* Ventilation–perfusion inequality in asymptomatic asthma. *Am Rev Respir Dis* 1978; 118: 511.

561 Kanagami H, Katsura T, Shiroishi K *et al.* Studies on the pulmonary diffusing capacity by the carbon monoxide breath-holding technique: II. Patients with various pulmonary diseases. *Acta Med Scand* 1961; 169: 595.

562 Ohman JL, Schmidt-Nowara W, Lawrence M *et al.* The diffusing capacity in asthma: effect of air flow obstruction. *Am Rev Respir Dis* 1973; 107: 932.

563 Gazioglu K, Condeni JJ, Hyde RW, Kaltreider NL. Effect of isoproterenol on gas exchange during air and oxygen breathing in patients with bronchial asthma. *Am J Med* 1971; 50: 185.

564 Lorriman G. The effects of bronchodilators on pulmonary ventilation and diffusion in asthma and emphysema. *Thorax* 1959; 14: 146.

565 McFadden ER, Lyons HA. Arterial blood gas tensions in asthma. *N Engl J Med* 1968; 278: 1027.

566 Karetsky MS. Blood studies in untreated patients with acute asthma. *Am Rev Respir Dis* 1975; 112: 607.

567 Permutt S. Physiologic changes in the acute asthma attack. In: Austen KF, Lichtenstein LM, eds. *Asthma: Physiology, Immunopharma-*

cology, and Treatment. New York: Academic Press, 1973: 15.

568 Crompton GK. Severe acute asthma. In: Barnes PJ, Rodger IW, Thomson NC, eds. *Asthma: Basic Mechanisms and Clinical Management*, 2nd edn. London: Academic Press, 1992.

569 Chappell AG. Painless myocardial infarction in asthma. *Br J Dis Chest* 1984; 78: 174.

570 Nogrady SG, Hartley JPR, Seaton A. Metabolic effects of intravenous salbutamol in the course of acute severe asthma. *Thorax* 1977; 32: 559.

571 Dale G, Fleetwood JA, Weddell A *et al.* B-endorphin: a factor in 'fun run' collapse. *Br Med J* 1987; 294: 1004.

572 Williams SJ, Seaton A. Intravenous or inhaled salbutamol in severe acute asthma? *Thorax* 1977; 32: 555.

573 Williams SJ, Winner SJ, Clark TJH. Comparison of inhaled and intravenous terbutaline in acute severe asthma. *Thorax* 1981; 36: 629.

574 Miller GJ, Davies BH, Cole TJ, Seaton A. Comparison of the bronchial response to running and cycling in asthma, using an improved definition of the response to work. *Thorax* 1975; 30: 306.

575 Jones RS. Assessment of respiratory function in the asthmatic child. *Br Med J* 1966; ii: 972.

576 Anderson S, Silverman M, Konig P, Godfrey S. Exercise-induced asthma. *Br Dis Chest* 1975; 69: 1.

577 Burge PS, O'Brien IM, Harries MG. Peak flow records in the diagnosis of occupational asthma due to colophony. *Thorax* 1979; 34: 308.

578 Hodson ME, Simon G, Batten JC. Radiology of uncomplicated asthma. *Thorax* 1974; 29: 296.

579 Petheram IS, Kerr IH, Collins JV. Value of chest radiographs in severe acute asthma. *Clin Radiol* 1981; 32: 281.

580 Hodson CJ, Trickey SE. Bronchial wall thickening in asthma. *Clin Radiol* 1960; 11: 183.

581 Horn BR, Robin ED, Theodore J, van Kessel A. Total eosinophil counts in the management of bronchial asthma. *N Engl J Med* 1975; 292: 1152.

582 Stretton TB, Lee HY. Asthma in the elderly. *Br Med J* 1972; iv: 93.

583 Brown HM. Treatment of chronic asthma with prednisolone. Significance of eosinophils in the sputum. *Lancet* 1958; ii: 1245.

584 Stenius B, Wide L, Seymour WM *et al.* Clinical significance of specific IgE to common allergens. 1. Relationship of specific IgE against *Dermatophagoides* spp and grass pollen to skin and nasal tests and history. *Clin Allergy* 1971; 1: 37.

585 Sethi TJ, Lessof MH, Kemeny DM *et al.* How reliable are commercial allergy tests? *Lancet* 1987; i: 92.

586 Burge PS. Problems in the diagnosis of occupational asthma. *Br J Dis Chest* 1987; 81: 105.

587 Seaton A, Cherrie B, Turnbull J. Rubber glove asthma. *Br Med J* 1988; 296: 531.

588 Burge PS. Aerosol challenge in lung disease. In: Clark SW, Pavia D, eds. *Aerosols and the Lung.* London: Butterworth, 1984: Chapter 10.

589 Denman AM. Diagnostic methods and criteria. In: Coombs RRA, ed. *Proceedings of First Food Allergy Workshop.* Oxford: Medical Education Services, 1980: 47.

35

ASTHMA: MANAGEMENT

GRAHAM CROMPTON

Asthma is a disease that affects people of all ages, in all parts of the world. Despite greatly increased knowledge of the immunopathological processes characteristic of the disease, and apparent improvements in treatment, morbidity (and in some countries mortality) is increasing rather than decreasing. It is extremely unlikely that a cure of asthma will be available for many years to come, but even without further pharmacological advance there is now great potential for improving the management of most asthmatic patients by encouraging more rational use of treatments already in existence. To encourage uniformity of asthma treatment, management plans and guidelines have been published in several countries. In general terms the contents of all the guidelines are similar, and it is hoped that a greater number of clinicians will become aware of these management recommendations in the future. A worldwide unified approach to the management of asthma would be the ideal. However, it is likely that the more wealthy nations will have to give the lead, since the resources necessary to educate patients and clinicians about management principles are considerable, and the financial burden of therapy would be too heavy for some of the less-developed nations.

The overall management of asthma has many similarities with that of diabetes, since in both diseases the aim is to allow the patient to be as independent as possible and to make treatment changes as appropriate to maintain clinical control. Professional advice should be readily available when self-management has not been successful, and for most patients there should be regular contact with a healthcare professional for review and advice.

Aims and principles of management

The aims of management are to:
- recognize asthma;
- abolish symptoms;
- restore normal or best possible long-term airway function;
- reduce the risk of severe attacks;
- enable normal growth to occur in children;
- minimize absence from school or work.
  The principles of management are:
- patient and family participation;
- avoidance of identified causes where possible;
- use of lowest effective doses of convenient medications minimizing short-term and long-term side-effects.

These aims and principles of management have been taken from British guidelines for the management of asthma [1] but are similar to statements in many other guidelines now in existence in many parts of the world. In general terms the major objectives are to allow all patients to lead symptom-free normal lives with the aid of treatments, free from side-effects, which can be adjusted and modified by informed patients themselves.

Patient participation

Efficient management of asthma requires a partnership between the patient and family and the healthcare professional. At the outset it should be made clear that cure or spontaneous remission of chronic asthma in adults is unlikely and therefore treatment and supervision are likely to be required over a prolonged period. Education is essential to allow sharing of information about the nature of the disease and its treatment and to enable the patient and family to acquire understanding and management skills. An important stage of the education process is allowing and encouraging the patient and family to express fears and concerns about the disease and treatment, and to discuss both the clinician's and the patient's expectations of the condition and its management. Patients and parents require both verbal and written advice; ideally all asthmatics with more than mild disease should have a guided self-management plan.

Self-management plans

All patients who have to make frequent decisions about the management of their asthma should be offered a

973

self-management plan, which in effect means most of those requiring treatment with an inhaled steroid in a dose of more than 800 μg daily. The common finding of controlled trials on patient education alone is that verbal, written, audio and video educational programmes can increase a patient's knowledge but without improvement in asthma morbidity [2–4]. Ideally the self-management plans should be written for, and tailored to, the needs of the individual patient, since these can be cost-effective in the short term if directed at those with moderate to severe disease [5]. However, this is rarely possible and standardized plans that can, in part, be tailored for each asthmatic are commonly used. The most popular plans are based on a three-colour system (green, amber and red) and carry advice about management actions depending upon symptoms and peak expiratory flow (PEF) values.

1 *Green*. Symptoms under control and PEF greater than 80% of predicted or best: continue to use steroid inhaler regularly in the same dose, and use bronchodilator inhaler as required.

2 *Amber*. Symptoms not well controlled or PEF less than 80% but greater than 50% of best or predicted: double dose of steroid inhaler and use bronchodilator inhaler as necessary or regularly every 4 h.

3 *Red*. Distressing symptoms not responding to the bronchodilator inhaler or PEF less than 50% of best or predicted: start oral steroid treatment immediately and obtain medical help.

Plans need to be tailored to individual patients and their local healthcare circumstances so that they know when to contact the general practitioner, call an ambulance by using the emergency telephone code, attend the nearest hospital emergency department or use a respiratory unit self-admission service [6–9]. Written personalized management plans are essential for patients with poorly controlled asthma; in these patients, if the three-colour system is used, it is probably appropriate to omit the amber zone to encourage early aggressive intervention in the event of deteriorating asthma. Written educational materials should be available to supplement self-management plans since these materials are likely to help patients accept their diagnosis and gain confidence in coping with its effects.

It is difficult to prove beyond doubt that self-management plans are effective in the long term. Controlled studies show evidence of benefit by their reduction of hospital admissions, courses of oral steroids and nebulized bronchodilators, although there are questions concerning 'enthusiast bias' compromising outcomes [10,11], i.e. patients who are perceived to be likely to benefit from plans tend to receive them and operate them [12,13]. This may be the explanation of the widespread clinical acceptance that self-management plans work despite the doubts raised by analysis of controlled trials [4,5]. It is likely that the success of management strategies depends to a considerable extent upon the healthcare professional who issues the self-management plan. He or she should be known and trusted by the patient, be readily accessible by telephone and ideally should be the person who reviews the patient at follow-up. Appropriately trained practice nurses with the time, enthusiasm and accessibility to patients could be the ideal choice [13], although it is appreciated that in many areas these individuals may not exist. The major problem in asthma management is translating the theory of good asthma care into everyday practice. There are marked differences between patients' self-management knowledge and their actual behaviour in an acute attack [14]. Self-management plans appear to be the best available option at present [15,16], although these alone are unlikely to overcome the major problem of compliance known to exist in a large number of patients with asthma [17,18].

Peak flow monitoring

The variable orifice PEF meter was introduced in 1959 [19]. Since then a number of lightweight PEF meters have become available, and are commonly used in both the diagnosis and management of asthma. In the last decade self-management plans using PEF monitoring have become widely used [11,13]. Peak flow monitoring is used for (i) diagnosis (see Chapter 34), (ii) monitoring the effect of treatment, particularly the effects of treatment changes, (iii) self-management plans, especially in patients with poor perception of symptom severity [20] and in the day-to-day management of the patient with brittle asthma, (iv) investigation of suspected occupational asthma (see Chapter 34) and (v) research.

Avoidance of causes and non-specific triggers and aggravating factors

Specific causes of asthma are rarely known except for some occupational sensitizers and aeroallergens. Physical factors, such as exercise, strong smells, cold, sudden changes in ambient humidity and temperature, cigarette smoking and smoky atmospheres, can trigger episodes of asthma or make chronic symptoms more troublesome. All patients should, of course, be encouraged not to smoke and also to avoid passive smoking if possible. Unfortunately a surprising number of asthmatics continue to smoke even though they realize it aggravates their symptoms. It is difficult to modify climatic conditions; however, any suggestions about modifications to the home environment should include the advice that ideally there should be, as far as possible, an even temperature and humidity in all rooms. The control of exercise-induced asthma requires therapeutic intervention rather than avoidance of exercise.

Allergy avoidance

The increase in prevalence and severity of asthma in westernized countries may be due partly to increase in exposure to indoor aeroallergens [21]. The logical approach to the treatment of asthma involves avoidance of allergens where possible, including occupational sensitizers, together with the early intervention of anti-inflammatory therapy, usually inhaled steroids. Evidence is now accumulating that aeroallergens, particularly the house-dust mite and animal danders, are major independent variables in the prediction of asthma in different populations [22,23]. Exposures during the neonatal period are thought to be critical in the development of atopic sensitization [24] and avoidance of perennial aeroallergens and/or food allergens during early life may delay or even prevent the onset of atopic sensitization and allergic manifestations [25,26]. An advance in the evaluation of allergen avoidance has been the identification and characterization of the major allergenic determinants of common perennial allergens, namely *Der p*I (dust mites), *Fel d*I (cats) and, more recently, *Can f*I (dogs). This has enabled the development of monoclonal antibodies that allow accurate measurement of major allergens in dust samples and airborne exposure [27–29]. Ideally the efficacy of any allergy avoidance measure should be assessed by measurement of the reduction or elimination of allergen as well as by clinical response [30,31]. Barrier bedding methods, removal of carpets, regular cleaning and application of liquid nitrogen to bedding and furnishing have been associated with a reduction in house-dust mite levels [32–35]. The value of acaricides in reducing mite allergen levels remains controversial [32,36] and on the evidence currently available these products cannot be recommended for routine use. In children, barrier bedding methods combined with regular cleaning and removal of carpets appear to be effective in reducing bronchial hyperresponsiveness [36,37], but unless these arduous and often expensive prophylactic measures can be carried out fastidiously they usually have little clinical benefit. Animal allergens are difficult to avoid and eradicate as long as the pets remain in the home. After the departure of a cat from a home environment, several months of vigorous cleaning is necessary in order to reduce cat allergen load to clinically acceptable levels [38]. Washing a cat every week for 4 weeks has been shown to reduce the airborne cat allergen levels when the washing was combined with vigorous cleaning measures and removal of bedroom carpets [39], although this cannot be regarded as a substitute for removal of the animal from the household environment. A major source of animal dander allergen is contaminated clothing. High levels of *Can f*I have been demonstrated on schoolroom desks and chairs but not on floors, suggesting contamination from children's clothing from pets at home [29].

It is impossible to avoid pollens. Simple advice includes wearing spectacles or sunglasses, remaining indoors during periods of high pollen counts and keeping windows closed particularly in high buildings and cars. Walking in open grassy spaces should be avoided, especially during the evening and night when pollen counts tend to be at their highest. However, these lifestyle modifications are often unacceptable, particularly by those whose atopic symptoms are not severe and easily controlled by pharmacological agents.

Those asthmatics who give a history of symptoms on allergen exposure and who have a positive skin-prick test to the same allergen should be given advice about appropriate allergen avoidance measures, although advice about pets is rarely taken [30,31]. Such advice should not be given because of a positive skin-prick test in the absence of historical evidence of allergen hypersensitivity. Negative skin tests are helpful in excluding an allergic basis for asthma, providing they have been performed correctly at a time when the patient has not been taking an antihistamine. Serum allergen-specific IgE concentrations by radioallergosorbent test provide an alternative to skin tests, but in general are more expensive and perhaps less sensitive. Recognition of an occupational sensitizer is of extreme importance, since removal from exposure may result in improvement or remission of asthmatic symptoms; unfortunately this does not occur in every case. Food and food additives are a much less common, although important, cause of asthma. When genuine food allergy exists it is usually readily detected and the offending item of diet can be avoided. Many patients believe that certain foods have caused or made their asthma worse and modify their diets or those of their children. With these patients it is often difficult or impossible to confirm or exclude food allergy. Milk products and eggs are commonly incriminated and in some patients with severe disease a strict exclusion diet can be tried in an attempt to establish whether or not foods are causing asthma. Although the problem appears to be rare in adults, there can be no doubt that food allergens during early life play some role in the onset of atopic sensitization and allergic manifestations [25,26].

Drug avoidance

All β-adrenoreceptor antagonists are absolutely contraindicated in all patients with asthma. Even eyedrops containing one of these drugs can precipitate severe acute asthma. Aspirin can also induce worsening of asthma, which can be severe and is sometimes, but by no means always, accompanied by urticaria. Aspirin-sensitive asthmatics are usually adults with a history of nasal symptoms often due to nasal polyps. Other nonsteroidal anti-inflammatory drugs can make asthma worse and all should be used with great caution in asthmatic individuals.

Patient compliance with treatment

Poor patient adherence to prescribed medications has been shown to be a widespread problem in asthma [40–42] and has been linked to increased morbidity [43] and mortality [44]. Poor compliance with treatment in general is difficult to identify by routine clinical assessment [45] and there does not appear to be any association between compliance and age, sex, socioeconomic group, personality traits or level of education [46]. Patients' attitudes to treatment are likely to influence how they cope with their illness and use their treatment [47]. Inappropriate overemphasis of the side-effects of corticosteroids leading to rapid reduction of dose or withdrawal of treatment could be a factor contributing to the deaths of some patients from severe acute asthma [15,44,48]. There is no simple method of improving treatment compliance in asthma, nor is there any way of identifying patients likely to benefit from intervention programmes. All patients must therefore be assumed to be poor compliers and all should receive similar, but individually tailored, self-management plans and education about the disease and the treatments used to control it.

Drug treatment

Avoidance of allergens and non-specific aggravating factors may result in the disappearance of symptoms in some patients but in the majority some form of drug treatment is also required. This may be intermittent in episodic or seasonal asthma, while in adults the disease is usually chronic and long-term treatment has to be planned. There are two principal aims in the treatment of all patients with chronic asthma: (i) the rapid achievement of symptom control and optimal or best lung function; and (ii) maintenance of symptom control and best lung function. Initially this usually requires the use of a steroid, either orally or by inhalation, to achieve rapid control of symptoms and best lung function. Once this has been achieved, a step-down of treatment is usually possible in all but those patients with very severe chronic disease. Long-term maintenance therapy in most patients has to be with an inhaled steroid since this is the most effective treatment available for the control of the asthmatic bronchial wall inflammation.

The drugs used in the treatment of asthma can be broadly split into two categories: the β_2-agonist bronchodilators, sometimes called 'relievers', and the antiasthma inflammatory agents, sometimes called 'preventers'. However, there are other bronchodilator drugs, such as the anticholinergics, which have a useful but less major role than the β_2 agonists, and theophylline. Traditionally, this drug has been classed as a bronchodilator but has now been found to have some anti-inflammatory activity in addition, though its role in the treatment of asthmatic inflammation has still to be established. The development of long-acting inhaled bronchodilators and the production of oral sustained-release preparations of shorter-acting drugs has made it more difficult to categorize drugs simply as relievers and preventers; nevertheless this naive classification is of value in the education of patients and in the production of management plans and educational literature.

Management of chronic asthma

Drugs used for the relief or suppression of symptoms (the relievers)

β_2 adrenoreceptor agonists

The β_2 agonists are bronchodilators that give symptomatic relief but have no major beneficial effects on the underlying bronchial wall pathology. Indeed regular use of short-acting β_2 agonists has been questioned because of the possibility that such treatment might have a detrimental effect on the control of asthma, possibly by increasing bronchial hyperresponsiveness either during treatment or soon after its withdrawal [49–53]. Since β_2 agonists only give symptomatic relief, there seems little reason to encourage patients to take them regularly. If regular treatment is necessary for relief of symptoms this should stimulate the prescription of an anti-inflammatory preparation or an increase in its dose.

Inhaled short-acting β_2 agonists

The β_2 agonists relax airway smooth muscle and enhance mucociliary clearance. They also decrease vascular permeability and may modulate mediator release from mast cells and basophils, but they do not have any clinically relevant beneficial effects on the underlying chronic inflammatory disorder of the asthmatic airways. Short-acting β_2 agonist inhalers should be used as necessary to relieve symptoms. Regular treatment with these compounds should be avoided wherever possible, unless the results of clinical trials now in progress show that such treatment is not harmful in terms of increasing bronchial hyperresponsiveness or adversely affecting the overall control and prognosis of asthma [49–54]. The International Consensus Report on Diagnosis and Management of Asthma [55] suggests that if a patient has to use a short-acting bronchodilator more often than three times a week this indicates asthma of sufficient severity to warrant regular treatment with an anti-inflammatory or prophylactic drug. The British guidelines [1] suggest that this form of treatment would be appropriate if a bronchodilator inhaler has to be used more than once a day. It follows therefore that inhaled bronchodilator therapy alone should only be used by patients with mild asthma. However, all patients able to use an inhaler should have one, to be used for symptom relief as necessary, irrespective of the other treatments required for their asthma. The inhalation of a short-acting bronchodilator prior to exercise is often necessary to prevent exercise-induced asthma.

All patients with asthma should be aware that a β_2 agonist bronchodilator inhaler only provides short-term relief of symptoms, and that the development of asthmatic symptoms leading to more frequent use of this inhaler is a sure sign of worsening of asthma, which usually requires extra anti-inflammatory therapy. Little, short-lived or no response to a bronchodilator inhaler heralds the onset of potentially life-threatening asthma. All patients should be aware of this and should know that in this situation they should seek medical help at once.

The most commonly used β_2 agonists are salbutamol, terbutaline and fenoterol. Fenoterol has recently lost some of its popularity because of the possibility that adverse effects may be more likely with this drug than other β_2 selective bronchodilators [53,56–59]. For the relief of mild to moderate symptoms, the doses of salbutamol and terbutaline usually recommended are 100–200 µg and 250–500 µg respectively. Considerably larger doses are necessary for the treatment of severe acute asthma. The duration of action of these drugs is 4–6 h and the onset of activity is rapid, maximum bronchodilatation being achieved within 15 min after inhalation. Rimiterol is a β_2 agonist with a shorter duration of action (1–2 h) because, unlike salbutamol and terbutaline, it is rapidly metabolized by the enzymes catechol-O-methyltransferase and monoamine oxidase. The recommended dose of this short-acting β_2 agonist is 200–400 µg as required for symptom relief.

Long-acting β_2 agonists

Slow-release oral formulations of salbutamol and terbutaline are available and these increase the duration of activity of these bronchodilators considerably compared with conventional oral tablets. Prodrugs are also now available which, when given orally, also greatly increase the duration of bronchodilatation (e.g. bambuterol is a prodrug of terbutaline, to which it is metabolized by hydrolysis). In general, however, inhaled therapy is preferable to oral since the inhaled route allows more rapid onset of bronchodilator activity and with a minute fraction of the dose necessary to achieve a similar clinical response via the oral route; this therefore reduces the risks of adverse effects [60].

The production of β_2 agonists with a long duration of action when administered by inhalation has created a new era of bronchodilator therapy [61]. Salmeterol has a molecule with a long lipophilic tail that adheres tightly to regions in the receptor or adjacent to it while its head engages the active site. Even when displaced by an antag-

onist its activity resumes after the antagonist is washed free [62]. Eformoterol is even more potent but less adherent, its high lipophilicity retaining it in the receptor region. These long-acting bronchodilators have the advantage of being effective when used twice daily, although their role in the routine management of the asthmatic patient is far from clear. They do not have any clinically relevant anti-inflammatory effects and therefore should not be used as primary treatment of asthma, since patients who require more than occasional use of a short-acting β_2 agonist should be treated with an anti-inflammatory drug, usually an inhaled corticosteroid [1,55,63]. Salmeterol has been shown to be effective in the treatment of asthma of almost all degrees of severity [62–69], and its long duration of action is obvious convenient for patients. However, the controversy about the possible dangers of regular treatment with short-acting β_2 agonists [49–59] must be considered before recommending the regular use of drugs like salmeterol and eformoterol. Indeed, it could be postulated that if short-acting β_2 agonists are in any way detrimental when given regularly in the long-term management of asthma, there could be greater problems with long-acting β_2 agonists because they are more potent bronchodilators [49,51,70]. The more effective and prolonged bronchodilator efficacy of drugs like salmeterol could allow more specific and non-specific bronchial insults with irritant or allergen triggers before bronchoconstriction breaks through and hence the resulting acute episode could be more severe than one prevented by short-acting bronchodilator therapy. This theoretical danger has not been a problem in clinical practice in postmarketing surveillance studies of salmeterol; nevertheless the drug's use should be restricted to patients whose asthmatic symptoms are not controlled by inhaled corticosteroid therapy in doses unlikely to be associated with long-term adverse effects. The major debate about long-acting inhaled bronchodilator treatment is whether to start salmeterol or eformoterol if asthma is not well controlled with low-dose or high-dose inhaled corticosteroid therapy [71]. It has been pointed out that the much-publicized asthma guidelines [1,55,63] vary somewhat with regard to recommendations about drug use as well as classification of asthma severity [72]. Salmeterol is recommended for patients who have local laryngeal or oropharyngeal adverse effects of inhaled corticosteroids that do not allow high-dose therapy to be used [1]. Also, it would appear to be sensible to use this form of treatment once daily at night for patients already on an inhaled corticosteroid but who continue to have more than occasional nocturnal symptoms [60]. The addition of salmeterol to the treatment of patients whose asthma was not well controlled by treatment with a low dose of inhaled beclometasone (beclomethasone) dipropionate (200 µg twice daily) has been shown to be at least as effective as increasing the dose of inhaled beclometasone (500 µg twice daily) [71]. Studies are now in progress in which attempts are being made to assess the control, or the suppression, of markers of inflammation by low-dose inhaled corticosteroid therapy plus long-acting inhaled β_2 agonists compared with high-dose inhaled corticosteroid therapy in the treatment of patients with asthma whose symptoms are not well controlled by inhaled corticosteroid treatment in conventional low doses. The preliminary results of these studies suggest that long-acting inhaled β_2-agonist bronchodilator preparations are not associated with adverse effects. The role of eformoterol is likely to be more controversial than that of salmeterol because it has a much more rapid onset of bronchodilator activity and could therefore be used as a relief inhaler with a long duration of activity.

Side-effects of β_2 agonists

Large doses of β_2 agonists can produce adverse metabolic and cardiovascular effects [73–75]. However, these events only occur when very large doses are used and even then are rarely of clinical importance. The β_2 agonists are extremely safe drugs even when large doses are used, especially when given by inhalation and with oxygen. Unwanted cardiovascular effects include tachycardia, increased cardiac output, inotropism and ECG changes. Cardiac dysrhythmias are usually asymptomatic and rarely occur in patients who do not have pre-existing heart disease. General systemic effects include hypokalaemia and hyperglycaemia, increased free fatty acids, hypomagnesaemia, increased blood lactate and uterine relaxation. The only general unwanted effect that often causes patient concern is skeletal muscle tremor which, while not serious, can be distressing [76]. The individual response to tremor is highly variable but to some extent is dose dependent and, unlike bronchodilatation, tachyphylaxis occurs rapidly in the majority of patients. Tremor therefore is usually only a problem when β_2 agonists are being given for the first time.

The predictable physiological adverse effects of β_2 agonists rarely cause any serious clinical events. Most depend on route of administration and dose. Conventional doses administered by an inhaler for 'as-necessary' relief of the symptoms of chronic asthma can be assumed to be free from all unwanted effects, except for tremor in a few patients. Larger doses given orally, by inhalation or intravenously are associated with demonstrable unwanted effects, but only rarely are these of clinical significance. High-dose treatment for the control of chronic persistent asthma should of course be avoided; however, large doses of β_2 agonists, usually by inhalation, are essential for the treatment of severe acute asthma and patients should not be denied this treatment simply because of the theoretical risks of adverse effects.

Theophylline

In the USA in the 1970s and early 1980s, theophylline (1,3-dimethylxanthine) was the most commonly prescribed bronchodilator. Detailed study of its pharmacokinetics and the development of sustained-release preparations, often monitored by theophylline serum levels, improved the therapeutic value of this drug by increasing its efficacy and decreasing its adverse effects. However, emphasis on the importance of anti-inflammatory therapy coupled with the simplicity and assumed safety of inhaled β_2 agonists led to a decline in its use. It still has a role in the management of nocturnal asthma resistant to other forms of treatment, and is prescribed for many patients with severe chronic asthma in an attempt to avoid oral corticosteroid therapy. Paediatricians use theophylline more often than clinicians treating adult patients with asthma, mainly because it is easier for children to be treated with oral preparations, because many are unable to use inhalers and perhaps also because young children are less likely to be aware of side-effects. Theophylline relaxes smooth muscle by inhibition of phosphodiesterase and probably via other mechanisms [77]. A serum theophylline concentration of 10–20 μg/mL was recommended, since below this range bronchodilatation is unlikely and above it symptoms of toxicity are common [78,79]. A dose–response relationship can be shown in chronic stable asthma with increasing serum concentrations of theophylline up to 20 μg/mL, serum concentrations of 15 and 20 μg/mL achieving bronchodilatation similar to that of conventional doses of salbutamol administered by metered dose inhaler (MDI) [80]. In most patients there is also a direct relationship between serum theophylline levels and side-effects, the most troublesome being nausea, vomiting, headache, nervousness and irritability. Because these toxic effects are common, the popularity of theophylline has declined markedly. There is an additive bronchodilator effect when theophylline is given in combination with β_2 agonists [81–83], and in an attempt to decrease adverse effects low doses of theophylline preparations have been used in combination with salbutamol or terbutaline. However, this therapeutic approach requires regular β_2 agonist, which should be avoided in the treatment of asthma whenever possible. Theophylline has been shown to increase the contractility of the diaphragm and render it less susceptible to fatigue [84], and also to increase maximal transdiaphragmatic pressure [85]. However, these actions of the drug are not likely to be of much clinical significance in asthma, except perhaps in severe acute episodes. Of much more interest recently has been the discovery that theophylline has anti-inflammatory properties, although the relevance of these to the treatment of asthma is far from clear. Type IV phosphodiesterase inhibitors, including theophylline, have been shown to effect changes in the activity and function of macrophages

[86,87] and lymphocytes [88,89]. Theophylline has been shown to reduce eosinophil infiltration of the airway [90] and to produce a reduction in eosinophil activity after prolonged treatment [91]. Also, unlike β_2 agonists, theophylline modulates the late asthmatic response [92–95]. It has been suggested that theophylline may provide clinical effects comparable to those of low-dose inhaled corticosteroids in selected asthmatics [96,97]. The evidence suggests that theophylline has anti-inflammatory properties at doses lower than those necessary to achieve the conventional therapeutic serum level (10–20 µg/mL) required for optimal bronchodilatation. However, the role of theophylline in the treatment of the basic underlying eosinophilic inflammation of asthma has yet to be determined, and may be minimal. In the future, low-dose theophylline in combination with other drugs may become more established in the management of mild to moderate chronic asthma, although until more knowledge of the efficacy of such treatment is available oral theophylline therapy should be reserved for patients whose asthma is not controlled with conventional doses of inhaled corticosteroids. However, intravenous aminophylline continues to have an important role in the management of patients with severe acute asthma.

Anticholinergic agents

The drugs of this category (muscarinic antagonists) most widely used in the treatment of reversible airways disease are ipratropium bromide and oxitropium bromide. It is generally accepted that they are more effective in chronic obstructive pulmonary disease, i.e. chronic bronchitis and emphysema, than in chronic asthma [61]. In chronic stable asthma, ipratropium bromide produces a smaller response of delayed onset compared with salbutamol [98], although older asthmatics may respond better to anticholinergic agents than do younger patients [99,100]. In chronic asthma these drugs are usually reserved for use in patients who have not responded to conventional doses of an inhaled corticosteroid, when they are added to the treatment regimen as regular inhaled therapy (ipratropium bromide 20–40 µg three or four times daily, or oxitropium bromide 200 µg two or three times daily). Ipratropium bromide is of much greater value in the treatment of the severe acute episode than it is in the routine treatment of most patients with chronic asthma.

Drugs with anti-inflammatory properties used to influence the underlying inflammatory mechanisms of asthma (the preventers)

Sodium cromoglycate (cromoglycate) and nedocromil sodium

Sodium cromoglycate was first synthesized and its use in asthma reported in a small trial in 1967 [101]. Its clinical efficacy was established in both adults and children in a series of clinical trials performed in different parts of the world [102–111], although in recent years its use has been almost completely restricted to the treatment of childhood asthma [112–114]. In the main this has been due to the often irrational fears of treating children with inhaled corticosteroids, sodium cromoglycate being preferred because it is virtually free from side-effects. This drug continues to be prescribed as first-choice treatment for atopic asthmatic children, particularly those with exercise-induced asthma, despite reports of early treatment failure and greater efficacy of low-dose inhaled corticosteroids [115–119]. To be optimally effective it has to be taken regularly at least four times daily and this very frequently leads to problems with compliance, which may be the explanation of treatment failure in some patients. Sodium cromoglycate has no role in the treatment of severe acute asthma.

Nedocromil has an extremely good safety record, although some patients find its taste unpleasant. An attempt to disguise this has been made by adding mint flavouring to the inhaler. The role of this drug in the management of chronic asthma is difficult to define [120–123]. It has little place in primary treatment, since its anti-inflammatory properties and clinical efficacy are inferior to those of inhaled corticosteroids. However, it may be of value in patients not well controlled by conventional doses of an inhaled corticosteroid and should be used as a corticosteroid-sparing agent in patients on oral and high-dose inhaled corticosteroids [124,125]. Compared with sodium cromoglycate, the evidence suggests that it is at least as good, or even superior, in the treatment of adult chronic asthmatics [126–128]. Like sodium cromoglycate it has no role in the treatment of severe acute asthma.

H_1-receptor antagonists

Although effective in the treatment of allergic rhinitis, antihistamines have little place in the treatment of asthma. The evidence for and against the use of these drugs in asthma has been extensively reviewed and it is apparent that the few patients who may benefit from these compounds are young atopic individuals with mild seasonal symptoms [129].

Ketotifen is a commonly used drug, especially in underdeveloped countries. It is a non-competitive H_1-receptor antagonist and *in vitro* has an inhibitory effect on mast cells similar to that of sodium cromoglycate. In challenge studies ketotifen has an immediate bronchoprotective effect, although there are no convincing clinical trial data to confirm its value in the long-term treatment of asthma. Like many of the early antihistamines, the most common side-effect of ketotifen is drowsiness, which occurs in over 20% of patients [129].

Inhaled corticosteroids

Corticosteroids have been used in the treatment of asthma for nearly half a century [130,131]. The early treatment of both acute and chronic asthma was with adrenocorticotrophin (ACTH). However, following the development of a number of glucocorticosteroids, prednisolone became the standard oral therapy, and hydrocortisone and methylprednisolone have become established as the most commonly chosen corticosteroids for intravenous administration. The treatment of asthma with systemic corticosteroids in sufficiently high doses to control symptoms led to the development in many patients of numerous adverse effects, which ironically were all outside the respiratory tract. This stimulated the pharmaceutical search for a drug that was locally active in the control of asthma when inhaled but not absorbed from the lungs or gastrointestinal tract in sufficient quantities to have the same degree of systemic side-effects. The breakthrough came in the early 1970s when beclomethasone dipropionate and betamethasone valerate were found to have high topical activity in the bronchi with low systemic availability. Very soon after this, triamcinolone acetonide and flunisolide were found to possess similar pharmacokinetic profiles, and almost a decade later budesonide was introduced as a corticosteroid with a higher topical activity than those already established in the treatment of chronic asthma. Recently, approximately a decade further on, fluticasone propionate was marketed as a more potent drug than budesonide. The role of this drug has yet to be established since it appears to have greater topical activity than budesonide in terms of control of asthmatic symptoms, but may also have greater systemic activity when absorbed from the lungs.

There can be no doubt that the development of inhaled corticosteroids revolutionized asthma therapy. In the early 1970s there were enthusiastic reports of the efficacy of inhaled corticosteroids assessed in uncontrolled studies [132,133], followed by confirmation of efficacy by the publication of the results of well-designed placebo-controlled studies [134–136]. These showed that withdrawal of oral prednisolone and substitution with an inhaled corticosteroid did not result in poorer control of asthmatic symptoms but did allow worsening of atopic nasal and skin problems, thus confirming the topical, rather than systemic, activity of inhaled corticosteroid therapy. Beclomethasone dipropionate was first introduced into clinical practice in a recommended dose of 400 µg daily (100 µg four times daily). The careful controlled clinical trials in which this drug was substituted for oral prednisolone indicated that this four-times-daily dose of beclomethasone dipropionate, and also betamethasone valerate, was equivalent to 7 or 8 mg of prednisolone [137]. The introduction of topical inhaled corticosteroid therapy thus allowed withdrawal of systemic corticosteroid therapy in the majority of patients previously treated with these drugs and allowed a considerable reduction in dose in those patients with very severe disease requiring treatment with high doses of prednisolone.

Inhaled glucocorticosteroids have now become first-line therapy for the treatment of chronic asthma in most countries. They are the most effective therapy available and have been shown to have beneficial effects on bronchial wall inflammation and airway hyperresponsiveness as well as symptoms. Bronchial biopsies of patients being treated with inhaled corticosteroids have shown a reduction in the number and activation of inflammatory cells in the airway [138–141] and also restoration of the disrupted epithelium and normalization of the ratio of ciliated cells to goblet cells [138]. Inhaled corticosteroids reduce airway responsiveness to both direct and indirect stimuli. In acute challenge studies, the late response to allergen and the accompanying increase in airway responsiveness is reduced [142] and prolonged therapy protects against the early asthmatic response [143]. A single dose of inhaled corticosteroid fails to protect against exercise-induced asthma, but more prolonged therapy does [144,145]. Chronic treatment reduces airway responsiveness to inhaled histamine and methacholine, although this may take up to 3 months or even longer [143,145–150]. Corticosteroids presumably improve airway responsiveness by reducing the underlying inflammation, although any component of the airways disease caused by structural changes in the bronchial wall, such as thickening of the basement membrane and airway muscle hypertrophy, may be irreversible. Indeed there is now evidence which suggests that if inhaled corticosteroid therapy for asthma is delayed the response, as judged by objective measurements of pulmonary function, is less good than when this treatment is given quickly after the diagnosis has been made [151–153]. It has not yet been established whether prolonged therapy with inhaled corticosteroids can overcome this problem, or whether this indicates irreversible bronchial wall changes that cannot be remodelled. One study showed that there was no 'catch up' in the delayed treatment group after 1 year [151]. These findings have led to the concept of early intervention with inhaled corticosteroids in the treatment of asthma.

Numerous controlled clinical trials have now established that corticosteroids are effective in controlling symptoms of asthma and in reducing the number and severity of exacerbations. This proven efficacy of inhaled corticosteroids, coupled with our knowledge that inflammation is found even in patients with very mild asthma, has indeed led to the use of these drugs at a much earlier stage in treatment [154]. A low dose of an inhaled corticosteroid (e.g. budesonide 200 µg daily) is effective in mild asthma [155], as is once-daily therapy [156]. The various guidelines for asthma therapy recommend this form of treatment for any patient symptomatic enough to require the use of a bronchodilator inhaler more than once daily [1,55,157].

High-dose inhaled corticosteroid is now frequently used in many countries for treatment of patients with more severe disease [158]. This significantly reduces the need for maintenance oral corticosteroids, and many patients with 'difficult to control' chronic asthma have benefited from this treatment [158–161], although the value of high-dose compared with low-dose therapy has been questioned [162]. Inhaled corticosteroids are effective in the treatment of asthma because they control bronchial wall inflammation, although this may take many weeks to be achieved [138]. When treatment is withdrawn, there is usually an increase in airway responsiveness and recurrence of symptoms to pretreatment levels presumably because of recurrence of bronchial inflammation [147,163–165]. The longer treatment is given, the more likely the possibility of a prolonged remission; indeed, the ultimate aim of treatment is the induction of a complete remission by inhibition of the inflammatory process, or of prolonged remissions by intermittent courses of therapy. A clinically worthwhile prolonged remission is more likely in mild asthmatics treated soon after the onset of their disease. Early treatment is also important since it has been shown that objective response to inhaled corticosteroid therapy is significantly better in patients treated soon after the onset of symptoms compared with treatment delayed by 2 years or more [151–153]. The evidence that there is a better objective response when inhaled corticosteroids are given early after the onset of asthmatic symptoms suggests that irreversible and permanent pathological changes, possibly fibrosis in the bronchial wall, occur at an early stage even in patients with mild asthma. Theoretically this treatment should reduce the irreversible component of airway narrowing seen in patients with more severe poorly controlled disease [166–168]. Whether inhaled corticosteroids reduce the mortality from asthma remains to be demonstrated. The Saskatchewan study of asthma deaths and near-death attacks [169] suggested that this therapy does have this effect, although the numbers studied were too small to reach a firm conclusion.

Although most patients with asthma respond to corticosteroids, there is a small minority who appear to be resistant or much less responsive to these drugs. Disease of this type has been called steroid-resistant asthma [170]. This problem is not explained by pharmacokinetic abnormalities such as impaired absorption or rapid elimination of oral corticosteroids. Compared with normal individuals and corticosteroid-sensitive asthmatics, these patients have been found to have a significantly different response to beclomethasone dipropionate applied to their skin [171], suggesting that this phenomenon is not organ-specific. Corticosteroid-resistant asthma can be defined as a less than 15% improvement in forced expiratory

volume in 1 s (FEV_1) or PEF to treatment with oral prednisolone in a daily dose of 40 mg given for a period of at least 2 weeks in a patient in whom all other exacerbating asthma factors have been excluded or removed. Patients with asthma resistant to the beneficial effects of corticosteroids have been the focus of much *in vitro* research and abnormalities of peripheral blood cell behaviour have been detected [172]. It is anticipated that if the crucial defect in these patients can be determined, this will lead to the discovery of how corticosteroids exert their beneficial effects in asthma and thus to a focused approach in searching for a cure of this common disease. Corticosteroid-resistant asthma has been comprehensively reviewed [172].

Local side-effects

The most frequent side-effects of inhaled corticosteroids are local effects on the upper airways caused directly by oropharyngeal deposition; these are discussed below.

Oropharyngeal candidiasis

The reported incidence of oropharyngeal candidiasis has varied greatly (5–77%) because of the different criteria used for diagnosis, ranging from a throat swab positive on culture for *Candida albicans* to clinical thrush requiring treatment, and also whether cross-sectional or cumulative analyses have been made [173–177]. Oropharyngeal candidiasis is much less common in children than it is in adults [178,179]. The incidence of thrush is related to the daily dose of inhaled corticosteroid and possibly also to dosing frequency [177,180,181]. The combined use of oral and inhaled corticosteroids does not appear to increase the incidence of candidiasis [173,174,181]. The use of large-volume spacer attachments to the conventional MDI appears to offer some protection against the development of thrush [182,183]. Oropharyngeal candidiasis tends to develop more readily in patients who have a positive *C. albicans* throat swab [184] but is seldom a major clinical problem, can usually be controlled with topical treatment using nystatin or amphotericin, and rarely necessitates withdrawal of inhaled corticosteroid therapy [185]. Oesophageal candidiasis is a very rare complication of inhaled corticosteroid therapy [186]. Candidiasis of the lower respiratory tract has not been reported to have been caused by inhaled corticosteroid treatment.

Dysphonia

Dysphonia or hoarseness of the voice is a much more common problem than candidiasis in patients being treated with inhaled corticosteroids. It occurs to some degree in one-third to half of patients [177,187] and has been reported to be due to a local corticosteroid myopathy of the vocal cord muscles, which is reversible after withdrawal of treatment [188] but which, unlike thrush, tends to recur when treatment is restarted [189]. The occurrence of dysphonia is related to the total daily dose of inhaled corticosteroid but not to dose frequency [177,187]. Large-volume spacers do not provide any protection against the development of voice problems [180,187], since they increase rather than decrease drug deposition in the region of the larynx and could therefore theoretically make the problem worse. There is some evidence that dry powder inhalers (DPIs) cause fewer voice problems than conventional pressurized MDIs with or without spacer attachments [190,191].

Cough and throat irritation

Cough and non-specific throat irritation are also common complaints of patients using inhaled corticosteroids [187]. Corticosteroid inhaler-induced cough is much more common with pressurized MDIs than with DPIs and is more often caused by the additives in the inhaler, such as surfactants, rather than the drugs [192,193]. Inhaler-induced cough is often associated with bronchoconstriction [192,194] and pressurized aerosol inhalers should be changed to dry powder systems whenever patients have this problem [193]. Non-specific throat irritation is quite common in patients being treated with inhaled corticosteroids [187], although this is rarely of more than nuisance value and tends to be less of a problem when DPIs are used.

Other local side-effects

There is no evidence to suggest an increase in infections, including tuberculosis, of the lower respiratory tract after prolonged use of inhaled corticosteroids [178,179], and this treatment does not adversely influence pre-existing colonization of the bronchi with *Aspergillus fumigatus* in patients with allergic bronchopulmonary aspergillosis [195]; indeed it is useful in the long-term management of this condition [196]. Biopsy studies have failed to demonstrate any bronchial mucosal abnormalities, even after treatment for over 10 years [138,197].

Systemic side-effects

Inhaled corticosteroid treatment was first introduced in a recommended dose of 100 µg four times daily. Subsequently it was found that a dose regimen of 200 µg twice daily was as effective as administration four times daily in maintaining control of chronic asthma. In low doses of up to 400 µg daily it is possible to detect evidence of systemic absorption and activity by assessment of hypothalamic–pituitary–adrenal (HPA) axis function [198], although these minor changes are of no clinical

importance even after prolonged therapy [178]. Indeed the lack of systemic activity allows recurrence of disorders such as eczema and allergic rhinitis when beclomethasone dipropionate or betamethasone valerate is substituted for oral steroids in atopic asthmatics. Despite initial fears regarding the potential side-effects of long-term inhaled corticosteroids, only the minor local upper respiratory problems of oropharyngeal candidiasis and dysphonia have occurred [178].

In recent years, however, much larger doses of inhaled corticosteroids have been used in the treatment of asthmatic patients whose symptoms are not controlled by low-dose therapy, and high doses of these drugs are inevitably associated with systemic effects. These arise from absorption of drug from the lung and the gastrointestinal tract. Adverse effects from swallowed drug depend upon first-pass liver metabolism. Budesonide is more efficiently inactivated by the liver than is beclomethasone dipropionate. The recently introduced fluticasone propionate is almost completely inactivated by the liver when ingested [199] but, like all corticosteroids clinically effective in the treatment of asthma by the inhaled route, gives rise to systemic effects from the fraction deposited in the lung. This is because drug reaching the lung is very rapidly absorbed without metabolism and is consequently available for systemic activity [200]. Therefore, all inhaled corticosteroid preparations in clinical use give rise to systemic effects if high enough doses are inhaled. The differentiation between 'low-dose' and 'high-dose' therapy is now generally accepted. In effect this separates therapy assumed to be safe (low dose) and free from systemic effects from high-dose therapy that might be associated with unwanted systemic corticosteroid effects if given long term. However, the advantages and disadvantages of long-term low-dose and high-dose inhaled corticosteroid therapy are somewhat controversial [201]. It is generally accepted that in adults total daily doses of beclomethasone dipropionate or budesonide up to and including 800 µg are safe and are defined as 'low dose', while 'high-dose' therapy is 800–2000 µg daily [1]. Long-term treatment with doses in excess of 2000 µg (or 1000 µg of fluticasone propionate) should be assumed to be able to cause systemic adverse effects in some of the patients. However, it must be emphasized that, in the main, the amount of drug absorbed from the lung determines the magnitude of systemic activity, and the pulmonary deposition efficiency of different inhalation delivery systems varies considerably. Hence, it is inappropriate to assume that the nominal doses of different inhalers achieve similar therapeutic and adverse effects. Thus, a clinically very effective inhaler must also be expected to have a higher systemic effect than a device that achieves a lower pulmonary deposition [154]. There is a great need for the equivalence of inhaled drugs to be assessed in order to lessen the confusion in this important area of asthma management [202,203].

HPA axis function

A large number of studies have assessed the effects of inhaled corticosteroids on HPA axis function. Researchers have focused on the HPA axis because assessments of its function are very much more simple to make than any other estimation of the systemic activity of corticosteroid treatment. However, it is not possible to use HPA axis function abnormalities induced by exogenous corticosteroid treatment to assess the risk of other adverse effects of long-term treatment, such as osteoporosis. Few studies have compared the effects on HPA axis function of the various inhaled corticosteroid preparations available for clinical use, and the findings of these studies are conflicting [154]. However, as one would expect, there appears to be a dose-dependent effect and it has to be assumed that the risk of all systemic adverse effects is dose dependent. Undoubted improvement in HPA function has been established when oral corticosteroid therapy has been replaced by inhaled treatment with beclomethasone dipropionate or budesonide in doses of up to 2000 μg daily [204–206]. Considering all the published data on beclometasone dipropionate and budesonide and HPA axis function, it can be assumed that clinically significant HPA suppression is unlikely to occur with daily doses up to and including 1500 μg in adults and 400–800 μg in children [154].

Osteoporosis

One of the most feared unwanted effects of systemic corticosteroids is osteoporosis [207]. Although low-dose inhaled therapy in adults has been proved to be safe (except perhaps in patients who have received oral corticosteroid treatment prior to substitution with inhaled drugs), the recent increased use of inhaled drugs in high dose has given rise to some doubt about its effect upon bone metabolism. The effects of inhaled corticosteroids on biochemical markers of bone metabolism, such as bone-specific serum alkaline phosphatase, serum osteocalcin, urinary hydroxyproline, calcium and pyridinium cross-links, have been assessed in many short-term studies, even though the relevance of these markers to the risk of development of osteoporosis in the distant future is far from clear. The results of long-term studies of bone density in patients being treated with different doses of different inhaled corticosteroids will have to be awaited before any conclusions about the risks of high-dose therapy and osteoporosis can be made. Clinical trial data so far available raise the possibility of clinically significant osteoporosis developing as a result of long-term high-dose inhaled corticosteroid treatment, although skeletal fracture has not yet been reported as a direct result of such treatment [154]. Those patients at greatest risk are postmenopausal women, the inactive and smokers.

Growth in children

Knemometry studies have made it possible to measure accurately linear growth velocity of the lower leg over short periods of time. However, the relationship of this measurement to long-term statural growth has not been determined. However, knemometry is a sensitive method of assessing systemic activity of corticosteroid treatments. It has been shown that budesonide delivered via a large-volume spacer in a dose of 400 μg does not adversely affect lower leg growth velocity [208–210]. Knemometry is extremely sensitive since it has been found that prednisolone in the small dose of 2.5 mg totally suppresses short-term lower leg growth [211]. However, this emphasizes the fact that knemometry is not a measurement of statural growth since although small doses of prednisolone may suppress growth, complete suppression is unlikely. Long-term treatment with budesonide in doses of 400–800 μg daily does not suppress statural growth in children [152].

Other systemic effects

The increased risk of the development of subcapsular cataracts in patients being treated with systemic corticosteroids is well known, although despite isolated reports there is no convincing evidence that inhaled corticosteroids cause cataracts in adults or children [154]. Similarly, although minor metabolic effects can be detected, there is no evidence that inhaled corticosteroids result in clinically significant changes in glucose or lipid metabolism.

Leukotriene antagonists

Several orally administered leukotriene antagonists have recently been released on the market, and it is likely that other variants will soon be available. It is possible that they may have a role in the treatment of mild asthma or as corticosteroid-sparing drugs, although it is premature to assess their therapeutic role or safety in long-term use. Their actions are considered in Chapter 9.

Systemic corticosteroids

Corticosteroids are used in asthma on account of their anti-inflammatory properties, and it is unfortunate that no drug has yet been synthesized that separates these from the metabolic effects responsible for many of their side-effects. The drugs act in a common way. Steroids diffuse through the cell membrane and bind to intra-cytoplasmic (rather than membrane) receptors. The steroid–receptor complex binds with nuclear chromatin, inducing the production of an mRNA that promotes the synthesis of an effector protein responsible for the steroid actions. The anti-inflammatory actions include reduction in permeability and dilatation of blood vessels and suppression of accumulation of neutrophils; other effects include reduction in the numbers of circulating monocytes, eosinophils and basophils and extravascular sequestration of lymphocytes, together with inhibition of fibroblast proliferation. Steroids are considered in more detail in Chapter 9.

Oral corticosteroids, usually prednisolone, are the mainstay for aborting and treating acute exacerbations of asthma. Most patients who have suffered a severe attack can recognize the early signs, especially increasing tightness in the chest and failure to respond other than partially to their usual bronchodilator. Such patients should be provided with a supply of prednisolone and told to take it as soon as they realize an attack is starting. The dose may be judged on the patient's size and experience of previous attacks, although it is the author's practice to advise 30–60 mg daily until the chest feels normal, then reducing by 5 mg daily. This is discussed further in the section on acute exacerbations.

Oral corticosteroids are also necessary for the long-term management of patients with chronic asthma. Attempts should always be made to avoid this by maximizing other treatment and by using short intermittent courses, but in some patients control is impossible without regular prednisolone. When this is necessary, the dose should be kept as low as possible and periodic attempts should be made to wean the patient from the drug. The patient should be given a 'steroid card', on which is recorded the dose, duration of treatment, name and telephone number of the doctor and a brief list of emergency instructions. In many subjects this form of treatment is far from satisfactory, requiring as it does a balance between acceptable control of the disease and limitation of side-effects. Hospital asthma clinics are unfortunately full of patients with steroid facies, cataracts, osteoporotic vertebral crush fractures, bruised fragile skin, hypertension and diabetes; some alternative to this treatment is therefore highly desirable.

Parenteral hydrocortisone is used primarily in the management of the acute severe attack. The drug takes at least several hours to have a measurable effect on the airways, presumably depending on the severity of the mucosal inflammation and plugging of the lumen. Depending on an assessment of the severity of the condition at presentation, the dose varies from 100 mg to as high as 1 g. This is usually then repeated either in a constant infusion or as 6-hourly pulses until recovery occurs. This is discussed further in the section on acute severe asthma.

Other uses of parenteral steroids are in the occasional management of chronic severe asthma and patients incapable of taking their medicines reliably (see below). In addition, intermittent injections of ACTH have been used in the management of severe childhood asthma in the hope of avoiding long-term adrenal suppression.

Fortunately the need for this therapy has been much reduced by the advent of cromoglycate and inhaled corticosteroids.

As stated above, patients on long-term steroids should be maintained on the smallest dose consistent with proper control of the asthma. This is judged from the history of symptoms and from regular assessment of PEF or FEV_1, and no attempt should be made to wean patients from steroids without such careful monitoring. If it seems possible that a patient will manage without long-term steroids, the daily dose should be reduced very gradually (by 1 mg prednisolone each week) and adrenal function assessed periodically by short Synacthen tests. If the patient is successfully weaned from the drugs, he or she should be warned of possible adrenal hypofunction at times of future stress (e.g. operations) and should be told that future acute attacks of asthma will undoubtedly require short courses of steroids. Such patients are understandably reluctant to restart these drugs, and tragic deaths have occurred as a consequence.

In order to prevent the major side-effects of long-term treatment, patients with a history of indigestion should have concomitant therapy with an H_2 antagonist and considered for eradication therapy if there is evidence of *Helicobacter pylori* infection. Postmenopausal women should be encouraged to keep physically active and considered for hormone replacement therapy or other measures to prevent osteoporosis (discussed in Chapter 9).

General principles of drug use in the treatment of chronic asthma

The principles of management are based on the guidelines produced by the British Thoracic Society [1], the International Consensus Report on the Diagnosis and Management of Asthma [55] and Australian guidelines [63].

The stepwise approach to the treatment of asthma is based on the use of corticosteroids. It is now common practice to use long-acting β_2 agonists at an earlier stage than step 3 or 4, although it is accepted that they should always be used in combination with an inhaled corticosteroid. A rare exception to this would be the patient with severe dysphonia or, if less serious, interfering with their occupation, for example a professional singer. The initial management of asthma should be based on the principal aim of achieving optimal lung function and symptom control as quickly as possible initially, and subsequently deciding on the therapy required to maintain symptom control. On many occasions this would require the use of oral prednisolone or high-dose inhaled corticosteroid treatment initially with a subsequent titrated step-down thereafter according to symptoms and PEF recordings. PEF monitoring is essential in the early management of asthma especially when prednisolone or high-dose inhaled corticosteroid therapy is being used to achieve optimal asthma control.

Step 1

Occasional use of inhaled short-acting β_2-agonist bronchodilators. If more than occasional use (more than once daily or three times each week) is necessary, treatment with inhaled drugs that have a beneficial effect on the underlying asthmatic inflammatory process should be prescribed (Step 2 treatment). Treatment with an inhaled β_2 agonist alone is recommended if it is only used occasionally by a patient with mild asthma who is leading a normal active life and who is free from nocturnal and exercise-induced symptoms.

Step 2

Regular inhaled corticosteroid in a low dose of up to 800 µg daily (or 400 µg of fluticasone propionate) together with an inhaled β_2 agonist to be used as required. Alternatively, sodium cromoglycate or nedocromil sodium can be used instead of an inhaled corticosteroid, although these drugs are rarely as effective. Sodium cromoglycate is mainly used in the treatment of asthma in childhood.

Step 3

Inhaled short-acting β_2 agonist as required plus an inhaled corticosteroid in the dose range 800–2000 µg daily (or 400–1000 µg daily for fluticasone propionate). Large-volume spacers are recommended for use with the conventional pressurized MDI in order to reduce both local and systemic corticosteroid side-effects. The alternative to high-dose inhaled corticosteroid therapy is addition of a long-acting bronchodilator to low-dose inhaled corticosteroid.

Step 4

Inhaled short-acting β_2 agonist as required with an inhaled corticosteroid (800–2000 µg daily) plus a sequential therapeutic trial of one or more of (i) an inhaled long-acting β_2 agonist such as salmeterol xinafoate or eformoterol, (ii) a sustained-release theophylline, (iii) inhaled ipratropium bromide or oxitropium bromide, (iv) a long-acting oral β_2 agonist such as bambuterol, (v) nedocromil sodium or sodium cromoglicate or (vi) high-dose inhaled bronchodilators.

Step 5

The addition of oral corticosteroid (prednisolone) therapy to high-dose inhaled corticosteroid therapy and the other drug(s) found to be of benefit during the sequential therapeutic trial in step 4.

Increasing the dose of inhaled corticosteroid

Doubling the dose of inhaled corticosteroid irrespective of the actual maintenance dose appears to be an effective way of controlling minor exacerbations of asthma. This advice is given to most patients even though there is no clinical trial evidence to prove its effectiveness.

Short-course oral prednisolone treatment

Short courses of 'rescue' prednisolone are often required to regain control of symptoms during exacerbations. Prednisolone in a dose of 30–40 mg daily can be given to adults until 2 or 3 days after symptom control has been regained. Tapering of the dose is not necessary unless treatment has been required for more than 3 weeks [212].

Management of severe acute asthma

The clinical features of acute severe asthma are described in Chapter 34. The presentation can range from the moribund patient who has developed respiratory arrest to the apparently distressed breathless asthmatic whose disease is not life-threatening but who is hyperventilating in response to relatively mild airflow obstruction. It is therefore extremely important that an accurate assessment of the degree of severity of the acute episode is made, since the treatment necessary depends on the severity.

General measures

The majority of patients with severe acute asthma are frightened and distressed by their breathing difficulties, and this may stimulate the uninitiated to attempt relief by the administration of some form of sedative or anxiolytic drug. This is the most culpable mistake that can be made in the management of the distressed asthmatic [213,214]. Sedation must be avoided in all patients outside an intensive care area. Patients suffering a severe acute episode of asthma breathe with maximally efficient use of their respiratory muscles and despite this are unable to maintain normal arterial blood gas tensions. To suppress ventilation with any form of sedation is therefore likely to lead to deterioration. Very occasionally a patient with a mild attack of asthma can become excessively agitated and distressed and this can lead to inappropriate hyperventilation. In this situation the judicious use of a benzodiazepine by the experienced clinician may be of benefit, after the severity of the patient's asthma has been fully assessed objectively. In general terms, however, sedation of any type is contraindicated in severe acute asthma.

Prolonged severe asthma can lead to dehydration

because of lack of intake coupled with an increase in obligatory fluid loss. While intravenous replacement is rarely necessary, it is wise to have an intravenous access in all sick patients, the main purpose of this being to provide a route for drug administration should this become necessary, perhaps unexpectedly.

Electrolyte imbalance is theoretically possible in many patients because of side-effects of drug therapy but, like dehydration, is rarely a clinically significant problem. In particular, hypokalaemia should always be kept in mind since this can be induced by β_2-agonist and corticosteroid therapy in the doses used to treat some patients with severe acute asthma; this can be made worse by the overzealous use of potassium-free solutions for the treatment of theoretical dehydration or for the delivery of intravenous drugs such as aminophylline.

Physiotherapy is of no benefit in the treatment of the severe acute episode unless the patient also has another condition requiring a physiotherapist's assistance, such as bronchiectasis perhaps as a result of coexisting allergic bronchopulmonary aspergillosis. Even then the physiotherapy used must be gentle since the gymnastic rituals of treatments such as postural drainage are absolutely contraindicated in the distressed asthmatic.

Antibiotic treatment is very rarely necessary in the treatment of severe acute asthma, even though a majority of patients are prescribed an antibiotic such as amoxicillin (amoxycillin). Many exacerbations of asthma are triggered by upper respiratory tract viral infections and this often induces the clinician to prescribe antibiotic treatment. However, antibiotics are rarely necessary even if the patient produces scanty apparently purulent sputum. Bronchoconstriction itself, no matter what has triggered it, causes retention of bronchial secretions that might appear to be purulent, either because of minor bacterial infection or because of the presence of large numbers of eosinophils. In either case, treatment should be aimed at improving bronchoconstriction in order to allow the retained bronchial secretions to expectorated.

Specific treatment

There is no precise order for listing the essential treatments for severe acute asthma, since in critically ill patients most drugs and oxygen should be given at the same time. In the less severely ill, bronchodilator therapy alone may be the only treatment necessary. However, the majority of patients require a combination of treatments. Assessment of the degree of severity of the episode is essential and response to treatment must be assessed carefully with both clinical and objective measurements. The response to treatment of all patients with severe acute asthma should, when possible, include measurement of arterial blood gases (if abnormal initially) and PEF.

Oxygen

All dangerously ill patients with severe acute asthma are hypoxaemic, or are capable of suddenly becoming hypoxaemic, and oxygen treatment should therefore be routine. Patients with asthma become hypoxaemic and then hypercapnic because of asphyxia caused by severe airflow obstruction and not because of any pre-existing brainstem abnormality of response to oxygen or carbon dioxide (unlike the patient with severe chronic obstructive pulmonary disease). Oxygen should therefore be given by face mask in high concentration, and should only be adjusted according to Pao_2 measurements irrespective of any degree of carbon dioxide retention and respiratory acidosis. The most severely ill asthmatic, prior to death, has respiratory acidosis because of carbon dioxide retention as a result of alveolar hypoventilation caused by severe diffuse airways narrowing leading to asphyxia. These moribund patients are also hypoxaemic for the same reason (asphyxia) and are in need of treatment with oxygen in high concentrations, which unfortunately they are often denied because of the false assumption that high-concentration oxygen therapy in the presence of carbon dioxide retention in asthmatics is dangerous.

The aim should be to maintain a Pao_2 of at least 9 kPa (70 mmHg) and therefore blood gas monitoring of treatment is essential in all patients whose first blood gas analysis is abnormal. When hypoxaemia persists and hypercapnia worsens despite drug treatment (see below), assisted ventilation may be required. Most distressed asthmatics dislike closely fitting face masks and should be treated with masks designed to use the Venturi principle, or even nasal prongs if face masks cannot be tolerated. Those delivering 35% oxygen should be the ones used in the initial treatment of severe acute asthma, and masks delivering higher oxygen concentrations may be necessary. Oxygen tents may have to be used for the treatment of young children.

The administration of bronchodilator drugs, particularly when given intravenously, can theoretically result in worsening of hypoxaemia [215,216] and it is therefore prudent to administer oxygen before, during and after such treatment. Oxygen should be given in the ambulance during transfer from home to hospital, and general practitioners should be encouraged to give oxygen to sick asthmatics whenever possible.

β_2 Agonists

Nebulized administration of β_2 agonists has now become established as first-line treatment of severe acute asthma [217]. A large dose of one of these preparations, nebulized in oxygen, is at least as effective as the same drug given intravenously but is associated with less unwanted effects [218–220]. The dose of intravenous salbutamol required to achieve a better response than nebulized treatment is associated with unacceptable side-effects [221]. However, in one study of the early management of acute severe asthma in children, intravenous salbutamol was found to be more effective than when given by the nebulized route [222]. In most circumstances a combination of nebulized and intravenous administration of the same drug should be avoided; similarly, because of the unpredictable onset of activity of a subcutaneously injected β_2 agonist, this route of administration should also be avoided. Large doses of salbutamol (5 mg) or terbutaline (10 mg) should be nebulized as initial treatment, since the actual amount of drug reaching the bronchi is unpredictable. In patients who have the most severe airflow obstruction, the amount of drug reaching their bronchi is likely to be less than in those with less severe disease and it is therefore illogical to give all patients the same dose of inhaled β_2 agonist. The dose and frequency of administration should be tailored to disease severity and adherence to a strict drug–dose protocol must be avoided. Indeed, continuous nebulization may be successful in patients in whom repeated single treatments have failed [223]. Treatment with a nebulized β_2 agonist is unlikely to result in worsening of hypoxaemia [224], but oxygen therapy should not be interrupted during treatment of the hypoxaemic patient. Therefore ultrasonic nebulizers and air compressors driving jet nebulizers should not be used in hospitals for the treatment of severe acute asthma. Aerosol therapy delivered by intermittent positive-pressure breathing has no advantages over simple jet nebulizer treatment [225]. The response to a large dose of a nebulized β_2 agonist is rapid, and continued improvement of ventilatory function should not be expected to occur for more than 10–20 min [224,225]. Hence, if a patient remains unwell 10–20 min after this treatment, it should be repeated, possibly in combination with ipratropium bromide; in the very ill asthmatic, intravenous aminophylline should also be considered.

Large-volume spacers designed for use with the conventional MDI provide an alternative to the jet nebulizer for administration of large doses of β_2 agonists in the treatment of severe acute asthma [226]. Spacer devices can be used for the treatment of severe acute asthma outside hospital. Face masks allow young children to use large-volume spacers.

Occasionally it is necessary to give therapy intravenously. Salbutamol (4 μg/kg) or terbutaline (250–500 μg) can be given by slow intravenous injection and also by continuous intravenous infusion.

Anticholinergic agents

The quaternary ammonium compound ipratropium bromide is of limited therapeutic value in the treatment of chronic asthma but has an important role in the management of severe acute asthma. The onset of bronchodilator action of this drug is considerably slower than that of an inhaled β_2 agonist but it is as effective as salbutamol [227,228]. Because of the slow onset of action of ipratropium bromide it should not be used alone as primary treatment of a severe attack; when used in conjunction with a β_2 agonist, there is evidence that this combination is at least as good as, or better than, either drug given alone [227–231]. The value of this combination therapy has been questioned [232–234], although its use is recommended for patients whose asthma does not respond well to initial treatment with a nebulized β_2 agonist [1]. The dose of ipratropium most commonly used is 0.5 mg and there does not appear to be additional benefit if the dose is increased [235]. There are no data available to indicate how long ipratropium bromide should be continued in the treatment of severe acute asthma. However, it is unlikely that it needs to be used for more than 24 h in patients who respond satisfactorily to conventional therapy in the first few hours. Ipratropium bromide is usually given regularly every 4–6 h in combination with salbutamol or terbutaline.

Xanthine derivatives

Aminophylline has been used for many years in the treatment of severe acute asthma. However, nebulized β_2-agonist therapy has replaced intravenous theophyllines as first-line treatment of severe asthma for reasons of efficacy and safety. Aminophylline is of value in the moribund asthmatic and in the less severely ill patient who does not respond rapidly to treatment with oxygen, parenteral corticosteroids and nebulized bronchodilator therapy. An aminophylline infusion is recommended in a dose of 0.5–0.9 mg/kg/h, or 750 mg over 24 h in small patients and 1500 mg over 24 h in large individuals if the weight of the patient is unknown [1]. In the very severely ill patient a loading dose may be necessary (250 mg by slow intravenous injection, preferably over 20 min), although this should be avoided in the patient known to be taking an oral theophylline preparation. Lower doses may be needed in patients with liver or heart disease and in those taking cimetidine and most quinolone and macrolide antibiotics. Higher doses may be appropriate in smokers. If intravenous aminophylline therapy is necessary for more than a few hours, the dose should be adjusted according to theophylline blood levels.

Corticosteroids

The value of corticosteroid therapy in the management of severe asthma was first reported in 1949 [236] and confirmed by clinical trial in 1956 [237]. The value of these drugs in the treatment of the severely ill asthmatic has rarely been questioned [238] and their use should be routine in all patients who do not rapidly respond fully to bronchodilator therapy [239,240]. Large doses of intravenous hydrocortisone or methylprednisolone are usually given empirically since short-course high-dose systemic corticosteroid therapy is rarely responsible for adverse effects, except in the diabetic or patient with cardiac failure. Very high doses of these drugs are probably not necessary [241,242] and might occasionally give rise to an acute steroid myopathy [243]. Occasionally, patients on such doses also develop steroid psychosis, requiring rapid reduction of the dose. Doses of hydrocortisone producing blood levels that exceed stress-induced physiological levels have been recommended [244], i.e. 3–4 mg/kg loading dose followed by the same dose by intravenous infusion every 6 h. However, standard empirical doses of 100 or 200 mg every 4–6 h are used most frequently, intravenous therapy being rapidly replaced with prednisolone in doses of 40 or 60 mg daily. Oral prednisolone is usually given immediately at the same time as hydrocortisone and may be as effective as intravenous therapy in all but the most extremely ill patients [245].

Assisted ventilation

Assisted mechanical ventilation is rarely necessary but has to be used as a life-saving procedure in some patients who are either moribund on admission to hospital or deteriorate even though they have been treated as outlined above. The indications for assisted ventilation are difficult to define, since they range from the elective decision to ventilate because of lack of response to standard treatment in a patient who is becoming exhausted to the acute emergency resuscitation of the patient who has had a respiratory arrest. The generally accepted indications for the institution of mechanical ventilation include:
1 $Paco_2$ of more than 6.6 kPa (50 mmHg) and rising;
2 Pao_2 of less than 6.6 kPa (50 mmHg) and falling;
3 pH of 7.3 or less and falling;
4 intolerable respiratory distress;
5 exhaustion because of lack of response to conventional treatment;
6 respiratory arrest;
7 cardiorespiratory arrest.
The clinically dramatic indications for assisted ventilation in asthma, such as respiratory arrest, are obvious, although mechanical assistance of breathing should also be considered in the less obvious emergency. Physical exhaustion, especially when associated with systemic hypotension, is a dangerous combination and when there is any doubt about the necessity for assisted ventilation the safest course of action must be to ventilate rather than to procrastinate. When a patient with severe asthma has to be ventilated, there is some controversy about the method of assisted ventilation that should be employed. The use of high inflation pressures can theoretically cause baro-

trauma, and the use of controlled hypoventilation carries the risks of prolonged assisted mechanical ventilation [246–249]. The debate about the advantages and disadvantages of adopting policies of planned hypoventilation or the more aggressive approach of trying to normalize arterial blood gas tensions as quickly as possible will continue, and the decisions will depend upon local expertise and facilities available. However, there appears to be no doubt about the dangers of therapeutic lavage of asthmatic patients requiring assisted ventilation [250].

Inhalation delivery systems

Inhaled remedies have been used for centuries in the treatment of respiratory disorders and bronchodilator aerosols have been used for the treatment of asthma since at least 1935 [251]. In the early days, a number of ways were used to allow the inhalation of medicaments and aerosol inhalation was achieved by hand-held nebulizers driven by air generated by squeezing a rubber bulb. The conventional pressurized MDI was introduced into clinical practice as long ago as 1956 and its basic design has changed little in the last four decades.

Pressurized metered-dose inhaler

The pressurized MDI is the most commonly prescribed inhaler. It consists of a canister and a plastic actuator. When the canister is depressed into the actuator a measured amount of aerosol is released, the amount of which is determined by the valve in the actuator into which the canister nozzle is seated. Within the canister is drug either as a suspension or as a solution in volatile propellants under pressure (approximately 303 kPa in the case of chlorofluorocarbon, CFC, propellants). The canister of most inhalers also contains a dispersant or lubricant to ensure accurate dose delivery by the valve during multiple actuations of the inhaler. When the valve is actuated, the propellants and drug leave the inhaler at high velocity. The propellants evaporate very rapidly as soon as they leave the canister and this 'flashing' breaks up the liquid stream into droplets that continue to evaporate as they move away from the valve. Because of the high velocity of the aerosol cloud, together with the anatomical structure of the upper respiratory tract and the physical characteristics of the drug particles, the majority of the drug impacts in the oropharynx even when the pressurized MDI is used efficiently. Less than 25% of drug reaches the lung [252,253].

The most efficient way of using a pressurized MDI is as follows [254].
1 Shake the canister thoroughly (after removing the mouthpiece cover).
2 Place the mouthpiece of the actuator between the lips.
3 Breathe out steadily.

4 Release the dose while taking a slow, deep breath in.
5 Hold the breath in while counting to 10.

These instructions appear to be simple but many, if not the majority, of adults cannot use a pressurized MDI efficiently if the only instruction they receive is the manufacturer's package insert [255–259]. Also, more than 10% of patients develop an inefficient technique with prolonged use of the pressurized MDI [255,259], the majority of these being those who had some difficulty in using the device when it was first prescribed [260]. The main problem experienced is the coordination of dose release during inspiration [259], although a significant number of patients cannot continue to inhale through the mouth when the propellants are released into the mouth ('cold freon effect') [259]. It is rarely possible to teach these patients how to overcome this problem unless a spacer attachment to the pressurized MDI is used. Young children and the elderly experience the greatest difficulties using the conventional pressurized MDI, and for many of these patients spacers or holding chambers have to be used with the pressurized aerosol or alternative inhalation devices have to be prescribed.

Until recently all pressurized MDIs used CFCs as propellants, but because of the effect of these compounds on the ozone layer 80 nations agreed to ban their use before the beginning of the twenty-first century [261]. In some Western countries this ban was brought forward to 1995, with a temporary exemption for medicinal aerosols. Alternative propellants, such as tetrafluoroethane, have been produced and are now in clinical use or undergoing clinical trials. It is likely that because of the enforced change in the contents of the pressurized MDI brought about by the CFC ban, the opportunity will be taken to change or reduce the amounts of lubricants/surfactants in these inhalers, since these have been shown to produce cough and bronchoconstriction in a high proportion of patients [187,192–194].

Spacers or holding chambers

The principle behind the use of spacers is the fact that the drug aerosol cloud released from a pressurized MDI remains in suspension for many seconds before it is dispersed by gravity and other factors. Also the droplet size of aerosols is dependent on the distance from the actuator orifice. Experiments with tubes and holding chambers of different sizes led to the discovery that these devices could result in an increase in drug availability to the lungs and at the same time decrease the unwanted drug deposition in the oropharynx [262–264]. Large-volume spacers have proved to be of greater clinical value than small 'tube spacer' devices [263,265,266]. A one-way valve at the mouthpiece of a large-volume spacer enables it to contain the aerosol cloud before inhalation, and this overcomes the problem of coordinating dose-release and inhalation,

which therefore do not have to be synchronized when using spacer systems. The efficiency of spacer devices in terms of increasing pulmonary deposition of drug depends upon many factors, including their size, the presence or absence and characteristics of the one-way valve, the electrostatic charge of the plastics used to manufacture the device and the hygroscopic properties of the drug particles. The amount of drug available from the many different spacer systems varies enormously and it is recommended that each device be evaluated for each drug used [267–271]. Large-volume spacers decrease oropharyngeal deposition of drug and their use is recommended for inhaled corticosteroids in order to decrease systemic side-effects (if they are not inactivated by first-pass liver metabolism when swallowed) and also to minimize the risk of oropharyngeal candidiasis [1,182,272–276]. The use of spacers for inhalation of corticosteroids does not cause too much inconvenience, since most treatment regimens are twice daily, although bulky spacer devices are much less convenient for the 'as-required' use of a bronchodilator. Spacers are now most often used in the treatment of children with asthma. In adults their main use is when corticosteroid therapy via the pressurized MDI has to be taken in high dose [1]. However, they can be used as alternatives to nebulizers in chronic [277,278] and severe [226] asthma. Spacers do not decrease the amount of drug deposited in the region of the larynx and do not protect against dysphonia, the most common local side-effect of inhaled corticosteroids [187,251].

Breath-actuated metered-dose inhaler

The conventional pressurized MDI has been made easier to use by making it breath-actuated. The canister is completely enclosed within the body of the actuator and, depending on the design, is primed by opening a hinged mouthpiece cover or lifting a latching lever on top of the device. When primed, the valve is actuated by a low inspiratory flow in the region of 30 L/min. These devices are easier to use than the conventional pressurized MDI [279,280] and can be triggered by patients with severe airflow obstruction [281].

Dry powder inhalers

DPIs depend entirely upon the patient's inspiratory effort and are generally easier to use than the conventional pressurized MDI [260]. The first DPIs to be introduced were single dose (Spinhaler soon followed by the Rotahaler) and had to be reloaded with a cartridge/capsule containing micronized drug in a large particle carrier powder, usually lactose.

The second generation of DPIs carry multiple doses (range 4–200) and are more convenient than single-dose inhalers. The four-dose and eight-dose Diskhalers have to be reloaded after all the foil blisters on the Rotadisk have been punctured; other devices such as the Accuhaler, which like the Diskhaler uses the aluminium foil blister system, are disposable after its 60 doses have been used. The multidose DPIs that use a drug reservoir from which drug is fed by gravity into the dosing mechanism, such as the Turbohaler (Turbuhaler in the USA) and Klickhaler, contain up to 200 doses and are discarded when empty.

DPIs are less bulky than spacers and are as easy to use as the breath-actuated pressurized MDI, although some DPIs are less convenient because of the need to reload capsules/cartridges or discs frequently. Clinical comparisons of different DPIs indicate that patients prefer multidose devices to single-dose inhalers [282,283], and a meta-analysis of all available studies showed that 58% of 530 patients preferred a multidose DPI to the pressurized MDI [284]. The major drawback of DPIs is that their efficient use depends upon the patient being able to generate sufficient inspiratory flow to allow the drug to reach the lungs in therapeutic amounts. The various DPIs have vastly different inspiratory resistances, but there have been few comparisons of intrapulmonary drug deposition and clinical efficacy of these devices used at different inspiratory flow rates. This makes it difficult to give informed recommendations about the advantages and disadvantages of the numerous DPIs now available [260]. Children under the age of 6 years may not be able to generate sufficient inspiratory flow to use the Turbuhaler; the younger the child, the more likely this is the case [285]. It is known that the Turbuhaler is less efficient at an inspiratory flow rate of 30 L/min than at 60 L/min [285,286], and the Rotahaler has only about 10% of its maximum bronchodilator effect at inspiratory flow rates of 40 L/min [287]. Until direct comparisons of all DPIs have been made and data about optimal inspiratory flow rates are available, it has to be assumed that, unlike the pressurized MDI, the most efficient way of using a DPI is to breathe in through the device from residual volume as quickly and as deeply as possible. There is a need for more research on DPIs, especially with regard to the proportion of the dose reaching the lung, since this is extremely important when corticosteroid preparations are being inhaled. There is already evidence that the Turbuhaler is twice as efficient as the pressurized MDI for the inhalation of budesonide [288], while another study has suggested that another DPI is only about half as efficient as the pressurized MDI [253]. Immediately after DPIs are used for corticosteroid administration, gargling and mouth rinsing should be advised since this has been shown to decrease systemic effects from drug deposited in the oropharynx [289].

Nebulizers

Nebulizers are of two types: jet and ultrasonic. Jet nebulizers have widely differing characteristics with regard to the generation of particles within the respirable range [290] and the performance of individual nebulizers is influenced by many factors, such as the flow rate of the driving gas (air or oxygen), the nature of the drug solution or suspension, the fill-volume of the nebulizer chamber and, of course, the nebulization time [290–295]. For basic clinical purposes it is essential to be familiar with the characteristics of one nebulizer system, particularly the flow rate at which it functions most efficiently. For most clinical purposes jet nebulizers are more efficient than ultrasonic nebulizers. An ultrasonic nebulizer should be chosen for the administration of hypertonic saline to induce the production of sputum. For full details concerning the use of nebulizers the publication produced by the British Thoracic Society is recommended [296].

Immunotherapy

The treatment of asthma by antigen injection goes back to 1911, before its allergic basis was described, and such treatment remains in widespread and often uncritical use in some countries [297]. This continued use without clear evidence of value, together with the success achieved by bronchodilator drugs, has given immunotherapy a reputation of unorthodoxy. Nevertheless, there is evidence of efficacy in certain cases and it would be a pity if further research in this subject were to cease [298,299].

The principle of immunotherapy is to give initially small, then increasing, doses of pure antigen to a patient who is sensitive to that antigen in the hope of producing interference with the IgE–antigen-mediated reaction responsible for the symptoms. Whether this effect, when it occurs, is due to IgG blocking-antibody formation, a decrease in the sensitivity of mast cells to challenge or some other mechanism is not known [300,301]. Success of such therapy might therefore be expected to depend on selection of a patient in whom the symptoms are entirely or very largely due to the antigen in question and on the availability of a sufficiently pure form of the antigen in the vaccine. In keeping with these criteria, there is no evidence of the efficacy of immunotherapy in non-atopic asthma, asthma associated primarily with infection or in asthma with multiple allergic factors. The use of blunderbuss-type vaccines is strongly to be condemned, as is the use of vaccines in circumstances where treatment for anaphylactic reactions is not readily available. Indeed, use of such vaccines outside hospitals has been effectively prohibited in the UK [297].

There is some evidence of efficacy of immunotherapy in the treatment of hay fever and asthma associated with grass pollen and ragweed sensitivity, rhinitis and asthma associated with house-dust mite sensitivity, and similar symptoms related to exposure to cats and laboratory animals [302–308]. However, it has to be admitted that several equally well-controlled studies have failed to show differences between groups treated with active and placebo preparations, and a strong placebo effect has been present in most investigations [309,310]. It is to be expected that research will lead to the production of increasingly pure vaccines that, in turn, will increase the range of allergies treatable and the overall efficacy of the treatment.

At present, it is recommended that treatment be reserved for those few patients with clear evidence of sensitivity to house-dust mites or grass pollen (or ragweed pollen) in whom drug therapy proves ineffective or unacceptable. Such patients usually have conjunctival and nasal symptoms as well as asthma. Careful explanation of the likely outcome is advisable before starting: it is reasonable to predict an evens chance of some improvement and a small chance of a big improvement. Epinephrine (adrenaline) should be available for anaphylaxis and the patient should remain under observation for 2 h after the injection, although almost all reactions occur immediately. If the injections cause worsening of the asthma or any other suspicious symptoms, it is very unwise to continue the course. Use of such treatment for other allergic factors in asthma is best confined to allergy specialists engaged in research.

Miscellaneous problems in asthma management

Bronchopulmonary aspergillosis

The clinical manifestations of this syndrome vary from asthma associated with very occasional episodes of pulmonary eosinophilia to a severe progressive condition leading to lung fibrosis and bronchiectasis (see Chapter 34). Treatment should be judged by the response of the individual and not on the basis of studies that have shown average effects or lack of effects on groups of patients. Thus it is perfectly possible to maintain patients with milder manifestations on inhaled bronchodilators and inhaled steroids, so long as they are taught to treat exacerbations early with courses of high-dose oral steroids [196]. Asymptomatic episodes of pulmonary eosinophilia do occur in patients not on long-term oral steroids but only very rarely. If these are occurring, they may be detected at annual clinic visits by evidence of radiographic and functional deterioration. Such episodes, or frequent symptomatic attacks, or persistent presence of hyphae in the sputum require long-term oral steroids, again with increase in dose to cover exacerbations. It is in such patients, where the persisting antigenic stimulus due to survival and germination of the fungus in the airways leads to chronic disease, that consideration should be given to eradication of the organism. Newer oral antifungals are available (see Chapter 21) and promising results

have been reported with ketaconazole [311]. In severe cases where there is a risk of high-dose steroids leading to invasive disease, a course of amphotericin should be considered. A patient treated successfully with antifungal drugs would of course still remain sensitized to *A. fumigatus* and therefore liable to an exacerbation next time adequate numbers of spores are present in the air. Trials of pulsed antifungal therapy are ongoing, the aim being to eradicate the fungus with the first treatment and then to prevent recolonization with shorter courses of treatment every few months. The long-term outlook, and the effect of antifungal treatment on it, must therefore remain uncertain, although experience suggests that many such patients can be maintained well and without deterioration in lung function for many years on routine treatment of chronic asthma. It is probable that early diagnosis, before significant lung damage has occurred, is the secret of successful management.

Pregnancy

Many young female patients with asthma are understandably anxious about the effects of their illness on pregnancy and vice versa. Three problems merit discussion: the effects of asthma on pregnancy, the effects of drugs on the child and the chances of having an asthmatic child. The course of asthma during pregnancy is impossible to predict but usually is no different to that when the patient is not pregnant, improving in a few cases and requiring additional treatment in others [312,313]. It is wise to reassure the patient and to make oneself available for help with attacks should they occur. It is possible that very high steroid doses may have a deleterious effect on the early fetus, although it is likely that a severe asthma attack could have similar consequences. Either or both seem to increase the risk of mild pre-eclampsia [313]. The patient should be encouraged to use steroids in adequate dose early, so as to avoid the large doses that might be required in hospital. The other drugs used in asthma are not known to be toxic to the fetus, although clearly it is wise to confine treatment to inhaled drugs as far as possible except during acute exacerbations. Finally, patients who have had severe asthma are often worried that their children will suffer the same problem. It has to be admitted that this is possible, though the severity of asthma in several affected members is usually very different. There is no good genetic reason for an asthmatic patient to deny herself children.

Having discussed these matters, the management of asthma in pregnancy should be exactly as in the non-pregnant state. Care should be taken to explain this to the patient, who has a natural tendency to withdraw treatment and avoid drugs for the exacerbations that may ensue as a result. As always, time spent explaining this to the patient is time well spent.

Heart disease

The asthma patient who develops angina or hypertension is at risk of having β-blocking drugs prescribed and thus being made worse, sometimes acutely. Alternatives for hypertension are diuretics, methyldopa, reserpine, captopril, prazosin or nifedipine. For angina, vasodilators such as nitrates, verapamil or nifedipine are acceptable. From the cardiologist's point of view, drugs used in asthma may be undesirable; β$_2$ agonists in high dose may worsen angina and steroids commonly promote fluid retention and hypertension. Judgement is therefore necessary in deciding on an optimal dose.

Surgery

The majority of patients with asthma have no problems even with thoracic surgery, so long as they, the surgeon and the anaesthetist are adequately prepared. The patient should be treated vigorously for a week or two preoperatively in order to achieve normal or near-normal flow rates, and appropriate inhaled medications continued over the postoperative period. Corticosteroid cover should be provided if the patient is likely to have suppressed adrenal function and acute exacerbations of asthma should be treated along routine lines.

Other problems

An asthmatic on oral corticosteroids who develops tuberculosis and is given rifampicin probably needs to double the dose of steroid to obtain the same effect, because of drug interaction. Senile, psychotic or retarded patients cause particular problems with drug compliance. Treatment should be kept as simple as possible and supervised by a nurse or relative. Those requiring long-term oral steroids may sometimes be most reliably treated with depot injections. Visually impaired patients should be provided with inhalers that have different shapes for different functions.

References

1 British Thoracic Society. The British guidelines on asthma management: 1995 review and position statement. *Thorax* 1997; 52 (Suppl 1): S1.

2 Hilton S, Sibbald B, Anderson MR, Freeling P. Controlled evaluation of the effects of patient education on morbidity in general practice. *Lancet* 1986; i: 26.

3 Jenkinson D, Davison J, Jones S, Martin P. Comparison of effects of a self management booklet and audio cassette for patients with asthma. *Br Med J* 1988; 297: 267.

4 Bernard-Bonian AC, Stachenko S, Bonin D, Chasette C, Rousseau E. Self management teaching programs and control of paediatric asthma: a meta-analysis. *J Allergy Clin Immunol* 1995; 95: 34.

5 Lindgren B. The importance of self-management. *Eur Respir Rev* 1996; 6: 108.

6 Osman L, Adalla M, Beattie J *et al.* Reducing hospital admission through computer supported education for asthma patients. *Br Med J* 1994; 308: 568.

7 Lloyd BW, Ali MH. How useful do parents find home peak flow monitoring for children with asthma? *Br Med J* 1992; 305: 1128.

8 Kendrick AH, Higgs CMB, Whitfield MJ, Laslo G. Accuracy of perception of severity of asthma: patients treated in general practice. *Br Med J* 1993; 307: 422.

9 Crompton GK, Grant IWB, Bloomfield P. Edinburgh Emergency Asthma Admission Service: report on 10 years' experience. *Br Med J* 1979; ii: 1199.

10 Fireman P, Friday GA, Gira C, Veirthaler WA, Michaels L. Teaching self management skills to asthmatic children and their parents in an ambulatory care setting. *Pediatrics* 1981; 68: 341.

11 Beasley R, Cushley M, Holgate ST. A self management plan in the treatment of adult asthma. *Thorax* 1989; 44: 200.

12 Hayward SA, Levy M. Self management of asthma. *Br J Gen Pract* 1990; 40: 166.

13 Charlton I, Charlton G, Broomfield J, Mullee MA. Evaluation of peak flow and symptoms only self management plans for control of asthma in general practice. *Br Med J* 1990; 301: 1355.

14 Kolbe J, Vamos M, Fergusson W, Elkind G, Garrett J. Differential influences on asthma self-management knowledge and self-management behavior in acute severe asthma. *Chest* 1996; 110: 1463.

15 Brewis RAL. Patient education, self management plans and peak flow measurements. *Respir Med* 1991; 85: 457.

16 Partridge MR. Asthma: guided self management. *Br Med J* 1994; 308: 547.

17 Cochrane GM. Therapeutic compliance in asthma: its magnitude and implications. *Eur Respir J* 1992; 5: 122.

18 Cochrane GM. Compliance in asthma: a European perspective. *Eur Respir Rev* 1995; 5: 116.

19 Wright BM, McKerrow CB. Maximum forced expiratory flow rate as a measure of ventilatory capacity with a description of a new portable instrument for measuring it. *Br Med J* 1959; ii: 1041.

20 Sly PD, Landau LI, Weymouth R. Home recording of peak expiratory flow rates and perception of asthma. *Am J Dis Child* 1985; 139: 479.

21 von Mutius E, Fritzsch C, Weiland SK, Röll G, Magnussen H. Prevalence of asthma and allergic disorders among children in united Germany: a descriptive comparison. *Br Med J* 1992; 305: 1395.

22 Sears MR, Hervison GP, Holdaway MD, Hewitt CJ, Flannery EM, Silva PA. The relative risks of sensitivity to grass pollen, house dust mite, and cat dander in the development of childhood asthma. *Clin Exp Allergy* 1989; 19: 419.

23 Sporik R, Holgate S, Platts-Mills TAE, Cogswell J. Exposure to house dust mite allergen (*Der p*1) and the development of asthma in childhood. *N Engl J Med* 1990; 323: 502.

24 Holt P, McMenamin C, Nelson D. Primary sensitisation to inhalant allergens during infancy. *Pediatr Allergy Immunol* 1990; 1: 3.

25 Arshad SH, Matthews S, Grant C, Hide DW. Effect of allergen avoidance on development of allergic disorders in infancy. *Lancet* 1992; 339: 1493.

26 Sloper KS, Wadsworth J, Brostoff J. Children with atopic eczema. 1. Clinical response to food elimination and subsequent double-blind food challenge. *Q J Med* 1991; 80: 677.

27 Chapman MD, Hayman PW, Wilkins R, Brown MB, Platts-Mills TAE. Monoclonal immunoassays for the major dust mite (*Dermatophagoides*) allergens *Der p*1 and *Der f*1 and quantitative analysis of the allergen content of mite and house dust extracts. *J Allergy Clin Immunol* 1987; 80: 184.

28 Luczynska CM, Li Y, Chapman MD, Platts-Mills TAE. Airborne concentrations and particle size distribution of allergen derived from domestic cats (*Felis domesticus*): measurement using cascade impactor, liquid impinger and two site monoclonal antibody assay for *Fel d*1. *Am Rev Resp Dis* 1990; 141: 361.

29 Munir AKM, Einarsson R, Schou C, Dreborg SKG. Allergens in school dust. *J Allergy Clin Immunol* 1993; 91: 1067.

30 Coren S. Allergic patients do not comply with doctors' advice to stop owning pets. *Br Med J* 1997; 314: 517.

31 Crompton GK. How I manage the difficult asthmatic. *Proc R Coll Physicians Edinb* 1997; 27: 194.

32 Collof MJ, Ayers J, Carswell F *et al.* The control of allergens of dust mites and domestic pets: a position paper. *Clin Exp Allergy* 1992; 22 (Suppl 2): 1.

33 Owen S, Morgenstern M, Hepworth J, Woodcock A. Control of house dust mite antigen in bedding. *Lancet* 1990; 335: 396.

34 Walshaw MJ, Evans CC. Allergen avoidance in house dust mite sensitive adult asthma. *Q J Med* 1986; 58: 199.

35 Dorward AJ, Colloff MJ, Mackay NS, McSharry C, Thomson NC. Effect of house dust mite avoidance measures in adult atopic asthma. *Thorax* 1988; 43: 98.

36 Ehnert B, Lau-Schadendorf S, Weber A, Buettner P, Schou C, Wahn V. Reducing domestic exposure to dust mite allergen reduces bronchial hyperreactivity in sensitive children with asthma. *J Allergy Clin Immunol* 1993; 90: 135.

37 Murray AB, Fergusson AC. Dust free bedroom in the treatment of asthmatic children with house dust mite allergy: a controlled trial. *Pediatrics* 1983; 91: 418.

38 Wood RA, Mudd KE, Eggleston PA. The distribution of cat allergen on vertical surfaces. *J Allergy Clin Immunol* 1990; 85: 226.

39 de Blay F, Chapman MD, Platts-Mills TAE. Airborne cat levels (*Fel d*1). Environmental control with the cat *in situ*. *Am Rev Respir Dis* 1991; 143: 1334.

40 Mawhinney H, Spector SL, Kinsman RA *et al.* Compliance in clinical trials of two nonbronchodilator, antiasthma medications. *Ann Allergy* 1991; 66: 294.

41 Rand CS, Wise RA, Nides M *et al.* Metered-dose adherence in a clinical trial. *Am Rev Respir Dis* 1992; 146: 1559.

42 Bosley CM, Parry DT, Cochrane GM. Patient compliance with inhaled medication: does combining beta-agonists with corticosteroids improve compliance? *Eur Respir J* 1994; 7: 504.

43 Horn CR, Clark TJH, Cochrane GM. Compliance with inhaled therapy and morbidity from asthma. *Respir Med* 1990; 84: 66.

44 British Thoracic Association. Death from asthma in two regions of England. *Br Med J* 1982; 285: 1251.

45 Cochrane GM. Compliance in asthma: a European perspective. *Eur Respir Rev* 1995; 26: 116.

46 Blackwell B, Gutmann MC. Compliance. In: Bulpitt CJ, ed. *Handbook of Hypertension, Vol 6, Epidemiology of Hypertension*. Amsterdam: Elsevier Science Publishers, 1985, p. 35.

47 Hilton S, Sibbald B, Anderson JR, Freeling P. Controlled evaluation of the effects of patients' education on asthma morbidity in general practice. *Lancet* 1986; i: 26.

48 Pretet S, Perdrizet S, Poisson N, Pujet JCM, Marsac J. Treatment compliance and self-medication in France. *Eur Respir J* 1989; 2: 303.

49 Kraan J, Koëter GH, van der Mark TW, Sluiter HJ, de Vries K. Changes in bronchial hyperreactivity induced by 4 weeks of treatment with anti-asthmatic drugs in patients with allergic asthma: a comparison between budesonide and terbutaline. *J Allergy Clin Immunol* 1985; 76: 628.

50 Vathenen AS, Knox AJ, Higgins BG, Britton JR, Tattersfield AE. Rebound increase in bronchial responsiveness after treatment with inhaled terbutaline. *Lancet* 1988; i: 554.

51 Kerrebijn KF, Essen-Zandvliet EEM, Neijens HJ. Effect of long-term treatment with inhaled corticosteroids and beta-agonists on the bronchial responsiveness in children with asthma. *J Allergy Clin Immunol* 1987; 79: 653.

52 van Schayck CP, Graafsma SJ, Visch MB, Dompeling E, van Weel C, van Herwaarden CLA. Increased bronchial hyperresponsiveness after inhaling salbutamol during one year is not caused by subsensitisation to salbutamol. *J Allergy Clin Immunol* 1990; 86: 793.

53 Sears MR, Taylor DR, Print CG *et al.* Regular inhaled beta-agonist treatment in bronchial asthma. *Lancet* 1990; 336: 1391.

54 van Schayck CP, Dompeling E, van Herwaarden CLA. Bronchodilator treatment in moderate asthma or chronic bronchitis: continuous or demand. A randomised control trial. *Br Med J* 1991; 303: 1426.

55 National Heart, Lung and Blood Institute, National Institutes of Health. International Consensus Report on Diagnosis and Management of Asthma. *Eur Respir J* 1992; 5: 601.

56 Pearce N, Grainger M, Crane J *et al.* Case-control study of prescribed fenoterol and death from asthma in New Zealand, 1977–1981. *Thorax* 1990; 45: 170.

57 Spitzer WO, Suissa S, Ernst P *et al.* The use of beta-agonists and the risk of death and near-death from asthma. *N Engl J Med* 1992; 326: 501.

58 Löfdahl C-G, Svedmyr N. Beta-agonists: friends or foes? *Eur Respir J* 1991; 4: 1161.

59 Ernst P, Habbick B, Suisa S *et al.* Is the association between inhaled beta-agonists and life-threatening asthma because of confounding by severity. *Am Rev Respir Dis* 1992; 148: 75.

60 Tattersfield AE, Britton JR. β_2-Adrenoreceptor agonists. In: Barnes PJ, Rodger IW, Thomson NC, eds. *Asthma: Basic Mechanisms and Clinical Management*. London: Academic Press, 1992: 527.

61 Jenne JW. Bronchodilators. In: O'Byrne P, Thomson NC, eds. *Manual of Asthma Management*. London: WB Saunders, 1995: 291.

62 Nials AT, Sumner MT, Johnson M, Coleman RA. Investigation into factors determining the duration of action of the β_2-adrenoreceptor agonist, salmeterol. *Br J Pharmacol* 1993; 108: 507.

63 National Asthma Education Program. *Asthma Management Handbook*. Melbourne: National Asthma Campaign, 1993.

64 Ulman A, Svedmyr N. Salmeterol, a new long acting inhaled β_2-adrenoreceptor agonist: a comparison with salbutamol in adult asthmatic patients. *Thorax* 1988; 43: 674.

65 Dahl R, Earnshaw JS, Palmer JBD. Salmeterol: a four week study of a long-acting beta-adrenoreceptor agonist for the treatment of reversible airways disease. *Eur Respir J* 1991; 4: 1178.

66 Palmer JBD. Salmeterol in clinical practice. *Eur Respir J* 1991; 4: 297.

67 Britton MG, Earnshaw JS, Palmer JBD. A twelve month comparison of salmeterol with salbutamol in asthmatic patients. *Eur Respir J* 1992; 5: 1062.

68 Pearlman DS, Chervinsky P, LaForce C *et al.* A comparison of salmeterol with albuterol in the treatment of mild-to-moderate asthma. *N Engl J Med* 1992; 327: 1420.

69 Palmer JBD, Stuart AM, Shepherd GL, Viskum K. Inhaled salmeterol in the treatment of patients with moderate to severe reversible obstructive airways disease: a 3 month comparison of the efficacy and safety of twice daily salmeterol (100μg) with salmeterol (50μg). *Respir Med* 1992; 86: 409.

70 Jack D. A way of looking at agonism and antagonism: lessons from albuterol, salmeterol, and other β-adrenoreceptor agonists. *Br J Clin Pharmacol* 1991; 31: 501.

71 Greening AP, Ind PW, Northfield M, Shaw G. Added salmeterol versus higher-dose corticosteroid in asthma patients with symptoms on existing inhaled corticosteroid. *Lancet* 1994; 344: 219.

72 Meijer RJ, Kerstjens HAM, Postma DS. Comparison of guidelines and self-management plans in asthma. *Eur Respir J* 1997; 10: 1163.

73 Lipworth BJ, McDevitt DG, Struthers AD. Systemic β-adrenoreceptor responses to salbutamol given by metered-dose inhaler alone and with pear shaped spacer attachment: comparison of electrocardiographic, hypokalaemic and haemodynamic effects. *Br J Clin Pharmacol* 1989; 27: 837.

74 Lipworth BJ, Tregaskis BF, McDevitt DG. β-Adrenoreceptor responses to inhaled salbutamol in the elderly. *Br J Clin Pharmacol* 1989; 28: 725.

75 Kendall MJ, Haffner C. The acute unwanted effects of beta$_2$ receptor agonist therapy. In: Beasly R, Pearce NE, eds. *The Role of Beta Receptor Agonist Therapy in Asthma Mortality*. Boca Raton, Florida: CRC Press, 1993: 163.

76 Jenne JW, Ridley DF, Marcucci R, Druz WS, Rook JC. Objective and subjective tremor responses to oral beta-2 agents on first exposure. *Am Rev Respir Dis* 1982; 126: 607.

77 Jenne JW. Physiology and pharmacodynamics of theophylline. In: Jenne JW, Murphy S, eds. *Drug Therapy for Asthma: Research and Clinical Practice*. New York: Marcel Dekker, 1987: 297.

78 Jenne JW, Wyse E, Rood BS, MacDonald FM. The pharmacokinetics of theophylline. Application to adjustment of the clinical dose of aminophylline. *Clin Pharmacol Ther* 1972; 13: 349.

79 Hendeles L, Weinberger M, Johnson G. Monitoring serum theophylline levels. *Clin Pharmacokinet* 1978; 3: 294.

80 Racineux JL, Troussier J, Tureant A. Comparison of bronchodilator effects of salbutamol and theophylline. *Bull Eur Physiopathol Respir* 1981; 17: 799.

81 Wolfe JD, Tashkin DP, Calvarese B, Simmons M. Bronchodilating effects of terbutaline and aminophylline alone and in combination in asthmatic patients. *N Engl J Med* 1978; 298: 363.

82 Billing B, Dahlquist R, Gal M. Separate and combined use of terbutaline and theophylline in asthmatics. *Eur J Respir Dis* 1982; 63: 399.

83 Svedmyr K, Svedmyr N. Does theophylline potentiate inhaled β$_2$-agonists? *Allergy* 1982; 37: 101.

84 Aubier M, de Troyer A, Sampson M, Macklem PT, Roussos C. Aminophylline improves diaphragmatic contractility. *N Engl J Med* 1981; 305: 249.

85 Murciano D, Aubier M, Lecocguic Y, Pariente R. Effects of theophylline on diaphragmatic strength and fatigue in patients with chronic obstructive pulmonary disease. *N Engl J Med* 1984; 311: 349.

86 Calhoun WJ, Stevens CA, Lambert SB. Modulation of superoxide production of alveolar macrophages and peripheral blood mononuclear cells by beta-agonists and theophylline. *J Lab Clin Med* 1991; 117: 514.

87 Dent G, Giembycz MA, Rabe KF. Theophylline suppresses human alveolar macrophage respiratory burst through phosphodiesterase inhibition. *Am J Respir Cell Mol Biol* 1994; 10: 565.

88 Limatibul S, Shore A, Dosch HM, Gelfand

EW. Theophylline modulation of E-rosette formation: an indicator of T-cell maturation. *Clin Exp Immunol* 1978; 33: 503.

89 Bruserud O. The effect of theophylline on T-lymphocyte activation *in vitro*. *Clin Immunol Immunopathol* 1984; 32: 111.

90 Sullivan PJ, Bekir S, Jaffar Z, Page CP, Costello JF. Anti-inflammatory effects of low dose oral theophylline in atopic asthma. *Lancet* 1995; 343: 1006.

91 Venge P, Dahl R, Karlstrom R, Pedersen B, Peterson CGB. Eosinophil activity in asthma in a one year double-blind trial with theophylline and two doses of inhaled budesonide. *J Allergy Clin Immunol* 1992; 89: 181.

92 Pauwels R, van Renterghem D, van der Straeten M, Johannesson N, Persson CGA. The effect of theophylline and enprofylline on allergen-induced bronchoconstriction. *J Allergy Clin Immunol* 1985; 76: 583.

93 Crescioli S, Spinazzi A, Plebani M *et al.* Theophylline inhibits early and late asthmatic reactions induced by allergens. *Ann Allergy* 1991; 66: 245.

94 Hendeles L, Harman E, Huang D *et al.* Alteration of allergen induced airways hyperactivity and late responses by theophylline. *Eur Respir J* 1991; 4: 481.

95 Hendeles L, Harman E, Huang D, O'Brien R, Blake K, Delafuente J. Theophylline attenuation of airways responses to allergen: comparison with cromolyn metered dose inhaler. *J Allergy Clin Immunol* 1995; 95: 505.

96 Matthys H, Muller S, Herceg R. Theophylline versus budesonide in the treatment of mild to moderate asthma. *Respiration* 1994; 61: 241.

97 Tinkleman DG, Reed CE, Nelson KS, Offord KP. Aerosol beclomethasone dipropionate compared with theophylline as primary treatment of chronic, mild to moderately severe asthma in children. *Pediatrics* 1993; 92: 64.

98 Ruffin RE, Kitzgerald JD, Rebuck AS. A comparison of the bronchodilator activity of Sch 1000 and salbutamol. *J Allergy Clin Immunol* 1977; 59: 136.

99 Ullah MI, Newman GB, Saunders KB. Influence of age on response to ipratropium and salbutamol in asthma. *Thorax* 1981; 36: 523.

100 van Schayck CP, Folgering H, Harbers H, Maas KL, van Weel C. Effect of allergy and age on responses to salbutamol and ipratropium bromide in moderate asthma and chronic bronchitis. *Thorax* 1991; 46: 355.

101 Howell JBL, Altounyan REC. A double-blind trial of disodium cromoglycate in the treatment of allergic bronchial asthma. *Lancet* 1967; ii: 539.

102 Smith JM, Devey GF. Clinical trial of disodium cromoglycate in treatment of asthma in children. *Br Med J* 1968; ii: 340.

103 Shioda H, Murano J, Mishima K, Iikura Y, Tanaka F, Izeki M. Disodium cromoglycate (Intal) in the treatment of bronchial asthma in children. *Acta Allergol* 1970; 25: 221.

104 Engstrom I, Kraepelien S. The corticosteroid sparing effect of disodium cromoglycate in children and adolescents with bronchial asthma. *Acta Allergol* 1971; 26: 90.

105 Brompton Hospital/Medical Research Council Collaborative Trial. Long-term study of disodium cromoglycate in treatment of severe extrinsic or intrinsic bronchial asthma in adults. *Br Med J* 1972; iv: 383.

106 Silverman M, Connolly NM, Balfour-Lynn L, Godfrey S. Long-term trial of disodium

cromoglycate and isoprenaline in children with asthma. *Br Med J* 1972; 3: 378.

107 Northern General Hospital, Bromptom Hospital and Medical Research Council Collaborative Trial. Sodium cromoglycate in chronic asthma. *Br Med J* 1976; i: 361.

108 Eigen H, Reid JJ, Dahl R *et al.* Evaluation of the addition of cromolyn sodium to bronchodilator maintenance therapy in the long-term management of asthma. *J Allergy Clin Immunol* 1987; 80: 612.

109 Smith JM, Pizzarro YA. Observations on the safety of disodium cromoglycate in long-term use in children. *Clin Allergy* 1972; 2: 143.

110 Hiller EJ, Milner AD. Betamethasone 17 valerate aerosol and disodium cromoglycate in severe childhood asthma. *Br J Dis Chest* 1975; 69: 103.

111 Mitchell I, Paterson IC, Cameron SJ, Grant IWB. Treatment of childhood asthma with sodium cromoglycate and beclomethasone dipropionate aerosol singly and in combination. *Br Med J* 1976; ii: 457.

112 Shapiro GG, Sharpe M, de Rouen TA *et al.* Cromolyn versus triamcinolone acetonide for youngsters with moderate asthma. *J Allergy Clin Immunol* 1991; 88: 742.

113 Ng SH, Dash CH, Savage SJ. Betamethasone valerate compared with sodium cromoglycate in asthmatic children. *Postgrad Med J* 1977; 53: 315.

114 Francis RS, McEnery G. Disodium cromoglycate compared with beclomethasone dipropionate in juvenile asthma. *Clin Allergy* 1984; 14: 537.

115 Silverman M, Andrea T. Time course of effect of disodium cromoglycate on exercise-induced asthma. *Arch Dis Child* 1972; 47: 419.

116 Bar-Yishay E, Gur I, Levy M *et al.* Duration of action of disodium cromoglycate on exercise-induced asthma: comparison of 2 formulations. *Arch Dis Child* 1983; 58: 624.

117 Rohr AS, Siegel SC, Katz RM *et al.* A comparison of inhaled albuterol and cromolyn in the prophylaxis of exercise-induced bronchospasm. *Ann Allergy* 1987; 59: 107.

118 Godfrey S, Balfour-Lynn L, König P. The place of cromolyn sodium in the long-term management of childhood asthma based on a 3–5 year follow-up. *J Pediatr* 1975; 87: 465.

119 Østergaard PA, Pedersen S. The effect of inhaled disodium cromoglycate and budesonide on bronchial responsiveness to histamine and exercise in asthmatic children. In: Godfrey S, ed. *Glucocorticosteroids in Childhood Asthma.* Amsterdam: Exerpta Medica, 1987: 55.

120 Brogden RN, Sorkin EM. Nedocromil sodium. An updated view of its pharmacological properties and therapeutic efficacy in asthma. *Drugs* 1993; 45: 693.

121 Konig P, Hordvik NL, Kreutz C. The preventative effect and duration of action of nedocromil sodium and cromolyn on exercise-induced asthma (EIA) in adults. *J Allergy Clin Immunol* 1987; 79: 64.

122 North American Tilade Study Group. A double-blind multicentre group comparative study of nedocromil sodium in the management of asthma. *Chest* 1990; 97: 1299.

123 Rebuck AS, Kesten S, Boulet LP *et al.* A 3-month evaluation of the efficacy of nedocromil sodium in asthma: a randomized, double-blind, placebo-controlled trial of nedocromil sodium conducted by a Canadian multicentre study group. *J Allergy Clin Immunol* 1990; 85: 612.

124 Bone MF, Kubik MM, Keaney NP *et al.* Nedocromil sodium in adults with asthma dependent on inhaled corticosteroids: a double blind, placebo controlled study. *Thorax* 1989; 44: 654.

125 Boulet LP, Cartier A, Cockcroft DW *et al.* Tolerance to reduction of oral steroid dosage in severely asthmatic patients receiving nedocromil sodium. *Respir Med* 1990; 84: 317.

126 Cartier A. Anti-allergic drugs. In: O'Byrne P, Thomson NC, eds. *Manual of Asthma Management.* London: WB Saunders, 1995: 254.

127 Lal S, Dorow PD, Venho KK, Chatterjee SS. Nedocromil sodium is more effective than cromolyn sodium for the treatment of chronic reversible obstructive airways disease. *Chest* 1993; 104: 438.

128 Boldy DA, Ayres JG. Nedocromil sodium and sodium cromoglycate in patients aged over 50 years with asthma. *Respir Med* 1993; 87: 517.

129 Rafferty P, Holgate ST. Anti-allergic drugs. In: Barnes PJ, Rodger IW, Thomson NC, eds. *Asthma: Basic Mechanisms and Clinical Management.* London: Academic Press, 1992: 519.

130 Report to the Medical Research Council by the Subcommittee on Clinical Trials in Asthma. Controlled trial of effects of cortisone acetate in chronic asthma. *Lancet* 1956; i: 798.

131 Fletcher CM. The use of corticosteroids in the treatment of asthma and related conditions. *Postgrad Med J* 1958; 34: 310.

132 Brown HM, Storey G, George WS. Beclomethasone dipropionate: a new steroid aerosol for the treatment of allergic asthma. *Br Med J* 1971; i: 585.

133 Clark TJH. Effect of beclomethasone dipropionate delivered by aerosol in patients with asthma. *Lancet* 1972; i: 1361.

134 Cameron SJ, Cooper EJ, Crompton GK, Hoare MV, Grant IWB. Substitution of beclomethasone aerosol for oral prednisolone in the treatment of chronic asthma. *Br Med J* 1973; iv: 205.

135 Hodson ME, Batten JC, Clarke SW, Gregg I. Beclomethasone dipropionate aerosol in asthma. Transfer of steroid-dependent asthmatic patients from oral prednisolone to beclomethasone dipropionate aerosol. *Am Rev Respir Dis* 1974; 110: 403.

136 British Thoracic and Tuberculosis Association. A controlled trial of inhaled corticosteroids in patients receiving prednisolone tablets for asthma. *Br J Dis Chest* 1976; 70: 95.

137 Brogden RN. Inhaled steroids: studies in adult and childhood asthma. In: Clark TJH, ed. *Steroids in Asthma: a Reappraisal in the Light of Inhalation Therapy.* Auckland: ADIS Press, 1983: 135.

138 Latinen LA, Latinen A, Haahtela T. A comparative study of the effects of an inhaled corticosteroid, budesonide, and of a β_2-agonist, terbutaline, on airway inflammation in newly diagnosed asthma. *J Allergy Clin Immunol* 1992; 90: 32.

139 Djukanovic R, Wilson JW, Britten YM. Effect of an inhaled corticosteroid on airway inflammation and symptoms of asthma. *Am Rev Respir Dis* 1992; 145: 669.

140 Jeffery PK, Godfrey RW, Ädelroth E *et al.* Effect of treatment on airway inflammation and thickening of basement membrane reticular collagen in asthma. *Am Rev Respir Dis* 1992; 145: 890.

141 Ädelroth E, Rosenhall L, Johansson S-Å,

Linden M, Venge P. Inflammatory cells and eosinophilic activity in asthmatics investigated by bronchoalveolar lavage. *Am Rev Respir Dis* 1990; 142: 91.

142 Cockroft DW, Murdoch KY. Comparative effects of inhaled salbutamol, sodium cromoglycate and BDP on allergen-induced early asthmatic responses, late asthmatic responses and increased bronchial responsiveness to histamine. *J Allergy Clin Immunol* 1987; 79: 734.

143 De Baets FM, Goetyn M, Kerrebijn KF. The effect of two months treatment with inhaled budesonide on bronchial responsiveness to histamine and house-dust mite antigen in asthmatic children. *Am Rev Respir Dis* 1990; 142: 581.

144 Henriksen JM, Dahl R. Effects of inhaled budesonide alone and in combination with low-dose terbutaline in children with exercise induced asthma. *Am Rev Respir Dis* 1983; 128: 993.

145 Molema J, van Herwaarden CLA, Folgering HTM. Effect of long-term treatment with inhaled cromoglycate and budesonide on bronchial hyperresponsiveness in children with allergic asthma. *Eur Respir J* 1989; 2: 308.

146 Kerrebijn KF, van Essen-Zandvliet EEM, Neijens HL. Effect of long-term treatment with inhaled corticosteroids and beta-agonists on bronchial responsiveness in asthmatic children. *J Allergy Clin Immunol* 1987; 79: 653.

147 Dutoit JI, Salome CM, Woolcock AJ. Inhaled corticosteroids reduce the severity of bronchial hyperresponsiveness in asthma, but oral theophylline does not. *Am Rev Respir Dis* 1987; 136: 1174.

148 Juniper EF, Kline PA, van Zieleshem MA *et al.* Long-term effects of budesonide on airway responsiveness and clinical asthma severity in inhaled steroid-dependent asthmatics. *Eur Respir J* 1990; 3: 1122.

149 Haahtela T, Jarvinen M, Kava T *et al.* Comparison of a β₂-agonist terbutaline with an inhaled steroid in newly detected asthma. *N Engl J Med* 1991; 325: 388.

150 Groot CAR, Lammers J-WJ, Festen J, van Herwaarden CLA. Effect of inhaled beclomethasone and nedocromil sodium on bronchial hyperresponsiveness to histamine and distilled water. *Eur Respir J* 1992; 5: 1075.

151 Haahtela T, Järvinen M, Kava T *et al.* Effects of reducing or discontinuing inhaled budesonide in patients with mild asthma. *N Engl J Med* 1994; 331: 700.

152 Agertoft L, Pedersen S. Effects of long-term treatment with an inhaled corticosteroid on growth and pulmonary function in asthmatic children. *Respir Med* 1994; 88: 373.

153 Selroos O, Pietinahlo A, Löfroos A-B, Riska H. Effect of early vs late intervention with inhaled corticosteroids in asthma. *Chest* 1995; 108: 1228.

154 Barnes PJ, Pedersen S. Efficacy and safety of inhaled corticosteroids in asthma. *Am Rev Respir Dis* 1993; 148: S1.

155 Lorenzon S, Boe J, Eriksson G, Persson G. Use of inhaled corticosteroids in mild asthma. *Thorax* 1990; 45: 733.

156 Jones AH, Langdon CG, Lee PS *et al.* Pulmicort® Turbohaler® once daily as initial prophylactic therapy for asthma. *Respir Med* 1994; 88: 293.

157 Hargreave FE, Dolovich J, Newhouse MT. The assessment and treatment of asthma: a conference report. *J Allergy Clin Immunol* 1990; 85: 1098.

158 Toogood JH. High dose inhaled steroid therapy for asthma. *J Allergy Clin Immunol* 1989; 83: 528.

159 Laursen LC, Taudorf E, Weeke B. High-dose budesonide in treatment of severe steroid-dependent asthma. *Eur J Respir Dis* 1986; 68: 19.

160 Salmeron S, Guerin J-C, Godard P *et al.* High doses of inhaled corticosteroids in unstable chronic asthma. *Am Rev Respir Dis* 1989; 140: 167.

161 Lacronique J, Renon D, Georges D, Henry-Amar M, Marsac J. High-dose beclomethasone: oral steroid-sparing effect in severe asthmatic patients. *Eur Respir J* 1991; 4: 807.

162 Hummel S, Lehtonen L. Comparison of oral steroid sparing by high-dose and low-dose inhaled steroid in maintenance treatment of severe asthma. *Lancet* 1992; 340: 1483.

163 Kraan J, Koeter GH, Van de Mark TW, Sluiter HJ, De Vries K. Changes in bronchial hyperreactivity induced by 4 weeks of treatment with antiasthmatic drugs in patients with allergic asthma: a comparison between budesonide and terbutaline. *J Allergy Clin Immunol* 1985; 76: 628.

164 Vathenen AS, Knox AJ, Wisniewski A, Tattersfield AE. Time course of change in bronchial reactivity with an inhaled corticosteroid in asthma. *Am Rev Respir Dis* 1991; 143: 1317.

165 Juniper EF, Kline PA, Vanzielegmem MA, Hargreave FE. Reduction of budesonide after a year of increased use: a randomised controlled trial to evaluate whether improvements in airways responsiveness are maintained. *J Allergy Clin Immunol* 1991; 87: 483.

166 Brown JP, Greville WH, Finucane KE. Asthma and irreversible airflow obstruction. *Thorax* 1984; 39: 131.

167 Peat JK, Woolcock AJ, Cullen K. Rate of decline of lung function in subjects with asthma. *Eur J Respir Dis* 1987; 70: 171.

168 Dompeling E, van Schayck CP, Molema J *et al.* Inhaled beclomethasone improves the course of asthma and COPD. *Eur Respir J* 1992; 5: 945.

169 Ernst P, Spitzer WD, Suissa S *et al.* Risk of fatal and near fatal asthma in relation to inhaled corticosteroid use. *JAMA* 1992; 268: 3462.

170 Carmichael J, Paterson IC, Diaz P, Crompton GK, Kay AB, Grant IWB. Corticosteroid resistance in chronic asthma. *Br Med J* 1981; 282: 1419.

171 Brown PH, Teelucksingh S, Matusiewicz SP, Greening AP, Crompton GK, Edwards CRW. Cutaneous vasoconstrictor responses to glucocorticoids in asthma. *Lancet* 1991; 337: 576.

172 Barnes PJ, Greening AP, Crompton GK. Glucocorticoid resistance in asthma. *Am J Respir Crit Care Med* 1995; 152: S125.

173 Milne JR, Crompton GK. Beclomethasone dipropionate and oropharyngeal candidiasis. *Br Med J* 1974; 3: 797.

174 Willey RF, Milne JR, Crompton GK, Grant IWB. Beclomethasone dipropionate aerosol and oropharyngeal candidiasis. *Br J Dis Chest* 1976; 70: 32.

175 Davis G, Thomas P, Broder I *et al.* Steroid-dependent asthma treated with inhaled beclomethasone dipropionate. A long-term study. *Ann Intern Med* 1977; 86: 549.

176 Brompton Hospital/Medical Research Council Collaborative Trial. Double-blind trial comparing two dose schedules of beclomethasone dipropionate in the treatment of chronic bronchial asthma. *Lancet* 1974; ii: 303.

177 Toogood JH, Jennings B, Greenway RW, Chung L. Candidiasis and dysphonia complicating beclomethasone treatment of asthma. *J Allergy Clin Immunol* 1980; 65: 145.

178 Brogden RN, Heel RC, Speight TM, Avery GS. Beclomethasone dipropionate. A reappraisal of its pharmacodynamic properties and therapeutic efficacy after a decade of use in asthma and rhinitis. *Drugs* 1984; 28: 99.

179 Brogden RN, McTavish D. Budesonide. An updated review of its pharmacological properties and therapeutic efficacy in asthma and rhinitis. *Drugs* 1992; 44: 375.

180 Toogood JH, Jennings B, Baskerville J, Andersson J, Johansson SA. Dosing regimen of budesonide and occurrence of oropharyngeal complications. *Am Rev Respir Dis* 1989; 140: 624.

181 Smith MJ, Hodson ME. High-dose beclomethosone inhaler in the treatment of asthma. *Lancet* 1983; i: 265.

182 Toogood JH, Baskerville J, Jennings B. Use of spacers to facilitate inhaled corticosteroid treatment of asthma. *Am Rev Respir Dis* 1984; 129: 723.

183 Salzman GA, Mszczynski DR. Oropharyngeal candidiasis in patients treated with beclomethasone dipropionate delivered by metered-dose inhaler alone and with Aerochamber. *J Allergy Clin Immunol* 1988; 81: 424.

184 Spector SL, Wangaard C, Bardana EJ. The use of cultures and immunological procedures to predict oropharyngeal candidiasis in patients on steroid aerosols. *Clin Allergy* 1982; 12: 269.

185 Crompton GK. Local adverse effects of inhaled corticosteroids: oropharyngeal candidiasis and dysphonia. *Prescribers' J* 1995; 35: 59.

186 Sievert W, Holmes P, King RWF. Oesophageal candidosis in patients on high-dose inhaled steroids. *Lancet* 1992; 339: 1551.

187 Williamson I, Matusiewicz S, Brown PH, Greening AP, Crompton GK. Frequency of voice problems and cough in patients using pressurized aerosol inhaled steroid preparations. *Eur Respir J* 1995; 8: 590.

188 Williams AJ, Baghat MS, Stableforth DE, Cryton RM, Shenos PM, Skinner C. Dysphonia caused by inhaled steroids: recognition of a characteristic laryngeal abnormality. *Thorax* 1983; 38: 813.

189 Settipane GA, Kalliel DE, Klein DE. Rechallenge of patients who developed oral candidiasis or hoarseness with beclomethasone dipropionate. *N Engl Reg Allergy Proc* 1987; 8: 95.

190 Selroos SO, Backman R, Forsen K-O *et al.* Local side-effects during 4 years treatment with inhaled corticosteroids: a comparison between metered dose inhaler and Turbuhaler. *Allergy* 1994; 49: 888.

191 Dewar MH, Matusiewicz SP, Ning A *et al.* Comparison of pMDI plus Nebuhaler® and Turbuhaler® in asthmatic patients with dysphonia. *Thorax* 1996; 51 (Suppl 3): A74.

192 Shim CS, Williams MH. Cough and wheezing from beclomethasone dipropionate aerosol are absent after triamcinolone acetonide. *Ann Intern Med* 1987; 106: 700.

193 Engel T, Heinig JH, Malling H-J, Scharing B, Nikander K, Masden F. Clinical comparison

of inhaled budesonide delivered either by pressurized metered dose inhaler or Turbuhaler. *Allergy* 1989; 44: 220.

194 Yarbrough J, Lyndon RN, Mansfield E, Ting S. Metered dose inhaler induced bronchospasm in asthmatic patients. *Ann Allergy* 1985; 55: 25.

195 Crompton GK. Inhaled beclomethasone dipropionate in allergic bronchopulmonary aspergillosis. Report to Research Committee of British Thoracic Association. *Br J Dis Chest* 1979; 73: 349.

196 Seaton A, Seaton RA, Wightman AJA. Management of allergic bronchopulmonary aspergillosis without maintenance oral corticosteroids: a fifteen-year follow-up. *Q J Med* 1994; 87: 529.

197 Lundgren R, Söderberg M, Horstedt P, Stenling R. Morphological studies on bronchial mucosal biopsies from asthmatics before and after ten years treatment with inhaled steroids. *Eur Respir J* 1988; 1: 883.

198 Law CM, Preece MA, Warner JO. Nocturnal adrenal suppression in children inhaling beclomethasone dipropionate. *Lancet* 1986; i: 321.

199 Harding SM, Daniel M. The clinical pharmacology of fluticasone propionate. *Eur Respir J* 1990; 3 (Suppl 10): 250S.

200 Szefler S. Glucocorticoid therapy for asthma: clinical pharmacology. *J Allergy Clin Immunol* 1991; 88: 147.

201 Geddes DM. Inhaled corticosteroids: benefits and risks. *Thorax* 1992; 47: 404.

202 Rogers DF, Ganderton D. Workshop report. Determining equivalence of inhaled medications. *Respir Med* 1995; 89: 253.

203 Fuller RW, Hallett C, Dahl R. Assessing equivalence of inhaled drugs. *Respir Med* 1995; 89: 525.

204 Maberly DJ, Gibson GJ, Butler AG. Recovery of adrenal function after substitution of beclomethasone dipropionate for oral corticosteroids. *Br Med J* 1973; i: 778.

205 Tarlo SM, Broder I, Davies GM, Lenzoff A, Minz S, Corey PN. Six month double-blind controlled trial of high dose, concentrated beclomethasone dipropionate in the treatment of severe chronic asthma. *Chest* 1988; 93: 998.

206 Stiksa G, Nemcek K, Glennow C. Adrenal function in asthmatics treated with high-dose budesonide. *Respiration* 1985; 48: 91.

207 Luengo M, Picado C, Del Rio L, Gunabens N, Montserrat JM, Setoain J. Vertebral fractures in steroid dependent asthma and involutional osteoporosis: a comparative study. *Thorax* 1991; 46: 803.

208 Wolthers O, Pedersen S. Growth of asthmatic children during treatment with budesonide: a double blind trial. *Br Med J* 1991; 303: 163.

209 Wolthers O, Pedersen S. A controlled study of linear growth in asthmatic children during treatment with inhaled glucocorticosteroids. *Pediatrics* 1992; 89: 839.

210 Wolthers O, Pedersen S. Growth in asthmatic children treated with budesonide. *Pediatrics* 1993; 90: 517.

211 Wolthers O, Pedersen S. Short term linear growth in asthmatic children during treatment with prednisolone. *Br Med J* 1990; 301: 145.

212 Webb J, Clark TJH. Recovery of plasma corticotrophin and cortisol levels after a three-week course of prednisolone. *Thorax* 1981; 36: 22.

213 Benatar SR. Fatal asthma. *N Engl J Med* 1986; 314: 423.

214 Eason SR, Markowe HLJ. Controlled investigation of deaths from asthma in hospitals in the North East Thames Region. *Br Med J* 1987; 294: 1255.

215 Wagner PD, Dantzker DR, Iacovoni VE, Tomlin WC, West JB. Ventilation–perfusion inequality in asymptomatic asthma. *Am Rev Respir Dis* 1978; 118: 511.

216 Ingram RH, Krumpe PE, Duffell GM, Maniscalco B. Ventilation–perfusion changes after aerolised isoproterenol in asthma. *Am Rev Respir Dis* 1970; 101: 364.

217 O'Driscoll BR, Cochrane GM. Emergency use of bronchodilator drugs in British hospitals. *Thorax* 1987; 42: 491.

218 Fitchett DH, McNicol MW, Riordan JF. Intravenous salbutamol in the management of status asthmaticus. *Br Med J* 1975; i: 53.

219 Bloomfield P, Carmichael J, Petrie GR *et al.* Comparison of salbutamol given intravenously and by intermittent positive pressure breathing in life-threatening asthma. *Br Med J* 1979; i: 848.

220 Swedish Society of Chest Medicine. High dose inhaled versus intravenous salbutamol compared with theophylline in severe acute asthma. A multicentre study of 176 patients. *Eur Respir J* 1990; 3: 163.

221 Cheong B, Reynolds SR, Rajan G, Ward MJ. Intravenous beta agonist in severe acute asthma. *Br Med J* 1988; 297: 448.

222 Browne GJ, Penna AS, Phung X, Michael S. Randomised trial of intravenous salbutamol in the early management of acute severe asthma in children. *Lancet* 1997; 349: 301.

223 Kelly HW, McWilliams B, Katz R, Crowley M, Murphy S. Safety of frequent high dose nebulized terbutaline in children with acute asthma. *Ann Allergy* 1990; 64: 229.

224 Douglas JG, Rafferty P, Fergusson RJ *et al.* Nebulised salbutamol without oxygen in severe acute asthma: how effective and how safe? *Thorax* 1985; 40: 180.

225 Fergusson RJ, Carmichael J, Rafferty P *et al.* Nebulised salbutamol in life-threatening asthma: is IPPB necessary? *Br J Dis Chest* 1983; 77: 255.

226 Morgan MDL, Singh BV, Frame MH, Williams SJ. Terbutaline aerosol given through pear spacer in acute severe asthma. *Br Med J* 1982; 285: 849.

227 Ward MJ, Fentem PH, Roderick Smith WH, Davies D. Ipratropium bromide in acute asthma. *Br Med J* 1981; i: 589.

228 Leahy BC, Gomm SA, Allen SC. Comparison of nebulised salbutamol with nebulised ipratropium bromide in acute asthma. *Br J Dis Chest* 1983; 77: 159.

229 Rebuck AS, Chapman KR, Abboud R *et al.* Nebulised anticholinergic and sympathomimetic treatment of obstructive airways disease in the emergency room. *Am J Med* 1987; 82: 59.

230 Watson WT, Becker AB, Simons FE. Comparison of ipratropium solution, fenoterol solution, and their combination administered by nebulizer and face mask to children with acute asthma. *J Allergy Clin Immunol* 1988; 82: 1012.

231 O'Driscoll BR, Taylor RJ, Horsby MG, Chambers DK, Bernstein A. Nebulised salbutamol with and without ipratropium bromide in acute airflow obstruction. *Lancet* 1989; ii: 1418.

232 Higgins RM, Stradling JR, Lane DJ. Should ipratropium bromide be added to beta-agonists in treatment of severe asthma? *Chest* 1988; 94: 718.

233 Summers QA, Tarala RA. Nebulised ipratropium in the treatment of acute asthma. *Chest* 1990; 97: 430.

234 Karpel JP, Schacter EN, Fanta C *et al.* A comparison of ipratropium and albuterol vs albuterol alone for treatment of acute asthma. *Chest* 1996; 110: 611.

235 Whyte KF, Gould GA, Jeffrey AA, Airlie MA, Flenley DC, Douglas NJ. Dose of nebulized ipratropium bromide in acute severe asthma. *Respir Med* 1991; 85: 517.

236 Bordley JE, Carey RA, Harvey AM *et al.* Preliminary observations on the effect of adreno-corticotrophic hormone (ACTH) in allergic diseases. *Bull Johns Hopkins Hosp* 1949; 85: 396.

237 Medical Research Council. Controlled trial of effects of cortisone acetate in status asthmaticus. *Lancet* 1956; ii: 803.

238 Luksza AR. Acute severe asthma treated without steroids. *Br J Dis Chest* 1982; 76: 15.

239 Anon. Acute asthma. *Lancet* 1986; i: 131.

240 Fanta CH, Rossing TH, McFadden ER. Glucocorticoids in acute asthma: a critical controlled trial. *Am J Med* 1983; 74: 845.

241 Britton MG, Collins JV, Brown D *et al.* High-dose corticosteroids in severe acute asthma. *Br Med J* 1976; ii: 73.

242 Tanaka RM, Santiago SM, Kuhn GJ *et al.* Intravenous methylprednisolone in adults in status asthmaticus. *Chest* 1982; 82: 438–40.

243 Shee CD. Risk factors for hydrocortisone myopathy in acute severe asthma. *Respir Med* 1990; 84: 229.

244 Collins JV, Clark TJH, Brown D, Townsend J. Intravenous corticoids in the treatment of acute bronchial asthma. *Lancet* 1970; ii: 1047.

245 Harrison BDW, Stokes TC, Hart GJ *et al.* Need for intravenous hydrocortisone in addition to oral prednisolone in patients admitted to hospital with severe asthma without ventilatory failure. *Lancet* 1986; i: 181.

246 Darioli R, Perret C. Mechanical controlled hypoventilation in status asthmaticus. *Am Rev Respir Dis* 1984; 129: 385.

247 Karetzky MS. Asthma mortality: an analysis of one year's experience, review of the literature and assessment of current modes of therapy. *Medicine* 1975; 54: 471.

248 Branthwaite MA. The management of severe asthma. In: Baderman H, ed. *Management of Medical Emergencies.* Tonbridge Wells: Pitman Medical, 1978: 48.

249 Higgins B, Greening AP, Crompton GK. Assisted ventilation in severe acute asthma. *Thorax* 1986; 41: 464.

250 Luksza AR, Smith P, Coakley J *et al.* Acute severe asthma treated by mechanical ventilation: 10 years' experience from a district general hospital. *Thorax* 1986; 42: 459.

251 Greaser JB, Rowe AH. Inhalation of epinephrine for relief of asthmatic symptoms. *J Allergy* 1935; 6: 415.

252 Newman SP, Morén F, Pavia D, Sheahan NF, Clarke SW. Deposition of pressurised aerosols in the human respiratory tract. *Thorax* 1981; 36: 52.

253 Melchor R, Biddiscome MF, Mak VHF, Short MD, Spiro SG. Lung deposition patterns of directly labeled salbutamol in normal subjects and in patients with reversible airflow obstruction. *Thorax* 1993; 48: 506.

254 Newman SP, Pavia D, Clarke SW. How

should a pressurized β-adrenergic bronchodilator be inhaled? *Eur J Respir Dis* 1981;
62: 3.

255 Paterson IC, Crompton GK. Use of pressurised aerosols by asthmatic patients. *Br
Med J* 1976; i: 76.

256 Orehek J, Gayrard P, Grimaud CH, Charpin
J. Patient error in use of bronchodilator
metered aerosols. *Br Med J* 1976; i: 76.

257 Epstein SW, Manning CPR, Ashley MJ,
Corey PN. Survey of the clinical use of pressurized aerosol inhalers. *Can Med Assoc J*
1979; 120: 813.

258 Gayrard P, Orehek J. Inadequate use of pressurized aerosols by asthmatic patients. *Respiration* 1980; 40: 47.

259 Crompton GK. Problems patients have
using pressurized aerosol inhalers. *Eur J
Respir Dis* 1982; 63 (Suppl 119): 101.

260 Crompton GK. Delivery systems. In:
O'Byrne PM, Thomson NC, eds. *Manual of
Asthma Management*. London: WB Saunders,
1995: 341.

261 Newman SP. Metered dose pressurized
aerosols and the ozone layer. *Eur Respir J*
1990; 3: 495.

262 Morén F. Drug deposition of pressurized
inhalation aerosols. 1. Influence of actuator
tube design. *Int J Pharm* 1978; 1: 205.

263 Lindgren SB, Formgren H, Morén F.
Improved aerosol therapy of asthma: effect
of actuator tube size on drug availability.
Eur J Respir Dis 1980; 61: 56.

264 Newman SP, Morén F, Pavia D, Little F,
Clark SW. Deposition of pressurized suspension aerosols inhaled through extension
devices. *Am Rev Respir Dis* 1981; 124: 318.

265 Tobin MJ, Jenouri G, Danta I, Kim C, Watson
H, Sackner MA. Response to bronchodilator
drug administration by a new reservoir
aerosol delivery system and a review of
other auxiliary delivery systems. *Am Rev
Respir Dis* 1982; 126: 670.

266 Newman SP, Millar AB, Lennard-Jones TR,
Morén F, Clarke SW. Improvement of pressurized aerosol deposition with Nebuhaler
spacer device. *Thorax* 1984; 39: 935.

267 Barry PW, O'Callaghan C. Inhalation drug
delivery from seven different inhalers.
Thorax 1996; 51: 835.

268 Bisgaard H. Drug delivery from inhaler
devices. *Br Med J* 1996; 313: 895.

269 O'Callaghan C, Barry P. Spacer devices in
the treatment of asthma. *Br Med J* 1997; 314:
1061.

270 Wildhaber JH, Devadason SG, Hayden MJ
et al. Electrostatic charge on a plastic spacer
device influences the delivery of salbutamol. *Eur Respir J* 1996; 9: 1943.

271 Woodcock A. Use of spacers with metered
dose inhalers. *Lancet* 1997; 349: 446.

272 Prahl P, Jensen T. Decreased adreno-cortical
suppression utilising the Nebuhaler for the
inhalation of steroid aerosols. *Clin Allergy*
1987; 17: 393.

273 Brown PH, Blundell G, Greening AP,
Crompton GK. Do large, spacer devices
reduce the systemic effects of high dose
inhaled corticosteroids? *Thorax* 1990; 45: 736.

274 Farrer M, Francis AJ, Pearce SJ. Morning
serum cortisol concentrations after 2mg
inhaled beclomethasone dipropionate in
normal subjects: effect of a 750ml spacing
device. *Thorax* 1990; 45: 740.

275 Brown PH, Matusiewicz SP, Shearing C,
Greening AP, Crompton GK. Systemic

effects of high dose inhaled steroids: comparison of beclomethasone dipropionate
and budesonide in healthy subjects. *Thorax*
1993; 48: 967.

276 Toogood JH, Jennings B, Baskerville J,
Newhouse M. Assessment of a device for
reducing oropharyngeal complications
during beclomethasone treatment of
asthma. *Am Rev Respir Dis* 1981; 123: 113.

277 O'Reilly JF, Buchanan DR, Sudlow MF. Pressurised aerosol with conical spacer is an
effective alternative to nebuliser in chronic
stable asthma. *Br Med J* 1983; 286: 1548.

278 Prior JG, Nowell RV, Cochrane GM. High-
dose inhaled terbutaline in the management
of chronic severe asthma: comparison of wet
nebulisation and tube-spacer delivery.
Thorax 1982; 37: 300.

279 Crompton GK, Duncan J. Clinical assessment of a new breath-actuated inhaler. *Practitioner* 1989; 233: 268.

280 Newman SP, Weisz AWB, Talaee N, Clarke
SW. Improvement of drug delivery with a
breath actuated pressurised aerosol for
patients with poor inhaler technique. *Thorax*
1991; 46: 712.

281 Fergusson RJ, Lenny J, McHardy GJR,
Crompton GK. The use of a new breath-
actuated inhaler by patients with severe
airflow obstruction. *Eur Respir J* 1991; 4: 172.

282 Crompton GK. New inhalation devices. *Eur
Respir J* 1988; 1: 679.

283 Anani A, Higgins AJ, Crompton GK. Breath-
actuated inhalers: comparison of terbutaline
Turbohaler with salbutamol Rotahaler. *Eur
Respir J* 1989; 2: 640.

284 Sininghe Damsté HEJ, Oostringaa P,
Heeringa A. Clinical comparison of inhaled
bindesoride administered via a pressurised
metered close inhaler via Tuibuhaler® in
patients with branchial asthma. *Ein Respir J*
1989: 2(Suppl 8): 861.

285 Pedersen S, Hansen OR, Fugsland G.
Influence of inspiratory flow rate upon the
effect of a Turbuhaler. *Arch Dis Child* 1990;
65: 308.

286 Dolovich M, Vanzieleghem M, Hidinger K-
G, Newhouse MT. Influence of inspiratory
flow rate on the response to terbutaline sulphate inhaled via the Turbuhaler. *Am Rev
Respir Dis* 1988; 137: A433.

287 Pedersen S. How to use a Rotahaler. *Arch Dis
Child* 1986; 61: 11.

288 Thorsson L, Edsbäcker S, Conradson T-B.
Lung deposition of budesonide from Turbuhaler is twice that from a pressurized
metered-dose inhaler p-MDI. *Eur Respir J*
1994; 7: 1839.

289 Selroos O, Halme M. Effect of a Volumatic
spacer and mouth rinsing on systemic
absorption of inhaled corticosteroids from a
metered dose inhaler and dry powder
inhaler. *Thorax* 1991; 46: 891.

290 Hardy JG, Newman SP, Knoch M. Lung
deposition from four nebulisers. *Respir Med*
1993; 87: 461.

291 Clay MM, Pavia D, Newman SP, Clarke SW.
Factors influencing the size distribution of
aerosols from jet nebulisers. *Thorax* 1983; 38:
755.

292 Clay MM, Pavia D, Newman SP, Lennard-
Jones T, Clarke SW. Assessment of jet nebulisers for lung aerosol therapy. *Lancet* 1983;
ii: 592.

293 Newman SP, Pellow PGD, Clarke SW. The
flow–pressure characteristics of compres-

sors used for inhalation therapy. *Eur J Respir
Dis* 1987; 71: 122.

294 Department of Health and Social Security.
*Health Equipment Information. An evaluation
of powered nebulisers*. London: HMSO, 1988.

295 Smith EC, Denyer J, Kendrick AH. Comparison of twenty three nebulizer/compressor
combinations for domiciliary use. *Eur Respir
J* 1995; 8: 1214.

296 British Thoracic Society. Current best practice for the use of nebulisers. *Thorax* 1997; 52
(Suppl 2): S1.

297 Committee on Safety of Medicines. CSM
update: desensitizing vaccines. *Br Med J*
1986; 293: 948.

298 Warner JO, Kerr IW. Hyposensitization. *Br
Med J* 1987; 294: 1179.

299 Lichtenstein LM, Valentine MD, Norman
PS. A re-evaluation of immunotherapy for
asthma. *Am Rev Respir Dis* 1984; 129: 657.

300 Sadan N, Rhyne MB, Mellits ED *et al.*
Immunotherapy of pollenosis in children:
an investigation of the immunological basis
of clinical improvement. *N Engl J Med* 1969;
280: 623.

301 Sobotka AK, Valentine MD, Ishizaka K,
Lichtenstein LM. Measurement of IgG
blocking antibodies: development and
application of an immunoassay. *J Immunol*
1976; 117: 84.

302 Frankland AW, Augustin R. Prophylaxis of
summer hay fever and asthma: a controlled
trial comparing crude grass pollen extracts
with the isolated main protein component.
Lancet 1954; i: 1055.

303 Smith AP. Hyposensitization with *Dermatophagoides pteronyssinus* antigen: trial in
asthma induced by house dust. *Br Med J*
1971; iv: 204.

304 Zeiger RS, Schatz M. Immunotherapy of
atopic disorders. *Med Clin North Am* 1981;
65: 987.

305 Lichtenstein LM, Norman PJ, Winken-
werder WL. A single year of immunotherapy for ragweed hay fever. *Ann Intern
Med* 1971; 75: 663.

306 Warner JO, Price JF, Soothill JF, Hey EN.
Controlled trial of hyposensitization to *Dermatophagoides pteronyssinus* in children with
asthma. *Lancet* 1978; ii: 912.

307 Wahn U, Siraganian RP. Efficacy and specificity of immunotherapy with laboratory
animal allergen extracts. *J Allergy Clin
Immunol* 1980; 65: 413.

308 Taylor WW, Ohman JL, Lowell FC.
Immunotherapy in cat induced asthma.
Double blind trial with evaluation of
bronchial responses to cat allergen and histamine. *J Allergy Clin Immunol* 1978; 61: 283.

309 Bruce CA, Norman PS, Rosenthal RR,
Lichtenstein LM. The role of ragweed pollen
in autumnal asthma. *J Allergy Clin Immunol*
1977; 59: 449.

310 Forgacs P, Swan AD. Treatment of house
dust allergy: a report from the research committee of the British Tuberculosis Association. *Br Med J* 1968; iii: 774.

311 Shale DJ, Faux JA, Lane DJ. Trial of ketoconazole in non-invasive pulmonary
aspergillosis. *Thorax* 1987; 42: 26.

312 Gluck JC, Gluck PA. The effects of pregnancy on asthma: a prospective study. *Ann
Allergy* 1976; 37: 164.

313 Stenius-Aarniala B, Piiriala P, Teramo K.
Asthma and pregnancy: a prospective study
of 198 pregnancies. *Thorax* 1988; 43: 12.

36

REACTIVE AIRWAYS DYSFUNCTION SYNDROME

ANTHONY SEATON

Exposure of the respiratory tract to irritant gases or fumes may lead to one or more of a number of adverse consequences, although in the majority of cases no long-term harm ensues. To some extent, the site of pathological change is determined by the solubility of the gas, in that the most soluble exert their effects proximally in the nose, throat and main airways while the less soluble cause damage more distally in the acinus. These different responses and the agents that most frequently cause them are discussed in Chapter 54 and summarized in Table 36.1. It is important to recognize that in practice such responses may occur in combination and mixed syndromes, not fitting neatly into any one classification, are quite common.

Of all the possible lung responses, the one most frequently seen is an asthmatic type of reaction that has acquired the name of reactive airways dysfunction syndrome (RADS). Asthma has been recognized for many years as an occasional consequence of accidental exposure to high concentrations of airborne irritants, and such exposure was included by Gandevia in 1970 [1] as one of the causes of occupational asthma, although he did not regard this as true asthma. From the late 1970s a series of papers reported the development of asthma after exposure to sulphur dioxide, ammonia and chlorine [2–5], and in 1985 the term RADS was coined to describe the syndrome and to draw attention to it as a response to a wide range of toxic inhalation episodes [6].

Definition

There is an obvious danger in defining any disease, since it results in an arbitrary cut-off between health and normality in what is often a continuum. It thus leads to exclusion of individuals with obvious ill-health who do not quite fit into the definition. Definition should therefore be specific to the purpose for which it is intended and should not be used for other purposes. When Brooks and colleagues [6] first defined RADS, they correctly indicated the criteria that they had used to identify their cases in

order to clarify their methods for the reader. These criteria were:

1 a documented absence of previous respiratory complaints;
2 onset of symptoms occurring after a specific exposure incident or accident;
3 exposure to a gas, smoke, fume or vapour present in high concentration and with irritant properties;
4 onset of symptoms occurring within 24 h of the exposure and persisting for at least 3 months;
5 symptoms simulating asthma, with cough, wheeze and dyspnoea;
6 pulmonary function tests 'may show airflow obstruction';
7 other pulmonary disease ruled out.

Since that time there has been debate about the possibility of RADS occurring after repeated or chronic relatively low exposures [7]; it is also clear that someone with pre-existing asthma or airways disease may worsen after an exposure to irritant chemicals [8]. The above criteria should not therefore be looked upon as a definition of the disease. Rather, it is appropriate to define RADS for clinical purposes simply and broadly as non-allergic asthma occurring following exposure to airborne irritant chemicals. For a discussion of the definition of asthma see Chapter 34.

Clinical features

In the classical case, a patient who has been well previously is exposed to a spill of irritant chemical, for between seconds and hours, and within the next few days develops cough, wheeze and breathlessness. The symptoms at first are often rather mild and may be dismissed by the patient and doctors as unimportant, but as time goes by they become more rather than less troublesome [6,9]. Cough is often the most prominent symptom and may cause disturbed sleep. The patient usually complains that laughing, raising the voice, exertion and exposure to smoke or strong scents precipitates cough and wheeze. Severe

Table 36.1 Syndromes associated with exposure to irritant substances.

Site of lesion	Pathological response
Nose	Rhinitis
Larynx	Acute laryngitis, laryngeal oedema
Trachea	Tracheitis
Bronchi	Acute bronchitis, asthma, irritable airways
Bronchioles	Obliterative bronchiolitis
Alveoli	Pulmonary oedema

attacks of asthma may occur, although these are usually confined to the first few weeks after the exposure.

Lung function testing often, though not always, shows a reduction in forced expiratory volume in 1s (FEV_1) and an increase in residual volume. The airflow obstruction is usually partially reversible. A methacholine challenge test would be expected to be positive, and this has been viewed by some as a necessity for making the diagnosis [8,10]. In general, diffusing capacity is normal, although different patients may show different patterns of abnormality in keeping with the combination of syndromes that follow toxic gas exposure [11]. The chest radiograph is normal in the absence of pulmonary oedema.

As time passes, personal experience suggests that the majority of patients find their symptoms less troublesome, though adequate follow-up studies unclouded by litigation issues are few. One such study reported the examination and lung funtion testing of 20 patients up to 12 years after exposure to a spill of chlorine in a pulp mill [12]. All had suffered acute symptoms including dry cough and none had been treated with corticosteroids. In general, they had shown an obstructive pattern of lung function immediately after the episode, with raised residual volume. Thereafter, the FEV_1 improved initially and then showed a slow decline, while the residual volume progressively declined, suggesting that the long-term consequences were not trivial and that some permanent damage to small airways had occurred. In another study of 64 workers exposed repeatedly to chlorine over several months in another pulp mill, 58 had symptoms, 16 airflow obstruction and 29 bronchial hyperreactivity when examined 18–24 months after exposure had ceased [8].

Because of the paucity of good long-term studies, it is necessary to rely on personal experience to comment on the outcome and this is inevitably coloured by one's practice and local referral patterns. The large majority of workers exposed to irritant gases or fumes never present for specialist care and make a full recovery after a few hours or days of coughing and perhaps a visit to the local accident department, as indicated by the relatively small proportion of those subjects reported by occupational

physicians to the SWORD project (see below) who develop asthma [13]. Those seen by a specialist present the more typical features described above and are usually treated for asthma with satisfactory results. They slowly recover and can often stop their medications over the course of a couple of years. However, some present more severe symptoms, never respond adequately to antiasthma medication and become progressively more breathless with irreversible airflow obstruction; these patients fall into the classification of obliterative bronchiolitis (see Chapter 29). Between the two extremes are a few patients who continue with persistent and typical asthma.

In the author's opinion, the chest physician should keep an open mind about the possibility of a similar syndrome occurring as a response to repeated lower-dose exposures to irritant fumes or gases. Recent studies have confirmed that cigarette smoking is, after a family history of atopic disease, the most important risk factor for adult-onset wheezy illness [14]. It would not be surprising if similar consequences occasionally followed long-term exposure to other irritants, and the author's experience suggests that this is so. Several reports in the literature support this view. For example, Kippen and colleagues [7] described 32 patients seen in an occupational clinic with asthma, of whom seven had classical RADS while 10 had a similar syndrome following low-dose exposure on a frequent basis. Chia and colleagues [15] showed that regular firefighters were more likely to show increased airway reactivity after experimental exposure to smoke than were recruits, suggesting that recurrent exposure had rendered them more susceptible. The construction workers described by Bhérer and colleagues [8] who developed bronchial hyperreactivity from working in a pulp mill gave a history of recurrent exposures to chlorine rather than a single severe exposure. All these examples suggest that increased airway reactivity may follow a wide range of types of airway irritant damage apart from that caused by inhaling tobacco smoke.

Frequency

The best indication of the frequency of the syndrome to date comes from the UK SWORD project, in which respiratory and occupational physicians report clinical diagnoses of occupational and work-related diseases [16]. Among these are two categories, inhalation accidents and occupational asthma, the latter being divided into allergic and RADS. Approximately 180 inhalation accidents are reported each year, leading to an estimated annual incidence of about 230 [17]. This probably represents a minimum figure, as it is likely to exclude many of those treated by non-respiratory physicians and of those occurring in industries without an occupational physician. One study of these reports has shown that of

623 patients, 50 developed asthma lasting for a month or more [13]. Among 47 of these cases in whom data were available, 34 were confirmed as having developed asthma as a consequence of the exposure. Thus, some 5–6% of people reported as having had an exposure to toxic gases or fumes in the UK seem to develop asthma. In addition, among the reports of occupational asthma, some 15% appear to be ascribed to irritants rather than to allergens, suggesting that around 110 such cases are reported each year. In total, therefore, about 150–200 patients develop asthma severe enough to be reported to the SWORD scheme each year, from a total UK workforce of about 20 million, or 1 per 100000 per annum. This might be regarded as a minimum incidence of the condition.

In a survey in 1978 by the US Social Security Administration, a question was asked about work-related ill-health. The survey was biased towards people with disabilities. Of the 6000 respondents 7.7% said they had asthma, most of whom reported a physician diagnosis [18]. This prevalence was roughly double that recorded in a contemporary national health survey. Of those with asthma, 15% attributed it to bad working conditions. These would have included many with true allergic occupational asthma but presumably some had asthma due to irritants. If this proportion approximates to that in the SWOKD study, it suggests that some 2 per 1000 respondents might have had RADS. In view of the deliberate bias in sampling towards disabled people, this is a substantial overestimate of the prevalence in the working population. In a survey in the UK in 1990, a random sample of adults in 60000 households was asked if they had any illness that they related to their work [19]. From the responses it was estimated that about 30000 people believed that they had work-caused asthma, and on the same 15% basis this suggests that some 5000 may have RADS, or 2–3 per 10000 of the current workforce.

In practical terms for those who see patients with asthma, it has been reported that of 154 patients referred to an occupational medicine clinic with a possible diagnosis of occupational asthma, the diagnosis was confirmed in 59, in 10 of whom it had been induced by high-dose exposure to irritant chemicals [20]. This experience tallies with that of the SWORD project in suggesting that some one in five or six people with occupational asthma have it as a consequence of exposure to irritants rather than sensitizers.

Causes

On reading the literature one is struck by the wide range of exposures reported as having led to RADS, and personal experience supports this. In the original paper by Brooks and colleagues [6], the illness was reported after exposure to uranium hexafluoride, floor sealant, ammonia, smoke,

and various fumigating and surface coat-removing substances. The most common reported causes are spills of strong acid and alkali, escape of chlorine and ammonia, and sulphur dioxide. However, any irritant smoke or fume seems able to initiate the process, and it is not uncommon to see patients with it after inadvertent mixing of household cleansing chemicals. Some well-known sensitizers, such as isocyanates, are also irritants in high concentrations and exposures may lead to either RADS or true sensitization [21].

Pathology

There are few reports of the pathology of RADS. In the original description, bronchial biosies in two cases showed some epithelial desquamation and primarily lymphocytic inflammation [6]. More recently, Gautrin and colleagues [22] have reported on the bronchial biopsies in five subjects with RADS, in whom they showed focal epithelial desquamation, squamous cell metaplasia, some subepithelial fibrosis, thickening of the basement membrane and mainly lymphocytic inflammation. Bronchoalveolar lavage fluid showed mainly lymphocytes. They considered these changes to be consistent with the generally reduced reversibility and lability of the airflow obstruction in such patients compared to those with sensitization, and therefore concluded that the two types of occupational asthma are pathologically distinct.

Management

There are no clear guidelines for either acute or long-term management of RADS. Since airway inflammation is the basis of the initial pathological damage, it would seem sensible to treat patients who are symptomatic following acute irritant exposure with high-dose oral corticosteroids. Once RADS has developed, it is usual to treat it along conventional lines for asthma, and partial reversibility is to be expected. Progressive irreversible obstruction suggests obliterative bronchiolitis and in these circumstances high-dose steroids should be continued until it becomes apparent that no benefit is occurring.

In the majority of patients treated personally, slow improvement from RADS has occurred, the need for inhaled steroids and bronchodilators progressively diminishing. Ultimately, most are able to lead a normal life with only intermittent episodes of wheeze provoked by infections or further exposure to irritants. Long-term oral steroids have not been of benefit in either those with RADS or those with obliterative bronchiolitis.

References

1 Gandevia B. Occupational asthma. *Med J Aust* 1970; ii: 332.

2 Charan NB, Myers CG, Lakshminarayan S, Spencer TM. Pulmonary injuries associated with acute sulfur dioxide inhalation. *Am Rev Respir Dis* 1979; 119: 555.

3 Hasan FM, Geshman A, Fuleihan FJD. Resolution of pulmonary dysfunction following acute chlorine exposure. *Arch Environ Health* 1983; 38: 76.

4 Flury KE, Ames DE, Rodarte JR, Rodgers R. Airway obstruction due to inhalation of ammonia. *Mayo Clin Proc* 1983; 58: 389.

5 Härkönen H, Nordman H, Korhonen O, Winblad I. Long-term effects of exposure to sulfur dioxide. *Am Rev Respir Dis* 1983; 128: 890.

6 Brooks SM, Weiss MA, Bernstein IL. Reactive airways dysfunction syndrome. Persistent asthma syndrome after high level irritant exposure. *Chest* 1985; 88: 376.

7 Kippen HM, Blume R, Hutt D. Asthma experience in an occupational and environmental medicine clinic. Low dose reactive airways dysfunction syndrome. *J Occup Med* 1994; 36: 1133.

8 Bhérer L, Cushman R, Courteau J-P *et al.* Survey of construction workers repeatedly exposed to chlorine over a three to six month period in a pulpmill. II. Follow up of affected workers by questionnaire, spirometry, and assessment of bronchial responsiveness 18–24 months after exposure ended. *Occup Environ Med* 1994; 51: 225.

9 Watt MM, Watt SJ, Seaton A. Episode of toxic gas exposure in sewer workers. *Occup Environ Med* 1997; 54: 277.

10 Kern DG. Outbreak of the reactive airways dysfunction syndrome after a spill of glacial acetic acid. *Am Rev Respir Dis* 1991; 144: 1058.

11 Gilbert R, Auchincloss JH. Reactive airways dysfunction syndrome presenting as a reversible restrictive defect. *Lung* 1989; 167: 55.

12 Schwartz DA, Smith DD, Lakshminarayan S. The pulmonary sequelae associated with accidental inhalation of chlorine gas. *Chest* 1990; 97: 820.

13 Ross DJ, McDonald JC. Asthma following inhalation accidents reported to the SWORD project. *Ann Occup Hyg* 1996; 40: 645.

14 Ross S, Godden DJ, Abdalla M *et al.* Outcome of wheeze in childhood: the influence of atopy. *Eur Respir J* 1995; 8: 2081.

15 Chia KS, Jeyaratnam J, Chan TB, Lim TK. Airway responsiveness of firefighters after smoke exposure. *Br J Ind Med* 1990; 47: 524.

16 Keynes HL, Ross DJ, McDonald JC. SWORD '95: surveillance of work-related and occupational respiratory disease in the UK. *Occup Med* 1996; 46: 379.

17 Sallie B, McDonald JC. Inhalation accidents reported to the SWORD surveillance project 1990–1993. *Ann Occup Hyg* 1996; 40: 211.

18 Blanc P. Occupational asthma in a national disability survey. *Chest* 1987; 92: 613.

19 Health and Safety Commission. *Annual Report 1991/92.* London: HMSO, 1992: 96.

20 Tarlo SM, Broder I. Irritant induced asthma. *Chest* 1989; 96: 297.

21 Boulet L-P. Increases in airway responsiveness following acute exposure to respiratory irritants. Reactive airway dysfunction syndrome or occupational asthma? *Chest* 1988; 94: 476.

22 Gautrin D, Boulet L-P, Boulet M *et al.* Is reactive airways dysfunction syndrome a variant of occupational asthma? *J Allergy Clin Immunol* 1994; 93: 12.

37

HYPERSENSITIVITY LUNG DISEASES

ANTHONY SEATON

The history of hypersensitivity lung diseases goes back to 1932, when Campbell [1] described acute respiratory symptoms in farmers after work with hay and Tower and colleagues [2] described similar symptoms in maple bark peelers. The association of the conditions with inhalation of microbial spores was recognized and, in the case of maple bark disease, it was speculated that the pathogenesis might be a form of hypersensitivity reaction to *Cryptostroma corticale*. Farmer's lung was subsequently shown to be due to the inhalation of spores of thermophilic actinomycetes (now classified as bacteria) and of species of *Aspergillus*. The finding of precipitating antibody to such organisms led to the concept that the disease was an example of a pulmonary type 3 allergic reaction, although study of lung biopsies, animal models and bronchoalveolar lavage (BAL) fluid has shown that cell-mediated reactions are also crucial to the development of the condition.

Study of the pathogenesis of farmer's lung led to considerable interest in other possible causes of hypersensitivity pneumonitis; bagassosis had been described (as a bronchiolitis) in 1946 [3] and it became apparent that this disease was similar in aetiology to farmer's lung. The occurrence of similar syndromes in response to animal antigen was recognized when bird fancier's lung was described in 1960 [4,5], while more recently sporadic examples of a similar condition have been described in response to exposure to certain chemicals of relatively low molecular weight [6–8]. A very large number of causes, mostly related to inhalation of fungal spores, have been recorded and undoubtedly more remain to be described.

It is important to recognize that the syndrome of hypersensitivity pneumonitis covers a range of reactions, varying from the classical severe acute episodes of farmer's lung to a much more chronic illness such as occurs most frequently in response to bird antigen. In addition, variations on the theme occur in people exposed to aerosols from air conditioners and humidifiers, to dust in grain silos and to sewage sludge. These other conditions are discussed further in Chapter 54. Moreover, very similar reactions may occur in response to treatment with certain drugs and these are discussed in Chapter 55.

Clinical features

The classical acute presentation occurs mainly in individuals exposed to high doses of microbial spores, as seen typically in farmers feeding cattle with mouldy hay [9,10]. The onset of symptoms is about 4–9 h after exposure, with chills, dry cough and an influenzal feeling. Rigors may occur and the patient notices breathlessness on normal exertion. Severe attacks may result in profound dyspnoea but in most cases general malaise is the predominant symptom. The main findings on examination are repetitive mid- and late-inspiratory crackles and tachypnoea. Polyphonic wheezes may be heard and should not deter one from making the diagnosis. Precipitating antibodies are commonly found in the blood.

Such acute attacks usually settle after 48 h. However some episodes may be much more persistent and the patient may remain ill and breathless for several weeks. In very rare instances the acute attack may be fatal [11]. Another variant, related to the removal of mouldy grain from the tops of silos prior to emptying the silage, presents with cough, fever, chest tightness, malaise and headache about 2–8 h after exposure [12,13]. Crackles are less frequent and precipitins are absent. This syndrome has been called mycotoxicosis or organic dust toxicity. However, despite differences in immunopathogenesis, its similar aetiological, clinical and pathological features to farmer's lung suggest that it should be regarded as a variant of that form of hypersensitivity pneumonitis.

At the other extreme of the spectrum of clinical presentation is the usual response to budgerigar (parakeet) antigen. Such patients present with insidious malaise, breathlessness, unproductive cough and sometimes loss of weight, often over months or even years [14,15]. Again, repetitive inspiratory crackles are the characteristic physical sign. Polyphonic wheezes may also occur and, in the more chronic cases, a high-pitched, short, late inspiratory squeak is often heard [16]. This sign, which also occurs in other chronic pulmonary fibroses and in rheumatoid bronchiolitis, usually follows an inspiratory crackle and is probably caused by vibration in the wall of a bronchiole as it opens following abnormal closure. The presence of such signs of airway disease serves as a reminder that so-called allergic alveolitis affects bronchioles as well as alveoli.

A proportion of patients with allergic alveolitis of any sort may progress to a chronic form of the disease, characterized particularly by increasing exertional dyspnoea over years [9,17]. Inspiratory crackles are usually present but some of these patients may develop the clinical, radiological and physiological features of generalized emphysema. Patients with chronic allergic alveolitis may progress to fatal cardiorespiratory failure [11]. Finger clubbing is not a feature at any stage. In contrast, some patients who continue to be exposed to antigen despite medical advice do not progress to chronic disease and may even show evidence of spontaneous desensitization.

In most patients with allergic alveolitis, the most important diagnostic clues come from the history and the finding of inspiratory crackles. Acute episodes bear a clear relationship to exposures to antigen, such as mouldy hay, pigeons or work in maltings. If a more insidious type is suspected, attention should be paid in history-taking to exposure on a regular basis to known causes. Periodicity of symptoms is important; in Japan, *Trichosporon cutaneum* commonly grows in damp wooden houses and sporulates in the warm summer temperatures, causing outbreaks of seasonal alveolitis [18]. Patients with budgerigars improve when they (or the budgerigars) leave home for a while, and work-related symptoms may improve over holidays.

Allergic alveolitis may occur at any age; children who help their parents on farms or in pigeon lofts or who are exposed to antigen in the house may present with the disease. In several surveys cigarette smokers have been shown to be less susceptible than non-smokers [19,20].

Radiographic features

In acute episodes, the chest radiograph commonly shows a bilateral, diffuse, micronodular infiltrate, usually denser towards the hila (Fig. 37.1). An irregular and linear infiltrate may also be present in the lower zones. In severe attacks it may mimic acute pulmonary oedema, *Mycoplasma* pneumonia or pneumonitis due to inhalation of toxic gases, although it should be noted that in some of the precipitin-negative cases occurring in workers clearing the tops of silos the radiograph remains normal even when the systemic illness is quite severe. The changes usually resolve rapidly on removal from exposure and treatment with corticosteroids. As mentioned above, in

some cases resolution is slow, taking several weeks and giving rise to diagnostic difficulties. If the patient is a farmer, silo-filler's lung (pneumonitis due to nitrogen dioxide) needs to be considered in the differential diagnosis and lung biopsy may be necessary. *Mycoplasma* or other atypical pneumonia may also be confused clinically and radiologically, especially as such patients occasionally produce false-positive precipitating antibody to farmer's lung antigens [21].

In less acute cases, the radiographic signs may be more subtle and sometimes even absent. A very sparse micronodular infiltrate, perhaps indistinguishable from a normal film, should not prevent the diagnosis in the presence of an appropriate history and the finding of inspiratory crackles. Some patients, particularly those with disease related to inhalation of chemicals, may present with dense, patchy consolidation easily confused with an infective pneumonia. The first patient described as having alveolitis due to isocyanates presented in this way [6] (Fig. 37.2).

Chronic allergic alveolitis may progress to pulmonary fibrosis, which characteristically affects upper zones predominantly. Coarse, irregular shadows extend from hila to apices with attendant bronchiectatic change, retraction upwards of pulmonary vessels and, often, well-marked emphysema in the lower zones (Fig. 37.3). In some of these patients the fibrosis may be invisible radiologically, the appearances being indistinguishable from those of cigarette-related emphysema [9]. In the more usual type, the radiological appearances resemble those of old tuberculosis, chronic sarcoidosis, ankylosing spondylitis lung or accelerated silicosis. High-resolution CT may assist in the differential diagnosis by showing a peribronchiolar or centriacinar distibution of nodular change [22].

Pulmonary function

The typical changes in an acute attack are reductions in lung volumes, carbon monoxide diffusing capacity and Po_2 [9,23]. In milder cases, only a slight fall in diffusing capacity and Po_2 during exercise may be found. If compliance is measured it is found to be decreased, as would be expected. The reduction in diffusing capacity is a more sensitive test of acinar disease than the chest radiograph, and in the more subacute syndromes (e.g. in people exposed to budgerigars) it is often present when the radiograph is normal. Sometimes the patients with the so-called organic dust toxicity syndrome or mycotoxicosis have normal chest films and lung function, showing only slight oxygen desaturation [13].

In most patients with acute episodes the volumes, codiffusion and Po_2 abnormalities recover over a few days or weeks, though increases in diffusing capacity may still occur after a year [24]. However, in those with subacute or chronic disease recovery may be slow and incomplete,

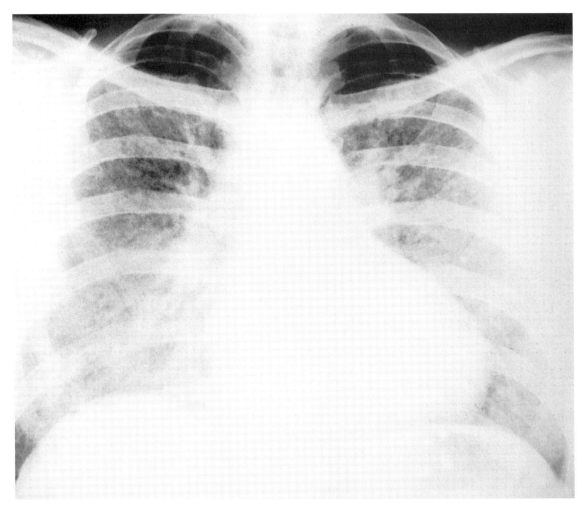

Fig. 37.1 Diffuse bilateral ground-glass appearance of acute farmer's lung.

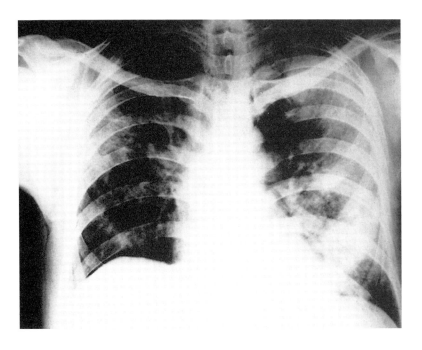

Fig. 37.2 Dense pneumonic infiltrates throughout left lung and in right mid zone. This proved to be an acute hypersensitivity reaction to toluene diisocyanate.

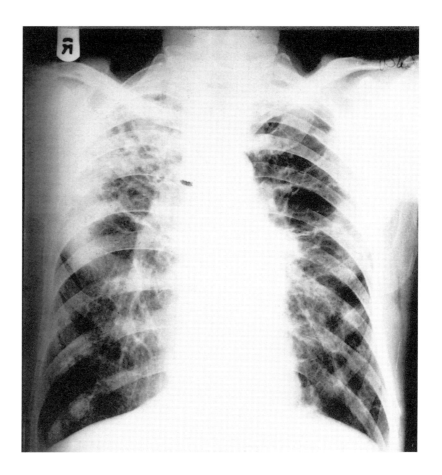

Fig. 37.3 Irregular upper zone fibrosis in patient with chronic farmer's lung.

leaving the patient with chronic impairment of function. Evidence of airflow obstruction may be present in a number of these patients, not always explicable on the basis of smoking or concomitant asthma [25]. While bronchiolitis is the likely explanation in some, up to one-third of patients with well-developed chronic allergic alveolitis develop a pattern of irreversible airflow obstruction, reduction in diffusing capacity and pathological emphysema [9,26,27].

Pathology

In keeping with the inhalational route of exposure, the pathological changes in acute allergic alveolitis are most marked at the centre of the acinus and least at the periphery [10,27]. When a biopsy shows non-specific changes, this pattern of distribution may be an important clue as to aetiology. In the very acute cases described as mycotoxicosis, intense inflammatory change with polymorphonuclear leucocytes has been noted in bronchioles [12], although one such patient studied personally has also shown typical non-caseating granulomas. In typical acute cases, the alveolar inflammation extends to the bronchioles where it is somewhat less marked, and is usually characterized by a lymphocytic and granulomatous reaction. Sometimes this may occlude the smallest airways. In

addition, non-caseating granulomas including Langhans-type giant cells, lymphocytes and plasma cells are found predominantly at the centre of the acinus (Fig. 37.4). The alveolar walls are thickened, with oedema and chronic inflammatory cells; foamy macrophages may fill the alveoli. Fibrin deposition may be demonstrated and, depending on the length of the illness, it is not uncommon to see some mature collagen in alveolar walls. In contrast to immune complex disease, vascular changes do not normally occur. In a unique case, a lady with allergic alveolitis due to dust from sea snail shells was shown to have deposition of amyloid in her alveolar septa [28]. Ultrastructural studies show swelling of alveolar epithelial cells and disruption of basement membrane in association with the inflammation [29].

In chronic disease, the granulomatous changes may disappear. The lungs become fibrosed and secondary cystic change due to bronchiolectasis occurs. The fibrosis is usually more marked in upper zones and secondary emphysema is common. Secondary vascular changes reflect the pulmonary hypertension.

Pathogenesis

Despite its relative rarity and the ease with which the condition may be treated and prevented, the pathogenesis of

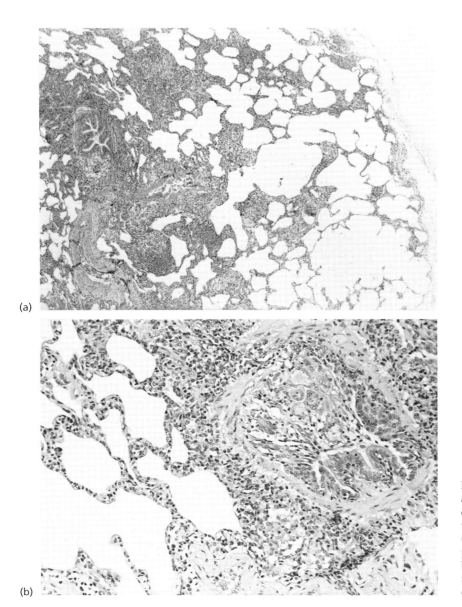

(a)

(b)

Fig. 37.4 Histological appearances of acute allergic alveolitis: (a) centriacinar distribution of mononuclear cell infiltrate with poorly formed granulomas (haematoxylin & eosin ×25); (b) higher power demonstrating granuloma within the bronchiolar wall as well as the interstitial mononuclear cell infiltrate (haematoxylin & eosin ×115)

hypersensitivity pneumonitis has attracted a huge amount of interest among immunologists [30]. Nevertheless, the mechanisms of the disease remain obscure. The earliest concept of pathogenesis was that allergic alveolitis was an example of a type 3, complement-fixing, immune complex reaction in the lung [31]. In support of this concept was the frequent finding of precipitating antibodies to the inhaled antigen in the blood of farmers, pigeon fanciers and others with the disease. However, many patients, especially among those exposed to budgerigars, did not show such antibodies, while they were found in a suprising number of exposed but well subjects [32,33]. Moreover, the histopathological features suggested that the aetiology was more complex, since vasculitis was usually absent and granulomas were present. Interest therefore started to centre on cell-mediated reactions and, in particular, on the roles of macrophages and lympho-

cytes [34]. The popularization of the technique of BAL allowed study of the cellular reactions within the acinus, including studies of the functional status of cells so obtained. Even so, the precise immunological or para-immunological mechanisms have still not been clearly defined.

Features that seem to be usual in patients with allergic alveolitis are a response to inhalational challenge with the offending antigen in terms of fever, polymorphonuclear leucocytosis with fall in total blood lymphocyte count, and evidence of impairment of acinar lung function [35]. Bronchial washings in patients with active allergic alveolitis (Fig. 37.5) show an increased proportion of lymphocytes up to about 80% of the total count and averaging about 60% [36,37]. Studies of T-cell subtypes in BAL fluid have shown findings similar to those in peripheral blood, with a relative excess of suppressor CD8 over helper CD4

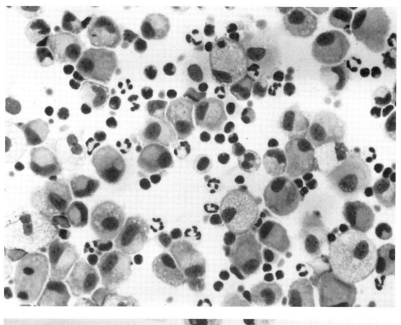

(a)

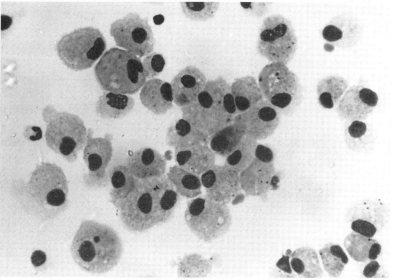

(b)

Fig. 37.5 Bronchoalveolar lavage from (a) patient with allergic alveolitis showing large numbers of lymphocytes together with macrophages and some polymorphonuclear leucocytes and (b) from normal subject showing macrophages.

T lymphocytes [38]. Curiously, exposed but unaffected subjects have also been shown to have raised lymphocyte counts and proportions in their alveolar fluid [39]. However, functional tests of BAL lymphocytes *in vitro* have shown that those from symptomatic subjects with bird fancier's lung increase markedly in blastogenic activity when stimulated with phytohaemagglutinin or pigeon serum compared with the response of cells from exposed but asymptomatic subjects [40]. A soluble protein associated with suppressor T lymphocytes, sCD8, has been shown to augment proliferation of lymphocytes when stimulated with relevant antigen [41], while the proinflammatory cytokines macrophage inhibitory factor and interleukin (IL)-8 (which attract CD8 T lymphocytes and neutrophils respectively) have been demonstrated in high concentrations in BAL fluid from patients with allergic

alveolitis [42]. Other macrophage cytokines identified in various animal models include IL-1 and tumour necrosis factor γ and various growth factors [30], some of which can be released by immune complexes and lead to the formation of granulomas.

In addition to increased numbers of lymphocytes in BAL fluid of exposed subjects, those with disease may also show high counts of mast cells, up to about 5% of the total cell count [43–45]. In different studies, the proportions of these cells have been shown to fall to normal, but the absolute numbers to rise, when exposure ceases [43,44]. Increases in neutrophil leucocytes, averaging 10% of the total cells, may also be observed in the exposed individual, falling when exposure ceases. Indeed, a transient and often severe bronchoalveolar neutrophil leucocytosis has been shown to be an important component of the initial response to bronchial challenge, appearing within 24 h of exposure and clearing within a week [46]. Finally, plasma cells may be found in BAL fluid from patients with acute allergic alveolitis and are rarely found in any other condition [47,48]. They may therefore be of some diagnostic value.

The evidence suggests that people exposed to these organic antigens may develop a complement-fixing, IgG-mediated reaction detectable by precipitating antibodies in serum. In addition, and despite remaining perfectly well, they may have a lymphocytic alveolitis following release of cytokines from alveolar macrophages challenged by the antigen. In those in whom disease develops, the functional activity of the lymphocytes is altered; it may be that this is responsible for the formation of granulomas, since these cells produce lymphokines that inhibit macrophage migration. Furthermore, the T cell may also produce other lymphokines and leukotrienes that attract mast cells and cause them to release their mediators [49,50]; this would provide an alternative explanation to a type 3 reaction for the oedema, though the absence of eosinophils in the pathology of the disease is a point against an important role for mast cells. Nevertheless, degranulation of mast cells may contribute towards the disease [44,45].

Bronchoalveolar neutrophil leucocytosis seems to be a common response to inhalation of a number of irritant and toxic particles. The histology of so-called mycotoxicosis shows neutrophils and, as mentioned above, many subjects with acute allergic alveolitis have blood and bronchoalveolar neutrophilia early in the course of the disease. There is good evidence that in some subjects activation of the alternative pathway of complement may occur in response to dust inhalation; it may be that this could be important in some of the more acute, precipitin-negative cases [51].

The question remains why some exposed individuals develop neither disease nor immunological response, some develop the response in terms of antibodies and/or lymphocytic alveolitis but no disease, and some develop disease with striking changes in both proportions and functions of alveolar inflammatory cells. Dose of antigen exposure probably plays a part [52], as does the immunomodulatory (in this case, suppressive) effect of cigarette smoke [53]. Genetic factors have not yet been identified and, despite the sacrifice of many rats, mice and rabbits, the question remains unanswered. It is perhaps fortunate that satisfactory management of the condition does not depend on understanding its mechanisms.

Diagnosis

A physician scanning the literature on allergic alveolitis might get the impression that diagnosis is complicated and requires the use of many sophisticated and, for the patient, uncomfortable tests. Happily this is not so, as in most cases the diagnosis can be made by taking a competent history and by the use of stethoscope, simple laboratory tests, chest radiograph and lung function testing, supplemented if necessary by a visit to the site of the suspected antigen source. Only occasionally are challenge testing, bronchoscopy with lavage and transbronchial biopsy necessary.

History

Acute episodes usually bear a clear relationship to the exposure and are recognized by the patient. The more subacute presentation is often regarded as recurrent bronchitis or asthma by the primary care physician and is more difficult to pin down to antigen exposure. All patients with respiratory symptoms suggestive of allergic alveolitis should be asked about exposures at work or home to dusts and moulds, birds and small animals, and volatile chemicals (as well as drugs, see Chapter 55). One potential source of antigen that may be overlooked is feathers in cushions or pillows. This was the proven cause of chronic allergic alveolitis in the first patient with the condition investigated by the author many years ago, and a similar case resulting from exposure to goose feathers in a duvet has been described more recently [54,55]. Attention should be paid to any improvement in symptoms that may occur with the season or on holiday. However, apart from suggesting a possible source of antigen, the history in subacute and chronic allergic alveolitis is often of non-specific respiratory symptoms with little or no diurnal variation.

Physical examination

The crucial finding is of repetitive inspiratory crackles. If these are persistent, they indicate disease and justify further investigation. They are virtually always present in acute, subacute and chronic disease and their absence should cast doubt on the diagnosis, tipping the scales in favour of sarcoidosis. Other causes of such crackles in the relatively young and middle-aged people who predominantly suffer from allergic alveolitis are nowadays quite uncommon. The finding of finger clubbing is a strong pointer against allergic alveolitis and towards cryptogenic pulmonary fibrosis.

Blood tests

In someone with appropriate clinical features, the finding of precipitins to the suspected antigen in the serum can normally be taken to clinch the diagnosis. The straightforward gel diffusion test may not be adequate to detect antibody in a number of subjects, and many laboratories now favour a quantitative radioimmunoassay [56]. This technique is more sensitive but detects antibody in a higher proportion of exposed but unaffected subjects. However, the higher the titre, the greater the likelihood that disease is present, and in the clinical setting sensitivity is invaluable in a test used to complement clinical findings.

Radiology and lung function testing

As stated before, the chest radiograph may be misleadingly normal in subacute disease; indeed the presence of a relatively normal film in a patient with diffuse inspiratory crackles should alert the physician to the possibility of allergic alveolitis as a diagnosis. In acute episodes the film is usually convincingly abnormal, and here the problem is differentiating allergic alveolitis from other causes of diffuse shadowing. To this extent, the radiographic changes are non-specific. The usual abnormality of lung function, a reduced carbon monoxide diffusing capacity, is also non-specific but is a useful indication of parenchymal disease justifying further investigation. The chief value of chest radiography and lung function testing lies in follow-up of the patient after removal from exposure in order to assess response.

More complex investigations

In most patients the cause of the disease is clear from the above investigations, and the physician is able to plan appropriate management monitored by the same tests. Occasionally, however, the cause is not clear and further investigations are necessary. The first essential is to establish the diagnosis and to exclude other causes of interstitial lung disease. This may be done by biopsy or immunological testing. Biopsy requires an adequate specimen and the transbronchial method is rarely satisfactory in this respect; increasingly, surgeons are offering thoracoscopic biopsy, enabling several good-sized specimens to be taken with control of bleeding and air leaks by stapling [57]. It seems likely that this method will displace all others where appropriate surgical expertise is available. However, biopsy does not always enable a certain diagnosis of allergic alveolitis, especially if a granuloma is not included in the sample or in more chronic cases, and never helps establish the cause. It therefore has its main application in patients in whom there is a serious likelihood of some other disease being present. BAL is frequently performed as part of the investigation, although the usually lymphocytic alveolitis (with a ratio of suppressor to helper T cells greater than unity and with plasma cells sometimes present) is no more than a guide to the diagnosis without usually giving specific aetiological information. However, if a likely antigen has been identified it can then be used not only to search for precipitating antibodies in the blood but also to look at specific proliferative responses of bronchoalveolar lymphocytes to antigen stimulation [58]. It can also be used in challenge testing, where a small dose is administered to the subject by nebulizer and response measured in terms of white cell count, temperature and lung function tests (see later).

If an antigen is suspected but unknown, a visit to likely sources is worth while. Search of a patient's house for fungi, air conditioners or exotic pets may sometimes be revealing, as may a careful look around the workplace. In doing this, the physician should not confine the search to seeking known antigens; any organic material capable of generating particles of respirable size should come under suspicion, including dusts that might contain fungi or animal material, and fumes at work. Particular attention should be paid to stored organic matter that could have become damp and mouldy, to damp places or rotten wood where fungi could sporulate and to ducted or blown air conditioning or heating systems. Furnishings may contain feathers or straw; the author has diagnosed allergic alveolitis in a housewife due to feathers in cushions, as mentioned above, and also in an upholsterer due to contaminated straw in antique furniture. If a source of antigen is detected in a workplace, further study of all those exposed using epidemiological techniques is usually desirable. Ultimate confirmation of the diagnosis may depend on demonstration of a response to either withdrawal from exposure or challenge with the suspected antigen. The simplest procedure, and that most usually practised, is to remove the antigen source or to have the patient change his or her work practice and to follow the response in terms of lung function. A slow but steady improvement would be anticipated, although complete recovery may never occur in more chronic disease. Alternatively, a challenge test may be carried out. The simplest form of this is to expose the subject to antigen in the normal way, for example a farmer is exposed to mouldy hay or a worker exposed to the suspect fumes or dust in the workplace, and appropriate measurements made. Alternatively, the exposure may take place in the laboratory, either to crude antigen or to purified extracts. The latter is appropriate if the subject is exposed to a known antigen but if it is not certain whether or not the disease is present.

Laboratory challenge tests require decisions about dose of exposure. It is always wise to precede them with a skin-prick test, since if immediate hypersensitivity is present a severe bronchial reaction may occur. The dose of antigen may be estimated very roughly from the history, in terms of severity of reaction, and may be adjusted by time, by concentration or both. For example, using budgerigar or pigeon serum it is usual to challenge first with a 1/100 dilution, then (if no reaction occurs) on another day with a 1/20 dilution and finally with a 1/5 dilution of 1 mL neat serum. Similar dilutions can be made of mouldy hay extract and of fungal antigens. Clearly, laboratory

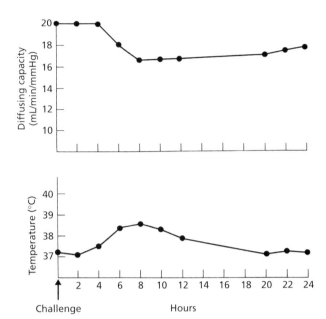

Fig. 37.6 Rise in temperature and fall in lung diffusing capacity following challenge with budgerigar antigen. Ideally, a smaller dose might have been given to avoid too great a fall in diffusing capacity.

Table 37.1 Response to challenge testing [35].

Test	Change	Specificity (%)	Sensit-ivity (%)
Exercise minute ventilation	>+25%	94	40
Exercise respiratory frequency	>+25%	94	30
Body temperature	>37.2°C	95	78
Neutrophil count	+2.5×10⁹/L	96	68
Lymphocyte count	>−0.5×10⁹/L*	97	52
Vital capacity	>−15%	97	48

*When combined with absolute lymphocyte count of <1.5×10⁹/L.

challenge testing is not an exact science and should be approached with caution. The subject should remain in hospital under observation for 36 h and corticosteroids should be available to treat severe reactions. The response to challenge tests may not be as clear-cut as one would anticipate. The most obvious response is a feeling of malaise, with fever, aches and exertional dyspnoea (Fig. 37.6). These are associated with a rise in exercise ventilation, temperature, neutrophil count in the blood and respiratory frequency during exercise, together with a fall in circulating lymphocytes and forced vital capacity [35]. Changes in diffusing capacity and the chest radiograph may occur, but only in severe reactions that are best avoided. Criteria for a positive response proposed by Hendrick and colleagues are shown in Table 37.1. If three or more of these tests are positive within 36 h of the challenge test, there is a high likelihood that the antigen has been found. A scheme for the investigation of suspected allergic alveolitis is given in Fig. 37.7.

Management

Acute episodes of allergic alveolitis may require hospitalization and oxygen therapy to help the patient during the reaction; occasionally hypoxaemia may be so severe and the lungs so stiff as to necessitate assisted ventilation. Corticosteroids should be given for all but the mildest attacks, in a dose of 40 mg prednisolone daily until lung function and Po_2 have improved to clinically adequate levels. A controlled trial in acute farmer's lung

has shown that an 8-week course of corticosteroids speeded functional recovery but that longer-term lung function did not differ between the active and placebo groups [59].

Further exposure to antigen should if possible be prevented. In the case of exposure to birds, the creatures must be removed if possible. Unfortunately, for financial and social reasons, many pigeon breeders are unwilling to do this; in such cases effective oronasal respirators should be used whenever the loft is entered. Cross-reactivity occurs, so that pigeon breeders may get exacerbations when they visit houses with budgerigars and they should be warned of this possibility. It should be noted that after a bird has been removed from a patient's house it may find a home with a relative whom the patient visits; in the author's experience this has caused recurrent disease, sometimes manifesting as quite severe attacks. Moreover, bird antigen may persist for months in a room after the bird has been removed, despite careful cleaning, and this may explain persisting symptoms in some very sensitive patients [60]. Farmers often require respirators, but should also be given advice about keeping hay dry or changing to making silage (though this may require some education also on avoidance of silo-filler's lung and mycotoxicosis). Colleges of agriculture can usually give appropriate advice, as can the Health and Safety Executive in the UK.

The use of respirators requires some comment [61,62]. These should be well fitting and well maintained. Filters should be changed regularly and should be adequate to exclude respirable-sized particles; in the UK and the USA, they are subject to testing against standards and should not allow penetration of more than 1–2% of a standard aerosol. If a subject is advised to obtain a respirator, an appropriate one should be recommended and the patient instructed in its fitting, use and maintenance. Care should be taken to ensure that one is chosen that provides a good seal without too much discomfort or respiratory resistance. Powered helmet-type respirators, as opposed to

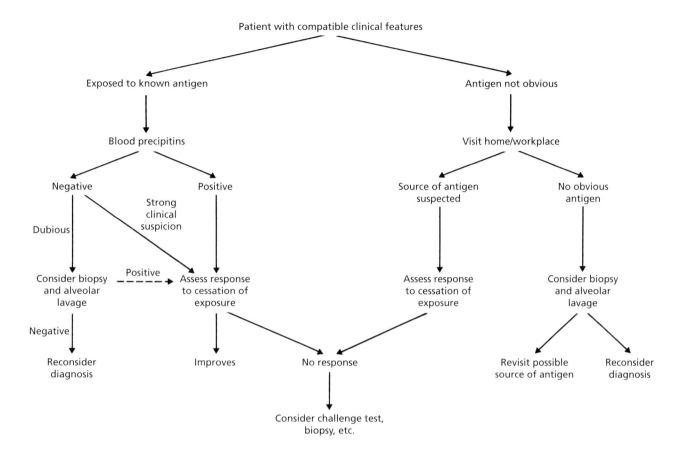

Fig. 37.7 Investigation of suspected allergic alveolitis.

mask types, may be adequate, depending on the efficiency of the filter and the sensitivity of the patient to antigen. Before the subject purchases a respirator, it is wise to test its efficacy in preventing symptoms under normal exposure conditions. Chronic allergic alveolitis should be treated with a prolonged course of corticosteroids, usually for several months, until it is clear that no further functional improvement will occur. The drugs should then be stopped, assuming that further exposure can be prevented. The airways' obstructive component does not respond adequately to corticosteroids, and there is no point in continuing these drugs long term in the hope that it will. However, it should be remembered that asthma sometimes coexists with allergic alveolitis and trials of antiasthma therapy are always justified in such patients.

Causes of allergic alveolitis

The causes of allergic alveolitis may be separated into three main types: microbial, animal and chemical. In addition there is a small group in which the antigens have not been identified. The main causes are listed in Table 37.2.

Microbial causes

Farmer's lung

Farmer's lung commonly presents in the acute form, although chronic cases may go unrecognized for long periods [9,10,27]. It is usually caused by inhalation of spores of thermophilic actinomycetes, higher bacteria of a filamentous appearance that grow in hay or other organic matter that has been stored in a damp condition. The two most usual organisms in the UK are *Micropolyspora faeni* (now known as *Faenia rectivirgula*) and *Thermoactinomyces vulgaris*, though other organisms including fungi of *Aspergillus* species may sometimes cause the syndrome. The spores are liberated into the air when the dried mouldy hay is fed to cattle, usually in the winter. The condition occurs most commonly in countries where rain is frequent at harvest time and among farmers unaware of the problem. Studies of the epidemiology have shown a prevalence of 3–5% of farmers in agricultural areas of Britain and the USA, most cases occurring in the areas of highest rainfall [20,32,63,64]. Precipitating antibodies in the absence of disease are found in approximately twice as many subjects, and can therefore only be taken as an indication of exposure unless the farmer has appropriate symptoms and signs as well. As with other types

Table 37.2 Principal causes of allergic alveolitis.

Antigen source	Disease
Microbial	
Thermophilic actinomycetes	Farmer's lung
(*Micropolyspora faeni*,	Bagassosis
Thermoactinomyces vulgaris)	Mushroom worker's lung
	Air conditioner lung
Aspergillus clavatus	Maltworker's lung
Aspergillus fumigatus	Allergic aspergillosis
Aspergillus versicolor	Doghouse disease
Alternaria spp., *Trichoderma*	Wood-pulp worker's lung
koningii	
Aureobasidium pullulans,	Sequoiosis
Graphium sp.	
Cryptostroma corticale	Maple bark stripper's lung
Penicillium frequentens	Suberosis
Merulius lacrimans	Dry rot lung
Mucor spp.	Paprika splitter's lung
Penicillium casei, P. roqueforti	Cheeseworker's lung
Lycoperdon spp.	Puff-ball lung
Trichosporon cutaneum	Summer pneumonitis
Bacillus subtilis	Washing powder lung
Bacillus cereus, Cephalosporium	Humidifier lung
acrimonium,	
Klebsiella oxytoca	
Animal	
Budgerigar, pigeon, hen,	Bird fancier's lung
turkey, owl, etc.	
Fish protein	Fishmeal lung
Animal pituitary	Pituitary snuff-taker's lung
Animal pancreas	Enzyme worker's lung
Rodents	Rodent handler's lung
Wheat weevil	Weevil alveolitis
Chemical	
Bordeaux mixture	Vineyard sprayer's lung
Cobalt	Hard-metal disease
Isocyanates	Isocyanate alveolitis
Pauli's reagent	Pauli's reagent alveolitis
Pyrethrum	Insecticide lung
Trimellitic anhydride,	Acid anhydride lung
hexahydrophthalic anhydride	
Uncertain	
Lake water	Sauna lung
Hut thatch	New Guinea lung
Boxwood	Ramin lung

Table 37.3 Respiratory diseases of farmers.

Farmer's lung, farmer's fever	Actinomycetes
Mycotoxicosis	Fungi
Asthma/rhinitis	Fungi, storage mites
Swine fever	?Endotoxin in excreta
Silo-filler's disease	Nitrogen dioxide
Organophosphate poisoning	Insecticides

under conditions of intensive rearing, they may be subject to alveolitis or febrile reactions due to excreta and their contaminants [68], while chemical pneumonitis may occur as a result of exposure to oxides of nitrogen in silos [69]. To make life more difficult for the clinician, they may also present like anyone else with *Mycoplasma* pneumonia, which mimics either farmer's lung or silo-filler's lung [21]. A febrile illness like farmer's lung but without the pulmonary component has been described [70] and farm workers are of course at risk of poisoning by organophosphorus compounds, which can in severe cases lead to neuromuscular paralysis.

The diagnosis of farmer's lung is usually easy; indeed it is often made by the patient. If it is made sufficiently early in the course of the disease, preventive measures should be effective and progression should not occur. However, continued exposure is associated with a high risk of progression [71]. Only in difficult, precipitin-negative cases are further investigations necessary, and these should usually be preceded by a visit to the farm to make sure there is no other source of antigen that has been overlooked in the history.

Management is as discussed above. Since farmers are rarely able to retire or change jobs, it is important that they be educated in preventive measures. Equally, they should not simply hand over the dusty job to their wife or other assistant, as that is likely to produce a second case. Transfer from hay to silage, proper drying of damp hay and use of a respirator when exposure cannot be prevented [72] are the principles of management. In the UK, employed farmers with the disease (not self-employed, who have to make their own insurance arrangements) are eligible for industrial injuries benefit under the national social security scheme.

Mushroom worker's lung

Mushrooms are grown commercially on compost, often made of straw and horse droppings that is allowed to ferment, which is then heated in moist air to just below 60°C. While these conditions suit the mushroom mycelia with which it is seeded, they are also ideal for the growth of thermophilic actinomycetes. Workers may be exposed to spores when compost and mycelia are mechanically mixed or when the sheds are being cleaned. The manifes-

of allergic alveolitis, smokers are less likely to have the disease than non-smokers [64].

It is worth noting that farmers are subject to a number of respiratory disorders as a result of their work [65] (Table 37.3). Farmer's lung, both acute and chronic, may be associated also with asthma due to hay or its contaminants. On the acute side, with negative precipitins, farmer's lung merges into the acute organic dust (mycotoxicosis) syndrome [13]. Farmers may also have asthma and rhinitis due to exposure to fungi in harvesting grains and to mites in stored grains [66,67]. If they keep livestock

tations of the disease are clinically indistinguishable from those of farmer's lung [73–76].

Bagassosis

Bagasse is the residue after sugar is extracted from cane. It is a fibrous material used in the manufacture of paper, boards and building materials. Typically it becomes contaminated with thermophilic actinomycetes when lying in the hot and humid conditions of Louisiana, the West Indies and other tropical and subtropical areas where sugar cane is processed. Although the disease commonly affects workers handling the bagasse in these countries, it may also occur wherever mouldy material is imported [77–79]. Indeed, it was first described in London, in workers handling bagasse imported from Louisiana [3]. Again, the disease is a variant of farmer's lung.

Air conditioner and humidifier lung
(see also Chapter 54)

Many workers exposed to 'conditioned' air (air in which the humidity and temperature have been controlled to produce comfortable conditions) suffer mild general malaise known as humidifier fever [80,81], particularly on the first day of the week; however, some develop a true allergic alveolitis [82–86]. Various organisms have from time to time been incriminated, since conditions differ in different conditioning and humidifying systems, leading to preferential growth of different organisms. In some episodes, thermophilic actinomycetes have been thought to be responsible, in some *Aspergillus* spp., in others *Penicillium* spp. and thermotolerant bacteria resembling *Bacillus cereus* [87], while in some the cause has not been identified [88]. In general, humidifier fever, in which the predominant antigen source is *Naegleria gruberi* or other amoebae, is not associated with evidence of interstitial lung disease, although at least one patient with typical radiological and physiological changes has been described [86].

This spectrum of responses, from classical allergic alveolitis to humidifier fever, results from exposure to droplets from humidifying systems in which the water is sprayed into a moving stream of air. The drops that fall and the larger droplets removed by a baffle are collected in a sump and then recirculated and sprayed again. The sump and the baffle plates form a culture medium for microorganisms, and a food chain develops depending on temperature and nutrients. In theory this can be prevented by spraying steam or fresh (rather than recirculated) water, although these options are often expensive. Alternatively, the incoming and outgoing air can be filtered and/or subjected to ultraviolet light and biocides can be added to the water. Measures taken depend on the system and on economic factors, but must include regular cleaning of the whole system. If the water is heated, the temperature should also be raised above 60°C in order to discourage the growth of *Legionella* spp. (see Chapter 13).

An identical range of syndromes may occur from exposure to contaminated aerosol from home ultrasonic nebulizers. An outbreak in Japan has been asssociated with an aerosol containing *Cephalosporium* and *Candida* spp. [89], while one in the USA has been caused by *Klebsiella oxytoca* [90].

Maltworker's lung

Malt is used as a source of carbohydrate for fermentation in the manufacture of whisky. It is barley that has been dried, stored and then rehydrated and allowed to germinate in conditions of controlled temperature and humidity. The process may take place on the floor of a large room, the maltings, where the material is turned regularly to allow carbon dioxide to escape. Alternatively, it can be carried out in rotating drums. In the former situation, the malt may become contaminated with *Aspergillus clavatus* and workers may inhale spores of this organism [91–93]. The condition has been shown to cause a farmer's lung-like illness in up to 5% of those workers who turn the malt.

Woodworker's lung

Allergic alveolitis has been described in several different groups of woodworkers. Indeed, maple bark stripper's lung was described in the same year as farmer's lung [2]. These workers were exposed to the spores of *Cryptostroma corticale*, a fungus that grows under the bark and which is pathogenic to the tree [94]. The spores are liberated when the bark is mechanically removed in lumber mills [95–97]. The incidence of the disease may be controlled by hygiene measures, such as extract ventilation and spraying of the dusty process. Similar illnesses have been described in workers in paper mills due to inhalation of spores of *Alternaria* spp. [98], in sawyers of redwood (sequoiosis) due to *Graphium* spp. or *Aureobasidium pullulans* [99], in other sawmill workers due to *Trichoderma koningii* [100], and in workers making cork (suberosis) due to *Penicillium frequentans* [101,102]. One subject working with ramin dust has also been described as developing allergic alveolitis, probably due to the wood dust itself rather than to a fungus [103].

Aspergillosis

Allergic bronchopulmonary aspergillosis is discussed in detail in Chapter 34 and other diseases related to *Aspergillus* spp. in Chapter 21. Since *Aspergillus* spp. grow on dead organic matter, they can be found in mouldy hay and in compost heaps and may therefore cause episodes of allergic alveolitis in farmers and market gardeners. A severe episode, requiring assisted ventilation, occurred in a patient as a result of changing straw contaminated with *A. versicolor* in her dog's kennel [104].

Cheeseworker's disease

This relatively mild and chronic form of allergic alveolitis was described originally in Swiss cheese washers, whose job was to wash off mould that had grown on the surface of some cheeses aged in damp cellars. On the basis of blood serology the condition was thought to be due to sensitization to *Penicillium casei* [105–107]. Although the condition was thought unlikely to occur in industries in which cheese was aged by wrapping in plastic, it has subsequently been described in a worker in the USA who was engaged in crumbling blue cheese in the production of salad dressing; in this case the organism was the *P. roqueforti* used to give the cheese its distinctive flavour [108].

Japanese summer pneumonitis and other domestic causes

A distinctive type of allergic alveolitis, in which the symptoms occur in the patient's home during the summer months, has been described in Japan where it is the commonest form of allergic alveolitis [18,109,110]. This is caused by *Trichosporon cutaneum* in the houses, particularly in bird droppings, which enhance the organism's growth. In one case, the mould was growing in bedclothes. As with other forms of allergic alveolitis, the condition is less common in cigarette smokers [53]. Immunological studies in these cases have shown antibodies cross-reacting with *Cryptococcus neoformans*, a related yeast, and a particular rise in IgA antibodies to *T. cutaneum* in both blood and BAL fluid [111,112]. The antigen has been characterized as a polysaccharide with glucuronic acid residues on side-chains forming the epitope [113].

It would not be surprising if other episodes of alveolitis occur as a result of exposure to fungi in houses. Several such have been described, including reactions to the dry rot fungus, *Merulius lacrimans*, and to *Penicillium* spp. growing in wet rot [114,115]. *Bacillus subtilis* growing in rotten wood has also been shown to cause the disease in a family [116].

Other causes

An entomologist who developed allergic alveolitis in response to workplace exposure to antigen of *Penicillium* spp. and from humidifiers has been described [117]. Some of the workers exposed to *B. subtilis* in the manufacture of biological washing powders may have developed alveoli-

tis as well as asthma; certainly precipitating antibodies were found in their blood [118,119]. Workers splitting red peppers, or paprika, used to be exposed to heavy doses of spores of *Mucor* spp. and several cases of what was probably alveolitis were described among them [120]. An alveolitis associated with fever was also described in children using inhalation of puff-ball (*Lycoperdon*) spores to stop nose bleeds [121]. This last case report made the interesting suggestion that the disease could be prevented if the puff-balls were picked when young, sautéed in butter and garlic, and eaten rather than inhaled!

Animal causes

Bird fancier's lung

This condition was first described in 1960 in people plucking ducks and those exposed to budgerigars, and in 1965 in people breeding pigeons [4,5,122,123]. Chicken and turkey farmers may occasionally develop the disease and it has also been described in a bird ringer [124–126]. The presentation in people who keep the birds in their houses is often insidious and may be mistaken for neurosis, recurrent chest infections or asthma. In children, loss of weight or failure to thrive may be the presenting feature. Acute attacks occur most commonly in pigeon breeders, following visits to the loft. Re-exposure to a bird after exposure has ceased may also provoke a severe attack, and cross-reactivity may mean that a pigeon fancier suffers an attack on visiting a house where a budgerigar is kept. Otherwise the symptoms do not differ from those associated with other types of allergic alveolitis, shortness of breath, cough, malaise, wheeze and fever being the important ones [127]. The radiograph is often within normal limits in the more chronic cases, although crackles are usually audible at the bases. Lung function commonly shows a restrictive pattern with reduced diffusing capacity, but an obstructive syndrome can occur [128–130].

The frequency with which the condition occurs depends on the prevalence of bird exposure and the extent of that exposure; this is presumably why budgerigars (kept in some 12% of British homes) and pigeons are the most common sensitizers, since exposure to budgerigar antigen is unavoidable if the creature lives in the house while pigeon fanciers have intimate contact with their animals. Among pigeon fanciers, alveolitis has been estimated to occur in about 10–20% of those regularly visiting the lofts [131]. While precipitating antibodies often occur in exposed people without disease [132], the intensity of IgG response measured by radioimmunoassay is a good guide to the likelihood of disease being present [133].

The sensitized patient has precipitating antibody to bird serum protein and droppings. At least in pigeons, IgA seems to be the most important antigen; it was originally thought that this would be inhaled in dried bird faeces, although it now seems likely that bloom from feathers is the principal source [134,135]. Bloom consists of <1.0-μm spherical particles of keratin coated with IgA that cover the feathers and give them their glossy appearance (Fig. 37.8). It relates to the appearance of the bird and its ability to fly efficiently, and is therefore abundant on the wings of ornamental and sporting birds.

Two practical problems may occur in the diagnosis of bird fancier's lung. Firstly, false-positive titres of viral complement-fixing antibodies may be found due to either polyclonal stimulation of antibody formation or cross-reactions with proteins in the egg on which the virus was grown, leading to confusion with viral pneumonia [15,136]. Secondly, patients with coeliac disease may have precipitins in their serum to bird antigen, probably derived from egg protein in their food [137]. However, it appears that there is an association between bird fancier's lung and coeliac disease as well, and therefore the coincidence of coeliac disease with interstitial lung disease is one situation where inhalation challenge may be invaluable [138–140].

Management of bird fancier's lung is by preventing further exposure. Usually this may be achieved by removal of the birds; if this involves serious financial or

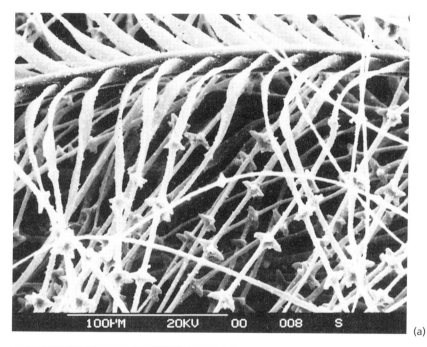

(a)

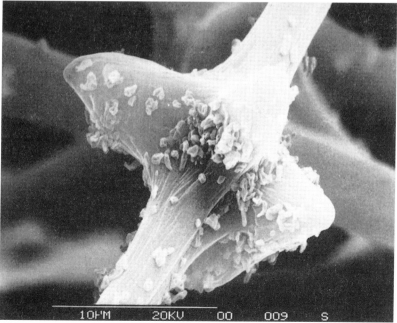

(b)

Fig. 37.8 Scanning electron micrographs of pigeon feather: (a) low power showing structure of the feather; (b) high power showing particles of bloom. The bars at the bottom show the scale. (Courtesy of Dr Gavin Boyd.)

emotional hardship, use of effective respirators may be a compromise [62]. As noted above, residual antigen in rooms vacated by birds may persist for months despite cleaning [60], and patients should be advised to keep out of the room in which the bird has been kept if possible. All patients should be warned of the dangers of irreversible pulmonary fibrosis if they are contemplating continued exposure. Corticosteroids are effective treatment for acute episodes and bring about partial improvement in most chronic cases if exposure is stopped.

Other animal causes

Apart from those caused by birds, episodes of allergic alveolitis due to exposure to animal protein have been described rarely. Small laboratory mammals frequently provoke asthma as a consequence of sensitization to urinary protein, and an occasional case of allergic alveolitis has been described in people exposed to rats and gerbils [141,142]. A granulomatous interstitial pneumonitis (probably of foreign body rather than immunological aetiology) has been described in a person handling animal furs [143], and a patient exposed to the wheat weevil, *Sitophilus granarius*, developed alveolitis as well as the more typical asthmatic reaction [144]. Workers making fishmeal as animal food may become sensitized and develop allergic alveolitis [145].

Alveolitis has been described in the production and use of two therapeutic substances. Pituitary snuff-taker's lung occurred in patients with diabetes insipidus taking extracts of porcine or bovine pituitary by nasal insufflation [146,147]. The particles of this were mostly below 50 μm, and some were small enough to reach alveoli and cause a chronic allergic alveolitis. Sensitization was usually to contaminating ox or pig protein but in one case was to the hormone itself [148]. Since synthetic vasopressin has been introduced the problem has not recurred. More recently, workers producing pancreatic extract have been described as developing alveolitis [149]. This substance has been known to cause asthma and is under suspicion of provoking emphysema in exposed workers, although one report has also documented a late alveolitic reaction to challenge testing and radiological evidence of interstitial disease in a few people employed in its production [149].

Chemical causes

In view of the relatively large numbers of subjects who develop asthma as a consequence of exposure to volatile reactive chemicals, it is surprising that so few have been described as developing alveolitis. This is particularly remarkable because the atopic state is not an important determinant of occupational asthma due to low molecular weight chemicals and their particle size is such that deposition is not likely to be preferentially in airways. Nevertheless, few chemical causes of alveolitis have been described and few patients have suffered these effects. Several volatile isocyanates have caused alveolitis, combined in some subjects with asthma [6,8,150–153]. A haemorrhagic pneumonitis has been associated with exposure to trimellitic anhydride, and allergic alveolitis and haemorrhagic rhinitis associated with IgG antibodies with exposure to hexahydrophthallic anhydride, acid anhydrides used in epoxy resin systems [154,155]. Typical allergic alveolitis and asthma have occurred in a laboratory technician using Pauli's reagent (sodium diazobenzene sulphonate) in chromatography [7]. Cobalt, to which workers in the hard-metal industry may be exposed because of its presence in coolant sprays in grinding and also in small amounts in the tungsten carbide metal itself, may cause both asthma and alveolitis, the latter sometimes leading to pulmonary fibrosis [156,157]. Pyrethrum, an extract of autumn crocus used in insecticides, has caused alveolitis in one subject [158], and exposure to Bordeaux mixture (copper sulphate neutralized with lime) in spraying vines has also caused a similar reaction [159].

Possible causes and some non-causes

Chronic lung disease in Papua New Guinea, though probably usually due to smoke inhalation, may occasionally be an allergic alveolitis due to inhalation of fungi or other contaminants in thatch [160]. Lake water constituents may be the cause of alveolitis described in Finland in people using saunas [161]. Three possible episodes of alveolitis have now been discounted: smallpox worker's lung turned out to have been a pneumonia modified by vaccination [162]; coffee worker's lung was a pulmonary fibrosis in association with rheumatoid disease [163]; and blackfat tobacco smoker's lung turned out to be a lipid pneumonia [164]. As mentioned above, furrier's lung seems likely to have been a foreign body granulomatous, rather than allergic, reaction.

References

1 Campbell JM. Acute symptoms following work with hay. *Br Med J* 1932; ii: 1143.
2 Tower JW, Sweany HC, Huron WH. Severe bronchial asthma apparently due to fungus spores found in maple bark. *JAMA* 1932; 99: 453.
3 Hunter D, Perry KMA. Bronchiolitis resulting from the handling of bagasse. *Br J Ind Med* 1946; 3: 64.
4 Plessner MM. Une maladie des trieurs de plumes: la fièvre de canard. *Arch Mal Prof* 1960; 21: 67.
5 Pearsall HR, Morgan EH, Tesluk H, Beggs D. Parakeet dander pneumonitis. Acute psittaco-keratopneumoconiosis. *Bull Mason Clin* 1960; 14: 127.
6 Charles J, Bernstein A, Jones B *et al.* Hypersensitivity pneumonitis after

exposure to isocyanates. *Thorax* 1976; 31: 127.

7 Evans WV, Seaton A. Hypersensitivity pneumonitis in a technician using Pauli's reagent. *Thorax* 1979; 34: 767.

8 Baur X. Hypersensitivity pneumonitis (extrinsic allergic alveolitis) induced by isocyanates. *J Allergy Clin Immunol* 1995; 95: 1004.

9 Hapke EJ, Seal RME, Thomas GO. Farmer's lung. A clinical, radiographic, functional and serological correlation of acute and chronic stages. *Thorax* 1968; 23: 451.

10 Emanuel DA, Wenzel FJ, Bowerman Cl Lawton BR. Farmer's lung. Clinical, pathologic and immunologic study of 24 patients. *Am J Med* 1984; 37: 392.

11 Kokkarinen J, Tukiainen H, Terho EO. Mortality due to farmer's lung in Finland. *Chest* 1994; 106: 509.

12 Emanuel DA, Wenzel FJ, Lawton BR. Pulmonary mycotoxicosis. *Chest* 1975; 67: 293.

13 May JM, Stallones L, Darrow D, Pratt DS. Organic dust toxicity (pulmonary mycotoxicosis) associated with silo unloading. *Thorax* 1986; 41: 919.

14 Hargreave FE, Pepys J, Longbottom JL, Wraith DG. Bird breeder's (fancier's) lung. *Lancet* 1966; i: 445.

15 Boyd G, Dick HW, Lorimer AR, Moran F. Bird breeder's lung. *Scott Med J* 1967; 12: 69.

16 Earis JE, Marsh K, Pearson MG, Ogilvie CM. The inspiratory 'squawk' in extrinsic allergic alveolitis and other pulmonary fibroses. *Thorax* 1982; 37: 923.

17 Barbee RA, Callies Q, Dickie HA, Rankin J. The long term prognosis in farmer's lung. *Am Rev Respir Dis* 1968; 97: 223.

18 Shimazu K, Ando M, Sakara T *et al.* Hypersensitivity pneumonitis induced by *Trichosporon cutaneum. Am Rev Respir Dis* 1984; 130: 407.

19 Warren CPW. Extrinsic allergic alveolitis: a disease commoner in non-smokers. *Thorax* 1977; 32: 567.

20 Morgan DC, Smyth JT, Lister RW *et al.* Chest symptoms in farming communities with special reference to farmer's lung. *Br J Ind Med* 1975; 32: 228.

21 Davies BH, Edwards JH, Seaton A. Crossreacting antibodies to *Micropolyspora faeni* in *Mycoplasma pneumoniae* infection. *Clin Allergy* 1975; 5: 217.

22 Buschman DL, Gamsu G, Waldron JA, Klein JS, King TE. Chronic hypersensitivity pneumonitis: use of CT in diagnosis. *Am J Roentgenol* 1992; 159: 957.

23 Rankin J, Kobayashi M, Barbee RA, Dickie HA. Pulmonary granulomatoses due to inhaled organic antigens. *Med Clin North Am* 1967; 51: 459.

24 Kokkarinen JI, Tukiainen HO, Terho EO. Recovery of pulmonary function in farmer's lung. A five-year follow-up study. *Am Rev Respir Dis* 1993; 147: 793.

25 Selman-Lama M, Perez-Padilla R. Airflow obstruction and airway lesions in hypersensitivity pneumonitis. *Clin Chest Med* 1993; 14: 699.

26 Lalancette M, Carrier G, Laviolette M *et al.* Farmer's lung. Long-term outcome and lack of predictive value of bronchoalveolar lavage fibrosing factors. *Am Rev Respir Dis* 1993; 148: 216.

27 Seal RME, Hapke EJ, Thomas GO *et al.* The pathology of the acute and chronic stages of farmer's lung. *Thorax* 1965; 23: 469.

28 Orriols R, Aliaga JL, Rodrigo MJ, Garcia F, Royo L, Morrell F. Localised alveolar-septal amyloidosis with hypersensitivity pneumonitis. *Lancet* 1992; 339: 1261.

29 Planes C, Valeyre D, Loiseau A, Bernaudin JF, Soler P. Ultrastructural alterations of the blood–air barrier in sarcoidosis and hypersensitivity pneumonitis and their relation to lung histopathology. *Am J Respir Crit Care Med* 1994; 150: 1067.

30 Salvaggio JE, Millhollon BW. Allergic alveolitis: new insights into old mysteries. *Respir Med* 1993; 87: 495.

31 Pepys J, Riddell RW, Citron KM *et al.* Clinical and immunological significance of *Aspergillus fumigatus* in the sputum. *Am Rev Respir Dis* 1959; 80: 167.

32 Grant IWB, Blythe W, Wardrop VE *et al.* Prevalence of farmer's lung in Scotland: a pilot study. *Br Med J* 1972; i: 530.

33 do Pico GA, Reddan WG, Chmelik F *et al.* The value of precipitating antibodies in screening for hypersensitivity pneumonitis. *Am Rev Respir Dis* 1976; 113: 451.

34 Burrell R, Rylander R. A critical review of the role of precipitins in hypersensitivity pneumonitis. *Eur J Respir Dis* 1981; 62: 332.

35 Hendrick DJ, Marshall R, Faux JA, Krall JM. Positive 'alveolar' responses to antigen inhalation provocation tests: their validity and recognition. *Thorax* 1980; 35: 415.

36 Semenzato G, Chilosi M, Ossi E *et al.* Bronchoalveolar lavage and lung histology. Comparative analysis of inflammatory and immunocompetent cells in patients with sarcoidosis and hypersensitivity pneumonitis. *Am Rev Respir Dis* 1985; 132: 400.

37 Leatherman JW, Michael AF, Schwartz BA, Hoidal JR. Lung T cells in hypersensitivity pneumonitis. *Ann Intern Med* 1984; 100: 390.

38 Costabel U, Bross KJ, Marxien J, Matthys H. T lymphocytosis in bronchoalveolar lavage fluid of hypersensitivity pneumonitis. Changes in profile of T-cell subsets during the course of disease. *Chest* 1984; 85: 515.

39 Cormier Y, Belanger J, Beaudoin J *et al.* Abnormal bronchoalveolar lavage in asymptomatic dairy farmers. Study of lymphocytes. *Am Rev Respir Dis* 1984; 130: 1046.

40 Keller RH, Swartz S, Schleuter DP *et al.* Immunoregulation in hypersensitivity pneumonitis: phenotypic and functional studies of bronchoalveolar lavage lymphocytes. *Am Rev Respir Dis* 1984; 130: 766.

41 Hamagami S, Miyagawa T, Ochi T, Tsuyuguchi I, Kishimoto S. A raised level of soluble CD8 in bronchoalveolar lavage fluid in summer-type hypersensitivity pneumonitis in Japan. *Chest* 1992; 101: 1044.

42 Denis M. Proinflammatory cytokines in hypersensitivity pneumonitis. *Am J Respir Crit Care Med* 1995; 151: 164.

43 Haslam P, Dewar A, Butchers P *et al.* Mast cells, atypical lymphocytes and neutrophils in bronchoalveolar lavage in extrinsic allergic alveolitis. Comparison with other interstitial lung diseases. *Am Rev Respir Dis* 1987; 135: 35.

44 Soler P, Nioche S, Valeyre D *et al.* Role of mast cells in the pathogenesis of hypersensitivity pneumonitis. *Thorax* 1987; 42: 565.

45 Miadonna A, Pesci I, Tedeschi A, Bertorelli G, Arquati M, Oliveri D. Mast cell and histamine involvement in farmer's lung disease. *Chest* 1994; 105: 1184.

46 Fournier E, Tonnel AB, Gosset P *et al.* Early neutrophil alveolitis after antigen inhalation

in hypersensitivity pneumonitis. *Chest* 1985; 88: 563.

47 Drent M, Wagenaar S, van Velzen-Blad H, Mulder PG, Hoogsteden HC, van den Bosch JMM. Relationship between plasma cell levels and profile of bronchoalveolar lavage fluid in patients with subacute extrinsic allergic alveolitis. *Thorax* 1993; 48: 835.

48 Drent M, van Velzen-Blad H, Diamant M, Wagenaar SS, Donckerwolck-Bogaert M, van den Bosch JM. Differential diagnostic value of plasma cells in bronchoalveolar lavage fluid. *Chest* 1993; 103: 1720.

49 Ihle JN, Keller J, Oroszlan S *et al.* Biologic properties of homogeneous interleukin 3. *J Immunol* 1983; 131: 282.

50 Ezeamuzie IC, Assem ESK. A study of histamine release from human basophils and lung mast cells by products of lymphocyte stimulation. *Agents Actions* 1983; 13: 222.

51 Edwards JH, Wagner JC, Seal RME. Pulmonary responses to particulate materials capable of activating the alternative pathway of complement. *Clin Allergy* 1976; 6: 155.

52 Malmberg P, Rask-Andersen A, Rosenhall L. Exposure to microorganisms associated with allergic alveolitis and reactions to mold dust in farmers. *Chest* 1993; 103: 1202.

53 Arima K, Ando M, Ito K *et al.* Effect of cigarette smoking on prevalence of summer-type hypersensitivity pneumonitis caused by *Trichosporon cutaneum. Arch Environ Health* 1992; 47: 274.

54 Haitjema T, van Velzen-Blad H, van den Bosch JMM. Extrinsic allergic alveolitis caused by goose feathers in a duvet. *Thorax* 1992; 47: 990.

55 Seaton A. Allergic alveolitis due to goose feathers in a duvet (letter). *Thorax* 1993; 48: 411.

56 McSharry C, Banham SW, Lynch PP, Boyd G. Antibody measurement in extrinsic allergic alveolitis. *Eur J Respir Dis* 1984; 65: 259.

57 Bentzon N, Adamsen S, Jacobsen B, Eriksen C, Hansen OH. Videothoracoscopic lung biopsy by a stapling technique. *Eur J Surg* 1994; 160: 543.

58 Moore VL, Pederson GM, Hauser WC, Fink JN. A study of lung lavage materials in patients with hypersensitivity pneumonitis: *in vitro* response to mitogen and antigen in pigeon breeder's disease. *J Allergy Clin Immunol* 1982; 65: 365.

59 Kokkarinen JI, Tukiainen HO, Terho EO. Effect of corticosteroid treatment on the recovery of pulmonary function in farmer's lung. *Am Rev Respir Dis* 1992; 145: 3.

60 Craig TJ, Hershey J, Engler RJ, Davis W, Carpenter GB, Salata K. Bird antigen persistence in the home environment after removal of the bird. *Ann Allergy* 1992; 69: 510.

61 Boehlecke B. Respiratory protection. In: Morgan WKC, Seaton A, eds. *Occupational Lung Diseases*, 3rd edn. Philadelphia: WB Saunders, 1995, p. 182.

62 Hendrick DJ, Marshall R, Faux JA, Krall JM. Protective value of dust respirators in extrinsic allergic alveolitis: clinical assessment using bronchial provocation tests. *Thorax* 1981; 36: 917.

63 Wenzel FJ, Gray RL, Emanuel DA. Farmer's lung: its geographic distribution. *J Occup Med* 1970; 12: 493.

64 Madsen D, Klock LE, Wenzel FJ *et al.*

The prevalence of farmer's lung in an agricultural population. *Am Rev Respir Dis* 1976; 113: 171.

65 do Pico GA. Hazardous exposure and lung disease among farm workers. *Clin Chest Med* 1992; 13: 311.

66 Cuthbert OD, Brostoff J, Wraith DG, Brighton WD. 'Barn allergy.' Asthma and rhinitis due to storage mites. *Clin Allergy* 1979; 9: 229.

67 Ingram CG, Jeffrey IG, Symington IS, Cuthbert OD. Bronchial provocation studies in farmers allergic to storage mites. *Lancet* 1979; ii: 1330.

68 Donham KJ, Rubino M, Thedell TD, Kammermeyer J. Potential health hazards to agricultural workers in swine confinement buildings. *J Occup Med* 1977; 19: 383.

69 Horvath EP, do Pico GA, Barbee RA, Dickie HA. Nitrogen dioxide-induced pulmonary disease: five new cases and a review of the literature. *J Occup Med* 1978; 20: 103.

70 Cormier Y, Fournier M, Laviolette M. Farmer's fever. Systemic manifestation of farmer's lung without lung involvement. *Chest* 1993; 103: 632.

71 Braun SR, do Pico GA, Tsiatis A *et al.* Farmer's lung disease: long-term clinical and physiologic outcome. *Am Rev Respir Dis* 1979; 119: 185.

72 Gourlay CA, Braidwood GD. The use of dust respirators in the prevention of recurrence of farmer's lung. *Trans Soc Occup Med* 1971; 21: 93.

73 Bringhurst LS, Byrne RN, Gershon-Cohen J. Respiratory disease of mushroom workers. Farmer's lung. *JAMA* 1959; 171: 15.

74 Sakula A. Mushroom worker's lung. *Br Med J* 1987; iii: 708.

75 Stewart CJ. Mushroom worker's lung-two outbreaks. *Thorax* 1974; 29: 252.

76 Chan-Yeung M, Grzybowski S, Schonell M. Mushroom worker's lung. *Am Rev Respir Dis* 1972; 105: 819.

77 Buechner HA, Prevatt AL, Thompson J, Blitz O. Bagassosis. A review with further historical data, studies of pulmonary function, and results of adrenal steroid therapy. *Am J Med* 1958; 25: 234.

78 Weill H, Buechner HA, Gonzalez E *et al.* Bagassosis: a study of pulmonary function in 20 cases. *Ann Intern Med* 1966; 64: 737.

79 Hearn CED, Holford-Strevens V. Immunological aspects of bagassosis. *Br J Ind Med* 1968; 25: 283.

80 MRC, Symposium. Humidifier fever. *Thorax* 1977; 32: 653.

81 Pickering CAC, Moore WKS, Lacey J *et al.* Investigation of a respiratory disease associated with an air conditioning system. *Clin Allergy* 1976; 6: 109.

82 Banaszak EF, Thiede WH, Fink JN. Hypersensitivity pneumonitis due to contamination of an air conditioner. *N Engl J Med* 1970; 283: 271.

83 Fink JN, Banaszak EF, Thiede WH, Barbonak JJ. Interstitial pneumonitis due to hypersensitivity to an organism contaminating a heating system. *Ann Intern Med* 1971; 74: 80.

84 Burke GW, Carrington CB, Strauss R *et al.* Allergic alveolitis caused by home humidifiers. *JAMA* 1977; 238: 2705.

85 Arnow PM, Fink JN, Schleuter DP *et al.* Early detection of hypersensitivity pneumonitis in office workers. *Am J Med* 1978; 64: 236.

86 Anderson JK, McSharry CP, Boyd G. Radiographic changes in humidifier fever. *Thorax* 1985; 40: 312.

87 Kohler PF, Gross G, Salvaggio J, Hawkins J. Humidifier lung: hypersensitivity pneumonitis related to thermotolerant bacterial aerosols. *Chest* 1976; 69 (Suppl): 294.

88 Robertson AS, Burge PS, Wieland GA, Carmalt MHB. Extrinsic allergic alveolitis caused by a cold water humidifier. *Thorax* 1987; 42: 32.

89 Suda T, Sato A, Ida M, Gemma H, Hayakawa H, Chida K. Hypersensitivity pneumonitis associated with home ultrasonic humidifiers. *Chest* 1995; 107: 711.

90 Kane GC, Marx JJ, Prince DS. Hypersensitivity pneumonitis secondary to *Klebsiella oxytoca*. A new cause of humidifier lung. *Chest* 1993; 104: 627.

91 Riddell HVF, Channell S, Blythe W *et al.* Allergic alveolitis in a malt worker. *Thorax* 1968; 23: 271.

92 Channell S, Blythe W, Lloyd M *et al.* Allergic alveolitis in maltworkers. A clinical, mycological and immunological study. *Q J Med* 1969; 38: 351.

93 Grant IWB, Blackadder ES, Greenberg M, Blythe W. Extrinsic allergic alveolitis in Scottish maltworkers. *Br Med J* 1976; i: 490.

94 Gregory PH, Waller S. *Cryptostroma corticale* and sooty bark disease of sycamore (*Acer pseudoplantanus*). *Br Mycol Soc Trans* 1951; 34: 579.

95 Emanuel DA, Lawton BR, Wenzel FJ. Maple bark disease: pneumonitis due to *Coniosporium corticale*. *N Engl J Med* 1962; 266: 333.

96 Emanuel DA, Wenzel FJ, Lawton Br. Pneumonitis due to *Cryptostroma corticale* (maple bark disease). *N Engl J Med* 1966; 274: 1413.

97 Wenzel FJ, Emanuel DA. The epidemiology of maple bark disease. *Arch Environ Health* 1967; 14: 385.

98 Schlueter DP, Fink JN, Hensley GT. Wood pulp worker's disease: hypersensitivity pneumonitis caused by *Alternaria*. *Ann Intern Med* 1972; 77: 907.

99 Cohen HI, Merigan TC, Kosek JC, Eldridge F. Sequoiosis. A granulomatous pneumonitis associated with redwood sawdust inhalation. *Am J Med* 1967; 43: 785.

100 Halpin DM, Graneek BJ, Turner-Warwick M, Newman-Taylor AJ. Extrinsic allergic alveolitis and asthma in a sawmill worker: case report and review of the literature. *Occup Environ Med* 1994; 51: 160.

101 Avilar R, Villar TG. Suberosis. Respiratory disease in cork workers. *Lancet* 1968; i: 620.

102 Avilar R, Lacey J. The role of *Penicillium frequentans* in suberosis (respiratory disease in workers in the cork industry). *Clin Allergy* 1974; 4: 109.

103 Howie AD, Boyd G, Moran F. Pulmonary hyper-sensitivity to Ramin (*Gonystylus bancanus*). *Thorax* 1976; 31: 585.

104 Rhudy J, Burrell RG, Morgan WKC. Yet another cause of allergic alveolitis. *Scand J Respir Dis* 1971; 52: 177.

105 de Weck AL, Gutersohn J, Butikofer E. La maladie des laveurs de fromage (Kaserwascherkrankheit): une forme particulière du syndrome du poumon du fermier. *Schweiz Med Wochenschr* 1969; 99: 872.

106 Minnig H, de Weck AL. Das Kaserwascherkrankheit. Immunologische epidemiologische Studien. *Schweiz Med Wochenschr* 1972; 102: 1205, 1251.

107 Schleuter DP. Cheesewasher's disease: a new occupational hazard? *Ann Intern Med* 1973; 78: 606.

108 Campbell JA, Kryda MJ, Treuhaft MW *et al.* Cheese worker's hypersensitivity pneumonitis. *Am Rev Respir Dis* 1983; 127: 495.

109 Miyagawa T, Ochi T, Takahashi H. Hypersensitivity pneumonitis with antibodies to *Cryptococcus neoformans*. *Clin Allergy* 1978; 8: 501.

110 Kawai T, Tamura M, Murao M. Summer-type hypersensitivity pneumonitis. A unique disease in Japan. *Chest* 1984; 85: 311.

111 Soda K, Ando M, Shimazu K *et al.* Different classes of antibody activities to *Trichosporon cutaneum* antigen in summer-type hypersensitivity pneumonitis by enzyme-linked immunosorbent assay. *Am Rev Respir Dis* 1986; 133: 83.

112 Ando M, Yoshida K, Soda K, Araki S. Specific bronchoalveolar lavage IgA antibody in patients with summer-type hypersensitivity pneumonitis induced by *Trichosporon cutaneum*. *Am Rev Respir Dis* 1986; 134: 177.

113 Mizobe T, Ando M, Yamasaki H, Onoue K, Misaki A. Purification and characterisation of the serotype-specific polysaccharide antigen of *Trichosporum cutaneum* serotype II: a disease-related antigen of Japanese summer-type hypersensitivity pneumonitis. *Clin Exp Allergy* 1995; 25: 265.

114 O'Brien IM, Bull J, Creamer B *et al.* Asthma and extrinsic allergic alveolitis due to *Merulius lacrymans*. *Clin Allergy* 1978; 8: 535.

115 Fergusson RJ, Milne WR, Crompton GK. *Penicillium* allergic alveolitis: faulty installation of central heating. *Thorax* 1984; 39: 294.

116 Johnson CL, Bernstein IL, Gallagher JS *et al.* Familial hypersensitivity pneumonitis induced by *Bacillus subtilis*. *Am Rev Respir Dis* 1980; 122: 339.

117 Solley GO, Hyatt RE. Hypersensitivity pneumonitis induced by *Penicillium* species. *J Allergy Clin Immunol* 1980; 65: 65.

118 Newhouse ML, Tagg B, Pocock SJ, McEwan AC. An epidemiological study of workers producing enzyme washing powders. *Lancet* 1970; i: 689.

119 Franz T, McMurrain KD, Brooks S, Bernstein IL. Clinical, immunologic and physiologic observations in factory workers exposed to *B. subtilis* enzyme dust. *J Allergy* 1971; 47: 170.

120 Hunter D. *The Diseases of Occupations*, 6th edn. London: Hodder & Stoughton, 1978: 1061.

121 Strand RD, Neuhauser EBD, Sornberger CF. Lycoperdonosis. *N Engl J Med* 1967; 277: 89.

122 Reed CE, Sosman A, Barbee RA. Pigeon breeder's lung. A newly observed interstitial pulmonary disease. *JAMA* 1965; 193: 261.

123 Barboriak JJ, Sosman AJ, Reed CE. Serological studies in pigeon breeder's disease. *J Lab Clin Med* 1965; 65: 600.

124 Warren CPW, Tse KS. Extrinsic allergic alveolitis owing to hypersensitivity to chickens: significance of serum precipitins. *Am Rev Respir Dis* 1974; 109: 672.

125 Boyer RS, Klock LE, Schmidt CD *et al.* Hypersensitivity lung disease in the turkey raising industry. *Am Rev Respir Dis* 1974; 109: 630.

126 Kokkarinen J, Tukiainen H, Seppa A, Terho EO. Hypersensitivity due to native birds in a bird ringer. *Chest* 1994; 106: 1269.

127 Research Committee of the British Thoracic Society. A national survey of bird fancier's

lung: including its possible association with jejunal villous atrophy. *Br J Dis Chest* 1984; 78: 75.

128 Schleuter DP, Fink J, Sosman AJ. Pulmonary function in pigeon breeder's disease. A hypersensitivity pneumonitis. *Ann Intern Med* 1969; 70: 457.

129 Allen DH, Williams DV, Woodcock AJ. Bird breeder's hypersensitivity pneumonitis: progress studies of lung function after cessation of exposure to the presenting antigen. *Am Rev Respir Dis* 1976; 114: 555.

130 Warren CPW, Tse KS, Cherniack RM. Mechanical properties of the lung in extrinsic allergic alveolitis. *Thorax* 1978; 33: 315.

131 Christensen LT, Schmidt CD, Robbins L. Pigeon breeder's disease: a prevalence study and review. *Clin Allergy* 1975; 5: 417.

132 Barboriak JJ, Fink JN, Sosman AJ, Dhaliwal KS. Precipitating antibody against pigeon antigens in sera of asymptomatic pigeon breeders. *J Lab Clin Med* 1973; 82: 372.

133 Banham SW, McSharry C, Lynch PP, Boyd G. Relationships between avian exposure, humoral immune response, and pigeon breeder's disease among Scottish pigeon fanciers. *Thorax* 1986; 41: 274.

134 Boyd G, McSharry CP, Banham SW, Lynch PP. A current view of pigeon fancier's lung. A model for extrinsic allergic alveolitis. *Clin Allergy* 1982; 12 (Suppl): 53.

135 Banham SW, McKenzie H, McSharry C *et al.* Antibody against a pigeon bloom extract: a further antigen in pigeon breeder's lung. *Clin Allergy* 1982; 12: 173.

136 Newman Taylor AJ, Taylor P, Bryant DH *et al.* False positive complement fixation tests with respiratory virus preparations in bird fanciers with allergic alveolitis. *Thorax* 1977; 32: 563.

137 Faux JA, Hendrick DJ, Anand BS. Precipitins to different avian serum antigens in bird fancier's lung and coeliac disease. *Clin Allergy* 1978; 8: 101.

138 Hood J, Mason AMS. Diffuse pulmonary disease with transfer defect occurring with coeliac disease. *Lancet* 1970; i: 445.

139 Berrill WT, Eade OE, Fitzpatrick PF *et al.* Bird fancier's lung and jejunal villous atrophy. *Lancet* 1975; ii: 1006.

140 Hendrick DJ, Faux JA, Anand B *et al.* Is bird fancier's lung associated with coeliac disease? *Thorax* 1976; 33: 425.

141 Carroll KB, Pepys J, Longbottom JL *et al.* Extrinsic allergic alveolitis due to rat serum proteins. *Clin Allergy* 1975; 5: 443.

142 Korenblat P, Slavin R, Winzenburger P *et al.* Gerbil-keeper's lung: a new form of hypersensitivity pneumonitis. *Ann Allergy* 1977; 38: 437.

143 Pimentel JC. Furrier's lung. *Thorax* 1970; 25: 387.

144 Lunn JA, Hughes DTD. Pulmonary hypersensitivity to the grain weevil. *Br J Ind Med* 1967; 24: 158.

145 Avilar R. Extrinsic allergic alveolitis in workers exposed to fish meal and poultry. *Clin Allergy* 1971; 1: 343.

146 Mahon WE, Scott DJ, Ansell G *et al.* Hypersensitivity to pituitary snuff with miliary shadowing in the lungs. *Thorax* 1967; 22: 13.

147 Butikofer E, deWeck AL, Scherrer M. Pituitary snuff taker's lung. *Schweiz Med Wochenschr* 1970; 100: 97.

148 Harper LO, Burrell RG, Lapp NL, Morgan WKC. Allergic alveolitis due to pituitary snuff. *Ann Intern Med* 1970; 73: 581.

149 Wiessmann K-J, Baur X. Occupational lung disease following long-term inhalation of pancreatic extracts. *Eur J Respir Dis* 1985; 66: 13.

150 Fink JN, Schleuter DP. Bathtub refinisher's lung: an unusual response to toluene diisocyanate. *Am Rev Respir Dis* 1978; 118: 955.

151 Zeiss CR, Kanellakes TB, Bellone JD *et al.* Immunoglobulin E-mediated asthma and hypersensitivity pneumonitis with precipitating anti-hapten antibodies due to diphenyldimethane isocyanate (MDI) exposure. *J Allergy Clin Immunol* 1980; 65: 346.

152 Malo J-L, Zeiss CR. Occupational hypersensitivity pneumonitis after exposure to diphenylmethane isocyanate. *Am Rev Respir Dis* 1982; 125: 113.

153 Vandenplas O, Malo J-L, Saetta M, Mapp CE, Fabbri LM. Occupational asthma and extrinsic allergic alveolitis due to isocyanates: current status and perspectives. *Br J Ind Med* 1993; 50: 213.

154 Ahmad D, Morgan WKC, Patterson R *et al.* Pulmonary haemorrhage and haemolytic anaemia due to trimellitic anhydride. *Lancet* 1979; ii: 328.

155 Grammer LC, Shaughnessy MA, Lowenthal M, Yarnold PR. Risk factors for immunologically mediated respiratory disease from hexahydrophthallic anhydride. *J Occup Med* 1994; 36: 642.

156 Davison AG, Haslam PL, Corrin B *et al.* Interstitial lung disease and asthma in hard metal workers: bronchoalveolar lavage, ultrastructural, and analytical findings and results of bronchial challenge tests. *Thorax* 1983; 38: 119.

157 Sjorgren I, Hillerdal G, Andersson A, Zetterstrom O. Hard metal lung disease: importance of cobalt in coolants. *Thorax* 1980; 35: 653.

158 Carlson JE, Villaveces JW. Hypersensitivity pneumonitis due to pyrethrum. *JAMA* 1977; 237: 1718.

159 Pimental JC, Marques F. Vineyard sprayer's lung: a new occupational disease. *Thorax* 1969; 24: 678.

160 Blackburn CRB, Green W. Precipitins against extracts of thatched roofs in the sera of New Guinea natives with chronic lung disease. *Lancet* 1966; ii: 1396.

161 Muittari A, Kuusisto P, Virtanen P *et al.* An epidemic of extrinsic allergic alveolitis caused by tap water. *Clin Allergy* 1980; 10: 77.

162 Ross PJ, Seaton A, Foreman HM, Morris Evans WH. Pulmonary calcification following smallpox handler's lung. *Thorax* 1974; 29: 659.

163 van den Bosch JMM, van Toorn DW, Wagenaar SS. Coffee-worker's lung: reconsideration of a case report. *Thorax* 1983; 38: 720.

164 Miller GJ, Ashcroft MT, Beadnell HMSG *et al.* The lipid pneumonia of blackfat tobacco smokers in Guyana. *Q J Med* 1971; 40: 457.

38

PULMONARY EOSINOPHILIAS

A. GORDON LEITCH

Definition

The term 'pulmonary eosinophilia' was originally applied as a general one to a group of diseases in which lung shadows were observed radiologically and were accompanied by a blood eosinophilia. Resolving pneumonia, sarcoidosis, hydatid disease and Hodgkin's disease were excluded [1]. Some workers have used the term 'pulmonary infiltration with eosinophilia' (PIE syndrome) [2] and because eosinophilic infiltration of the lung can exist in the absence of blood eosinophilia, it has been suggested that the term 'the eosinophilic pneumonias' might be even more appropriate [3]. The terms are interchangeable but pulmonary eosinophilia is retained in this chapter for historical reasons.

Opinions vary on the level of blood eosinophil count that constitutes eosinophilia. In one study 95% of healthy non-allergic subjects had eosinophil counts of less than 0.27×10^9/L, whereas counts of greater than 0.35×10^9/L were usually seen in patients with active asthma [4]. Total eosinophil counts of greater than 0.5×10^9/L (and often much higher) are usually seen in patients with pulmonary eosinophilia.

The eosinophil

The eosinophil polymorphonuclear leucocyte is 12–15 µm in diameter, containing a bilobed nucleus, rich endoplasmic reticulum, an active Golgi complex and two types of eosinophilic granules (Fig. 38.1). The larger granules, of which there are about 200 in each cell, are 1×0.6 µm in size and comprise an electron-dense crystalloid matrix in which are found a number of enzymes, including a unique peroxidase [5], β-glucuronidase, acid phosphatase and histaminase [6–8]; 25–50% of the mass of the granules consists of the major basic protein (MBP), a 13.8-kDa protein [7,9]. In addition the granules contain eosinophil cationic protein (ECP) (18–21 kDa) [10] and eosinophil protein X (eosinophil-derived neurotoxin) (18 kDa) [11]. The smaller granules, which are more prominent in mature eosinophils, measure 0.2×0.2 µm and are rich in arylsulphatase B and acid phosphatase. The cell membrane contains lysolecithinase, an enzyme that spontaneously forms Charcot–Leyden crystals in tissues and fluids [12] (Fig. 38.2).

Eosinophils are produced in the bone marrow, circulate for 4–10h and then localize in the tissues, being most prominent in the submucosal sites of the respiratory, gastrointestinal and genitourinary tracts [13]. Their behaviour is influenced by chemotactic factors, chemokinetic factors and deactivation factors. Chemotactic factors cause migration towards a cell-sensed concentration gradient, while chemokinetic factors enhance random motility. Deactivation factors induce unresponsiveness to subsequent chemotactic stimuli, a property that localizes and immobilizes eosinophils in the tissues. Both complement-derived products C3a, C5a and C567 (which may be generated by the classical or alternative pathways [14]) and the mast-cell derived products ECF-A and ECF-A oligopeptide [15] demonstrate the combination of chemotactic and deactivation activities. Chemotactic activity is also shown by lipoxygenase pathway products, such as several of the monohydroxyeicosatetraenoic acids and leukotriene B_4, which may be generated by several cell types [16]. Eosinophils may therefore be attracted to tissues by many mechanisms, including mast cell activation, complement activation, lymphocyte-derived products and generation of arachidonic products via the lipoxygenase pathway by a variety of cells.

Blood eosinophil counts are depressed by glucocorticosteroids, which also inhibit eosinophil chemotaxis and facilitate eosinophil margination and tissue destruction [17]. Propranolol induces a modest peripheral blood eosinophilia in many patients, suggesting direct β-adrenergic control of eosinophil levels [18].

Function

The eosinophil is equipped to modulate mast cell-dependent reactions by virtue of the enzymes that it

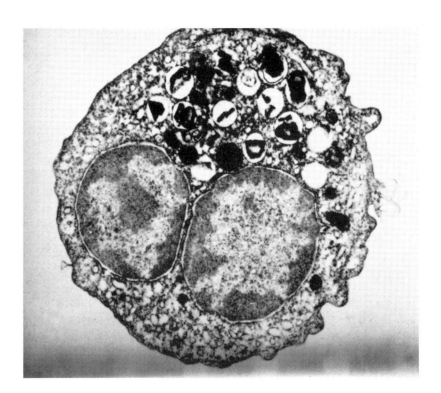

Fig. 38.1 Electron micrograph of an eosinophil showing bilobed nucleus, endoplasmic reticulum and prominent intracytoplasmic granules.

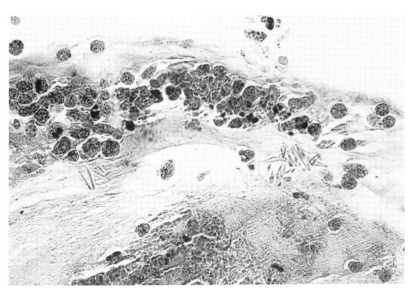

Fig. 38.2 Mucous plug from asthmatic airway showing eosinophils and Charcot–Leyden crystals (haematoxylin & eosin × 335).

produces [19]; histaminase degrades histamine, phospholipase D degrades platelet-activating factor and, in addition, the eosinophil can ingest mast cell granules and IgE–antigen complexes. An eosinophil-derived inhibitor of histamine release, which is probably prostaglandin E_2, also exists [20]. The marked eosinophilia found in many parasitic conditions suggests a role for the eosinophil in the destruction of parasites [21]. This has been shown to be the case in schistosomiasis, in which eosinophils inflict IgG antibody-dependent damage on the schistosomula [22]. Complement also enhances this process and mast

cells enhance both complement and IgG-dependent eosinophil-mediated schistosomular killing *in vitro* [23]. The eosinophil may function similarly in other parasitic diseases.

Not all the activities of the eosinophil are beneficial. Prolonged hypereosinophilia may be associated with tissue damage and a possible mechanism for this adverse effect has now been identified. Low concentrations of eosinophil MBP have been shown to damage a wide variety of mammalian cells and organs [24]. Concentrations of MBP comparable to those found in the sputum of patients with asthma have been shown to be ciliostatic and to damage tracheal mucosal cells [25]. Furthermore, using immuno-fluorescent techniques, MBP has been localized to areas of mucosal damage in the bronchi of patients with asthma [26]. It seems possible that deposition of MBP in the interstitium or vascular tree could cause pulmonary parenchymal or vascular damage in a similar fashion. Other constituents of the eosinophil that could exert a pathogenic effect include superoxide, lysosomal hydrolase, ECP, eosinophil protein X and the inflammatory products of arachidonic acid [27,28].

While knowledge of the factors regulating eosinophil behaviour and function continues to grow, it would be wrong to conclude that more than a start has been made in uncovering the mechanisms that underly the several varieties of pulmonary eosinophilia.

Classification

In the fourth edition of this book, the pulmonary eosinophilic disorders were classified into seven categories largely on the basis of clinical manifestations. Since then, acute eosinophilic pneumonia has been described [29,30] and the present classification of pulmonary eosinophilias is as shown in Table 38.1 [31].

Loeffler's syndrome or simple pulmonary eosinophilia

Definition

Originally described by Loeffler in 1932 [32], this syndrome is characterized by transient radiographic shadows and by blood eosinophilia that is usually relatively slight, although high counts have been recorded. The illness usually lasts less than 2 weeks and always less than 1 month and is related to the passage of parasitic larvae, most commonly *Ascaris lumbricoides*, through the lung.

Aetiology

The life cycle of *A. lumbricoides* in humans begins with

Table 38.1 Classification of pulmonary eosinophilias.

Loeffler's syndrome or simple pulmonary eosinophilia
Asthmatic pulmonary eosinophilia
Drug-induced pulmonary eosinophilia
Tropical pulmonary eosinophilia
Chronic or prolonged pulmonary eosinophilia
Churg–Strauss syndrome
Hypereosinophilic syndrome
Acute eosinophilic pneumonia

the ingestion of eggs and subsequent development of larvae in the intestine. Some 10–14 days after ingestion the larvae migrate to the liver and the lung, thence to the alveoli and up the bronchial tree to be swallowed into the intestine where they develop into the mature roundworm.

Koino, a Japanese investigator, swallowed 2000 ripe *Ascaris* eggs and 6 days later developed pneumonia with dyspnoea, cyanosis, eosinophilia and pyrexia that lasted for 7 days. The sputum was profuse from day 11 to day 16 and contained *Ascaris* larvae, of which 202 were counted. By 50 days after infection, 667 *Ascaris* worms were voided in the faeces [33].

The passage of larvae through the lung is associated with an allergic reaction that was well studied in four Canadian students who developed pulmonary eosinophilia 10–14 days after eating a meal maliciously seasoned with *A. suum* ova [34]. Asthma occurred in all four students and urticaria was also a feature of the illness. Studies of immunoglobulin and eosinophil levels in the course of the illness showed that peak humoral antibody levels of IgM and IgE occurred before peak eosinophil levels, which were found in the recovery phase of the illness. The authors concluded from their observations that the high IgE levels were responsible, via a type I hypersensitivity reaction, for the asthma and urticaria and that the pulmonary infiltrates were due to a type III reaction following deposition of IgM–antigen complexes in the lung, perhaps facilitated by the changes in vasopermeability occasioned by release of mast cell mediators. It is of interest that high levels of IgE have been demonstrated in children infected with *A. lumbricoides* [35].

Other parasites implicated in this form of pulmonary eosinophilia include *Paragonimus westermani* [36] and *Ancylostoma braziliense* (see Chapter 22).

Pathology

Histopathological sections of lung from a patient dying from Loeffler's syndrome showed that the bronchi and bronchioles were dilated and filled with a neutrophil and eosinophil polymorphonuclear infiltrated exudate [37]. Charcot–Leyden crystals were seen in some areas. In some of the bronchioles one or more portions of nematode larvae were demonstrated. The pulmonary interstitium was also infiltrated with eosinophils and areas of atelectasis were seen.

Clinical features

Over 23% of Loeffler's original cases were detected during routine radiography and were asymptomatic. Symptoms when present are usually mild and may include cough, malaise, anorexia, rhinitis, night sweats, slight fever and occasionally wheezing and dyspnoea [33,34]. Urticaria can occur. Sputum when present may contain eosinophils and, exceptionally, larvae. High fever may occur. Frequently there are no abnormal physical signs in the chest, although impairment of percussion note, a few crepitations or wheezes may be heard. Symptoms and physical signs usually disappear in a few days and almost always within a fortnight.

Radiology

The chest radiograph almost invariably shows bilateral involvement, with considerable variation in the extent and location of the pulmonary infiltrates [38]. These are usually scattered soft densities, a few centimetres in size, that tend to be discrete, without any clear-cut segmental distribution and often concentrated in the perihilar regions. In severe cases the densities may coalesce to create more extensive areas of consolidation. The opacities usually disappear within 6–12 days and almost always within a month.

Investigations and diagnosis

The white count is usually normal or high normal with a relatively low eosinophilia. Higher counts, with a total eosinophil count of greater than 5×10^9/L or even as high as 16.5×10^9/L, have been recorded. IgE and IgM levels are elevated in the acute phase of the illness but this is little aid to diagnosis [34].

Sputum should be examined for eosinophils and larvae and stools should be examined for parasites. Since the larvae of *Ascaris* only become adult some 6–8 weeks after infestation, eggs are unlikely to be found in the stools before this time. Stools should therefore be re-examined some 2–3 months after the onset of symptoms.

The main diagnostic problem arises from the radiographic abnormality, which needs to be differentiated from pneumonia, tuberculosis and pulmonary infarction. The transient nature of the shadows excludes tuberculosis; microbiology should help to exclude pneumonia; and pulmonary infarction, although it may cause similar pulmonary shadows, is not associated with eosinophilia unless there is a contemporaneous chronic parasitic infection.

Treatment

As the condition is usually mild, no specific therapy for the pulmonary eosinophilia is required. With severe manifestations oral corticosteroid therapy is extremely effective [34]. The *Ascaris* infestation may be treated with piperazine citrate 4 g in a single oral dose given after the larvae have developed into adult worms.

Asthmatic pulmonary eosinophilia or allergic bronchopulmonary aspergillosis

Definition

Asthmatic pulmonary eosinophilia is characterized by asthmatic symptoms, recurrent shadows on the chest radiograph and blood eosinophilia. The expectoration of inspissated mucus in the form of pellets or bronchial casts is relatively common.

Aetiology

This is by far the most common cause of pulmonary eosinophilia and it is seen worldwide. The paucity of cases in North America [39] has been attributed more to failure of recognition than to a true difference in prevalence [40]. The disease may be seen at any age, more commonly in women than men. Most cases are associated with type I hypersensitivity to *Aspergillus fumigatus*, hence the name [41–46]. Of 143 cases of pulmonary eosinophilia reported by McCarthy and Pepys [41], 111 had allergic bronchopulmonary aspergillosis; in a more recent series, 33 of 65 patients with pulmonary eosinophilia met the criteria for this condition [46]. The condition is now well recognized as a serious complication of cystic fibrosis [47,48]. The suggested criteria for a diagnosis of allergic bronchopulmonary aspergillosis are shown in Table 38.2. Other cases may be due to hypersensitivity to *Candida* antigens and individual cases due to hypersensitivity to *Pseudomonas aeruginosa*, *Aspergillus terreus*, *Helminthosporium* and *Curvularia lunata* have been reported [49–53].

The presence of high serum IgE levels in such patients, with marked elevations of IgE during acute episodes of pulmonary eosinophilia, suggests an important contribution from a type I hypersensitivity reaction and the acute rises may represent a response to an increased burden of *Aspergillus* antigen. The occurrence of late skin reactions to *Aspergillus* in many patients has also suggested that type III hypersensitivity mechanisms may be involved. However, it must be confessed that a complete understanding of the immunological mechanisms involved, which are surely more complex than those suggested above, is not yet available. A full account of the

Table 38.2 Diagnostic criteria for allergic bronchopulmonary aspergillosis.

Asthma
Chest X-ray
Peripheral blood eosinophilia
Positive skin-prick test for *Aspergillus* antigen
Positive serum *Aspergillus* precipitins
Raised serum IgE levels

Table 38.3 Drugs causing pulmonary eosinophilia.

Ampicillin [54]
Beclometasone dipropionate (inhaled) [55]
Bleomycin [56]
Carbamazepine [57]
Chlorpromazine [58]
Chlorpropamide [59]
Clofibrate [60]
Cocaine (inhaled) [61]
Disodium cromoglicate (inhaled) [62]
Diclofenac [63]
Febarbamate [64]
Fenbufen [65]
Glafenine [66]
Granulocyte–macrophage colony-stimulating factor [67]
Heroin (inhaled) [68]
Ibuprofen [69]
Imipramine [70]
Interleukin 2 [71]
Interleukin 3 [72]
Iodinated contrast dye [73]
L-tryptophan [74,75]
Mephenesin carbamate [76]
Methotrexate [77]
Methylphenidate [78]
Minocycline [79]
Naproxen [80]
Nickel [81]
Nitrofurantoin [82]
Para-aminosalicylic acid [83]
Penicillin [84]
Penicillamine [85]
Pentamidine (inhaled) [86]
Phenytoin [87]
Pyrimethamine [88]
Rapeseed oil [89]
Sulfadimethoxine [90]
Sulfadoxine [91]
Sulfasalazine [92,93]
Sulindac [94]
Tetracycline [95]
Tolazamide [96]
Tolfenamic acid [97]
Vaginal sulfonamide cream [98]

manifestations, diagnosis and treatment of allergic bronchopulmonary aspergillosis is given in Chapter 34.

Drugs and pulmonary eosinophilia (see Chapter 55)

A large number of drugs have been associated with pulmonary eosinophilic episodes (Table 38.3). The pulmonary shadowing usually develops within several days of starting therapy with the drug and resolves within 1 week of stopping the drug, although occasionally episodes may persist for longer periods of time. Recurrence is only seen following rechallenge with the drug. The clinical and radiological features are similar to those of Loeffler's syndrome in the majority, although some cases more closely resemble the severe and prolonged illness of chronic eosinophilic pneumonia. Some reactions are self-limiting but therapy with corticosteroids is often employed to hasten resolution.

Tropical pulmonary eosinophilia

Weingarten [99] first described the condition of spasmodic bronchitis associated with leucocytosis, marked eosinophilia and a dramatic response to organic arsenicals in India.

Aetiology

The condition has been reported in India, Sri Lanka, Burma, Malaysia, Indonesia, tropical Africa, South America and the southern Pacific [100,101] and may give rise to diagnostic difficulties when seen in immigrants in non-endemic countries [102]. There is little doubt that it represents a hypersensitivity reaction to filarial infestation because:
1 microfilariae have been demonstrated in the lung, liver and lymph nodes of typical cases [103];
2 high antifilarial antibody titres are found in patients and the titre diminishes after cure [104–106];
3 histamine release from basophils challenged with filarial antigen is much higher in patients with pulmonary eosinophilia than in patients with other manifestations of filarial infection [107];
4 the condition responds dramatically to antifilarial treatment.

Pathological features

In the early weeks of the disease, histiocyte infiltrates in alveolar spaces give way to eosinophilic bronchopneumonia and eosinophilic abscesses [106,108]. After several months, eosinophils, histiocytes and lymphocytes often organize into nodular patterns, progressively evolving to predominantly histiocytic granulomatous responses marked by increasing fibrosis.

Clinical features

Males comprise 80% of patients. The onset is often insidious with cough, sputum, wheeze, dyspnoea and chest pain [100,106,109]. Fever, weight loss and fatigue are common. These symptoms may continue for weeks or months with remissions and recurrences. Auscultation may reveal rhonchi and/or crepitations.

Radiographic abnormalities

The chest film may be normal, although the typical appearance is of bilateral indefinite mottling uniformly distributed in both lung fields and involving the middle and lower zones [100,106]. Increased bronchovascular markings may be noted and occasionally mottled shadows become confluent to produce a pneumonic appearance [110]. Cavitation and pleural effusion have also been recorded [111,112].

Other investigations

There is nearly always an absolute eosinophil count of greater than $3\times10^9/L$, the usual range being $5–60\times10^9/L$ [109]. The filarial complement test is positive. The sputum may contain predominantly eosinophils as does bronchoalveolar lavage fluid [113]. A marked increase in IgE concentration occurs, the IgE concentration appearing to be related to the degree of eosinophilia [105,114]. IgE levels are threefold higher in relapsing disease than in the primary disease [114].

Pulmonary function tests have shown an obstructive pattern in the early stages of the disease, progressing to a predominantly restrictive pattern with a decrease in D_{LCO} in untreated long-standing cases [115–117].

Treatment

Diethylcarbamazine in a dose of 6–8 mg/kg daily should be given orally in three divided doses for 10–14 days or for as long as 4 weeks [100]. Relief of symptoms occurs within a few days, and improvement of pulmonary function tests towards normal is detected in those who are treated early [100,115,116]. Clinical, haematological, radiological and physiological concomitants of the disease may still persist but continue to improve after the completion of 1 month of treatment with diethylcarbamazine [118]. Prolonged delay in treatment may result in irreversible pulmonary fibrosis.

Chronic eosinophilic pneumonia or cryptogenic pulmonary eosinophilia

This category of pulmonary eosinophilia is characterized by more severe clinical manifestations and, in the absence of treatment, persistence of radiographic abnormalities.

Aetiology

The aetiology is unknown. Some drugs, notably sulphonamides [119], nitrofurantoin [82] and chlorpropamide [59], have been implicated. In three patients the illness was associated with desensitization for allergic rhinitis [120]. In one case an associated immune complex vasculitis of skin was detected [121]; in others the pathological findings of microgranulomas and vasculitis with many degranulated eosinophils [122] has led to the suggestion that a cell-mediated reaction with release of lymphokines, which summon and activate eosinophils,

results in cellular damage largely mediated by the components of the eosinophil granules. The disease has been seen in association with an exacerbation of long-standing rheumatoid arthritis [123] and with coccidioidal infections [124].

Pathology

The histological findings are of interstitial and alveolar infiltration with eosinophils and histiocytes [125–127] (Fig. 38.3). The histiocytes contain eosinophil proteins and Charcot–Leyden crystals [128], and ECP is strikingly increased in bronchoalveolar lavage fluid [129]. Eosinophilic abscesses and multinucleated giant cells may be seen; mast cells, many partly degranulated, may be present. In some biopsy specimens, bronchiolitis obliterans, microgranuloma formation and vasculitis have been observed, indicating that the tissue response is not restricted to the alveoli [120–122]. Progression to lung fibrosis has been reported [130].

Clinical features

The syndrome can occur at any age, although most patients are middle-aged women (female/male ratio, 2 : 1). Onset in pregnancy has been reported [131] and, although heredity is not considered a factor, the disease has been reported in identical twins [132]. The onset is usually insidious, with an average symptom duration of 7.7 months before diagnosis [133]. Patients may be moderately to severely ill, with cough and mucoid sputum, dyspnoea, malaise, weight loss, night sweats and high fever. Haemoptysis may be present and the clinical picture may mimic that of tuberculosis [125–127,133–136]. If asthma is present it is frequently of recent onset [120]. In the absence of treatment these symptoms may have persisted for weeks or months. Spontaneous remissions and recurrences have been recorded [120,137].

Radiographic abnormalities

Radiographs typically show dense opacities, with ill-defined margins and without lobar or segmental distribution, arranged peripherally apposed to the pleura [1,120,125,126,133,137]. The opacities are usually axillary or apical but may be basal and mimic loculated pleural effusions. Opacities may disappear and recur in the same or different situations. Peculiar oblique or vertical lines without reference to the hilum or anatomical divisions may appear during resolution of the pneumonia. Gaensler and Carrington [120] described the changes as resembling the photographic negative of pulmonary oedema (Fig. 38.4), although this appearance may also occur in other conditions such as sarcoidosis [138] and bronchiolitis obliterans with organizing pneumonia [139]. Unilateral

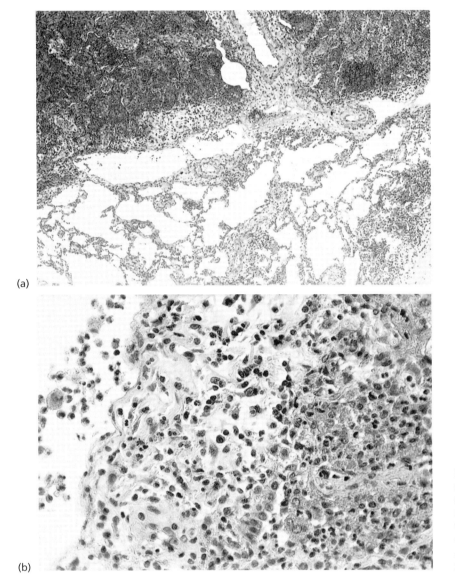

(a)

(b)

Fig. 38.3 Lung biopsy of patient with eosinophilic pneumonia: (a) intra-alveolar and interstitial infiltration with inflammatory cells (haematoxylin & eosin ×25); (b) bilobed eosinophils with granular cytoplasm, together with some histiocytes and lymphoid cells (haematoxylin & eosin ×170).

chest radiographic abnormalities have also been seen [135].

CT (Fig. 38.5) may show peripheral airspace disease, not always apparent on the chest radiograph [133,140]. Inapparent mediastinal adenopathy may also be detected by CT [140,141].

Other investigations

In as many as one-third of cases, peripheral blood eosinophilia may not occur [120]. The white blood cell count may be increased and eosinophilia of over 2.5×10^9/L has been recorded [133]. Anaemia is not uncommon [137] and an erythrocyte sedimentation rate (ESR) as high as 100 mm in the first hour is a frequent finding [126,137,142]. Eosinophils may be seen in the sputum [126]. Bronchoalveolar lavage in one patient showed 42%

eosinophils and 48% macrophages prior to therapy, with a normal cell differential count 13 weeks after steroid therapy was instituted [143]. Dynamic lung volumes usually indicate a restrictive pattern and D_{LCO} is decreased. Hypoxaemia, with an increased alveolar–arterial Po_2 difference, may occur [125,144] and type II respiratory failure has been described [145]. IgE concentrations are normal or only slightly increased [126,135].

Diagnosis

In most cases the radiographic and clinical appearances are so typical that a trial of corticosteroid therapy is indicated [120]. When there is doubt about the diagnosis, bronchoalveolar lavage or even open lung biopsy may be indicated to establish the diagnosis and exclude other possibilities.

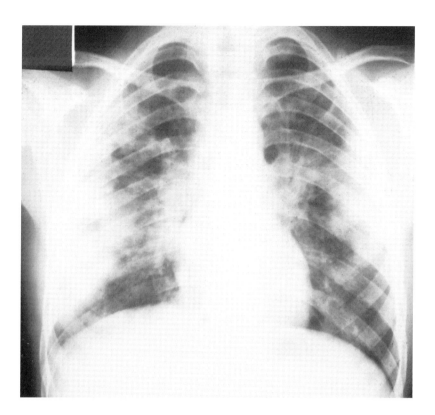

Fig. 38.4 Chest film of patient with chronic eosinophilic pneumonia before treatment with corticosteroids showing mainly peripheral areas of consolidation. His eosinophil count was $2 \times 10^9/L$.

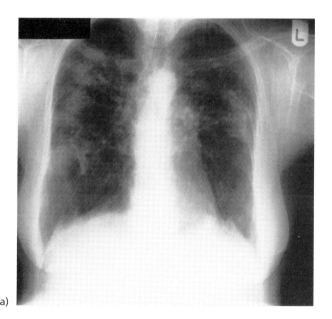

(a)

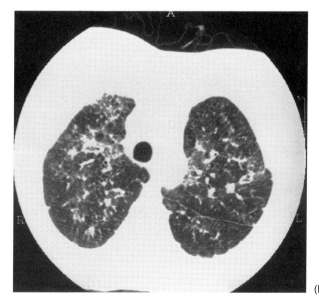

(b)

Fig. 38.5 (a) Chest radiograph of 50-year-old woman with patchy peripheral consolidation due to drug-induced chronic pulmonary eosinophilia. (b) High-resolution CT of the same patient showing patchy alveolitis and early fibrotic change. (Courtesy of Dr Lesley Gomersal.)

Treatment

Typically, clinical improvement occurs rapidly within 2–3 days of instituting therapy with 30–40 mg of prednisolone daily. Radiographic clearing should be evident after 2–3 days and the chest film is usually normal within 10–14 days [120]. Occasionally higher doses of prednisolone are required. Decrease in the dose and withdrawal of steroids should be possible after recovery, although recurrences requiring reinstitution of steroid therapy may occur. It is recommended that steroids should be continued in a maintenance dose of 5–20 mg daily for at least 6 months. The author usually tapers the dose slowly from the initial treatment dose over this period of time. A report of 12 cases followed for a mean interval of 10 years identified relapse (often multiple) in a majority when corticosteroids were discontinued or tapered; prompt resolution occurred with the reinstitution of therapy. A minority remained disease-free when treatment was discontinued [135]. Clearly, an attempt should be made to discontinue treatment, provided the possibility of recurrence is borne in mind.

Polyarteritis nodosa and allergic granulomatosis (Churg–Strauss syndrome)

Definition

Classical polyarteritis nodosa is characterized by a necrotizing vasculitis of small and medium-sized muscular arteries with involvement of multiple organ systems. Eosinophilia and granulomas are not characteristic of this disease and the lung and spleen are usually not involved [146–149]. Allergic granulomatosis (Churg–Strauss syndrome [146–148]) strongly resembles classical polyarteritis nodosa but has some obvious distinguishing features. An allergic diathesis, particularly severe asthma, is usual and, unlike the classical disease, lung involvement is a *sine qua non* of this syndrome. Other features include peripheral blood eosinophilia, eosinophilic tissue infiltration and granulomatous reactivity. Histologically, in addition to involvement of small and medium-sized muscular arteries, small vessels such as capillaries and venules may be affected by the pathological process. To complicate matters further an 'overlap syndrome', with features of both classical polyarteritis nodosa and allergic granulomatosis, is now recognized.

Aetiology

In cases with pulmonary involvement the sex incidence is approximately equal. The disease is found at all ages, with a mean age at onset of 38 years [31]. The disease may prove to be an immune complex vasculitis due to type III hypersensitivity to an external or internal antigen. Immune complexes have certainly been demonstrated with vasculitis and hepatitis B antigenaemia [150,151]. When immune complexes are trapped on a vessel basement membrane, complement is activated leading to an accumulation of polymorphonuclear leucocytes that cause damage and necrosis of the vessel wall by release of lysosomal enzymes. An alternative cell-mediated mechanism, which would explain the granuloma formation, postulates that macrophages are recruited to the vessel wall by lymphokines released from sensitized lymphocytes. The macrophages may be activated (possibly by immune complexes) to release lysosomal enzymes, with resultant vessel wall damage; at the same time the macrophages have the potential to transform into epithelioid cells with the formation of granulomas [146].

Studies using monoclonal antibodies have revealed large amounts of ECP and eosinophil protein X in the granulomas of Churg–Strauss syndrome. Activated and degranulating eosinophils are a feature of the pathological lesions and it would appear that these cytotoxic eosinophil proteins may play an active part in the development of the lesions [152].

In one large series [149] approximately one-quarter of the patients had received various drugs, most often sulphonamides, before the onset of their illness, and it has been suggested in the past that a real decrease in the incidence of polyarteritis was associated with a decline in the use of sulphonamides [153].

Pathological features

Macroscopically, necrotic lesions, infarcts and bronchiectasis may be found in the lungs [147–149]. The necrotic lesions may be nodular and cavitated and may give rise to areas of intra-alveolar haemorrhage. Microscopically, the necrotic areas are surrounded by giant cells, lymphocytes, plasma cells and neutrophils and there may be diffuse eosinophil infiltration. In the pulmonary arteries and veins, there is proliferation of intimal connective tissue and infiltration with eosinophils and neutrophils. The media particularly of the arteries often shows fibrinoid change, sometimes with giant cells, and granulomatous reactions are found in connective tissue and vessel walls (Fig. 38.6).

Clinical features

Patients with Churg–Strauss syndrome almost invariably have an illness presenting with respiratory symptoms [31,147,154]. These symptoms may precede other evidence of systemic involvement by a number of years. Asthma is the most common presenting symptom and is usually chronic and severe. Upper airway involvement may manifest as rhinitis, sinusitis or nasal polyps. In one series, asthma preceded the vasculitis in 80% of cases and the mean duration of this preceding asthma was 8 years [154]. Incidents of 'pneumonia' with cough and blood-stained sputum may occur and sputum may contain numerous eosinophils. There may be fever [154] and other systemic symptoms, including weakness, malaise, arthralgia, night sweats, myalgia and loss of weight. A diagnosis of tuberculosis may initially be considered (Fig. 38.7).

In patients with involvement of other systems, symptoms and signs referable to these systems may be noted.

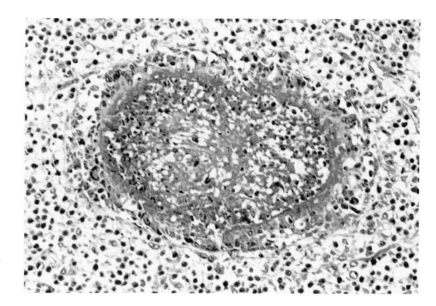

Fig. 38.6 Small artery from necropsy specimen in patient with Churg–Strauss syndrome showing a florid necrotizing vasculitis with thrombosis and inflammatory cells in the occluded lumen (haematoxylin & eosin ×170).

These include heart failure, pericarditis and hypertension [155,156]. The gastrointestinal tract may be involved, resulting in abdominal pain, diarrhoea or bleeding [31]. Skin lesions are found in 70% of patients and may include petechiae, purpura, nodules or urticaria. Mononeuritis multiplex occurs in 66% and central nervous system involvement in 29% [31]. Reversible exophthalmos and hearing loss have been reported [157].

Radiographic features

In the chest film, patchy pneumonic consolidation often resembling chronic eosinophilic pneumonia is found and the shadows may have the same migratory characteristics [154,158,159]. Diffuse interstitial shadows may occur (Fig. 38.7) and nodules, which may cavitate, are frequently seen. Pleural effusion has been recorded. The clinical and radiographic presentation may be confused with tuberculosis.

Other investigations

Anaemia and leucocytosis are common and eosinophilia occurs [31,147,154], with absolute counts higher than 5×10^9/L in one series [149]. The ESR is usually markedly elevated and a high plasma globulin fraction is found. IgE levels are elevated in most patients [160,161]. Antineutrophil cytoplasmic antibochies of the *P* type are commonly present [162,163]. Pulmonary function tests show obstructive defects. The diagnosis is established by biopsy of involved organs. Transbronchial lung biopsy is inadequate and open or thoracoscopic lung biopsy is preferred.

Treatment

Without treatment the course of the disease is progressive,

with exacerbations and partial remissions. In one series [149], 70% of those beginning with a respiratory illness were dead within 1 year. The treatment of choice is corticosteroids and large doses, such as 40–60mg of prednisolone daily, are often needed initially and should be continued for several weeks to ensure remission of the vasculitis [31]. With remission of symptoms and establishment of a normal ESR, the dose can be tapered to a maintenance level which, typically, is continued for at least 1 year. In the Mayo Clinic series of 30 cases treated with high-dose corticosteroids, 15 patients nevertheless died with a mean time to death of 4 years [154]. In cases resistant to corticosteroid therapy, remission may be induced by the addition of azathioprine [164] or cyclophosphamide [165]. Methylprednisolone pulse therapy has been used successfully in patients failing to respond to oral prednisolone [166,167].

Hypereosinophilic syndrome

This rare syndrome is characterized by marked peripheral blood eosinophilia and by eosinophilic infiltration of many organs in the absence of a known cause [168,169]. Suggested criteria for the diagnosis are:
1 persistent peripheral eosinophilia of greater than 1.5×10^9/L for longer than 6 months;
2 signs and symptoms of organ involvement;
3 no evidence of allergic, parasitic, vasculitic, neoplastic or other known cause of eosinophilia [168].

Clinical features

The cause of the hypereosinophilic syndrome is unknown. Onset is usually in the third or fourth decade and males predominate [170]. The clinical presentation may

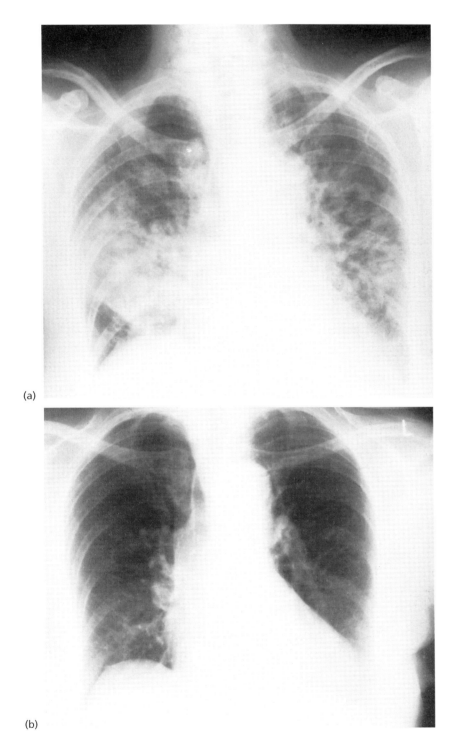

(a)

(b)

Fig. 38.7 Churg–Strauss syndrome: the patient presented with fever, arthralgia, dyspnoea and haemoptysis. Chest film showed diffuse patchy consolidation (a) that responded rapidly to high-dose corticosteroids (b).

superficially resemble that of eosinophilic pneumonia, with systemic symptoms including fever, night sweats, anorexia, malaise, weight loss, pruritus and cough. However, a profound peripheral eosinophilia is usually present, with eosinophils comprising 30–70% of a normal or increased white count [168]. IgE levels are often high. Eosinophils are present in large numbers in the bone marrow, and eosinophilic metamyelocytes, myelocytes and even myeloblasts may be found in the peripheral blood [168].

Pulmonary involvement, typically presenting as cough that is worse at night, may be seen in up to 40% of patients. Chest radiographs may show interstitial infiltrates and pleural effusions are common [168]. Bronchoalveolar lavage shows high percentages of eosinophils [171].

Cardiovascular involvement is the major cause of morbidity and mortality [172,173]. Endocardial fibrosis, restrictive cardiomyopathy, valvular damage and mural thrombus formation may occur. Arterial (and venous) thromboembolic disease is common. Splinter haemorrhages are frequent but infarction of the kidney, spleen, cerebrum and retina are also seen; deep vein thrombosis and other peripheral vascular occlusions such as femoral artery embolism have been recorded. Finally, eosinophil infiltration of the kidney, skin, gastrointestinal tract, joints and muscles may also give rise to symptoms.

Serum levels of interleukin-2 receptors appear to correlate with disease activity and severity [174].

Treatment

About 50% of patients respond to extended initially high-dose oral corticosteroid therapy beginning with 60 mg of prednisolone daily [175]. It has been suggested [175] that treatment should be reserved for those with demonstrable end-organ damage due to the hypereosinophilia. Other drugs that have been used successfully include hydroxy-carbamide (hydroxyurea), cyclophosphamide, azathioprine, interferon α, cyclosporin, etoposide and vincristine [168,170,176–178].

Acute eosinophilic pneumonia

Diagnostic criteria

This relatively new entity was first described in 1989 [179,180]; the diagnostic criteria are given in Table 38.4 [31].

Clinical features

Patients may be of any age or sex and typically present with an acute febrile illness of several days' duration with associated myalgia, pleurisy and hypoxaemia often requiring ventilatory support. There may be a history of allergic rhinitis [136]. Physical examination confirms fever, respiratory distress and diffuse inspiratory crepitations, usually without wheeze, on auscultation. There may be signs of pleural effusion.

Table 38.4 Diagnostic criteria for acute eosinophilic pneumonia [31].

Acute febrile illness of <5 days' duration
Hypoxaemic respiratory failure
Diffuse alveolar or mixed alveolar interstitial chest radiographic infiltrates
Bronchoalveolar lavage eosinophils >25%
Absence of parasitic, fungal or other infection
Prompt and complete response to corticosteroids
Failure to relapse after discontinuing steroids

Radiology

The chest radiograph typically shows diffuse alveolar or alveolar–interstitial infiltrates. Peripheral infiltrates (unlike chronic eosinophilic pneumonia) are unusual. Kerley B lines are common. Small to medium pleural effusions are often seen and, if tapped, show a high percentage of eosinophils [181].

Other investigations

Peripheral blood eosinophilia is not usually found; in striking contrast, the eosinophil count in bronchoalveolar lavage fluid is high with an average of 42% in one early series [179]. Serum IgE levels have been elevated in some but not all patients. Pulmonary function studies show a restrictive pattern with a low diffusing capacity [181]. Lung biopsy confirms the presence of a non-vasculitic eosinophilic pneumonia [182].

Treatment

Hypoxaemia may be severe enough to require ventilatory support. Treatment is with high-dose (60–125 mg daily) prednisolone or methylprednisolone until respiratory failure resolves. The lowest effective initial dose has yet to be determined, although it has been established that continuation therapy with 40–60 mg daily for 2–4 weeks with a subsequent tapering of dosage to zero over a further 2–4 weeks does not occasion relapse. The cause of this condition, if indeed it is a separate entity, remains to be determined. An acute hypersensitivity phenomenon has been suggested [179].

References

1 Crofton JW, Livingstone JL, Oswald NC, Roberts ATM. Pulmonary eosinophilia. *Thorax* 1952; 7: 1.
2 Reeder WH, Goodrich BE. Pulmonary infiltration with eosinophilia (PIE syndrome). *Ann Intern Med* 1952; 36: 1217.
3 Liebow AA, Carrington CB. The eosinophilic pneumonias. *Medicine* 1969; 48: 251.
4 Horn BR, Robin ED, Theodore J, Van Kessel A. Total eosinophil counts in the manage-

ment of bronchial asthma. *N Engl J Med* 1975; 292: 1152.
5 Carlson MGCh, Peterson CGB, Venge P. Human eosinophil peroxidase: Purification and characterisation. *J Immunol* 1985; 134: 1875.
6 Venge P. The eosinophil in inflammation. In: Venge P, Lindbom A, eds. *Inflammation.* Stockholm: Almquist and Wiksell, 1985: 85.
7 Gleich GJ, Adolphson CR. The eosinophil

leucocyte: structure and function. *Adv Immunol* 1986; 39: 177.
8 Spry CJF. *Eosinophils. A Comprehensive Review and Guide to the Scientific and Medical Literature.* Oxford: Oxford University Press, 1988.
9 Wasmoen TL, Bell MP, Loegering DA *et al.* Biochemical and amino acid sequence analysis of human eosinophil granule major basic protein. *J Biol Chem* 1988; 263: 12259.
10 Gleich GJ, Loegering DA, Bell MP *et al.*

Biochemical and functional similarities between human eosinophil derived neurotoxin and eosinophil cationic protein: homology with ribonuclease. *Proc Natl Acad Sci USA* 1986; 83: 3146.

11 Slifman NR, Venge P, Peterson CGB, McKean DJ, Gleich GJ. Human eosinophil derived neurotoxin and eosinophil protein X are likely the same protein. *J Immunol* 1989; 143: 2317.

12 Weller PF, Goetzl EJ, Austen KF. Identification of human eosinophil lysophospholipase as a constituent of Charcot–Leyden crystals. *Proc Natl Acad Sci USA* 1980; 77: 7440.

13 Schatz M, Wasserman S, Patterson R. The eosinophil and the lung. *Arch Intern Med* 1982; 142: 1515.

14 Kay AB, Shin HS, Austen KF. Selective attraction of eosinophils and synergism between eosinophil chemotactic factor of anaphylaxis (ECF-A) and a fragment cleaved from the fifth component of complement (C5a). *Immunology* 1973; 24: 969.

15 Kay AB, Stechschulte DJ, Austen KF. An eosinophil leucocyte chemotactic factor of anaphylaxis. *J Exp Med* 1971; 133: 602.

16 Leitch AG. Leukotrienes and the lung. *Clin Sci* 1984; 67: 153.

17 Altman LC, Hill JS, Hairfield WM, Mullarkey MF. Effects of corticosteroids on eosinophil chemotaxis and adherence. *J Clin Invest* 1981; 67: 28.

18 Koch-Weser J. Beta-adrenergic blockade and circulating eosinophils. *Arch Intern Med* 1968; 121: 255.

19 Butterworth AE, David JR. Eosinophil function. *N Engl J Med* 1981; 304: 154.

20 Hubscher T. Role of the eosinophil in allergic reactions. *J Immunol* 1975; 114: 1379.

21 Kay AB. The eosinophil in infectious diseases. *J Infect Dis* 1974; 129: 606.

22 Butterworth AE, Sturrock RF, Houba V *et al.* Eosinophils as mediators of antibody dependent damage to schistosomula. *Nature* 1975; 256: 727.

23 McLaren DJ. The role of eosinophils in tropical disease. *Semin Hematol* 1982; 19: 100.

24 Gleich GJ, Loegering DA, Frigas E *et al.* The major basic protein of the eosinophil granules: physicochemical properties, localisation and function. In: Mahmoud AAF, Austen KF, eds. *The Eosinophil in Health and Disease.* New York: Grune and Stratton, 1980: 79.

25 Gleich GJ, Frigas E, Leogering DA *et al.* Cytotoxic properties of the eosinophil major basic protein. *J Immunol* 1979; 123: 2925.

26 Filley WV, Kephart GM, Gleich GJ. Localisation of the eosinophil granules major basic protein (MBP) in the bronchi of patients with asthma. *J Allerg Clin Immunol* 1981; 67 (Suppl): 54.

27 Venge P. What is the role of the eosinophil? *Thorax* 1990; 45: 161.

28 Kroegel C, Warner JA, Virchow J-C, Matthys H. Pulmonary immune cells in health and disease: the eosinophil leucocyte (part II). *Eur Respir J* 1994; 7: 743.

29 Badesch DB, King TE, Schwarz MI. Acute eosinophilic pneumonia: a hypersensitivity phenomenon? *Am Rev Respir Dis* 1989; 139: 249.

30 Allen JN, Pacht ER, Gadek JE, Davis WB. Acute eosinophilic pneumonia as a reversible cause of respiratory failure. *N Engl J Med* 1989; 321: 569.

31 Allen JN, Davis WB. Eosinophilic lung diseases. *Am J Respir Crit Care Med* 1994; 150: 1423.

32 Loeffler W. Zur differential-diagnose der lungen infiltierungen: Uber fluchtige succedan-infiltraten (mit eosinophilie). *Beitr Klin Tuberk* 1932; 79: 368.

33 Koino A. Quoted in: Manson-Bahr PEC, Apted FIC, eds. *Manson's Tropical Diseases.* London: Baillière Tindall, 1982: 182.

34 Phills JA, Harrold AJ, Whiteman GV, Perelmutter L. Pulmonary infiltrates, asthma and eosinophilia due to *Ascaris suum* infection in man. *N Engl J Med* 1972; 286: 965.

35 Johansson SGO, Mellbin T, Vahlquist B. Immunoglobulin levels in Ethiopian preschool children with special reference to high concentrations of immmunoglobulin E (IgND). *Lancet* 1968; i: 1118.

36 Bahk YW. Pulmonary paragonimiasis as a cause of Loffler's syndrome. *Radiology* 1962; 78: 598.

37 Beaver PC, Danaraj TJ. Pulmonary ascariasis resembling eosinophilic lung. *Am J Trop Med Hyg* 1958; 7: 100.

38 Gelpi AP, Mustafa A. *Ascaris* pneumonia. *Am J Med* 1968; 44: 377.

39 Slavin RG, Stanczyk DJ, Lonigro AJ, Brown JD. Allergic bronchopulmonary aspergillosis: a North American rarity. *Am J Med* 1969; 47: 306.

40 Hoehne KFW, Reed CE, Dickie HA. Allergic bronchopulmonary aspergillosis is not rare. *Chest* 1973; 63: 177.

41 McCarthy DS, Pepys J. Allergic bronchopulmonary aspergillosis: clinical immunology. 1. Clinical features. *Clin Allergy* 1971; 1: 261.

42 Hinson KFW, Moon AJ, Plummer NS. Bronchopulmonary aspergillosis: a review and report of eight new cases. *Thorax* 1952; 7: 317.

43 Scadding JG. Eosinophilic infiltrations of the lung in asthmatics. *Proc R Soc Med* 1971; 64: 381.

44 Pepys J, Simon G. Asthma, pulmonary eosinophilia and allergic alveolitis. *Med Clin North Am* 1973; 57: 573.

45 Middleton WG, Patterson IC, Grant IWB, Douglas AC. Asthmatic pulmonary eosinophilia: a review of 65 cases. *Br J Dis Chest* 1977; 71: 115.

46 Chapman BJ, Capewell S, Gibson R *et al.* Pulmonary eosinophilia with and without allergic bronchopulmonary aspergillosis. *Thorax* 1989; 44: 919.

47 Mroueh S, Spock A. Allergic bronchopulmonary aspergillosis in patients with cystic fibrosis. *Chest* 1994; 105: 32.

48 Marchant JL, Warner JO, Bush A. Rise in total IgE as an indicator of allergic bronchopulmonary aspergillosis in cystic fibrosis. *Thorax* 1994; 49: 1002.

49 Pepys J, Faux JA, Longbottom JL *et al.* *Candida albicans* precipitins in respiratory disease in man. *J Allergy* 1968; 41: 305.

50 Gordon DS, Hunter RG, O'Reilly RJ, Conway BP. *Pseudomonas aeruginosa* allergy and humoral antibody mediated hypersensitivity pneumonia. *Am Rev Respir Dis* 1973; 108: 127.

51 Laham MN, Carpenter JL. *Aspergillus terreus*, a pathogen capable of causing infective endocarditis, pulmonary mycetoma and allergic bronchopulmonary aspergillosis. *Am Rev Respir Dis* 1982; 125: 769.

52 Hendrick DJ, Ellithorpe DB, Lyon F *et al.* Allergic bronchopulmonary helminthosporiosis. *Am Rev Respir Dis* 1982; 126: 935.

53 Halwig JM, Brueske DA, Greenberger PA *et al.* Allergic bronchopulmonary curvulariosis. *Am Rev Respir Dis* 1985; 132: 186.

54 Poe RH, Condemi JJ, Weinstein SS, Schuster RJ. Adult respiratory distress syndrome related to ampicillin sensitivity. *Chest* 1980; 77: 449.

55 Mollura JL, Bernstein RA, Fine SR *et al.* Pulmonary eosinophilia in a patient receiving beclomethasone diproprionate aerosol. *Ann Allergy* 1979; 42: 326.

56 Yousem SA, Lifson JD, Colby TV. Chemotherapy induced eosinophilic pneumonia. *Chest* 1985; 88: 103.

57 Lewis IJ, Rosenbloom L. Glandular fever like syndrome, pulmonary eosinophilia and asthma associated with carbamazepine. *Postgrad Med J* 1982; 58: 100.

58 Shear MK. Chlorpromazine induced PIE syndrome. *Am J Psychiatry* 1978; 135: 492.

59 Bell RJM. Pulmonary infiltration with eosinophils caused by chlorpropamide. *Lancet* 1964; i: 1249.

60 Hendrickson RM, Simpson F. Clofibrate and eosinophilic pneumonia. *JAMA* 1982; 247: 3082.

61 Nadeem S, Nasir N, Israel RI. Löffler's syndrome secondary to crack cocaine. *Chest* 1994; 105: 1599.

62 Lobel H, Macktey I, Eldror MY. Pulmonary infiltrates with eosinophilia in an asthmatic patient treated with disodium cromoglycate. *Lancet* 1972; ii: 1032.

63 Khalil H, Molinary E, Stoller JK. Diclofenac (Voltaren) induced eosinophilic pneumonitis. Case report and review of the literature. *Arch Intern Med* 1993; 153: 1649.

64 Gali JM, Vilanova JL, Mayos M *et al.* Febarbamate induced pulmonary eosinophilia: a case report. *Respiration* 1986; 49: 231.

65 Burton GH. Rash and pulmonary eosinophilia associated with fenbufen. *Br Med J* 1990; 300: 82.

66 Gheysens B, Van Mieghern W. Pulmonary infiltrates with eosinophilia due to glafenine. *Eur J Respir Dis* 1984; 65: 456.

67 Gonzales-Chambers R, Rosenfeld C, Winkelstein A, Dameshek L. Eosinophilia resulting from administration of recombinant granulocyte–macrophage colony stimulating factor (rh GM-CSF) in a patient with T-γ lymphoproliferative disease. *Am J Hematol* 1991; 36: 157.

68 Brander PE, Tukiainen P. Acute eosinophilic pneumonia in a heroin smoker. *Eur Respir J* 1993; 6: 750.

69 Goodwin SD, Glenny RW. Non-steroidal anti-inflammatory drug associated pulmonary infiltrates with eosinophilia. *Arch Intern Med* 1992; 152: 1521.

70 Cutler NR, Anderson TJ. Proven asymptomatic eosinophilia with imipramine. *Am J Psychiatry* 1977; 134: 1296.

71 van Haelst Pisani C, Kovach JS, Kita H *et al.* Administration of interleukin-2 (IL-2) results in increased plasma concentrations of IL-5 and eosinophilia in patients with cancer. *Blood* 1991; 78: 1538.

72 Lindermann A, Ganser A, Hermann F *et al.* Biologic effects of recombinant human interleukin-3 *in vivo*. *J Clin Oncol* 1991; 9: 2120.

73 Jennings CA, Deveckis J, Azumi N, Yeager H. Eosinophilic pneumonia associated with reaction to radiographic contrast medium. *South Med J* 1991; 84: 92.

74 Kaufman LD, Seidman RJ, Gruber BL. L-Tryptophan associated eosinophilic perimyositis, neuritis and fasciitis. A clinicopathologic and laboratory study of 25 patients. *Medicine* 1990; 69: 187.

75 Campagna AC, Blanc PD, Criswell LA *et al.* Pulmonary manifestations of the eosinophilia–myalgic syndrome associated with tryptophan ingestion. *Chest* 1992; 101: 1274.

76 Rodman T, Fraimow W, Myerson RM. Löffler's syndrome: report of a case associated with administration of mephenesin carbamate (Tolseram). *Ann Intern Med* 1958; 48: 668.

77 Clarysse AM, Cathey WJ, Cartwright GE, Wintrobe MM. Pulmonary disease complicating intermittent therapy with methotrexate. *JAMA* 1969; 209: 1861.

78 Wolf J, Fein A, Fehrenbacher L. Eosinophilic syndrome with methylphenidate abuse. *Ann Intern Med* 1978; 89: 224.

79 Sitbon O, Bidel N, Dussopt C *et al.* Minocycline induced eosinophilic pneumonitis. An analysis in 5 patients. *Am Rev Respir Dis* 1993; 147: A76.

80 Nader DA, Schillaci RF. Pulmonary infiltrates with eosinophilia due to naproxen. *Chest* 1983; 83: 280.

81 Gray J. Löffler's syndrome following ingestion of a coin. *Can Med Assoc J* 1982; 127: 999.

82 Hailey FJ, Gluscock HW, Hewitt WF. Pleuropneumonic reaction to nitrofurantoin. *N Engl J Med* 1969; 281: 1087.

83 Wold ED, Zahn DW. Allergic (Löffler's) pneumonitis occurring during antituberculous chemotherapy. *Am Rev Tuberc* 1950; 74: 445.

84 Riechlin S, Loveless MH, Kane EG. Löffler's syndrome following penicillin therapy. *Ann Intern Med* 1953; 38: 113.

85 Davies D, Lloyd-Jones JK. Pulmonary eosinophilia caused by penicillamine. *Thorax* 1980; 35: 957.

86 Dupon M, Malou M, Regnes AM, Lacut JY. Acute eosinophilic pneumonia induced by inhaled pentamidine isethionate. *Br Med J* 1993; 306: 109.

87 Mahatma M, Haponik EF, Nelson S, Lopez A, Summer WR. Pheynytoin induced acute respiratory failure with pulmonary eosinophilia. *Am J Med* 1989; 87: 93.

88 Davidson AC, Bateman C, Shovlin C *et al.* Pulmonary toxicity of malaria prophylaxis. *Br Med J* 1988; 297: 1240.

89 Kilbourne EM, Rigan-Perez JG, Heath CW *et al.* Clinical epidemiology of toxic oil syndrome: manifestations of a new illness. *N Engl J Med* 1983; 309: 1408.

90 Fiegenberg DS, Weiss H, Kirschman H. Migratory pneumonia and eosinophilia associated with sulphonamide administration. *Arch Intern Med* 1967; 120: 85.

91 Daniel PT, Holzschuh J, Berg PA. Sulfadoxine specific lymphocyte transformation in a patient with eosinophilic pneumonia induced by sulfadoxine–pyrimethamine (Fansidar). *Thorax* 1989; 44: 307.

92 Anon. Sulphasalazine induced lung disease. *Lancet* 1974; ii: 504.

93 Sullivan SN. Sulfasalazine lung: desensitisation to sulfasalazine with acrylic coated 5-ASA and azodisalicylate. *J Clin Gastroenterol* 1987; 9: 461.

94 Fein M. Sulindac and pneumonitis. *Ann Intern Med* 1981; 95: 245.

95 Ho D, Tashkin DP, Bein ME, Sharma O. Pulmonary infiltrates with eosinophilia associated with tetracycline. *Chest* 1979; 76: 33.

96 Bondi E, Slater S. Tolazamide induced chronic eosinophilic pneumonia. *Chest* 1981; 80: 652.

97 Strömberg C, Palva E, Alhava E, Aranko K, Idänpään-Heikkilä J. Pulmonary infiltrates induced by tolfenamic acid. *Lancet* 1987; ii: 685.

98 Donlan CJ, Scutero JV. Transient eosinophilic pneumonia secondary to use of a vaginal cream. *Chest* 1975; 67: 232.

99 Weingarten RJ. Tropical eosinophilia. *Lancet* 1943; i: 103.

100 Udwadia FE. Tropical eosinophilia: a review. *Respir Med* 1993; 87: 17.

101 Islam N. *Tropical Eosinophilia*. Chittagong: Anwar, Islam, 1964.

102 Jones DA, Pillai DK, Rathbone BJ, Cookson JB. Persisting 'asthma' in tropical pulmonary eosinophilia. *Thorax* 1983; 38: 692.

103 Webb JKG, Job CK, Gault EW. Tropical eosinophilia: demonstration of microfilariae in lung, liver and lymph nodes. *Lancet* 1960; i: 835.

104 Danaraj TJ. The treatment of eosinophilic lung (tropical eosinophilia) with diethylcarbamazine. *Q J Med* 1958; 27: 243.

105 Danaraj TJ, Da Silva LS, Schacher JF. The serological diagnosis of eosinophilic lung (tropical eosinophilia) and its etiological implications. *Am J Trop Med Hyg* 1959; 8: 151.

106 Neva FA, Ottesen EA. Current concepts in parasitology: tropical (filarial) eosinophilia. *N Engl J Med* 1978; 298: 1129.

107 Ottesen EA, Neva FA, Paranjape RS *et al.* Specific allergic sensitisation to filarial antigens in tropical eosinophilia syndrome. *Lancet* 1979; i: 1158.

108 Udwadia FE, Joshi VV. A study of tropical eosinophilia. *Thorax* 1964; 19: 548.

109 Spry CJF, Kumaraswami V. Tropical eosinophilia. *Semin Hematol* 1982; 19: 107.

110 Jain VK, Beniwal OP. Unusual presentation of tropical pulmonary eosinophilia. *Thorax* 1984; 39: 634.

111 Viswanathan R. Pulmonary eosinophilosis. *Q J Med* 1948; 17: 257.

112 Nath J, Vain VK. Atypical presentation of pulmonary eosinophilia. *Ind J Chest Dis All Sci* 1978; 20: 141.

113 Pinkston P, Vijayan VK, Nutman TB *et al.* Acute tropical pulmonary eosinophilia: characterisation of the lower respiratory tract inflammation and its response to therapy. *J Clin Invest* 1987; 80: 216.

114 Ray D, Saha K. Serum immunoglobulin and complement levels in tropical pulmonary eosinophilia and their correlation with primary and relapsing stages of the illness. *Am J Trop Med Hyg* 1978; 27: 503.

115 Udwadia FE. Tropical eosinophilia: a correlation of clinical, histiopathologic and lung function studies. *Dis Chest* 1967; 52: 531.

116 Nesarajali MS. Pulmonary function in tropical eosinophilia before and after treatment with diethylcarbamazine. *Thorax* 1975; 30: 574.

117 Vijayan VK, Kuppurao KV, Venkateson P, Sankaran K, Prabhakar R. Pulmonary membrane diffusing capacity and capillary blood volume in tropical eosinophilia. *Chest* 1990; 97: 1386.

118 Vijayan KV, Kappurao KV, Sankaran K, Venkatesan P, Prabhakar R. Tropical eosinophilia: clinical and physiological response to diethylcarbamazine. *Respir Med* 1991; 85: 17.

119 Feinman L. Drug induced lung disease: pulmonary eosinophilia and sulphonamides. *Proc R Soc Med* 1975; 68: 440.

120 Gaensler EA, Carrington CB. Peripheral opacities in chronic eosinophilic pneumonia: the photographic negative of pulmonary oedema. *Am J Roentgenol* 1977; 128: 1.

121 Chan NH, Boybo WJ, Schellenberg RR *et al.* A case of eosinophilic pneumonia. Unusual immune complex vasculitis in the skin. *Chest* 1982; 82: 113.

122 Fox B, Seed WA. Chronic eosinophilic pneumonia. *Thorax* 1980; 35: 570.

123 Payne CR, Connellan SJ. Chronic eosinophilic pneumonia complicating long standing rheumatoid arthritis. *Postgrad Med J* 1980; 56: 519.

124 Lombard CM, Tazelaar HD, Krasne DL. Pulmonary eosinophilia in coccidioidal infections. *Chest* 1987; 91: 734.

125 Carrington CB, Addington WW, Goff AM *et al.* Chronic eosinophilic pneumonia. *N Engl J Med* 1969; 280: 787.

126 Turner-Warwick M, Assen ESK, Lockwood M. Cryptogenic pulmonary eosinophilia. *Clin Allergy* 1976; 6: 135.

127 Kanner RE, Hammar SP. Chronic eosinophilic pneumonia. *Chest* 1977; 71: 95.

128 Janin A, Torpier J, Courtin P *et al.* Segregation of eosinophil proteins in alveolar macrophage compartments in chronic eosinophilic pneumonia. *Thorax* 1993; 48: 57.

129 Shijubo N, Shigehara K, Hirasowa H, Inuzuka M, Abe S. Eosinophil cationic protein in chronic eosinophilic pneumonia and eosinophilic granuloma. *Chest* 1994; 106: 1481.

130 Yoshida K, Shijubo N, Koba H *et al.* Chronic eosinophilic pneumonia progressing to lung fibrosis. *Eur Respir J* 1994; 7: 1541.

131 Dothager DW, Kollef MH. Post-partum pulmonary infiltrates with peripheral eosinophilia. *Chest* 1991; 99: 463.

132 Barnes N, Gray BJ, Heaton R, Costello JF. Pulmonary eosinophilia in identical twins. *Thorax* 1983; 38: 318.

133 Jederlinic PJ, Sicilian L, Gaensler EA. Chronic eosinophilic pneumonia: a report of 19 cases and review of the literature. *Medicine* 1988; 67: 154.

134 Capewell S, Chapman BJ, Alexander F, Greening AP, Crompton GK. Pulmonary eosinophilia with systemic features: therapy and prognosis. *Respir Med* 1992; 86: 485.

135 Naughton M, Fahy J, Fitzgerald MX. Chronic eosinophilic pneumonia. A long term follow-up of 12 patients. *Chest* 1993; 103: 162.

136 Hayakawa H, Sato A, Toyoshima M, Imokawa S, Taniguchi M. A clinical study of idiopathic eosinophilic pneumonia. *Chest* 1994; 105: 1462.

137 Pearson DJ, Rosenow EC III. Chronic eosinophilic pneumonia (Carrington's). A follow up study. *Mayo Clin Proc* 1978; 53: 73.

138 Glazer HS, Levitt RG, Shackelford GD. Peripheral pulmonary infiltrates in sarcoidosis. *Chest* 1984; 86: 741.

139 Bartler T, Irwin RS, Nash G, Balikian JP, Hollingsworth HH. Idiopathic bronchiolitis obliterans organising pneumonia with peripheral infiltrates on chest roentgenogram. *Arch Intern Med* 1989; 149: 273.

140 Mayo JR, Muller NL, Road J, Sisler J, Lillington G. Chronic eosinophilic pneumonia: CT findings in six cases. *Am J Roentgenol* 1989; 153: 727.

141 Onitsuka H, Onitsuka S, Yokomizo Y, Matsuura K. Computed tomography of chronic eosinophilic pneumonia. *J Comput Assist Tomogr* 1983; 7: 1092.

142 Lindesmith L. Prolonged pulmonary infiltration with eosinophilia. *N C Med J* 1964; 25: 466.

143 Dejaegher P, Demedts M. Bronchoalveolar lavage in eosinophilic pneumonia before and during corticosteroid therapy. *Am Rev Respir Dis* 1984; 129: 631.

144 Rogers RM, Christiansen JR, Walson JJ, Patterson CD. Eosinophilic pneumonia. *Chest* 1975; 68: 665.

145 Libby DM, Murphy TF, Edward A *et al.* Chronic eosinophilic pneumonia: an unusual cause of respiratory failure. *Am Rev Respir Dis* 1980; 122: 497.

146 Fauci AS. The spectrum of vasculitis. *Ann Intern Med* 1978; 89: 660.

147 Churg J, Strauss L. Allergic granulomatosis, allergic angiitis and periarteritis nodosa. *Am J Pathol* 1952; 27: 277.

148 Alarcon-Segovia D. The necrotising vasculitides: a new pathogenetic classification. *Med Clin North Am* 1977; 61: 241.

149 Rose GA, Spencer H. Polyarteritis nodosa. *Q J Med* 1957; 26: 43.

150 Gocke DJ, Hsu K, Morgan C *et al.* Association between polyarteritis and Australia antigen. *Lancet* 1970; ii: 1149.

151 Michalak T. Immune complexes of hepatitis B surface antigen in the pathogenesis of periarteritis nodosa. *Am J Pathol* 1978; 90: 619.

152 Tai P-C, Holt ME, Denny P *et al.* Deposition of eosinophil cationic protein in granulomas in allergic granulomatosis and vasculitis: the Churg–Strauss syndrome. *Br Med J* 1984; 289: 400.

153 Symmers WStC. The occurrence of angiitis and of other generalised diseases of connective tissue as a consequence of the administration of drugs. *Proc R Soc Med* 1962; 55: 20.

154 Chumbley LC, Harrison EG, Deremee RA. Allergic granulomatosis and angiitis (Churg–Strauss syndrome). Report and analysis of 30 cases. *Mayo Clin Proc* 1977; 52: 477.

155 Davison AG, Thompson PJ, Davies J *et al.* Prominent pericardial and myocardial lesions in the Churg–Strauss syndrome (allergic granulomatosis and angiitis). *Thorax* 1983; 38: 793.

156 Kozak M, Gill EA, Green LS. The Churg–Strauss syndrome. A case report with angiographically documented cardiac involvement and a review of the literature. *Chest* 1995; 107: 578.

157 Sale S, Patterson R. Recurrent Churg–Strauss vasculitis with exophthalmus, hearing loss, nasal obstruction, amyloid deposits, hyperimmunoglobulin E and circulating immune complexes. *Arch Intern Med* 1981; 141: 1363.

158 Levin DC. Pulmonary abnormalities in the necrotising vasculitides and their rapid response to steroids. *Radiology* 1970; 97: 521.

159 Hueto-Perez-de-Heredia J-J, Dominguez-del-Valle F-J, Garcia E, Gomez M-L, Gallego J. Chronic eosinophilic pneumonia as a presenting feature of Churg–Strauss syndrome. *Eur Respir J* 1994; 7: 1006.

160 Kus J, Bergin C, Miller R *et al.* Lymphocyte sub-populations in allergic granulomatosis and angiitis (Churg–Strauss syndrome) *Chest* 1985; 87: 826.

161 Lanham JG, Elkon KB, Pusey CD, Hughes GR. Systemic vasculitis with eosinophilia and asthma: a clinical approach to the Churg–Strauss syndrome. *Medicine* 1984; 63: 65.

162 Tervaert JWC, Goldschmeding R, Elema JD, Von Dem Borne AEGK, Kallenberg CGM. Antimyeloperoxidase antibodies in the Churg–Strauss syndrome. *Thorax* 1991; 46: 70.

163 Higgs CMB. Anti-neutrophil cytoplasmic antibodies. *Respir Med* 1992; 86: 367.

164 Cooper BJ, Bacal E, Patterson R. Allergic angiitis and granulomatosis: prolonged remission induced by combined prednisone–azathioprine therapy. *Arch Intern Med* 1978; 138: 367.

165 Fauci AS, Doppmann JL, Wolff SM. Cyclophosphamide induced remission in advanced polyarteritis nodosa. *Am J Med* 1978; 64: 890.

166 Neild GH, Lee HA. Methylprednisolone pulse therapy in the treatment of polyarteritis nodosa. *Postgrad Med J* 1977; 53: 382.

167 McFadyen R, Tron V, Keshmiri M, Road TD. Allergic angiitis of Churg and Strauss syndrome. Response to pulse methyl prednisolone. *Chest* 1987; 91: 629.

168 Chusid MJ, Dale DC, West BC, Wolff SM. The hypereosinophilic syndrome. Analysis of 14 cases with review of the literature. *Medicine* 1975; 54: 1.

169 Fauci AS, Harley JB, Roberts WC *et al.* The idiopathic hypereosinophilic syndrome: clinical, pathophysiologic and therapeutic considerations. *Ann Intern Med* 1982; 97: 78.

170 Spry CJF, Davies J, Tai PC *et al.* Clinical features of fifteen patients with the hypereosinophilic syndrome. *Q J Med* 1983; 205: 1.

171 Winn RE, Kollef MH, Meyer JL. Pulmonary involvement in the hypereosinophilic syndrome. *Chest* 1994; 105: 656.

172 Parrillo JE, Borer JS, Henry WL *et al.* The cardiovascular manifestation of the hypereosinophilic syndrome. *Am J Med* 1979; 67: 572.

173 Spry CJF. The hypereosinophilic syndrome: clinical features, laboratory findings and treatment. *Allergy* 1982; 37: 539.

174 Prin L, Plumas J, Gruart V *et al.* Elevated serum levels of soluble interleukin-2 receptor: a marker of disease activity in the hypereosinophilic syndrome. *Blood* 1991; 78: 2626.

175 Parrillo JE, Fauci AS, Wolff SM. Therapy of the hypereosinophilic syndrome. *Ann Intern Med* 1978; 89: 167.

176 Zielinski RM, Lawrence WD. Interferon-α for the hypereosinophilic syndrome. *Ann Intern Med* 1990; 113: 716.

177 Smit AJ, Van Essen LH, De Vries EGE. Successful long-term control of hypereosinophilic syndrome with etoposide. *Cancer* 1991; 67: 2826.

178 Zabel P, Schlaak M. Cyclosporin for hypereosinophilic syndrome. *Ann Haematol* 1991; 62: 230.

179 Badesch DB, King TE, Schwarz MI. Acute eosinophilic pneumonia: a hypersensitivity phenomenon? *Am Rev Respir Dis* 1989; 139: 249.

180 Allen JN, Pacht ER, Gadek JE, Davis WB. Acute eosinophilic pneumonia as a reversible cause of non-infectious respiratory failure. *N Engl J Med* 1989; 321: 569.

181 Ogawa H, Fujimura M, Matsuda T *et al.* Transient wheeze. Eosinophilic broncho-bronchiolitis in acute eosinophilic pneumonia. *Chest* 1993; 104: 493.

182 Buchheit J, Eid N, Rodgers G, Feger T, Yakoub O. Acute eosinophilic pneumonia with respiratory failure: a new syndrome? *Am Rev Respir Dis* 1992; 145: 716.

39
SARCOIDOSIS

A. GORDON LEITCH

Definition

Until the precise cause of sarcoidosis is known, the following descriptive paragraph prepared by the Seventh International Conference on Sarcoidosis will continue to be useful in place of a definition:

> Sarcoidosis is a multisystem granulomatous disorder of unknown aetiology most commonly affecting young adults and presenting most frequently with bilateral hilar lymphadenopathy, pulmonary infiltration and skin or eye lesions. The diagnosis is established most securely when clinicoradiographic findings are supported by histological evidence of widespread non-caseating epithelioid granulomas in more than one organ or a positive Kveim–Siltzbach skin test. Immunological features are depression of delayed-type hypersensitivity, suggesting impaired cell-mediated immunity, and raised or abnormal immunoglobulins. There may also be hypercalciuria with or without hypercalcaemia. The course and prognosis may correlate with the mode of onset: an acute onset with erythema nodosum heralds a self-limiting course and spontaneous resolution, while an insidious onset may be followed by relentless progressive fibrosis. Corticosteroids relieve symptoms and suppress inflammation and granuloma formation [1].

Since this description was published in 1976, substantial advances in the understanding of the immunology of sarcoidosis have resulted from the application of the technique of bronchoalveolar lavage (BAL) via the fibreoptic bronchoscope. These advances are described in detail later in the chapter and considerably enhance the outline of the immunological abnormalities given in the above description.

Historical background

In 1936 Hunter [2] suggested that a case seen by Hutchinson in 1869 and reported in 1877 [3] may have been an example of the condition subsequently described by Hutchinson in 1898 as Mortimer's malady. It now seems clear that Hutchinson did not himself identify the 1869 case as one of Mortimer's malady, making any claim to priority dubious [4]. In 1889 Besnier gave a detailed account of a patient with the clinical features of lupus pernio [5] and 3 years later Tenneson [6] described a similar case in which the histology was studied and the typical granulomatous lesion found.

Hutchinson in 1898 described skin lesions that principally affected the face, arms and hands and which were referred to for a long time as 'Mortimer's malady', a tribute to the lady who was the first of a series of patients with these manifestations. In his comment on four cases, Hutchinson showed remarkable foresight when he wrote 'the truth is probably that the various pathogenetic influences are capable of the most various combinations and that we have, on all sides, connecting links between maladies which have gained distinctive names'. Over the next few years, Boeck, Heerfordt and Jungling, unaware of the unitary nature of the disease, described clinical pictures that were regarded as disease entities and given eponymous designations [3,5,7–15] (Table 39.1). The term 'sarcoid' was introduced by Boeck because of a superficial resemblance of a skin lesion to sarcoma.

In 1914 Schaumann recognized the relation between the various recorded presentations and in an essay entitled 'Sur le lupus pernio' (for some reason not published until 1934) emphasized the systemic nature of the disease [13]. In 1917 he suggested the term 'lymphogranuloma benigna' [14]. This was something of a euphemism considering that Schaumann himself stated that 'the most usual course is that a classical tuberculosis manifests itself in the lungs, peritoneum, etc. causing death'. He clearly favoured a tuberculous aetiology. He felt that the benignity of the disease 'should be regarded as only relative and referred to the protracted course of the disease and, for a long time, its insignificant effect on general condition'. Apart from tuberculosis, death frequently occurred from 'debility, usually combined with severe dyspnoea and cardiac weakness'. It should, of course, be remembered

Table 39.1 Historical background of sarcoidosis.

Date	Author	Description
1869	Hutchinson [3]	'Anomalous disease of skin of fingers' (papillary psoriasis)
1889	Besnier [5]	Lupus pernio
1898	Hutchinson [7]	Lupus vulgaris multiplex non-ulcerans (Mortimer's malady)
1899	Boeck [8]	Multiple benign sarcoid
1904	Kriebich [9]	Bone changes ('chronic osteomyelitis') in cases of lupus pernio
1905	Boeck [10]	Benign miliary lupoid
1906	Darier & Roussy [11]	Subcutaneous sarcoid
1909	Heerfordt [12]	Uveoparotid fever
1914	Schaumann [13]	'Sur le lupus pernio'
1917	Schaumann [14]	Benign lymphogranuloma
1920	Jungling [15]	Ostitis tuberculous multiplex cystica
1940+		Universal acceptance of term 'sarcoidosis'

that it was mainly the chronic form of the disease that was being recognized and that many cases were erroneously treated in tuberculosis sanatoria with inevitable exposure to infection.

With the introduction of mass miniature radiography during the Second World War, it soon became apparent that the hilar glands and lungs were affected, that many cases were asymptomatic and that spontaneous resolution was the rule in the vast majority of cases.

The relationship between erythema nodosum, bilateral hilar lymphadenopathy and sarcoidosis was first properly defined by Lofgren to give us the syndrome that bears his name [16,17]. In the 1940s the term 'sarcoidosis' was universally accepted as the name for this condition. It soon became obvious that many patients with sarcoidosis had previously been wrongly classified as tuberculosis, a situation that probably still exists in many developing countries today [18].

Epidemiology

Incidence and prevalence

There are considerable difficulties in obtaining reliable prevalence figures for sarcoidosis that allow valid comparisons between different geographical areas. The nature of the disease is such that many asymptomatic cases escape detection, particularly in countries where radiographic screening programmes are not available. Presentation may be to any one of a wide range of medical specialties, with all the resulting problems of collating medical records. Finally, there may be different degrees of awareness of the disease in different countries and probably also variation in diagnostic criteria.

Mass radiography studies

The results of an international study of pulmonary sarcoidosis detected by mass radiography are shown in Table 39.2 [19]. There is considerable disparity in prevalence figures for the various countries, with a range from 0.2 per 100000 in Poland and Brazil to 64 per 100000 in Sweden. A more recent study from Sweden in which 64% of the population over 15 years were screened at 3-yearly intervals gave a prevalence of 19 per 100000, which extrapolated to 24 per 100000 assuming 100% screening [20,21]. A similar recent survey from Finland reported a prevalence of 15 per 100000 in those over 15 years [22]. The wide range of reported prevalences may reflect a distinctive geographical pattern for the disease and suggest that sarcoidosis is an entity determined by a specific environmental factor or factors. Other factors that may contribute to geographical differences, other than the sources of error referred to in the introduction, are the age and sex structure of the population, ethnic groups and genetic factors, which are discussed later in this section.

Data from diagnostic records

Where special efforts are made to identify all cases presenting to medical practitioners including general practitioners, the incidence is more likely to reflect the true state of affairs. A recent study of this kind in the Isle of Man [23] found a mean annual incidence of 15 per 100000 over the years 1977–83 compared with 3.5 per 100000 in the preceding 15 years when less intensive searching had been carried out.

A similar intensive study was conducted in four areas of the UK by the British Thoracic and Tuberculosis Association from 1961 to 1966 in predominantly Caucasian populations [24]. This found a range of annual incidences of 2.1–4.5 per 100000 for men and 3.5–4.5 per 100000 for women, with an increase in incidence from north to south. Peak incidence was in the age group 25–34 years. In the US Army, based on records of disability and death, the incidence of cases was found to be 11 per 100000, with the peak incidence in the 25–29 age group [25]. The rates for Blacks were 16 times the rates for all other groups.

In developing countries, comparable figures are not easily obtained but where the disease has been sought, as in the Bantu, it has been found and is 10 times more common than in the white population [18]. In other countries where the incidence is believed to be low, such as China, South-East Asia and South America, it is still not clear whether this represents a real finding or is the result of a combination of confounding factors, such as misdiagnosis, inadequate diagnostic facilities and continuing confusion with tuberculosis [4].

Despite geographical variations in incidence of disease,

Table 39.2 Prevalence of pulmonary sarcoidosis. (From Proceedings of the Third International Conference on Sarcoidosis 1963 [19].)

Country	Reporter	No. of cases examined (thousands)	No. of sarcoid cases			Prevalence per 100 000
			Total	Males	Females	
Scandinavia						
Finland	Patiala	1430	111			8.1
	Riska & Selroos	155	8			5.1
Norway	Riddervold	1448	387	181	206	26.7
Sweden	Bauer & Wijkstrom (I)	1873	1023	453	570	55*
	Bauer & Wijkstrom (II)	1351	867	396	471	64
UK and Eire						
London	James	868	160	87	73	19
Scotland	Douglas	1709	141	59	82	8.2 (6.5–18)
N. Ireland	Milliken	1448	149	60	89	10.3
Eire	Logan	383				33.3
Europe						
Czechoslovakia	Levinsky & Altmann	3436	118	53	65	3.4
France	Turiaf	207	20			*c.* 10
Germany						
W. Berlin	Fried	(2200†)	319	114	205	14.5
Leipzig	Lindig	1017	134	48	86	13.3
Hungary	Mandi & Kelemen	*c.* 91	5			5
Italy	Muratore	17	2			(11.6)
The Netherlands	Orie & Brugge	4591	994	370	624	21.6
Poland	Jaroszewicz	93	10			10.7
Portugal	Villar	*c.* 3500	6			0.2
Switzerland	Sommer	3161	515			16.3
Yugoslavia	LaGrasta	277	33	6	27	11.9
America						
Canada	Pollak	*c.* 77	>8			>10.5
Argentina	Rey	340‡	17			5.0
	Castells	695	7			1.0
Brazil	Certain & de Paula	1810	4			0.2
Uruguay	Purriel	1839	8			0.4
Asia						
Israel	Rakower	422	7	6	1	1.6
Japan	Hosoda & Nobechi	193	11			5.6
Australia and New Zealand						
Australia	Marsham	1571	145	66	79	9.2
New Zealand	Reid	1081	171	88	83	16 (6.1–24.3)

*I, II, two surveys.
†Population.
‡University students.

the pattern of disease in different countries is remarkably similar [26] (Table 39.3), with a few important exceptions. Patients most commonly present with respiratory symptoms, ocular or skin disease or because of a routine chest radiograph.

Age and sex incidence

Most studies have shown the highest incidence in the third and fourth decades [24–30], with a variable female predominance [27,31,32]. Children and the aged are not immune but the disease is uncommon at the extremes of life. It is of interest that in Japan, where children over

Table 39.3 Involvement of various tissue systems (%) in 3676 patients with sarcoidosis. (From James *et al.* [26].)

City	Intrathoracic	Reticuloendothelial*	Eyes	Skin	Erythema nodosum	Parotid	Nervous system	Bone
London	84	40	27	25	31	6	7	4
New York	92	55	20	19	11	8	4	9
Paris	94	32	11	12	7	6	4	4
Los Angeles	93	46	11	27	9	6	2	4
Tokyo	87	24	32	12	4	5	4	2
Reading	89	30	16	13	32	5	9	1
Lisbon	88	29	6	18	12	2	4	13
Edinburgh	94	39	11	7	33	5	3	1
Novi Sad	90	14	15	4	11	3	1	11
Naples	99	0	0	0.4	6	0	0	0
Geneva	97	17	12	6	11	2	1	3
Total	87	28	15	9	17	4	4	3

*Reticuloendothelial, spleen and peripheral lymph nodes.

8 years of age are included in a comprehensive mass radiography programme, the prevalence rates for schoolchildren have ranged from 1 to 2 per 100 000 [33].

Ethnic factors

As already mentioned, sarcoidosis is 16 times more common in Black compared with non-Black US soldiers and is also much commoner in the Bantu compared with the white South African population [18,25]. In London, the annual incidence of sarcoidosis was shown to be 20 per 100 000 in Black people per 100 000 in Asians and 1.5 per 100 000 in Caucasians [34]. As reported previously from London and the USA, erythema nodosum is relatively uncommon in Black people, who tend to have more extrathoracic and severe disease requiring steroid therapy [35,36]. The clinical picture in Asians and Puerto Ricans more closely resembles that in West Indians and Black people than in Caucasians [34,36].

Familial factors

A British Thoracic Society Research Committee investigation reported 59 families in Britain with more than one case of sarcoidosis [37]. There were three families with more than two cases, giving a total of 62 instances made up of five twins (four monozygotic and one dizygotic), 28 siblings, 22 parent–child and seven husband–wife. The total number of patients was 121, comprising 46 males and 75 females. A review of 160 published instances of familial sarcoidosis also showed a marked excess of monozygotic over dizygotic twins (13 : 1), supporting a genetic influence. The most striking features of these were the significantly larger proportions of like sex over unlike sex pairs among both siblings and parent–child instances and the excess of mother–child over father–child associations. The conclusions were valid even when account was taken of

the known higher incidence of sarcoidosis in females [24]. Other published reports also show a marked excess of mother–child over father–child relationships but only a slight excess of like sex over unlike sex pairs [38,39]. An Irish study described 114 index cases of sarcoidosis with a total sibling pool of 534 [40]. Of the index cases, 11 had siblings with a diagnosis of sarcoidosis giving a prevalence of sarcoidosis among siblings of 2.2%. This may suggest that genetic influences are determinants for the development of sarcoidosis. Nevertheless, the demonstration in the Isle of Man of space–time clustering of the disease is also consistent with sarcoidosis being a communicable disease [41,42].

Human leucocyte antigens

A number of studies of human leucocyte antigens (HLA) in sarcoidosis have been undertaken and the evidence that HLA type does not influence susceptibility to sarcoidosis is reviewed by Scadding and Mitchell [4].

There is evidence that HLA type does influence the pattern of disease. A high incidence of HLA-B8 has been found in London patients with arthropathy or erythema nodosum [43]. Two other studies have confirmed this association [44,45]: of 107 white patients with sarcoidosis, 40% had HLA-B8, while the percentages among those with arthropathy and erythema nodosum were 62% and 89% respectively. In 19 Swedish patients with acute-onset sarcoidosis (all having bilateral hilar lymphadenopathy and arthropathy and seven erythema nodosum), HLA-B8 was present in 67% and HLA-DR3 in 90% compared with frequencies of 24% and 26% in the Swedish population [46]. These authors noted that HLA-B1, -B8 and -DR3 occur in linkage disequilibrium and that this haplotype has been associated with abnormal immune responsiveness [46]. A more recent study in English Caucasians and Black West Indians with sarcoidosis has found an increased frequency of HLA-Cw7 in the Caucasians and that HLA-DR3 and the B8/Cw7/DR3 haplotype were associated with a good prognosis in the Caucasians. No significant associated good prognostic indices were found in the West Indians [47]. In Japan, increased frequencies of HLA-DRw52 and -DR5J have been found in sarcoidosis patients, the latter being especially significant in unresolved cases [48–50].

It would appear from studies to date that HLA-B8, -Cw7 and -DR3 are associated with the hilar lymphadenopathy/erythema nodosum/arthopathy form of the disease, which carries a good prognosis. This association may explain the correlation between the frequencies of HLA-B8 and sarcoidosis with erythema nodosum in different populations, for example the frequency of HLA-B8 is 29% in London, 16% in New York and 2% in Tokyo and the percentage of patients with sarcoidosis and erythema nodosum in these cities is 31%, 11% and 4%, respectively [45].

Aetiology

The cause of sarcoidosis is unknown. A number of aetiologies, including exposure to pine pollen or beryllium and infection with *Mycobacterium*, viruses and fungi, have been suggested and rejected as reviewed by Scadding and Mitchell [4]. Animal inoculation studies have suggested the possibility of an unidentified transmissible agent [51], as have the Isle of Man studies [41,42].

Possible role of an unidentified transmissible agent

In 1969 Mitchell and Rees [51] reported the results of a controlled experiment in which an attempt was made to demonstrate a transmissible agent from sarcoid material. Sarcoid and non-sarcoid lymph node homogenates were inoculated into the footpads of normal and immunologically deficient mice. The early and late changes in the footpads were assessed microscopically. A substantial proportion of the mice receiving sarcoid homogenate showed the histological characteristics typical of sarcoidosis in humans, which evolved fully after a period of 6–8 months following inoculation. Kveim tests were carried out and positive results were confined to a proportion of those mice given sarcoid homogenates and were all associated with sarcoid granulomas in the footpad. Conversely, the inflammatory lesions seen in the footpads of mice inoculated with non-sarcoid homogenates were negative. The authors concluded from this preliminary work that an agent, as yet unidentified, may have been transmitted to the mice from human sarcoid tissue; however, an alternative explanation might be that they were demonstrating the reactivity of mice to a factor, or factors, common to granulomatous reactions in general. They obtained

similar results with tissues from Crohn's disease [52]; normal human lymph node extracts used as controls did not give rise to footpad granulomas or positive Kveim tests.

The work on induction of granulomas in mice by injection of human sarcoid and ileitis homogenates has been confirmed and extended by other workers and allows the speculation that the affected lymph nodes of sarcoidosis and regional ileitis and ileitis bowel may harbour transmissible agents that play a role in granuloma formation [53–56].

Later work by Mitchell and Rees [55] found that granulomas could be produced in normal or immunologically deficient mice by footpad, intraperitoneal or intravenous injections with fresh whole sarcoid homogenates, fresh supernatants or fresh 0.22-μm filtered supernatants. In contrast, no granulomas were seen in response to identically prepared non-sarcoid tissue homogenates. Successful passage was also achieved following the inoculation of both filtered and unfiltered 'sarcoid' mouse tissue homogenates into secondary hosts [56]. The agent could be inactivated by autoclaving or by irradiation with cobalt-60 [57].

In 1983 Mitchell and Rees [58] reported that although the human tissues used had been negative microscopically and culturally for *Mycobacterium*, acid-fast bacilli had been seen in granulomatous tissues of mice passaged from sarcoid tissues of six patients. These were found in mouse lungs and spleen 17 months or more after the injection of homogenate or supernatant filtrate of mouse granulomatous tissue on first to third passage from the original injection of human sarcoid tissue 3–9 years before. *Mycobacterium tuberculosis* was grown from pooled homogenates of lungs and spleen from mice in two of these serial passages. This has fuelled interest in the suggestion originally made by Burnet in 1959 [59] that a protoplast or L form of the tubercle bacillus may be a cause of sarcoidosis.

The implication that *M. tuberculosis* might have a pathogenetic role in sarcoidosis has been further explored by sophisticated and very sensitive molecular biological techniques, including polymerase chain reaction (PCR) for the mycobacterial DNA sequence known as IS6110 [60–62]. In one UK study, *M. tuberculosis* DNA was found by PCR in half the patients with sarcoidosis, one-third of the patients with inactive tuberculosis and in 60% of patients with active tuberculosis [61]. In contast, a meticulously controlled North American study found DNA from *M. tuberculosis* in only a minority of patients with sarcoidosis [62]. An accompanying editorial [63] emphasizes that for most patients with sarcoidosis PCR analysis of their cells or tissues is unable to detect any DNA from *M. tuberculosis* at a level of sensitivity of 15 organisms per million human cells. The sensitivity of PCR for *M. tuberculosis* is fraught with hazard, particularly with regard to contamination [63]. At present, the jury does not have enough evidence to implicate mycobacteria in sarcoidosis. It may be that detected DNA simply represents previous mycobacterial infection. Studies in patients with sarcoidosis from countries with dramatically differing prevalences of tuberculosis may resolve this issue.

Transplantation and sarcoidosis

Recurrence of disease in the pulmonary allografts of patients treated for end-stage pulmonary sarcoidosis by lung transplantation has been recorded [64,65] and is consistent with current thinking about the immunopathogenesis of the disease (see below). Recurrence was limited to transbronchial biopsy evidence of granulomas within months of transplantation in one report [64] and to radiological and biopsy evidence of sarcoid infiltrates 13 months after transplantation in the other [65]. Disease

recurred despite immunosuppression and responded to an increased dose of oral prednisolone [65].

Pathology

The histological reaction in active sarcoidosis (Figs 39.1 and 39.2) consists essentially of nodular collections of large closely packed, pale-staining histiocytes (epithelioid cells). In early lesions the nodules are all characteristically at the same stage of development. A few multinucleated giant cells are usually seen among the histiocytes and some lymphocytes are often present at the periphery of the nodule. Three different types of inclusion bodies may be found in the cytoplasm of the epithelioid and giant cells.

1 Schaumann bodies, which are round or oval and vary in size from that of a leucocyte to about 100 μm in diameter. The larger of these bodies (sometimes referred to as con-

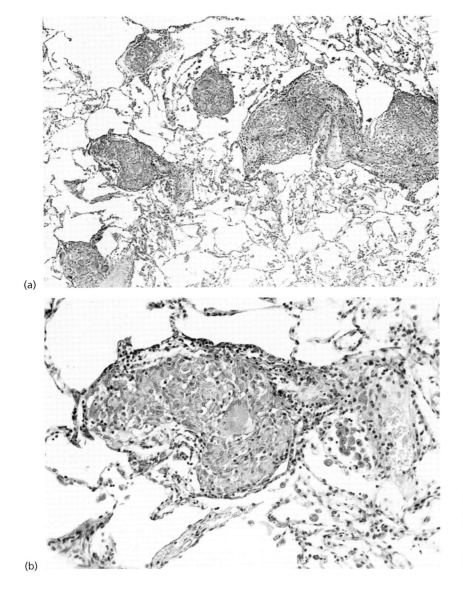

(a)

(b)

Fig. 39.1 Resected lung from patient with sarcoidosis: (a) small, compact epithelioid and giant cell interstitial granulomas (haematoxylin & eosin ×15); (b) epithelioid and giant cells in the granuloma (haematoxylin & eosin ×35).

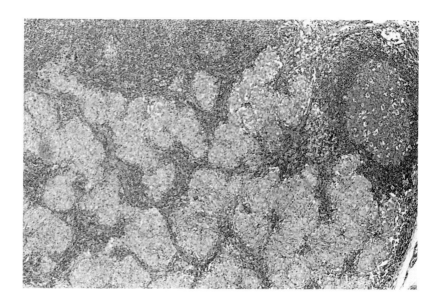

Fig. 39.2 Lymph node from same patient as in Fig. 39.1 showing multiple non-caseating granulomas (haematoxylin & eosin ×35).

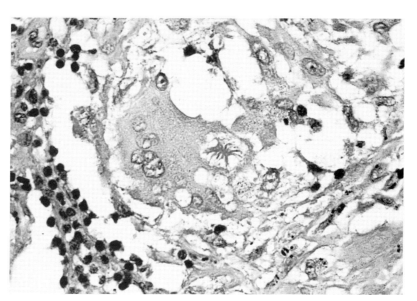

Fig. 39.3 Multinucleate giant cell from a sarcoid granuloma containing a typical asteroid body (haematoxylin & eosin ×350).

choid bodies) seem to be formed of basophilic concentric lamellae that appear to contain calcium and iron.

2 Doubly refractile crystalline inclusion bodies are 1–20 μm in diameter and may take up stains for calcium and iron.

3 Asteroid bodies consist of a central mass 2.3–3 μm in diameter with radiating straight or centred spinous projections, the whole being 5–25 μm in diameter (Fig. 39.3).

Necrosis does not occur in the sarcoid nodule, or is only minimal. In consequence the reticulin between the histiocytes and around the nodules remains intact. Where present, this is an important point of distinction from the tuberculous follicular reaction. No acid-fast bacilli are found in the sections or can be cultured from them, with rare exceptions that may be explained by pre-existing, coexisting or consequential independent infection.

The epithelioid cells are large mononuclear cells about 20 μm in diameter with round or oval nuclei and are derived from macrophages. They are poorly phagocytic but highly secretory, producing acid phosphatase, cathepsin, β-glucuronidase, collagenase, elastase, cytolytic factors, lysozyme and angiotensin-converting enzyme [66–71]. Giant cells are up to 300 μm in diameter, containing as many as 30 nuclei usually arranged peripherally. Giant cells occur by the fusion of macrophages, which are constantly arriving, dividing and ageing. Spector [72] points out that the macrophages in sarcoid granulomas are not only metabolically active but are turning over rapidly, in contrast to macrophages in granulomas produced by relatively inert materials such as carbon. Soler and colleagues [73] have studied serial sections of a pulmonary sarcoid granuloma by electron microscopy and noted that epithelioid cells tend to be central and macrophages peripheral. This supports Spector's concept of the constant arrival of macrophages into a granuloma pool of mixed young and old macrophages, epithelioid and giant cells. The inclusion bodies are all non-specific end-products of the active metabolism and secretion that has taken place. As the lesion ages, reticulin fibres ramify between epithelioid cells, gradually thicken and eventually become converted into collagen. It loses its outline and becomes a solid amorphous eosinophilic mass of hyaline material.

The lymphocytes associated with the granulomas are larger than usual and morphologically appear activated [73]. Lymphocyte accumulations are more common in active lesions, when they are predominantly CD4 T-helper cells. As activity declines CD8 T-suppressor cells become more common [74]. Relatively large numbers of B cells and plasma cells are also present, suggesting that immunoglobulin production is also occurring at sites of granuloma formation [75].

Sarcoid follicles may resolve completely. When healing occurs in long-standing cases, the cellular nodules become replaced by fibrous tissue. In chronic sarcoidosis, follicles with the characteristic appearance may exist among masses of avascular fibrous tissue. Sclerosis of a follicle usually begins at the periphery with the formation of discrete hyaline clumps, which fuse to girdle the nodule; hyalinosis proceeds in a centripetal fashion until the follicle is wholly involved [76].

Several electron microscope studies have been made of Kveim and sarcoid lesions [77–82]. The epithelioid cells are seen by the electron microscope to be closely packed. At their margin, there is much plication and interdigitation of the various cells [78]. All the cells have large numbers of mitochondria indicating high metabolic activity. Certain cells show small dark bodies that are some kind of granule and may include large, pale vacuole-like bodies which probably contain protein. Very dark fibrillar material between the cells has the appearance of collagen. The giant cells show irregular peripheral nuclei and have numerous mitochondria, consistent with high metabolic activity.

The histological features of the sarcoid lesion are not specific and may occur in tuberculosis as well as leprosy, tertiary syphilis, brucellosis, primary biliary cirrhosis, hypogammaglobulinaemia, fungal infection and berylliosis [83–86]. A localized sarcoid reaction of the same histological pattern is sometimes observed in the vicinity of lesions due to carcinoma (especially in regional lymph nodes), lymphomas, fungal infections [87], trauma and chemical injury. Zirconium, a constituent of deodorant sticks, has been shown to cause a chronic axillary dermatosis via the development of a specific hypersensitivity reaction. These local tissue sarcoid reactions can usually be distinguished from systemic sarcoidosis by the absence of depressed or negative delayed-type hypersensitivity reactions and a negative Kveim test [88]. Lack of evidence of sarcoid lesions in other tissues or organs is another distinguishing feature.

Immunology

The granulomas of pulmonary sarcoidosis are now thought to be the consequence of activation of lymphocytes and macrophages within the lung, with resultant release of potent mediators that play a critical part in the pathogenesis of the disease [89–92] (Fig. 39.4). The stimulus for activation is unknown, although the state of activation of lung mononuclear cells is characteristic of that due to antigen stimulation and it may be that an unknown antigen is involved. In support of an unknown antigen is the finding of circulating immune complexes, particularly in the early stages of the disease [93–97]. Major advances in understanding the pathogenesis of sarcoidosis have come from studies on cells obtained by BAL using the fibreoptic bronchoscope [98]. Studies that have compared lavage with biopsy cell populations, including typing of T cells, suggest that cells obtained by lavage are representative of those found in biopsies from the same patient [99–101]. The total number of cells recovered at BAL is increased, with striking increases in the absolute numbers of macrophages and lymphocytes, although the percentage of macrophages decreases while the lymphocyte percentage increases (Fig. 39.5).

Lung lymphocytes

In active sarcoidosis the vast majority of lavage lymphocytes are T lymphocytes and of these most are CD4 T-helper cells, these cells outnumbering T-suppressor cells by 10 to 1. The T cells are activated, as demonstrated by increased rosetting with sheep erythrocytes at 37°C, and have been shown to release a number of lymphokines [101–105]. These include interleukin (IL)-2, a 15-kDa glycoprotein known to induce T-cell activation and replication [106]. Such activated T cells release other lymphokines that produce polyclonal B-cell activation and increased immunoglobulin production resulting in hyperglobulinaemia [106–108]. In addition, activated T cells release monocyte chemotactic factor and migration inhibition factor that act together to attract, immobilize and activate monocytes, the building blocks of granuloma formation [109].

Lung macrophages

The macrophage population in the lung is increased in active sarcoidosis and consists of alveolar macrophages and young macrophages that are probably freshly recruited monocytes [90]. The macrophages are activated, as shown by increased uptake of gallium-67 [110] and the

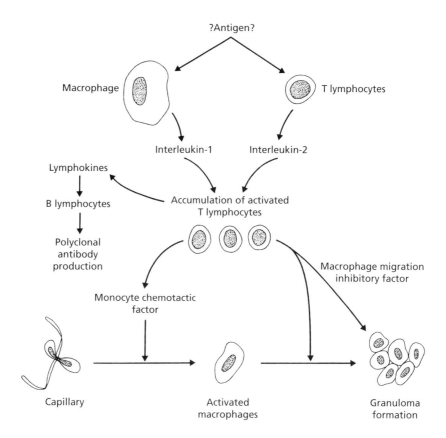

Fig. 39.4 Pathogenesis of granuloma formation (see text for explanation).

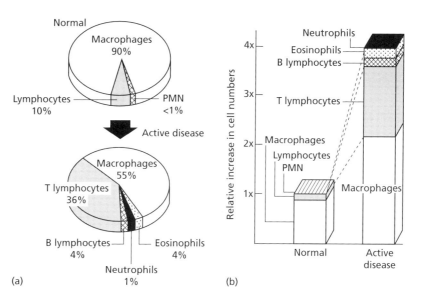

Fig. 39.5 Proportions (a) and total numbers (b) of cells obtained by bronchoalveolar lavage in normal subjects and in active sarcoidosis. (From Crystal *et al.* [90].)

(a)   (b)

release of mediators. IL-1 is released and leads to T-cell activation [111,112]. In addition, the release of interferon γ, fibronectin and alveolar macrophage-derived growth factor may promote fibroblast recruitment, attachment and proliferation and lead to fibrosis [89,113]. Transforming growth factor β_1 can also be demonstrated in the sarcoid granuloma [114].

Blood

In striking contrast to the findings in the lung, peripheral blood in sarcoidosis usually shows a lymphopenia with a lower than normal ratio of T-helper to T-suppressor cells [115–117]. Where the ratio of T-helper to T-suppressor cells is low, blood lymphocytes show diminished phytohaemagglutinin responsiveness [116]. These findings may explain the depression of delayed-type hypersensitivity that has long been noted as a feature of sarcoidosis. Thus, reactions to tuberculin, mumps virus antigen, *Candida albicans* antigen and trichophytin have all been shown to be depressed in patients with sarcoidosis [118–122]. The hyperglobulinaemia that is a feature of chronic active sarcoidosis is largely due to overproduction of predominantly IgG and IgA at sites of disease activity [95,108].

Modes of presentation

The diversity of the possible clinical manifestations is such that a practitioner in almost any branch of medicine may be called upon to make the diagnosis. All kinds of combinations of organ involvement are possible [123] (Table 39.4). With the exception of the pleura, the serous membranes are rarely involved but only the adrenals appear to be sacrosanct. No authenticated adrenal involvement has been reported apart from a suggested but unproven case in one series [124].

Sarcoidosis would be relatively unimportant if not for the fact that it can affect vital organs in a chronic fashion, with the development of irreversible fibrosis resulting in functional impairment. Involvement of the eyes can lead to blindness and death can occur from cardiac, respiratory or renal failure.

Thoracic sarcoidosis

Clinical features

The hilar glands and the lungs are the organs most commonly affected in sarcoidosis and intrathoracic involvement is the most frequent accompaniment of sarcoidosis affecting other organs (see Table 39.3). By convention thoracic sarcoidosis is classified in four stages on the basis of the appearances of the chest radiograph. Stage I represents hilar lymphadenopathy (Fig. 39.6), stage II hilar adenopathy plus pulmonary opacities (Fig. 39.7) and stage III pulmonary opacities only. Stage IV represents the development of irreversible pulmonary fibrosis.

Hilar lymphadenopathy

Enlargement of hilar lymph glands with or without paratracheal lymphadenopathy is the commonest manifestation of sarcoidosis (Fig. 39.6). Usually, the glands are bilaterally and symmetrically involved, although rarely hilar enlargement may appear unilateral [125,126]. Many cases of hilar lymphadenopathy due to sarcoidosis undoubtedly go unrecognized because of the absence of symptoms.

In the UK, the most common association that may suggest the diagnosis is erythema nodosum [127]. Sarcoidosis is now the most likely cause of erythema

Table 39.4 Possible presentations of sarcoidosis.

Chest physician
Hilar glands
Diffuse pulmonary opacities
Breathlessness

Ophthalmologist
Uveitis: anterior and posterior
Conjunctivitis
   Non-specific
   Phlyctenular
Keratoconjunctivitis
Enlarged lacrimal glands
Sjögren-like syndrome (when salivary glands involved)
Glaucoma

Neurologist
Peripheral neuropathy
Eye change
Meningitis
Isolated cranial nerve lesions
Space-occupying lesions
Pituitary involvement (usually posterior)
Transverse myelitis

Rheumatologist
Subcutaneous tissue swellings
Polyarthralgia
Bone cysts

Gastroenterologist
Hepatomegaly
Splenomegaly

Dermatologist
Erythema nodosum
Plaques
Papules
Nodules
Lupus pernia
Scars

Cardiologist
Pulmonary heart disease
Myocarditis and congestive cardiac failure
Conduction disorders

Surgeon
Diagnostic lymph node biopsy

ENT surgeon
Nasal granuloma
Laryngeal granuloma

General physician
All above, for 'sorting out'
Atypical mumps
Hypercalcaemia
Renal calculi
Impaired renal function

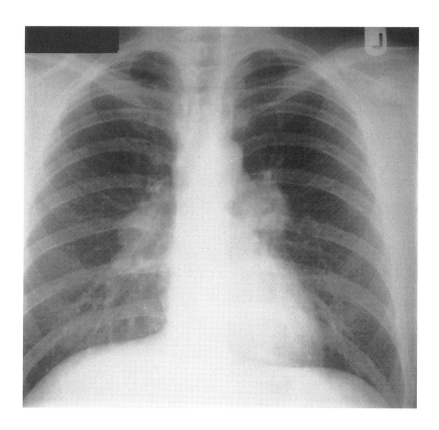

Fig. 39.6 Extensive bilateral hilar lymphadenopathy in a 31-year-old man with biopsy-proven sarcoidosis.

nodosum in the 20–40 age group in this country and its occurrence should always prompt further investigation by chest radiography. The association of erythema nodosum with sarcoidosis varies throughout the world. It is common in Scandinavia [128] and the UK but is an unusual manifestation in the USA in the white as well as the black population. In North America a generation ago erythema nodosum was apparently equally uncommon as a complication of primary tuberculosis [129]. In a worldwide study of sarcoidosis, erythema nodosum was more commonly the mode of onset in the three British series than elsewhere, with a frequency of about one-third of all presentations compared with about 10% elsewhere [26]. At the extremes, the incidence in Edinburgh was 33% and in Tokyo zero.

Polyarthralgia affecting principally the knees, ankles, wrists and elbows is a frequent accompaniment of erythema nodosum and may precede the skin rash. The joint symptoms commonly subside in 3–6 weeks and joint effusions are unusual. Other presenting symptoms may include cough, dyspnoea, chest pains [130], loss of weight, malaise or excessive fatigue.

The differential diagnosis of bilateral hilar adenopathy includes tuberculosis (usually unilateral with high tuberculin sensivity), coccidioidomycosis and histoplasmosis (USA), lymphoma (may be pain and usually systemic upset), leukaemia (blood count diagnostic), beryllium disease (occupational history), hypogammaglobulinaemia (recurrent infections) and enlarged

pulmonary arteries (characteristic appearances on CT scans).

The hilar lymphadenopathy syndrome with or without erythema nodosum is most commonly a benign manifestation. In the Edinburgh series of 230 cases of stage I disease, 80% resolved spontaneously in the first year and a further 10% showed spontaneous resolution in the second year [26]. In the worldwide study of 1865 cases of stage I disease, resolution ranged from 46 to 90% with an overall average of 65% [26]. The average time for the chest film to become normal is about 8 months [31]. About 1 in 10 cases of hilar lymphadenopathy develop chronic sarcoidosis with or without the development of further manifestations such as pulmonary opacities. In general, the older the age at onset, the greater the chance of chronicity. In a few of the cases that resolve spontaneously, transient pulmonary opacities may develop when the glands begin to regress and clear spontaneously thereafter [31]. Plaque-like or eggshell calcification may develop in persistently enlarged hilar and mediastinal glands [131,132] (Fig. 39.8).

Pulmonary disease

Pulmonary opacities

Most patients with pulmonary opacities present with stage II or stage III disease, although occasionally a patient presents with chronic progressive dyspnoea due to stage

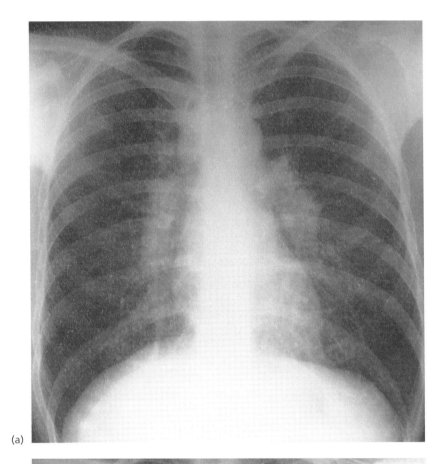

(a)

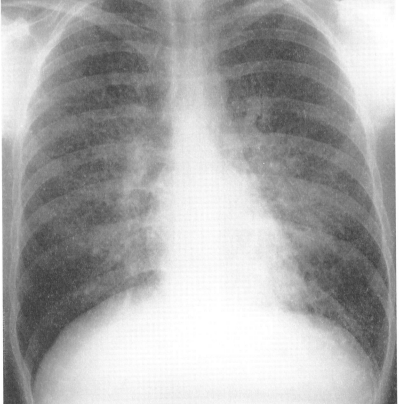

(b)

Fig. 39.7 (a) Chest radiograph of a 25-year-old man showing bilateral hilar and paratracheal lymph node enlargement (stage I sarcoidosis). (b) The same patient 18 months later showing the development of marked pulmonary shadowing (stage II sarcoidosis).

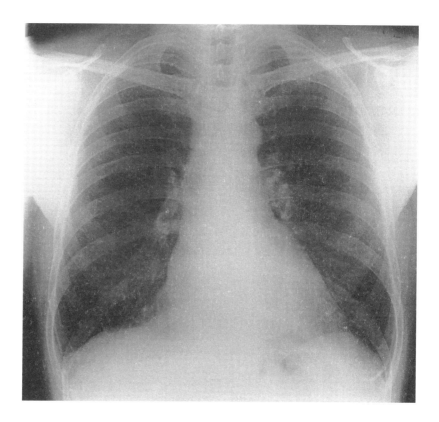

Fig. 39.8 Calcified hilar nodes in a patient with previous sarcoid hilar lymphadenopathy. (Courtesy of Dr James Choo-Kang.)

IV disease. There are often no symptoms but there may be those already outlined for hilar adenopathy. Many types of abnormality may be seen on the chest film and these may be classified as follows:

1 disseminated miliary lesions (Fig. 39.9);

2 disseminated nodular lesions (Fig. 39.10);

3 linear type of infiltration extending fan-wise from the hilum;

4 diffuse and confluent patchy shadows;

5 diffuse fibrosis (Fig. 39.11);

6 diffuse fibrosis with cavitation [133];

7 diffuse ground-glass shadowing [134];

8 changes similar to chronic tuberculosis as regards location and distribution;

9 bilateral confluent massive opacities resembling areas of pneumonia;

10 atelectasis.

Of the varieties of pulmonary change, cavitation and atelectasis are the least common. Aspergillomas may rarely develop in cavities, apparently more commonly in men [135].

The differential diagnosis of sarcoidosis with pulmonary opacities (in which there is usually a disparity between the minimal symptoms and signs and the marked radiographic abnormalities) includes extrinsic allergic alveolitis, fibrosing alveolitis and carcinomatous infiltration (in which dyspnoea may be disproportionate to the radiographic abnormality), pneumoconiosis (occupational history), miliary tuberculosis (fever, systemic symptoms, choroidal tubercles), metastatic malignancy (primary source may be evident), alveolar cell carcinoma (usually associated with dyspnoea if bilateral), eosinophilic granuloma (may be bone cysts on radiograph), honeycomb lung (in which evidence of mesodermal dysplasia or eosinophilic granuloma may be found) and talc granulomatosis [136].

In the Edinburgh series, 60% of pulmonary opacities showed spontaneous clearing. Half of these had cleared within 1 year, 80% within 2 years and the remaining 20% in periods from 3 to 7 years. Excluding those cases taking more than 2 years to clear, the average time for spontaneous resolution of pulmonary opacities was around 11 months.

Of patients with pulmonary opacities for whom corticosteroid therapy was considered necessary, some 50% showed clearing without any rebound phenomena after the withdrawal of treatment so that overall 80% of pulmonary opacities cleared either spontaneously or with corticosteroids and did not recur. These patients obviously belonged to a transient group of sarcoidosis and the duration of corticosteroid therapy must have coincided with the period of waning of the disease. A few patients who, for a variety of reasons, were not treated with corticosteroids early in the disease progressed to serious respiratory disability as a result of pulmonary fibrosis and many have developed the features of chronic bronchitis and airflow obstruction over the years.

In the Edinburgh series, about 1 in 10 patients with

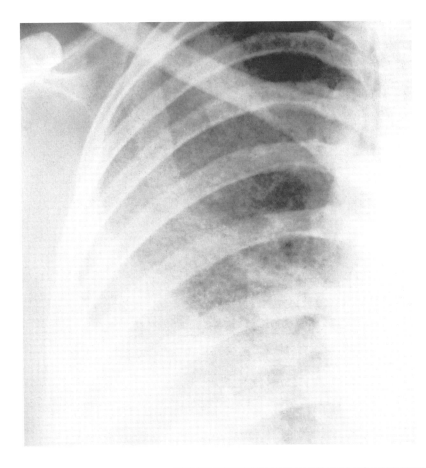

Fig. 39.9 Miliary shadowing on the chest radiograph of a 21-year-old woman with sarcoidosis.

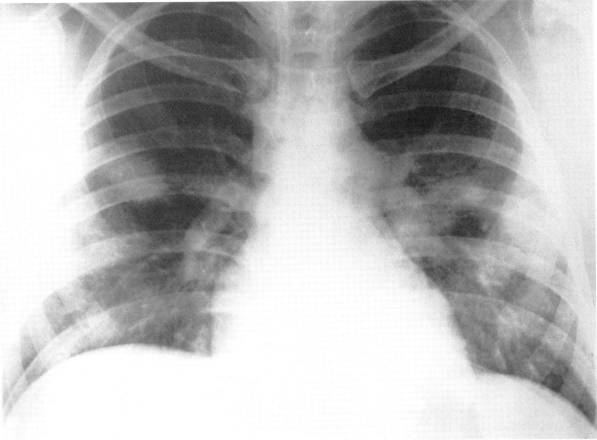

Fig. 39.10 Bilateral coarse nodular shadows in a 40-year-old man with sarcoidosis.

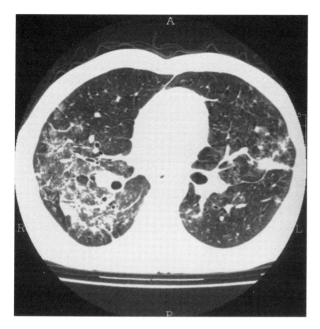

Fig. 39.11 High-resolution CT of a patient with chronic sarcoidosis showing irregular diffuse fibrosis. The patient showed no response to corticosteroids.

pulmonary involvement proved to have chronic disease, as in the hilar gland group. Males fared worse than females as far as the tendency to chronicity was concerned; fortunately, the use of long-term corticosteroid therapy would seem to have prevented major disability in the majority [137]. Of the 130 patients with stage II disease and 62 with stage III disease reported from Edinburgh, radiographic resolution, spontaneous or after treatment, occurred in 79% and 42% respectively. In the worldwide study, the percentage resolution varied quite markedly from centre to centre, with overall figures of 49% for stage II and 20% for stage III disease [26].

Bronchial sarcoidosis

The bronchi may be involved in sarcoidosis through external compression by glands, resulting in atelectasis in a very few cases [138]. Sarcoid lesions may actually be present in the bronchi and it would seem that the more often bronchial lesions are sought the more commonly they are found [139,140]. Stenosis of major airways may result [141]. Bronchial hyperreactivity to methacholine may be demonstrated but not usually in patients with normal spirometric values [142,143].

Pleural sarcoidosis

Pleural sarcoidosis is uncommon but has been reported [144–146]. In one review of the literature, pleural involvement was found in 0.8% of 2410 patients from 10 large series [147]. In contrast, in a review of 227 biopsy-proven

cases of sarcoidosis, Wilen and colleagues [145] described pleural effusion and/or thickening in 23 (10%). Pleural effusions were noted in 15 and in all of these the disease progressed to stage II or beyond. However, 87% of the patients in this series were Black and such patients are well recognized to have more florid expressions of the disease.

The effusion may be a transudate or an exudate and may appear early or late in the course of the disease. It may be blood-stained and the predominant cell is usually the lymphocyte, although eosinophilic effusion has been reported [148]. Pleural biopsy may show thickened fibrous pleura interspersed with non-caseating granuloma. Rarely, presentation may occur with acute pleuritic pain [149].

Rare thoracic manifestations of sarcoidosis

Superior vena cava obstruction has been reported in sarcoidosis due to enlarged nodes compressing the superior vena cava [150]. There has been one report of a young woman who died with progressive pulmonary hypertension and was found to have non-caseating granulomas obliterating the pulmonary veins as well as granulomas in the hilar lymph nodes and liver [151]. The author has seen a similar patient.

Extrathoracic sarcoidosis

Clinical features

Lymphatic system

The lymph nodes most frequently affected in sarcoidosis are those of the hilar and paratracheal groups. Of the superficial nodes, those of the right scalene group are most commonly affected but enlargement of any of the superficial nodes may be found. The involvement of superficial lymph nodes provides readily accessible tissue for biopsy.

Eyes

Ocular manifestations have been reported in as many as 25% of patients with sarcoidosis [32,152–155]. The eyes should be examined routinely, preferably with a slit lamp, in all cases since mild asymptomatic eye involvement may be commoner than is suspected. Uveitis is the most frequent manifestation of eye involvement causing symptoms. It develops acutely with pain in the eyes and misty vision in about one-third of patients, while the remainder show the chronic form that develops insidiously. Anterior uveitis is usual in self-limiting sarcoidosis, while posterior uveitis is typical of the chronic form of the disease. Acute conjunctivitis, sometimes of the phlyctenular type, may occur particularly in early sarcoidosis and conjunctival biopsy may provide proof of the diagnosis. Keratoconjunctivitis sicca results in dryness of the eyes; a Sjögren-like syndrome may be encountered if the salivary glands are also involved. The lacrimal glands may also be enlarged.

Skin

The most common skin manifestation in sarcoidosis is erythema nodosum, which in severe cases may be associated with prolonged fever [156]. Recurrent episodes of erythema nodosum may occur sometimes over many years [157]. Maculopapular eruptions, subcutaneous nodules, plaques and lupus pernio are other lesions that may be found. Occasionally old scars, including tattoos, may become infiltrated with sarcoid tissue (Fig. 39.12). The clinical examination of a case of suspected sarcoidosis should include inspection of previous traumatic, operation and vaccination scars for the development of lividity, which suggests infiltration. Women appear to be more prone to chronic skin lesions. Rarely the site of a previous Mantoux test may become infiltrated with sarcoid tissue.

Sarcoidosis of the upper respiratory tract carries a 50% risk of the development of lupus pernio within 2–3 years [158]. The early use of corticosteroid therapy may prevent this complication.

Upper respiratory tract

Sarcoidosis of the upper respiratory tract is an uncommon but disabling manifestation of the disease affecting the nose, nasopharyngeal mucosa and the larynx [158–160]. Disease of the nasal mucosa results in crusting, obstruc-tion and discharge in varying degrees. The septum and inferior turbinates are most commonly involved, although sometimes the lesions are more widespread. The mucosa is erythematous and granular, with associated polypoid hypertrophy causing nasal obstruction that is aggravated when stagnation and crusting leads to suppuration, purulent discharge and rarely epistaxis.

Disease of the laryngeal and pharyngeal mucosa may coexist with, or be independent of, nasal lesions. Hoarseness, cough, dysphagia and dyspnoea secondary to upper airway obstruction may occur [160]. Inspection reveals erythema and oedema with or without punctate nodules and mass lesions.

A patient presenting with sarcoidosis of the upper respiratory tract has a 50% chance of developing lupus pernio, although one feature may be present without the other. Sarcoidosis of the upper respiratory tract and lupus pernio are nearly six times more common in women in the child-bearing years of life. Both are indicators of chronic fibrotic sarcoidosis, developing insidiously and progressing indolently over the years with associated chronic lesions of the lungs, skin or bone.

Nasal septal or palatal perforations may complicate untreated sarcoidosis of the upper respiratory tract. Misguided submucous resection in this condition almost certainly results in septal perforation. The Kveim test is almost always positive, and this assists in the differential diagnosis of granulomas in the upper respiratory tract, which includes Wegener's granulomatosis, tuberculosis and leprosy.

Alimentary system

Involvement of the salivary glands and liver is common, while affection of the pancreas and gastrointestinal tract is

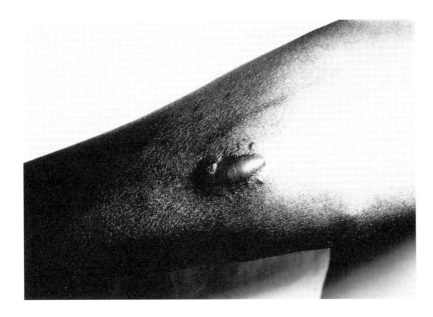

Fig. 39.12 Subcutaneous nodules and infiltration of biopsy scar with sarcoid tissue in a Black patient.

rare. Pancreatitis has been reported [161,162], and bloody ascites secondary to granulomatous involvement of the peritoneum has been described in two cases [163]. There is no evidence that Crohn's disease is a manifestation of sarcoidosis and the Kveim test has been shown to be negative in such cases [164–168]. Liver involvement, though frequent as judged by the results of biopsy, does not usually cause symptoms unless there is gross enlargement, when discomfort may occur.

Uveoparotid fever

Uveoparotid fever was first described by Heerfordt in 1909 [12] as a febrile illness characterized by uveitis and swelling of the parotids, accompanied frequently by facial palsy. At first thought to be a mild form of tuberculosis, it is now recognized as one of the curious combinations of organ involvement that can occur in sarcoidosis. Parotid enlargement is bilateral in more than half the cases and may be mistaken for mumps [169]. Unlike mumps, however, the swollen parotids are not painful (Fig. 39.13). Enlargement of the lacrimal and other salivary glands may sometimes accompany the uveoparotid syndrome.

Haemopoietic system

Enlargement of the spleen is relatively common in sarcoidosis and is usually symptomless, although gross enlargement may give rise to abdominal discomfort. Spontaneous rupture of the spleen has been recorded [170]. Hypersplenism is rare but, like haemolytic anaemia, has been described [170,171].

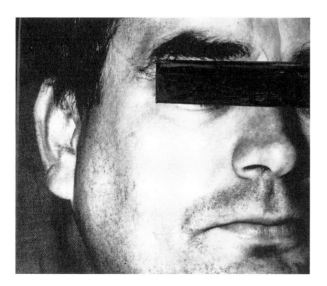

Fig. 39.13 Enlarged parotid glands as a presenting feature in sarcoidosis.

Nervous and endocrine systems

Sarcoidosis affecting the nervous system by infiltration or sarcoid deposits may result in a variety of clinical pictures [172–190]:

1 peripheral neuropathy or mononeuritis multiplex;
2 cranial neuropathy, most commonly of the seventh cranial nerve (sarcoidosis is the commonest cause of bilateral facial nerve palsy);
3 lymphocytic meningitis, in which the cerebrospinal fluid shows pleocytosis, increased protein and decreased glucose levels;
4 meningoencephalitis;
5 space-occupying lesions;
6 epilepsy;
7 brainstem and spinal syndromes are rare but may masquerade as multiple sclerosis, amyotrophic lateral sclerosis or spinal tumour.

Left recurrent laryngeal nerve palsy due to compression of the nerve by enlarged mediastinal nodes has been reported as the presenting symptom of sarcoidosis [189,190].

In most series, the majority of patients have presented with the neurological abnormalities; in only a minority did neurological signs develop in patients with an established diagnosis of sarcoidosis. The reported series illustrate the infinite variety of the clinical expression of central nervous system (CNS) sarcoidosis (and the difficulty in making the diagnosis in the absence of evidence of sarcoidosis in other systems), the chronicity of this form of the disease in most instances, and its variable and often poor prognosis even when corticosteroid therapy is employed [177,191,192].

The affinity of sarcoid granulomas for cerebral vessels has been stressed by many authors and may offer one explanation for the variable response to corticosteroid therapy. Areas of cerebral ischaemia and infarction have been described in relation to granulomatous angiitis. The development of meningeal fibrosis is another feature that may determine progression of neurological phenomena and limit response to corticosteroid therapy and may sometimes compel surgical intervention for relief of hydrocephalus or intractable epilepsy.

Sarcoid invasion of the posterior pituitary or hypothalamus may result in diabetes insipidus. It is rare for sarcoidosis to involve the anterior pituitary or other endocrine glands sufficiently to disturb function. Hypothalamic hypothyroidism has been described and it is important to be aware of this possible complication of CNS sarcoidosis because of the therapeutic implications [173]. In addition to diabetes insipidus and hypopituitarism, hypothalamic involvement can result in other diverse manifestations, including marked somnolence, hypothermia, personality changes, central alveolar hypoventilation, loss of libido, amenorrhoea and cessation of normal sexual development. These hypothalamic syndromes have been reviewed extensively [193–195].

Musculoskeletal system

Bone involvement in sarcoidosis most commonly affects the terminal phalanges of the hands and feet, although the proximal limb bones are occasionally involved in severe cases. Radiologically, the punched-out bone cysts initially noted by Kriebich [9] and later studied in detail by Jungling [15] are the most typical of the skeletal changes, although diffuse infiltration of the phalangeal shaft and destruction of cortical and medullary bone are occasionally seen. It is not uncommon for a single digit to be wholly spared while others on the same hand or foot are severely involved. The bone lesions are not affected by treatment with corticosteroids [196]. They were present in only 3% of the Edinburgh series [26].

Subcutaneous tissue swellings affecting several of the fingers or toes are frequently associated with bone involvement and add to the disability resulting from progressive disorganization of the terminal phalanges. It is unusual to find radiographic bone changes without clinical evidence of abnormality in the digits. Unlike the bone lesions, the subcutaneous swellings are usually improved by corticosteroid therapy. Skin sarcoids commonly coexist.

In one series of 29 patients with sarcoidosis of bone observed for up to 43 years, the hands and/or feet were affected in 26 patients, the nasal bone in three and in one each the hard palate and temporal bones were involved [197]. There were three types of bone lesion: lytic in 25 patients, permeative in nine and destructive in three. Lytic lesions are minute defects of the cortex, or larger defects of both cortex and medulla, and are usually rounded. With the passage of time, the larger defects may form the characteristic appearances of cysts. Permeative lesions show 'tunnelling' of the cortex of the shaft of the phalanx, leading to distortion of the normal cortical and trabecular pattern, which is replaced by a fine or coarse reticular pattern. Destructive lesions are rapidly progressive, with multiple fractures of devitalized cortex, sequestrum formation and local deformity. In this series, soft tissue swelling preceded the radiographic abnormality for up to 4 years in 10 patients, accompanied it twice, followed it once and was absent in 16 (55%). Bone involvement was usually an incidental finding when sarcoidosis presented elsewhere. Other features included intrathoracic sarcoid (86%), lupus pernio (48%), skin plaques (41%), ocular lesions (48%), nasal mucosal disease (24%), hepatomegaly (13%), splenomegaly (10%) and parotid enlargement (10%). Pulmonary infiltration with or without lymphadenopathy was present in three-fifths and hilar adenopathy alone in one-third of patients. Abnormalities in the chest radiographs of patients with bone sarcoid resolved in only 20%, underlining the chronicity of the sarcoid process in these patients.

Sarcoid granulomas may occur in skeletal muscle, most commonly affecting the pectoral, shoulder, arm and calf muscles [198–204]. The muscle foci are usually symptomless, but exceptionally there may be pain, weakness, atrophy or even pseudohypertrophy [205]. Only very rarely can nodules be palpated in muscles; they can be more often detected in tendon sheaths. Respiratory muscle weakness due to sarcoid involvement has been reported [206,207]. Serum creatine phosphokinase may be elevated [208].

Sarcoid arthritis independent of erythema nodosum has been described [209]. In the vast majority of cases, however, the polyarthralgia of sarcoidosis is simply a feature of the erythema nodosum syndrome.

Genitourinary system

Sarcoidosis may affect the kidneys in two ways, both of which can cause varying degrees of functional impairment [210–213]. There may be either invasion of the organ by sarcoid granulomas or deposition of calcium in and around the renal tubules (nephrocalcinosis) secondary to hypercalcaemia or, more commonly, hypercalciuria [214]. The reported incidence of hypercalcaemia has varied greatly. One large series found persistent hypercalcaemia in only 8 of 364 patients (2.2%) and only in association with severe and widespread sarcoidosis [215]. The disturbance in calcium metabolism in sarcoidosis is due to an unexplained increase in sensitivity to vitamin D, which results in increased absorption of calcium from the gut. The value of corticosteroid drugs in reversing this effect is well established; they are thought to act by accelerating the already delayed clearance of 1,25-dihydroxyvitamin D_3 from the blood [216]. It has been shown that exposure to sunlight increases the degree of hypercalcaemia, and there is an impression that hypercalcaemia in sarcoidosis is commoner in sunny climes [217]. The symptoms include tiredness, muscular weakness, thirst, polyuria, vomiting and constipation. There may be deposition of calcium in the kidneys, cornea and subcutaneous tissues [217]. When direct sarcoid involvement of the kidney is suspected renal biopsy is justified [218].

Renal calculi are a rare but not unknown presenting feature of sarcoidosis; in an Italian series 1% of patients presented with renal calculi [219]. Glomerulonephritis may also rarely occur in sarcoidosis [220]. Sarcoidosis of the epididymis has been reported [221].

Cardiovascular system

The cardiovascular system may be affected by sarcoidosis in two ways. Extensive pulmonary fibrosis can lead to cor pulmonale, while actual involvement of the myocardium may result in dysrhythmias, conduction disorders, heart failure or sudden death [222–225]. Pericarditis has been recorded [224,226]. ECG abnormality in the absence of cardiac symptoms is a frequent finding during the course of sarcoidosis [227,228].

There is good reason for believing that involvement of the heart in sarcoidosis is more frequent than was once thought [226]. A clinicopathological study of 84 unselected patients demonstrated myocardial involvement in 25% [229]. Most often only a small part of the myocardium is involved, explaining the absence of clinical features. Occasionally angina may result from granulomatous myocardial disease [230,231]. In a UK series of 163 patients with cardiac involvement, 70 had died at an average age of 47 years [224]; 45 deaths were sudden and in 26 of these sarcoidosis was previously undiagnosed. Other principal manifestations were ventricular extrasystoles or tachycardia in 64, complete heart block in 31, lesser heart block in 56, supraventricular tachycardia in 35 and myocardial disease in 34. If suspected, a 24-h ECG, echocardiogram, exercise ECG and thallium imaging should be performed and treatment with corticosteroids and antiarrhythmics initiated for any significant dysrhythmia [224,225]. Cyclophosphamide therapy may be effective in steroid-unresponsive disease [232]. Combined heart and lung transplantation is the ultimate effective therapy [233] for life-threatening cardiac sarcoidosis and lives may be saved in the waiting period by employing implantable pacemakers or automatic cardiac defibrillators [234]. Endomyocardial biopsy has been successfully used to establish the diagnosis [235].

Investigations

Pulmonary function tests

There have been numerous studies of abnormalities of pulmonary function associated with the various stages of intrathoracic sarcoidosis [236–243]. Functional impairment cannot be predicted from the radiographic appearances [242]. A patient whose chest film has become normal may still have significant pulmonary sarcoidosis as judged by reduction in static lung volumes, decreased pulmonary compliance and a reduction in carbon monoxide diffusing capacity [243]. Conversely, extensive shadowing may sometimes be associated with little impairment of function. The most subtle indication of lung function abnormality appears to be a decrease in $D_{L}CO$, which may only be evident on exercise studies. Reduced $D_{L}CO$ has been demonstrated in patients whose radiograph only shows hilar adenopathy.

Evidence of airflow obstruction is common in patients with sarcoidosis; two separate studies of black North American and British white patients found airflow obstruction in over 60% [244], indicating that this is the commonest physiological abnormality in pulmonary sarcoidosis. Airflow obstruction was found at all stages of disease, was unrelated to smoking history and was not reversible with bronchodilators [244,245]. It seems likely that this finding reflects the common occurrence of airway involvement in sarcoidosis [246] and is consistent with the presence of bronchial hyperreactivity [142,247].

Abnormal oxygen uptake responses to exercise in patients with mild pulmonary sarcoidosis have been reported and have been attributed to possible subclinical impairment of right-sided cardiac function [248].

Kveim test

It is now well established that particulate saline suspensions of sarcoid tissue contain, in varying amounts, some component that when injected intradermally in a patient with active sarcoidosis can provoke the slow development of an epithelioid cell granuloma of sarcoid type. This is the basis of the Kveim test [249–252] and for over two decades a steady accumulation of data has resulted in a wide acceptance of the test as a reliable and clinically useful aid to diagnosis. Unfortunately, shortage of suitable tissue and fears of transmission of viral infection have caused the test to be abandoned is most centres.

Value of the test

False-positive reactions are rare, only 1–2% [168,249], and a positive test can be regarded as virtual proof of active sarcoidosis. The more active the disease, the greater the likelihood of the test being positive. Its highly specific nature makes it an invaluable tool in the elucidation of atypical cases and often obviates the need for more traumatic forms of biopsy. Unfortunately, even with the best test substances presently available, positive results are obtained in only 75% of patients with clinical evidence of the disease [32,253].

Nature of the test substance

Sarcoid tissue suitable for preparation of Kveim test substance must meet the following criteria [254]:
1 it must have a sufficiently high concentration of the active principle;
2 it must have a sufficiently low concentration of substances giving non-specific, inflammatory responses;
3 it must be free from agents of transmissible disease;
4 there must be sufficient tissue to provide adequate supplies to prove these points and to be available for general diagnostic use.
The details of the preparation of Kveim test substance are of prime importance in relation to both the activity and specificity of the material; monitoring of bulk test material for activity and specificity should be a continuous process [166,255,256]. Douglas and colleagues [250] have described in detail a technique used in Edinburgh for the preparation of two test suspensions that have satisfied all the criteria when subjected to worldwide validation.

The Kveim test substance is remarkably stable; its activity is only destroyed by autoclaving or exposure to alkali. It can stand boiling for 30 min [257]. Freeze-dried test material kept for several months at room temperature retains its potency and specificity [253,258]. The active principle is particulate [259]. It is not water soluble and is not contained in the nucleoprotein or the lipid fraction of the material [260,261], and its precise nature is still unknown. Similar skin reactions can be induced in patients with sarcoidosis by the injection of non-viable autologous BAL cell preparations [262]. Other substances can produce local sarcoid reactions in systemic sarcoidosis (e.g. killed tubercle bacilli) but none so reliably as sarcoid tissue.

Studies with subcellular fractions (nuclear, mitochondrial, microsomal and submicrosomal) prepared by homogenization and differential ultracentrifugation have shown that results equal to those of the whole homogenate can be obtained by all fractions except the submicrosomal. These results tend to support the view that the active principle in sarcoid tissue that evokes the epithelioid granulomatous response is of particle form and is concentrated in the membrane-containing elements [250,251].

Method of testing

The test is performed by injecting intradermally 0.1–0.2 mL of a suspension of human sarcoid tissue, usually obtained from a cervical gland. Rarely, splenectomy for splenomegaly due to sarcoidosis allows the preparation of large quantities of test substance. Within 2–3 weeks a positive test shows a purplish-red nodule at the site of injection. Biopsy at 4–6 weeks reveals sarcoid tissue on histological examination (Fig. 39.14).

The forearm is usually used as the site of injection but, for cosmetic reasons, the upper and outer thigh may be used in females. Biopsy is made with a Hayes–Martin drill, which can remove a small core of skin without leaving a significant scar.

Coincident corticosteroid therapy depresses the reaction and, if at all possible, treatment should not be given until the test is read.

Nature of the Kveim reaction

The epithelioid granuloma of the Kveim reaction shares the histological, histochemical, immunofluorescent and ultrastructural features of the granuloma found within affected organs in sarcoidosis, and it has been supposed that the substances and mechanisms involved in the development of both granulomas are the same [249,252,263]. Two theories, which are not mutually exclusive, have been proposed. On the one hand, some believe that the Kveim test detects a specific aetiological agent, some component of which is present in the sarcoid tissue from which the test substance is made. Others have felt that it simply demonstrates a specific form of tissue reactivity common to sarcoid patients. Despite the increasing sophistication of immunological studies, it is still not known which of these two theories, if either, is correct. Siltzbach has supported the unitarian concept of sarcoidosis, using as evidence the fact that the spleen of a single sarcoid patient has provided a test substance that has been shown to produce specific reactions in sarcoid patients all over the world, suggesting that 'a primary inciting agent may be at work' [254]. The uniformity of response to Kveim testing in all geographical areas has been taken to support the concept of a single disease rather than a syn-

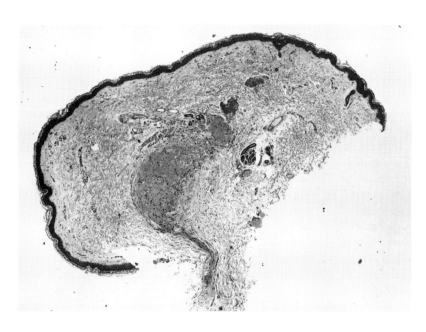

Fig. 39.14 Kveim biopsy showing typical sarcoid granuloma.

drome, and a single aetiology rather than a multiple one. It might equally mean that the test is detecting a specific form of reactivity. The Kveim 'reaction' remains an immunological puzzle [252].

Tissue biopsy procedures

Tissue biopsy is often crucial to the diagnosis of sarcoidosis. Strictly speaking, an absolute diagnosis of sarcoidosis cannot be made on suggestive clinical and radiographic findings alone because of the similarity between sarcoidosis and other conditions such as tuberculosis and reticulosis. Similarly, a biopsy report describing sarcoid tissue is of itself insufficient for absolute diagnosis since this might simply represent a local sarcoid tissue reaction. When typical clinical and radiographic findings are supported by histological proof of the sarcoid granulomatous process and tuberculosis has been excluded by the tuberculin test and by bacteriology, the diagnosis of sarcoidosis can be confidently made.

The desirability of histological confirmation of the disease in every case was undoubted in the years when the patterns of disease were being evaluated. However, we have now reached the stage when the quest for demonstrable sarcoid tissue must be tempered by the knowledge concerning the presentation and behaviour of sarcoidosis that has accrued over the last three decades. In the UK, a young woman with erythema nodosum, bilateral hilar lymphadenopathy and a negative tuberclin test has sarcoidosis for all practical purposes and physicians would hesitate to employ any biopsy procedure in these circumstances. On the other hand, obscure bilateral pulmonary changes may justify biopsy, including scalene node biopsy, mediastinoscopy or preferably transbronchial lung biopsy via the fibreoptic bronchoscope. If potent Kveim reagent is not available, the decision whether to perform diagnostic biopsy exercises the physician's judgement.

The tissues found to be useful for biopsy in sarcoidosis have increased in number with the years (Table 39.5) and now include superficial lymph nodes, mediastinal glands, skin, palate, bronchus, lung, liver, conjunctiva, gastrocnemius muscle, bone marrow and old scars with evidence of infiltration. The wide range of positivity for scalene fat-pad biopsy is probably explained by failure to distinguish between biopsy of palpable nodes and 'blind' biopsy.

Transbronchial biopsy of lung and bronchial wall via the flexible fibreoptic bronchoscope is the procedure of choice in the diagnosis of diffuse pulmonary abnormality of probable sarcoid aetiology and is employed especially if there are cogent reasons for securing a diagnosis earlier than can be expected from the Kveim test [264,265]. A minimum of four lung biopsies by this method optimizes the chances of securing a diagnosis.

Table 39.5 Results of biopsy in sarcoidosis (several authors). Figures in parentheses indicate percentage positive.

Readily accessible abnormalities
Epitrochlear lymph nodes (100)
Enlarged parotid glands (100)
Nasal mucosal lesions (100)
Subcutaneous nodules (100)
Cutaneous lesions (including livid scars) (90)
Palpable scalene lymph nodes (90)
Inguinal lymph nodes (90)
Axillary lymph nodes (80)
Enlarged tonsils (80)
Bronchial mucosa (visible abnormality) (80)
Conjunctival lesions (75)

Less readily accessible abnormalities
Mediastinal lymph nodes (100)
Lung (open biopsy) (100)
Lung (transbronchial biopsy) (80)
Liver (80)
Scalene fat pad (40–75)
Gastocnemius muscle (70)
Palate (40)
Bronchial mucosa (no visible abnormality) (30–40)
Bone marrow (30)

Tuberculin testing

Numerous studies have shown that about two-thirds of patients with active sarcoidosis fail to react to 100 TU; about one-quarter react to 100 TU, less than one-tenth to 10 TU and less than 1 in 20 to 1 TU.

Serum angiotensin-converting enzyme

Lieberman was the first to report that serum angiotensin-converting enzyme (ACE) was elevated in patients with sarcoidosis compared with controls, giving rise to the hope of a relatively simple method for confirming the diagnosis [266]. Serum ACE has been reported to be elevated in 75% of patients with active sarcoidosis, with higher levels in Blacks than whites [267]. The enzyme probably originates from active epithelioid and giant cells and is elevated in BAL fluid of patients with active sarcoidosis compared with that of controls and patients with inactive sarcoidosis [268–270]. Serum ACE may be elevated in conditions other than sarcoidosis, such as Gaucher's disease, leprosy and atypical mycobacterial infection [267]. In other conditions, the combined false-positive rate for non-sarcoid patients has been reported to be as high as 20% in one series [271].

A number of studies have reported falls in serum ACE levels following steroid therapy and also in association with clinical improvement in the natural course of the disease [267,272–275]. Nevertheless, clinical or radiographic deterioration may occur without an associated rise in serum ACE, and clinical or radiographic improvement may occur without any fall in elevated serum ACE levels [274–276].

In summary, there is evidence that serum ACE is elevated in a majority of patients with sarcoidosis and that its measurement may therefore be of value in substantiating a diagnosis in a difficult case. Elevated serum ACE is neither sensitive nor specific for sarcoidosis. Serial measurements do not necessarily predict activity of disease or outcome as assessed clinically, radiographically or in terms of respiratory function and are therefore unnecessary in routine clinical management, although possibly of interest in research studies [274].

Gallium-67 scanning

Gallium-67 is concentrated in metabolically and mitotically active tissues, where it binds to granulocytes and macrophages [110,277]. Sarcoid and other inflammatory tissue avidly accumulate gallium and gallium scanning may be used to delineate it. Following an intravenous injection of 11×10^7 Bq of gallium-67 citrate, simultaneous anterior and posterior scans of the thorax are performed 3 days later [278]. The pattern of uptake is generally diffuse and involved nodes may be well defined. In one study, 65% of patients with sarcoidosis had increased uptake of gallium-67 with little correlation between degree of uptake and clinical, physiological and radiographic findings [279]. Close correlations between gallium uptake and the total number of lymphocytes, or T lymphocytes recovered by BAL and serum ACE levels, have been reported [279,280]. Gallium uptake diminishes with spontaneous or steroid-induced improvement in sarcoidosis but, as with serum ACE, abnormal values may be found even in the presence of a normal chest film and pulmonary function [273,274,279]; positivity of the initial gallium scan appeared to have no predictive value for outcome in one prospective study [274].

In summary, increased gallium-67 uptake by the lungs is found in the majority of patients with pulmonary sarcoidosis but is not specific for this condition. It is an expensive investigation involving a substantial radiation dose to the patient and cannot at present be justified in the routine investigation of this disease. A possible role in the diagnosis of atypical cases of sarcoidosis has been suggested [281] but awaits further evaluation.

Bronchoalveolar lavage

As already mentioned, BAL fluid from patients with pulmonary sarcoidosis contains increased numbers of T lymphocytes, with a high ratio of CD4 to CD8 T cells, and increased macrophages in comparison with control fluid. This finding may be used to support but not prove a diagnosis of sarcoidosis [90,98]. The first 20 mL of the BAL

specimen should be discarded and cell counts made on subsequent specimens [282,283].

Measurements in blood, urine and sputum

Serum calcium should be measured as well as 24-h urinary calcium. Serum globulins may be elevated, although this finding is of little diagnostic or prognostic significance. Routine examination of the peripheral blood is of no value in diagnosis. If sputum production is a feature, acid-fast bacilli should be sought by direct smear or culture.

CT of the thorax

CT of the thorax is usually unnecessary in sarcoidosis. It may be of value, when used with contrast, in differentiating hilar enlargement due to lymphadenopathy from enlargement of the pulmonary vessels. Hilar and mediastinal lymphadenopathy are usually found to be more extensive than the plain chest radiograph indicates. Pulmonary abnormalities may include irregular linear opacities, ground-glass shadowing (particularly related to bronchovascular bundles, interlobar septa and in subpleural areas) and nodular or ill-defined shadows with a similar distribution. CT is frequently abnormal in the presence of apparently normal lungs on the chest radiograph [284–286].

Strategy for investigation of suspected sarcoidosis

As already mentioned, where bilateral hilar lymphadenopathy and erythema nodosum occur together in a tuberculin-negative young woman it is probably excessive to pursue a tissue diagnosis. However, in the case of obscure pulmonary infiltrates where sarcoid is suspected, initial investigations should include a baseline measurement of lung volumes and $D_{L}CO$ and tuberculin testing. If corticosteroid therapy is not obviously imminently indicated, a Kveim test may establish the diagnosis within 6 weeks. If early therapeutic intervention seems likely to be necessary or if Kveim test reagent is unavailable, the diagnosis is most likely to be established at fibreoptic bronchoscopy, when at least four transbronchial lung biopsies (with or without endobronchial mucosal biopsies) should be taken to search for epithelioid granulomas. Serum and 24-h urinary calcium should be measured.

The role of BAL has been investigated in two careful studies. Keogh and colleagues [287] reported 19 patients with pulmonary sarcoidosis, of whom 80% were initially classified as having 'low-intensity alveolitis' (BAL T cells <28% of total and/or gallium scan negative) and 20% as having 'high-intensity alveolitis' (BAL T cells >28% of total and gallium scan positive). Clinical, radiological and physiological assessment did not predict the intensity of the alveolitis. With serial assessments of these parameters they showed that 75% of patients with high-intensity alveolitis reverted to low-intensity alveolitis spontaneously, whereas the reverse phenomenon occurred in 12% of patients with low-intensity alveolitis. An episode of high-intensity alveolitis was associated with deterioration in pulmonary function in 87%. They suggested that staging the intensity of alveolitis in these patients might aid therapeutic decision-making. Turner-Warwick and colleagues [274] have repeatedly staged 32 patients with gallium scans, BAL and serum ACE while withholding the information from the clinicians who managed the individual patients on the basis of clinical, radiological and functional parameters. Initial values for gallium uptake, BAL lymphocyte count and serum ACE were not predictive of the outcome in individual patients. Although these parameters tended to normalize with clinical improvement in disease, poor concordance with clinical, radiological and functional parameters was observed. This would suggest that in the routine investigation of pulmonary sarcoidosis, measurement of serum ACE, gallium uptake and BAL lymphocyte count are of little help in planning the future management of the patient.

In extrapulmonary sarcoidosis, attention should be directed to obtaining biopsy material from the most accessible involved site (see Table 39.5).

Treatment

In nearly every case, corticosteroid therapy can suppress the manifestations of active sarcoidosis, a possible exception being CNS sarcoidosis. Although there is considerable debate about the indications for corticosteroid therapy in thoracic sarcoidosis, most are agreed that steroid therapy is indicated when vital organs are involved or if there are significant symptoms.

Thoracic sarcoidosis

Bilateral hilar lymphadenopathy alone is not an indication for corticosteroid therapy since the vast majority resolve spontaneously with the passage of time. The associated arthralgia may necessitate treatment with non-steroidal anti-inflammatory drugs; exceptionally, when systemic upset is severe with persisting or recurring erythema nodosum, a few weeks of corticosteroid therapy may be required to suppress symptoms.

There is no universal agreement about the indications for corticosteroid therapy in stage II and stage III thoracic sarcoidosis [288]. One extreme view would be that in a disease which may have a mortality of 5–10% and significant disability due to fibrosis in 3–20% if left untreated [288], it is mandatory to treat all patients with pulmonary shadowing due to sarcoidosis. At the other extreme, it can be argued that corticosteroids are unnecessary in the man-

agement of stage II and III sarcoidosis since controlled trials show that although there may be early (e.g. at 6 months) significant differences in chest radiography or lung function in the treated versus the control group, in the longer term (1–15 years) there are no significant differences between the treated and control groups [289–295]. By the nature of their design, however, these trials of necessity exclude patients for whom corticosteroid therapy was considered clinically indicated and the patients studied therefore presumably had a relatively good prognosis. There is no doubt that if all patients with stage II and stage III sarcoidosis were treated with corticosteroids many would be unnecessarily exposed to the risk of side-effects.

Our own policy is to treat patients with significant symptomatology, most commonly dyspnoea. In asymptomatic patients, baseline assessment of lung volumes and D_{LCO} is undertaken and the patient then observed with repeated radiographic and functional assessment at regular intervals for 6–12 months. Treatment may be initiated if significant symptoms develop, if there is significant radiographic or functional deterioration or if at the end of the observation period there has been no significant improvement. There is evidence to suggest that serial assessment of gallium uptake, serum ACE or BAL lymphocyte counts does not contribute any additional advantage to such a management plan [273]. A recent report from the USA of the management of 98 patients endorses the view that the use of simple clinical criteria augmented by simple radiographic and pulmonary function tests minimizes the number of patients exposed to corticosteroid therapy and results in no adverse outcomes [296]. Treatment, when required, is initiated with prednisolone 20–40 mg in daily or alternate-day regimens and is continued for 3–6 months, when a slow and graduated reduction in dosage may be attempted while clinical, radiographic and functional status is monitored. If relapse is to occur, it is commonly seen when the prednisolone dose is reduced below 7.5–15 mg; this necessitates a return to a higher dose and a further period (6–12 months) on a continuing maintenance dose, commonly 10 mg daily, before further reduction in dosage is attempted. In the Edinburgh series, corticosteroid therapy was given to 260 patients; this was discontinued in 80% in 2 years and their follow-up was uneventful [137]. This experience contrasts with that found in a predominantly black American population where relapses occurred in the majority on reduction of prednisolone dosage below 10–15 mg and the majority required more than 2 years of treatment, perhaps reflecting the greater severity and chronicity of the disease in this population [297]. Although most patients respond satisfactorily to the dosage regimen outlined above, individual relatively unresponsive patients may require higher doses of prednisolone initially to suppress activity, and a small proportion of patients are found to require long-term treatment with corticosteroids. Despite this, some progress remorselessly to chronic pulmonary fibrosis.

Anecdotal experiences and accounts, including our own, of the benefits of high-dose inhaled corticosteroids in the management of pulmonary sarcoidosis, often in patients who reject systemic corticosteroid therapy, are beginning to be addressed by controlled trials [298]. At present the precise role of this intervention in replacing, or reducing the dose of, systemic corticosteroids remains to be determined [299,300].

There has been a report of successful treatment of pulmonary sarcoidosis with cyclosporin in three patients, two of whom were unresponsive to steroids and one in whom corticosteroids were contraindicated [301]. Cyclosporin was a logical choice since it acts by suppressing T-helper lymphocytes and there may be a case for further studies of its use in different clinical situations. Chlorambucil has also been used successfully in corticosteroid-resistant sarcoidosis [302].

Extrathoracic sarcoidosis

Treatment with the same dosage schedule of oral corticosteroids is also indicated in the management of eye involvement uncontrolled by topical steroids and in persistent hypercalcaemia or hypercalciuria to prevent the development of nephrocalcinosis and renal failure. CNS, symptomatic muscle and myocardial sarcoidosis are all indications for corticosteroid therapy, although CNS sarcoidosis may be unresponsive even to high doses of prednisolone. In one such case of unresponsive sarcoid meningitis, improvement was recorded following whole brain irradiation [303]. Disfiguring skin lesions may justify treatment, as may parotid and lacrimal gland enlargement and symptomatic splenic involvement.

References

1 James DG, Turiaf J, Hosoda Y *et al*. Description of sarcoidosis: Report of the subcommittee on classification and definition. *Ann N Y Acad Sci* 1976; 278: 742.

2 Hunter FT. Hutchinson–Boeck's disease (generalised sarcoidosis). *N Engl J Med* 1936; 214: 346.

3 Hutchinson J. *Illustrations of Clinical Surgery*. London: J & A Churchill, 1877: 42.

4 Scadding JG, Mitchell DN. *Sarcoidosis*, 2nd edn. London: Chapman & Hall, 1985.

5 Besnier E. Lupus pernio de la face. *Ann Derm Syph Paris* 1889; 10: 333.

6 Tenneson H. Lupus pernio. *Ann Derm Syph Paris* 1892; 3: 1142.

7 Hutchinson J. Cases of Mortimer's malady. *Arch Surg Lond* 1898; 9: 307.

8 Boeck C. Multiple benign sarkoid of the skin. *J Cutan Dis* 1899; 17: 543.

9 Kreibich K. Uber lupus pernio. *Arch Derm Syph Wien* 1904; 71: 3.

10 Boeck C. Fortgesetze Untersuchungen uber das multiple benigne Sarkoid. *Arch Derm Syph Wien* 1905; 73: 301.

11 Darier J, Roussy G. Des sarcoides souscutanees. *Arch Med Exp* 1906; 18: 1.

12 Heerfordt CF. Uber eine 'Febris uveoparotidea subchronica'. *von Graefes Arch Ophthal* 1909; 70: 254.

13 Schaumann J. Sur le lupus pernio. Memoire presenté en Novembre 1914 a la Societé Francoise de Dermatologie et de Syphiligraphie pour le prix Zambo, Stockholm, 1934.

14 Schaumann J. Etudes sur le lupus pernio et ses rapports avec les sarcoides et la tuberculose. *Ann Derm Syph Paris* 1917; 5: 357.

15 Jungling O. Ostitis tuberculosa multiplex cystica (eine eigenartige Form der Knockentuberculose) *Fortschr Röentgenstr* 1920; 27: 375.

16 Lofgren S. Erythema nodosum: studies on etiology and pathogenesis in 185 adult cases. *Acta Med Scand* 1946; Suppl 174.

17 Lofgren S. Primary pulmonary sarcoidosis. *Acta Med Scand* 1953; 145: 424, 465.

18 Morrison JGL. Sarcoidosis in the Bantu. *Br J Dermatol* 1974; 90: 649.

19 Proceedings of the Third International Conference on Sarcoidosis, 1963. *Acta Med Scand* 1964; Suppl 425.

20 Hillerdal G, Nou E, Osterman K, Schmekel B. Sarcoidosis: epidemiology and prognosis. *Am Rev Respir Dis* 1984; 130: 29.

21 Anon. Sarcoidosis in the long-term. *Lancet* 1984; ii: 674.

22 Poukkula A, Huhti E, Lilja M, Saloheimo M. Incidence and clinical picture of sarcoidosis in a circumscribed geographical area. *Br J Dis Chest* 1986; 80: 138.

23 Parkes SA, Baker SBdec, Bourdillon RE *et al*. Incidence of sarcoidosis in the Isle of Man *Thorax* 1985; 40: 284.

24 British Thoracic and Tuberculosis Association. Geographical variations in the incidence of sarcoidosis in Great Britain: a comparative study of four areas. *Tubercle* 1969; 50: 211.

25 Cooch JW. Sarcoidosis in the United States Army, 1952 through 1956. *Am Rev Respir Dis* 1961; 84 (Suppl): 103.

26 James DG, Neville E, Siltzbach LE *et al*. A worldwide review of sarcoidosis. *Ann N Y Acad Sci* 1976; 278: 321.

27 Douglas AC. Sarcoidosis in Scotland. *Am Rev Respir Dis* 1961; 84 (Suppl): 143.

28 Douglas AC. Sarcoidosis. *Proc R Soc Med* 1967; 60: 983.

29 Israel HL. Sarcoidosis. *Basics RD* 1978; 7: 1.

30 Lofgren S. Some aspects of the relationship between tuberculosis and sarcoidosis. Transactions of NAPT Fourth Commonwealth Health and Tuberculosis Conference. London: National Association for the Prevention of Tuberculosis, 1955.

31 Douglas AC. The prognosis of early sarcoidosis. *Acta Med Scand* 1964; Suppl 425: 284.

32 Israel HL, Sones M. Sarcoidosis. *Adv Tuberc Res* 1961; 11: 214.

33 Hosoda Y, Hirga Y, Furuta M *et al*. Epidemiology of sarcoidosis in Japan. In: Iwai K, Hosoda Y, eds. *Proceedings of the Sixth International Conference on Sarcoidosis*. Tokyo: University Press, 1974: 297.

34 Edmonstone WM, Wilson AG. Sarcoidosis in Caucasians, Blacks and Asians in London. *Br J Dis Chest* 1985; 79: 27.

35 Honeybourne D. Ethnic differences in the clinical features of sarcoidosis in south-east London. *Br J Dis Chest* 1980; 74: 63.

36 Teirstein AS, Siltzbach LE, Berger H. Patterns of sarcoidosis in three population groups in New York City. *Ann N Y Acad Sci* 1976; 278: 371.

37 British Thoracic and Tuberculosis Association Research Committee Investigation. Familial associations in sarcoidosis. BTTA review. *Tubercle* 1972; Suppl 3: 41.

38 Headings VE, Weston D, Young RC, Hackney RL. Familial sarcoidosis with multiple occurrences in eleven families: a possible mechanism of inheritance. *Ann N Y Acad Sci* 1976; 278: 377.

39 Sharma OP, Neville E, Walker AN, James DG. Familial sarcoidosis: a possible genetic influence. *Ann N Y Acad Sci* 1976; 278: 386.

40 Brennan NJ, Crean P, Long JP, Fitzgerald M. High prevalence of familial sarcoidosis in an Irish population. *Thorax* 1984; 39: 14.

41 Parkes SA, Baker SBdec, Bourdillon RE *et al*. Epidemiology of sarcoidosis in the Isle of Man. 1. A case controlled study. *Thorax* 1987; 42: 420.

42 Hills SE, Parkes SA, Baker SBdec. Epidemiology of sarcoidosis in the Isle of Man. 2. Evidence for space–time clustering. *Thorax* 1987; 42: 427.

43 Brewerton DA, Cockburn C, James DCO *et al*. HLA antigens in sarcoidosis. *Clin Exp Immunol* 1977; 27: 227.

44 Neville E. HLA antigens and disease. *J Mt Sinai Hosp* 1977; 44: 772.

45 Neville E, James DG, Brewerton DA *et al*. HLA antigens and clinical features of sarcoidosis. In: Jones Williams W, Davies BH, eds. *Proceedings of the Eighth International Conference on Sarcoidosis and other Granulomatous Diseases*. Cardiff: Alpha Omega, 1980: 201.

46 Hedfors E, Lindstrom F. HLA-B8/DR3 in sarcoidosis. *Tissue Antigens* 1983; 22: 200.

47 Gardner J, Kennedy HG, Hamblin A, Jones E. HLA-associations in sarcoidosis: a study of two ethnic groups. *Thorax* 1984; 39: 19.

48 Abe S, Yamaguchi E, Makimura S *et al.* Association of HLA-DR with sarcoidosis. *Chest* 1987; 92: 488.

49 Kunikane H, Abe S, Tsuneta Y *et al.* Role of HLA-DR antigens in Japanese patients with sarcoidosis. *Am Rev Respir Dis* 1987; 135: 688.

50 Ina Y, Takada K, Yamamoto M *et al.* HLA and sarcoidosis in the Japanese. *Chest* 1989; 95: 1257.

51 Mitchell DN, Rees RJW. A transmissible agent from sarcoid tissue. *Lancet* 1969; ii: 81.

52 Mitchell DN, Rees RJW. Agent transmissible from Crohn's disease tissue. *Lancet* 1970; ii: 168.

53 Iwai K, Takahashi S. Transmissibility of sarcoid-specific granulomas in the footpads of mice. *Ann N Y Acad Sci* 1976; 278: 249.

54 Taub RN, Sachar DB, Janowitz H, Siltzbach LE. Induction of granulomas in mice by inoculation of tissue homogenates from patients with inflammatory bowel disease and sarcoidosis. *Ann N Y Acad Sci* 1976; 278: 56.

55 Mitchell DN, Rees RJW. The nature and physical characteristics of a transmissible agent from human sarcoid tissue. *Ann N Y Acad Sci* 1976; 278: 233.

56 Mitchell DN, Rees RJW, Goswami KKA. Transmissible agent from human sarcoid and Crohn's disease tissues. *Lancet* 1976; ii: 761.

57 Mitchell DN, Bradstreet CMP, Dighero MW *et al.* Irradiated Kveim suspensions. *Lancet* 1974; i: 734.

58 Mitchell DN, Rees RJW. The nature and physical characteristics of transmissible agents from human sarcoid and Crohn's disease tissues. In: *Proceedings of the Ninth International Conference on Sarcoidosis.* Oxford: Pergamon Press, 1983: 132.

59 Burnet FM. *The Clonal Selection Theory of Acquired Immunity.* Cambridge: Cambridge University Press, 1959: 160.

60 Mitchell IC, Turk JL, Mitchell DN. Detection of mycobacterial rRNA in sarcoidosis with liquid-phase hybridisation. *Lancet* 1992; 339: 1015.

61 Saboor SA, Johnson NMcI McFadden J. Detection of mycobacterial DNA in sarcoidosis and tuberculosis with polymerase chain reaction. *Lancet* 1992; 339: 1012.

62 Bocart D, Lecossier D, DeLassence A *et al.* A search for mycobacterial DNA in granulomatous tissues from patients with sarcoidosis using the polymerase chain reaction. *Am Rev Respir Dis* 1992; 145: 1142.

63 Anon. 'Tastes great, less filling.' The debate about mycobacteria and sarcoidosis. *Am Rev Respir Dis* 1992; 145: 986.

64 Johnson BA, Duncan SR, Ohori NP *et al.* Recurrence of sarcoidosis in pulmonary allograft recipients. *Am Rev Respir Dis* 1993; 148: 1373.

65 Martinez FJ, Orens JB, Deeb M. Recurrence of sarcoidosis following bilateral allogeneic lung transplantation. *Chest* 1994; 106: 1597.

66 Werb Z, Gordon S. Secretion of a specific collagenase by stimulated macrophages. *J Exp Med* 1975; 142: 346.

67 Werb Z, Gordon S. Elastase secretion by stimulated macrophages. *J Exp Med* 1975; 142: 361.

68 Gallily K, Ben-Ishay Z. Immune cytolysis of mono- macrophages *in vitro. J Reticuloendothelial Soc* 1975; 18: 44.

69 Mebom H, Sanner T, Seljelid R. Macrophage cytolytic factor: some observations on its physicochemical properties and mode of action. *Exp Cell Res* 1975; 94: 221.

70 McLelland DBL, Van Furth R. *In vitro* synthesis of lysozyme by human and mouse tissues and leucocytes. *Immunology* 1975; 28: 1099.

71 Hinman LM, Stevens CA, Matthay RA, Gee JBL. Angiotensin convertase activities in human alveolar macrophages: the effects of cigarette smoking and pulmonary sarcoidosis. *Science* 1979; 205: 202.

72 Spector WG. Epithelial cells, giant cells and sarcoidosis. *Ann N Y Acad Sci* 1976; 278: 3.

73 Soler P, Bassett F, Bernaudin JF, Chretien JF. Morphology and distribution of sarcoid granuloma: ultrastructural study of serial sections. *Ann N Y Acad Sci* 1976; 278: 147.

74 Semenzato G, Zezzutto A, Pizzola G *et al.* Immunohistological study in sarcoidosis: evaluation at different sites of disease activity. *Clin Immunol Immunopathol* 1984; 30: 29.

75 Fazel SB, Howie SEM, Krajewski AS, Lamb D. B lymphocyte accumulations in human pulmonary sarcoidosis. *Thorax* 1992; 47: 964.

76 Uehlinger EA. The morbid anatomy of sarcoidosis. *Am Rev Respir Dis* 1961; 84 (Suppl): 6.

77 Basset F, Collet A, Chrétien J *et al.* Etude ultra-microscopique des cellules de la réaction de Kveim. In: Turiaf J, Chabot J, eds. *Proceedings of the Fourth International Conference on Sarcoidosis 1966.* Paris: Masson, 1967: 89.

78 Douglas AC. Electron microscopy of Kveim and sarcoid lesions. In: Turiaf J, Chabot J, eds. *Proceedings of the Fourth International Conference on Sarcoidosis 1966.* Paris: Masson, 1967: 117.

79 Douglas SD, Siltzbach LE. Electron microscopy of Kveim biopsies in sarcoidosis. In: Iwai K, Hosoda Y, eds. *Proceedings of the Sixth International Conference on Sarcoidosis.* Tokyo: University Press, 1974: 54.

80 Hirsch JG, Fodorko ME, Dwyer CM. The ultrastructure of epithelioid and giant cells in positive Kveim test sites and sarcoid granulomata. In: Turiaf J, Chabot J, eds. *Proceedings of the Fourth International Conference on Sarcoidosis 1966.* Paris: Masson, 1967: 59.

81 Kalifat SR, Bouteille M, Delame J. Etude ultrastructurale des alterations cellulaires et extracellulaires dans le granulome sarcoidosique. In: Turiaf J, Chabot J, eds. *Proceedings of the Fourth International Conference on Sarcoidosis 1966.* Paris: Masson, 1967: 71.

82 Wanstrup J. On the ultrastructure of granuloma formation in sarcoidosis. In: Turiaf J, Chabot J, eds. *Proceedings of the Fourth International Conference on Sarcoidosis 1966.* Paris: Masson, 1967: 110.

83 James DG, Jopling WH. Sarcoidosis and leprosy. *Trop Med Hyg* 1961; 64: 42.

84 Kooij R. Sarcoidosis or leprosy? *Br J Dermatol* 1964; 76: 203.

85 Jordan JW, Darke CS. Chronic beryllium poisoning. *Thorax* 1958; 13: 69.

86 Slavin P. Diffuse pulmonary granulomatosis in young women following exposure to beryllium compounds in the manufacture of radio tubes. *Am Rev Tuberc* 1949; 60: 755.

87 Lurie HL. Five unusual cases of sporotrichosis from South Africa showing lesions in muscles, bones and viscera. *Br J Surg* 1963; 50: 585.

88 Anderson R, James DG, Peters PM, Thomson AD. Local sarcoid tissue reactions. *Lancet* 1962; i: 1211.

89 Hunninghake GW, Garrett KC, Richerson HB *et al.* Pathogenesis of the granulomatous lung diseases. *Am Rev Respir Dis* 1984; 130: 476.

90 Crystal RG, Bitterman PB, Rennard SI *et al.* Interstitial lung diseases of unknown cause. *N Engl J Med* 1984; 310: 235.

91 Thomas PD, Hunninghake GW. Current concepts of the pathogenesis of sarcoidosis. *Am Rev Respir Dis* 1987; 135: 747.

92 Semenzato G. Immunology of interstitial lung disease: cellular events taking place in the lung of sarcoidosis, hypersensitivity pneumonitis and HIV infection. *Eur Respir J* 1991; 4: 94.

93 Daniele RP, Dauber JH, Rossman MD. Immunologic abnormalities in sarcoidosis. *Ann Intern Med* 1980; 92: 406.

94 Gupta RC, Kueppers F, Deremee RA *et al.* Pulmonary and extra-pulmonary sarcoidosis in relation to circulating immune complexes: a quantitation of immune complexes by two radioimmunoassays. *Am Rev Respir Dis* 1977; 116: 261.

95 Saint-Remy J-MR, Mitchell DN, Cole PJ. Variation in immunoglobulin levels and circulating immune complexes in sarcoidosis. *Am Rev Respir Dis* 1983; 127: 23.

96 Lambre CR, Maho SL, Dibella G *et al.* Bronchoalveolar lavage fluid and serum complement activity in pulmonary sarcoidosis. *Am Rev Respir Dis* 1986; 134: 238.

97 Schoenfeld N, Schmolke B, Schmitt M *et al.* Specification and quantitation of circulating immune complexes in the serum of patients with active pulmonary sarcoidosis. *Thorax* 1994; 49: 688.

98 Reynolds HY. Bronchoalveolar lavage. *Am Rev Respir Dis* 1987; 135: 250.

99 Campbell DA, Poulter LW, Dubois RM *et al.* Immunocompetent cells in bronchoalveolar lavage reflect the cell population in transbronchial biopsies in pulmonary sarcoidosis. *Am Rev Respir Dis* 1985; 132: 1300.

100 Semenzato G, Chilosi M, Ossi E *et al.* Bronchoalveolar lavage and lung histology. *Am Rev Respir Dis* 1985; 132: 400.

101 Paradis IL, Dauber JH, Rabin BS. Lymphocyte phenotypes in bronchoalveolar lavage and lung tissue in sarcoidosis and idiopathic pulmonary fibrosis. *Am Rev Respir Dis* 1986; 133: 855.

102 Hunninghake GW, Crystal RG. Pulmonary sarcoidosis: a disorder mediated by excess helper T lymphocyte activity at sites of disease activity. *N Engl J Med* 1981; 305: 429.

103 Ceuppens JL, Lacquet LM, Marien G *et al.* Alveolar T cell subsets in pulmonary sarcoidosis. *Am Rev Respir Dis* 1984; 129: 563.

104 Rossi GA, Sacco O, Cosulich E *et al.* Pulmonary sarcoidosis: excess of helper T lymphocytes and T cell sub-set imbalance at sites of disease activity. *Thorax* 1984; 39: 143.

105 Costabel U, Bross KJ, Ruhle KH *et al.* Ia-like antigens on T cells and their subpopulations in pulmonary sarcoidosis and in hypersensitivity pneumonitis. *Am Rev Respir Dis* 1985; 131: 337.

106 Hunninghake GW, Bedell GN, Zavala DC *et al.* Role of interleukin-2 release by lung T cells in active pulmonary sarcoidosis. *Am Rev Respir Dis* 1983; 128: 634.

107 Bauer W, Gorny MK, Baumann HR, Morell A. T lymphocyte sub-sets and immunoglobulin concentrations in bronchoalveolar lavage of patients with sarcoidosis and high and low intensity alveolitis. *Am Rev Respir Dis* 1985; 132: 1060.

108 Rankin JA, Naegel GP, Schrader CE *et al*. Air space immunoglobulin production and levels in bronchoalveolar lavage fluid of normal subjects and patients with sarcoidosis. *Am Rev Respir Dis* 1983; 127: 442.

109 Rossi GA, Sacco O, Cosulich E *et al*. Helper T lymphocytes in sarcoidosis. *Am Rev Respir Dis* 1986; 133: 1086.

110 Hunninghake GW, Line BR, Szapiel SV, Crystal RG. Activation of inflammatory cells increases the localisation of gallium-67 at sites of disease. *Clin Res* 1981; 29: 171A.

111 Hunninghake GW. Release of interleukin-1 by alveolar macrophages of patients with active pulmonary sarcoidosis. *Am Rev Respir Dis* 1984; 129: 569.

112 Hudspith BN, Flint KC, Geraint-James D *et al*. Lack of immune deficiency in sarcoidosis: compartmentalisation of the immune response. *Thorax* 1987; 42: 250.

113 Robinson BWS, Mclemore TL, Crystal RG. Gamma interferon is spontaneously released by alveolar macrophages and lung T lymphocytes in patients with pulmonary sarcoidosis. *J Clin Invest* 1985; 75: 1488.

114 Limper AH, Colby TV, Sanders MS *et al*. Immunohistochemical localization of transforming growth factor β-1 in the non-necrotizing granulomas of pulmonary sarcoidosis. *Am J Respir Crit Care Med* 1994; 149: 197.

115 Hunninghake GW, Fulmer JD, Young RC *et al*. Localisation of the immune response in sarcoidosis. *Am Rev Respir Dis* 1979; 120: 49.

116 Chailleux E, Bignon JD, Peyrat MA *et al*. Lymphocyte subsets, phytohaemagglutinin responsiveness of blood lymphocytes and interleukin-2 production in sarcoidosis. *Thorax* 1985; 40: 768.

117 Anon. The immune response in sarcoidosis. *Lancet* 1987; ii: 195.

118 Chusid EL, Shah R, Siltzbach LE. Tuberculin tests during the course of sarcoidosis in 350 patients. *Am Rev Respir Dis* 1971; 104: 13.

119 Friou GJ. Delayed cutaneous hypersensitivity in sarcoidosis. *J Clin Invest* 1952; 31: 630.

120 Citron KM. Skin tests in sarcoidosis. *Tubercle* 1957; 38: 33.

121 Friou GJ. A study of the cutaneous reaction to didiomycin, trichophytin and mumps skin test antigens in patients with sarcoidosis. *Yale J Biol Med* 1952; 24: 233.

122 Sones M, Israel HL. Altered immunologic reactions in sarcoidosis. *Ann Intern Med* 1954; 40: 260.

123 James DG. Diagnosis and treatment of sarcoidosis. *Br Med J* 1956; 2: 900.

124 Mayock RL, Bertrand P, Morrison CE, Scott JH. Manifestations of sarcoidosis. Analysis of 145 patients with a review of 9 series selected from the literature. *Am J Med* 1963; 35: 67.

125 Spann RW, Rosenow EC, Deremee RA, Miller WE. Unilateral hilar or paratracheal adenopathy in sarcoidosis: a study of 38 cases. *Thorax* 1971; 26: 296.

126 Williams MJ. Sarcoidosis presenting with unilateral hilar lymph node enlargement. *Scott Med J* 1961; 6: 18.

127 James DG. Erythema nodosum. *Br Med J* 1961; 1: 853.

128 Lofgren S. The concept of erythema nodosum revised. *Scand J Respir Dis* 1967; 48: 348.

129 Sones M, Israel HL. Course and prognosis of sarcoidosis. *Am J Med* 1960; 29: 84.

130 Anderson J, Boughton CR. The concept of mediastinal pain. *Br Med J* 1957; 1: 1490.

131 Israel HL, Sones M, Roy RL, Stein GN. The occurrence of intrathoracic calcification in sarcoidosis. *Am Rev Respir Dis* 1961; 84: 1.

132 Israel HL, Lenchner G, Steiner RM. Late development of mediastinal calcification in sarcoidosis. *Am Rev Respir Dis* 1981; 124: 302.

133 Lofgren S, Lindgren AG. Cavern formation in pulmonary sarcoidosis. *Acta Chir Scand* 1959; Suppl 245: 113.

134 Tazi A, Desfemmes-Baleyte T, Soler P *et al*. Pulmonary sarcoidosis with a diffuse ground glass pattern on the chest radiograph. *Thorax* 1994; 49: 793.

135 Wollschlager C, Khan F. Aspergillomas complicating sarcoidosis. A prospective study in 100 patients. *Chest* 1984; 86: 585.

136 Farber HW, Fairman RP, Glauser FL. Talc granulomatosis: laboratory findings similar to sarcoidosis. *Am Rev Respir Dis* 1982; 125: 258.

137 Middleton WG, Douglas AC. Prolonged corticosteroid therapy in pulmonary sarcoidosis. In: Jones Williams W, Davies BH, eds. *Proceedings of the Eighth International Conference on Sarcoidosis and Other Granulomatous Diseases*. Cardiff: Alpha Omega, 1980: 632.

138 Hsu JT, Cottrell TS. Pulmonary sarcoidosis: unilateral hilar adenopathy presenting as an endobronchial tumour. *Radiology* 1971; 98: 385.

139 Citron KM, Scadding JG. Stenosing non-caseating tuberculosis (sarcoidosis) of the bronchi. *Thorax* 1957; 12: 10.

140 di Benedetto RJ, Ribaudo C. Bronchopulmonary sarcoidosis. *Am Rev Respir Dis* 1966; 94: 952.

141 Miller A, Brown LK, Teirstein AS. Stenosis of main bronchi mimicking fixed upper airway obstruction in sarcoidosis. *Chest* 1980; 88: 244.

142 Bechtel JJ, Starr T, Dantzker DR, Bower JS. Airway hyper-reactivity in patients with sarcoidosis. *Am Rev Respir Dis* 1981; 124: 759.

143 Olafsson M, Simonsson BG, Hansson S-B. Bronchial reactivity in patients with recent pulmonary sarcoidosis. *Thorax* 1985; 40: 51.

144 Kovnat PJ, Donohue RF. Sarcoidosis involving the pleura. *Ann Intern Med* 1965; 62: 120.

145 Wilen SB, Rabinowitz JG, Ulreich S, Lyons HA. Pleural involvement in sarcoidosis. *Am J Med* 1974; 57: 200.

146 Nicholls AJ, Friend JAR, Legge JS. Sarcoid pleural effusion: three cases and review of the literature. *Thorax* 1980; 35: 277.

147 Chusid EL, Shah R, Siltzbach LE. Sarcoidosis of the pleura. In: Iwai K, Hosoda Y, eds. *Proceedings of the Sixth International Conference on Sarcoidosis*. Tokyo: University Press, 1974: 373.

148 Vital Durand D, Dellinger A, Guerin C *et al*. Pleural sarcoidosis: one case presenting with an eosinophilic effusion. *Thorax* 1984; 39: 468.

149 Gardiner IT, Uff JS. Acute pleurisy in sarcoidosis. *Thorax* 1978; 33: 124.

150 Morgans WE, Al-Jilahawi AN, Mbatha PB. Superior vena cava obstruction caused by sarcoidosis. *Thorax* 1980; 35: 397.

151 Hoffstein V, Ranganathan N, Mullen JBM. Sarcoidosis simulating pulmonary veno-occlusive disease. *Am Rev Respir Dis* 1986; 134: 809.

152 Ainslie D, James DG. Ocular sarcoidosis. *Br Med J* 1956; 1: 954.

153 Cowan CL. Ocular sarcoidosis. *J Natl Med Ass* 1959; 51: 371.

154 James DG. Ocular sarcoidosis. *Am J Med* 1959; 26: 331.

155 Nielsen RH. Ocular sarcoidosis. *AMA Arch Ophthalmol* 1959; 61: 455.

156 Nolan JP, Klatskin G. The fever of sarcoidosis. *Ann Intern Med* 1964; 61: 455.

157 MacFarlane JT. Recurrent erythema nodosum and pulmonary sarcoidosis. *Postgrad Med J* 1981; 57: 525.

158 Neville E, Mills RGS, Jash DK *et al*. Sarcoidosis of the upper respiratory tract and its association with lupus pernio. *Thorax* 1976; 31: 660.

159 Neville E, Mills RGS, James DG. Sarcoidosis of the upper respiratory tract and its relation to lupus pernio. *Ann N Y Acad Sci* 1976; 278: 416.

160 Bower JS, Belen JE, Weg JG, Dantzker DR. Manifestations and treatment of laryngeal sarcoidosis. *Am Rev Respir Dis* 1980; 122: 325.

161 Tsou E, Romano MC, Kerwin DM *et al*. Sarcoidosis of anterior mediastinal nodes, pancreas and uterine cervix: three unusual sites in the same patient. *Am Rev Respir Dis* 1980; 122: 333.

162 McCormick PA, Malone D, Fitzgerald MX, Fitzgerald O. Pancreatitis in sarcoidosis. *Br Med J* 1985; 290: 1472.

163 Wheeler JE, Rosenthal NS. Bloody ascites in sarcoidosis. *Chest* 1985; 88: 917.

164 Fletcher J, Hinton JM. Tuberculin sensitivity in Crohn's disease. *Lancet* 1967; ii: 753.

165 Phear DN. The relation between regional ileitis and sarcoidosis. *Lancet* 1958; ii: 1250.

166 Anon. Kveim–Siltzbach test vindicated. *Lancet* 1972; i: 188.

167 Middleton WG, Douglas AC. Further experience with Edinburgh prepared Kveim–Siltzbach suspensions. In: Jones Williams W, Davies BH, eds. *Proceedings of the Eighth International Conference on Sarcoidosis and Other Granulomatous Diseases*. Cardiff: Alpha Omega, 1980: 655.

168 Siltzbach LE. Kveim test in sarcoidosis. *JAMA* 1961; 178: 476.

169 Greenberg G, Anderson R, Sharpstow P, James DG. Enlargement of parotid gland due to sarcoidosis. *Br Med J* 1964; 2: 861.

170 Roberts JC, Rang MC. Sarcoidosis of liver and spleen. *Lancet* 1958; ii: 296.

171 Hirschman RJ, Johns CJ. Hemoglobin studies in sarcoidosis. *Ann Intern Med* 1965; 62: 129.

172 Aszkanazy CL. Sarcoidosis of the central nervous system. *J Neuropathol* 1952; 11: 392.

173 Campbell IW, Short AIK, Douglas AC. Hypothalamic manifestations of sarcoidosis – with particular reference to hypothalamic hypothyroidism. In: Jones Williams W, Davies BH, eds. *Proceedings of the Eighth International Conference on Sarcoidosis and Other Granulomatous Diseases*. Cardiff: Alpha Omega, 1980: 579.

174 Colover J. Sarcoidosis with involvement of the central nervous system. *Brain* 1948; 71: 451.

175 Cummins SD, Clark DH, Gandy TH. Boeck's sarcoid of the thyroid gland. *Arch Pathol* 1951; 51: 68.

176 Daum JJ, Canter HG, Katz S. Central

nervous system sarcoidosis with alveolar hypoventilation. *Am J Med* 1965; 38: 893.

177 Douglas AC, Maloney AFJ. Sarcoidosis of the central nervous system. *J Neurol Neurosurg Psychiatry* 1973; 36: 1024.

178 Fazlullah S. Sarcoidosis with involvement of the nervous system. *Dis Chest* 1962; 41: 685.

179 Goodson WH. Neurological manifestations of sarcoidosis. *South Med J* 1960; 53: 1111.

180 Hook O. Sarcoidosis with involvement of the nervous system: report of nine cases. *AMA Arch Neurol Psychiatry* 1954; 71: 554.

181 Jefferson M. Sarcoidosis of the nervous system. *Brain* 1957; 80: 540.

182 Jefferson M. The nervous system in sarcoidosis. *Postgrad Med J* 1958; 34: 259.

183 Jonasson JV. Sarcoidosis of the nervous system: report of four cases with interesting signs. *Acta Psychiatr Scand* 1960; 35: 182.

184 Matthews WB. Sarcoidosis of the nervous system. *Br Med J* 1959; 1: 267.

185 Nora JR, Levitsky JM, Zimmerman HJ. Sarcoidosis with panhypopituitarism and diabetes insipidus. *Ann Intern Med* 1959; 51: 1400.

186 Schonell ME, Gillespie WJ, Maloney AEJ. Cerebral sarcoidosis. *Br J Dis Chest* 1968; 62: 195.

187 Thompson JR. Sarcoidosis of the central nervous system: report of a case simulating intracranial neoplasm. *Am J Med* 1961; 31: 977.

188 Walker AG. Sarcoidosis of the brain and spinal cord. *Postgrad Med J* 1961; 37: 431.

189 El-Kassimi FA, Ashour M, Vijayaraghavan R. Sarcoidosis presenting as recurrent laryngeal nerve palsy. *Thorax* 1990; 45: 565.

190 Jaffe R, Bogomolski-Yahalom V, Kramer MR. Vocal cord paralysis as the presenting symptom of sarcoidosis. *Respir Med* 1994; 88: 633.

191 Pentland B, Mitchell JD, Cull RE, Ford MJ. Central nervous system sarcoidosis. *Q J Med* 1985; 56: 457.

192 Anon. Sarcoidosis of the nervous system. *Lancet* 1985; ii: 1048.

193 Winnacker JL, Becker KL, Katz S. Endocrine aspects of sarcoidosis. *N Engl J Med* 1969; 278: 483.

194 Delaney P. Neurologic manifestations in sarcoidosis. Review of the literature with a report of 23 cases. *Ann Intern Med* 1977; 87: 336.

195 Vesely DL, Maldonodo A, Levey GS. Partial hypopituitarism and possible hypothalamic involvement in sarcoidosis. Report of a case and review of the literature. *Am J Med* 1977; 62: 425.

196 James DG, Thomson AD. The course of sarcoidosis and its modification by treatment. *Lancet* 1959; i: 1057.

197 Neville E, Carstairs LS, James DG. Sarcoidosis of bone. *Q J Med* 1977; 46: 215.

198 Crompton MR, Macdermott V. Sarcoidosis associated with progressive muscular wasting and weakness. *Brain* 1961; 84: 62.

199 Dyken PR. Sarcoidosis of the skeletal muscle: a case report and review of the literature. *Neurology* 1962; 12: 643.

200 Harvey JC. A myopathy of Boeck's sarcoid. *Am J Med* 1959; 26: 356.

201 Powell LW. Sarcoidosis of the skeletal muscle. Report of 6 cases and review of the literature. *Am J Clin Pathol* 1953; 23: 881.

202 Rothfield B, Folk EE. Sarcoid myopathy. *JAMA* 1962; 179: 903.

203 Snorrason E. Myositis fibrosa progressiva.

204 Wallace SL, Lattes R, Malia JP, Ragan C. Muscle involvement in Boeck's sarcoid. *Ann Intern Med* 1958; 48: 497.

205 Douglas AC, MacLeod JG, Mathews JD. Symptomatic sarcoidosis of skeletal muscle. *J Neurol Neurosurg Psychiatry* 1973; 36: 1034.

206 Baydur A, Pandya K, Sharma OP, Kanel GC, Carlson M. Control of ventilation, respiratory muscle strength and granulomatous involvement of skeletal muscle in patients with sarcoidosis. *Chest* 1993; 103: 396.

207 Ost D, Yeldandi A, Cugell D. Acute sarcoid-myositis with respiratory muscle involvement. *Chest* 1995; 107: 879.

208 Ando DG, Lynch JP, Fantone JC. Sarcoid myopathy with elevated creatine phosphokinase. *Am Rev Respir Dis* 1985; 131: 298.

209 Kaplan H. Sarcoid arthritis. *Arch Intern Med* 1963; 112: 924.

210 Bell NH, Gill JR, Bartter FC. Calcium metabolism in sarcoidosis. *Am Rev Respir Dis* 1961; 84 (Suppl): 27.

211 Coburn JW, Hobbs C, Johnston GS *et al.* Granulomatous sarcoid nephritis. *Am J Med* 1967; 42: 273.

212 Lofgren S, Norbert R. Metabolic aspects of sarcoidosis. *Acta Tuberc Scand* 1959; Suppl 45: 40.

213 Lofgren S, Snellman B, Lindgren AG. Renal complications in sarcoidosis. *Acta Med Scand* 1957; 159: 296.

214 Ellman P, Parfitt AM. The resemblance between sarcoidosis with hypercalcaemia and hyperparathyroidism. *Br Med J* 1960; 2: 108.

215 Goldstein RA, Israel HL, Becker KL, Moore CF. The infrequency of hypercalcaemia in sarcoidosis. *Am J Med* 1971; 51: 21.

216 Sandler LM, Winearls CG, Fraher J *et al.* Studies of the hypercalcaemia of sarcoidosis: effect of steroids and exogenous vitamin D3 on the circulating concentrations of 1,25-dihydroxy vitamin D3. *Q J Med* 1984; 53: 165.

217 Taylor RL, Lynch HJ, Wysor WG. Seasonal influence of sunlight on the hypercalcaemia of sarcoidosis. *Am J Med* 1963; 34: 221.

218 Ogilvie RI, Kaye M, Moore S. Granulomatous sarcoid disease of the kidney. *Ann Intern Med* 1964; 61: 711.

219 Rizzato G, Fraioli P, Montemurro L. Nephrolithiasis as a presenting feature of sarcoidosis. *Thorax* 1995; 50: 555.

220 Akmal M, Sharma OP. Renal sarcoidosis: a reminder. *Chest* 1990; 97: 1284.

221 Ryan DM, Lesser BA, Crumley LA *et al.* Epididymal sarcoidosis. *J Urol* 1993; 149: 134.

222 Forbes G, Usher A. Fatal myocardial sarcoidosis. *Br Med J* 1962; 2: 771.

223 Anon. Sarcoid heart disease. *Br Med J* 1972; 4: 627.

224 Fleming HA. Sarcoid heart disease: a review and an appeal. *Thorax* 1980; 35: 641.

225 Sharma OP, Maheshwari A, Thaker K. Myocardial sarcoidosis. *Chest* 1993; 103: 253.

226 Stein E, Stimmel B, Siltzbach LE. Clinical course of cardiac sarcoidosis. *Ann N Y Acad Sci* 1976; 278: 470.

227 Mikhail JR, Mitchell DN, Ball KP. Abnormal electrocardiographic findings in sarcoidosis. In: Iwai K, Hosoda Y, eds. *Proceedings of the Sixth International Conference on Sarcoidosis.* Tokyo: University Press, 1974: 365.

228 Stein E, Jackler I, Stein W *et al.* Asymptomatic electrocardiographic alterations in 80 patients with sarcoidosis. In: Iwai K, Hosoda Y, eds. *Proceedings of the Sixth International Conference on Sarcoidosis.* Tokyo: University Press, 1974: 360.

229 Silverman KJ, Hutchins GM, Bulkley BH. Cardiac sarcoid: a clinicopathologic study of 84 unselected patients with systemic sarcoidosis. *Circulation* 1978; 58: 1204.

230 Wait JL, Movahed A. Anginal chest pain in sarcoidosis. *Thorax* 1989; 44: 391.

231 Anon. Cardiac sarcoidosis. *Thorax* 1989; 44: 371.

232 Demeter SL. Myocardial sarcoidosis unresponsive to steroids. Treatment with cyclophosphamide. *Chest* 1988; 94: 202.

233 Scott J, Higenbotham T. Transplantation of the lungs and heart for patients with severe complications from sarcoidosis. *Sarcoidosis* 1990; 7: 9.

234 Paz HL, McCormick DJ, Kutalek SP, Patchefsky A. The automated implantable cardiac defibrillator. Prophylaxis in cardiac sarcoidosis. *Chest* 1994; 106: 1603.

235 Ratner SJ, Fenoglio JJ, Ursell PC. Utility of endomyocardial biopsy in the diagnosis of cardiac sarcoidosis. *Chest* 1986; 90: 528.

236 Boushy SF, Kurtzman RS, Martin ND, Lewis BM. The course of pulmonary function in sarcoidosis. *Ann Intern Med* 1965; 62: 939.

237 Marshall R, Smellie HC, Baylis JH *et al.* Pulmonary function in sarcoidosis. *Thorax* 1958; 13: 48.

238 Marshall R, Karlish AJ. Lung function in sarcoidosis. *Thorax* 1971; 26: 402.

239 Sharma OP, Colp C, Williams MH. Course of pulmonary sarcoidosis with and without corticosteroid therapy as determined by pulmonary function studies. *Am J Med* 1966; 41: 541.

240 Svanborg N. Studies on cardiopulmonary function in sarcoidosis. *Acta Med Scand* 1961; Suppl 366.

241 Young RC, Carr C, Shelton TG *et al.* Sarcoidosis: relationship between changes in lung structure and function. *Am Rev Respir Dis* 1967; 95: 224.

242 Carrington CB, Gaensler EA, Mikus JP *et al.* Structure and function in sarcoidosis. *Ann N Y Acad Sci* 1976; 278: 265.

243 Bates DV, Macklem PT, Christie RV. Pulmonary sarcoidosis. In: *Respiratory Function in Disease*, 2nd edn.. London: WB Saunders, 1971: 287.

244 Sharma OP, Johnson R. Airway obstruction in sarcoidosis. A study of 123 non-smoking black American patients with sarcoidosis. *Chest* 1988; 94: 343.

245 Harrison BDW, Shaylor JM, Stokes TC, Wilkes AR. Airflow limitation in sarcoidosis: a study of pulmonary function in 107 patients with newly diagnosed disease. *Respir Med* 1991; 85: 59.

246 Armstrong JR, Radke JR, Kvale PA, Eichenhorn MS, Popvich J. Endoscopic findings in sarcoidosis. Characteristics and correlations with radiographic staging and bronchial mucosal biopsy yield. *Ann Otol* 1981; 90: 339.

247 Lewis MI, Horak DA. Airflow obstruction in sarcoidosis. *Chest* 1987; 92: 582.

248 Sietsema KE, Kraft M, Ginzton L, Sharma OP. Abnormal oxygen uptake responses to exercise in patients with mild pulmonary sarcoidosis. *Chest* 1992; 102: 838.

249 Douglas AC. The Kveim test and its

practical significance. *Scand J Respir Dis* 1972; Suppl 80: 61.

250 Douglas AC, Wallace A, Clark J *et al*. The Edinburgh spleen: source of a validated Kveim Siltzbach test material. *Ann N Y Acad Sci* 1976; 278: 670.

251 Middleton WG, Douglas AC. Further experience with Edinburgh prepared Kveim–Siltzbach test suspensions. In: Jones Williams W, Davies BH, eds. *Proceedings of the Eighth International Conference on Sarcoidosis and other Granulomatous Diseases*. Cardiff: Alpha Omega, 1980: 655.

252 Munro CS, Mitchell DN. The Kveim response: still useful, still a puzzle. *Thorax* 1987; 42: 321.

253 Douglas AC. Experience with the Kveim test: conventional and freeze dried test substance. *Acta Med Scand* 1964; Suppl 425: 189.

254 Siltzbach LE. Qualities and behaviour of satisfactory Kveim suspensions. *Ann N Y Acad Sci* 1976; 278: 665.

255 Anon. The Kveim controversy. *Lancet* 1971; ii: 750.

256 Siltzbach LE. Surveillance of Kveim test results. In: Iwai K, Hosoda Y, eds. *Proceedings of the Sixth International Conference on Sarcoidosis*. Tokyo: University Press, 1974: 79.

257 Nelson CT. The Kveim reaction in sarcoidosis. *J Chron Dis* 1957; 6: 158.

258 Kennedy WPU. An evaluation of freeze-dried Kveim reagent. *Br J Dis Chest* 1967; 61: 40.

259 Rife E, Izumi T, Kallner A *et al*. On the active principle in the Kveim suspension. *Scand J Respir Dis* 1973; 54: 111.

260 Chase MW, Siltzbach LE. Further studies on the fractionation of materials used in the intracutaneous diagnostic test for sarcoidosis. *Excerpta Med* 1961; 42: 58.

261 Rogers FJ, Haserich JR. Sarcoidosis and the Kveim reaction. *J Invest Dermatol* 1954; 23: 389.

262 Holter JF, Park KH, Sjoerdsma KW, Kataria YP. Non-viable autologous bronchoalveolar lavage cell preparations induce intradermal cell granulomas in sarcoidosis patients. *Am Rev Respir Dis* 1992; 145: 864.

263 Douglas AC. Kveim and Siltzbach. *Mt Sinai J Med* 1977; 44: 706.

264 Gilman MJ, Wang KP. Transbronchial lung biopsy in sarcoidosis. *Am Rev Respir Dis* 1980; 122: 721.

265 Polletti V, Patelli M, Spiga L *et al*. Transbronchial lung biopsy in pulmonary sarcoidosis. *Chest* 1986; 89: 361.

266 Lieberman J. Elevation of serum angiotensin-converting enzyme (ACE) levels in sarcoidosis. *Am J Med* 1975; 59: 365.

267 Lieberman J, Nosal A, Schleissner LA, Sastre-Foken A. Serum angiotensin converting enzyme for diagnosis and therapeutic evaluation of sarcoidosis. *Am Rev Respir Dis* 1979; 120: 329.

268 Silverstein E, Pertschuk LP, Friedland J. Immuno-fluorescent localisation of angiotensin converting enzyme in epithelioid and giant cells of sarcoidosis granulomas. *Proc Natl Acad Sci USA* 1979; 76: 6646.

269 Okabe T, Suzuki A, Ishikawa H *et al*. Cells originating from sarcoid granulomas *in vitro*. *Am Rev Respir Dis* 1981; 124: 608.

270 Mordelet-Dambrine MS, Stanislaus-Leguern GM, Huchon GJ *et al*. Elevation of the bronchoalveolar concentration of angiotensin-1 converting enzyme in sarcoidosis. *Am Rev Respir Dis* 1982; 126: 472.

271 Turton CWG, Grundy E, Firth G *et al*. Value of measuring serum angiotensin-1 converting enzyme and serum lysozyme in the management of sarcoidosis. *Thorax* 1979; 34: 57.

272 Deremee RA, Rohrbach MS. Normal serum angiotensin converting enzyme activity in patients with newly diagnosed sarcoidosis. *Chest* 1984; 85: 45.

273 Lawrence EC, Teague RB, Gottlieb MS *et al*. Serial changes in markers of disease activity with corticosteroid treatment in sarcoidosis. *Am J Med* 1983; 74: 747.

274 Turner-Warwick M, Mcallister W, Lawrence R *et al*. Corticosteroid treatment in pulmonary sarcoidosis: do serial lavage lymphocyte counts, serum angiotensin converting enzyme measurements, and gallium-67 scans help management. *Thorax* 1986; 41: 903.

275 Ueda E, Kawabe T, Tachibana T, Kokubu T. Serum angiotensin-converting enzyme activity as an indicator of prognosis in sarcoidosis. *Am Rev Respir Dis* 1980; 121: 667.

276 Baughman RP, Ploysongsang Y, Roberts RD, Srivastava L. Effect of sarcoid and steroids on angiotensin-converting enzyme. *Am Rev Respir Dis* 1983; 128: 631.

277 Gelrud LG, Arseneau JC, Milder MS *et al*. The kinetics of 67-gallium incorporation into inflammatory lesions: experimental and clinical studies. *J Lab Clin Med* 1974; 83: 489.

278 Nosal A, Schleissner LA, Mishkin FS, Lieberman J. Angiotensin-1 converting enzyme and gallium scan in non-invasive evaluation of sarcoidosis. *Ann Intern Med* 1979; 90: 328.

279 Line BR, Hunninghake GW, Keogh BA *et al*. Gallium-67 scanning to stage the alveolitis of sarcoidosis: correlation with clinical, studies pulmonary function studies and bronchoalveolar lavage. *Am Rev Respir Dis* 1981; 123: 440.

280 Cohen RD, Bunting PS, Meindok HO *et al*. Does serum angiotensin converting enzyme reflect intensity of alveolitis in sarcoidosis? *Thorax* 1985; 40: 497.

281 Israel HL, Albertine KH, Park CH, Patrick H. Whole-body gallium-67 scans. Role in diagnosis of sarcoidosis. *Am Rev Respir Dis* 1991; 144: 1182.

282 Winterbauer RH, Wu R, Springmeyer SC. Fractional analysis of the 120-ml bronchoalveolar lavage. Determination of the best specimen for diagnosis of sarcoidosis. *Chest* 1993; 104: 344.

283 Winterbauer RH, Lammert J, Selland H *et al*. Bronchoalveolar lavage cell populations in the diagnosis of sarcoidosis. *Chest* 1993; 104: 352.

284 Lynch DA, Webb WR, Gamsu G, Stalbarg M, Golden J. Computed tomography in pulmonary sarcoidosis. *J Comput Assist Tomogr* 1989; 13: 405.

285 Brauer MW, Grenier P, Mompoint D, Lenoir S, De Cremoux H. Pulmonary sarcoidosis: evaluation with high resolution CT. *Radiology* 1989; 172: 467.

286 Muller NL, Miller RA. Computed tomography of chronic infiltrative lung disease. *Am Rev Respir Dis* 1990; 142: 1206.

287 Keogh BA, Hunninghake GW, Line BR, Crystal RG. The alveolitis of pulmonary sarcoidosis. *Am Rev Respir Dis* 1983; 128: 256.

288 Deremee RA. The present status of treatment of pulmonary sarcoidosis: a house divided. *Chest* 1977; 71: 388.

289 Young RL, Harkleroad LE, Lordon RE, Weg JG. Pulmonary sarcoidosis: a prospective evaluation of glucocorticoid therapy. *Ann Intern Med* 1970; 73: 207.

290 Harklebroad LE, Young RL, Savage PJ *et al*. Pulmonary sarcoidosis. Long term follow up of the side effects of steroid therapy. *Chest* 1982; 82: 84.

291 Israel HL, Fouts DW, Beggs RA. A controlled trial of prednisolone treatment of sarcoidosis. *Am Rev Respir Dis* 1973; 107: 609.

292 Mikami R, Hiraga Y, Iwai K *et al*. A double-blind controlled trial on the effect of corticosteroid therapy in sarcoidosis. In: Iwai K, Hosoda Y, eds. *Proceedings of the Sixth International Conference on Sarcoidosis*. Tokyo: University Press, 1974: 538.

293 Selroos O, Sellergren TL. Corticosteroid therapy of pulmonary sarcoidosis: a prospective evaluation of alternate day and daily dosage of Stage II disease. *Scand J Respir Dis* 1979; 60: 215.

294 Eule H, Roth I, Weide W. Clinical and functional results of a controlled clinical trial of the value of prednisolone therapy in sarcoidosis, Stage I and II. In: Jones Williams W, Davies BH, eds. *Proceedings of the Eighth International Conference on Sarcoidosis and Other Granulomatous Diseases*. Cardiff: Alpha Omega, 1980: 624.

295 Yamamoto M, Saito N, Tachibana T *et al*. Effects of an 18-month corticosteroid therapy on Stage I and II sarcoidosis patients (a controlled trial). In: *Proceedings of the Ninth International Conference on Sarcoidosis*. Oxford: Pergamon Press, 1983: 470.

296 Hunninghake GW, Gilbert S, Pueringer R *et al*. Outcome of the treatment for sarcoidosis. *Am J Respir Crit Care Med* 1994; 149: 893.

297 Johns CJ, Mcgregor MI, Zachary JB, Ball WC. Extended experience in the long term corticosteroid treatment of sarcoidosis. *Ann N Y Acad Sci* 1976; 278: 722.

298 Alberts C, Van Der Mark Thw Jansen HM *et al*. Inhaled budesonide in pulmonary sarcoidosis: a double blind placebo controlled study. *Eur Respir J* 1995; 8: 682.

299 Du Bois RM. Corticosteroids in sarcoidosis: friend or foe? *Eur Respir J* 1994; 7: 1203.

300 Kirsten D. Inhaled steroids for sarcoidosis? *Eur Respir J* 1995; 8: 679.

301 Rebuck AS, Stiller CR, Braude AC *et al*. Cyclosporin for pulmonary sarcoidosis. *Lancet* 1984; i: 1174.

302 Israel HL, Mccomb BL. Chlorambucil treatment of sarcoidosis. *Sarcoidosis* 1991; 8: 35.

303 Grizzants JN, Knapp AB, Sheeter AJ, Williams MH. Treatment of sarcoid meningitis with radiotherapy. *Am J Med* 1982; 73: 605.

40

PULMONARY LYMPHOCYTIC ANGIITIS AND GRANULOMATOSIS

ANTHONY SEATON

A number of conditions, originally grouped together because they share the common factors of a lymphocytic angiitis or vasculitis with a tendency to granuloma formation, may cause disease of the respiratory tract [1–9]. It is now recognized that despite their similar histological appearances they differ in clinical characteristics, natural history and aetiology, and several represent low-grade lymphocytic neoplasms. Nevertheless, their names have become familiar to chest physicians and since they all cause similar diagnostic problems they are considered together in this chapter. These conditions are:

1 classical Wegener's granulomatosis;
2 limited Wegener's granulomatosis;
3 midline granuloma;
4 lymphomatoid granulomatosis;
5 benign lymphocytic angiitis and granulomatosis;
6 necrotizing sarcoid granulomatosis;
7 bronchocentric granulomatosis.

Two other conditions characterized by eosinophilic granulomas, polyarteritis nodosa and allergic granulomatosis (Churg–Strauss syndrome), have been considered separately in Chapter 38.

Classical Wegener's granulomatosis

In 1931 Klinger [10] described a patient with destructive sinusitis, nephritis and disseminated vasculitis but it was not until 1936 that Wegener [11] clearly defined the triad as a distinct clinical and pathological entity. In 1954 a review by Godman and Churg [12] led to the establishment of firm criteria for the diagnosis. Classical generalized Wegener's granulomatosis is characterized by (i) necrotizing granulomas in the respiratory tract, (ii) generalized focal necrotizing vasculitis and (iii) focal necrotizing glomerulonephritis. In practical terms the demonstration of one or more of these in combination with positive serological evidence is now generally accepted as fulfilling the criteria. When one element of the triad is absent it is usually the renal or the upper respiratory tract component.

Frequency

Wegener's granulomatosis is more common than was once thought. Up to 1967 approximately 200 cases had been reported, although two series published in the 1980s matched this total number of cases [13–15]. Since then, the description of the antineutrophil cytoplasmic autoantibody as a marker of the disease, and the attention drawn to it at the International Symposium at the Mayo Clinic in 1986, have increased the rate at which it has been diagnosed, and it is now estimated to occur at a rate of about 5–12 new cases per million population per annum [16].

There is a slight male preponderance (male/female ratio 3:2) and most patients reported have been of Caucasian extraction. The condition may be found at any age including childhood, although the peak incidence is in the fourth and fifth decades [15,17]. There is a suggestion that, at least in England, the disease may present more frequently in the winter months [16].

Pathogenesis and antineutrophil cytoplasmic antibodies

The pathogenesis of Wegener's granulomatosis remains unclear. The finding of a significant increase in HLA-DR2 frequencies suggests that in some cases there may be a genetic predisposition to this disease [18], and the increased incidence in winter is consistent with Wegener's original hypothesis that infection may play an aetiological role. There are indications that deposition of circulating immune complexes in vessel walls initiates the vasculitis. The antibodies are usually of the IgG or IgM class. Following deposition, the immune complexes trigger the complement cascade thus generating potent chemotactic factors for polymorphonuclear leucocytes such as C5a [19]. Once attracted to the site, neutrophils release lysosomal enzymes, such as elastase and collagenase, with resultant necrosis of vessel walls [20]. In support of this concept is the finding of circulating immune complexes in patients with Wegener's granulomatosis, their correlation with disease activity or relapse and the probable beneficial therapeutic effect of plasmapheresis [13,21–25]. In addition IgG, IgM and complement deposition have been demonstrated in tissue from kidney, lung and the maxillary sinus of patients with Wegener's granulomatosis [23,24,26]. However, the failure to demonstrate deposition of immunoglobulins and complement in involved tissue [26–28] or the presence of circulating immune complexes in all patients [13] suggests that the phenomenon may be relatively transient or, alternatively, that the immune complex concept of pathogenesis may not be the whole story [29].

There is also evidence that cellular as well as humoral immune mechanisms play a part in pathogenesis. Immune complexes can cause granuloma formation [30]. Lymphocytes, mainly T cells, and monocytes are seen infiltrating vessels [27]. In addition, it is suggested that T lymphocytes can be sensitized to antigen and on contact with it release lymphokines, resulting in cellular infiltration, giant cell formation and tissue destruction [9]. After ingestion of immune complexes, macrophages may also release tissue-damaging lysosomal enzymes or transform into epithelioid cells and form granulomas.

In 1985 van der Woude and colleagues reported an association between Wegener's granulomatosis and the presence in the blood of antineutrophil cytoplasm antibodies (ANCA), and this finding has been replicated by a number of other investigators [31–33]. ANCA react with cytoplasmic granules in neutrophils and demonstrate one of two staining patterns: diffusely cytoplasmic (cANCA) or per-

inuclear (pANCA) (Fig. 40.1). The main target of cANCA appears to be proteinase C and that of pANCA myeloperoxidase [34,35]. Initial use of ANCA in an indirect immunofluorescence test suggested that they had a very high specificity and sensitivity for the diagnosis of Wegener's granulomatosis, based on studies from large specialized units. However, ANCA have been shown to occur in other diseases, including such common conditions as tuberculosis, lung cancer and human immunodeficiency virus (HIV) infection, and a recent audit of the results of the use of the test in a regional diagnostic service has shown a sensitivity of 65% and a specificity of 77% in patients with respiratory symptoms, cANCA being somewhat more sensitive [36]. False-positive results were found in other autoimmune diseases, cancer, pulmonary emboli and pulmonary fibroses. Since Wegener's granulomatosis is relatively rare, the positive predictive value of the test is quite low, at around 45%.

The role, if any, of ANCA in pathogenesis remains the subject of speculation, and it is debated whether they are a cause or consequence of some of the pathological features. In support of a pathogenic role, ANCA have been shown to cause neutophils to release free radicals and to injure endothelial cells, while T lymphocytes have been demonstrated to become sensitized to ANCA [37–39]. It has been proposed on the basis of *in vitro* studies that viral or other illnesses that lead to the release of cytokines, such as tumour necrosis factor, cause neutrophil enzymes to migrate to the surface of the cell from the primary granule and that presentation of these antigens at the cell surface leads to the development of the ANCA [37]. This in turn

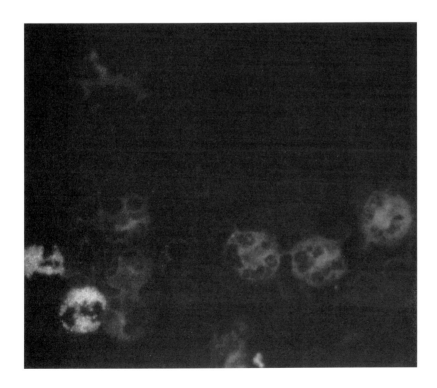

Fig. 40.1 Neutrophil leucocytes from a patient with Wegener's granulomatosis stained by immunofluorescent technique to show cytoplasmic antibodies.

may cause release of free radicals, damage vascular endothelium and recruit more neutrophils. On balance it seems likely that a condition characterized by granulomatous inflammation of lungs, nasal passages and kidneys is likely to have an environmental cause, the pathological changes being a consequence of inflammation resulting from secondary disturbances of the immune defences. This is in keeping with Wegener's original suggestion that the disease is an altered response to an infective organism. An outline of a proposed pathogenesis is shown in Fig. 40.2 [9].

Pathology

The pulmonary lesions are characterized by the presence of confluent or isolated areas of basophilic necrosis that frequently display cavities or crevices [40,41]. Communi-

cation with a sizeable bronchus may occur, resulting in evacuation of the necrotic material. The lesion may look distinctly suppurative, resembling an abscess or a septic infarct. Eosinophils are present throughout the lesion and are more numerous within the necrotic core where destructive angiitis of muscular arteries and veins can be seen (Fig. 40.3). The tissue around the foci of necrosis consists of fibroblastic and histiocytic proliferation with variable numbers of giant cells (Fig. 40.4). Scanty lymphocytes and plasma cells are also seen in the tissue surrounding the necrotic areas. Similar pathology may be seen in other affected organs.

The renal lesion is a focal necrotizing glomerulonephritis [26,28]. Fibrinoid necrosis with destruction of one or more glomerular capillary loops, along with a neutrophil infiltrate, is characteristic. Granulomatous change may be seen around affected glomeruli, as may necrotizing

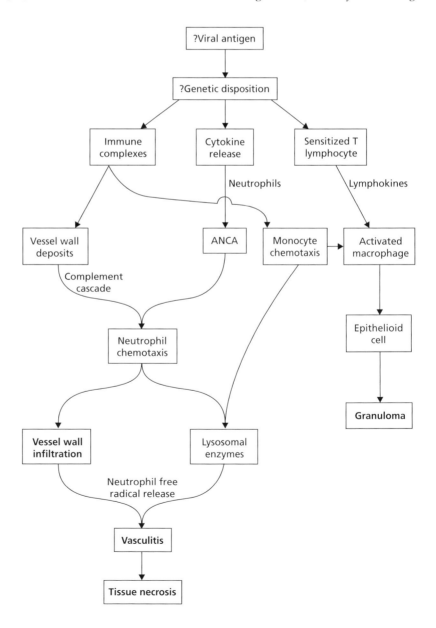

Fig. 40.2 Proposed pathogenesis of Wegener's granulomatosis. (Adapted from Leavitt & Fauci [9].)

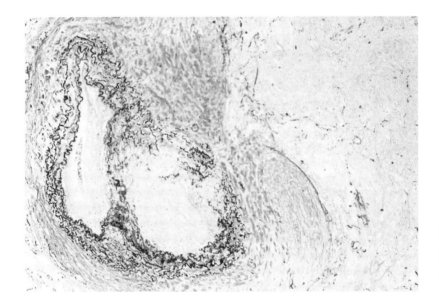

Fig. 40.3 Lung biopsy from Wegener's lesion stained for elastic tissue showing destruction and loss of elastic laminae and partial obliteration of lumen in artery adjacent to area of necrosis (elastic van Gieson ×35)

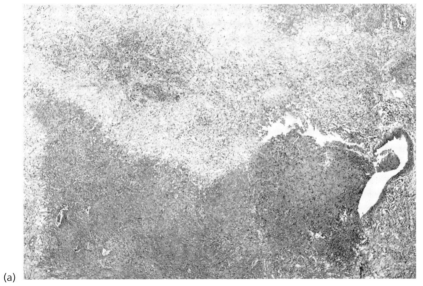

(a)

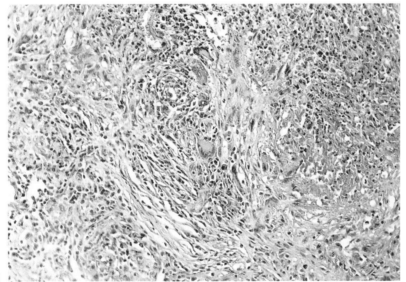

(b)

Fig. 40.4 (a) Open lung biopsy specimen from patient with Wegener's granulomatosis showing darkly stained area of necrosis with involvement of small airway (haematoxylin & eosin ×25). (b) Higher-power view of same lesion showing poorly formed granuloma with giant cells and chronic inflammatory cells (haematoxylin & eosin ×110)

vasculitis of small and medium-sized vessels. When healing occurs following treatment, the changes seen are hyalinization of affected areas, capsular adhesions and epithelial crescent formation in Bowman's capsule. With suitable immunofluorescent stains it is often possible to demonstrate immunoglobulin or complement deposition in the glomerular capillary membrane and/or mesangium.

Clinical features

The clinical expressions of Wegener's granulomatosis are diverse and the patient may present initially to practitioners from almost any branch of medicine [42,43]. Neither sex predominates. The course varies from a very acute systemic illness with dramatic pulmonary and renal manifestations to a much more chronic, often nasal, inflammatory condition, although acute presentations are more usual. Chronic courses are more frequent in those without renal involvement. In the large National Institutes of Health (NIH) series, most patients at presentation had evidence of upper airways involvement and fewer than half had lung involvement, although this developed in almost all eventually. Renal disease at presentation was relatively uncommon but developed in almost 80% within 2 years; similarly, eye involvement increased from 15 to 50% over the same period [43]. The main nasal symptoms are rhinorrhoea, nasal mucosal ulceration or sinusitis. To these may be added respiratory symptoms such as cough and haemoptysis. Alternative presentations are with systemic symptoms, such as anorexia, malaise, fever, weight loss and arthralgia, or with involvement of other organs such as the skin, eye or ear. When the diagnosis is suspected haematuria and proteinuria should always be sought as evidence of renal involvement. The most common systems involved are discussed below.

Upper respiratory tract

Nasopharyngeal lesions can include mucosal ulceration with crusting, perforation of the nasal septum and varying degrees of sinusitis. In chronic cases, saddle nose deformity may occur but erosion of skin or palate as seen in midline granuloma does not [15]. 'Strawberry gums' or hyperplastic gingivae that are red to purple in colour with many petechiae may be seen [44,45]. Radiographs of the nasal sinuses may show obliteration due to chronic bacterial infection, resulting in sinus wall thickening and new bone formation [46]. Biopsies usually show either acute or chronic inflammation, with granulomas or vasculitis in only 50% of cases [15].

Lower respiratory tract

Respiratory tract symptoms may lead to the finding of an abnormal chest film [47]. The most common finding is of solitary or multiple nodules 1–10 cm or more in diameter and these may cavitate (Fig. 40.5). Rarely, rupture of a cavitated nodule may result in pneumothorax; even more rarely a cavitated nodule may be colonized by an aspergilloma [48–50]. The radiological appearances are very variable [47,51]. Nodular and alveolar infiltrates are commonly seen on chest radiographs and may appear relatively insignificant. Such findings should not lull one into a false sense of security if other clinical features are present to suggest the diagnosis. Alveolar infiltrates may be due to intrapulmonary haemorrhage, which is more common that was once thought and may be detected by increases in diffusing capacity for carbon monoxide [52,53]. Small pleural effusions may occur. Endobronchial involvement is not uncommon and may result in large airway stenosis or lobar collapse [54,55]. CT may be helpful in providing evidence of vascular involvement, showing vessels leading into nodules and small peripheral densities suggestive of microinfarcts [56].

Functionally, patients with Wegener's granulomatosis frequently have decreased lung volumes and diffusing capacity, although airways obstruction is even more common and presumably reflects endobronchial disease [57]. The defects in pulmonary function improve with therapy but a persistent decrease in diffusing capacity is often found.

Urogenital

There may be no renal tract manifestations at the time of presentation. More commonly, microscopic or macroscopic haematuria with proteinuria is found. If renal failure is not established at presentation, it may develop rapidly and progressively and is the principal reason for seeking an urgent pathological diagnosis and initiating chemotherapy as soon as possible. Renal failure carries a poor prognosis but, even when established, recovery is possible with present-day therapy [25,58–60]. Other, uncommon urogenital manifestations include involvement of prostate, testes, ureter and penis [61].

Eyes

Eye manifestations are found eventually in some 60% of patients [15,43], including corneal/scleral ulceration, granulomatous keratitis or uveitis, conjunctivitis, proptosis, orbital pseudotumour, dry eyes, retinal vein occlusion and retinal artery thrombosis [62,63].

Ears

The ear is also involved in about 60% of patients [15]. The patient may present with serous or purulent otitis media, usually secondary to nasopharyngeal ulceration and obstruction of the eustachian tube [64,65]. The middle ear

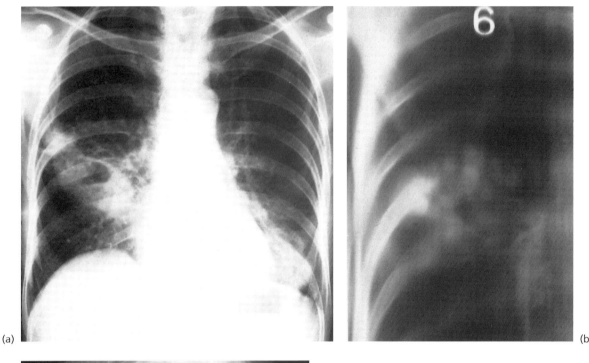

(a)

(b)

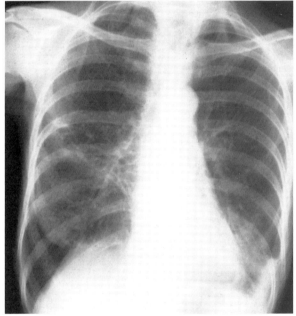

(c)

Fig. 40.5 Chest films of patient acutely ill with Wegener's granulomatosis: (a) cavities in consolidation in right mid zone and consolidation at left base; (b) tomography of one of the lesions just after commencement of treatment showing its nodular structure; (c) residual fibrosis after 1 month of prednisolone and cyclophosphamide.

and mastoid may be destroyed by granulomatous tissue, with associated lesions of cranial nerves, most commonly the fifth, seventh, ninth and twelfth [65,66]. Sensorineural hearing loss may occur due to cochlear inflammation [65].

Skin

Skin and mucosal involvement occurs in up to 50% of cases [15]. In one review of 75 patients with dermatological manifestations, the most frequent findings were palpable purpura and oral ulcers, with skin nodules, skin ulcers and necrotic papules occurring less commonly [67]. Other manifestations included gum hyperplasia, pustules, digital necrosis and livedo reticularis. In general the purpuric lesions were associated with vasculitic histopathology and the non-purpuric with granulomas.

Joints

Polyarthralgia is common and is seen in about 50% of cases [15]. In most series, true arthritis has been less common, although it was present in the majority of patients in one report, presumably representing selection bias [68].

Heart

Cardiac disease as a presenting manifestation of Wegener's granulomatosis must be very rare indeed, although subtle cardiac involvement in established cases is probably less so. The most frequent manifestations are pericarditis, myocarditis and dysrhythmias due to coronary vasculitis [15,69,70]. Aortitis and aortic valvulitis with sterile endocarditis have been reported [70,71]. The availability of ANCA allows the diagnosis to be made more readily than previously and the condition should be considered in cardiac disease of obscure aetiology.

Nervous system

Central nervous system involvement can occur with direct invasion by granulomatous tissue from ear or sinus, with resultant cranial nerve involvement. Remote granulomatous involvement of the brain is also recognized [72]. Vasculitic lesions of the peripheral nervous system may give rise to mononeuritis multiplex, while central nervous system vasculitis may result in thrombosis or haemorrhage in brain tissue.

Gastrointestinal system

Gastrointestinal involvement is not common but patients have been described presenting with features more typical of inflammatory bowel disease, and severe haemorrhage has been recorded in patients with vasculitis of bowel [73–75].

Investigations

Most patients have a normochromic, normocytic anaemia with a raised erythrocyte sedimentation rate, leucocytosis and hyperglobulinaemia. Plasma levels of C-reactive protein are raised and, although not specific for this disease, have been used as an index of activity [76]. As discussed above, a positive test for ANCA, especially those of the diffuse type (cANCA), in conjunction with consistent clinical features is as close as there is to a diagnostic test [31,77] (see Fig. 40.1).

Differential diagnosis

Where the clinical findings are suggestive, no time should be wasted before obtaining biopsies of the involved organs, most commonly the upper respiratory tract and the lungs. Renal biopsy should be considered even in the absence of renal manifestations, since early renal disease may be detected and confirm the diagnosis.

The differential diagnosis is wide-ranging and includes conditions as diverse as polychondritis and Behçet's disease. Other vasculitic diseases may need to be considered, such as polyarteritis, systemic lupus erythematosus and Churg–Strauss syndrome, other granulomatous diseases such as sarcoidosis and the infectious granulomatoses and neoplastic diseases such as nasopharyngeal lymphoma or pulmonary Hodgkin's disease. Finally, the other principal pulmonary–renal condition, Goodpasture's syndrome, frequently enters into the differential diagnosis. In children, diagnostic confusion with Henoch–Schönlein purpura has been recorded [17].

Treatment

The management of the condition may be tailored to the presenting clinical course. It has to be said that as the condition is rare, guidance on treatment at present is based on the results of case series rather than on controlled trials, and these are largely (and almost inevitably) derived from highly specialized centres where selection bias ensures that the case mix is atypical. There is therefore an important need for exercising good clinical judgement in interpreting the literature in relation to one's individual patient. Having said this, there is no real dispute about the management of ill patients with progressive lung or renal disease, who require to be treated vigorously with corticosteroids and cyclophosphamide in high dose in order to induce remission. The problem of how to treat arises mainly in those less ill patients in whom the course is slowly progressive and the diagnosis made early, the disease being primarily granulomatous and confined to lungs and upper airways. In such patients, co-trimoxazole may be effective in a dose of 960 mg twice daily [78,79]. If this does not bring about improvement within 6–8 weeks, prednisolone 40 mg on alternate days should be added, reserving the further addition of cyclophosphamide 2 mg/kg daily for those who still fail to respond [77].

In most cases the presentation warrants treatment with corticosteroids and cyclophosphamide. The NIH group originally reported 93% complete remission in 85 patients using an induction regimen of cyclophosphamide 2 mg/kg and prednisolone 1 mg/kg [15]. More recently they have reported improvement in 91% and complete remission in 75% of 180 patients, mostly treated with the same regimen though including some less severely affected patients treated with cyclophosphamide, other cytotoxic drugs or steroids alone or in combination [43]. However, 50% of remitting patients suffered relapse, although half of all remissions lasted at least 5 years. There was a 13% mortality, either from the disease itself or from side-effects of treatment, and almost all patients suffered some side-effects. Even after a 10-year remission, some 20% of patients relapse.

The usual starting dose of prednisolone of 1 mg/kg daily may be increased in severely ill patients. Once complete remission has been achieved, usually within about 4 weeks, the prednisolone is changed to an alternate-day regimen; if remission is maintained, the prednisolone is tapered to zero over about 1 year depending on the clinical response. Cyclophosphamide is usually started at 2 mg/kg daily or more in severe cases and continued for a year after complete remission has been achieved, when a slow but graduated reduction in dosage (25 mg every 2–3 months) can be made to zero if no relapse occurs. If relapse occurs, therapy has to be restarted or increased. Cyclophosphamide causes serious side-effects; cystitis occurred in 43% of the NIH series, bladder cancer in 3% and myelodysplasia in 2%. The dose may have to be reduced to ensure a leucocyte count of greater than 3×10^9/L, with a neutrophil count of 1×10^9/L. Other side-effects of cyclophosphamide include hair-thinning, an increased incidence of herpes zoster, gonadal dysfunction and rarely, but significantly, the later development of leukaemia or lymphoma [80–83]. The side-effects of the steroids are as expected and include a much increased risk of infections, though this can be reduced by alternate-day therapy.

The major challenge in treating Wegener's granulomatosis relates to prevention and management of side-effects. If these are unacceptable, therapy with methotrexate may be effective [84]. Azathioprine has also proved successful in occasional cases [85], but neither of these drugs has become established as first-line treatment. Other experimental therapies have included plasmapheresis and transfusion of pooled gamma globulin [22,25,76,86–88]. If renal failure develops, dialysis and even renal transplantation may be necessary [15].

There has been much discussion of the value of serial ANCA titres in monitoring response and detecting early relapse. There is a general relationship between level of antibodies, severity of disease and risk of relapse, and concentrations fall with successful treatment. However, the finding of high or rising ANCA in a patient on treatment is not a sure indication that relapse is imminent and should probably only be taken as a guide to more careful follow-up rather than as an indication for increasing the therapy [89,90]. As always, good clinical judgement should be used in a patient on treatment who shows rising ANCA, in balancing the risks of increasing the dose against those of side-effects; the patient's clinical status should generally be the main determinant of change in therapy.

Finally, the occasional mechanical complication may persist in large airways despite standard treatment. Such endobronchial obstruction has been shown to respond to radiotherapy and bougienage or to stenting [55,91].

Prognosis

The condition, when recognized, was uniformly fatal prior to the introduction of corticosteroids; these drugs alone made little long-term difference, with a mean survival of 5 months and 90% of patients dead within 2 years [92]. Better recognition of the condition allows diagnosis in a relatively benign category with a much better prognosis than that of the more common progressive disease, though one suspects that many of these, treated initially with co-trimoxazole, relapse later. Of those requiring standard cyclophosphamide and corticosteroid treatment, more than 80% can be expected to be alive at 5 years [43,93]. However, as noted above, there is a large cost in terms of therapeutic side-effects, including late development of lymphomas and bladder cancer. The patient is probably never free of the risk of relapse, even when complete and prolonged remission appears to have occurred, and life-long outpatient supervision is advisable [85].

Limited Wegener's granulomatosis

In 1966 Carrington and Liebow identified a group of 16 patients with otherwise typical Wegener's granulomatosis in whom renal disease was not present [94–96]. A positive ANCA test is less frequent than in the classical form of the disease. There may be involvement of other tissues such as the skin and eye [1,62,63]. The pulmonary lesions in this condition predominate in the lower lobes and the most common form is a discrete lesion greater than 1 cm in diameter. In two-thirds of cases the lesions are multiple and bilateral and in one-third cavitation occurs.

The patients usually present with lower respiratory tract symptoms with variable degrees of systemic upset, although a lesion may be discovered at routine radiographic examination of an asymptomatic patient. The disease appears to follow a less aggressive course than classical Wegener's granulomatosis, although relapse after treatment is not infrequent and may be in a more aggressive form with renal involvement [85]. A 20% 5-year mortality was reported prior to modern treatment [95]. Death has occurred from progressive involvement of the lung or massive haemorrhage from a cavitating lesion but is more likely now as a result of relapse to a more aggressive form.

This condition responds to steroids and should be treated with both cyclophosphamide or azathioprine and corticosteroids as for the classical form of the disease [1].

Midline granuloma (nasal T-cell lymphoma)

Midline granuloma is a localized process characterized by

a pansinusitis and destructive lesions of the nasal septum and soft and hard palate. The process is localized to the upper airway, although ulceration can occur through skin [97]. If left untreated, death eventually ensues from cachexia, haemorrhage, meningitis or infection [98]. Biopsies of involved tissue reveal acute and chronic inflammation with necrosis and it is unusual to see granulomas or vasculitis [99,100]. There is no associated systemic disease. It must be differentiated from Wegener's granulomatosis, nasal carcinoma and infectious diseases [100]. Recent evidence indicates that it is a locally invasive lymphoma of T-cell variety [101,102]. There are interesting geographical variations in its incidence and it is more common in the Orient. In many cases, Epstein–Barr virus has been demonstrated in the malignant T lymphocytes and may be causative [103–105]. Radiation therapy has proved successful in arresting the process, although management should be discussed with appropriate lymphoma specialists if possible [87,98,100].

Lymphomatoid granulomatosis

Pathology

Histologically, lymphomatoid granulomatosis is a necrotizing angiocentric and angiodestructive infiltrative process composed of small lymphocytes, plasma cells, histiocytes and atypical lymphoreticular cells. It predominantly involves the lungs, although infiltration of skin, kidney and the nervous system is not uncommon [1,106]. Upper airway lesions are unusual [106]. Recent evidence suggests that the pulmonary manifestation of this condition, in contrast to cutaneous and head and neck manifestations, may be predominantly an Epstein–Barr virus-associated B-cell lymphoma with a marked T-cell reaction leading to the vasculitis [107]. However, this hypothesis is based on study of small numbers of cases and it would not be surprising if other series showed different results in the future.

Clinical features

In a study of 152 patients there was a male/female ratio of 1.7:1 [106]. Most patients present with chest and/or systemic symptoms such as fever or malaise. Neurological signs, including peripheral neuropathy, are not uncommon. Laboratory investigations are generally unhelpful. The chest film shows a similar frequency and distribution of nodular masses, cavitation and migratory lesions as are seen in Wegener's granulomatosis [108]. However, reticulonodular changes are seen in lymphomatoid granulomatosis and not in Wegener's granulomatosis. A skin rash, most commonly raised and erythematous, and neurological signs are the most common extrapulmonary findings and renal involvement may occur.

Treatment and prognosis

The median survival of the 152 patients in the original series of Katzenstein and colleagues [106] was 14 months and 94% were dead by 3 years; 12% of all patients developed generalized evidence of lymphoma. The outcome appeared to be independent of any therapy employed, including steroid and cytotoxic drugs. Before the lymphomatous nature of the condition was recognized there were reports of response of localized disease to radiotherapy [109], and in one study 7 of 15 patients achieved complete remission for a mean of 5.2 years with cyclophosphamide 2 mg/kg and prednisolone 1 mg/kg [110]. Current advice would be to regard the condition as a low-grade lymphoma *ab initio* and treat it accordingly, bearing in mind the toxic effects of antineoplastic drugs and the relatively benign course of low-grade lymphomas [111].

Benign lymphocytic angiitis and granulomatosis

Pathology

This very rare clinical entity is characterized by pulmonary infiltrates consisting of lymphocytes, plasma cells and histiocytes, with lymphocytic infiltration of arteries and veins [41,112,113]. Compression or infiltration of the walls of the bronchioles that resembles bronchiolitis obliterans is commonly seen. The chest radiographic appearances are most frequently of a single nodule but may show other features similar to Wegener's granulomatosis. It is now regarded as a T-cell lymphoproliferative disease but is probably not a malignant lymphoma [114].

Clinical features

The condition may present with symptoms suggesting respiratory tract infection or be discovered incidentally on routine chest radiography. It is one of the lung conditions that may appear in HIV infection [115]. Extrapulmonary involvement is uncommon but skin and eye lesions have been reported.

Treatment and prognosis

It is frequent for the lung lesions to wax and wane and for opacities to clear spontaneously with minimal residual fibrosis, only to be followed by the development of fresh lesions elsewhere. Development into lymphomatoid granulomatosis has been described [5]. Corticosteroid therapy is ineffective, although cytotoxic drugs, particularly chlorambucil, have been reported to be effective in producing remission [40,41].

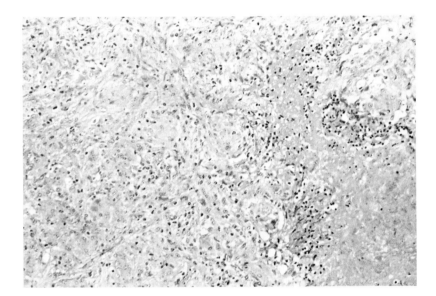

Fig. 40.6 Lung biopsy from patient with necrotizing sarcoid granulomatosis showing irregular necrosis to the right of a zone of confluent epithelioid granulomas (haematoxylin & eosin ×120).

Necrotizing sarcoid granulomatosis

Pathology

First described by Liebow in 1973 [1], this condition is characterized by pulmonary lesions with granulomatous vasculitis and pneumonitis against a background of sarcoid-like granulomas and parenchymal necrosis of variable extent (Fig. 40.6). Muscular pulmonary arteries and veins are infiltrated by histiocytes, spindled mononuclear cells, lymphocytes and giant cells, with a tendency towards marked involvement of the subintima [116,117].

Clinical features

The disease is three to five times more common in women than men and the average age at presentation is 50 years. Patients may be entirely asymptomatic or may present with chest pain, cough or dyspnoea with or without systemic features such as malaise, fever, night sweats, weight loss and lethargy [116–119]. Extrapulmonary involvement is unusual but granulomatous disease of the nervous system has been described.

The chest film most commonly shows bilateral nodules or nodular infiltrates, although solitary nodules have been seen (Fig. 40.7). Miliary shadowing, hilar lymphadenopathy and pleural effusions have been recorded.

Treatment and prognosis

The condition may resolve spontaneously [116] though in most cases resolution has been achieved either with corticosteroid therapy or surgical resection of a single lesion. It remains possible that this pathological entity is simply a variant of sarcoidosis since there are many immunological parallels [5,120]. The author has reviewed one case that progressed to a fatal conclusion, with widespread pulmonary arteritis and pulmonary hypertension, owing to a foolish medicolegal misdiagnosis of asbestosis.

Bronchocentric granulomatosis

Pathology

The characteristic feature of bronchocentric granulomatosis is a necrotizing granulomatous reaction centred around airways (Fig. 40.8). Large and small airways are involved but the most marked changes are in the periphery, where irregular necrotic lesions lie within collapsed consolidated lung tissue. The necrotic lesions consist of airways with ulceration of the surface epithelium and cellular debris within the lumen, often with irregular masses of eosinophils. Occasional true epithelioid granulomas are present in the tissues surrounding the necrotic lesions. There is a variable but often marked peribronchial inflammatory infiltrate in which eosinophils may be prominent. Proximal bronchi may show plugging by inspissated material and there may be chondritis and cartilage destruction within their walls. Pulmonary arteritis is not a major feature and when it occurs is secondary to the bronchial and parenchymal infiltration [1,121,122].

Clinical features

Patients with bronchocentric granulomatosis divide into two groups: those with and those without asthma [121,123]. The asthmatic patients present with chest-related symptoms such as cough, haemoptysis, dyspnoea, wheeze and chest pain, whereas the non-asthmatics tend to present with non-specific symptoms such as malaise, fever or fatigue.

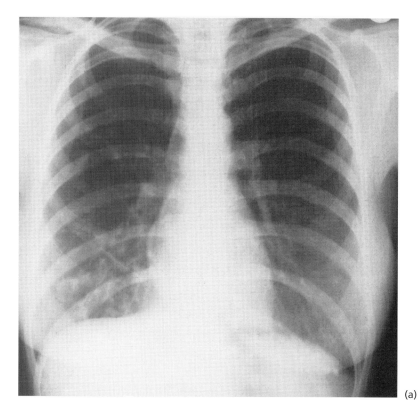

(a)

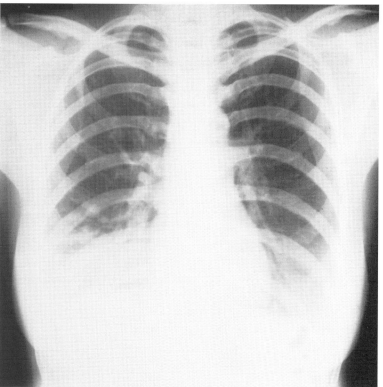

(b)

Fig. 40.7 Chest films of patient with necrotizing sarcoid granulomatosis: (a) nodular lesions in right lung, originally thought to be metastases; (b) 2 weeks later, showing increasing consolidation also at right base.

The radiological appearance is commonly that of a solitary mass lesion, most often in the upper lobe, although alveolar and reticulonodular infiltrates have also been described [124]. Adenopathy and cavitation are uncommon. Asthmatic patients tend to be younger and have peripheral blood eosinophilia, positive skin tests, and precipitins and elevated IgE levels to *Aspergillus fumigatus*. This organism may be present in sputum or lung biopsy

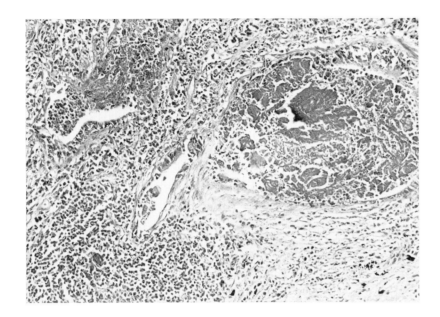

Fig. 40.8 Section of lung resected from patient with bronchocentric granulomatosis. Small bronchi are seen with walls partly destroyed by a florid infiltrate with lymphocytes and eosinophils and intraluminar cellular and granular debris (haematoxylin & eosin ×85).

specimens [121,122], and pathological appearances of bronchocentric granulomatosis are frequently present in lung specimens resected from patients with typical bronchopulmonary aspergillosis [125]. The asthmatics have an eosinophil pulmonary infiltrate, whereas the non-asthmatics have a predominance of neutrophils. It has been postulated that the main requirement for the development of bronchocentric granulomatosis is a sustained inflammatory insult within the lumen, often associated with proximal bronchial obstruction and distension of distal airways by retained secretions and cellular debris [122]. In the asthmatic, the allergic response to *Aspergillus* (or other fungus) provides the insult [121]. In the non-asthmatics the insult is usually unidentified though inter-esting case reports of bronchocentric granulomatosis in association with tuberculosis, echinococcosis, ankylosing spondylitis and seropositive arthritis suggest that it may be varied [126–130].

Treatment and prognosis

Most patients with this disease are diagnosed after thoracotomy and resection of the diseased lung effects a cure; some patients require corticosteroids for some time postoperatively [121,123,131]. For those with residual or recurrent disease, corticosteroid therapy is recommended with an initial dosage of 40 mg of prednisolone daily, tapering once remission is achieved.

References

1 Liebow AA. The J. Burns Amberson lecture: pulmonary angiitis and granulomatosis. *Am Rev Respir Dis* 1973; 108: 1.

2 Saldana MJ, Patchefsky AS, Israel HJ, Atkinson WG. Pulmonary angiitis and granulomatosis. The relationship between histological features, organ involvement and response to treatment. *Hum Pathol* 1977; 8: 391.

3 Fauci AS. The spectrum of vasculitis. *Ann Intern Med* 1978; 89: 660.

4 Edwards CW. Vasculitis and granulomatosis of the respiratory tract. *Thorax* 1982; 37: 81.

5 Churg A. Pulmonary angiitis and granulomatosis revisited. *Hum Pathol* 1983; 14: 868.

6 Fauci AS. Vasculitis. *J Allergy Clin Immunol* 1983; 72: 211.

7 Dreisin RB. Pulmonary vasculitis. *Clin Chest Med* 1982; 3: 607.

8 Vath RR, Alexander CB, Fulmer JD. The lymphocytic infiltrative lung diseases. *Clin Chest Med* 1982; 3: 619.

9 Leavitt RY, Fauci AS. Pulmonary vasculitis. *Am Rev Respir Dis* 1986; 134: 149.

10 Klinger H. Grenzformen der Periarteritis nodosa. *Frankfurt Z Pathol* 1931; 42: 455.

11 Wegener F. Uber generalisierte septische Geffasserkrankungen. *Verh Dtsch Pathol Ges* 1936; 29: 202.

12 Godman GC, Churg A. Wegener's granulomatosis: pathology and review of the literature. *Arch Pathol* 1954; 58: 533.

13 Fauci AS, Wolff SM. Wegener's granulomatosis: studies in eighteen patients and a review of the literature. *Medicine* 1973; 52: 535.

14 McDonald TJ, DeRemee RA. Wegener's granulomatosis. *Laryngoscope* 1983; 93: 220.

15 Fauci AS, Haynes BF, Katz P, Wolff SM. Wegener's granulomatosis: prospective clinical and therapeutic experience with 85 patients for 21 years. *Ann Intern Med* 1983; 98: 76.

16 Carruthers DM, Watts RA, Symmons DP, Scott DG. Wegener's granulomatosis: increased incidence or increased recognition? *Br J Rheumatol* 1996; 35: 142.

17 Hall SL, Miller LC, Duggan E *et al.*

Wegener's granulomatosis in pediatric patients. *J Pediatr* 1985; 106: 739.

18 Elkon KB, Sutherland DC, Rees AJ *et al.* HLA antigen frequencies in systemic vasculitis: increase in HLA-DR2 in Wegener's granulomatosis. *Arthritis Rheum* 1983; 26: 102.

19 Fernandez HN, Henson PM, Otani A, Hugli TE. Chemotactic response to human C3a and C5a anaphylotoxins. *J Immunol* 1978; 120: 109.

20 Daniele RP. Immune complex injury of the lung. *Am Rev Respir Dis* 1981; 124: 738.

21 Pinching AJ, Rees AJ, Pussell BA *et al.* Relapses in Wegener's granulomatosis: the role of infection. *Br Med J* 1980; 281: 836.

22 Cairns SA, Solomon LR, Loudon RA *et al.* Circulating immune complexes and the treatment of Wegener's granulomatosis. *Nephron* 1981; 29: 90.

23 Hui AN, Ehresmann GR, Quismorio FP *et al.* Wegener's granulomatosis: electron microscopic and immunofluorescent studies. *Chest* 1981; 80: 753.

24 Shasby DM, Schwarz MI, Forstot JZ *et al.* Pulmonary immune complex deposition in

Wegener's granulomatosis. *Chest* 1982; 81: 338.

25 Pinching AJ, Lockwood CM, Pussell BA *et al*. Wegener's granulomatosis: observations on 18 patients with severe renal disease. *Q J Med* 1983; 52: 435.

26 Novak RF, Christiansen RG, Sorenson ET. The acute vasculitis of Wegener's granulomatosis in renal biopsies. *Am J Clin Pathol* 1982; 78: 367.

27 Gephardt GN, Ahmad M, Tubbs RR. Pulmonary vasculitis (Wegener's granulomatosis). Immunohistochemical study of T and B cell markers. *Am J Med* 1983; 74: 700.

28 Weiss MA, Crissman JD. Renal biopsy findings in Wegener's granulomatosis. *Hum Pathol* 1984; 15: 943.

29 Ronco P, Verroust P, Mignon F *et al*. Immunopathological studies of polyarteritis nodosa and Wegener's granulomatosis: a report of 43 patients with 51 renal biopsies. *Q J Med* 1983; 52: 212.

30 Spector WG, Heesom N. The production of granulomata by antigen–antibody complexes. *J Pathol* 1969; 98: 31.

31 Van der Woude FJ, Rasmussen N, Lobatto S *et al*. Autoantibodies against neutrophils and monocytes: tool for diagnosis and marker of disease activity in Wegener's granulomatosis. *Lancet* 1985; i: 425.

32 Nolle B, Specks U, Ludemann MS, Rohrbach MS, DeRemee RA, Gross WL. Anticytoplasmic autoantibodies: their immunodiagnostic value in Wegener's granulomatosis. *Ann Intern Med* 1989; 111: 28.

33 Cohen Tervaert JW, van der Woude FJ, Fauci AS *et al*. Association between active Wegener's granulomatosis and anticytoplasmic antibodies. *Arch Intern Med* 1989; 149: 2461.

34 Ludemann J, Utecht B, Gross WG. Antineutrophil cytoplasmic antibodies in Wegener's granulomatosis recognise an elastolytic enzyme. *J Exp Med* 1990; 171: 357.

35 Ulmer M, Rautmann A, Gross WL. Immunodiagnostic aspects of autoantibodies against myeloperoxidase. *Clin Nephrol* 1992; 37: 161.

36 Davenport A, Lock RJ, WallingtonTB. Clinical relevance of testing for antineutrophil cytoplasm antibodies (ANCA) with a standard indirect immunofluorescence ANCA test in patients with upper or lower respiratory tract symptoms. *Thorax* 1994; 49: 213.

37 Falk RJ, Terrell RS, Charles LA. Antineutrophil cytoplasmic antibodies induce neutrophils to degranulate and produce oxygen radicals *in vitro*. *Proc Natl Acad Sci USA* 1990; 87: 4115.

38 Mayet WJ, Schwarting A, Zumbuschenfelde KHM. Cytotoxic effects of antibodies to proteinase 3 (c-ANCA) on human endothelial cells. *Clin Exp Immunol* 1994; 98: 458.

39 Brower E, Stegeman CA, Heistema MG, Limburg PC, Callenberg CGM. T cell reactivity to proteinase 3 and myeloperoxidase in patients with Wegener's granulomatosis. *Clin Exp Immunol* 1994; 98: 448.

40 Israel HL, Patchefsky AS, Saldana MJ. Wegener's granulomatosis, lymphomatoid granulomatosis and benign lymphocytic angiitis and granulomatosis of lung. *Ann Intern Med* 1977; 87: 691.

41 Saldana MJ, Patchefsky AS, Israel HL, Atkinson WG. Pulmonary angiitis and granulomatosis. The relationship between histological features, organ involvement and responses to treatment. *Hum Pathol* 1977; 8: 391.

42 DeRemee RA. Wegener's granulomatosis. In: James DG, ed. *Sarcoidosis and Other Granulomatous Disorders*. New York: Marcel Decker, 1994: 657.

43 Hoffman GS, Kerr GS, Leavitt RY *et al*. Wegener granulomatosis: an analysis of 158 patients. *Ann Intern Med* 1992; 116: 488.

44 Cohen PS, Meltzer JA. Strawberry gums. A sign of Wegener's granulomatosis. *JAMA* 1981; 246: 2610.

45 Handlers JP, Waterrnan J, Abrams AM, Melrose RJ. Oral features of Wegener's granulomatosis. *Arch Otolaryngol* 1985; 111: 267.

46 Paling MR, Roberts RL, Fauci AS. Paranasal sinus obliteration in Wegener's granulomatosis. *Radiology* 1982; 144: 539.

47 Farrelly CA. Wegener's granulomatosis: a radiological review of the pulmonary manifestations at initial presentation and during relapse. *Clin Radiol* 1982; 33: 545.

48 Epstein DM, Gefter WB, Miller WT *et al*. Spontaneous pneumothorax: an uncommon manifestation of Wegener granulomatosis. *Radiol J* 1980; 35: 327.

49 Aspan TJ, Davidson AM, Walker WC. Spontaneous pneumothorax in Wegener's granulomatosis. *Thorax* 1982; 37: 774.

50 Martens J. Pulmonary aspergilloma: an unusual complication in Wegener's granulomatosis. *Postgrad Med J* 1982; 58: 55.

51 Cordier JF, Valeyre D, Guillevin L, Loire R, Brechot JM. Pulmonary Wegener's granulomatosis: a clinical and imaging study of 77 cases. *Chest* 1990; 97: 906.

52 Stokes TC, McCann BG, Rees RT *et al*. Acute fulminating intrapulmonary haemorrhage in Wegener's granulomatosis. *Thorax* 1982; 37: 315.

53 Haworth SJ, Savage COS, Carr D *et al*. Pulmonary haemorrhage complicating Wegener's granulomatosis and microscopic polyarteritis. *Br Med J* 1985; 290: 1775.

54 Lampaman JH, Querubin R, Kondapalli P. Subglottic stenosis in Wegener's granulomatosis. *Chest* 1981; 79: 230.

55 Amin R. Endobronchial involvement in Wegener's granulomatosis. *Postgrad Med J* 1983; 59: 452.

56 Kuhlman JE, Hruban RH, Fishman EK. Wegener granulomatosis: CT features of parenchymal lung disease. *J Comput Assist Tomogr* 1991; 15: 948.

57 Rosenberg DM, Weinberger SE, Fulmer JD *et al*. Functional correlates of lung involvement in Wegener's granulomatosis. *Am J Med* 1980; 69: 387.

58 Berry S, Greene J, Park HS *et al*. Return of renal function after renal insufficiency with cyclosphosphamide therapy in Wegener's granulomatosis. *Arch Intern Med* 1981; 141: 544.

59 Van der Woude FJ, Hoorntje SJ, Weening JJ *et al*. Renal involvement in Wegener's granulomatosis. *Nephron* 1982; 32: 185.

60 Garrett PJ, Dewhurst AG, Morgan LS, Mason JC, Dathan JR. Renal disease associated with circulating antineutrophil cytoplasm activity. *Q J Med* 1992; 85: 731.

61 Huong DL, Papo T, Piette JC *et al*. Urogenital manifestations of Wegener granulomatosis. *Medicine* 1995; 74: 152.

62 Spalton DJ, Graham EM, Page NGR, Sanders MD. Ocular changes in limited forms of Wegener's granulomatosis. *Br J Ophthalmol* 1981; 65: 553.

63 Stavrou P, Deutch J, Rene C, Laws DE, Luqmani RA, Murray PI. Ocular manifestations of classical and limited Wegener's granulomatosis. *Q J Med* 1993; 86: 719.

64 Nicklasson B, Stangeland N. Wegener's granulomatosis presenting as otitis media. *J Laryngol* 1982; 96: 277.

65 Branley PJ. Wegener's granulomatosis of the ear. *J Laryngol Otol* 1983; 97: 623.

66 Illum P, Thorling K. Otological manifestations of Wegener's granulomatosis. *Laryngoscope* 1982; 92: 801.

67 Frances C, Du LT, Piette JC *et al*. Wegener's granulomatosis: dermatological manifestations in 75 cases with clinicopathologic correlation. *Arch Dermatol* 1994; 130: 861.

68 Brandwein S, Esdaile J, Danoff D, Tannenbaum H. Wegener's granulomatosis. Clinical features and outcome in 13 patients. *Arch Intern Med* 1983; 143: 476.

69 Schiavone WA, Ahmad M, Ockner SA. Unusual cardiac complications of Wegener's granulomatosis. *Chest* 1985; 88: 745.

70 Goodfield NE, Bhandari S, Plant WD, Morley-Davies A, Sutherland GR. Cardiac involvement in Wegener's granulomatosis. *Br Heart J* 1995; 73: 110.

71 Gerbracht DD, Savage RW, Scharff N. Reversible valvulitis in Wegener's granulomatosis. *Chest* 1987; 92: 182.

72 Oimomi M, Suehiro I, Mizuno N *et al*. Wegener's granulomatosis with intracerebral granuloma and mammary manifestations. *Arch Intern Med* 1980; 140: 853.

73 Sokol RJ, Farrell MK, MacAdams AJ. An unusual presentation of Wegener's granulomatosis mimicking inflammatory bowel disease. *Gastroenterology* 1984; 87: 426.

74 Haworth SJ, Pusey CD. Severe intestinal involvement in Wegener's granulomatosis. *Gut* 1984; 25: 1296.

75 Coward RA, Gibbons CP, Brown CB *et al*. Gastrointestinal haemorrhage complicating Wegener's granulomatosis. *Br Med J* 1985; 291: 865.

76 Winearls CG, Hind CRK, Mason P, Pepys MB. Treatment of Wegener's granulomatosis. *Lancet* 1984; i: 634.

77 DeRemee RA. Wegener's granulomatosis. *Curr Opin Pulm Med* 1995; 1: 363.

78 DeRemee RA. The treatment of Wegener's granulomatosis with trimethoprim–sulfamethoxazole: illusion or vision? *Arthritis Rheum* 1988; 31: 1068.

79 West BC, Todd JR, King JW. Wegener granulomatosis and trimethoprim–sulfamethoxazole: complete remission after a twenty-year course. *Ann Intern Med* 1987; 106: 840.

80 Cupps TR, Silverman GJ, Fauci AS. Herpes zoster in patients with treated Wegener's granulomatosis. *Am J Med* 1980; 69: 881.

81 Wheeler GE. Cyclophosphamide associated leukaemia in Wegener's granulomatosis. *Ann Intern Med* 1981; 94: 361.

82 Morton CE, Easton DJ. Cytotoxic therapy for Wegener's granulomatosis. *Lancet* 1984; i: 1411.

83 Ambrus JL, Fauci AS. Diffuse histiocytic lymphoma in a patient treated with cyclophosphamide for Wegener's granulomatosis. *Am J Med* 1984; 76: 745.

84 Sneller MC, Hoffman GS, Talar-Williams C, Kerr GS, Hallahan CW, Fauci AS. An

analysis of forty-two Wegener's granulomatosis patients treated with methotrexate and prednisolone. *Arthritis Rheum* 1995; 38: 608.

85 Gordon M, Luqmani RA, Adu D *et al.* Relapses in patients with a systemic vasculitis. *Q J Med* 1993; 86: 779.

86 Alpern RJ. Vasculitis: it's time to reclassify. *Am J Med Sci* 1995; 309: 235.

87 Jayne DRW, Davies MJ, Fox CJV, Black CM, Lockwood CM. Treatment of systemic vasculitis with pooled intravenous immunoglobulin. *Lancet* 1991; 337: 1137.

88 Anon. Wegener's granulomatosis. *Lancet* 1984; i: 260.

89 D'Oliviera J, Gaskin G, Dash A, Rees AJ, Pusey CD. Relationship between disease activity and anti-neutrophil cytoplasmic antibody concentration in long-term management of systemic vasculitis. *Am J Kidney Dis* 1995; 25: 380.

90 Kerr GS, Fleisher TA, Hallahan CW, Leavitt RY, Fauci AS, Hoffman GS. Limited prognostic value of changes in antineutrophil cytoplasmic antibody titer in patients with Wegener's granulomatosis. *Arthritis Rheum* 1993; 36: 365.

91 Daum TE, Specks U, Colby TV *et al.* Tracheobronchial involvement in Wegener's granulomatosis. *Am J Respir Crit Care Med* 1995; 151: 522.

92 Walton EW. Giant cell granuloma of the respiratory tract (Wegener's granulomatosis). *Br Med J* 1958; ii: 265.

93 Fauci AS, Haynes BF, Katz P, Wolff SM. Wegener's granulomatosis: prospective clinical and therapeutic experience with 85 patients for 21 years. *Ann Intern Med* 1983; 98: 76.

94 Carrington CB, Liebow AA. Limited forms of angiitis and granulomatosis of Wegener's type. *Am J Med* 1966; 41: 497.

95 Cassan SM, Coles DT, Harrison EG. The concept of limited forms of Wegener's granulomatosis. *Am J Med* 1970; 49: 366.

96 Luqmani RA, Adu D, Michael J *et al.* Limited Wegener's granulomatosis: mild disease or distinct entity? *Arthritis Rheum* 1990; 33: S135.

97 Fauci AS, Johnston RE, Wolff SM. Radiation therapy of mid-line granuloma. *Ann Intern Med* 1976; 84: 140.

98 Friedmann I. McBride and the mid-facial granuloma syndrome. *J Laryngol Otol* 1982; 96: 1.

99 Crissman JD, Weiss MA, Gluckman J. Midline granuloma syndrome. *Am J Surg Pathol* 1982; 6: 335.

100 Tsokos M, Fauci AS, Costa J. Idiopathic midline destructive disease (IMDD). A sub-

group of patients with the 'mid-line granuloma syndrome'. *Am J Clin Pathol* 1982; 77: 162.

101 Cleary KR, Batsakis JG. Sinonasal lymphomas. *Ann Otol Rhinol Laryngol* 1994; 103: 911.

102 Aosaza K, Ohsawa M, Tomita S, Tagawa S, Yamamura T. Polymorphic reticulosis is a neoplasm of large granular lymphocytes with CD3+ phenotype. *Cancer* 1995; 75: 894.

103 Mishima K, Horiuchi K, Kojya S, Takahashi H, Ohsawa M, Aozasa K. Epstein–Barr virus in patients with polymorphic reticulosis (lethal midline granuloma) from China and Japan. *Cancer* 1994; 73: 3041.

104 Chan JK, Yip TT, Tsang WY *et al.* Detection of Epstein–Barr viral DNA in malignant lymphoma of the upper aerodigestive tract. *Am J Surg Pathol* 1994; 18: 938.

105 Kanavaros P, Lescs MC, Briere J *et al.* Nasal T-cell lymphoma: a clinicopathologic entity associated with peculiar phenotype and Epstein–Barr virus. *Blood* 1993; 81: 2688.

106 Katzenstein A-LA, Carrington CB, Liebow AA. Lymphomatoid granulomatosis. A clinicopathologic study of 152 cases. *Cancer* 1979; 43: 360.

107 Guinee D, Jaffe E, Kingma D *et al.* Pulmonary lymphomatoid granulomatosis. Evidence for a proliferation of Epstein–Barr virus infected B-lymphocytes with a prominent T-cell component and vasculitis. *Am J Surg Pathol* 1994; 18: 753.

108 Wechsler RJ, Steiner RM, Israel HL, Patchefsky AS. Chest radiograph in lymphomatoid granulomatosis: comparison with Wegener granulomatosis. *Am J Roentgenol* 1984; 142: 79.

109 DeRemee RA, Weiland LH, McDonald TJ. Respiratory vasculitis. *Mayo Clin Proc* 1980; 55: 492.

110 Fauci AS, Haynes BF, Costa J *et al.* Lymphomatoid granulomatosis. *N Engl J Med* 1982; 306: 68.

111 Cordier JF, Chailleux E, Lauque D *et al.* Primary pulmonary lymphomas. A clinical study of 70 cases in nonimmunocompromised patients. *Chest* 1993; 103: 201.

112 Gracey DR, DeRemee RA, Colby TV, Unni KK, Weiland LH. Benign lymphocytic angiitis and granulomatosis: experience with three cases. *Mayo Clin Proc* 1988; 63: 323.

113 Tukiainen H, Terho EO, Syrjanen K, Sutinen S. Benign lymphocytic angiitis and granulomatosis. *Thorax* 1988; 43: 649.

114 Vergier B, Capron F, Trojani M *et al.* Benign lymphocytic angiitis and granulomatosis: a T-cell lymphoma? *Hum Pathol* 1992; 23: 1191.

115 Calabrese LH, Estes M, Yen-Lieberman B

et al. Systemic vasculitis in association with human immunodeficiency virus infection. *Arthritis Rhem* 1989; 322: 569.

116 Koss MN, Hochholzer L, Feigin DS *et al.* Necrotising sarcoid-like granulomatosis: clinical, pathologic and immunopathologic findings. *Hum Pathol* 1980; 11 (Suppl 5), 510.

117 Churg A, Carrington CB, Gupta R. Necrotising sarcoid granulomatosis. *Chest* 1979; 76: 406.

118 Beach RC, Corrin B, Scopes JW, Graham E. Necrotising sarcoid granulomatosis with neurological lesions in a child. *J Pediatr* 1980; 97: 950.

119 Singh N, Cole S, Krause PJ *et al.* Necrotising sarcoid granulomatosis with extrapulmonary involvement. *Am Rev Respir Dis* 1981; 124: 189.

120 Spiteri MA, Gledhill A, Campbell D, Clarke SN. Necrotising sarcoid granulomatosis. *Br J Dis Chest* 1987; 81: 70.

121 Katzenstein A-L, Liebow AA, Friedman PJ. Bronchocentric granulomatosis, mucoid impaction and hypersensitivity reactions to fungi. *Am Rev Respir Dis* 1975; 111: 497.

122 Clee MD, Lamb D, Clark RA. Bronchocentric granulomatosis: a review and thoughts on pathogenesis. *Br J Dis Chest* 1983; 77: 227.

123 Koss MN, Robinson RG, Hochholzer L. Bronchocentric granulomatosis. *Hum Pathol* 1981; 12: 632.

124 Robinson RG, Wehunt WD, Tsou E *et al.* Bronchocentric granulomatosis: roentgenographic manifestations. *Am Rev Respir Dis* 1982; 125: 751.

125 Bosken CH, Myers JL, Greenberger PA, Katzenstein AL. Pathologic features of allergic bronchopulmonary aspergillosis. *Am J Surg Pathol* 1988; 12: 216.

126 Maguire GP, Lee M, Rosen Y, Lyons HA. Pulmonary tuberculosis and bronchocentric granulomatosis. *Chest* 1986; 89: 606.

127 Den Hertog RW, Wagenaar Sj Sc Westermann CJJ. Bronchocentric granulomatosis and echinococcosis. *Am Rev Respir Dis* 1982; 126: 344.

128 Rohatgi PK, Turrisi BC. Bronchocentric granulomatosis and ankylosing spondylitis. *Thorax* 1984; 39: 317.

129 Berendsen HH, Hofstee N, Kapsenberg PD *et al.* Bronchocentric granulomatosis associated with seropositive polyarthritis. *Thorax* 1985; 40: 396.

130 Bonafede RP, Benatar SR. Bronchocentric granulomatosis and rheumatoid arthritis. *Br J Dis Chest* 1987; 81: 197.

131 Saldana MJ. Bronchocentric granulomatosis: clinicopathologic observations in 17 patients. *Lab Invest* 1979; 40: 281.

41

LUNG CANCER

RONALD J. FERGUSSON

Epidemiology

Size of the problem

During the twentieth century lung cancer has emerged as the most common form of malignant disease in the western world. In the UK after the Second World War there was a dramatic rise in the numbers of patients dying from lung cancer (Fig. 41.1) and for some time it has been the most common cause of cancer death in men. Around 40 000 new patients are now seen each year, accounting for more than 8% of all male deaths and 4% of all female deaths [1]. In the European Community, almost 160 000 new patients are registered each year as having lung cancer and in 1992 the Surgeon General reported 133 700 deaths from the disease in the USA [2].

The disease is more common in men than women, although this difference has become smaller; in the USA and the UK, the male/female ratio was approximately 5:1 in 1970 but fell to around 2.5:1 in 1982 [3]. Recently, mortality rates have been falling in men of all ages. In contrast, lung cancer is the most rapidly increasing cause of cancer death in women. Since 1984, deaths from lung cancer have exceeded those due to breast cancer among women in Scotland and in some parts of northern England, and lung cancer looks set to be the major cancer killer of women in other areas. Encouragingly, mortality rates have recently begun to decline in younger women in England and Wales (Fig. 41.1), although the incidence of the disease continues to climb in the older age groups.

Aetiological factors

Tobacco smoking

It has been known for many years that the smoking of tobacco cigarettes is by far the most common cause of lung cancer [4,5]. In England, Wales and the USA, it is estimated that 92–94% of lung cancer deaths are attributable to tobacco smoking in males, the figures in females being

78–80% [6]. The evidence for this association is derived from epidemiological studies, the earliest of which were retrospective. Doll and Hill [7] compared over 1300 lung cancer patients in hospital with a matched group of controls. It was found that there were very few non-smokers in the cancer group and this group contained many more heavy smokers than were found in the control group. Further support for the hypothesis that smoking causes lung cancer was provided by prospective studies. Doll and Peto [8] correlated the smoking habits of over 34 000 British doctors with lung cancer mortality over a period of 20 years and found a significant decline in both cigarette smoking and lung cancer mortality in this group. This was in contrast to the general male population in whom neither mortality rate from the disease nor tobacco consumption fell. These data were subsequently supported by studies of a large group of American physicians [9] and of British women doctors [10].

It has been estimated that cigarette smokers are 8–20 times more likely to develop lung cancer than lifelong non-smokers and that the extent of this risk correlates closely with the number of cigarettes smoked [11]. There is some evidence to suggest that the risk of lung cancer may be reduced by the use of filter tips and by lower tar yields [6,12]. Following cessation of smoking, the risk of developing carcinoma of the lung has been shown to decline progressively with time. However, even by 10–20 years the risk is still about 2.5 times that of non-smokers [13].

Unfortunately, smokers do not only increase their own risk of developing lung cancer, since there is evidence that the inhalation of other people's tobacco smoke (passive smoking) on a long-term basis is linked with an increased incidence of the disease. This risk was first noted in a study of non-smoking wives of heavy smokers in Japan [14]. It has now been shown that people who have been exposed to environmental tobacco smoke in their homes, both as children and adults, have an increased risk of lung cancer [15].

Pipe and cigar smokers have a slightly reduced risk of developing lung cancer compared with cigarette smokers,

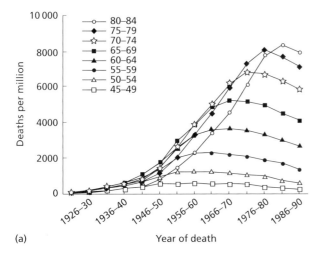

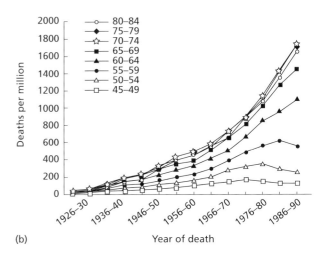

Fig. 41.1 Mortality from lung cancer by age and year of death, England and Wales 1921–90: (a) males, (b) females. (From Lung and Asthma Information Agency Factsheet 93/1, with permission of Professor Ross Anderson.)

probably because less smoke is inhaled [13]. It is also clear that of the principal histological types of lung cancer, squamous cell carcinoma and small-cell carcinoma have the clearest association with cigarette smoking, while adenocarcinoma is the commonest histological type in non-smokers who develop the disease [6].

Trends in smoking and lung cancer

In the UK, the consumption of cigarettes by men rose steadily throughout the first half of this century: the average annual consumption of cigarettes per man in 1905 was 800, rising to 4420 by 1945 [16]. Since then, and particularly in the last 20 years, consumption has fallen, reaching 2380 by 1985. The pattern of annual consumption in women has lagged behind that of men, starting with 13 in 1921, reaching 1250 in 1945 and peaking at 2630 in 1974. Since then consumption has fallen, but more slowly than that of men, reaching 1930 in 1985. The prevalence of cigarette smoking shows a similar trend, decreasing from 52% of men in 1972 to 31% in 1990; prevalence among women has fallen from 41% to 29% over the same time span [17]. If the current trends in the UK continue, smoking will soon be more common in women than in men. The clear link between tobacco consumption and lung cancer means that trends in the disease closely follow changes in cigarette consumption but with a lag period of approximately 20 years. Two important statistics concerning cigarette smoking will be reflected in the future pattern of lung cancer cases: (i) smoking problems among young women have increased in recent years; and (ii) most cigarette smokers are now in the less affluent socioeconomic groups in society [2]. At present the risk of an unskilled working

Table 41.1 World age-standardized rates per 100 000 (WASR) for selected cancer registries, cancer of the trachea, bronchus and lung (ICD-9 162), 1983–87.

Males		Females	
Country/registry	WASR	Country/registry	WASR
Scotland	88.1	Scotland	30.5
Netherlands, Eindhoven	87.2	USA, Connecticut, whites	29.9
Italy, Varese	82.3	Canada	23.9
Poland, Cracow	73.1	Denmark	23.1
Canada	68.5	England and Wales	20.5
England and Wales	65.4	China, Shanghai	18.1
USA, Connecticut, whites	62.5	Poland, Cracow	13.2
Denmark	58.5	Japan, Osaka	11.7
China, Shanghai	53.0	Italy, Varese	8.2
Spain, Zaragoza	42.2	Netherlands, Eindhoven	7.9
Japan, Osaka	41.5	Spain, Zaragoza	3.6
India, Bangalore	10.1	India, Bangalore	1.9

man dying of lung cancer is three times that of a professional man and it is likely that smoking habits are the major contributor to this difference. Table 41.1 shows the marked geographical variation in lung cancer mortality in different developed countries. The precise reasons for this variation are unclear; although socioeconomic, genetic and cultural differences exist, cigarette consumption must be important. While cigarette consumption is decreasing in all industrial societies it is extremely worrying that smoking is increasing in less developed countries, especially Africa and South America. Of the 10 nations with the highest smoking rates among males, eight are regarded as developing countries and of the top 30 only nine are industrialized [18]. If the current trends in tobacco consumption continue, it has been estimated that by the year 2025 80% of the projected 3.5 million cases of lung cancer per year will be in developing countries.

Atmospheric pollution

The role of environmental air pollution in the production of lung cancer is controversial and has certainly been far less important than the part played by cigarette smoking. Studies carried out to investigate the effect of environmental pollution and which have allowed for tobacco consumption show that urban dwellers have a risk of lung cancer that is 1.26–2.33 times greater than people living in the countryside [19,20]. Atmospheric pollution has also been used to explain the differences of incidence in lung cancer between two countries with similar cigarette consumption (Table 41.1). Recently there has been a lot of interest in the influence of residential radon exposure in the development of lung cancer. It is known that underground miners exposed to high levels of the radon progeny that decay from uranium have an increased risk of lung cancer [21]. Residential radon is the principal source of exposure to ionizing radiation in most countries. Studies from Sweden have suggested that residential exposure to radon is an important factor in the development of lung cancer in the general population, the interaction between radon exposure and smoking being almost a multiplicative effect [22,23].

Occupational factors

Certain occupations are associated with a higher than expected incidence of lung cancer. Table 41.2 lists a number of known causative agents and it is predictable that the list will grow with the ever-increasing complexity of industrial processes. In many instances the carcinogenic effect of the individual exposure is added to or multiplied by the effect of cigarette smoking, making the apportion-

Table 41.2 Occupational causes of lung cancer.

Cause	Occupation
Asbestos	Mining, processing, usage
Radioactivity (radon daughters)	Metal ore mining Uranium mining Fluorspar mining
Nickel	Refining
Chromium salts	Extraction, production, usage
Arsenic	Metal refining Chemical industry Insecticides
Chloroethers	Organic chemical industry
Mustard gas	Manufacture
Volatile coal products (?)	Coke oven workers
Printing ink (?)	Printing industry

ment of blame difficult in individual cases. Asbestos is particularly notable for its association with lung cancer. There is often a considerable latent period between exposure to asbestos and the onset of lung cancer. The risk rises until at least 30 years after first exposure, with an approximately linear relationship between the dose of asbestos and mortality and no detectable threshhold dose below which there is no increased risk of lung cancer. The interaction between asbestos exposure and smoking appears important [24], all longitudinal studies having shown that the interaction between these two risk factors is close to multiplicative [25].

The precise importance of asbestos exposure in the development of lung cancer in the general population is unknown. De Vos Irvine and colleagues [26] estimated that 5.7% of cases of lung cancer in the west of Scotland were asbestos-related. Extrapolating these figures to the whole of the UK would suggest that in excess of 2000 cases a year may be related to asbestos; however, this projection may not be appropriate since the west of Scotland has been an area with classically high exposures in shipyards and construction. Data from the SWORD surveillance scheme [27] suggest that comparatively few such cases are recognized, possibly because once the patient is identified as a tobacco smoker the physician does not enquire further into asbestos exposure. Also this exposure may appear trivial and have occurred many years before the presentation with lung cancer. Other aspects of asbestos-related disease are discussed in Chapters 43 and 54.

The increased risk of lung cancer described in workers extracting metal ores from deep mines is thought to be caused mostly by radioactivity rather than the metal being mined. This radioactivity emanates from radon gas, high concentrations of which can build up in poorly ventilated mines. Groups of workers in whom lung cancer has been described include uranium miners in various American states [28], fluorspar miners in Canada [29], iron ore miners in Sweden [30] and tin miners in Cornwall, England [31]. Other occupational exposures associated with lung cancer include nickel [32], the extraction and production of chromium salts [33], the use of arsenicals in the metal refining and chemical industries [34], the use of chloroethers in production of ion exchange resins [35] and coke oven work in the steel industry [36]. It is suspected that printing ink used in the newspaper industry may have been associated with lung cancer [37].

Pulmonary scarring

There have been reports of lung cancer occurring in close spatial relation to localized areas of pulmonary scarring and in patients with more diffuse lung fibrosis. The pathogenesis of these small numbers of 'scar cancers' is not established and in many cases the subject's tobacco smoking history may be highly relevant. This is particularly true in patients with asbestos exposure, as mentioned above. It used to be believed that lung cancer only occurred in asbestos-exposed individuals secondary to the lung fibrosis of asbestosis, and in the UK and several other countries compensation for asbestos-related disease recognized lung cancer as work-related only if there was radiological or pathological evidence of lung fibrosis [38,39]. However, Wilkinson and colleagues [40] studied the occupational histories of 271 patients with lung cancer and a suitable control group and showed that the risk of lung cancer from asbestos exposure was independent of radiologically apparent pulmonary fibrosis.

Cryptogenic fibrosing alveolitis (see Chapter 31) is also associated with cancer of the lung and, like asbestosis, an increased incidence of adenocarcinoma has also been noted in this group [26,41]. The incidence of lung cancer has also been found to be three times higher than anticipated in over 3500 patients with sarcoidosis [42]. It is not clear whether this was due to pulmonary fibrosis, although the histological distribution was no different from that in the general population upper lobe fibrosis due to tuberculosis may be associated with neoplastic change [43], adenocarcinoma being the usual cell type. A high proportion of cases of bronchioloalveolar carcinoma (a subtype of adenocarcinoma) occurs in areas of scarring [44] and this cell type has also been described in relation to congenital cystic lung disease [45].

Laboratory studies

Lung cancer is not a single entity but a generic term applied to a heterogeneous group of epithelial lung tumours that show varying degrees of malignancy in their different rates of progression and patterns of behaviour. Current laboratory evidence suggests that lung cancer starts with a single cell capable of developing into various pathological forms, including mixed tumours (Fig. 41.2). Clinicians recognize four major groups, namely squamous carcinoma, adenocarcinoma, large-cell carcinoma and small-cell carcinoma. Because of the markedly different growth rates and response to certain treatments of small-cell carcinomas, there is a tendency for investigators to simplify even further and to apply their treatment protocols to small-cell carcinoma and non-small-cell carcinoma groups. Although this approach may be pragmatic, it has the obvious shortcomings inherent in assigning several different pathological entities to a convenient clinical category.

Histological classification

The ideal classification of lung cancer should list histologically distinguishable groups of tumours according to clearly recognizable criteria so that different pathologists can reliably and independently arrive at the same diagnosis on the same piece of tissue. It should also be of value to physicians and surgeons who have to choose appropriate therapies and to investigators who seek to establish the value of different treatment regimens or the validity of possible aetiological links. The mere fact that several different classifications have been proposed is an indication that an ideal one has not yet been devised. The pathologist's difficulties are further increased by the now widespread submission of small quantities of biopsy material. Although the cellular characteristics of the same tumour may vary significantly in a standard section, these variations may not be detectable in a tiny fibreoptic bronchoscopy specimen or from a cytological preparation of a small number of malignant cells.

The 1981 World Health Organization (WHO) classification (Table 41.3) is still widely used [46]. Even at the time of its introduction it was criticized on the grounds that no account had been taken of differentiation and that some of the listed subtypes were of doubtful significance. It is also clear from immunoperoxidase and electron microscopic studies that lung cancers are heterogeneous in differentiation [47]. Well-differentiated squamous carcinoma may contain foci of adeno- or neuroendocrine differentiation, and tumours that are anaplastic on light microscopy may show glandular or squamous features at an ultrastructural level.

In an attempt to overcome these problems two new classifications of lung cancer have been suggested depending on the type of pathological specimen submitted. The first

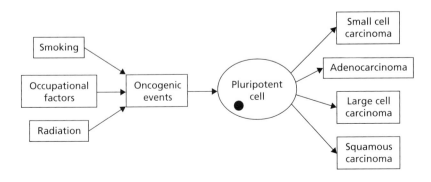

Fig. 41.2 Hypothesis for the development of different histological types of lung cancer from a single cell.

Table 41.3 World Health Organization (1981) classification of lung tumours. Group C: malignant epithelial tumours.

1 Squamous cell carcinoma (epidermoid carcinoma)
  Variants: *spindle cell (squamous) carcinoma*

2 Small-cell carcinoma
  (a) *Oat cell carcinoma*
  (b) *Intermediate cell type*
  (c) *Combined oat cell carcinoma*

3 Adenocarcinoma
  (a) *Acinar adenocarcinoma*
  (b) *Papillary adenocarcinoma*
  (c) *Bronchioloalveolar carcinoma*
  (d) *Solid carcinoma with mucus formation*

4 Large-cell carcinoma
  Variants: (a) *Giant-cell carcinoma*
       (b) *Clear-cell carcinoma*

5 Adenosquamous carcinoma

6 Carcinoid tumour

7 Bronchial gland carcinoma
  (a) *Adenoid cystic carcinoma*
  (b) *Mucoepidermoid carcinoma*
  (c) *Others*

8 Others

Table 41.4 Classification of lung cancer proposed for use with large biopsy specimens. (From Edwards [48].)

Type	Tumour
1/0	Squamous carcinoma
	1/1 Well differentiated
	1/2 Moderately differentiated
	1/3 Poorly differentiated
	1/4 Undifferentiated (squamoid)
2/0	Neuroendocrine carcinoma
	2/1 Carcinoid tumour
	2/2 Well-differentiated neuroendocrine carcinoma
	2/3 Large-cell neuroendocrine carcinoma
	2/4 Small-cell carcinoma
3/0	Adenocarcinoma
	3/1 Well differentiated
	3/2 Moderately differentiated
	3/3 Poorly differentiated
	3/4 Undifferentiated
4/0	Large-cell undifferentiated carcinoma
5/0	Miscellaneous carcinomas
	5/1 Tumours of mixed differentiation (i.e. adenosquamous carcinoma)
	5/2 Bronchial gland carcinomas
	5/3 Bronchioloalveolar carcinoma
	5/4 Giant-cell carcinoma
	5/5 Clear-cell carcinoma
	5/6 Carcinosarcoma
	5/7 Spindle cell carcinoma
6/0	Malignant epithelial tumours of uncertain type

Table 41.5 Classification proposed by the UK CCCR Lung Cancer Working Party for routine use in the diagnosis of small biopsy specimens. (From Thomas *et al.* [50].)

Category	Tumour
1	Squamous carcinoma
2	Small-cell carcinoma
3	Adenocarcinoma
4	Non-small-cell carcinoma of specified type
5	Non-small-cell carcinoma, not otherwise specified
6	Malignant tumour, not otherwise specified
7	Technical failure
8	Carcinoma, not otherwise specified

(Table 41.4) is proposed for use with large specimens (resections or large open biopsies) [48] and is an adaptation of the pioneering work of Lamb [49]. It can be seen that the degree of differentiation is important in both squamous carcinomas and adenocarcinomas, and that tumours of neuroendocrine type are grouped together. This classification is clearly unsuitable for small biopsies. In 1993 the Lung Cancer Working Party of the UK Coordinating Committee for Cancer Research (CCCR) highlighted the problems with small specimens in a study comparing the diagnosis made on biopsy with that made on the resected specimen [50]. A diagnostic accuracy of 75% was achieved for squamous cell carcinoma, 66% for small-cell carcinoma but only 50% for adenocarcinoma. A new simplified classification (Table 41.5) was proposed that should improve the diagnostic accuracy of small biopsy specimens. The results of clinical evaluation of both these classifications are awaited.

For most pathologists, four major subgroups of lung cancer still predominate and account for about 95% of cases: squamous cell carcinoma (40–60%), small-cell carcinoma (7–25%), adenocarcinoma (10–25%) and large-cell carcinoma (5–15%) [49]. Carcinoid tumours, which account for up to 10% of cases, are discussed with other rarer tumours in Chapter 42.

Squamous cell carcinoma

This is the most common type of lung cancer. It shows histological evidence of squamous differentiation, with stratification, the formation of intercellular bridges and intracellular keratinization (Fig. 41.3). The majority of squamous cell carcinomas are centrally situated, and those that are more differentiated grow more slowly and are less likely to give rise to extrathoracic metastases. Those squamous cell carcinomas that are more poorly differentiated tend to behave aggressively, extrathoracic metastases being more frequent. However, the relation-

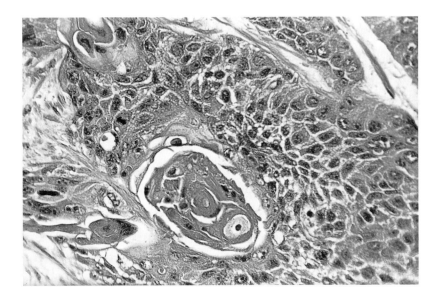

Fig. 41.3 Well-differentiated squamous carcinoma showing keratin pearl formation and intracellular cytoplasmic bridges (haematoxylin & eosin ×305).

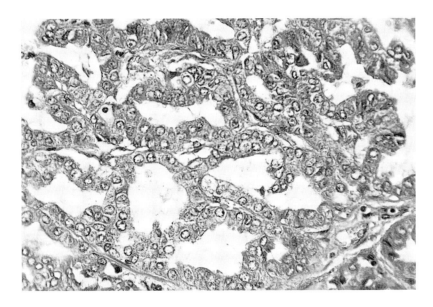

Fig. 41.4 Moderately differentiated adenocarcinoma showing a well-marked acinar pattern (haematoxylin & eosin ×305).

ship between differentiation and prognosis remains uncertain [51]. It is not uncommon for squamous cell carcinomas to cavitate.

Adenocarcinoma

Adenocarcinomas of the lung often present a wide variety of patterns. The WHO classification, which splits tumours into acinar or papillary types, is confusing since in practice these patterns may coexist in the same tumour [52] (Fig. 41.4). Both types tend to produce mucin. There appears to be quite a wide geographical variation in the incidence of adenocarcinoma and some evidence that it is becoming more common. These tumours, unlike squamous cell varieties, are less related to cigarette smoking and are usually situated in the periphery of the lung. Often they are unrelated to bronchi other than by spread.

The WHO classification includes bronchioloalveolar carcinoma (also known as alveolar cell carcinoma) along with other adenocarcinomas. Electron microscopic studies imply that these tumours are a heterogeneous group of peripheral lung tumours that arise from any epithelial cell within or distal to the terminal bronchioles [52]. They account for about 5% of all lung cancers. Apart from their lepidic mode of spread, they behave in a similar fashion to other malignant lung tumours. On gross inspection their margins are less well defined than other members of this group, often appearing as multiple pulmonary nodules or an area of peripheral 'pneumonic consolidation'. It is common for tumour cells to exfoliate and be detected in sputum (Fig. 41.5). Regional and more distant metastases may occur less commonly than is the case with other lung tumours. At the light microscopic level these tumours as well as other adenocarcinomas may be indistinguishable

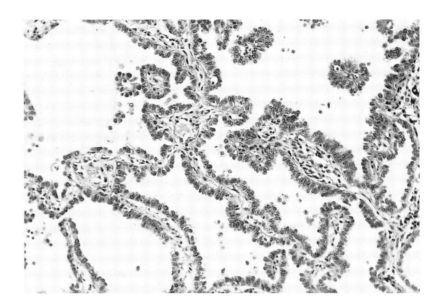

Fig. 41.5 Bronchioloalveolar carcinoma showing tumour cells lining alveolar walls, forming papillary structures with shedding of clumps of malignant cells into alveolar spaces (haematoxylin & eosin ×150).

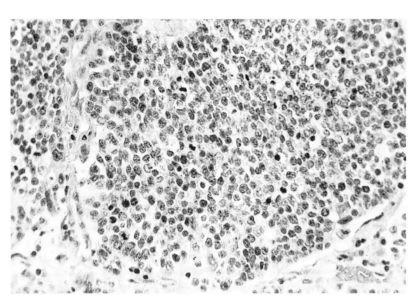

Fig. 41.6 Undifferentiated small-cell carcinoma showing many mitoses (haematoxylin & eosin ×305).

from metastatic adenocarcinoma arising from an extrathoracic primary site, the most common of which are pancreas, colon, breast, stomach and kidney.

Small-cell carcinoma

This group contains the most malignant tumours of the lung and accounts for 20–25% of cases. The WHO classification [46] divides small-cell carcinoma into three main types.

1 Small or oat-cell carcinomas characterized by a proliferation of cells with round or oval nuclei and scanty cytoplasm (high nuclear/cytoplasmic ratio) (Fig. 41.6). These cells are about twice the size of lymphocytes, which they superficially resemble.

2 The intermediate cell subtype, which contain cells less

regular in shape with more abundant cytoplasm. There is some evidence that this subtype containing some large cells is more resistant to chemotherapy.

3 A combined subgroup, which includes rare examples of small-cell carcinoma containing areas of squamous carcinoma or adenocarcinoma. Probably only about 1% of tumours fall into this category [53]. It is accepted that they should be managed as small-cell carcinoma and carry the same prognosis.

Small-cell carcinomas usually arise in central bronchi. They are often grouped with carcinoid tumours as they probably originate from common neuroendocrine precursor cells. Small-cell carcinomas grow rapidly and metastasize early and widely, so that disease is rarely limited to the chest at necropsy. At presentation over two-thirds of patients have evidence of extensive disease, the most important clinical sites of metastases being the liver, central nervous system (CNS) and bone. Other frequent sites include the abdominal lymph nodes, adrenals and other abdominal organs.

Large-cell carcinoma

These tumours account for about 15% of lung cancers. The group is somewhat heterogeneous and many authorities now regard it as a diagnostic wastebasket [48]. The tumours tend to be anaplastic, light microscopy showing no features of maturation and the presence of large, less well-differentiated, polygonal, spindle-shaped or oval cells with abundant cytoplasm (Fig. 41.7). Electron microscopy may show features of squamous cells or adenocarcinoma. Many authors feel that they may be undifferentiated examples of squamous carcinoma or adenocarcinoma in which only anaplastic material has been sampled. It is obviously significant that the entity of large-cell carcinoma does not exist in the UK CCCR proposed classification for the pathology of small biopsy specimens [50]. The majority of large-cell carcinomas arise towards the lung periphery and are bulky. The two variant forms in the WHO classification are rare. Clear-cell carcinoma contains large rounded cells with clear cytoplasm and is commonly mistaken for metastatic renal cancer.

Biology

The lack of progress in the treatment of lung cancer has led to a growth of interest in the biology of the disease, with the hope that an increase in knowledge could be translated into therapeutic advances. It is now possible to take tumour cells from a patient with lung cancer and grow them in the laboratory in the form of cell lines or as xenografts in immunosuppressed animals [53,54]. These models of human lung cancer have facilitated the study of the biology of the disease. The tumours can be maintained indefinitely and remain cytologically identical to the original biopsy specimen. There are a number of areas where advances in our understanding of basic mechanisms at the cellular level may soon be translated into benefits for the patient with lung cancer.

Growth factors

Growth factors are polypeptides that take part in the control of cell differentiation and proliferation. They act locally on tumour cells via growth factor receptors but may also be found in the circulation [55]. It has long been known that small-cell tumours are able to synthesize a wide range of peptides and hormones and that these substances can readily bind to cell receptors causing autocrine growth stimulation (Fig. 41.8). Bombesin/gastrin-releasing peptide has been shown to be an important growth factor both *in vitro* [56] and *in vivo* [57]. It has also been shown that the growth of small-cell lung cancer in the laboratory can be inhibited by a monoclonal antibody to bombesin [58]. Other important growth factors in small-cell lung cancer include vasopressin and bradykinin [59], opioids [60] and insulin-like growth factor 1. Numerous other substances have been shown to be secreted by small-cell lung cancer cells and have the potential to regulate their growth [55]. Non-small-cell lung cancer appears to have fewer recognized growth factors, although epidermal growth factor and transforming growth factor α have been shown to bind to specific cell receptors and to stimulate growth [55,61]. The expression of growth factors and their receptors in some non-small-cell lung cancers appears to be related to aggressive clinical behaviour and the increased likelihood of a

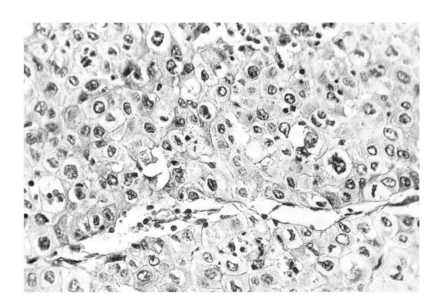

Fig. 41.7 Undifferentiated large-cell carcinoma showing large pleomorphic tumour cells (haematoxylin & eosin ×305).

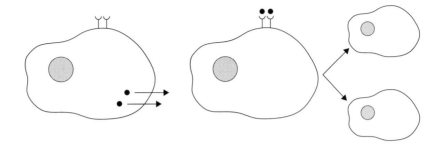

Fig. 41.8 Autocrine growth stimulation: a lung cancer cell produces a growth factor that binds to a receptor to stimulate proliferation.

response to chemotherapy. Results of clinical trials involving the manipulation of these autocrine growth factors are eagerly awaited.

Genetic abnormalities

It is surprising that only 15% of male smokers contract lung cancer, given the close association between smoking and the disease. It seems likely that the remaining 85% have an inherited resistance to the disease and that the small number of non-smokers who develop lung cancer may be inherently susceptible [62]. This has led to much interest in genetic abnormalities in patients with lung cancer and in laboratory models of the disease [63]. A plethora of genetic abnormalities has been detected and this has created some confusion as to their significance in the genesis and progression of the disease. One of the earliest and most consistent chromosomal deletions seen is the loss of the short arm of chromosome 3 (p14–p23) in small-cell lung cancer [64,65]. This suggests that loss of specific gene function may be a critical step in the development of lung cancer. This model certainly seems to fit for the development of another, rarer tumour, retinoblastoma, where a specific tumour suppressor gene is also lost from chromosome 3, and indeed there is a close association between small-cell lung cancer and retinoblastoma [66]. Similar genetic abnormalities are seen in tumour cells from non-small-cell cancers [67,68], although the situation is less striking and inactivation of the *CDKN2* gene on chromosome 9 may be more important in this histological subtype [69].

Oncogenes

Activation of small parts of the genetic code is seen in many cancers and the role of these oncogenes is unclear. Members of the *myc* gene family are often activated in lung tumours, particularly of small-cell type, and may be associated with increased aggressiveness of tumour growth [70]. The normal function of these genes has remained elusive and it is not clear how overexpression contributes to tumour growth. Activation of the K-*ras* oncogenes is usually detected in adenocarcinoma of the lung and patients carrying these mutations have been shown to have a more aggressive clinical course [71]. It is to be hoped that a greater understanding of the importance of oncogenes will lead to innovative therapies for the patient [63,70,72].

Tumour markers

Tumour markers are substances produced by tumour cells that are released into the bloodstream where they can be measured. They may be helpful in screening and in the early diagnosis of cancer, in an assessment of the extent of disease and in response to treatment. Many of these markers are produced by normal cells, for example neurone-specific enolase, creatine phosphokinase BB and carcinoembryonic antigen. A long list of tumour-associated antigens has also been discovered. However, despite the deliberations of large international workshops in this field [73], the large variations in sensitivity and specificity of all these compounds has made their precise clinical usefulness uncertain [74,75].

Clinical features

Common modes of presentation

Patients with lung cancer can present in many different ways. The majority of patients present as the result of the investigation of some new respiratory symptom or because their pre-existing respiratory state has worsened. A small percentage have no respiratory symptoms and the diagnosis is made by the chance finding of an opacity on a chest radiograph ordered for some other reason. A third group develop non-specific symptoms of malignancy, including malaise, anorexia and weight loss. A fourth group presents as a result of metastatic disease and usually have an extremely poor prognosis.

Central tumours

Three-quarters of patients with lung cancer have their primary disease in the central airway. This is especially true of squamous and small-cell carcinomas. The commonest symptoms at presentation are cough, haemoptysis, dyspnoea and chest pain, either alone or in combination. Cough is by far the most common symptom at presentation and any 'new' cough that persists longer than 2 weeks should be regarded with suspicion, especially in patients over the age of 40 years who are tobacco smokers. Unfortunately this group tend to have a chronic cough due to chronic bronchitis and this may often lead to some delay in diagnosis. Haemoptysis is usually an alarming symptom for the patient and one that should always be thoroughly investigated. It may amount to only minimal streaking of blood in mucoid sputum and the patient often presents in order to be reassured. Copious haemoptysis is uncommon. However, it should be recognized that most patients who have haemoptysis do not have lung cancer; nevertheless all patients with this symptom require investigation. Breathlessness may arise because of central airway narrowing or because of partial or complete collapse of a distal segment of lung. Poorly localized deep chest discomfort occurs in up to 60% of patients at diagnosis. The exact cause of this symptom in patients with centrally placed tumours is unclear but it may be due to involvement of peribronchial or perivascular nerves.

Peripheral tumours

Peripheral neoplasms, commonly adenocarcinoma or large-cell types, often have a different mode of presentation. They may cause no respiratory symptoms at the time of diagnosis, which may follow a chest radiograph taken for some other reason or as part of the investigation of non-specific symptoms. Cough and haemoptysis are less common than in central lesions. Cough with large amounts of mucoid sputum (bronchorrhoea) is described in 10% of cases of bronchioloalveolar carcinoma, although this is an unusual symptom [76]. Dyspnoea is also less common and if present is likely to be due to either pleural involvement with tumour or blockage of lymphatics in lymphangitis carcinomatosa. Pleural effusion also causes breathlessness if it is large enough to compress the lung. Adenocarcinoma is particularly noted for seeding the pleura. Spread beyond the pleura into the chest wall produces dull, continuous pain that commonly interferes with sleep.

Distant spread

Approximately one-third of patients with lung cancer present with symptoms due to metastatic spread outwith the thorax. Skeletal metastases, which are most commonly seen in small-cell and large-cell lesions, may present with bone pain and even pathological fractures. Cerebral metastases may present with progressive neurological symptoms and are common in patients with widespread disease. Cervical lymph gland and adrenal involvement are also common but do not usually produce symptoms.

Spread to the liver similarly rarely produces symptoms unless the metastases are large.

Common clinical findings at presentation

Frequently, physical examination of the chest in a patient with lung cancer reveals no abnormal signs. However, physical signs may be elicited that are helpful for not only reaching a diagnosis but also making a preliminary assessment of the extent of disease and determining the most appropriate sequence of further investigation and perhaps treatment in an individual case. For instance, if the patient is obviously breathless while undressing this is usually an indication of coexisting chronic obstructive airways disease, which may preclude attempts at surgical treatment.

The hoarse voice of vocal cord paralysis is easily detectable and may be the only complaint of the patient. When asked to cough the patient often produces a relatively ineffectual expiratory noise, the so-called 'bovine cough'. This lacks the explosive quality of a normal cough produced by proper juxtaposition of two fully adducted cords. The left recurrent laryngeal nerve is most commonly involved as it loops round the aortic arch where it passes over the left main bronchus, a site that may be involved directly by tumour or by mediastinal lymph node metastases. Involvement of the right recurrent laryngeal nerve indicates a thoracic inlet tumour or invasion of the cervical nodes since the nerve loops around the right subclavian artery in the root of the neck. Vocal cord paralysis is therefore only seen in irresectable tumours because of mediastinal involvement.

Clubbing of the fingers and toes is commonly seen, although in one series was not present in patients with small-cell lesions [77]. The cause is unknown and may be associated with hypertrophic osteoarthropathy (discussed below).

Lymphatic spread is common and the scalene and supraclavicular lymph glands are usually the first to become enlarged. Axillary lymph glands are rarely involved and indicate invasion of the chest wall. The palpation of a lymph node provides ready access for histological sampling and positive histological confirmation indicates inoperability also.

Narrowing of the trachea or a lesion in either main bronchus at the level of the carina may cause stridor, an easily audible sound during inspiration. With more distally placed obstructing tumours this sound assumes the quality of a wheeze, which may be audible without a stethoscope. It may persist despite coughing, implying the presence of a fixed mechanical obstruction. A central obstructing lesion may cause a decrease in the intensity of breath sounds over a lobe or entire lung. Such patients are likely to develop atelectasis of the affected portion of lung if treatment is delayed.

The presence of a pleural effusion in a patient with lung cancer is more likely to be due to neoplastic pleural involvement than to be secondary to complicating infection or some other process. A pleural friction rub may be heard over an area of pleuritic pain.

About 5–10% of patients may present with symptoms due to obstruction of the superior vena cava (SVC). The patient notices swelling of the face and neck with tightness around the collar, which may progress to gross oedema. Occasionally the patient may be misdiagnosed as having an allergic reaction, especially if persistent flushing of the face is seen. The earliest and most common sign is bilateral jugular venous engorgement and superficial varicosities over the area drained by the SVC. Obstruction of the SVC is caused by either mediastinal lymph node metastases or direct venous compression of a tumour in the right upper lobe.

Dullness to percussion at a lung base may be due to not only perfusion or collapse but also to a raised and paralysed hemidiaphragm. This may be confirmed radiologically or on ultrasound by the presence of paradoxical movement on sniffing and it may contribute significantly to dyspnoea. The majority of cases of phrenic nerve paralysis indicate widespread mediastinal involvement.

A palpably enlarged liver due to hepatic involvement is an unusual finding at presentation, as are the symptoms and signs of raised intracranial pressure resulting from cerebral spread. Dysphagia due to mediastinal node compression of the oesophagus is also a late symptom. The clinical features of superior sulcus (Pancoast) tumours and paraneoplastic syndromes are discussed below.

Investigation

Clinicians faced with the management of a patient with a likely bronchial carcinoma need to instigate investigations in order to allow a rational management plan for that patient (Fig. 41.9). The purpose of any investigations performed are to confirm the clinical diagnosis, including if possible the histological type, and also to assess the extent

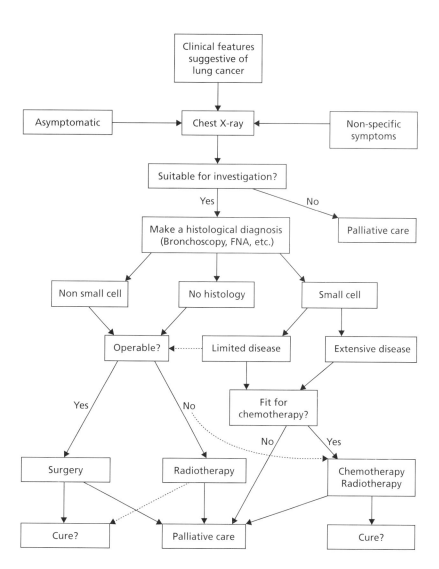

Fig. 41.9 Outline of the investigation and management of patients with lung cancer. (FNA, fine-needle aspiration.)

or stage of the disease in order to plan the most appropriate management. Clearly the complexity of investigations should correlate with the patient's suitability for active treatment. Lung cancer commonly presents at an advanced stage in predominantly older patients who often have other significant medical conditions related to cigarette smoking, and in the past there was a feeling that investigating these patients was not justified as effective treatment was not available. However it is now felt that obtaining a precise diagnosis helps patients come to terms with their disease and allows some indication concerning prognosis to be given to them and their families. In most countries the initial assessment of lung cancer patients is performed by respiratory physicians [78], and a case is now developing for recommending that all patients with the possible diagnosis should be assessed by a team involving respiratory physicians as well as clinicians who may be responsible for further treatment, such as cardiothoracic surgeons and oncologists.

Chest radiography

The chest radiograph is nearly always abnormal in patients with lung cancer at presentation [78]. Common early findings include slight prominence of a hilar shadow in the case of a central tumour and a small pulmonary nodule in the case of a peripheral tumour [79]. By the time the patient presents with symptoms there is more commonly obvious unilateral hilar or perihilar enlargement that is highly suggestive of a primary carcinoma or hilar lymph node spread (Fig. 41.10). Often it may be difficult to distinguish between a prominent hilar shadow due to a normal but prominent pulmonary vessel and an early central tumour.

More peripherally situated lung cancer usually produces a homogeneous mass shadow. The margins are often poorly defined so that they may be mistaken for inflammatory disease. The average diameter of rounded lesions at presentation is 3–4 cm; lesions of less than 1 cm in diameter are likely to be missed [80]. When central necrosis in the tumour occurs, cavitation may be evident and this is most commonly seen in squamous carcinomas [81]. Cavitation is not a feature of small-cell carcinoma. The inner lining of the cavity is often irregular and the shadow may be indistinguishable from that produced by a lung abscess, particularly if a fluid level is present

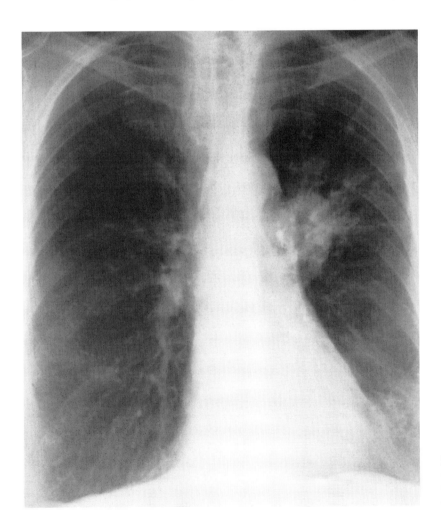

Fig. 41.10 Chest film of 60-year-old woman with left hilar squamous tumour arising at the origin of the upper lobe bronchus and causing some distal consolidation.

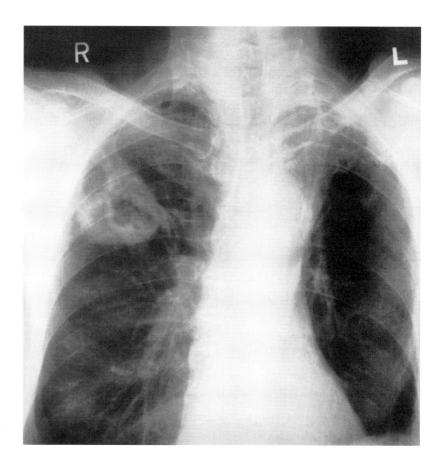

Fig. 41.11 Irregularly cavitated carcinoma in right upper lobe. The fibrosed left upper lobe was due to the after-effects of tuberculosis.

(Fig. 41.11). Bronchial obstruction by tumour may produce a true lung abscess, although consolidation without cavitation is more common.

Frequently the most striking radiographic features in lung cancer are the result of the mechanical effects of the tumour which, by obstructing a bronchus, may cause total or partial collapse of a segment, lobe or lung (Fig. 41.12). An ipsilateral unaffected lobe tends to overinflate, becoming more lucent as it expands to fill the additional space provided by the area of collapse, and characteristic displacement of interlobar fissures may be seen. Extensive atelectasis or consolidation may conceal the central causative lung cancer, as may a large pleural effusion.

Elevation of one or other hemidiaphragm may indicate phrenic nerve paralysis. This may be confirmed by fluoroscopy or ultrasound when paradoxical movement of the paralysed leaflet is seen on sniffing. Mediastinal lymph node involvement is often not radiographically visible on plain films unless very advanced, in which case widening of the mediastinum may be seen. In a few cases, lymphatic spread may extend from mediastinal or hilar nodes to pulmonary lymphatics, producing fine, lace-like shadows that may involve the whole of both lung fields, a form of dissemination known as lymphangitis carcinomatosa [82] (Fig. 41.13).

The radiographic features of bronchioloalveolar carcinoma are frequently indistinguishable from those of other histological types. However, this tumour may sometimes produce diffuse ill-defined fluffy infiltrates resulting from its tendency to spread along the airways at bronchiolar level [83] (Fig. 41.14). Radiographically this may resemble pneumonic consolidation but it obviously does not respond to standard antibiotic therapy.

Carcinomas at the extreme apex of the lung are known as Pancoast, thoracic inlet or superior sulcus tumours. In their early stages they may produce only a thin rim of shadowing at the apex that is indistinguishable from pleural thickening due to other causes. As these tumours enlarge, they may also erode and destroy adjacent ribs and infiltrate nerves of the brachial plexus to produce the familiar clinical syndrome (Fig. 41.15).

It is possible, although unusual, for a patient with lung cancer to have a normal chest radiograph [78,84]. This usually occurs when a primary tumour is small and central. Such patients require further investigation, usually by bronchoscopy, if there are other clinical features suggesting bronchial carcinoma, such as haemoptysis.

Sputum cytology

The examination of sputum expectorated by patients suspected of having lung cancer is a simple investigation to

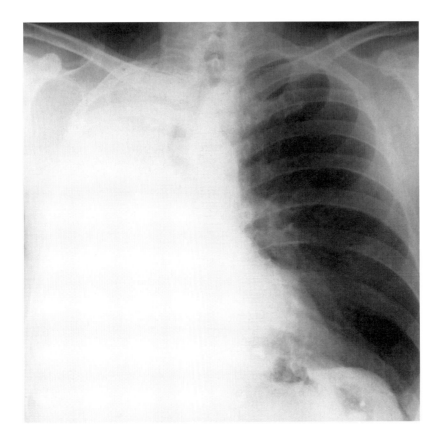

Fig. 41.12 Complete collapse of the right lung secondary to main bronchial tumour. Note tracheal deviation and absence of air bronchogram in right lung.

perform and often a valuable diagnostic aid. In experienced hands a definitive diagnosis of lung cancer may be made in 60–70% of all cases in whom the diagnosis is subsequently confirmed histologically [84]. The likelihood of this test being positive increases when the tumour is centrally placed, with increasing tumour size and when the lesion is situated in the lower lobe [85,86]. Not surprisingly, squamous and small-cell tumours, which are usually central, have a higher positive yield. Establishment of the correct histological group by sputum cytology has an accuracy of 50–80% depending on the degree of differentiation. Poorly differentiated tumours are more difficult to subtype [84].

The collection of adequate samples is extremely important. The first sputum in the morning or one produced after a bronchoscopy tends to produce a higher positive yield. The yield from a single sample in patients with lung cancer is approximately 40%, although this can be increased by repeated collections to in excess of 80% with four specimens [87]. In experienced hands, false-positive results do not usually exceed 1%.

Bronchoscopy

Bronchoscopy is the most useful investigation in the evaluation of a patient suspected of harbouring a lung cancer, as it can provide histological confirmation as well as information regarding the extent of the disease. The procedure itself is discussed fully in Chapter 8. Tumours that are situated centrally on a radiograph may be visible bronchoscopically as a neoplastic mass within the lumen. Frequently the presence of a tumour is indicated by bronchial stenosis or external compression due to surrounding tumour tissue or lymph node metastases.

Tumours that are beyond bronchoscopic vision may be biopsied using the transbronchial technique or by blind brushings and washings. Positive diagnoses have been made in 60% of such lesions when they are greater than 2 cm in diameter [88]. Techniques have also been developed for transbronchial needle aspiration of mediastinal nodes [89].

Bronchoscopic evidence of inoperability is provided by the endobronchial site of the tumour and any evidence of mediastinal involvement. Tumours confined to a lobar bronchus may be removed by a lobectomy but those growing to within 1 cm of the carina require pneumonectomy. Mediastinal involvement is suggested by a paralysed vocal cord and by widening of the main carina due to subcarinal lymph node enlargement. External compression of the lateral wall of the lower trachea by enlarged paratracheal lymph nodes also suggests inoperability, assuming that the lymph nodes are involved with tumour. Previously it was common practice for thoracic surgeons to repeat a physician's bronchoscopy prior to surgery. Modern bronchoscopic techniques involving video imaging may allow the surgeon to view the bronchoscopic

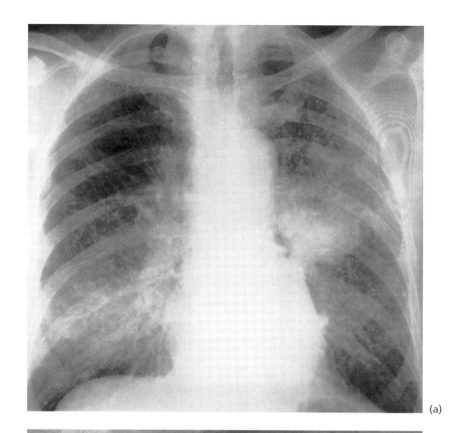

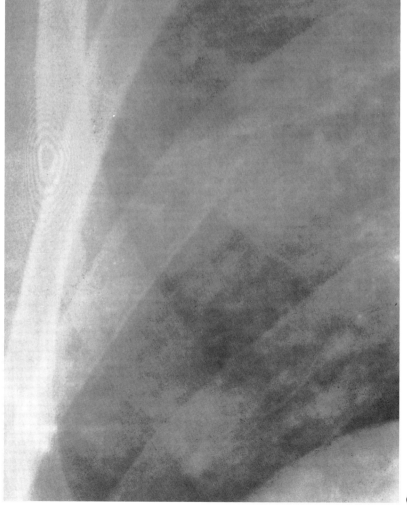

Fig. 41.13 (a) Bronchial carcinoma in left mid zone with lymphangitic spread. Note diffuse nodular change and Kerley's lines in lower zones. (b) Magnified view of right lower zone.

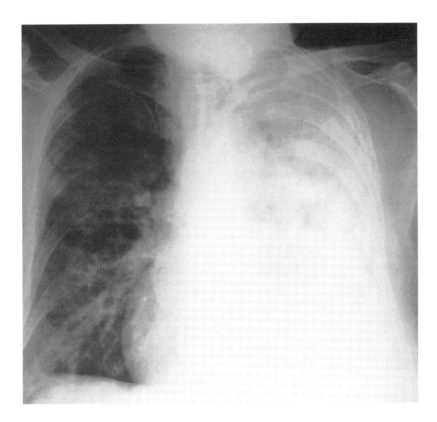

Fig. 41.14 Diffuse confluent shadowing through left lung and nodular lesions in right lung due to bronchioloalveolar carcinoma.

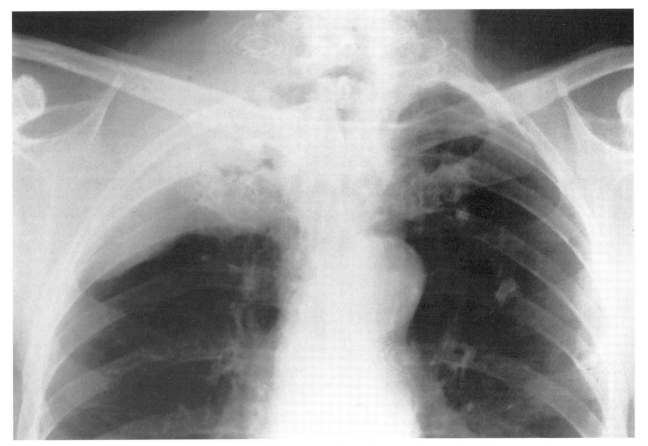

Fig. 41.15 Extensive pleural infiltration at right apex with destruction of first and second ribs together with the second transverse process: Pancoast tumour.

findings and perhaps save the patient from a repeat procedure.

Other initial investigations

The vast majority of patients have blood tests as part of their initial assessment [78]. These provide no diagnostic information, although they may point to hepatic involvement or the presence of a paraneoplastic endocrine syndrome (see below). In patients with peripheral lesions a definitive histological diagnosis may only be obtained by percutaneous needle biopsy of the lung or pleura, by aspiration of subcutaneous swellings, lymph nodes or pleural fluid, or by aspiration or biopsy of distant metastases in bones, liver, adrenals, etc. Intrathoracic disease may be confirmed at thoracoscopic lung biopsy, mediastinoscopy or thoracotomy (see below).

Determination of operability

Once a diagnosis has been made, the investigation of a patient with lung cancer is aimed at deciding the most appropriate therapy available for that individual. Surgical resection has the greatest impact on survival, although at the time of diagnosis the majority of patients are clearly inoperable. If the patient is a prospective surgical candidate, further evaluation has to be carried out in order to ensure that he or she is fit for an operation and that metastatic disease, which would render the patient incurable despite removal of the primary lesion, is excluded.

Assessment of fitness for surgery

It is common for the lung function of patients with carcinoma of the bronchus to be impaired, as a result of total or partial occlusion of a large bronchus by a central lesion and because of coexisting chronic bronchitis and emphysema which, like lung cancer, are causally related to cigarette smoking. Careful consideration must be given to the effect of the removal of *functional* lung tissue in the tumour-bearing lung in order to prevent, at worst, postoperative respiratory failure and even death or, at best, extreme and persistent dyspnoea that would greatly impair the patient's level of physical activity and quality of life.

The forced expiratory volume in 1 s (FEV_1) and forced vital capacity are simple to measure, reproducible and form the basis of the most reliable predictable measurement in the evaluation of suitability for lung resection. Studies have shown that the risk of postoperative chronic ventilatory insufficiency is high if the postoperative FEV_1 is less than 1 L [90], although allowance for the height of the patient should be made in view of the increasing numbers of women presenting with lung cancer. Spirome-

try is reduced by approximately 10–15% of predicted values as a result of lobectomy and by 20–30% with pneumonectomy; in general, patients with a preoperative FEV_1 exceeding 2 L tolerate surgery without severe postoperative breathlessness. Patients who are considered marginal for surgery require further investigation. A quantitative assessment of regional lung function may be useful in borderline patients. It may demonstrate that the patient has already undergone the physiological equivalent of a pneumonectomy or lobectomy by virtue of the tumour occluding a main or lobar bronchus. In such situations resection may do nothing to worsen lung function and may even produce physiological improvement by removing a major cause of ventilation–perfusion mismatch. There is no consensus about the best method of carrying out split lung function studies but most rely on radioisotopes [91,92].

Other useful tests that can be performed preoperatively include the measurement of diffusing capacity, since it is known that postoperative complications are more common if this is less than 40% of predicted before the operation [90]. Most clinicians place considerable reliance on the history of breathlessness and observation of the patient, for example, breathlessness while undressing is a good indication that the patient will be more breathless after surgery, unless of course the tumour has already caused a physiological pneumonectomy. The original lung function test prior to pneumonectomy, carried out by the pioneers of this operation, was to induce an artificial pneumothorax and observe the patient! Nowadays, a 6-min walking test gives a good indication of preoperative function, and difficulty completing this test at a reasonable pace should cause one to think twice before advising surgery.

Consideration also needs to be given to other medical conditions, such as ischaemic heart disease and peripheral vascular disease. Patients who have well-controlled angina usually need to undergo an exercise ECG test and any significant abnormality may need further evaluation with coronary angiography. Subjects whose exercise tolerance is limited by significant intermittent claudication are usually not deemed good surgical candidates.

Assessment of local spread

Evidence of spread of tumour into local structures and the mediastinum may be obvious from a history of dysphagia, hoarseness or obstruction of the SVC. A pleural effusion usually means that the subject is inoperable, although it should be further evaluated with pleural aspiration and biopsy. Some centres do not exclude patients if the effusion is small and does not contain malignant cells on repeated aspiration. However, results of surgery in these patients is poor.

The results of surgery correlate well with the extent of

mediastinal node involvement (see below) and assessment of the mediastinum is essential in all patients being considered for surgery. While the initial chest radiograph may show obvious mediastinal lymphadenopathy, a normal mediastinal appearance on a plain radiograph still requires the patient to undergo further mediastinal evaluation.

Computed tomography

Computed tomography (CT) (Fig. 41.16) is now established as the best non-invasive method for assessing the mediastinum in patients with lung cancer being considered for resection [93]. Technological advances over the last two decades, with the introduction of much faster scanners, have enhanced the sensitivity of the investigation (see Chapter 7). The most important limitation of preoperative CT is the fact that although it is good at detecting enlarged lymph nodes, it cannot distinguish between neoplastic and reactive nodes, nor can it tell whether a normal-sized lymph node contains microscopic deposits of tumour. Studies that have measured the sensitivity and specificity of preoperative CT compared with mediastinal node sampling at either mediastinoscopy or thoracotomy show considerable variability in sensitivity and specificity [94–96]. Earlier studies were limited by the technical ability of the available scanners, although many studies using modern machines have given comparable results. A meta-analysis of over 40 studies published in 1990 showed a sensitivity of 79% and a specificity of 86% [97]. The authors used 1 cm as the cut-off value for normality, while most reports assume a 1.5-cm diameter as the upper limit of normal. There is a correlation between nodal size and the likelihood of malignancy, although the association is fairly weak. In one study [94] only 13% of 336 nodes less than 1 cm in diameter contained metastases, while 36% of 78 nodes greater than 1 cm were malignant.

Even in the group with very large nodes (>2 cm in diameter) only two-thirds were subsequently found to contain tumour. While a normal-sized node may well contain a small focus of tumour cells, the predictive value of a negative result on CT has been shown to be in the order of 90%. However, a recent study [98] has questioned this value, finding mediastinal lymph node metastases in 19 of 90 patients (21%) with non-small-cell lung cancer who underwent thoracotomy and who had normal-sized nodes (<1 cm) on CT.

A consensus view about the place of preoperative CT in non-small-cell lung cancer is now emerging. Patients with abnormal scans require mediastinal lymph node sampling to confirm malignant involvement. This allows a significant number of patients to undergo successful thoracotomy who might otherwise have been denied surgery by the presence of enlarged lymph nodes on their scan. Patients with a negative scan who are otherwise operable should proceed directly to thoracotomy, although mediastinal lymph nodes should be sampled at the time of operation. CT may also be useful for identifying tumour invasion of the mediastinum and pleura [99] but its main role would appear to be in detecting which patients should have mediastinoscopy prior to surgery.

Magnetic resonance imaging (MRI) may be useful in assessing Pancoast tumours and chest wall invasion but appear to have no specific advantage over CT in the routine evaluation of a patient. Likewise the place of positron emission tomography has not been established in lung cancer [100] and it is not widely available to most clinicians.

The use of radioactive isotopes taken up by tumour cells, such as gallium, has been evaluated but adds nothing to the sensitivity or specificity of CT. A major advance in this field would be the discovery of a technique by which malignant tissue could be discriminated from non-malignant tissue, therefore allowing accurate documentation of tumour spread.

Mediastinoscopy

As stated above, patients who have abnormal mediastinal nodes on CT should have mediastinoscopy to confirm or refute the presence of metastatic spread. This allows for better selection of patients for surgery, since those with metastatic disease can be excluded and those with enlarged benign nodes can proceed to operation. Mediastinoscopy can thus improve the survival figures of surgical patients, although in the UK it is not universal practice among thoracic surgeons to sample the mediastinum preoperatively [78,101]. Mediastinoscopy cannot increase the number of patients cured by surgery but can prevent some futile operations being performed on some patients.

For anatomical reasons it is not possible for the surgeon to sample the whole of the mediastinum at medi-

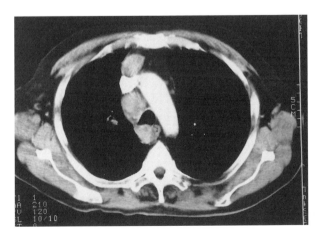

Fig. 41.16 Thoracic CT showing three enlarged lymph nodes at the level of the aortic arch.

astinoscopy and false-negative rates of around 10% are recorded [100]. Complications are not usually significant and mortality is rare. Some surgeons prefer to perform an anterior mediastinotomy if access is required to sample nodes draining into the left upper lobe or the anterior segment of the right upper lobe. It is also possible to sample periaortic and subaortic glands by this route.

Assessment of distal spread

Spread of bronchial carcinoma to a site outside the thorax, such as the brain, liver or skeleton, clearly makes a patient inoperable. Patients who have abnormal biochemical tests or specific symptoms that may point to evidence of distant spread should have further evaluation.

Liver metastases

The finding of an obviously enlarged, hard and irregular liver on physical examination is strong evidence of hepatic metastases. However, this is unusual at presentation, as is jaundice. Liver function tests should be requested routinely on all patients requiring staging of lung cancer. Although normal values do not exclude hepatic spread and elevated values may be due to non-metastatic liver disease, further investigations are required if the patient's management is likely to be affected as a result. Liver ultrasound and CT have a similar degree of accuracy in the detection of hepatic metastasis [102]. In the UK, it has become routine practice for radiologists to include the liver (and adrenal glands) when asked to perfrom CT of the thorax to assess operability. Occasionally, if there is doubt about the presence of hepatic involvement, histological clarification may be obtained by fine-needle aspiration or liver biopsy, either of which can be performed under ultrasound or CT guidance.

Bone metastases

The skeleton is a common metastatic site for bronchial carcinoma. Usually these metastases are symptomatic, and pain suggestive of a bony metastasis should lead to radiographs of the affected area. Lytic lesions are usually seen on these films. Isotope bone scanning is much more sensitive than conventional radiography in the detection of bony metastasis, false-negative rates being less than 2% (Fig. 41.17). The main disadvantage of bone scanning is its lack of specificity. False-positive rates of 40–50% have been reported, the increased uptake presumably being due to benign metabolic bone disease [103,104]. It is known that patients who are asymptomatic and have no biochemical abnormalities have a truly negative bone scan in more than 95% of cases [105]. It seems clear therefore that there is no place for routine bone scanning in all patients preoperatively and that this investigation should be reserved

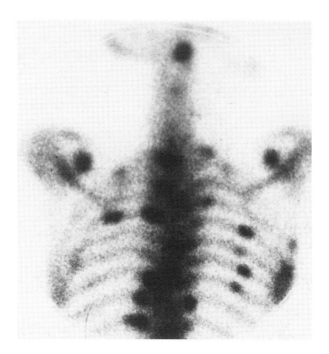

Fig. 41.17 Bone scan showing multiple spinal, shoulder girdle and rib metastatic deposits.

for those in whom there is clinical or biochemical evidence to suggest skeletal spread. As with liver metastases, occasionally it may be necessary to obtain further information with local biopsy.

Patients with small-cell carcinoma have a much higher incidence of bony metastases and in this situation scans may be useful to document both the extent of disease and its response to chemotherapy [106].

Brain metastases

Intracranial spread may come to light as a result of headache, vomiting, personality change or fits, or because of the development of focal neurological deficit. Occasionally, intracranial metastases present at a stage when the lung primary is neither symptomatic nor even radiologically apparent, the diagnosis being made retrospectively after craniotomy. When cerebral metastases are suspected as a result of these clinical features, the investigation of choice is CT with contrast enhancement. Routine CT of the brain in asymptomatic patients gives a very low yield (approximately 2%) [107] and is not indicated as a screening procedure.

The likelihood of detectable intracranial metastases being present at the time of diagnosis varies according to cell type, being most common in patients with small-cell carcinoma. In one necropsy study, the frequency of cerebral metastases varied from 14% in squamous cell tumours to 31% in small-cell lesions [108]. The clinician therefore may have a much lower threshold for requesting this investigation in patients with small-cell lesions.

A routine preoperative management plan

The assessment of suitability for resection is an important part of the management of lung cancer patients, as this form of treatment offers the best chance of significant prolongation of survival. The various steps in this management process are illustrated in Fig. 41.18. Patients should have a definite diagnosis, with histological subtype if possible, prior to evaluation. Those with small-cell lesions are usually more suitable for systemic treatment with chemotherapy (see below). The place of surgery in patients with small-cell lesions is controversial and clinicians considering this form of treatment in these patients should conduct a comprehensive search for metastatic disease.

Patients thought to be fit for surgery, with no symptoms or signs to suggest metastatic disease, should undergo CT of their thorax and upper abdomen. Those patients without significant mediastinal node enlargement (<1 cm) should proceed directly to thoracotomy. Those with mediastinal invasion or metastases are inoperable and should be assessed for other forms of therapy. Patients with enlarged lymph nodes should have mediastinal sampling at mediastinoscopy. Positive nodes at this stage make the patient inoperable. Patients with a negative mediastinoscopy should proceed to thoracotomy.

A more vexed question is the role of CT of the brain and bone in otherwise operable patients. Hillers and colleagues [109] performed a meta-analysis in order to determine the proportion of patients with potentially operable non-small-cell lung cancer who could have been spared thoracotomy by these investigations. They concluded that fewer than 5% of patients thought operable on previous CT of the thorax had evidence of distant metastases on

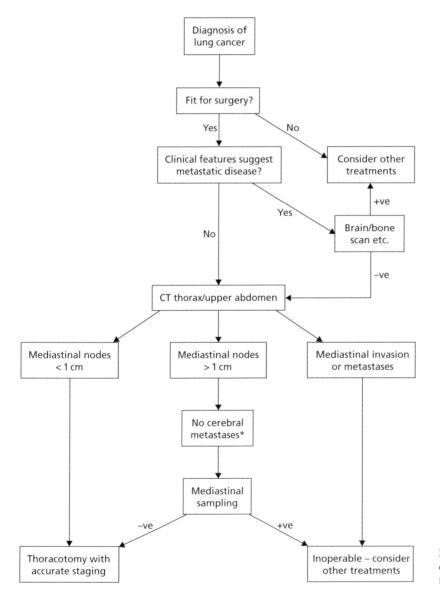

Fig. 41.18 Management of a potentially operable patient (see text on cerebral metastases).

scans. However, the likelihood of metastatic disease increases if the mediastinum has been found to be abnormal preoperatively. For instance in one study [107], 4% of patients with normal CT of the thorax had occult metastases compared with 32% who had an abnormal mediastinum on CT.

Muers, in his excellent reviews of the situation [110,111], concluded that patients with a normal mediastinum should not undergo routine brain and bone scanning as 95% of them are normal. Patients with enlarged mediastinal nodes should be investigated. They should have a bone scan if they have suggestive symptoms or biochemical abnormalities and he also recommends that they should have CT of the brain. Clearly the decision is between mediastinal sampling or scanning of distant organs. The latter is certainly cheaper and can be done on an outpatient basis. There is a clear need for large multicentre trials to try to clarify this situation.

Staging

The clinical staging of lung cancer is an attempt to define the anatomical extent of the tumour. Staging has been used primarily as a means of allowing management decisions to be based on published data relating to survival of clearly defined groups or 'stages'. Separate systems have evolved for non-small-cell and small-cell tumours.

Non-small-cell lung cancer

Patients with non-small-cell lung cancer are staged by the application of a process using 'T' for primary tumour, 'N' for regional lymph nodes and 'M' for distant metastases. Each letter is qualified by numerical suffixes that describe the size or local extent of the tumour, the extent of regional lymph node spread if present, and the presence or absence of distant extrathoracic metastases. The use of such a TNM system in non-small-cell lung cancer has shown that the stage of the tumour clearly influences prognosis [112]. The TNM staging classification currently in use was upgraded in 1997 and is presented in Table 41.6 [113]. The various TNM classifications have been divided into stages I–IV. Stage III is split into stage IIIA, which accommodates the potentially operable T3 and N2 patients, and stage IIIB, which contains inoperable patients whose disease may be controlled locally by thoracic radiotherapy. Stage I and II tumours are clearly operable, while patients in stage IV have distant metastases. It can be seen from Fig. 41.19 that this staging classification clearly separates the different prognostic groups and allows accurate prediction of survival at the time of diagnosis. The clinical methods used for establishing the stage of lung cancer have been described above. Providing that staging has been thorough, the number of patients found at thoracotomy to be

Table 41.6 TNM definitions in the international staging system for lung cancer. (From Mountain [113].)

Extent of primary tumour (T)

T0	No primary tumour detected.
Tis	Carcinoma *in situ*.
TX	Primary cannot be assessed/positive cytology only.
T1	A tumour 3 cm or less in greatest dimension, surrounded by lung or visceral pleura, not in main bronchus.
T2	A tumour more than 3 cm in size, or in main bronchus more than 2 cm from main carina, or invading visceral pleura, or associated with partial atelectasis (not entire lung).
T3	Involves any of following: chest wall (including superior sulcus), diaphragm, parietal pericardium, mediastinal pleura. In main bronchus less than 2 cm from main carina (but not involving it), atelectasis of entire lung.
T4	Invasion of mediastinum, heart/great vessels, trachea, carina, oesophagus, vertebral body. Separate nodules in same lobe as primary, malignant pleural or pericardial effusion.

Condition of regional lymph nodes (N)

NX	Regional lymph nodes cannot be assessed.
N0	No regional lymph node metastases.
N1	Ipsilateral peribronchial or hilar nodes involved.
N2	Ipsilateral mediastinal or subcarinal nodes involved.
N3	Contralateral hilar or mediastinal nodes involved, or any scalene/supraclavicular nodes involved.

Presence or absence of distant metastases (M)

MX	Distant metastases cannot be assessed.
M0	No distant metastases.
M1	Distant metastases, includes separate nodule in different lobe.

Stage groupings (5-year survival rates in parentheses)

Stage 0	Tis	N0	M0	(?)
Stage IA	T1	N0	M0	(60%)
Stage IB	T2	N0	M0	(38%)
Stage IIA	T1	N1	M0	(34%)
Stage IIB	T2	N1	M0	(24%)
	T3	N0	M0	(22%)
Stage IIIA	T1	N2	M0	(13%)
	T2	N2	M0	(13%)
	T3	N1–2	M0	(9%)
Stage IIIB	T4	N0–2	M0	(7%)
	T1–4	N3	M0	(3%)
Stage IV	Any T	Any N	M1	(1%)

inoperable should not exceed 5%. A few are found to have N2 disease when macroscopically involved mediastinal nodes are beyond the reach of the mediastinoscope. Such patients may still undergo surgery but have a 5-year survival of around 10% [113]. Although it is not widespread practice, it is recommended that surgeons should methodically sample and separately submit lymph nodes from differently numbered mediastinal gland groups and

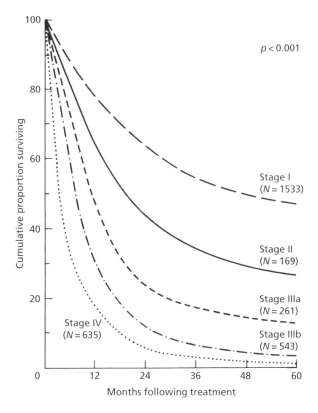

Fig. 41.19 Cumulative proportions of patients with lung carcinoma surviving 5 years, by clinical stage of disease. (From Mountain [113] with permission.)

from the hilum in order to allow pathological staging following thoracotomy. In general, pathological staging (pTNM) tends to downgrade the preoperative stage by finding previously undetected disease, and it is not surprising therefore that the median survival of pTNM subsets is much better than that of equivalent TNM stages based on clinical investigations [113].

Small-cell lung cancer

Small-cell lung cancers grow more aggressively and often metastasize earlier from a much smaller primary than other cell types; because of this, the TNM system of staging is irrelevant for small-cell tumours. Clinicians have adopted a simple staging system using the terms 'limited' and 'extensive' disease. Limited disease refers to a group of approximately 30% of patients who at presentation appear to have disease confined to the ipsilateral hemithorax (lung, pleura, and hilar, mediastinal and supraclavicular lymph nodes). Extensive disease refers to spread beyond these confines.

Since the majority of patients with small-cell tumours have inoperable disease at presentation, systemic therapy with drugs, to which the tumour is initially fairly sensitive, has become the mainstay of treatment. However,

there is a small subgroup of patients who do present with operable disease and they should be considered for operation in the standard way using routine staging procedures. It would seem reasonable to perform fairly intensive investigations for metastases in this group of patients, including CT of the thorax, upper abdomen and brain, as well as bilateral iliac crest marrow aspiration since bone marrow deposits are common in small-cell lung cancer. However, the natural history of small-cell lung cancer means that prolonged investigation delaying treatment may leave some patients unfit for active intervention.

In the same way as the TNM staging system gives a useful prognostic guide in non-small-cell lung cancer, disease extent (limited or extensive) is also a useful prognostic aid. Other factors influencing prognosis are a measure of the patient's ability to function (performance status) and a few simple biochemical investigations (serum sodium, and a measure of liver function such as lactate dehydrogenase or alkaline phosphatase). It can be seen therefore that in a patient with known small-cell cancer, taking a history, performing a clinical examination and arranging a simple blood test and chest radiograph are all that is required to give a fairly accurate guide to prognosis [114].

Treatment

When discussing the current treatments available for patients with lung cancer it is relevant to divide the subject into the management of non-small-cell and small-cell types. As stated above, these two groups of patients have different prognoses and their tumours respond differently to the currently available therapies. The majority of patients have non-small-cell tumours and the treatment modality that gives the best result is still surgery. However, most patients are inoperable and palliation is the aim of any treatment offered. In this respect radiotherapy is very helpful; indeed, some patients who are not suitable for surgery may be treated with radical radiation therapy. The role of chemotherapy in non-small-cell lung cancer is controversial but is gaining acceptance, especially in North America.

Chemotherapy gives the best hope of prolonged survival and improved quality of life in patients with small-cell lesions. The tumour is radiosensitive, although the exact place of radiotherapy is not clear. There is a small subgroup of patients who are operable and their survival is as good as that seen with the best chemotherapy results. However, long-term survival in patients with this tumour is rare.

The place of different treatment modalities in the overall management of patients with lung cancer is outlined in Fig. 41.9. For the majority of patients, an attempt at curative therapy is not possible and efforts should be directed towards palliation of the patient's symptoms. Quality of life is a term that is seen more commonly in studies of the treatment of lung cancer and is something that clinicians are now attempting to measure and to influence.

Non-small-cell lung cancer

The prognosis for patients diagnosed with non-small-cell lung cancer is poor, most large series of unselected patients giving an overall 5-year survival of less than 10% irrespective of treatment [115]. This figure has not changed over the last 30 years [116] and the best results are in patients treated with surgery.

Surgery

Although surgery is effective treatment for bronchial carcinoma, unfortunately the disease is only operable in a small minority of patients. Upwards of two-thirds of patients are inoperable at the time of presentation because of advanced age, poor respiratory function, other significant medical conditions or clinical evidence of tumour spread (see above). Of the remainder who are considered for surgery, 10–15% are rejected because of mediastinal involvement discovered at mediastinoscopy. Approximately 20–25% undergo surgery and up to 5% are found inoperable at thoracotomy. This means that only about 12–15% of all patients with non-small-cell tumours have a chance of receiving a potentially curable operation.

Types of operations

Pneumonectomy involves ligation of the pulmonary veins, division of the pulmonary artery and suturing or stapling of the bronchial stump at the level of the carina. At lobectomy, corresponding vessels may be ligated at segmental level. Hilar and accessible mediastinal nodes should be removed at operation and labelled according to their site of origin in order to enable more accurate pathological staging. Serosanguineous fluid is allowed to accumulate in the empty haemothorax of patients undergoing pneumonectomy and this tends to stabilize the mediastinum. Following lobectomy, underwater seal drainage is mandatory to prevent the accumulation of fluid and to allow full expansion of the remaining lobe or lobes. As an alternative to pneumonectomy, a variety of bronchoplastic procedures have been devised to remove tumour and yet conserve part of the lung subtended by the involved bronchus. The most common of these procedures is 'sleeve resection' of a tumour, extending from the right upper lobe bronchus into the right main and intermediate bronchi. Anatomical considerations make such procedures less common on the left side. When sleeve resections are carried out, facilities for frozen section are required at

operation to ensure that both ends of the sleeve are clear of tumour.

When a peripheral pulmonary opacity is found at thoracotomy to be small and confined to a bronchopulmonary segment, the more limited procedure of segmental resection may be carried out, and it may be possible to perform this operation using a thoracoscope [117]. This procedure, which permits 'keyhole surgery' in the chest, allows much quicker rehabilitation postoperatively and a much shorter perioperative period in hospital. There is no large thoracotomy wound and postoperative pain is less of a problem. Some surgeons are concerned that thoracoscopic resections may be incomplete in malignant disease, although modern techniques have allowed for pneumonectomies to be carried out and it is possible to sample nodes in the mediastinum with this instrument [118]. The results of studies of long-term survival of larger series of patients operated on in this way are awaited with interest.

Complications

Apart from the general complications that may beset any major surgical procedure, there are several problems peculiar to pulmonary resective surgery. Lower respiratory tract infection in residual lung tissue is common and requires treatment with appropriate antibiotics and physiotherapy. Postoperative infection of the resected space (empyema) can be a particularly difficult problem especially in an upper lobectomy. One or other of the phrenic nerves occasionally has to be sacrificed in a resection of a central tumour abutting the pericardium. The left recurrent laryngeal nerve may be similarly damaged during a left pneumonectomy.

Operative mortality has fallen over the years and is a reflection of better surgical techniques and the application of more stringent selection criteria. The intraoperative and 30-day postoperative mortality for over 2000 resections in 12 different North American centres carried out between 1979 and 1981 under the auspices of the Lung Cancer Study Group found the overall rate for pneumonectomy to be 6.2%, for lobectomy 2.9% and for segmental and wedge resections 1.4% [119]. Surgery in older patients used to be associated with a high mortality rate but published figures from the last decade have suggested an overall mortality of less than 6% [119,120]. The results of macroscopically complete resection in elderly patients justify active treatment, since the 5-year survival rate is about 35% [120]. It has become increasingly difficult to justify the decision that a patient is unsuitable for surgical resection on the grounds of age alone, provided the same careful staging procedures that are applied to younger patients are followed. It should also be remembered that the life expectancy in a developed country for a patient reaching the age of 70 is in excess of 10 years.

Results

Survival after resection for non-small-cell lung cancer is closely related to the stage and pathological type of disease. Stage I tumours (T1/T2N0M0) when treated surgically carry a 5-year survival rate of 40–60% [121,122]. In stage II tumours, the survival rate following operation falls to 20–50% depending on histology [122]. The survival of patients with stage IIIA disease is much poorer after surgery with between only 9 and 13% surviving for 5 years [123]. The overall 5-year survival figures for surgery for non-small-cell lung cancer is 35%. Patients with squamous cell tumours fare better than those with adenocarcinoma at all stages. Mountain [123] reported 4-year postoperative survival for stage IIB (T2N1) patients to be 53% for squamous carinoma and 25% for adenocarcinoma, and for (T3N0) 37% and 21% respectively.

It is depressing that the vast majority of patients who die after resection do so from recurrent disease. The pattern of recurrence in surgically treated stage I and II disease was analysed by the Lung Cancer Study Group in a retrospective review of 771 patients [124]; 70% occurred initially outside the chest, presumably from occult distant metastases present at the time of surgical resection of the primary tumour.

Radiotherapy

Radiotherapy is most commonly used to achieve symptomatic relief when given in low palliative doses to patients who are clearly inoperable and have appropriate symptoms due to their disease. Radical radiotherapy may offer the chance of cure in a small proportion of patients with non-small-cell lung cancer who are considered unsuitable for surgery on medical grounds but otherwise have 'operable' disease. Treatments are usually administered by means of a megavoltage linear accelerator, with some centres still using a cobalt-60 source for palliative treatments. The collimated beams of ionizing radiation are positioned to produce a tumoricidal dose in an area where the beams cross, with as much sparing of normal tissue as possible. Tissue absorption of radiation is measured in grays (Gy), 1 Gy being equivalent to 1 J of energy absorbed per kilogram of tissue; the relationship between the SI unit (Gy) and the old unit (rad) is shown in Table 41.7. Radiotherapy is the most frequently employed treatment in

Table 41.7 Units of absorbed radiation.

1 joule/kg	=	1 gray (Gy)
1 Gy	=	100 rad (old units)
1 cGy (centigray)	=	1 rad

patients with non-small-cell carcinoma of the bronchus [78].

Radical radiotherapy

This term implies an intention on the part of the radiotherapist to employ a relatively large dose of treatment in order to increase the patient's survival time or even to achieve a cure. Patients with stage I and II non-small-cell lung cancer are best treated by surgical resection; however, if this form of treatment cannot be followed, either because an operation has been declined or because of some medical contraindication, then radiotherapy does offer a small chance of cure. It should be recommended provided that the patient's general condition is good and that he or she has sufficient ventilatory capacity to survive the loss of functioning lung tissue that results from radiation damage to normal lung. Trials comparing radical radiotherapy with surgery in otherwise operable patients were performed more than 30 years ago. Initial results suggested that radical radiotherapy was the more effective treatment [125], although subsequent studies have not supported this and the place of surgery in these treatments is well established [126]. Patients who have stage IIIB (inoperable) disease have a much poorer outlook but may benefit from radical radiotherapy provided that their disease is limited to one hemithorax and can thus be encompassed by the radiotherapy field. This type of treatment is prolonged and requires the patient's performance status to be good; it is these fitter patients who seem to benefit most from this form of treatment.

A variety of techniques are employed in the delivery of radical radiotherapy, making comparison between reported studies difficult. The identification of those areas to be treated is determined from conventional chest radiographs and bronchoscopic findings. CT of the chest gives a much more precise location of the tumour, especially in the anteroposterior plane where lateral films may be difficult to interpret [127]. It is routine practice for the treatment field to include the primary tumour mass, ipsilateral and contralateral hilar lymph nodes and the mediastinum. Ipsilateral supraclavicular nodes may also be included and this is always the case in upper lobe tumours [128]. A dosemetric compromise has to be reached between delivery of a tumoricidal dose to this large area and the avoidance of injury to normal tissues, including the spinal cord, larynx and oesophagus.

In addition to planning the treatment field, the further important variables that have to be determined are the total dose of radiation, the number of fractions in which it is given and the duration of the course. In general, doses of 50–60 Gy over a period of 4–6 weeks are used. Trials from various centres using different scheduling techniques have demonstrated that survival is related to the dose of radiotherapy given. It has also been shown that small numbers of large fractions are less effective in controlling local tumour in the chest than large numbers of small fractions, even though the total dose remains the same [128]. Some workers have preferred split-course therapy, in which the same total dose is given in two half-dose courses with a 'rest period' of about 4 weeks between them, and have claimed similar results to continuous treatment [129]. Split-course treatment carries the added advantages of initial palliation due to tumour shrinkage with mild side-effects and a chance for further assessment of extrathoracic spread before the second course of treatment. This may allow the avoidance of unnecessary radical irradiation in patients with rapidly progressive disease. The argument against this form of therapy is that the design of treatment does not allow for initial local control, which could therefore deny an otherwise curable patient long survival.

The survival results of radical radiotherapy in inoperable patients are generally disappointing. Many authors report good 1-year survival figures (30–60%) but 5-year survival rarely exceeds 20% [129–131]. The subset of patients with stage I disease have a better outcome, some authors reporting up to 40% survival at 5 years [132,133]. Several factors make the results of radical radiotherapy difficult to evaluate. Firstly, the populations studied are not homogeneous as different cell types are usually lumped together as non-small-cell tumours. Also staging procedures differ within studies and by definition only inoperable patients are included. Patient survival time often reflects the spread of tumour beyond the radiotherapy field prior to treatment and need not indicate the success or failure of the local treatment. Lastly, radiotherapy itself may cause radiographic changes in normal lung that make the detection of local recurrence difficult to monitor. Despite this, the similarity of survival figures reported from various studies is striking and perhaps the most useful benchmark in a form of treatment where prolonged survival is the aim.

An interesting recent development in the scheduling of radical radiotherapy has taken into account evidence from cell kinetic studies that tumours may repopulate in the standard intervals between treatments. A regimen of continuous hyperfractionated accelerated radiotherapy (CHART) has been developed where treatment is given three times daily at intervals of 6 h for 12 consecutive days, including the weekend [134]. Although initial reports suggest that this may be a toxic regimen [135], the schedule has been modified and initial survival and local control results have been impressive [136]. CHART treatment was compared with conventional radical radiotherapy (60 Gy in 30 fractions over 6 weeks) in a randomized trial in patients with locally advanced non-small-cell lung cancer [137]. In the CHART group, there was a significant improvement in survival at 2 years (29% vs. 20%), especially in patients with squamous histology (33% vs. 19%). However more severe dysphagia (19% vs. 3%) was seen in the first 3 months with this treatment.

Palliative treatment

The majority of patients with non-small-cell lung cancer who have extrathoracic metastases die within 6 months of diagnosis, and when radiotherapy is used in these patients its only aim is to relieve distressing symptoms (Table 41.8). Since this may be achieved by restraining tumour growth rather than by attempting to eradicate it totally, lower doses of radiation are generally used. Many fractionation schemes are practised throughout the UK [138], usually with a total dose of 20–30 Gy given in up to 10 fractions. Randomized controlled trials carried out by the Medical Research Council (MRC) have shown that, for fit patients, two treatments of 8.5 Gy 7 days apart are of equal efficacy to 10 daily treatments of 3 Gy [139]. In patients with poor performance status, a similar study showed that one treatment of 10 Gy is as effective as two treatments of 8.5 Gy in palliating symptoms [140].

Treatable symptoms due to intrathoracic disease, including haemoptysis, may be relieved in over 80% of cases [139], distressing cough in about 60% [139,141] and breathlessness due to bronchial obstruction in 60% [139]. However, areas of atelectasis are not re-expanded in more than one-quarter of patients [128], and dyspnoea due to lymphangitis carcinomatosa is also unrelieved. Well-localized pain due to chest wall or rib involvement responds in over 70% of patients [139,141], although more diffuse chest discomfort is often not responsive. Obstruction of the SVC is reported to be relieved in 60–86% of cases [142] and dysphagia due to oesophageal compression by nodes responds in a similar proportion of patients.

Brain metastases are nearly always multiple, and symptomatic relief may be achieved in a significant group of patients by total brain irradiation using a 30-Gy dose given as 10 fractions over 2 weeks [143]. However, improvements may be small and dense neurological deficit rarely responds. The median survival time for untreated patients with cerebral metastases is about 3 months and therefore the fractionation scheme should be

Table 41.8 Palliative radiotherapy for distressing symptoms.

Haemoptysis
Pain: bony, chest wall, nerve root
Cough
Dyspnoea due to large bronchus obstruction
Mediastinal compression: obstruction of superior vena cava
Symptoms due to intracranial metastases
Symptoms due to spinal cord compression

as short as possible. The Royal College of Radiologists in a randomized controlled trial of patients with cerebral metastases due to various primaries showed that 12 Gy in two fractions was as useful as 30 Gy in 10 fractions. Median survival was 7 days longer in the second group (84 vs. 77 days), who required 8 days more treatment [144]. Dexamethasone, given initially in a dose of 16 mg daily, may also produce temporary relief by reducing intracranial pressure. Spinal cord compression due to tumour is a particularly distressing complication. Prompt treatment is required to prevent permanent neurological damage, which at worst may result in paraplegia with a sensory deficit and loss of sphincter control. In this emergency situation corticosteroids should be given and, if neurosurgery is not advised, urgent palliative radiotherapy is indicated. There is still debate about the optimal treatment schedule [145]. The spinal level involved may be indicated by clinical features and confirmed more precisely by plain radiography, CT and MRI.

Other extrathoracic metastatic disease that responds to palliative radiotherapy includes bony deposits, in which pain may be relieved in the vast majority of cases, and cervical lymph node enlargement. Radiotherapy is of no value in relieving systemic symptoms, such as malaise, anorexia or weight loss, nor can it reverse a recurrent laryngeal or other frank nerve palsy. The response of the paraneoplastic syndromes (see below) to radiotherapy is variable and unpredictable.

Side-effects

Side-effects tend to be dose-related and are therefore much more common in patients undergoing radical treatment. Since the aim of palliative radiotherapy is to relieve the patient's symptoms, any side-effects should be kept to a minimum. Cutaneous erythema is seen with large doses of radiotherapy but is not a serious problem. There may also be a general feeling of weakness and malaise. The patient should be warned to expect dysphagia, which is due to oesophagitis. This occurs after about 2 weeks of treatment and usually subsides spontaneously or with local anaesthetic preparations.

Radiation pneumonitis may occur following radical radiotherapy, the radiographic changes becoming evident 2–6 months after the completion of treatment. The changes are seen as a non-specific hazy infiltrate initially caused by inflammation but later as a result of fibrosis. The margin of the radiographic abnormality may be characteristically straight, matching the shielding around the radiotherapy portal. In the majority these changes are unaccompanied by symptoms, although 5–15% of patients may notice the insidious onset of breathlessness and a dry cough. The symptoms may respond to steroids but may be long-standing where progression to fibrosis occurs [146]. Radiation myelitis, potentially a most serious side-effect, may be

transient and self-limiting, in which case pain and paraesthesia occur about 3 months after radiotherapy only to disappear gradually over the space of a few weeks or months. These symptoms result from spinal cord vascular damage and demyelination. Fortunately, progression to complete paraplegia with loss of sphincter control is extremely unusual. It is estimated to occur in 1–5% of patients after a spinal cord dose of 50 Gy in 25 fractions over 5 weeks [147]. The risk is increased in shorter courses with higher dose fractions. Clearly it is important to exclude cord compression from recurrent tumour before making this diagnosis. Radiation pericarditis may occur 3–6 months after radiotherapy in about 4% of patients and is associated with sternal discomfort, breathlessness and ECG changes [148]. The condition is self-limiting and treatment is symptomatic.

Endobronchial treatments

Endobronchial techniques have evolved in the last two decades to help palliate symptoms such as haemoptysis and critical obstructions of main airways [149]. Most experience has been gained with laser therapy. A laser is an electrical device for producing an extremely powerful and narrow beam of light. Various types of laser are available and that most widely used in respiratory work is the Nd–Yag laser. The beam is transmitted endoscopically using fibreoptic techniques. The fibre can be passed down the suction channel of the fibreoptic bronchoscope and the beam is directed against tissue. Its energy evaporates moisture and coagulates blood in vessels to a depth of about 5 mm. At present laser therapy remains a palliative treatment, as most tumour is beyond bronchoscopic view and therefore beyond the reach of the laser. Its use is confined to symptomatic relief by debulking proximal endobronchial or tracheal tumour in the treatment of dyspnoea and the coagulation of vessels in order to relieve haemoptysis. However, results from laser therapy do not add much to standard palliative radiotherapy.

Modern endobronchial radiotherapy techniques deliver high-dose irradiation to the tumour via a catheter positioned next to the tumour at bronchoscopy. Treatment takes about 10–15 min and can relieve the symptoms of bronchial obstruction caused by tumour or of extraluminal pressure caused by nodes. Unfortunately, secondary haemorrhage appears to be an important complication of the procedure and studies comparing endobronchial radiotherapy with standard techniques have not yet been published.

Photodynamic therapy involves the intravenous administration of a light-sensitive drug (a haematoporphyrin derivative) that has an affinity for malignant tissue and is activated by laser light delivered at bronchoscopy. This produces necrosis of tumours in animals but its use in patients is not yet established. Another problem with these new techniques is that they are only available in a few centres in most countries.

Chemotherapy

The main limitation to the effectiveness of surgery and radiotherapy in patients with non-small-cell lung cancer is that evidence of metastatic spread at presentation may prevent treatment or that treatment may fail because of recurrent disease commonly occurring at distant sites. There is a clear need for 'systemic' treatment for the vast majority of patients and this has inevitably led to trials of cytotoxic drugs. Unfortunately, while chemotherapy is the mainstay of treatment of small-cell carcinoma of the lung, non-small-cell tumours are relatively resistant to the drugs currently available. Single-agent drugs have modest activity in terms of objective response rates (Table 41.9). Some authors have claimed prolonged survival for patients who respond compared with 'non-responders'. However, for such an approach to be valid, both groups must have the same prognosis with no treatment and this often cannot be assumed. Moreover, these drugs, either singly or in combination, are capable of considerable toxicity and the price paid in terms of quality of life for modest survival benefit has rarely been measured. Trials comparing chemotherapy with a control group of best supportive care have only recently appeared. Most have shown a modest survival advantage to chemotherapy treatment, although no study has accurately measured quality of life and therefore the effect of treatment on palliation of symptoms is not yet available. In a major meta-analysis published in 1995 [150], the Non-Small Cell Lung Cancer Collaborative Group analysed data published from 11 trials involving 1190 patients. Despite considerable statistical heterogeneity, the results suggested that the use of alkylating agents was detrimental to survival compared with best supportive care but that cisplatin-based regimens conferred benefits. A reduction in the risk of death of 27% was seen, equivalent to an absolute improvement in survival of 10% at 1 year. Although this may sound impressive, the overall increase in median survival was only 6 weeks. No measurements of the toxicity of the treatment were performed. Many enthusiasts are keen to extrapolate these findings to the millions of people worldwide who have this disease [151] while others, worried about toxicity with such little benefit, sound a note of caution [152]. Well-designed clinical studies examining the place of chemotherapy in the management of non-small-cell lung cancer are required. It may well be that chemotherapy has a place in a multimodality approach to the disease and future studies should consider this role for chemotherapy.

Combined modality treatment

Surgery and radiotherapy

The combination of radiotherapy and surgery was first reported in the early 1950s for tumours that were originally believed to be inoperable but which were subsequently resected after initial radiotherapy and tumour shrinkage [153]. However, no clear survival advantage has ever been shown for this scheduling of radiotherapy and surgery [154], and the concept of preoperative radiotherapy has largely been abandoned. The exception to this is with superior sulcus tumours (see below).

Compared with surgery alone, the use of *postoperative* radiotherapy for patients with N1 and N2 disease has been demonstrated to improve local control within the chest [155], and one study [156] has also shown a statistically significant survival benefit. However the exact effect of postoperative radiotherapy on survival has been questioned by a meta-analysis of nine trials showing worse survival in irradiated patients in the first 3 months [157]. This difference may be related to radiotherapy techniques (cobalt source vs. linear accelerator). It is common practice for thoracic surgeons to refer patients for postoperative radiotherapy when they know they have left disease in the chest postoperatively. These patients do particularly badly, and radiotherapy does not improve their survival.

Surgery and chemotherapy

A retrospective review performed by the Lung Cancer Study Group of the pattern of recurrences in 771 patients undergoing surgery showed that 70% initially recurred outside the chest, presumably from occult distant metastases present at the time of surgical resection of the primary tumour [124]. This has led to interest in combining good local control (surgical resection) with systemic treatment (chemotherapy) [158]. In the past chemotherapy was given postoperatively (adjuvant therapy). More recently, encouraging results have been obtained from the use of chemotherapy given before the operation (neoadjuvant) [159].

The meta-analysis conducted by the Non-Small Cell

Table 41.9 Activity of single-agent drugs in non-small-cell lung cancer.

Drug	Response rate (%)
Ifosfamide	26
Cisplatin	21
Mitomycin	20
Vindesine	18
Doxorubicin	13
Carboplatin	11
Etoposide	9

Lung Cancer Collaborative Group [150] examined 14 trials involving a total of 4357 patients that compared surgery alone with surgery plus postoperative chemotherapy. The results are very similar to those quoted above for surgery and radiotherapy. The earlier trials that used alkylating agents showed better survival in the patients treated with surgery alone, i.e. the use of this kind of postoperative chemotherapy was actually hazardous to the patient. However, for regimens containing cisplatin there was a survival advantage for postoperative treatment. This amounted to a 13% reduction in the risk of death, with an absolute benefit from chemotherapy of 3% at 2 years and 5% at 5 years. These results are encouraging, although postoperative chemotherapy is not routine practice at present and further good clinical trials are required to confirm the suggestion of any such benefit.

The results of surgical treatment on stage IIIA patients are disappointing, with 5-year survival usually less than 30%. A number of reports have described the use of chemotherapy given prior to surgery [160,161]. Most have shown a good response to therapy and some increased resectability. In 1994 the first two randomized studies comparing neoadjuvant chemotherapy plus surgery with surgery alone appeared [162,163]. Both were small studies but appeared to show a significant benefit for neoadjuvant treatment. Roth and colleagues [162] entered 60 patients thought to have resectable stage IIIA disease; 28 patients were randomized to receive preoperative chemotherapy with cyclophosphamide, etoposide and cisplatin every 4 weeks for a total of three cycles. Patients who responded to chemotherapy were given three cycles after surgery. The objective response rate to chemotherapy was 35% including one complete response. Only 15% progressed while receiving chemotherapy. The resectability rate did not differ significantly between the two groups. Only 39% of patients in the chemotherapy group and 31% in the surgery alone group achieved complete resection. The estimated median survival in the chemotherapy group was 64 months compared with 11 months for surgery alone. In a similar study from Spain [163], 30 patients at a similar stage received mitomycin, ifosfamide and cisplatin prior to surgery. An identical number had an operation alone. Both groups received mediastinal radiotherapy following surgery. A higher proportion of patients had a complete resection compared with the first study. Median overall survival in patients receiving surgery and radiotherapy alone was 8 months compared with 26 months for the group receiving chemotherapy in addition. This trial has provoked a lot of comment. Patients in the control group did very poorly, none of the 30 patients surviving more than 20 months. The trials are small and larger studies are required to see whether this is an appropriate use of chemotherapy in this disease. Two interesting points arise: firstly, patients did not become inoperable while receiving chemotherapy for a number of weeks

prior to surgery and, secondly, the Spanish group identified the K-*ras* oncogene as a significant prognostic indicator in resected specimens. It is possible that in the future the use of this marker may be helpful in identifying which patients require adjuvant therapy [164].

Radiotherapy and chemotherapy

The aim of combined chemotherapy and radiotherapy is to optimize local control and to control distant metastases. In general, studies comparing radical radiotherapy alone with radiotherapy and chemotherapy have been performed in inoperable patients who have a poor prognosis. In the 1995 meta-analysis of chemotherapy [150], 22 trials involving 3033 patients were assessed. There was a definite benefit for combined therapy compared with radiation therapy alone. Cisplatin-containing regimens gave an absolute benefit of 4% at 2 years and 2% at 5 years. The optimal sequence of chemotherapy before or during radiotherapy is not known. There is evidence that platinum-based chemotherapy before radiotherapy gives a modest survival advantage, possibly in its role in controlling micrometastases, and that concurrent treatment can improve local control [165]. As with most combinations involving chemotherapy, there would appear to be more unanswered questions than answers and further randomized clinical trials are required [166].

Small-cell lung cancer

Of all patients with bronchial carcinoma, 25% have small-cell tumours. These lesions grow more aggressively and patients usually present with a short history and evidence of metastases. As explained above, the disease is usually staged in terms of limited and extensive groups. Without treatment the median survival for patients with limited disease is 6–8 weeks and patients with extensive disease fare even worse [167]. At presentation more than 70% of patients have extensive disease. An outline for the management of patients with small-cell tumours is illustrated in Fig. 41.20.

Chemotherapy

Unlike non-small-cell lung cancer, small-cell tumours have been found to be more sensitive to chemotherapy and this is now the accepted modality of treatment for most patients with the disease [167,168]. Many drugs have been found to have activity against this tumour, although if used singly their duration of action is brief with minimal impact on long-term survival. Responses in the range of 15–40% are seen with drugs such as cyclophosphamide, doxorubicin, vincristine, cisplatin, ifosfamide and etoposide when given alone, but fewer than 5% of patients gain a complete response [168]. Not surprisingly, when agents

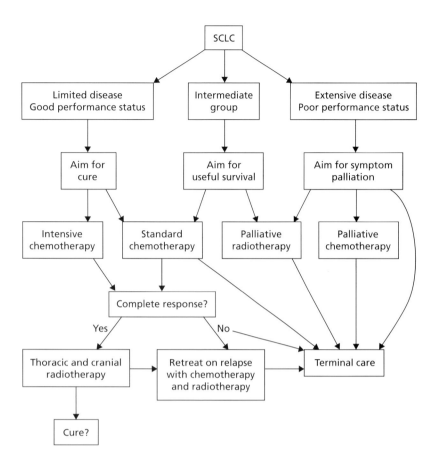

Fig. 41.20 Management of patients with small-cell carcinoma (SCLC, small-cell lung cancer).

are added together and given as combination treatments the results are more encouraging. In the last two decades combination chemotherapy has improved the prognosis significantly. The median survival time in patients with limited disease is now 14–16 months and in those with extensive disease 8–10 months. The disease may show an objective response (partial and complete) to therapy in up to 90% of patients treated, and those who do respond live longer than those who do not. Drug regimens that have been well used and which have predictable results include cyclophosphamide/doxorubicin/vincristine, doxorubicin/cyclophosphamide/etoposide and cisplatin/etoposide. However, Fig. 41.21 shows the poor survival even in patients who have an apparent complete response to chemotherapy. Of 100 patients with small-cell lung cancer treated with combination chemotherapy, perhaps half a dozen survive for over 2 years, this number representing 15–20% of those with limited disease and less than 2% of those with extensive disease [169].

It is conventional to administer these combination drug regimens to the patient every 3–4 weeks. This can largely be done on an outpatient basis. Treatment with platinum requires careful hydration and antiemetic therapy and should only be given in specialized units. Patients should be assessed for response to treatment after a minimum of two or three cycles unless the disease is obviously progressive or the patient cannot tolerate the treatment. Oncologists often measure activity of treatment in terms of response rates. An objective response to therapy may be either partial or complete. In a partial response, shrinkage of the tumour by at least 50% in a measurable diameter must have occurred. A partial response is not recorded if tumour at another site is progressing. It is clear that there must be inaccuracies in this form of assessment. Measuring a shadow on a chest film gives definitive data but it is often not known whether the radiographic opacity is due to tumour or perhaps to atelectasis or consolidation behind the tumour. Clearly, opening up a small endobronchial lesion may cause dramatic 'improvement' on a chest film when in fact the response of the tumour may be minimal. Complete responses, seen in approximately half the patients with limited disease and one-quarter of the patients with extensive disease [168], are defined as the total removal of all tumour as evaluated by physical examination, radiography, scanning or bronchoscopy.

Although the early results of drug treatment in small-cell carcinoma were very promising, the survival of patients with 'conventional' treatment has reached a plateau with little change over the last decade [170]. A variety of different therapeutic manoeuvres have been tried in order to improve this situation.

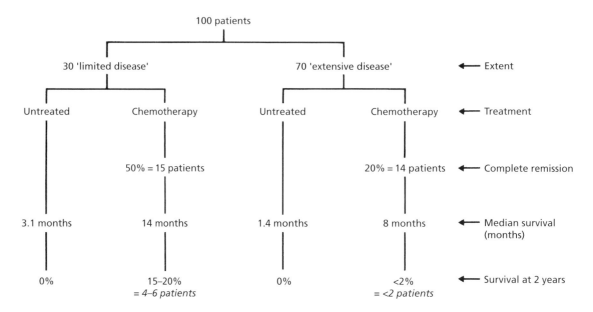

Fig. 41.21 Probable results in 100 patients with small-cell lung cancer.

High-dose chemotherapy

It is known that combinations of two and three drugs have much more activity than single-drug therapy in gaining a remission and it is likely therefore that a definite dose–response relationship exists in the treatment of this disease. Several strategies have been tried to increase the initial dose of induction chemotherapy in order to try to prevent later relapses. The main problem with increasing the intensity of drug treatment is that the toxicity experienced by the patient is also increased. In a typical early study of high-dose chemotherapy, fit patients with limited disease were prospectively randomized to either a double dose ($1.5\,g/m^2$) or a standard dose ($0.75\,g/m^2$) of cyclophosphamide in a regimen also containing methotrexate and lomustine at conventional doses. The high-dose group had a significantly increased median survival rate of 56 weeks compared with 42 weeks for standard therapy. This was at the expense of 'a life-threatening complication' rate of 53% compared with 7% and a drug-related death rate of 4% vs. 1% [171]. The toxicity of this treatment is clearly unacceptable for the small benefit in survival.

The principal drug-related toxicity that threatens life is myelosuppression. Two strategies have been developed to try to overcome this problem. Autologous bone marrow transplantation [172] involves taking marrow from a patient prior to chemotherapy, giving high doses of chemotherapy that would normally cause complete marrow failure, and managing this by replacement with the patient's own harvested bone marrow. High doses of chemotherapy can be given with this technique, although complete eradication of the disease rarely occurs. One potential problem with this method is that malignant cells may be harvested as well as normal marrow cells; thus when marrow cells are reinjected after chemotherapy, the patient also receives untreated cancer cells. Attempts have been made to overcome this by 'cleansing' the bone marrow after harvesting. The other strategy involves the use of haematopoietic growth factors that can stimulate normal haematopoiesis [173]. Granulocyte colony-stimulating factor can be produced by recombinant DNA techniques and allows clinicians to increase the production of bone marrow cells by patients after myelotoxic chemotherapy. The results of randomized studies using this technique to allow higher doses of chemotherapy are awaited.

In intensive regimens it is important to be aware that there may well be a selection bias, with patients whose general condition is poor being excluded as they would be unable to tolerate the rigours of high-dose chemotherapy. Valid comparisons can only be drawn if the performance status, the extent and size of the tumour, and the age of the patient are known.

Scheduling

Several randomized trials have attempted to determine the minimum number of courses of chemotherapy that can be given without compromising survival, aiming to minimize toxicity and improve the quality of life of the patient. The MRC reported a trial in 265 patients who had responded to induction chemotherapy (six courses of etoposide, cyclosphosphamide, methotrexate and vincristine). Patients were then randomized to receive a further six courses of the same chemotherapy (maintenance chemotherapy) or no further treatment until relapse. No overall survival advantage was seen for maintenance chemotherapy [174]. The same researchers have compared six courses of the same treatment to three courses in a randomized study of 458 patients [175]. There appeared to be a marginal survival advantage for the six-course regimen.

In an interesting study reported by the London Lung Cancer Group [176], 616 patients were randomized to receive either four or eight courses of chemotherapy (etoposide, cyclophosphamide and vincristine) and at relapse to receive either symptomatic treatment or further chemotherapy with new agents (methotrexate and doxorubicin). The results showed that patients receiving only four courses of chemotherapy and then symptomatic treatment at relapse had a much poorer median survival compared with the other three treatment groups (30 weeks vs. 39–42 weeks). There was no advantage to relapse chemotherapy in the group given eight courses initially.

The concept of introducing at relapse further combinations of new drugs to which the residual tumour cells would not be resistant has been tried before. Many studies have compared alternating (crossover) regimens but consistent benefit in terms of increased median survival has not been shown. As with high-dose induction chemotherapy, this strategy has largely been abandoned. In summary therefore it seems that patients given chemotherapy for small-cell lung cancer should receive, if possible, no less than four but no more than six courses of induction therapy. Maintenance chemotherapy is of no value but retreatment on relapse is worth while.

Complications

The main agents currently used in combination chemotherapy for small-cell lung cancer may produce significant toxicity. Myelosuppression may lead to bleeding problems and infections. Febrile episodes in neutropenic patients are associated with infection in about 60% of cases [177,178] and require immediate broad-spectrum antibiotic treatment. Likely pathogens include *Staphylococcus aureus*, *Pseudomonas aeruginosa* and *Escherichia coli*. Although treatment may be modified in the light of subsequent microbiological culture, it is inadvisable to withhold antibiotics pending these results [179]. Nausea and vomiting commonly accompany treatment with cytotoxic drugs, especially platinum compounds. Pharmacological techniques have been developed to counteract this, with the use of intravenous antiemetics such as metoclopramide and ondansetron. Patients often express fears of alopecia. However this is transient and is best managed by early counselling and an appropriate wig.

In general it is clear that chemotherapy is best given by experts. Oncology units are obviously well geared to support patients both physically and psychologically through chemotherapy, and most of the clinical trials of treatment in this condition are conducted by oncologists rather than respiratory physicians. However, patients with lung cancer are almost always referred to respiratory physicians who are keen to give chemotherapy themselves. Once again, a team approach involving interested clinicians would appear to be in the patient's best interests.

Palliative effects

Patients with small-cell lung cancer have a dreadful prognosis if untreated and in general the results of chemotherapy in terms of long-term prolongation of survival are poor. Some clinicians take the view that the use of chemotherapy is not always justified because of toxicity and the adverse effects of treatment. For many years there was a feeling that it was cruel to inflict treatment on old and ill patients and that any prolongation in life would be of poor quality. Is this protective attitude by clinicians reasonable or does active treatment have any palliative benefit? In the MRC trial comparing three and six courses of chemotherapy [175], effects of the treatment on the patient's symptoms were recorded. Good relief of local symptoms was seen, the vast majority of patients reporting palliation and, in many, disappearance of symptoms. Also, systemic problems such as anorexia were greatly improved, a feature not seen with local treatment such as radiotherapy.

Some clinicians believe that patients who are well at diagnosis should be left until they develop symptoms, which should then be palliated. This approach was compared with standard immediate treatment in an MRC trial [180]. Patients given immediate treatment had much better survival and, although adverse effects of treatment were more common in this group, other aspects of quality of life as recorded by clinicians were better. Other authors have also shown that patients who respond to chemotherapy have improvement in symptoms and quality of life [176], and it can be concluded that if patients are fit to have chemotherapy it should not be withheld since good control of disease and good palliation go together.

A more difficult decision can be whether to treat patients who have extensive disease and poor performance status. Obviously it is important that chemotherapy is not given to a patient for whom there is no realistic prospect of useful palliation or improvement in the quality of life. Recently, many groups have been investigating the use of simple more 'gentle' chemotherapy regimens that have minor side-effects but adequate anti-tumour activity. This would allow outpatient treatment, with modest improvement in survival and good palliation of symptoms without the cost, toxicity and need for in-patient care of more intensive regimens. Oral treatment with etoposide often forms the basis of these regimens [181]. Pharmacokinetic studies with this drug have shown that it is much more active when given in a chronic schedule, which makes its oral administration more attractive than intravenous use. Its safety and efficacy have been demonstrated in a large phase II trial in elderly patients [182]. Etoposide capsules were administered for 5 days to a total dose of 800 mg/m². A response rate in excess of 70% and a median survival of 9.5 months was seen, results comparable with the efficacy of more toxic and complicated combination chemotherapy regimens. Haematological and gastrointestinal toxicities were minimal and admissions to hospital for treatment related to toxicity were seldom necessary. However when oral etoposide was compared to 'standard' combination intravenous chemotherapy in a randomized trial it was found to be less effective in terms of survival [183]. Its place in the management of this disease is thus uncertain as it appears to be reasonably tolerated but relatively 'weak' therapy.

Radiotherapy

As with chemotherapy, small-cell tumours are in general more radiosensitive than non-small-cell varieties. However, the precise role for radiotherapy in small-cell tumours remains undefined. It may fulfil a useful palliative role in the treatment of distressing symptoms such as haemoptysis, localized pain and intractable cough, as well as those symptoms arising from CNS metastases, bone secondaries and obstruction of the SVC. What is the place of radiotherapy in patients with small-cell carcinoma in whom the ultimate yet remote objective is to cure or at least further prolong survival significantly?

Primary tumour control

It is clearly evident that radiotherapy, like surgery, is a local treatment and is therefore unlikely to be successful in disease that disseminates widely at an early stage. Since chemotherapy has the theoretical potential to treat disseminated disease and radiotherapy that of augmenting any effect the drug treatment has on more bulky localized intrathoracic disease, many centres have investigated the place of thoracic radiotherapy as an adjunct to chemotherapy. The primary site is by far the most common location for disease to relapse after failure of chemotherapy and therefore it is to be expected that combining radiotherapy with chemotherapy might improve survival. Almost all studies comparing chemotherapy and thoracic radiotherapy with chemotherapy alone have shown a reduction in local recurrence rate, from an average of 80% to about 30%, although few have shown much impact on survival [184–187]. It has taken two large meta-analyses [188,189]

involving more than 2000 patients in more than a dozen randomized trials to show any impact on survival for the addition of radiotherapy to combination chemotherapy in patients with limited small-cell lung cancer. More modern chemotherapeutic regimens using platinum drugs have not been reported or included in these meta-analyses [190] nor has the optimal dose and scheduling of radiotherapy been established. Reports from a French study [137,191], where dose escalation was performed, have shown that at least 40 Gy are required for a clinical response but that toxicity with this kind of treatment is common. The scheduling effect is also important since it is known that the therapeutic ratio of radiotherapy improves with division of the total dose into fractions (see above). A larger-than-standard fraction dose (>2 Gy) produces a larger kill of tumour cells but causes an increased risk of late effects to normal tissues. Dividing the total daily dose into smaller doses (hyperfractionation) improves this therapeutic index. Accelerated fractionation allows for frequent treatments in a shorter time span. The interval between treatments allows some repair of the damage to both cancer and normal tissues. The theory behind hyperfractionation and accelerated schedules is to optimize the effects of radiotherapy on tumour cells while allowing normal cells to recover. The precise sequencing of radiotherapy with chemotherapy is important, although an optimal schedule could not be discerned from the recent meta-analyses [188,189]. Two studies looking at early radiotherapy or late treatment, i.e. at the end of chemotherapy, have shown conflicting results [192,193].

It is generally accepted that if patients are to be submitted to thoracic radiotherapy as an adjunct to chemotherapy they should have limited disease at presentation, show a complete regression with chemotherapy or have local symptoms attributable to the disease. The optimal dose, fractionation and timing in relation to chemotherapy are undetermined and combined modality treatment may produce substantial toxicity [194].

Prophylactic cranial irradiation

The use of prophylactic cranial irradiation (PCI) in order to prevent the emergence of intracranial metastases is controversial. The reasons for its use are (i) the brain is a common site for spread of small-cell carcinoma, (ii) cytotoxic drugs in general do not cross the blood–brain barrier and (iii) the incidence of brain metastases increases as survival is prolonged by chemotherapy. In a meta-analysis of 11 studies, Pedersen [195] calculated that about 10% had CNS metastases at diagnosis of small-cell lung cancer, while a further 20% developed these during therapy. At autopsy the frequency was found to be approximately 50%. The small group of patients surviving for more than 2 years after diagnosis has been shown to have a probability of developing brain metastases of 50–80% [195,196]. Brain metastases are associated with considerable morbidity for the patient and distress for the relatives. Patients are often hospitalized [197] and their survival is short. Irradiation of the brain does not of course prevent new metastases in a relapsed patient and therefore strictly speaking the term 'prophylactic' is inappropriate.

By 1995, 11 trials that randomized patients into groups receiving and not receiving PCI had been published [198]. All showed a significant reduction in the CNS relapse rate, from approximately 25% to 5%, but none showed a significant survival advantage favouring PCI. In the largest recorded study [199], in which 219 patients with limited disease were randomized to either PCI with 30 Gy over 10 fractions ($n=107$) or no brain therapy ($n=112$), the CNS relapse rate was reduced from 20% to 5% by PCI but there was no impact on survival.

The adverse effects of PCI may also be significant. An acute organic syndrome, with memory loss, confusion and additional neurological deficits, can be seen 6–8 weeks after treatment in a small proportion of patients [200]. Late neurological toxicity has been reported in retrospective series of long-term survivors who have received PCI [201]. There appears to be a link between these effects and the timing and dose of radiotherapy. In summary therefore PCI is not advised as routine treatment and should only be given to patients with limited stage disease who are in complete remission following chemotherapy [202].

However, palliative cranial irradiation is often helpful in relieving distressing symptoms due to cerebral metastases. Dexamethasone is also useful in these patients and their response to this treatment is often taken as a guide to whether cranial irradiation should be attempted. The results from patients who have been treated show an intracranial response rate of approximately 70%, with 40% having a clinically complete remission [198]. Patients presenting with intracranial metastases from small-cell lung cancer have been shown to respond to systemic chemotherapy and this should still be part of the primary treatment [203].

Surgery

The early MRC studies on the treatment of small-cell carcinoma compared surgery unfavourably with radiotherapy and found no long-term survivors after operative treatment [204]. This led to a widespread belief that small-cell lung cancer was a 'systemic' disease regardless of clinical stage at presentation and that surgery was contraindicated in all patients. The early promise of chemotherapy in the 1970s led to its emergence as the standard form of treatment and physicians largely forsook surgery as a treatment option. However, this was not true of those many thoracic surgeons who had seen cures following operation. In the last decade chemotherapy results have

reached a plateau (see above) and manipulations of combination chemotherapy and radiotherapy seem to have had little or no further impact on survival. These observations, coupled with reports of occasional long-term survival following surgical treatment, has led to questioning of the dogma that small-cell carcinomas are inoperable. The Veterans Administration Surgical Oncology Group entered over 2000 patients into a study to evaluate the role of adjuvant chemotherapy in patients with resected non-small-cell lung cancer [205]. It was found that 148 patients with early-stage small-cell lung cancer were inadvertently included. Review of these patients showed remarkable 5-year survival rates: patients with T1N0 tumours had 60% survival, those with T2N0 27.9% and those with T1N1 31.3%. The overall 5-year survival rate, which included patients with T3 and N2 disease, was 23%.

Other workers have shown that when solitary pulmonary nodules removed from asymptomatic patients were subsequently found to be small-cell carcinomas, and when no obvious lymph node metastases were present, the 5-year survival rate was about 36% [206]. Although fewer than 5% of patients with small-cell carcinoma are found to have stage I disease after extensive staging, those that do so comprise a small subgroup that may benefit from surgical resection.

Patients with limited small-cell lung cancer treated with chemotherapy and thoracic radiotherapy have a high incidence of local recurrence, and this has led a number of investigators to re-explore the role of surgery in combination with other treatment in limited small-cell lung cancer [207,208]. Three uncontrolled studies in small groups of patients with limited small-cell lung cancer treated with preoperative chemotherapy followed by attempted surgical resection have shown that combined modality therapy is possible. All studies showed a high local control rate and, perhaps more interestingly, a high incidence of mixed histology or a conversion to non-small-cell histology following chemotherapy [208–210]. This presumably reflects the emergence of a chemoresistant clone of cells in mixed tumours and explains the poor eventual results of chemotherapy.

The largest study that has evaluated the role of surgery in small-cell lung cancer was by a group from Toronto [211]; 119 patients with limited disease were treated with combined modality therapy including surgical resection. The projected 5-year survival in stage I patients was 51%, stage II 28%, stage III 19% and the overall survival was 39%. The pattern of recurrence showed good local control, with local recurrence only in 8.3%. The Lung Cancer Study Group has performed the only prospective randomized trial evaluating the role of surgery in patients with limited small-cell lung cancer [212]; patients with stage I disease were excluded. All patients were treated with standard chemotherapy and were then randomized to receive radiotherapy (thoracic and PCI) with or without thoracotomy. The resectability rate was 83%, 19% had a complete pathological response and 9% of patients had no residual small-cell lung cancer but only non-small-cell lesions. The 2-year survival was 20% irrespective of whether an operation was performed.

It is appropriate in the present stage of knowledge for limited small-cell lung cancer to be further classified using the TNM system and for peripheral lesions to be assessed for surgery. Mediastinoscopy should be performed even when CT is normal and the patient should probably undergo bone and brain scanning. The question of whether postoperative adjuvant chemotherapy is beneficial is at present unanswered but the reports so far show no favourable impact on survival. However, results of surgical treatment in this very select group of patients with small-cell lung cancer is certainly as good as chemotherapy alone.

Paraneoplastic syndromes

The term 'paraneoplastic syndrome' encompasses a variety of non-metastatic metabolic or neuromuscular manifestations of lung cancer [213,214]. Although such syndromes may occur with all major types of lung cancer, they are most frequently associated with small-cell carcinoma, which commonly elaborates ectopic hormones from neurosecretory granules within its cells. In healthy subjects, these peptide hormones (Table 41.10) are produced not only in neural tissue, including the hypothala-

Table 41.10 Peptide hormones detected in small-cell lung cancer. (After Maurer [213].)

Hormone	Normal site of production
Thyrotropin releasing hormone Somatostatin	Hypothalamus
Thyrotropin Growth hormone β-Melanocyte stimulating hormone Adrenocorticotropin β-Endorphin β-Lipotropin Pro-opiomelanocortin	Anterior pituitary
Vasopressin Oxytocin VP-HNP OT-HNP	Posterior pituitary
Bombesin Neurotensin Glucagon	Gut–brain
Calcitonin	C-cells (thyroid)

mus and pituitary, but also in gut-derived tissues and are therefore sometimes referred to as gut–brain peptides. Although increasing numbers of these peptides are being detected by sensitive radioimmunoassay techniques, most of them are unassociated with gross clinical disturbances. However, a number of metabolic paraneoplastic syndromes are well recognized clinically. The mechanisms by which the paraneoplastic neuromuscular syndromes arise remain for the most part obscure. These syndromes may antedate discovery of a tumour by months or even years [215].

Hypercalcaemia

Malignant neoplastic disease is the most common cause of hypercalcaemia in the hospital population, accounting for about 60% of cases. Approximately 8% of patients with lung cancer are found to have hypercalcaemia and the majority of these have squamous cell carcinoma [216]. The most common cause of malignant hypercalcaemia is destruction of bone by osteolytic metastatic disease, but it may also result from the production of abnormal circulating factors by the tumour. True ectopic parathyroid hormone production is extremely rare [217], although lung cancers, especially squamous carcinoma, can produce parathyroid-like hormones that cause hypercalcaemia via increased mobilization of calcium from bones and by increased renal tubular absorption [218]. Hypercalcaemia produces polyuria, nocturia and thirst that if persistent result in dehydration, hypovolaemia and ultimately renal failure. The patient may experience malaise, weakness, anorexia, nausea, vomiting and constipation. Mental slowing, confusion, drowsiness and ultimately coma may mislead the physician into supposing that intracranial metastases are present. The symptoms may develop insidiously or so rapidly that the patient presents as a medical emergency.

In advanced or terminal malignancy, a decision not to treat hypercalcaemia may be taken with justification. However, if it is felt that the patient's quality of life would benefit from lowering the serum calcium, then treatment should be vigorous. If there are no obvious bony metastases it can be assumed that the tumour is producing parathyroid hormone-like substance. Treatment of the primary should therefore result in biochemical improvement, and resection or radiotherapy should be planned in the usual way, first correcting the biochemical disturbance by medical means.

The mainstay of medical treatment is correction of associated dehydration with intravenous saline. Renal function should be closely monitored and adequate potassium supplementation given. Mild hypercalcaemia (<3 mmol/ L) may respond to this alone but when hypercalcaemia is more severe, or does not respond to simple rehydration, a loop diuretic such as furosemide (frusemide) should be given in addition to intravenous fluids. If hypercalcaemia persists despite these measures, agents can be used that inhibit calcium resorption from bones. Intravenous and oral bisphosphonates have an important role to play in the management of malignancy-associated hypercalcaemia and may cause fairly dramatic falls in serum calcium [219]. The cytotoxic antibiotic mithramycin is no more effective and is rarely used due to toxic effects. Oral steroids have an unreliable calcium-lowering activity in hypercalcaemia associated with bronchial carcinoma, but are often used nevertheless.

Syndrome of inappropriate antidiuretic hormone secretion

When significant hyponatraemia (plasma sodium <120 mmol/L) occurs in association with lung cancer, it is usually part of the syndrome of inappropriate secretion of antidiuretic hormone (SIADH). This nearly always occurs in small-cell carcinoma, and SIADH is the most frequently encountered paraneoplastic syndrome associated with this cell type, being reported in 5–22% of patients [213]. SIADH is characterized by dilutional hyponatraemia, so that plasma sodium is low in the presence of abnormal water retention, resulting in low plasma osmolality (usually <260 mosmol/kg of water). There is continued urinary loss of sodium at a level inappropriate for the plasma sodium concentration so that urine osmolality is disproportionately high, being at least twice that of plasma. The syndrome is due to uncontrolled secretion of ADH by the tumour, and the diagnosis is made by measurement of urine and plasma osmolality.

The patient may be asymptomatic or may complain of anorexia, weakness, nausea, vomiting and headache. As hyponatraemia worsens, impaired concentration with forgetfulness and confusion may develop. With a plasma sodium concentration of less than 115 mmol/L, seizures and coma may occur.

The cornerstone of treatment of SIADH is water deprivation [220], 500–750 mL of fluid being given daily in addition to the losses in the previous 24 h. This water deprivation may be unpleasant for the patient, and where compliance is difficult, or where treatment has proved unsuccessful, the antibiotic demeclocycline may be given orally [221,222]. This drug competes for ADH binding sites in the renal tubule and is given in a maintenance dose of 600–900 mg daily. It undergoes hepatic metabolism and is best avoided in patients with renal insufficiency or liver disease, otherwise nephrotoxicity may result. It may also cause a photosensitivity reaction.

As with other ectopic hormone production, treatment of the primary tumour (usually with chemotherapy) may produce a prompt response [223]. However, many chemotherapeutic agents used in the management of small-cell lung cancer, such as cyclophosphamide, vincristine and cisplatin, can produce SIADH themselves [224].

Ectopic adrenocorticotrophin secretion

Abnormalities of cortisol metabolism may be found in almost 50% of patients with small-cell carcinoma. Raised concentrations of immunoreactive adrenocorticotrophin (ACTH) can be detected and there is a loss of diurnal variation or failure of cortisol to suppress following dexamethasone [225,226]. Despite this, the clinical syndrome of ectopic ACTH secretion has been found to be present in only 5% of patients with small-cell carcinoma and is even less common in other cell types [213,225]. Patients do not usually develop the signs associated with Cushing's syndrome such as moon face, central obesity and cutaneous striae, presumably because the relatively short natural history of the small-cell carcinoma does not allow the development of these abnormalities. Indeed it has been shown that ectopic ACTH secretion seems to carry a poor prognosis [225].

The diagnosis is usually made when symptoms such as anorexia, mental slowing and muscle weakness, which may be profound, are associated with a hypokalaemic metabolic alkalosis due to urinary loss of potassium. The most common physical findings are oedema (83%) and proximal myopathy (61%) [227]. Progressive cutaneous pigmentation is sometimes a feature of the syndrome and results from associated β-melanocyte stimulating hormone production. Confirmation of the diagnosis is made by finding an elevated cortisol level that fails to fall following dexamethasone administration. Plasma ACTH assay also shows elevated levels.

The most effective treatment of this syndrome is treatment of the tumour itself. This usually takes the form of chemotherapy of small-cell carcinoma, although successful resolution has occasionally resulted from resection [228]. Inhibition of adrenal steroid synthesis with the antifungal agent ketoconazole has been shown to be beneficial [229], and this drug should be administered to patients with the syndrome while a response to chemotherapy is awaited.

Hypertrophic pulmonary osteoarthropathy

Hypertrophic pulmonary osteoarthropathy (HPOA) is a syndrome characterized by periostitis of long bones, most commonly affecting the tibia, fibula, radius and ulna at their distal ends. The patient complains of bony pain in these involved areas, which are often hot and tender to touch, and there may be associated pain and swelling of the wrists, ankles and knee joints [230]. Clubbing of the digits is found in over 90% of cases, and is often gross [231].

The pathogenesis of the condition remains obscure but

lung cancer is by far the most common cause. Although some authors believe that HPOA is usually associated with adenocarcinoma [232], other workers have shown an equal distribution between major cell types with the exception of small-cell carcinoma [233]. HPOA is closely associated with finger clubbing and has been recorded in a variety of other malignant and non-malignant conditions associated with clubbing. It has been shown that blood flow to the calf and forearm is increased in HPOA and that this hyperaemia is directed particularly towards connective tissue and bone. The increased vascularity of subcutaneous tissues and periosteum leads to periostitis, resulting in loosely packed new bone being laid down outside the original cortex [234] and this produces the characteristic bony radiographic changes.

The mechanism by which lung cancer produces HPOA remains obscure. There is some evidence to support a role for vagally mediated afferent neural output from the tumour-bearing lung, as it was noted in the 1950s that division of the vagal branches around the hilum during unsuccessful attempts to resect lung cancer resulted in symptomatic relief, whereas 'open and shut' thoracotomy without nerve section produced no relief [235]. A number of possible pathogenic mechanisms have been put forward but none are universally accepted. When the diagnosis is suspected, radiographs of the lower ends of the radius, ulna, tibia and fibula, and of the hands are indicated. If the knees are painful, radiography of the proximal tibia and fibula and distal femoral shaft should be performed. The characteristic radiographic finding is a 1–2 mm line shadow running parallel to the cortex starting a few centimetres beyond the wrist or ankle joint and running for a variable distance along the shaft of the bone (Fig. 41.22). The active deposition of new bone along the inner aspect of the periosteum can be demonstrated on bone scans by the avid uptake of technetium in affected areas, although this investigation is seldom necessary in clinical practice.

Despite the reported success of vagotomy [235], this invasive procedure is unjustified unless thoracotomy is undertaken for an attempt to cure. In cases where successful resection of tumour is achieved, HPOA responds dramatically. Most other cases respond gratifyingly to treatment with a non-steroidal anti-inflammatory drug and corticosteroids may produce similar relief.

Other endocrine and metabolic complications

Gynaecomastia

This may occasionally occur in association with lung cancer, most frequently with large-cell and adenocarcinoma types. The mechanism is thought to involve the production of human chorionic gonadotrophin by tumour cells, this substance resulting in overproduction of testicu-

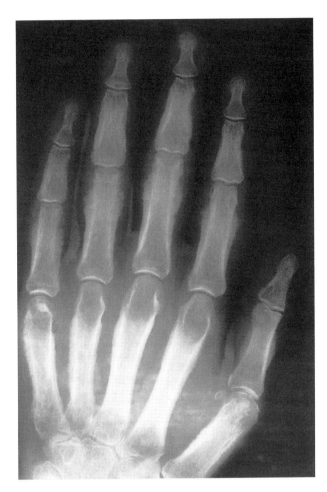

Fig. 41.22 Hand of patient with hypertrophic pulmonary osteoarthropathy showing subperiosteal new bone formation on metacarpals and phalanges.

lar oestrogen [236]. Drug-induced gynaecomastia (e.g. with spironolactone, cimetidine, digoxin) should be excluded before this physical sign is attributed to a tumour; however, when lung cancer is the cause, successful surgical resection also deals with the complication. If resection is not possible, then an antioestrogen such as tamoxifen may be effective in relieving symptoms.

Eosinophilia

As association between bronchial carcinoma and blood eosinophilia has been described [237]. This phenomenon, which may result from increased marrow production, prolonged eosinophil survival time or the production of an eosinophil chemotactic factor, is characterized by a high total white cell count and neutrophilia as well as eosinophilia [238]. It tends to be associated with advanced and rapidly progressive disease.

Non-metastatic neuromuscular syndromes

Paraneoplastic neurological syndromes have long been

recognized in lung cancer and these disorders are now thought to result partly from the cross-reaction of anti-tumour antibodies with antigens also present in neural tissue [239]. A variety of neuromuscular syndromes are recognized.

1 A peripheral neuropathy, which may be motor, sensory or mixed, accompanied by muscle weakness and wasting with loss of tendon reflex and stocking and glove hypoaesthesia. An autonomic neuropathy has also been described that may result in postural hypotension or disturbances of gastrointestinal motility, including intestinal pseudo-obstruction (Ogilvie's syndrome) [240]. Patients with sensory neuropathy usually have small-cell lung cancer and often have high titres of antibody to the nuclear-associated HuD protein [241]. However, the pathogenesis of neural injury is uncertain [227].

2 Neuromuscular junction and muscle syndromes include polymyositis/dermatomyositis, typified by proximal muscle weakness, pain and tenderness with a variety of systemic symptoms and a characteristic facial helio-trope rash. The myasthenic (Eaton–Lambert) syndrome is reported to occur in up to 6% of patients with small-cell lung cancer. In contrast to myasthenia gravis, the patient's muscle weakness improves with repeated efforts. The syndrome is thought to result from autoantibody-mediated functional blockade of the voltage-gated calcium channels involved in the release of acetylcholine at nerve terminals [227].

3 Cerebellar ataxia, with nystagmus, impaired coordination and dysarthria, has been described in a small group of patients with small-cell lesions [242].

Paraneoplastic neurological syndromes associated with small-cell lung cancer often precede discovery of the underlying tumour. Apart from patients with Eaton–Lambert myasthenic syndrome, immunosuppression including plasmapheresis has not been shown to be particularly beneficial, even in patients with detectable antineural antibodies. Similarly, the neurological syndromes generally do not respond to cytotoxic chemotherapy, even when there is a gratifying antitumour effect [227].

Special problems

Obstruction of the SVC

Over 85% of all cases of obstruction of the SVC are caused by malignant disease. Bronchial carcinoma is responsible for over 60% of cases, about 20% being accounted for by other tumours such as lymphoma, mesothelioma and metastatic mediastinal lymphadenopathy. The few remaining cases are caused by rare benign conditions, including granulomatous disease, cryptogenic mediastinal fibrosis, intrathoracic goitre or aneurysm, or as a complication of central venous catheterization [243]. Small-cell carcinoma is the commonest histological type of lung cancer involved and up to 10% of small-cell lesions present in this way [244]. The tumour usually compresses the vessel from without but occasionally invades its wall. Intraluminal thrombosis sometimes occurs and may be responsible for failure of treatment.

Diagnosis

The diagnosis is usually obvious from the symptoms and signs, with swelling of the face and upper torso and distension of veins and venules across the chest, upper arms and neck. The next step is to obtain histological confirmation. Some hold the view that it is more important to initiate immediate treatment with radiotherapy before obtaining histology, but this approach has several pitfalls. Firstly, radiotherapy may be administered to a patient with a benign condition, thus subjecting the individual to the potential toxicity of treatment without any chance of benefit. Secondly, if radiotherapy is administered first it may make a subsequent histological diagnosis difficult or impossible, and in those patients whose survival is prolonged the subsequent management becomes increasingly problematical. Thirdly, if the tumour responsible is small-cell carcinoma, this responds well to chemotherapy and radiotherapy may not be required at all [244]. Obstruction of the SVC, although unpleasant, is unlikely to result in mortality but the underlying cause is and it is therefore important to determine this cause as accurately as possible. Histological diagnosis is usually obtained by bronchoscopy where a central pulmonary tumour is evident or by exploration of the mediastinum via mediastinoscopy or mediastinotomy. The risks of uncontrollable bleeding as a result of raised venous pressure proximal to the obstruction have probably been overstated and in practice routine biopsies should be performed [245]. In patients without an endobronchial lesion at bronchoscopy, mediastinotomy is almost always diagnostic and carries the potential advantage of providing larger tissue samples, which may be important in lymphoma and in more unusual causes.

CT with contrast venography may be helpful in determining the extent of the disease although usually adds little to clinical examination and chest radiography. Some radiotherapists claim to have found venography helpful in determining how far to extend the treatment field and this procedure is also required if stenting of the SVC is contemplated [246].

Treatment

Treatment in cases due to cancer of the lung depends on whether histology is consistent with small-cell carcinoma or not. In a patient with small-cell carcinoma in whom a decision to use chemotherapy as primary treatment has been taken, the additional use of radiotherapy appears to confer no extra benefit [244,247]. In non-small-cell carcinoma, chemotherapy has not been shown to produce any relief over and above that resulting from treatment with radiotherapy [248]. Studies with more modern drugs (e.g. cisplatin) in patients with obstruction of the SVC due to non-small-cell carcinoma have not been performed. Corticosteroids are frequently used but have not been convincingly shown to be of benefit.

Radiotherapy is the mainstay of treatment in cases due to non-small-cell lung cancer. The high initial dose of radiotherapy followed by a lower daily dose to a total of approximately 20 Gy spread over 1–2 weeks is claimed to be more effective than initial low-dose treatment increased by gradual increments [248]. Symptoms usually begin to improve rapidly with signs diminishing more gradually, so that 90% of patients are free from oedema by 3 weeks. Radiotherapy in the treatment of obstruction of the SVC due to lung cancer is a palliative procedure and the ultimate prognosis depends on the cell type, the extent of the disease and the performance status. It has been reported that those who do not show a rapid response to radiotherapy die sooner than those who do, approximately 25% of patients overall surviving for 1 year [244,249]. In small-cell lung cancer, obstruction of the SVC is not in itself a poor prognostic indicator [244], and patients who relapse with obstruction of the SVC following initial chemotherapy should be treated with radiotherapy as there is a good chance of at least a partial response to both symptoms and signs.

Endovascular treatment of obstruction of the SVC has also been tried. Initial attempts using simple balloon angioplasty was occasionally successful in benign disease but recurrence rates in malignant disease are very high due to inability of the central veins to resist external compression. Since the first report of the successful placement of an intravascular stent in 1986 [250], there have been several reported series documenting the value of this technique [246,251,252]. So far its use appears to be confined to patients with malignant obstruction of the SVC who have failed to respond to conventional treatment or who require urgent relief of symptoms. Results of this form of treatment are impressive, with a primary clinical success rate in the region of 90% of patients [252]. There is no clear consensus on the need for thrombolysis or anticoagulation following stent insertion. There is no evidence that anticoagulation is required in patients in whom there is a good blood flow through the stent at the end of the procedure [246]. Thrombosis in the SVC is not a contraindication to stenting as this can be dealt with by local thrombolysis or dispersed with a mechanical device [253]. Few complications have been reported following stent insertion. Migration of stent into the right ventricle from the SVC has not been reported. The argument against stenting is its cost (approximately £1000 in 1998).

Superior sulcus tumours

Pancoast [254] used the term 'superior pulmonary sulcus tumour' to describe a carcinoma situated at the extreme apex of the lung. The Pancoast syndrome comprises pain in the lower part of the shoulder and inner aspect of the arm (C8, T1 and T2 distribution) that may be severe and unremitting. It may be accompanied by sensory loss in the same distribution and wasting and weakness of the small muscles of the hand and of the medial forearm, wrist and finger flexors. It is caused by involvement of the lower part of the brachial plexus by tumour. A further neurological component is involvement of the sympathetic chain at or above the T1 (stellate ganglion) level to produce Horner's syndrome (ipsilateral partial ptosis, the appearance of enophthalmos, a small pupil and hypohidrosis of the face). The two radiological components of the syndrome are the presence of an apical mass shadow on the chest radiograph and local evidence of bone destruction, usually of the first and second ribs and/or a vertebral body or transverse process (see Fig. 41.15). Any histological type of lung cancer can occur in this situation and clearly incomplete forms of this syndrome are found.

Management

The diagnosis is obvious where all components of the syndrome are present, although other diseases such as tuberculosis may occasionally produce confluent apical shadowing that is difficult to distinguish from tumour. In this situation bronchoscopy should be carried out, with the submission of washings for cytology and mycobacterial staining and culture, although the immediate results are often inconclusive. If this is the case and the lesion is thought to be an inoperable tumour, as most are by virtue of neurological or vertebral involvement, then percutaneous needle biopsy may provide histological confirmation of the diagnosis.

The best form of treatment for superior sulcus tumours remains the subject of controversy. These lesions were originally regarded as uniformly inoperable. In 1961 encouraging results were reported for radiotherapy followed by surgical removal of the tumour, usually by lobectomy [255]. This approach, with the addition of refinements such as completion of radiotherapy after surgical healing or placement of radioactive implants if the tumour is found to be unresectable at thoracotomy, continues to find favour in some places [256]. However, the evidence that preoperative radiotherapy improves either resectability or 5-year survival rate is weak [257] and requires confirmation with randomized prospective studies. Some take the view that if the lesion appears resectable after staging, surgery should proceed directly; if the tumour is deemed unresectable, radiotherapy should be given as a single course. A good result is achieved in over 70% of cases when radiotherapy is given palliatively for pain relief [258]. Patients treated with radiotherapy alone or combined with surgery have a reported 5-year survival rate of 20–30% [257,258].

Malignant pleural effusion

The presence of a malignant pleural effusion, whose origin has been determined by either pleural fluid cytology or pleural biopsy [259], indicates both incurability and a short life expectancy, survival rarely extending beyond 1 year with a median survival of approximately 6 months [260]. Once the diagnosis is certain, aspiration is necessary only if the pleural fluid is of sufficient volume to cause breathlessness. If reaccumulation is rapid or if repeated aspiration is required, then a chemical pleurodesis can be performed using one of a variety of available agents (see Chapter 43). When tetracycline is used for this purpose it may be mixed with local anaesthetic in order to reduce the pleural pain associated with the procedure [261].

Intracranial metastases

The diagnosis of intracranial metastases and the frequency with which they occur have been discussed previously. It is notable that in non-small-cell carcinoma, intracranial metastases are found more commonly with adenocarcinomas and large-cell carcinomas than with squamous cell lesions [262].

Cerebral metastases may present with symptoms of raised intracranial pressure such as headache and vomiting. A personality change or impaired intellectual function is an unusual presentation. Focal or generalized seizures may occur. A motor or sensory deficit or impairment of coordination may become manifest.

Management

If intracranial metastases become clinically evident in a patient who is clearly dying of advanced metastatic bronchial carcinoma, adequate narcotic analgesia may be the most appropriate treatment. Sometimes the general condition of the patient requires more active supportive treatment, even though the prognosis may only be a few months. Improvement is often obtained with oral corticosteroids given in a high initial dose, such as dexamethasone 16 mg daily, thereafter gradually reducing according to response. The results of treatment with cranial irradiation are discussed above, symptomatic relief being seen in up to 80% of patients.

Surgical treatment has a small role in the management of intracranial or brain metastases [263] when the disease can be shown to take the form of a solitary deposit that has arisen following an otherwise successful surgical resection for primary lung cancer of non-small-cell origin. Before such neurosurgery is undertaken, evidence of other metastatic disease should be excluded by a careful search. This approach is justified since intracranial metastatic disease may be the only extrathoracic site of spread in a few patients [264]. Indeed sometimes the neurosurgery is performed as the primary treatment when the primary bronchial carcinoma remains occult within the chest. Prolonged survival has been seen in a group of patients who subsequently proceeded to thoracotomy [264].

However, the prognosis for the great majority of patients with intracranial metastatic lung cancer is very poor, the overall median survival being variously reported as between 3 and 5 months [143,144]. Those whose symptoms respond to radiotherapy survive twice as long as those who do not [265], but only 14% of all patients are alive at 1 year [266].

Tracheal tumours

The trachea may be involved by direct extension of adjacent tumour or, rarely, may be the site of primary malignancy [267], of which the slow growing and locally invasive adenoid cystic carcinoma is probably the most common type [268]. Tracheal malignancy may occur at any age and may be mistaken for other common disorders such as asthma, the increasing stridor of a few weeks' duration in a young or middle-aged adult being misinterpreted as wheeze. Haemoptysis may also occur.

The chest film is frequently normal but clinical suspicion may be heightened by the characteristic appearance of the flow–volume loop (see Chapter 2). The tumour may be demonstrated by conventional or computed tomography of the trachea (Fig. 41.23). Confirmation is by bronchoscopy, although caution should be exercised in the choice of instrument since the fibreoptic bronchoscope may occlude an already narrowed opening. Where the stenosis is critical, biopsy using either instrument may result in complete occlusion of a small orifice.

Ideally, treatment of tracheal tumours is by complete surgical excision. This may not be possible because of the involvement of surrounding mediastinal structures. However, if the disease is apparently confined to the trachea, complete excision has been achieved in some centres using tracheobronchoplastic procedures [269]. Other methods of treatment frequently have to be employed, including radiotherapy, which may be administered externally or endotracheally [270], and laser devices [271]. One series described the use of an Nd–Yag laser in 21 patients with tracheal tumours, of which almost half were primary [272]. The majority were treated as emergencies for impending asphyxia and showed symptomatic benefit, allowing time to be gained for fuller diagnostic evaluation and treatment planning, including the use of further laser treatment, surgery or radiotherapy.

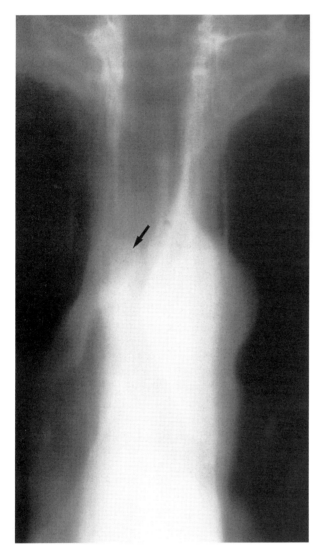

Fig. 41.23 Tracheal tomogram showing carcinoma (arrowed) arising from right lateral wall above bifurcation.

Sometimes patients with tracheobronchial obstruction not amenable to curative surgery and not helped by radiotherapy may benefit from the insertion of a prosthetic stent [273].

Quality of life

Traditionally, the outcome of treatment for patients with lung cancer has been measured in terms of the extent and duration of tumour response and patient survival, although differences between treatments as measured by these indices have been small. Since the vast majority of patients with lung cancer are treated with palliative intent, it has become increasingly more relevant to individual patient care and to policy-making to compare the cost, in both human and economic terms, of any gain achieved. Clinicians have therefore turned their attention to trying to measure not only the length of their patient's survival but also the quality of any such extension of life. This aspect of lung cancer management has recently been comprehensively reviewed [274–276]. The concept of quality of life is largely subjective, varying from individual to individual, and many clinicians regard it as a 'soft science' that is impossible to define or measure scientifically. It is generally agreed that quality of life is multidimensional and involves a number of components, including the impact of disease symptoms, the side-effects of treatment, the ability of the patient to function and their psychosocial well-being. Attempts to measure quality of life should therefore reflect all these domains if possible and emphasis should be placed on the subjective experience of the patient whose quality of life is in question. Recently, attention has focused particularly on the development of questionnaires completed by patients themselves.

Methods for measuring quality of life

Measurements of a patient's level of physical ability (performance status) and the response to treatment and its toxic effects are generally assessed by physicians. The Karnofsky Performance Index [277] has been in use for many years and is still widely favoured as a prognostic indicator. The WHO [278] and Eastern Cooperative Oncology Group [279] scales share many of the same limitations, scoring being influenced by whether the evaluation is performed at home or in hospital, with poor interindividual reliability. These instruments all neglect psychosocial variables and to this extent remain unsatisfactory as measures of quality of life (Table 41.11).

A bewildering array of questionnaires that attempt to measure different aspects of the patient's experience of quality of life [275] has been developed specifically for patients with cancer. These involve visual analogue self-assessment scales, diary cards [180] and, more recently, a modular approach where questions covering general cancer-related features are combined with those specific to lung cancer. The European Organization for Research on the Treatment of Cancer has developed such an instrument over several years [280]. This has a 30-item self-reporting questionnaire for use in cancer clinical trials, with a 13-item module specifically relevant to patients with lung cancer, for example covering cough, dyspnoea, pain and treatment-related side-effects [281]. The instrument is responsive to clinical change and has proved acceptable to patients. Other quality-of-life instruments that have proved popular and valid in the management of patients with lung cancer include the Rotterdam Symptom Checklist [282] and the Hospital Anxiety and Depression Scale [283].

There are surprisingly few reports of quality-of-life measurements in patients undergoing treatment for lung cancer, although things are improving [275]. As most

Table 41.11 Comparison of Karnofsky [277], European Cooperative Oncology Group (ECOG) [279] and World Health Organization (WHO) [278] scales used to measure performance status.

Karnofsky scale		ECOG/WHO scale	
Status	Score	Score	Status
Normal; no complaints or evidence of disease	100	0	Able to carry out normal activity
Able to carry on normal activity; minor signs or symptoms of disease	90	1	Restricted in physically strenuous activity but ambulatory and capable of light work
Normal activity with effort; some signs or symptoms of disease	80		
Cares for self; unable to carry on normal activity or to do active work	70	2	Ambulatory and capable of all self-care. Unable to work. Up and about >50% of waking hours
Requires occasional assistance but is able to care for most personal needs	60		
Requires considerable assistance and frequent medical care	50	3	Capable of only limited self-care, confined to bed or chair >50% of waking hours
Disabled; requires special care and assistance	40		
Severely disabled; hospitalization is indicated, although death not imminent	30	4	Completely disabled. Cannot carry out self-care. Confined to bed or chair
Very sick; hospitalization and active supportive treatment necessary	20		
Moribund; fatal processes progressing rapidly	10		

patients can only expect some palliation rather than significant prolongation of survival, there would appear to be a strong case for including measurements of quality of life in any future study. Indeed, there is an argument that measurement of quality of life should be part of the routine assessment of patients undergoing any form of intervention and that quality of life should be used to evaluate treatment outcomes in clinical trials. The data obtained could provide an objective basis for informed decision-making for individual patients and for making the case for allocation of appropriate resources to medical and supportive services [284,285].

Prognosis

It is evident that lung cancer is not a single disease and any discussion of prognosis therefore requires qualification. However, if all types of lung cancer are considered together, the overall survival 5 years after diagnosis is 5–15% [122,286]. More meaningful results include details such as tumour histology, surgical stage, the type of treatment used, the performance status of the patient and the length of follow-up.

Some authors take the view that the growth of micro-

scopic lung cancer is approximately exponential, duration of survival being a function both of the size of the tumour at diagnosis and its doubling time [287,288]. Doubling time can be crudely calculated using a mathematical equation [289]: for small-cell carcinoma it is approximately 50 days, for squamous and large-cell carcinoma approximately 100 days and for adenocarcinoma about 180 days [290,291]. The shorter doubling time for small-cell carcinoma is in keeping with its poor overall prognosis, although the longer doubling time of adenocarcinoma appears to give it no prognostic advantage over squamous and large-cell carcinoma. A tumour cell with a diameter of 10 μm produces a 1-cm diameter nodule weighing approximately 1 g after 30 doublings. It is therefore clear that in the lifespan of a tumour the majority of doublings must take place before the tumour is either clinically or radiographically detectable [292]. If exponential growth rates are assumed and if the tumour has arisen from a single cell, it is possible to extrapolate backwards to show that slow-growing tumours such as adenocarcinoma and squamous carcinoma may have been present for about 8–15 years prior to diagnosis and small-cell lesions for up to 3 years [288]. The natural history of lung cancer therefore is one of years of unrecognized growth from a single cell, with the tumour becoming clinically apparent just prior to death. The clinician thus has very little chance of having any impact on what is the end stage of a condition. It is extremely disappointing that methods are not available to detect the disease in the preclinical state and large screening studies that have attempted to do this have had no impact on survival [293–296].

Non-small-cell carcinoma

The overall prognosis for patients presenting with non-small-cell lung cancer is poor and survival rates have not changed over the last several decades. In large series of unselected patients, 5-year survival rates for this group of patients lie between 4 and 7%, irrespective of whether the patient received surgery, radiotherapy or chemotherapy [115,297].

The results of treatment in non-small-cell lung cancer have been well documented. Stage I tumours (T1/T2N0M0) when treated surgically carry a 5-year survival rate of 30–60% [122,298]. Unfortunately only about 20% of lung cancers are found to be stage I and the prognosis worsens as the stage advances. Thus for stage II tumours treated surgically, the survival rate falls to 20–40% at 5 years [122]. Studies that have examined radiotherapy as an alternative treatment to surgery in stage I and stage II non-small-cell lung cancer suffer from the disadvantage of lacking accurate pathological typing and staging, which is more easily achieved in surgically treated patients. Results reported show survival rates ranging from 6% at 4 years [126] to 40% at 5 years [146].

More extensive disease, where surgery is more difficult, carries an exceptionally poor overall outlook irrespective of treatment. Survival at 12, 24 and 60 months for stage IIIA disease is 37.7%, 12.7% and 6.1%, respectively, whereas for stage IIIB it is only 31.8%, 10.8% and 3.9% [299]. Patients with the least dismal outlook in this group are those with good pretreatment performance status and those with squamous histology. In the presence of distant metastases (stage IV disease), 1-year and 2-year survival is 19.8% and 5.4% respectively.

Other prognostic factors

An analysis of prognostic factors in lung cancer found that for some surgically inoperable non-small-cell tumours the dominant factors were initial performance status and extent of the disease as determined by staging [300]. Other factors, such as anorexia, significant weight loss (>10% of body weight) and breathlessness, were relevant to a lesser degree. For operable non-small-cell lung cancer the most important prognostic factors were the stage of disease and, to a much lesser degree, the histological type and degree of differentiation [301]. The prognosis in so-called scar carcinomas is dependent upon the stage and histological type of the tumour, the associated scar being of aetiological rather than prognostic significance [44].

Small-cell carcinoma

Untreated patients with small-cell lung cancer have a median survival of 2.8 months [302,303]. Those who have limited disease (i.e. confined to one hemithorax including ipsilateral supraclavicular nodes) have a median survival of 3.1 months compared with 1.4 months for the remaining majority (70%) who have more extensive disease. Aggressive chemotherapy extends the median survival for limited and extensive disease to about 14 and 8 months respectively; 15–20% of those with limited disease treated in this fashion survive for more than 2 years compared with less than 2% for those with extensive disease [167–169]. A very small proportion (<5%) may have stage I disease and 5-year survival rates of around 30% have been reported for these patients when treated surgically [205].

It is disappointing that there has been little change in the prognosis of all patients with lung cancer over the last three decades. This is almost certainly due to the fact that most patients present with advanced disease and effective systemic therapy is not available. While effective anti-smoking campaigns would have a profound effect on the incidence of the condition in the long term, what is urgently required is newer agents with activity in patients with established metastatic disease.

References

1 Cancer Research Campaign. Factsheet II: Lung cancer and smoking. Factsheet V: Cancer in the European Community. London: CRC, 1992.

2 Charlton A. Tobacco and lung cancer. In: Thatcher N, Spiro S, eds. *New Perspectives in Lung Cancer*. London: BMJ Publishing Group, 1994: 1.

3 Belcher JR. The changing pattern of bronchial carcinoma. *Br J Dis Chest* 1987; 81: 87.

4 Surgeon General. *The Health Consequences of Smoking*. Washington, DC: Government Printing Office, 1982.

5 Royal College of Physicians. *Health or Smoking?* London: Pitman Medical, 1983.

6 International Agency for Research on Cancer. *Tobacco Smoking*. Geneva: World Health Organization, 1986.

7 Doll R, Hill AB. A study of the aetiology of carcinoma of the lung. *Br Med J* 1952; 2: 1271.

8 Doll R, Peto R. Mortality in relation to smoking: 20 years' observations on male British doctors. *Br Med J* 1976; 2: 1525.

9 Enstrom JE. Trends in mortality among California physicians after giving up smoking: 1950–79. *Br Med J* 1983; 286: 1101.

10 Doll R, Gray R, Hafner B *et al*. Mortality in

relation to smoking: 22 years' observations on female British doctors. *Br Med J* 1980; 280: 967.

11 Kahn HA. *The Dorn Study of Smoking and Mortality among US Veterans: Report on 8$^1/_2$ Years of Observation*. Washington, DC: Government Printing Office, 1966.

12 Bross IDJ, Gibson R. Risks of lung cancer in smokers who switch to filter cigarettes. *Am J Public Health* 1968; 58: 1396.

13 Doll R, Hill AB. Mortality in relation to smoking: ten years' observations of British doctors. *Br Med J* 1964; 1: 1399, 1460.

14 Hirayama T. Cancer mortality in non-

smoking women with smoking husbands in a large scale cohort study in Japan. *Prev Med* 1984; 13: 680.

15 Janerich DT, Thompson WD, Varela LR *et al.* Lung cancer and exposure to tobacco smoke in the household. *N Engl J Med* 1990; 323: 632.

16 Wald N, Kiryluk S, Darby S *et al. UK Smoking Statistics.* Oxford: Oxford University Press, 1988.

17 Office of Population Censuses and Surveys. Cigarette smoking 1972–1990. In: *General Household Survey.* London: HMSO, 1991.

18 Stanley K, Stjernsward J. Lung cancer in developed and developing countries. In: Hansen HH, ed. *Basic and Clinical Concepts of Lung Cancer.* Boston: Kluwer Academic Publishers, 1989: 1.

19 Report of a Task Group. Air pollution and cancer: risk assessment methodology and epidemiological evidence. *Environ Health Perspect* 1978; 22: 1.

20 Doll R. Atmospheric pollution and lung cancer. *Environ Health Perspect* 1978; 22: 23.

21 Axelson O. Occupational and environmental exposure to radon: cancer risks. *Annu Rev Public Health* 1991; 12: 235.

22 Pershagen G, Liang ZH, Hrubec Z *et al.* Residential radon exposure and lung cancer in Swedish women. *Health Phys* 1992; 63: 179.

23 Pershagen G, Akerblom G, Axelson O *et al.* Residential radon exposure and lung cancer in Sweden. *N Engl J Med* 1994; 330: 159.

24 Saracci R. Asbestos and lung cancer: an analysis of the epidemiological evidence on the asbestos–smoking interaction. *Int J Cancer* 1977; 20: 323.

25 Hammond EC, Selikoff IJ, Seidman H. Asbestos exposure, cigarette smoking and death rates. *Ann N Y Acad Sci* 1979; 330: 473.

26 de Vos Irvine H, Lamont DW, Hole DJ *et al.* Asbestos in lung cancer in the West of Scotland. *Br Med J* 1993; 306: 1503.

27 Meredith SK, McDonald JC. Work related respiratory disease in the United Kingdom 1989–92: a report on the SWORD project. *Occup Med* 1994; 44: 183.

28 Samet JM, Cutvirt DM, Waxweiler RJ *et al.* Uranium mining and lung cancer in Navajo men. *N Engl J Med* 1984; 310: 1481.

29 De Villiers AJ, Windish JP. Lung cancer in a fluorspar mining community. 1. Radiation, dust and mortality experience. *Br J Ind Med* 1964; 21: 94.

30 Radford EPST, Clair Renard KG. Lung cancer in Swedish iron miners exposed to low doses of radon daughters. *N Engl J Med* 1984; 310: 1485.

31 Fox AK, Goldblatt P, Kinlen LJ. A study of the mortality of Cornish tin miners. *Br J Ind Med* 1981; 38: 378.

32 Doll R, Matthews ID, Morgan LG. Cancers of the lung and nasal sinuses in nickel workers: a reassessment of the period of risk. *Br J Ind Med* 1977; 34: 102.

33 Alderson MR, Rattun NE, Bustrup L. Health of workmen in the chromate-producing industry in Britain. *Br J Ind Med* 1981; 38: 117.

34 Lee AM, Fraumeni JF. Arsenic and respiratory cancer in man: an occupational study. *J Natl Cancer Inst* 1969; 42: 1045.

35 McCallam RL, Wooley V, Petrie A. Lung cancer associated with chloromethyl methyl ether manufacture: an investigation of two factories in the United Kingdom. *Br J Ind Med* 1983; 40: 384.

36 Hurley JF, Archibald RM, Collins PL *et al.* The mortality of coke workers in Britain. *Am J Ind Med* 1983; 4: 691.

37 Ask-Upmark E. Bronchial carcinoma in printing workers. *Dis Chest* 1955; 27: 427.

38 Browne K. Is asbestos or asbestosis the cause of the increased risk of lung cancer in asbestos workers? *Br J Ind Med* 1986; 43: 145.

39 Hughes JM, Weill H. Asbestosis as a precursor of asbestos related lung cancer: results of a prospective mortality study. *Br J Ind Med* 1991; 48: 229.

40 Wilkinson P, Hansell DM, Janssens J *et al.* Is lung cancer associated with asbestos exposure when there are no small opacities on the chest radiograph? *Lancet* 1995; 345: 1074.

41 Turner-Warwick M, Lebowitz M, Johnson A. Cryptogenic fibrosing alveolitis and lung cancer. *Thorax* 1980; 35: 496.

42 Brincker H, Wilbek E. The incidence of malignant tumours in patients with respiratory sarcoidosis. *Br J Cancer* 1974; 29: 247.

43 Chaudhuri MR. Primary pulmonary scar carcinomas. *Ind J Med Res* 1973; 61: 858.

44 Ochs RH, Katz AS, Edmunds LH *et al.* Prognosis of pulmonary scar carcinoma. *J Thorac Cardiovasc Surg* 1982; 84: 359.

45 Prichard MG, Brown PJE, Sterret GF. Bronchioloalveolar carcinoma arising in longstanding lung cysts. *Thorax* 1984; 39: 545.

46 World Health Organization. International histological classification of tumours, no. 1. In: *Histological Typing of Lung Tumours,* 2nd edn. Geneva: WHO, 1981.

47 Carter N, Nelson F, Gosney JR. Ultrastructural heterogeneity in undifferentiated bronchial carcinoma. *J Pathol* 1993; 171: 53.

48 Edwards CW. Current concepts in pathology: carcinoma of the lung. *Clin Oncol* 1994; 6: 319.

49 Lamb D. Histological classification of lung cancer. *Thorax* 1984; 39: 161.

50 Thomas JStJ, Lamb D, Ashcroft T *et al.* How reliable is the diagnosis of lung cancer using small biopsy specimens? Report a UK CCCR Lung Cancer Working Party. *Thorax* 1993; 48: 1135.

51 Carter D. Squamous cell carcinoma of the lung: an update. *Semin Diagn Pathol* 1984; 2: 226.

52 Edwards C. Pulmonary adenocarcinoma: a review of 106 cases and a proposed new classification. *J Clin Pathol* 1987; 40: 125.

53 Carney DN. Biology of small cell lung cancer. *Lancet* 1993; 339: 843.

54 Fergusson RJ, Smyth JF. Studying lung cancer in the laboratory. I. Development of model systems. *Thorax* 1989; 42: 753.

55 Woll PJ. Growth factors and lung cancer. In: Thatcher N, Spiro S, eds. *New Perspectives in Lung Cancer.* London: BMJ Publishing Group, 1994: 51.

56 Carney DN, Cuttita F, Moody TW, Minna JD. Selective stimulation of small cell lung cancer clonal growth by bombesin and gastric releasing polypeptide. *Cancer Res* 1987; 47: 821.

57 Alexander RW, Upp JR, Poston GJ *et al.* Effects of bombesin on growth of human small cell lung carcinoma *in vivo. Cancer Res* 1988; 48: 1439.

58 Cuttita F, Carney DN, Mulshine J *et al.* Bombesin like peptides can function as autocrine growth factors in human small cell lung cancer. *Nature* 1985; 316: 823.

59 Sethi T, Rozengurt E. Multiple neuro-

peptides stimulate clonal growth of small cell lung cancer: effects of bradykinin, vasopressin, cholecystokinin, galanin and neurotensin. *Cancer Res* 1991; 51: 3621.

60 Maneckjee R, Minna JD. Opioid and nicotine receptors affect growth regulation of human lung cancer cell lines. *Proc Natl Acad Sci USA* 1990; 87: 3294.

61 Putnam EA, Yen N, Gallick GE *et al.* Autocrine growth stimulation by TGF-alpha in human non-small cell lung cancer. *Surg Oncol* 1992; 1: 49.

62 Law MR. Genetic predisposition to lung cancer. *Br J Cancer* 1990; 61: 195.

63 Bench A, Rabbitts P. Genetic changes in lung cancer. In: Thatcher N, Spiro S, eds. *New Perspectives in Lung Cancer.* London: BMJ Publishing Group, 1994: 19.

64 Whang-Peng J, Bunn PAKAO, Shan CS *et al.* A non-random chromosomal abnormality, del 3p (14–23) in human small cell lung cancer (SCLC). *Cancer Genet Cytogenet* 1982; 6: 119.

65 Naylor SL, Johnson BE, Minna JD *et al.* Loss of heterozygosity of chromosome 3p markers in small cell lung cancer. *Nature* 1987; 329: 451.

66 Harbour JW, Lai S-L, Whang-Peng J *et al.* Abnormalities in structure and expression of the human retinoblastoma gene in SCLC. *Science* 1989; 241: 353.

67 Rabbits P, Douglas J, Daly M *et al.* Frequency and extent of the allelic loss in the short arm of chromosome 3 in non-small cell lung cancer. *Genes Chrom Cancer* 1989; 1: 95.

68 Yokoyama S, Yamakawa K, Tsuchiya E *et al.* Deletion mapping on the short arm of chromosome 3 in squamous cell carcinoma and adenocarcinoma of the lung. *Cancer Res* 1992; 52: 873.

69 Johnson BE, Kelley MJ. Biology of small cell lung cancer. *Lung Cancer* 1995; 12 (Suppl 3): S5.

70 Roth JA. Molecular events in lung cancer. *Lung Cancer* 1995; 12 (Suppl 2): S3.

71 Slebos RJC, Kibbelaar RE, Dalesio O *et al.* K-ras oncogene activation as a prognostic marker in adenocarcinoma of the lung. *N Engl J Med* 1990; 323: 561.

72 Anderson MLM, Spandidos DA. Oncogenes and onco-suppressor genes in lung cancer. *Respir Med* 1993; 87: 413.

73 Souhami RL, Beverley PCL, Bobrow LG *et al.* Results of central data analysis: 2nd International Workshop on Small Cell Lung Cancer Antigens. *J Natl Cancer Inst* 1991; 83: 609.

74 Ferrigno D, Buccheri G. Clinical applications of serum markers for lung cancer. *Respir Med* 1995; 89: 587.

75 Johnson PWM, Joel SP, Love S *et al.* Tumour markers for prediction of survival and monitoring of remission in small cell lung cancer. *Br J Cancer* 1993; 67: 760.

76 Manning JT, Spjurt HJ, Tschen JA. Bronchioloalveolar carcinoma. *Cancer* 1984; 54: 525.

77 Lam WK, So SY, YUDYC. Clinical features of bronchogenic carcinoma in Hong Kong: review of 480 patients. *Cancer* 1983; 52: 369.

78 Fergusson RJ, Gregor A, Dodds R *et al.* Management of lung cancer in South-East Scotland. *Thorax* 1996; 51: 569.

79 Weiss W, Boucot KR. The Philadelphia pulmonary neoplasm research project: early roentgenographic appearance of bronchogenic carcinoma. *Arch Intern Med* 1974; 134: 306.

80 Fontana RS, Sanderson DR, Woolner LB *et al.*

The Mayo lung project for early detection and localisation of bronchogenic carcinoma: a status report. *Chest* 1975; 67: 511.

81 Byrd RB, Carr DT, Miller WE *et al.* Radiographic abnormalities in carcinoma of the lung as related to histological cell type. *Thorax* 1969; 24: 573.

82 Harold JT. Lymphangitis carcinomatosa of the lungs. *Q J Med* 1952; 21: 353.

83 Watson WL, Farpour A. Terminal bronchiolar or 'alveolar cell' cancer of the lung: two hundred and sixty-five cases. *Cancer* 1966; 19: 776.

84 di Bonito L, Colautti I, Patriavca S *et al.* Cytological typing of primary lung cancer: study of 100 cases with autopsy confirmation. *Diagn Cytopathol* 1991; 7: 7.

85 Clee MD, Sinclair DJM. Assessment of factors influencing the result of sputum cytology in bronchial carcinoma. *Thorax* 1981; 36: 143.

86 Rosa UW, Prolla JL, Gastal ES. Cytology in diagnosis of cancer affecting the lung: results in 1000 consecutive patients. *Chest* 1973; 63: 203.

87 Evans DMD, Shelley G. Respiratory cytodiagnosis: study in observer variation and its relation to quality of material. *Thorax* 1982; 37: 259.

88 Radke JR, Conway WA, Eyler WR. Diagnostic accuracy in peripheral lung lesions: factors predicting success with flexible fiberoptic bronchoscopy. *Chest* 1975; 76: 176.

89 Wang KP, Marsh BR, Summer WE *et al.* Transbronchial needle aspiration for diagnosis of lung cancer. *Chest* 1981; 80: 48.

90 Gass GD, Olsen GN. Pre-operative pulmonary function testing to predict post-operative morbidity and mortality. *Chest* 1986; 89: 127.

91 Wernly JA, De Meester TR, Kirchner PT *et al.* Clinical value of quantitative ventilation–perfusion lung scans in the surgical management of bronchogenic carcinoma. *J Thorac Cardiovasc Surg* 1980; 80: 535.

92 Corris PA, Ellis DA, Hawkins T *et al.* Use of radionuclide scanning in the pre-operative estimation of pulmonary function after resection. *Thorax* 1987; 42: 285.

93 Kerr KM, Lamb D, Wathen CG *et al.* Pathological assessment of mediastinal lymph nodes in lung cancer: implications for non-invasive mediastinal staging. *Thorax* 1992; 47: 337.

94 McLeod TC, Bourgouin PM, Greenberg RW *et al.* Bronchogenic carcinoma: analysis of staging in the mediastinum with CT by correlative lymph node mapping and sampling. *Radiology* 1992; 182: 319.

95 Staples CA, Muller NL, Miller RR *et al.* Mediastinal nodes in bronchogenic carcinoma: comparison between CT and mediastinoscopy. *Radiology* 1988; 167: 367.

96 Webb WR, Gatson SC, Zerhouni E *et al.* CT and MR imaging in staging non-small cell bronchogenic carcinoma. Report of the Radiographic Diagnostic Oncology Group. *Radiology* 1991; 178: 705.

97 Dales RE, Stark R, Sanicaranarayanan R. Computed tomography to stage lung cancer: approaching a controversy using meta analysis. *Am Rev Respir Dis* 1990; 141: 1096.

98 Arita T, Kuramitsu T, Kawamura M *et al.* Bronchogenic carcinoma: incidence of metastases to normal sized lymph nodes. *Thorax* 1995; 50: 1267.

99 Goldstraw P, Kurzer M, Edwards D. Pre-operative staging of lung cancer: accuracy of computed tomography versus mediastinoscopy. *Thorax* 1983; 38: 10.

100 Lowe VJ, Naunheim KS. Current role of positron emission tomography in thoracic oncology. *Thorax* 1998; 53: 703.

101 Tsang GMK, Watson DCT. The practice of cardiothoracic surgeons in the pre-operative staging of non-small cell lung cancer. *Thorax* 1992; 47: 3.

102 Kunstek N, Cicin-Sain S, Kausic M *et al.* The ultrasonic diagnosis of focal liver lesions: findings compared to CT. *Recent Adv Ultrasound* 1981; 3: 320.

103 Hooper RG, Beechler CR, Johnson MC. Radioisotope scanning in the initial staging of bronchogenic carcinoma. *Am Rev Respir Dis* 1978; 118: 279.

104 Ramsdell JW, Peters RM, Taylor AT *et al.* Multi-organ scanning for staging lung cancer. *J Thorac Cardiovasc Surg* 1977; 73: 653.

105 Michel F, Soler M, Imhop E *et al.* Initial staging of non-small cell lung cancer. *Thorax* 1991; 46: 469.

106 Levenson RM, Sauerbrunn BJL, Ihde DC *et al.* Small cell lung cancer: radionuclide bone scans for assessment of tumor extent and response. *Am J Roentgenol* 1981; 137: 31.

107 Grant D, Edwards D, Goldstraw P. Computed tomography of the brain, chest and abdomen in the pre-operative assessment of non-small cell lung cancer. *Thorax* 1988; 43: 883.

108 Newman SJ, Hansen HH. Frequency, diagnosis and treatment of brain metastases in 247 consecutive patients with bronchogenic carcinoma. *Cancer* 1974; 33: 492.

109 Hillers TK, Sauve MD, Guyatt GH. Analysis of published studies on the detection of extrathoracic metastases in patients presumed to have operable non-small cell lung cancer. *Thorax* 1994; 49: 14.

110 Muers MF. Pre-operative screening for metastases in lung cancer. *Thorax* 1994; 49: 1.

111 Muers MF. How much investigation? In: Thatcher N, Spiro S, eds. *New Perspectives in Lung Cancer*. London: BMJ Publishing Group, 1994: 77.

112 Mountain CF, Carr DT, Anderson WAD. System for the clinical staging of lung cancer. *Am J Roentgenol* 1974; 120: 130.

113 Mountain CF. Revisions in the international system for staging lung cancer. *Chest* 1997; 111: 1710.

114 Rawson NBS, Peto J. An overview of prognostic factors in small cell lung cancer. A report from the sub-committee for the management of lung cancer of the UK CCCR. *Br J Cancer* 1990; 61: 597.

115 Edinburgh Lung Cancer Group. Patients presenting with lung cancer in South East Scotland. *Thorax* 1987; 42: 853.

116 Bignall JR, Martin M, Smithers DW. Survival of 6086 cases of bronchial carcinoma. *Lancet* 1967; i: 1067.

117 Walker WS, Carnochan FM, Tin M. Thoracoscopy assisted pulmonary lobectomy. *Thorax* 1993; 48: 921.

118 McKenna RJ. Lobectomy by video-assisted thoracic surgery with mediastinal node sampling for lung cancer. *J Thorac Cardiovasc Surg* 1994; 107: 879.

119 Ginsberg RJ, Hill LD, Eagen RT *et al.* Modern thirty-day operative mortality for surgical resections in lung cancer. *J Thorac Cardiovasc Surg* 1983; 86: 654.

120 Yellin A, Benfield JR. Surgery for bronchogenic carcinoma in the elderly. *Am Rev Respir Dis* 1985; 131: 197.

121 Mountain CF, Lukeman JM, Hammar SP *et al.* Lung cancer classification: the relationship of disease extent and cell type to survival in a clinical trial population. *J Surg Oncol* 1987; 35: 147.

122 Stanley KE. Experience of the Ludwig Lung Cancer Study Group. *Chest* 1986; 89 (Suppl 4): 343S.

123 Mountain CF. Expanded possibilities for surgical treatment of lung cancer: survival in stage IIIa disease. *Chest* 1990; 97: 1045.

124 Feld R, Rubenstein LV, Weisenberger TH. Sites of recurrence in resected stage I non-small cell lung cancer: a guide for future studies. *J Clin Oncol* 1984; 2: 1352.

125 Smart J, Hilton G. Radiotherapy of cancer of the lung: Results in a selected group of cases. *Lancet* 1956; i: 880.

126 Morrison R, Deeley TJ, Cleland WP. The treatment of carcinoma of the bronchus: a clinical trial to compare surgery and super-voltage radiotherapy. *Lancet* 1963; i: 683.

127 Dobbs HJ, Parker RP, Hodson NJ *et al.* The use of CT in radiotherapy treatment planning. *Radiother Oncol* 1983; 1: 133.

128 Cox JD. Non-small cell lung cancer, role of radiation therapy. *Chest* 1986; 89: 284S.

129 Lee RE, Carr DT, Childs DS. Comparison of split-course radiation therapy and continuous radiation therapy for unresectable bronchogenic carcinoma: 5 year results. *Am J Roentgenol* 1976; 126: 116.

130 Cox P, Kennelly GM. The role of curative radiotherapy in the treatment of lung cancer. *Cancer* 1980; 45: 698.

131 Deeley TJ, Singh SP. Treatment of inoperable carcinoma of the bronchus by megavoltage X-rays. *Thorax* 1967; 22: 562.

132 Graham PH, Gebski VJ, Langlands AO. Radical radiotherapy for early non small cell lung cancer. *Int J Radiat Oncol Biol Phys* 1996; 31: 261.

133 Gauden S, Ramsay J, Tripcony L. The curative treatment by radiotherapy alone of Stage I non small cell lung cancer. *Chest* 1995; 108: 1278.

134 Dische S. Continuous, hyperfractionated, accelerated radiotherapy (CHART). *Eur J Cancer* 1990; 26: 927.

135 Dische S, Saunders M. Continuous, hyperfractionated, accelerated radiotherapy (CHART). An interim report upon late morbidity. *Radiother Oncol* 1989; 16: 67.

136 Saunders M, Dische S, Grosch E *et al.* Experience with CHART. *Int J Radiat Oncol Biol Phys* 1991; 21: 871.

137 Saunders M, Dische S, Barrett A *et al.* Continuous hyperfractionated accelerated radiotherapy (CHART) versus conventional radiotherapy in non small cell lung cancer: a randomised multicentre trial. *Lancet* 1997; 350: 161.

138 Priestman TJ, Bullimore JA, Godden TP *et al.* The Royal College of Radiologists' Fractionation Survey. *Clin Oncol* 1989; 1: 39.

139 Medical Research Council. Inoperable non-small cell lung cancer. MRC randomised trial of palliative radiotherapy with 2 fractions or 10 fractions. *Br J Cancer* 1991; 63: 265.

140 MRC Lung Cancer Working Party. An MRC randomised trial of palliative radiotherapy with two fractions or a single fraction in patients with inoperable non-small cell lung

cancer (NSCLC) and poor performance status. *Br J Cancer* 1992; 65: 934.

141 Line D, Deeley TJ. Palliative therapy. In: Deeley TJ, ed. *Carcinoma of the Bronchus.* New York: Appleton-Century-Crofts, 1972.

142 Slawson RG, Scott RM. Radiation therapy in bronchogenic carcinoma. *Radiology* 1979; 132: 175.

143 Ryan GF, Ball DL, Smith JG. Treatment of brain metastases from primary lung cancer. *Int J Radiat Oncol Biol Phys* 1995; 31: 273.

144 Priestman TJ, Dunn J, Brada M *et al.* Final results of the Royal College of Radiologists' Trial comparing two different radiotherapy schedules in the treatment of cerebral metastases. *Clin Oncol* 1996; 8: 308.

145 Gilbert RW, Kim J, Posner JB. Epidural spinal cord compression from metastatic tumor: diagnosis and treatment. *Ann Neurol* 1978; 3: 40.

146 McBeth F. Radiotherapy in the treatment of lung cancer. *Br J Hosp Med* 1996; 55: 639.

147 Rubin P, Casarett GW. *Clincal Radiation Pathology.* Philadelphia: WB Saunders, 1968.

148 Lawson RAM, Ross WM, Gold RG *et al.* Post-radiation pericarditis: report on four more cases with special reference to bronchogenic carcinoma. *J Thorac Cardiovasc Surg* 1972; 63: 841.

149 Hetzel MR, Smith SGT. Endoscopic palliation of tracheobronchial malignancies. *Thorax* 1991; 46: 325.

150 Non-Small Cell Lung Cancer Collaborative Group. Chemotherapy in non-small cell lung cancer: a meta-analysis using updated data on individual patients from 52 randomised clinical trials. *Br Med J* 1995; 311: 899.

151 Vokes EE. Should non-small cell carcinoma of the lung be treated by chemotherapy? Pro: chemotherapy is for NSCLC. *Am J Respir Crit Care Med* 1995; 151: 1285.

152 White SR. Therapeutic empiricism: the case against chemotherapy in non-small cell lung cancer. *Am J Respir Crit Care Med* 1995; 151: 1288.

153 Bromley LL, Szur L. Combined radiotherapy and resection for carcinoma of the bronchus: experiences with 66 patients. *Lancet* 1955; ii: 937.

154 Warram J. Pre-operative irradiation of cancer of the lung: final report of a therapeutic trial, a collaborative study. *Cancer* 1975; 36: 914.

155 Weisenburger TH, Gail M for the Lung Cancer Study Group. Effects of post-operative mediastinal irradiation on completely resected stage II and stage III epidermoid cancer of the lung. *N Engl J Med* 1986; 315: 1377.

156 MRC Lung Cancer Working Party. Randomized trial of surgical resection with or without post-operative radiotherapy in NSCLC. *Lung Cancer* 1994; 11 (Suppl 1): 148.

157 PORT Meta-analysis Trialist Group. Post operative radiotherapy in non small cell lung cancer: systemic review and metanalysis of individual patient data from nine randomised controlled trials. *Lancet* 1998; 352: 257.

158 Jaklitsch MT, Strauss GM, Healey EA. An historical perspective of multi-modality treatment for resectable non-small cell lung cancer. *Lung Cancer* 1995; 12 (Suppl 2): S17.

159 Ginsberg RJ. Neoadjuvant (induction) treatment for non-small cell lung cancer. *Lung Cancer* 1995; 12 (Suppl 2): S33.

160 Burkes RL, Ginsberg RJ, Shepherd FA *et al.* Induction chemotherapy with mitomycin, vindesine and cisplatin for stage III unresectable non-small cell lung cancer: results of the Toronto Phase II trial. *J Clin Oncol* 1992; 10: 580.

161 Martini N, Kris MG, Flehinger BJ *et al.* Pre-operative chemotherapy for Stage IIIA (N2) lung cancer: the Memorial Sloan-Kettering experience with 136 patients. *Ann Thorac Surg* 1993; 55: 1365.

162 Roth JAQ, Fossella F, Komaki R *et al.* A randomized trial comparing peri-operative chemotherapy and surgery with surgery alone in resectable stage IIIA non-small cell lung cancer. *J Natl Cancer Inst* 1994; 86: 673.

163 Rosell R, Gomez-Codina J, Camps C *et al.* A randomized trial comparing pre-operative chemotherapy plus surgery with surgery alone in patients with non-small cell lung cancer. *N Engl J Med* 1994; 330: 153.

164 Milroy R, MacBeth F. Neoadjuvant chemotherapy in Stage IIIA non-small cell lung cancer. *Thorax* 1995; 50 (Suppl 1): S25.

165 Schaake-Konig C, Van Den Bogaert W, Dalesia O *et al.* Effects of concomitant cis-platin and radiotherapy on inoperable non-small cell lung cancer. *N Engl J Med* 1992; 326: 524.

166 Bishop JF. Scheduling of chemotherapy and radiotherapy in locally advanced non-small cell lung cancer. *Lung Cancer* 1995; 12 (Suppl 2): S53.

167 Leonard RCF. Small cell lung cancer. *Br J Cancer* 1989; 59: 487.

168 Spiro SG. Chemotherapy of small cell lung cancer. *Clin Oncol* 1985; 4: 105.

169 Oldham RK. Small cell lung cancer: a curable disease. *Clin Oncol* 1985; 4: 153.

170 Lassen UN, Hirsch FR, Osterlind K *et al.* Outcome of combination chemotherapy in extensive stage small-cell lung cancer: any treatment related progress? *Lung Cancer* 1998; 20: 151.

171 Mehta C, Vogl SE. High dose cyclophosphamide in the induction chemotherapy of small cell lung cancer: minor improvements in rate of remission and survival. *Proc Am Assoc Cancer Res* 1982; 23: 155.

172 Humblet Y, Symann M, Bosly A *et al.* Late intensification with autologous bone marrow transplantation for small cell lung cancer: a randomised trial. *Proc Am Soc Clin Oncol* 1985; 4: 176.

173 Thatcher N. Haematopoietic growth factors and lung cancer. *Thorax* 1992; 47: 119.

174 MRC Lung Cancer Working Party. Controlled trial of 12 versus 6 courses of chemotherapy in the treatment of small cell lung cancer. *Br J Cancer* 1989; 59: 584.

175 MRC Lung Cancer Working Party. A randomised trial of 3 or 6 courses of etoposide, cyclophosphamide, methotrexate and vincristine or 6 courses of etoposide and ifosfamide in small cell lung cancer I: survival and prognostic factors. *Br J Cancer* 1993; 68: 1150.

176 Spiro SG, Souhami RL, Geddes DM *et al.* Duration of chemotherapy in small cell lung cancer: a Cancer Research Campaign trial. *Br J Cancer* 1989; 59: 578.

177 Abeloff MD, Klastersky J, Drings PD *et al.* Complications of treatment of small cell carcinoma of the lung. *Cancer Treat Rep* 1983; 67: 21.

178 Feld R. Complications in the treatment of

small cell carcinoma of the lung. *Cancer Treat Rev* 1981; 8: 5.

179 Pizzo PA, Robichaud KJ, Gill FA *et al.* Duration of empiric antibiotic therapy in granulocytopenic patients with cancer. *Am J Med* 1979; 67: 194.

180 Bleehan NM, Fayers PM, Girling DJ *et al.* Survival, adverse reactions and quality of life during combination chemotherapy compared with selective palliative treatment for small cell lung cancer. *Respir Med* 1989; 83: 51.

181 Postmus PE, Smit EF. Oral therapy for small cell lung cancer. *Lung Cancer* 1995; 12 (Suppl 3): S63.

182 Carney DN, Grogan L, Smit EF *et al.* Single agent oral etoposide for elderly small cell lung cancer patients. *Semin Oncol* 1990; 17 (Suppl 2): 49.

183 MRC Lung Cancer Working Party. Comparison of oral etoposide and standard intravenous multidrug chemotherapy for small cell lung cancer: a stopped multicentre randomised trial. *Lancet* 1996; 348: 563.

184 Souhami RL, Geddes DM, Spiro SG *et al.* Radiotherapy in small cell cancer of the lung treated with combination chemotherapy: a controlled trial. *Br Med J* 1984; 288: 1643.

185 Perez CA, Einhorn L, Oldham FA *et al.* Randomised trial of radiotherapy to the thorax in limited small cell carcinoma of the lung treated with multiagent chemotherapy and elective brain irradiation: a preliminary report. *J Clin Oncol* 1984; 2: 1200.

186 Perry MC, Eaton WL, Propert KJ *et al.* Chemotherapy with or without radiation therapy in limited disease small cell carcinoma of the lung. *N Engl J Med* 1987; 316: 912.

187 Arriagada RLE, Chevalier T, Ruffie P *et al.* Alternating radiotherapy and chemotherapy in 173 consecutive patients with limited small cell lung carcinoma. *Int J Radiat Oncol Biol Phys* 1990; 19: 1135.

188 Pignon JP, Arriagada R, Ihde DC *et al.* A meta-analysis of thoracic radiotherapy for small cell lung cancer. *N Engl J Med* 1992; 327: 1618.

189 Warde P, Payne D. Does thoracic irradiation improve survival and local control in limited stage small cell carcinoma of the lung? A meta-analysis. *J Clin Oncol* 1992; 10: 890.

190 Turrisi AT. Combined platinum etoposide with radiation therapy in limited stage small cell lung cancer: an effective treatment strategy. *Lung Cancer* 1995; 12 (Suppl 3): S41.

191 Arriagada R, Kramer ALE, Chevalier T *et al.* Competing events determining relapse-free survival in limited small cell lung carcinoma. *J Clin Oncol* 1992; 10: 447.

192 Roth BJ, Johnson DH, Lawrence HE *et al.* Randomised study of cyclophosphamide, doxorubicin and vincristine versus etoposide and cisplatin versus alternation of these two regimens in extensive small cell lung cancer. A phase III trial of the South-Eastern Cancer Study Group. *J Clin Oncol* 1992; 10: 282.

193 Murray N, Coy P, Pater JL *et al.* Importance of timing for thoracic irradiation in the combined modality treatment of limited stage small cell lung cancer. *J Clin Oncol* 1993; 11: 336.

194 Brooks BJ, Seifter EJ, Walsh TE *et al.* Pulmonary toxicity with combined modality

therapy for limited small cell lung cancer. *J Clin Oncol* 1986; 4: 710.

195 Pedersen AG. Diagnosis of CNS metastases from SCLC. In: Hanson HH, ed. *Lung Cancer: Basic and Clinical Aspects.* Dordrecht: Martinus Nijhoff, 1986: 153.

196 Nujent JL, Bunn PA, Matthews M *et al.* CNS metastases in small cell bronchogenic carcinoma. Increasing frequency and changing pattern with lengthening of survival. *Cancer* 1979; 44: 1885.

197 Felletti R, Souhami RL, Spiro SG *et al.* Social consequences of brain or liver relapse in small cell carcinoma of the bronchus. *Radiother Oncol* 1985; 4: 335.

198 Kristjansen PEG, Hansen HH. Prophylactic cranial irradiation in small cell lung cancer: an update. *Lung Cancer* 1995; 12 (Suppl 3): S23.

199 Seydel HG, Greech R, Pagano M *et al.* Prophylactic versus no brain irradiation in regional small cell lung carcinoma. *Am J Clin Oncol* 1985; 8: 218.

200 Licciardello JTW, Cersosimo RJ, Karp DD *et al.* Disturbing central nervous system complications following combination chemotherapy and prophylactic whole brain irradiation in patients with small cell lung cancer. *Cancer Treat Rep* 1985; 69: 1429.

201 Turrisi AT. Brain irradiation and systemic chemotherapy for small cell lung cancer. Dangerous liaisons? *J Clin Oncol* 1990; 8: 196.

202 Arriagada RLE, Chevalier T, Borie F *et al.* Prophylactic cranial irradiation for patients with small cell lung cancer in complete remission. *J Natl Cancer Inst* 1995; 87: 183.

203 Kristensen CA, Kristjansen PE, Hansen HH. Systemic chemotherapy of brain metastases from small-cell lung cancer: a review. *J Clin Oncol* 1992; 10: 1498.

204 Fox W, Scadding JG. Medical Research Council comparative trial of surgery and radiotherapy for primary treatment of small-celled or oat-celled carcinoma of bronchus. Ten-year follow up. *Lancet* 1973; ii: 63.

205 Shields TW, Higgins GA, Matthews MJ *et al.* Surgical resection in the management of small cell carcinoma of the lung. *J Thorac Cardiovasc Surg* 1982; 84: 481.

206 Higgins GA, Shields TW, Keehn RJ. The solitary pulmonary nodule: ten year follow up of Veterans Administration–armed forces co-operation study. *Arch Surg* 1975; 110: 570.

207 Holmes EC. The role of surgery in small cell carcinoma of the lung (SCLC). *Lung Cancer* 1995; 12 (Suppl 3): S17.

208 Baker PB, Ettinger DS, Ruckdeschel JD *et al.* The role of surgery in the management of selected patients with small cell carcinoma of the lung. *J Clin Oncol* 1987; 5: 697.

209 Meyer JA, Gullo JJ, Ikins PM *et al.* Adverse prognostic effect of N2 disease in treated small cell carcinoma of the lung. *J Thorac Cardiovasc Surg* 1989; 97: 177.

210 Prager RL, Foster S, Hainsworth JD *et al.* The feasibility of 'adjuvant surgery' in limited stage small cell carcinoma: a prospective evaluation. *Ann Thorac Surg* 1984; 28: 622.

211 Shepherd FA, Ginsberg R, Patterson GA *et al.* Is there ever a role for salvage operations in limited small cell lung cancer? *J Thorac Cardiovasc Surg* 1991; 101: 196.

212 Ladd T, Piantadosi S, Thomas P *et al.* A prospective randomised trial to determine the benefit of surgical resection of residual disease following response of small cell lung cancer to combination chemotherapy. *Chest* 1994; 106: 3205.

213 Maurer LH. Ectopic hormone syndromes in small cell carcinoma of the lung. *Clin Oncol* 1985; 4: 67.

214 Posner JB. Non-metastatic effects of cancer on the nervous system. In: Wyngaarden JB, Smith LH, eds, *Textbook of Medicine.* Philadelphia: WB Saunders, 1982.

215 Henson RA, Urich H. Cancer and the nervous system. In: *The Neurological Manifestations of Systemic Malignant Disease.* Oxford: Blackwell Scientific Publications, 1982.

216 Rassam JW, Anderson G. Incidence of paramalignant disorders in bronchogenic carcinoma. *Thorax* 1975; 30: 86.

217 Stevenson JC. Malignant hypercalcaemia. *Br Med J* 1985; 291: 421.

218 Ralston SH, Fogelman I, Gardner MD *et al.* Hypercalcaemia of malignancy: evidence for a non-parathyroid humoral agent with an effect on renal tubular handling of calcium. *Clin Sci* 1984; 66: 187.

219 Ralston SH. Pathogenesis and management of cancer associated hypercalcaemia. *Cancer Surv* 1994; 21: 179.

220 Jamieson MJ. Hyponatraemia. *Br Med J* 1985; 290: 1723.

221 Forrest JN, Cox M, Hong C *et al.* Superiority of demeclocycline over lithium in the treatment of chronic syndrome of inappropriate secretion of antidiuretic hormone. *N Engl J Med* 1978; 298: 173.

222 Schrier RW. Treatment of hyponatremia. *N Engl J Med* 1985; 312: 1121.

223 Hainsworth JD, Workman R, Greco FA. Management of the syndrome of inappropriate antidiuretic hormone secretion in small cell lung cancer. *Cancer* 1983; 51: 161.

224 Littlewood TJ, Smith AP. Syndrome of inappropriate antidiuretic hormone secretion due to treatment of lung cancer with cisplatin. *Thorax* 1984; 39: 636.

225 Sheppard F, Laskey J, Evans W *et al.* Cushing's syndrome associated with ectopic corticotrophin production and small cell lung cancer. *J Clin Oncol* 1992; 10: 21.

226 Bondy PK, Gilby ED. Endocrine function in small cell undifferentiated carcinoma of the lung. *Cancer* 1982; 50: 2147.

227 Eisen T, Hickish T, Smith IE *et al.* Small cell lung cancer. *Lancet* 1995; 345: 1285.

228 Sachs BA, Becker N, Bloomberg AE *et al.* 'Cure' of ectopic ACTH syndrome secondary to adenocarcinoma of the lung. *J Clin Endocrinol Metab* 1970; 30: 590.

229 Hoffman D, Brigham B. The use of ketaconazole in ectopic adrenocorticotrophic hormone syndrome. *Cancer* 1991; 67: 1447.

230 Schumacher HR. Articular manifestations of hypertrophic pulmonary osteoarthropathy in bronchogenic carcinoma. *Arthritis Rheum* 1976; 19: 629.

231 Hammarsten JF, O'Leary J. The features and significances of hypertrophic osteoarthropathy. *Arch Intern Med* 1957; 99: 431.

232 Green N, Kurohara SS, George FW, Crews QE. The biologic behavior of lung cancer according to histologic type. *Radiol Clin Biol* 1972; 41: 160.

233 Yacoub MH. Relation between the histology of bronchial carcinoma and hypertrophic pulmonary osteoarthropathy. *Thorax* 1965; 20: 537.

234 Gall EA, Bennett GA, Bauer W. Generalised hypertrophic osteoarthropathy: a pathologic study of seven cases. *Am J Pathol* 1951; 27: 349.

235 Flavell G. Reversal of pulmonary hypertrophic osteoarthropathy by vagotomy. *Lancet* 1956; i: 260.

236 Rabson AS, Rosen SW, Tashjian AH *et al.* Production of human chorionic gonadotrophin *in vitro* by a cell line derived from a carcinoma of the lung. *J Natl Cancer Inst* 1973; 50: 669.

237 Healy TM. Eosinophilia in bronchogenic carcinoma. *N Engl J Med* 1974; 291: 794.

238 Knox AJ, Johnson CE, Page RL. Eosinophilia associated with thoracic malignancy. *Br J Dis Chest* 1986; 80: 92.

239 Kornguth S. Neuronal proteins and paraneoplastic syndromes. *N Engl J Med* 1989; 321: 1607.

240 Schuffler MD, Baird HW, Fleming CR *et al.* Intestinal pseudo-obstruction as the presenting manifestation of small cell carcinoma of the lung. *Ann Intern Med* 1983; 98: 129.

241 Szabo A, Dalman J, Manley G *et al.* HuD: a paraneoplastic encephalomyelitis antigen, contains RNA-binding domains and is homologous to Elar and sex lethal. *Cell* 1991; 67: 325.

242 Satoyoshi E, Kowa H, Fukunaga N. Subacute cerebellar degeneration and Eaton–Lambert syndrome with bronchogenic carcinoma. *Neurology* 1973; 23: 764.

243 Schraufnagel DE, Hill R, Leech JA *et al.* Superior vena caval obstruction: is it a medical emergency. *Am J Med* 1981; 70: 1169.

244 Spiro SG, Shah S, Harper PG *et al.* Treatment of obstruction of the superior vena cava by combination chemotherapy with or without irradiation in small cell carcinoma of the bronchus. *Thorax* 1983; 38: 501.

245 Jahangiri M, Taggart D, Goldstraw P. Role of mediastinoscopy in superior vena caval obstruction. *Cancer* 1993; 71: 3006.

246 Jackson JE, Brooks DM. Stenting of superior vena caval obstruction. *Thorax* 1995; 50 (Suppl 1): S31.

247 Ostler PJ, Clarke DP, Watkinson AF *et al.* Superior vena cava obstruction: a modern management strategy. *Clin Oncol* 1997; 9: 83.

248 Armstrong B, Perez C, Simpson J *et al.* Role of irradiation in management of superior vena cava syndrome. *Int J Radiat Oncol Biol Phys* 1987; 13: 531.

249 Perez C, Presant CA, Van Amberg AL. Management of superior vena cava syndrome. *Semin Oncol* 1978; 5: 123.

250 Charnsangavej C, Carrasco CH, Wallace S *et al.* Stenosis of the vena cava: preliminary assessment of treatment with expandable metallic stents. *Radiology* 1986; 161: 295.

251 Watkinson AF, Hansell DM. Expandable Wallstent for the treatment of obstruction of the superior vena cava. *Thorax* 1993; 48: 915.

252 Gaines PA, Belli A-M, Anderson PB *et al.* Superior vena caval obstruction managed by the Gianturco Z stent. *Clin Radiol* 1994; 49: 202.

253 Robinson L, Jackson J. New approach to superior vena cava obstruction. *Br Med J* 1994; 308: 1697.

254 Pancoast HK. Superior pulmonary sulcus tumor. *JAMA* 1932; 99: 1391.

255 Shaw RR, Paulson DL, Kee JL. Treatment of the superior sulcus tumor by irradiation followed by resection. *Ann Surg* 1961; 154: 29.

256 Hilaris BS, Martini N. Multimodality

therapy of superior sulcus tumors. *Adv Pain Res Ther* 1982; 4: 113.

257 Neal CR, Amdur RJ, Mendenhall WM *et al.* Pancoast tumor: radiation therapy alone versus preoperative radiation therapy and surgery. *Int J Radiat Oncol Biol Phys* 1991; 21: 651.

258 Komaki R, Roh J, Cox JD, Lopes DA, Conceicao A. Superior sulcus tumors: results of irradiation of 36 patients. *Cancer* 1981; 48: 1563.

259 Walshe AD, Douglas JG, Kerr KM *et al.* An audit of the clinical investigation of pleural effusion. *Thorax* 1992; 47: 734.

260 Martini N, Bains MS, Beattie EJ. Indications for pleurectomy in malignant effusion. *Cancer* 1975; 35: 734.

261 Wallach HW. Intrapleural tetracycline for malignant pleural effusions. *Chest* 1975; 68: 510.

262 Cox JD, Yesner RA. Adenocarcinoma of the lung: recent results from the Veterans Administration Lung Group. *Am Rev Respir Dis* 1979; 120: 1025.

263 Tarnoff JF, Calinog TA, Byla JG. Prolonged survival following cerebral metastasis from pulmonary cancer. *J Thorac Cardiovasc Surg* 1976; 72: 933.

264 Mussi A, Janni A, Pistolesi M *et al.* Surgical treatment of primary lung cancer and solitary brain metastases. *Thorax* 1985; 40: 191.

265 Borgelt B, Gelber R, Kramer S *et al.* The palliation of brain metastases: final results of the first two studies by the Radiation Therapy Oncology Group. *Int J Radiat Oncol Biol Phys* 1980; 6: 1.

266 Deeley TJ, Rice-Edwards JM. Radiotherapy in the management of cerebral secondaries from bronchial carcinoma. *Lancet* 1968; i: 1209.

267 Baraka ME. Malignant tumours of the trachea. *Ann R Coll Surg Engl* 1984; 66: 27.

268 Pearson FG, Thompson DW, Weissberg D *et al.* Adenoid cystic carcinoma of trachea. *Ann Thorac Surg* 1974; 18: 16.

269 Stalpaert G, Deneffe G, Van Maele R. Surgical treatment of adenoid cystic carcinoma of the left main bronchus and trachea by left pneumonectomy, resection of 7.5 cm trachea, and direct reanastomosis of right lung. *Thorax* 1979; 34: 554.

270 Macha HN, Koch K, Stadler M *et al.* New technique for treating occlusive and stenosing tumours of the trachea and main bronchi: endobronchial irradiation by high dose iridium-192 combined with laser canalisation. *Thorax* 1987; 42: 511.

271 George J. Endoscopic laser resection for tracheobronchial malignancy. *Lung Cancer Therapy* 1996; 13: 437.

272 George PJM, Garrett CPO, Hetzel MR. Role of the neodymium YAG laser in the management of tracheal tumours. *Thorax* 1987; 42: 440.

273 Westaby S, Jackson JW, Pearson FG. A bifurcated silicone rubber stent for relief of tracheobronchial obstruction. *J Thorac Cardiovasc Surg* 1982; 83: 414.

274 Fergusson RJ, Cull A. The measurement of quality of life in patients undergoing treatment for lung cancer. *Thorax* 1991; 46: 671.

275 Montazeri MPH, Gillis CR, McEwen J. Quality of life in patients with lung cancer. A review of the literature from 1970 to 1995. *Chest* 1998; 113: 467.

276 Bernhard J, Ganz PA. Psychosocial issues in lung cancer patients. *Chest* 1991; 99: 216.

277 Karnofsky DA, Abelmann WH, Craver LF *et al.* The use of nitrogen mustards in the palliative treatment of carcinoma. *Cancer* 1948; 1: 634.

278 World Health Organization. *Handbook for Reporting Results of Cancer Treatment.* Geneva: WHO, 1979.

279 Zubrod CG, Schneiderman M, Frei E *et al.* Appraisal of methods for the study of chemotherapy of cancer in man. *J Chron Dis* 1960; 11: 7.

280 Aaronson NK, Ahmedzai S, Bergmann B *et al.* The EORTC QLQ-C30: a quality of life instrument for use in international clinical trials in oncology. *J Natl Cancer Inst* 1993; 85: 365.

281 Bergman B. The EORTC QLQ Lung Cancer Module: a preliminary analysis. Internal report to the EORTC Qualify of Life Study Group, 1992.

282 de Haes KJM, Van Knippenberg FCE, Neijt JP. Measuring psychological and physical distress in cancer patients: structure and application of the Rotterdam Symptom Checklist. *Br J Cancer* 1990; 62: 1034.

283 Zigmond AS, Snaith RD. The Hospital Anxiety and Depression Scale. *Acta Psychiatr Scand* 1983; 67: 361.

284 Greenberg ER, Chute CG, Stukel T *et al.* Social and economic factors in the choice of lung cancer treatment. *N Engl J Med* 1988; 318: 612.

285 Jennett B, Buxton M. When is treatment for cancer economically justified? Discussion paper. *J R Soc Med* 1990; 83: 25.

286 Huhti E, Sutinen S, Saloheimo M. Survival among patients with lung cancer: an epidemiologic study. *Am Rev Respir Dis* 1981; 124: 13.

287 Chahinian AP, Israel L. Rates and patterns of growth of lung cancer. In: Israel L, Chahinian AP, eds. *Lung Cancer: Natural History, Prognosis, and Therapy.* New York: Academic Press, 1976.

288 Geddes DM. The natural history of lung cancer: a review based on rates of tumour growth. *Br J Dis Chest* 1979; 73: 1.

289 Meyer JA. The concept and significance of growth rates in human pulmonary tumors. *Ann Thorac Surg* 1972; 14: 309 1983.

290 Strauss MJ. Growth characteristics of lung cancer. In: Strauss MJ, ed. *Lung Cancer: Clinical Diagnosis and Treatment.* New York: Grune & Stratton, 1983.

291 Joseph WL, Morton DL, Adkins PC *et al.* Prognostic significance of tumour doubling times in evaluating operability in pulmonary metastatic disease. *J Thorac Cardiovasc Surg* 1971; 61: 23.

292 Collins VP, Loeffler RK, Tivey H. Observations on growth rates of human tumors. *Am J Roentgenol* 1956; 76: 988.

293 Bailar JC. Screening for lung cancer: where are we now? *Am Rev Respir Dis* 1984; 130: 545.

294 Berlin NI, Buncher CR, Fontana RS *et al.* The National Cancer Institute co-operative early lung cancer detection program; results of the initial screen (prevalence); early lung cancer detection: introduction. *Am Rev Respir Dis* 1984; 130: 545.

295 Frost JK, Ball WC, Levin ML *et al.* Early lung cancer detection: results of the initial (prevalence) radiologic and cytologic screening in the Johns Hopkins study. *Am Rev Respir Dis* 1984; 130: 549.

296 Fontana RS, Sanderson DR, Taylor WF *et al.* Early lung cancer detection: results of the initial (prevalence) radiologic and cytologic screening in the Mayo Clinic study. *Am Rev Respir Dis* 1984; 130: 561.

297 Bignall JR, Martin M, Smithers DW. Survival in 6086 cases of bronchial carcinoma. *Lancet* 1967; i: 1067.

298 National Cancer Institute. *Cancer Patient Survival Report No. 5.* Bethesda, Maryland: National Cancer Institute, 1976.

299 Mountain CF. Value of the new TNM staging system for lung cancer. *Chest* 1989; 96 (Suppl 1): 47S.

300 Albain KS, Crowley JJ, Leblanc M *et al.* Survival determinants in extensive stage non-small cell lung cancer: the Southwest Oncology Group experience. *J Clin Oncol* 1991; 91: 1618.

301 Ludwig Lung Cancer Study Group. Prognostic factors in operable non-small cell lung cancer. In: *Proceedings of the UICC Conference on Clinical Oncology.* Geneva: International Union Against Cancer, 1981.

302 Kato Y, Ferguson TB, Bennett DE *et al.* Oat cell carcinoma of the lung. *Cancer* 1969; 23: 517.

303 Hyde L, Yee J, Wilson R, Patno ME. Cell type and the natural history of lung cancer. *JAMA* 1965; 193: 140.

42

OTHER PULMONARY NEOPLASMS AND RELATED CONDITIONS

ANTHONY SEATON

The previous chapter describes the various types of bronchial and alveolar cell carcinomas. Apart from metastases, all other lung tumours are relatively rare, in one series from the Mayo Clinic comprising less than 1% of all primary lung tumours [1]. In that series, the most common were non-Hodgkin's lymphoma, carcinosarcoma and mucoepidermoid carcinoma, representing 41, 20 and 15%, respectively. This chapter deals with these other primary lung tumours, both benign and malignant, and also gives a brief account of the different patterns of lung metastases from tumours of other organs. It includes a description of some diseases that, though not strictly neoplastic, are related to the tumours described. An attempt is made to classify the primary tumours according to the tissue from which their cell type originates, although in a number of cases this is uncertain. The classification adopted is given in Table 42.1. For further pathological information on the many different types of lung tumour, the reader is referred to the bibliography of Whimster [2].

Tumours of the blood and reticuloendothelial system

Hodgkin's lymphoma

The clinical syndrome described by Thomas Hodgkin in 1832 is now taken to be confined to a particular histological type of lymphoma characterized by destruction of lymph node architecture, proliferation of large abnormal cells derived from monocytes and, usually, Reed–Sternberg cells (Fig. 42.1). It may be subclassified into four histological types: nodular sclerosing, lymphocyte-predominant, mixed cellular and lymphocyte-depleted. Nodular sclerosing Hodgkin's lymphoma tends to be the most benign variant, the other types often progressing from lymphocyte-predominant through mixed to lymphocyte-depleted. It is usual to classify Hodgkin's disease according to its extent, the tissues involved and the presence of systemic symptoms [3], this classification

being used in prognosis and in the planning of treatment (Table 42.2).

Clinical features

Hodgkin's disease primarily affects adults, with an annual incidence of 2–3 per 100000, and peaks at the ages of 25 and 60–70. It is more common in men. Only occasionally does it present as a primary intrathoracic lesion, when it is usually found as a result of investigation of enlarged hilar nodes. They are usually asymmetrically enlarged, in contrast to those of sarcoidosis, and the disease commonly extends into the mediastinal and paratracheal nodes (Fig. 42.2). More frequently, these features are part of a more generalized lymphadenopathy. The patient may be free of symptoms or may have evidence of systemic disease, with fever, loss of weight or night sweats. Symptoms referable to intrathoracic disease may include pleuritic pain, cough due to bronchial or tracheal compression, stridor, hoarseness due to recurrent laryngeal involvement, facial swelling due to vena caval obstruction, or breathlessness due to pulmonary infiltration [4]. Very rarely, the first presentation of the disease may be a diffuse intrapulmonary infiltrate without node enlargement [5,6]. Again, it is more usual for pulmonary infiltration to be found as part of a generalized disease, and usually associated with involvement of the hilar and mediastinal lymph nodes. In one review of 284 patients with Hodgkin's disease, 52% were found to have intrathoracic involvement; in 43% this was in the lung, in 34% hilar nodes, in 23% mediastinal nodes and in 11% pleura [7]. Thus node involvement is not essential for the diagnosis of pulmonary Hodgkin's, the disease manifesting itself wherever there is lymphatic tissue in the lung [8].

Apart from mediastinal and hilar node involvement, the radiological features of intrathoracic Hodgkin's disease most frequently show peribronchial infiltration. Direct extension from involved nodes is the next most frequent appearance, while patchy infiltrates, diffuse pneumonic consolidation and nodular lesions occur rather less often

Table 42.1 Classification of lung tumours and related conditions.

Blood and reticuloendothelial system
Hodgkin's lymphoma
Non-Hodgkin's lymphoma
Leukaemias
Plasmacytoma
Histiocytic conditions
Lymphoproliferative conditions

Vascular tissue
Haemangiopericytoma
Intravascular bronchioloalveolar tumour
Angiosarcoma
Lymphangioleiomyoma
Tuberous sclerosis
Arteriovenous malformations
Lymphangiectasis

Neural tissue
Neurofibroma
Neurilemmoma
Neurosarcoma
Chemodectoma

Epithelium
Carcinoid
Cylindroma
Mucoepidermoid tumour
Melanoma
Papilloma
Clear-cell tumour
Adenoma
Sclerosing pneumocytoma

Muscle and connective tissue
Leiomyoma (sarcoma)
Rhabdomyosarcoma
Fibroma (sarcoma)
Lipoma (sarcoma)
Chondroma (sarcoma)
Myxoma

Mixed-cell origin
Teratoma
Hamartoma
Carcinosarcoma
Blastoma

Table 42.2 Staging of lymphoma.

Stage I	Involvement of a single lymph node region (I) or of a single extralymphatic organ or site (I_E)
Stage II	Involvement of two or more lymph node regions on same side of the diaphragm (II) or localized involvement of extralymphatic organ or site and of one or more lymph node regions on the same side of the diaphragm (II_E)
Stage III	Involvement of nodes on both sides of the diaphragm (III). There may also be splenic involvement (III_S), localized involvement of extralymphatic organ or site (III_E) or both (III_{ES})
Stage IV	Diffuse or disseminated involvement of one or more extralymphatic organs or tissues with or without associated lymph node enlargement
	Each stage is divided into A, those with no systemic symptoms, and B, patients with night sweats, loss of more than 10% of body weight in 6 months or unexplained fever above 38°C

[7] (Fig. 42.3). Pleural effusion and direct spread into ribs may occur. All histological types of Hodgkin's disease may involve the lung, although the lymphocyte-predominant type does so less frequently than do the others. Involvement of the lung, as opposed to intrathoracic nodes, tends to be a later feature of Hodgkin's disease, though it is found at presentation in about one-third of patients [7]. It generally appears between 1 and 4 years after presentation, albeit the early use of chemotherapy may well prevent its development in many cases.

The diagnosis of intrathoracic Hodgkin's disease is made by biopsy of appropriate tissue. The main differen-tial diagnosis is sarcoidosis (see Chapter 39), which also commonly presents with hilar, mediastinal and other node enlargement but less frequently causes systemic symptoms, fever and weight loss. At first presentation, it is usual to be able to obtain a node from a more accessible part of the body; however, if the disease is confined to the thorax, mediastinoscopy, mediastinotomy or thoracotomy is necessary, since needle biopsies are insufficient for proper histological assessment. Assuming the diagnosis can be made from an involved node, it may not be necessary to biopsy lung as well. However, if thoracotomy is performed, it is sensible to take a lung biopsy as well as a node. If the disease presents as a primary intrapulmonary lesion, biopsy is necessary, as it is if the lung shadowing occurs after the start of treatment. In this case, differentiation has to be made from other causes of lung infiltration that may affect people immunosuppressed by drugs, radiotherapy or the primary disease, including infections by *Pneumocystis carinii*, fungi and mycobacteria. Transbronchial biopsy with brushing and lavage have proved to be the investigations of choice in this situation. Other rare pulmonary complications of Hodgkin's disease include Langerhans' cell histiocytosis (histiocytosis X) and veno-occlusive disease [9,10].

Treatment and prognosis

Treatment is planned on the basis of a staging procedure that usually includes CT, unless the disease is clearly stage IIIB or IV. Laparotomy and splenectomy were widely used in the past but probably confer no survival advantages and carry definite risks, so are rarely used nowadays.

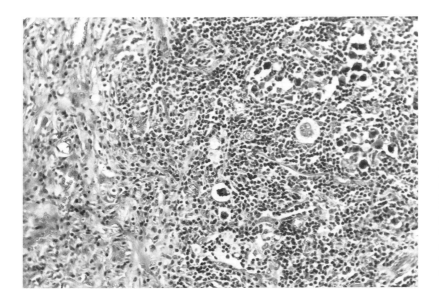

Fig. 42.1 Histological appearances of pulmonary deposit of nodular sclerosing Hodgkin's disease showing fibrosis to the left and a nodular tumour deposit to the right. This contains a background of small cells/lymphocytes, eosinophils and plasma cells mixed with large pleomorphic cells. One Reed–Sternberg cell is present in the centre of the nodule (haematoxylin & eosin ×150).

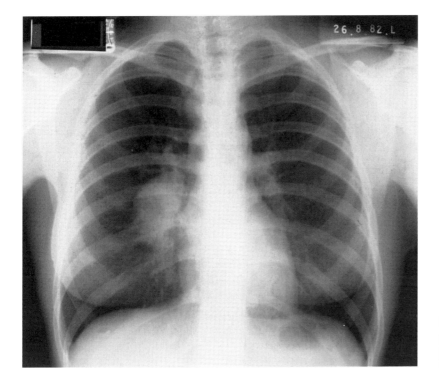

Fig. 42.2 Enlarged right hilar and paratracheal nodes in 18-year-old girl that proved to be due to nodular sclerosing Hodgkin's disease.

Intrathoracic disease is rarely stage I. Stage IA and IIA disease are usually managed by megavoltage radiotherapy, although clear-cut symptoms of B disease lead to treatment with chemotherapy. Stages III and IV are treated with chemotherapy, usually without radiotherapy. Treatment differs in different centres, although chemotherapy is normally started with a combination of nitrogen mustard, vincristine or vinblastine, procarbazine and prednisolone, given for at least six courses. The different regimens and their immediate and long-term side-effects are best managed by a specialist oncologist [11]. Patients receiving both radiotherapy and chemotherapy are known to have a much increased risk of developing other neoplasms [12]. In a recent series from The Netherlands, a second tumour occurred in 146 of 1939 patients over a mean follow-up of 9 years, over three times the expected rate [13]. The tumours with highest relative risks were leukaemia, non-Hodgkin's lymphoma, sarcoma and melanoma.

The prognosis in treated intrathoracic Hodgkin's disease is no worse than when any other part of the body is involved; at 10 years, some 75% of patients with stage II disease, 58% with stage III and 40% with stage IV may expect to be alive, most without relapse.

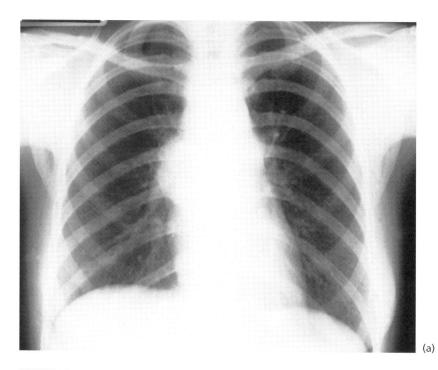

(a)

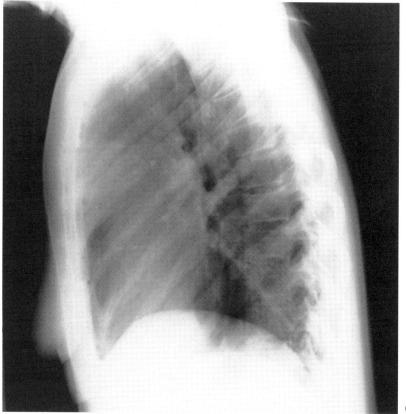

(b)

Fig. 42.3 Posteroanterior (a) and left lateral (b) chest films of 20-year-old girl with anterior mediastinal Hodgkin's disease. There was spread of lymphoma into the lingula anterior to the left hilum.

Non-Hodgkin's lymphoma

The term 'non-Hodgkin's lymphoma' includes several other malignant lymphoproliferative conditions that do not show the pathological features of Hodgkin's disease, including those previously known as lymphosarcoma and reticulum cell sarcoma. Their classification (there are several in use) is confusing to the non-specialist but one, the Kiel classification [14], is given in Table 42.3. This is based on cell-marker and cytological studies and has some

Table 42.3 Simplified classification of non-Hodgkin's lymphomas.

Low-grade B cell
Lymphocytic (including chronic lymphatic leukaemia)
Lymphoplasmacytoid (immunocytoma)
Plasmacytic
Follicle cell, centrocytic
Centroblastic/centrocytic (follicular or diffuse)
Centrocytic

High-grade B cell
Centroblastic
Lymphoblastic
Immunoblastic
Large cell anaplastic
Burkitt's lymphoma

Low-grade T cell
Lymphocytic (including chronic lymphocytic leukaemia)
Small cerebriform cell
Lymphoepithelioid
Angioimmunoblastic
Pleomorphic, small cell

High-grade T cell
Pleomorphic, medium and large cell
Immunoblastic
Large cell anaplastic
Lymphoblastic

Unclassified rare types

---

value prognostically, in that the high-grade tumours are the more malignant.

Clinical features

Non-Hodgkin's lymphoma is characteristically a disease of older people, with a peak incidence in those aged 60–80. Little is known of its pathogenesis, though it may affect people who have immune disturbances as a result of either disease, such as Sjögren's syndrome and coeliac disease, or immunosuppressive drugs. Epstein–Barr virus may be responsible in some cases, probably acting with another factor such as persistent stimulation of the immune system by another infection. In other cases infection with human T-cell leukaemia virus (HTLV)-1 may be responsible. Thoracic involvement most commonly takes the form of enlarged hilar and mediastinal nodes, although intrapulmonary involvement may occur, appearing as diffuse consolidation, peribronchial infiltration or single or multiple nodular lesions [15]. Pleural effusion is not infrequent. Altogether, intrathoracic involvement occurs in 20–25% of cases [16,17], with node enlargement and pleural effusion in about 20% and lung involvement in about 25%. Enlarged nodes may occur in any of the pathological types; however, lung infiltration is most frequent with the low-grade lymphocytic type

whereas nodular lesions occur, probably as blood-borne metastases, in the high-grade lymphoblastic types [17].

Primary lung involvement by non-Hodgkin's lymphoma is very rare. It presents with non-specific symptoms, including cough, breathlessness, chest pain and loss of weight [18,19]; finger clubbing and hypertrophic osteoarthropathy have been described [20]. Occasionally a lesion is found on routine radiography of a fit patient. The chest film usually shows a single area of diffuse infiltration, which may be nodular or involve as much as a whole lung [18]. Pathologically these are often low-grade lymphoplasmacytoid lesions (immunocytomas) [21].

The diagnosis of non-Hodgkin's lymphoma is made in the same way as that of Hodgkin's disease, i.e. an adequate piece of tissue is required for proper assessment. If the lung is involved at first presentation together with other organs, no further pulmonary investigation may be necessary, at least until there has been no response to antibiotics (in case of a pneumonic complication) and chemotherapy. However, sputum cytology is a useful non-invasive investigation [22]. If the only manifestation of disease is an intrathoracic lesion, mediastinoscopy and thoracotomy may well be necessary. Indeed, long-term remission has followed surgical removal of lymphocytic lymphoma confined to the lung [23].

In the case of lung infiltration occurring after diagnosis and initiation of treatment, other diagnostic measures are necessary, as the lesion may be due to opportunist infection. Transbronchial biopsy, together with brushing and local lavage, are the best techniques short of the more invasive procedures of thoracotomy or video-controlled thoracoscopy [24].

Treatment and prognosis

This is a matter for the specialist oncologist. In general, non-Hodgkin's lymphomas have a poorer outlook than the Hodgkin's type, and patients with the less-differentiated high-grade tumours, especially when they present with systemic symptoms, tend not to survive more than 2 years. However, in the few such patients who do respond to treatment, cure is possible; paradoxically at present, it is probable that low-grade tumours almost never respond completely to treatment [25]. The aim of management should therefore be to treat low-grade tumours with the minimum therapy necessary to relieve symptoms and ensure a good quality of life, whereas high-grade tumours should be treated with combination chemotherapy. Stage I disease and low-grade tumours, including chronic lymphatic leukaemia, have a much better prognosis, with 70% survival at 3 years [26]. Pulmonary infiltration occurring after the start of chemotherapy not surprisingly carries a worse prognosis than if it is found to be present *ab initio*. Treatment of stage I disease is usually with local radiotherapy. Low-grade lymphomas are often treated with cyclophosphamide or chlorambucil alone, and some are not treated at all; the age of the patient, the course and cell type of the disease and the potential toxicity of the drugs are all factors that should be taken into account when planning treatment. Pulmonary involvement almost always requires treatment and this is usually radiotherapy combined with chemotherapy. The higher-grade lymphomas would normally be treated with combinations such as cyclophosphamide, vincristine and prednisolone, with or without doxorubicin and bleomycin. It should be remembered that these drugs themselves can be the cause of diffuse pulmonary infiltrates (see Chapter 55).

Leukaemias

Chronic lymphatic leukaemia is now regarded generally as a variant of low-grade lymphocytic lymphoma in which the abnormal cells are found in the bloodstream. Involvement of intrathoracic nodes and of lung may occur, as discussed above [17]. Hilar adenopathy may occur in acute leukaemias as part of a generalized lymphadenopathy. Acute and chronic myeloid leukaemia may involve the lung secondarily, but usually only with microscopic

infiltration [27,28]. Thus the finding of pulmonary infiltrates in a patient with leukaemia should arouse the suspicion of either opportunist infection or lung haemorrhage. In acute leukaemias there is a strong case for instituting empirical treatment without further investigation, since such patients with pulmonary infiltrates usually die very rapidly (discussed further in Chapter 52). Briefly, treatment entails the administration of platelets if the platelet count is low and broad-spectrum antibiotics, including high-dose co-trimoxazole and amphotericin. If investigation is to be carried out, bronchoalveolar lavage or transtracheal aspiration is probably the safest and least traumatic [29,30].

Plasmacytoma

The respiratory system is rarely involved in multiple myeloma, although deposits may occasionally be found presenting as tumours of trachea or bronchi [31,32]. Even less frequently, a solitary lung plasmacytoma may be the only manifestation of the disease [33]. A more usual presentation to the chest physician is an osteolytic lesion of rib or sternum associated with an intrathoracic extension of tumour (Fig. 42.4).

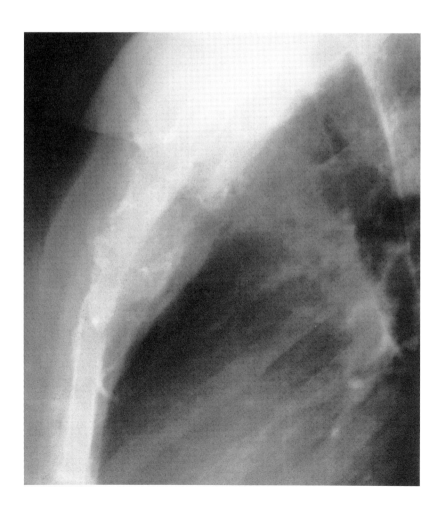

Fig. 42.4 Expansion and irregular destruction of sternum due to myeloma.

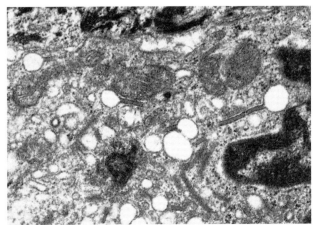

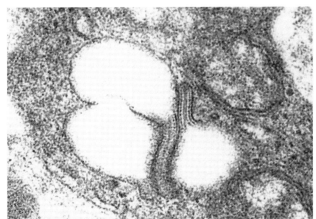

(a)

(b)

Fig. 42.5 (a) Electron micrograph of Langerhans' cell from patient with Langerhans' cell histiocytosis showing multiple characteristic tennis racquet or Birbeck bodies (uranyl acetate and lead citrate ×33700). (b) High-power view of three Birbeck bodies showing their tubular structure and terminal dilatation (×63500).

The finding of a monoclonal band of immunoglobulin on electrophoresis of serum proteins is characteristic of myeloma, and such a band would be expected with solitary plasmacytoma of lung. However, it should be remembered that monoclonal gammopathies may be associated with other lesions, especially lymphoma, and may occur without obvious cause in association with a range of pulmonary diseases [34].

A solitary plasmacytoma is likely to be diagnosed at bronchial biopsy. The treatment of choice is probably excision, which has been associated with prolonged remission. Disseminated disease may occur subsequently but is not inevitable. Treatment of generalized myeloma with lung involvement would probably include local radiotherapy and chemotherapy with melphalan and prednisone. Multiple-drug therapy is not yet established as having substantial advantages, although in some patients with aggressive disease vincristine, doxorubicin and dexamethasone or similar combinations have been used to produce a remission.

Histiocytoses

A number of conditions are characterized by abnormal proliferation of histiocytes; although not all are neoplastic, they are considered together here. All are extremely uncommon. Their classification has been changed frequently and at present they are differentiated into Langerhans' cell histiocytosis, histiocytoses of non-Langerhans' phagocytic cells, malignant histiocytoses, and a mixed bag of other histiocytoses. Langerhans' cell histiocytosis is the agreed name for the syndrome previously known by several names: histiocytosis X, eosinophilic granuloma, Hand–Schüller–Christian syndrome and Letterer–Siwe

disease [35]. Lung involvement is not uncommon and is described below. Malignant histiocytosis as described in the literature, a disease predominantly of young people and which may arise in the gastrointestinal tract of patients with coeliac disease, would probably now be regarded as histiocytic lymphoma. Lung involvement with diffuse acinar infiltrates is not uncommon at some stage in the course of the disease and occasionally pulmonary symptoms may be the presenting feature [36–38]. Lung disease is not a feature of the other histiocytoses.

Langerhans' cell histiocytosis

Langerhans' cell histiocytosis was originally thought to be a lipid storage disease but is now classified as a condition of histiocytic proliferation [39]. Langerhans' cells are derived from the bone marrow and normally found in the skin. They secrete interleukin (IL)-1 and prostaglandin E and promote secretion of IL-2 and interferon γ by T lymphocytes. Pathologically, the disease is characterized by proliferation of histiocytes with vesicular and lobulated nuclei, basophilic nucleoli and eosinophilic cytoplasm. Tissue necrosis and infiltration with lymphocytes, plasma cells and eosinophils are also seen. The histiocytes may be seen on electron microscopy to contain characteristic Birbeck or tennis racquet bodies [40,41] (Fig. 42.5). Deposits of lipid material may be seen in the cytoplasm of the histiocytes. A spectrum of appearances may be present in lesions, from histiocytic infiltrates through granulomas and lipid-containing lesions to fibrosis.

Clinically, the disease affects infants and children primarily but may present as late as the fifth decade [42]. Its peak incidence is in the first few years of childhood and becomes progressively less frequent thereafter. The three original names reflect three characteristic clinical groups: group 1, in which there is primarily bone involvement (eosinophilic granuloma); group 2, in which bone and other organs such as lung, lymph nodes and liver are involved (Hand–Schüller–Christian disease); and group 3, in which skin, viscera and bone are involved (Letterer–

Siwe disease). However, there is considerable overlap between the three. In general group 1 lesions have the best prognosis and group 3 the worst. Age is also an important prognostic factor, very young children having a bad prognosis [43]. The condition is uncommon, having been estimated to occur in 1 per 350 000 annually in the UK [44].

The symptoms vary depending on the site of disease. Skin lesions present as papular and vesicular eruptions. Bone lesions often involve the skull, ribs and femur and may be palpable as subcutaneous lumps. Radiology shows punched-out lytic areas (Fig. 42.6). Granulomatous polyps may present in the external auditory meatus or in the orbit causing exophthalmos. Diabetes insipidus is a rare feature due to infiltration of the hypothalamus. When the lung is involved in the generalized disease, the prognosis has usually been thought to be bad [43]; however, a more recent study in which special efforts were made to detect subtle evidence of lung involvement suggests that this is not necessarily the case [45]. Involvement of the lung alone, primary pulmonary Langerhans' cell histiocytosis, may occur at any age but is seen most commonly in young male adults and seems to be associated with smoking [46]. All forms of the disease have a natural tendency to burn out, leaving fibrosis in the case of lung involvement, and the primary lung form is not necessarily associated with a fatal prognosis [47]. The onset is insidious, with cough, shortness of breath and loss of weight. Pneumothorax may be a presenting feature and is a frequent complication of all stages of the disease [48], often occurring repeatedly.

The radiographic appearances are of a diffuse pulmonary infiltration with a mixture of small nodular and irregular reticular shadows [49] (Fig. 42.7). There is no characteristic distribution, except that several zones of both lungs are involved and the costophrenic angles are often spared. Cyst formation is common and becomes a more marked feature as the disease progresses; some patients develop diffuse emphysematous changes. There is a tendency for nodular opacities to progress to cysts, reflecting histological changes from granuloma to fibrosis. High-resolution CT may show a characteristic combination of nodules and cystic change in keeping with these pathological features (see Fig. 7.49) [46]. Pleural effusion and mediastinal node involvement are rare [50,51].

The diagnosis is usually made by lung biopsy, although electron microscopy of lavaged bronchoalveolar cells may show the characteristic X bodies [41] (see Fig. 42.5). Monoclonal antibodies have been shown to be of value in the histological diagnosis [52–54]. Clinically, the diagnosis is suspected in a young male with diffuse reticulonodular radiographic change, especially if associated with pneumothorax; sarcoidosis is the disease most likely to cause confusion. Pulmonary function tests usually show reduced diffusing capacity but normal or increased lung volumes [40].

There is no consensus on treatment of Langerhans' cell histiocytosis. Spontaneous remissions may occur or the disease may pursue a rapidly downhill course over 2 years. The primary pulmonary type, as opposed to pulmonary involvement in the generalized disease, may often appear to arrest or, more usually, to progress rather slowly to diffuse honeycombing or emphysema and pulmonary hypertension. Survivals up to 20 years from diagnosis have been reported. In the present state of knowledge, it is probably wise to review the patient several times over a few months, with careful radiographic and functional assessment of any progression, before starting treatment [55]. The first line should probably be a course of high-dose prednisolone [56]. If this is ineffective over 3–4 months, consideration should be given to chemotherapy with chlorambucil, methotrexate, vincristine or, possibly, interferon α [44,57]. If the disease has already reached the fibrotic stage, treatment is unlikely to be of value; in suitable patients transplantation may be considered, though recurrence after this procedure has been reported [58,59]. Pneumothoraces are often recurrent and pleurodesis may be necessary.

Histiocytoma

Although the nomenclature of histiocytomas is confusing, there is a very rare benign tumour, which may be a neoplasm or possibly a granulomatous reaction, composed predominantly of histiocytes that occurs in the lung or bronchus [60,61]. The lesion may contain mast cells and spindle cells, and has also been called xanthoma or mast

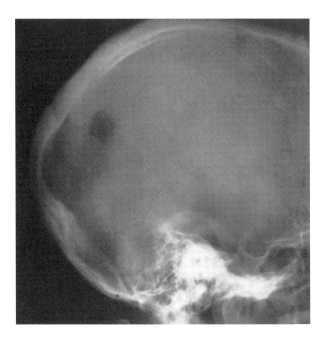

Fig. 42.6 Skull radiograph of patient with Langerhans' cell histiocytosis showing punched-out lesion in occiput.

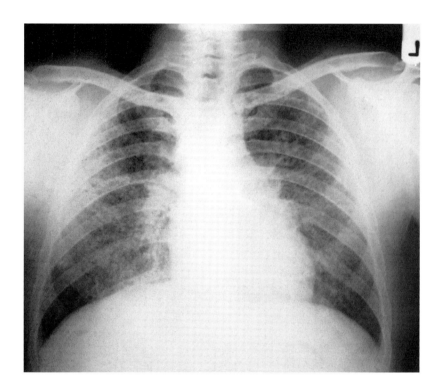

Fig. 42.7 Diffuse fine nodular and irregular infiltrates in a patient with Langerhans' cell histiocytosis.

cell granuloma. In addition, a fibrous histiocytoma has been described that usually presents as a small round lung lesion and which may occasionally metastasize [62,63]. It also is very rare and is probably analogous to the more common fibrous histiocytoma of the skin. One study of the pathology of these pulmonary tumours has distinguished benign, borderline and unequivocally malignant fibrohistiocytomas [64], and has reviewed the clinical correlates. Recurrence occurred occasionally after resection in the benign and intermediate groups as well as in the malignant. Pathological features of the malignant tumour linked to a poor prognosis included necrosis, bizarre giant cells, frequent mitoses and high cellularity. Those subjects with malignant tumours had a significant mortality. The niceties of diagnosis of these lesions and their cell of origin, if they are all indeed neoplastic, depend on electron microscopy and special histochemical techniques.

Lymphoproliferative conditions

Several conditions characterized by proliferation of lymphocytes within the lung have been described. These include lymphoid interstitial pneumonia and pseudolymphoma, lymphomatoid granulomatosis (see Chapter 40) and plasma cell granuloma. The first two appear to be monoclonal proliferations of B lymphocytes and are therefore properly classified as low-grade lymphomas [65,66]. They may be associated with paraproteinaemia [67]. Evolution to clinically progessive lymphoma occurs but usually over a long time-scale, such that malignant change

often does not become apparent in the adult. The conditions are recognized complications of Sjögren's syndrome [68], human immunodeficiency virus (HIV) infection [69,70], bone marrow transplantation [71], primary biliary cirrhosis [72] and agammaglobulinaemia [73], and occasionally occur in families [74].

Lymphoid interstitial pneumonia

This condition may cause no symptoms or may present with cough and shortness of breath. Chest films show a diffuse interstitial infiltrate, often bilateral but occasionally localized to a lobe or segment, when it may be mistaken for an infective pneumonia. The patient is often found to have paraproteinaemia. It may be associated with enlargement of the liver and peripheral lymph nodes. Histologically, the lung shows a diffuse infiltration of alveolar walls with mature lymphocytes and some plasma cells and histiocytes [75] (Fig. 42.8). The condition rarely if ever progresses to diffuse fibrosis, though evolution to malignant lymphoma [67] and lymphomatoid granulomatosis [76] has been described. It may respond to treatment with high-dose corticosteroids; if these are not successful, cyclophosphamide, chlorambucil or azathioprine may be effective [23,75]. Occasionally, as in one patient with acquired immune deficiency [69], spontaneous remission may occur; if the patient is symptom-free and without serious pulmonary impairment, a case may be made for withholding treatment and observing progress, as with other low-grade B-cell lymphomas.

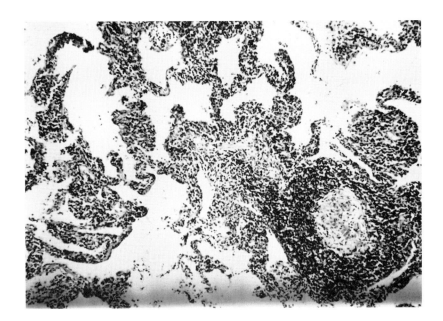

Fig. 42.8 Lung biopsy of patient with lymphoid interstitial pneumonia showing accumulation of lymphocytes in alveolar walls with follicle formation (haematoxylin & eosin ×45).

Pseudolymphoma

These tumours are probably best regarded as the early stage of lymphocytic interstitial pneumonitis, where the disease process is still confined to the bronchial mucosal lymphoid tissue. They are thus sometimes referred to as MALT or BALT tumours. They are differentiated from malignant lymphoma by the presence of infiltration of lung by mature lymphocytes, true germinal centres and the absence of local node involvement [23,77]. They may present, usually in the middle-aged, with fever, breathlessness and general malaise [78], although they may be an incidental finding on a chest radiograph as a solitary lesion, a pneumonic infiltrate or as several discrete lesions. While they appear generally benign, change to (or subsequent development of) malignant lymphoma has been described [79,80]. Surgical removal has been followed by relief of symptoms [23] and this is the most likely method of management since most are removed under suspicion of being carcinomas. Otherwise they should be managed conservatively as other B-cell lymphomas.

Plasma cell granuloma

This lesion, not to be confused with the rare primary plasmacytoma or with metastatic myelomatous deposits, is probably not a true neoplasm. It usually presents as a symptomless coin lesion on chest radiography but may cause bronchial obstruction and distal collapse or even diffuse lobar infiltration. It occurs predominantly in children and young adults and usually arises from a bronchus. Histologically it is composed of plasma cells, lymphocytes and histiocytes in a fibrous stroma [23,81]. Variations in this pattern may cause it to be confused with

other conditions, such as plasmacytoma or histiocytoma; however, plasma cell granuloma is always benign.

Tumours of epithelium

These tumours, sometimes in the past loosely and misleadingly termed pulmonary adenoma, comprise 1–2% of pulmonary neoplasms. The most common is carcinoid tumour, followed by cylindroma. The others are very uncommon indeed.

Carcinoid tumour

This is not only the most common of the tumours originally grouped as bronchial adenoma but also the least rare of the primary lung tumours presenting in childhood [82–85]. It arises usually from a main or segmental bronchus and can often be seen bronchoscopically as an intraluminal tumour, generally covered with intact epithelium. This may be associated with spread into adjacent lung, so that the tumour may be larger than at first appears. Occasionally the tumour arises in peripheral lung. It is a neoplasm of the bronchial endocrine or APUD cell (see Chapter 1) derived from the primitive gut and therefore has the potential, rarely realized in bronchial carcinoid, to secrete substances responsible for various paraneoplastic syndromes. Histologically, it is composed of sheets or aggregates of small cells with dark central nuclei and pale cytoplasm in a vascular stroma. Often a pseudoglandular pattern is seen [86] (Fig. 42.9). So-called atypical carcinoid tumours show increased mitotic activity, irregular nuclei and prominent nucleoli, and areas of tissue necrosis [87]. These may have a greater potential to metastasize and are more difficult to distinguish from oat-cell

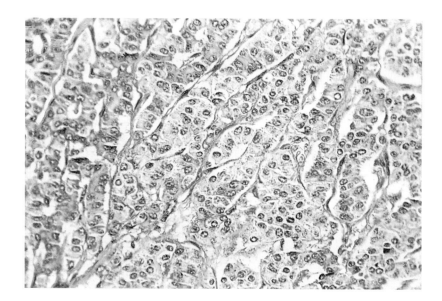

Fig. 42.9 Histology of pulmonary carcinoid tumour showing regular polygonal cells with small round nuclei, forming regular trabeculae (haematoxylin & eosin ×300).

carcinoma. Occasionally, amyloid material [88] or bone [82] may be laid down in the stroma of carcinoid tumours. When histological diagnosis is difficult, special stains may demonstrate the various neuropeptides [85] and electron microscopy may be helpful, showing the neurosecretory material as dense rounded granules (Fig. 42.10).

Clinical features

Carcinoid tumours, being predominantly slow-growing intrabronchial lesions, usually present with haemoptysis or symptoms due to bronchial obstruction [89,90]. They occur equally in either sex, usually at a younger age than bronchogenic carcinoma; the median age is between 40 and 50. About half of patients present with episodes of recurrent infection in the same lobe, one-third with haemoptysis, and small proportions with chest pain, cough, wheeze or shortness of breath [82]. The tumour may also be found on routine chest radiography in a symptom-free individual, especially if it is a peripheral one.

Important clinical features may be recurrent pneumonia, sometimes over several years [91], unilateral monophonic wheeze and signs of obstructive emphysema (see Chapter 6) [92]. These signs, which may be as subtle as slight reduction in movements and breath sounds over the affected lobe associated with a normal percussion note, are particularly important for detecting central tumours where the radiograph may not show an obvious abnormality.

Most patients have an abnormal radiograph at presentation [82], usually showing segmental or lobar collapse or consolidation. Discrete tumour may be seen in about one-quarter of cases and, especially in patients presenting with wheeze, the only abnormality may occasionally be lobar hyperinflation related to obstructive emphysema [92]; if

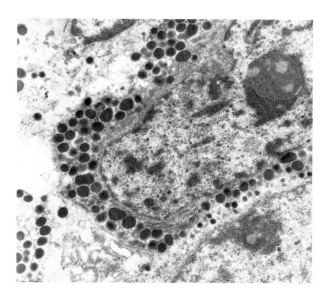

Fig. 42.10 Electron micrograph of carcinoid cell showing dense rounded granules of neurosecretory material (lead citrate and uranyl acetate ×4860).

this is suspected, it may be confirmed by taking a film on expiration. All three features may be mimicked by bronchial carcinoma or other endobronchial lesions and inhaled foreign bodies, so diagnosis requires biopsy. This would normally be carried out at fibreoptic bronchoscopy, although caution should be used in interpretation of any such biopsies as there is much scope for confusion with oat-cell carcinoma when only small pieces of tissue are available to the pathologist. If the suspicion of carcinoid is raised, it is probably wise to obtain a larger biopsy via the rigid bronchoscope, since surgical treatment may well differ depending on which of these two neoplasms is present.

Very rarely, carcinoid may present with diffuse multicentric endobronchial lesions [88] or as multiple periph-eral tumours [93], often associated with bronchiectasis and scarring. These latter lesions have been called tumourlets [94].

All forms of carcinoid have the potential to metastasize, though this probably occurs in fewer than 10% of treated cases. Metastasis may occur to local nodes, to liver and to bone particularly; in bone the lesions tend to be osteoblas-tic. Metastases may present clinically many years after surgical removal of the primary tumour, although when they do so the patient may still survive several years, with or without treatment.

The carcinoid syndrome, characterized by attacks of intense flushing, tachycardia, occasionally wheeze, and hypotension, occurs in approximately 1% of patients with bronchial carcinoid [95,96]. Other features may be abdominal cramps and profuse watery diarrhoea, oedema of the face and arms, symptoms of pellagra and stenotic or regurgitant lesions of the pulmonary and tricuspid valves [97]. Pulmonary carcinoid has been reported to cause mitral valve disease on one occasion [98]. This syndrome seems to be related in part to the carcinoid cell's role in tryptophan metabolism, the amino acid being converted to 5-hydroxytryptophan and then decarboxylated to 5-hydroxytryptamine (serotonin). Release of this substance into the blood may be a cause of the wheeze and diar-rhoea, while competition by the tumour for tryptophan may be responsible for the symptoms of pellagra. Subse-quent conversion of serotonin to 5-hydroxyindoleacetic acid occurs in the liver; this substance is then excreted in urine where it provides the basis of a useful test for diag-nosis of the syndrome. The flush does not seem to be related to serotonin but may be provoked by alcohol, excitement or intravenous norepinephrine (noradrena-line), and may be due to secretion of kinins or vasoactive peptides by the tumour [99]. These substances may also be responsible for fibrous damage to the heart valves, though how this occurs is not clear.

Carcinoid tumour of the lung has also been reported to be associated with Cushing's syndrome [96], acromegaly [100], pluriglandular adenomatosis [101] and hypercal-caemia [102]. These rare occurrences are presumably related to the potential of the APUD cell to secrete hor-mones or hormone precursors.

Treatment and prognosis

Carcinoid tumours should be removed surgically [82,83]. At operation it is unusual to find metastases in nodes, although the nodes may be enlarged due to associated infection and frozen section may be advisable. If the tumour is confined to a bronchus, it may be possible to remove it by sleeve resection; otherwise lobectomy or pneumonectomy may be necessary. In general, surgery should be as conservative as possible. After successful

resection, the prognosis is very good, with a better than 90% 10-year survival rate. If endocrine symptoms are present, these are relieved by successful tumour resection. However, metastasis may present even as late as 16 years after resection.

Liver metastases may be treated, and the attendant symptoms palliated, by selective hepatic arterial embolization [82,103]. If symptoms of the carcinoid syn-drome are associated with an irresectable or metastasized tumour, which is very rarely the case with lung tumours, control of diarrhoea, flushing and wheeze may be obtained with serotonin antagonists (methysergide or cyproheptadine) and α-adrenergic blocking drugs. Valvu-lar heart lesions may require surgical treatment, while pel-lagra may be treated with supplemental nicotinamide. Since the prognosis of carcinoid tumour is relatively pro-longed, even when associated with such symptoms and metastases, control of symptoms with this treatment may be an important part of the patient's management.

Cylindroma (adenoid cystic carcinoma)

This tumour represents only about 15% of so-called bronchial adenomas [104], although it is probably the most common primary malignant tumour of the trachea [105]. Histologically, it originates from bronchial glands and is composed of small round cells with dark nuclei arranged in a cribriform manner, with larger paler cells forming clumps and pseudoacini [96] (Fig. 42.11). The bronchial mucosa usually remains intact.

Clinical features

Cylindromas may occur at any age and cause haemoptysis and symptoms of bronchial obstruction [96,106]. They should be suspected particularly if a young or middle-aged adult presents with increasing stridor of a few weeks' or months' duration. Radiology of the chest may show a hilar tumour or distal collapse or consolidation; if the tumour arises in the trachea, the film is usually normal. Diagnosis is made by bronchial biopsy, and bronchogra-phy may be used to delineate the extent of a central tumour. The tumour may rarely metastasize to nodes and liver, but more commonly invades local structures widely.

Treatment and prognosis

Ideally, treatment is by excision, although owing to the usually central situation of the tumour this may not be fea-sible. In some centres, tracheal reconstruction procedures have allowed complete removal [107]. If resection proves impossible, radiotherapy often produces prolonged remission and relief of symptoms where tracheal obstruc-tion is threatening life [108]. The use of laser therapy holds promise of controlling the obstruction if resection is

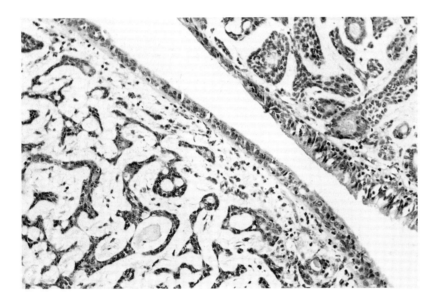

Fig. 42.11 Resected bronchial tumour showing bronchial lumen compressed from both sides by infiltrating submucosal adenoid cystic carcinoma (haematoxylin & eosin × 150).

impossible. The tumour grows slowly, but nevertheless has a considerably worse prognosis than carcinoid [109,110].

Mucoepidermoid tumour

These salivary gland-type tumours are even less common than cylindromas, which they resemble in clinical features [106,111–113]. They may occur at any age, and like all slow-growing intrabronchial tumours may initially be misdiagnosed as asthma [114]. Pathologically they may be divided into high-grade and low-grade types, the former having a greater propensity to metastasize and invade locally. They arise from glandular structures, usually in trachea and major bronchi, and histologically consist of squamous elements and mucus-secreting acini. A papillary variant has been described [115]. Treatment is by surgical resection if possible [113,116].

Bronchial melanoma

Malignant melanomas may metastasize to bronchi but more commonly to lung parenchyma. Very rarely, primary melanoma arises in bronchi where it is usually clinically indistinguishable from bronchial carcinoma [117], although pigmentation may be seen bronchoscopically or on sputum cytology [118]. The prognosis is poor, metastasis occurring to local nodes and by haematogenous dissemination; nevertheless, long-term survival has been reported following pneumonectomy [119]. The origin of the tumour is presumed to be from neuroectodermal melanoblasts that have migrated to the bronchial mucosa during embryonic development, since melanocytes are not a normal feature of the respiratory epithelium.

Bronchial papilloma

Papillomas are quite frequently seen on the larynx, but are rare tumours of trachea and bronchi. They may occur as solitary lesions [120,121] or as multiple tracheobronchial papillomatosis [122]. The latter seem to occur predominantly in middle-aged men. All papillomas should be regarded as having the potential to undergo malignant change to squamous carcinoma [123] and should be excised. Histologically they resemble papillomas elsewhere, with a vascular stroma surrounded by stratified keratinizing squamous epithelium. They are not to be confused with inflammatory polyps that may sometimes be seen in bronchiectasis or asthma [124].

Clear-cell tumour

This benign tumour is composed of sheets of cells with small nuclei and foamy or clear cytoplasm [125,126]. It usually appears as a small peripheral nodule on chest radiography. The cell of origin is not known and it has not been described as undergoing malignant change. It is not to be confused with metastatic renal carcinoma or with the clear-cell subdivision of large-cell anaplastic bronchial carcinoma.

True bronchial adenoma

Benign adenomas, which may occur at any age, may arise from several different cells in bronchial glands [127]. All are exceedingly rare. Mucous gland [128], serous [129], pleomorphic (derived from myoepithelial cells) [130], oncocytic (from a cell in the region of the collecting ducts) [131] and mixed cell types have been described. Diagnosis is normally made after excision, which would be expected to be curative.

Sclerosing pneumocytoma (sclerosing haemangioma)

This peripheral tumour occurs predominantly in women and may present at any age. It is usually small, subpleural and polypoid and may be associated with cough, haemoptysis or no symptoms [132,133]. It seems more common in Chinese women, and electron microscope studies have suggested that it is not a tumour of endothelial cells but of type II pneumocytes [134]. Malignant change has not been described.

Tumours of vascular tissue

A group of rare tumours originate in vascular tissue, including capillary haemangioma and haemangiomatosis [135], haemangiopericytoma, intravascular bronchioloalveolar tumour and angiosarcoma. Sclerosing haemangioma seems to be derived from type II epithelial cells in a number of cases (see above), although variants have been thought to be of endothelial origin [134]. Two non-neoplastic vascular anomalies, arteriovenous malformation and pulmonary telangiectasia, are discussed here for convenience, as are tumours arising from lymphatic tissue.

Haemangiopericytoma

This tumour arises from capillary pericytes, pluripotential cells associated with the vascular basement membrane [136]. It presents as a peripheral radiographic shadow, which may be very large and involve a whole lobe. Growth rate is very variable and it may both metastasize widely and invade locally. However, removal of a small or early lesion may be curative; if this is not possible, radiotherapy may be effective. Similar tumours may occur in other organs of the body.

Intravascular bronchioloalveolar tumour

This is a multicentric lung tumour that arises in either vascular pericytes or endothelial cells and which is more common in women [137,138]. It may occur at any age, half the reported tumours having presented before the age of 40. It is usually found incidentally on chest radiography, when it appears as multiple small nodules, but may present in a form that mimics pulmonary embolic disease with pulmonary hypertension [139]. Excision of these tumours shows collections of vesicular cells with nodules of eosinophilic hyaline material. The cells protrude into alveoli and bronchioles and invade arteries and veins. There is often central necrosis. Metastasis occurs occasion-

ally, but the course of the disease is usually characterized by slow extension of the tumour throughout the lungs until the patient dies in respiratory failure. No treatment has so far been shown to induce remission, although transplantation would presumably be an option.

Angiosarcoma (Kaposi's sarcoma)

This malignant tumour is derived from vascular endothelium [140]. Its cells secrete multiple cytokines that probably sustain the tumour's growth. It was very rarely recognized in the lung prior to the arrival of AIDS in the USA but now appears commonly in subjects with sexually acquired disease; however, it is still rare in those in whom AIDS was acquired through blood transfusion or intravenous drug abuse, suggesting that another infection together with immunosuppression is necessary for its pathogenesis. Recently a new herpes virus has been found in a proportion of these tumours [141]. Previously it was more familiar as a rather indolent skin tumour in Africans [142] or occasionally as a more aggressive disseminated disease [143]. Now, however, its most frequent presentation is in people suffering from AIDS [144], in one series being present in the skin at death in 59% of patients and in the lungs in 36% [145]. The tumour presents with diffuse nodular and patchy infiltrates throughout both lungs [146,147] (Fig. 42.12); the patient has often been unwell for some time previously and may have generalized lymphadenopathy. The radiograph shows gradually increasing diffuse nodular infiltrates that have a tendency to coalesce and become more profuse over several months, although the disease may be present with a normal radiograph [148,149]. Pleural involvement with effusion may occur. The diagnosis may be made by transbronchial [150] or open lung [144] biopsy, though until there is reasonably effective treatment for the tumour the latter procedure is rarely justified. However, there is therapeutic justification for the use of bronchoscopy for differentiating Kaposi's sarcoma from other diffuse infiltrative conditions that afflict AIDS sufferers, and future treatment possibilities, such as the use of combination chemotherapy, interferon α or liposomal agents [151–153], may make aggressive diagnostic procedures more worth while (see Chapter 52).

The pathological appearances are of multiple discrete haemorrhagic nodules throughout the lung parenchyma. Bronchi and vessels may be invaded. Histological appearances vary from thin fibrous septa with malignant epithelium in a lake of blood to solid sheets of spindle cells with inconspicuous vascular spaces [146] (Fig. 42.13).

Many combinations of antiviral and chemotherapeutic agents have been tried and temporary remission may be obtained [152,153]; the use of liposomal drug preparations to deliver adequate doses with minimal side-effects seems a promising approach. However, no regimen has been shown to be sufficiently effective and free of toxicity to

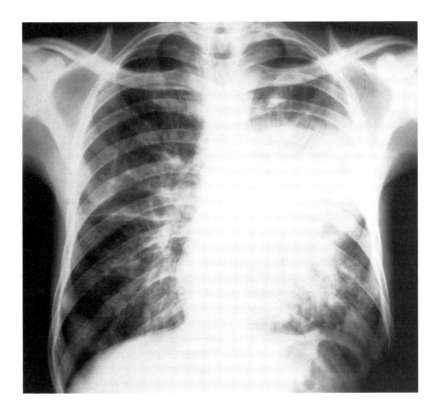

Fig. 42.12 Radiograph of African patient with AIDS and extensive pulmonary infiltration by Kaposi's sarcoma. (Courtesy of Dr Dwight McLeod.)

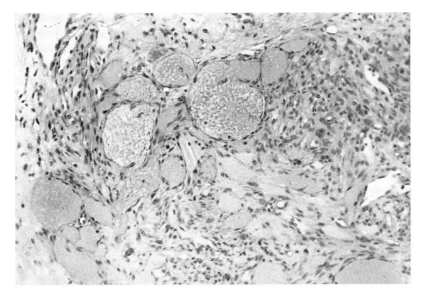

Fig. 42.13 Histological appearance of Kaposi's sarcoma showing ectatic vascular channels admixed with malignant spindle cells, infiltrating connective tissue stroma (haematoxylin & eosin ×150).

become established treatment, and usually the patient passes from having no respiratory symptoms to death from respiratory failure over the course of a few months.

Lymphangioleiomyoma

This is a condition affecting women [154–156], almost always of child-bearing age, though occasional cases have been described after the menopause [157]. The patient often presents initially with haemoptysis, pneumothorax and a chylous pleural effusion. Initially the chest radio-graph may be normal, but subsequently there is often a fine reticulonodular shadowing, sometimes associated with septal lines. The changes are more marked at the bases and are seldom profuse. In addition, or sometimes alternatively, there is evidence of overinflation or frank emphysema and this combination in a premenopausal woman should always raise the possibility of lymphangi-oleiomyomatosis. The patient may often have other mani-festations of systemic disease, such as lymphoedema and leiomyomas of kidney or uterus.

Unlike many conditions where the radiograph shows a

fine infiltrate, lung function testing usually shows an obstructive pattern and hyperinflation. Sometimes there may be a considerably higher thoracic gas volume (measured by plethysmography) than total lung capacity (measured by helium dilution); this probably represents air trapped in cysts by peribronchiolar muscle hypertrophy.

It is easy to miss the diagnosis of lymphangioleiomyomatosis because of the way it mimics emphysema. Chylous effusion and recurrent pneumothorax are clues, as is irreversible airways obstruction in a non-smoking woman. Lung biopsy shows the characteristic histology [158,159]; the lungs show diffuse cystic change with apparent intervening fibrosis. Microscopically, there is proliferation of spindle-shaped primitive smooth muscle cells around lymphatics throughout the lungs and pleura (Fig. 42.14). The airways obstruction is probably related to smooth muscle proliferation around bronchioles, leading to air trapping and cyst formation. Rupture of these cysts causes pneumothorax, while haemoptysis is probably explained by capillary congestion due to perivenular muscle hypertrophy.

The course of the disease is one of progressive increase in dyspnoea over about 10 years, culminating in death from respiratory failure. In postmenopausal women it may be more slowly progressive, suggesting that it is hormone-dependent [157]; indeed progesterone and oestrogen receptors have been demonstrated on lung biopsy material [160]. The condition may deteriorate in response to oral contraceptives, and remit or progress less rapidly after oophorectomy [161] or treatment with progesterone [162]. Because of this hormone dependence, it has been suggested that the use of oral contraceptives may be an aetiological factor, although a case–control study has not supported this hypothesis [163]. If the diagnosis is

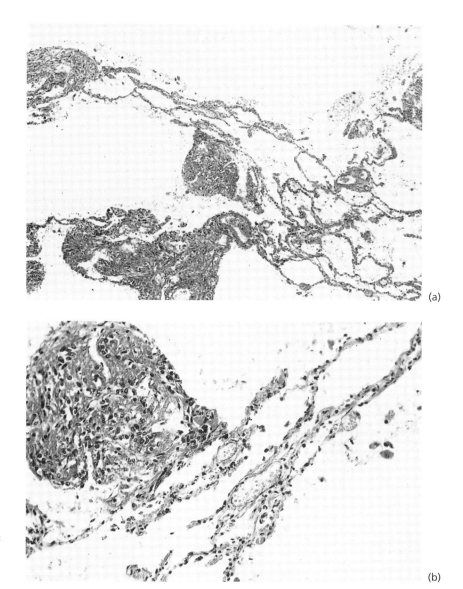

(a)

(b)

Fig. 42.14 Necropsy specimen from lung of a woman who died apparently of emphysema but who proved to have lymphangioleiomyoma. (a) Dilated airspaces with proliferating smooth muscle in remaining alveolar walls (haematoxylin & eosin ×50). (b) A higher-power view showing the proliferating smooth muscle cells (haematoxylin & eosin ×150).

made in life, progesterone or oophorectomy would be appropriate treatment, especially if instituted at an early stage of the condition, and lung transplantation would now be an option.

Tuberous sclerosis

This inherited disorder usually presents with mental retardation or slowly progressive dementia, associated with epilepsy and skin changes comprising patchy depigmentation, warty elevations on the face (adenoma sebaceum) and patches of elevated rough yellowish skin on the back (shagreen patch) [164]. It affects males and females equally. It may be associated with a nodular infiltrate on chest radiography that leads to cystic change. Pathologically the lesions are multiple leiomyomas, though probably based on blood vessels rather than lymphatics. Similar smooth muscle tumours are found in other organs. Sometimes the tumours are described as being angiomyolipomas, and this lesion has also been described in the lung in the absence of other evidence of tuberous sclerosis [165]. The pulmonary condition may be complicated by recurrent pneumothorax [166] or by pleural effusion [167]. The pathological condition overlaps with that of lymphangioleiomyomatosis and airflow obstruction with reduced diffusing capacity are physiological features also [168]. In view of this, hormonal treatment has been tried in female patients with some limited evidence of response.

Arteriovenous malformations and telangiectasia
(see also Chapter 50)

These lesions represent a developmental anomaly rather than a tumour and consist of abnormal connections between pulmonary artery and vein, probably due to persistence of the short fetal capillary anastomoses. Pathologically they appear as a thin-walled labyrinth of vessels connecting a rather dilated artery and vein [169,170]. Occasionally they may be supplied by more than one artery and there may be associated anomalies of pulmonary venous drainage.

Clinical features

Patients with this condition may present with one or several rounded radiological opacities [171]. In some cases there may be a fine diffuse nodularity of the lower zones, when the condition is known as pulmonary telangiectasia [172,173]. Discrete lesions, which may be single or multiple, are not necessarily associated with symptoms or signs [174]; the presence of these depends on the size of the shunt. If it is large, finger clubbing and cyanosis may be apparent and a systolic bruit, sometimes accentuated by inspiration, may be heard over the lesion [175]. In up to

half of all cases, evidence of hereditary telangiectasia (Osler–Weber–Rendu disease) elsewhere may be present [176], the patient having had nose or gastrointestinal bleeds and showing small telangiectases on tongue, face and lips (see Fig. 50.14). In pulmonary telangiectasia, the patient presents with cyanosis, finger clubbing and increasing breathlessness [172]. Faints or fits due to cerebral hypoxaemia may occur.

The discrete type of arteriovenous malformation may present at almost any age but is most frequent in the third decade and after. Telangiectasia is more frequently seen in young children, since it always causes cyanosis and symptoms, although the diagnosis may not be made until adult life. The radiological appearances of the discrete lesions are of rounded or lobulated shadows, usually in lower zones. The feeding and draining vessels may be apparent on the radiograph; if not, they can usually be demonstrated by tomography (Fig. 42.15). They gradually increase in size over several years. The diagnosis should be confirmed by pulmonary angiography, especially if removal is planned, as smaller lesions not seen on chest radiography may then become apparent [171]. Pulmonary hypertension is not normally present, because of low vascular resistance, but has been described [177]. In pulmonary telangiectasia the chest radiograph shows a diffuse lower zone nodularity that may be easily mistaken for pulmonary fibrosis (Fig. 42.16). The associated marked cyanosis and relative lack of breathlessness (relative to that of a patient with cyanosis at rest with pulmonary fibrosis) should alert the physician to the correct diagnosis. The nodular shadows may be quite small but tend to increase in size as time goes by. Pulmonary angiography demonstrates the lesions if they are large enough, although minute ones may not be seen.

The only physiological abnormality in patients with the discrete lesions may be slight hypoxaemia and failure of the arterial blood fully to saturate on breathing oxygen. With multiple lesions, a low carbon monoxide diffusing capacity is usual, due to diversion of blood from the pulmonary capillary bed. Paradoxically, in diffuse telangiectasia, breathing of 100% oxygen may lead to full saturation because oxygen is able to diffuse into the small abnormal vessels sufficiently rapidly [172]. On catheterization, dye curves do not show the two peaks of an intracardiac shunt but a decreased transit time with rapid reappearance of dye. Radiolabelled macroaggregates of albumin may be used to confirm the diagnosis in telangiectasia [173,178].

Management and prognosis

The solitary lesion should generally be removed [179,180], since the shunt increases progressively and complications such as brain abscess or bacterial infection of the angioma itself may occur. Before removal, angiography should be carried out to look for additional smaller lesions. Even if

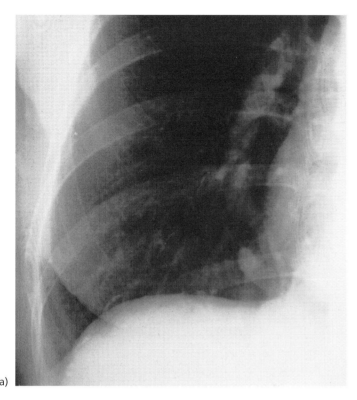

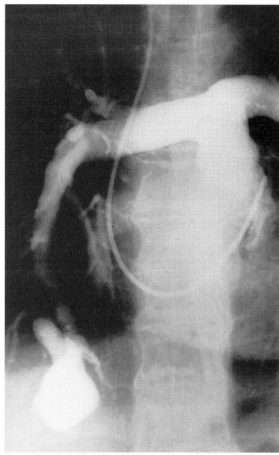

Fig. 42.15 (a) Penetrated film showing arteriovenous malformation in right lower lobe, in cardiophrenic angle. (b) Pulmonary arteriogram of the same patient.

these are undetected, there is a risk that other shunts may gradually become apparent after the operation and these in turn may need removal [172]. For this reason, surgery should if possible avoid resection of lung. If the lesions are multiple, as is the case in about 20% of patients, it may not be practicable to remove them and in such patients embolization with detachable balloons or coils passed through a catheter is now the treatment of choice (see Chapter 50) [172]. In the absence of such treatment these patients become progressively more cyanosed and breathless, eventually dying of the effects of hypoxaemia and high-output cardiac failure. Transplantation may be necessary in patients with telangiectasia [181]. While most such patients do not survive their fourth decade, the author has made the diagnosis for the first time in a patient of 58 whose symptoms dated back to childhood [182].

Pulmonary capillary haemangiomatosis

This is an exceedingly rare locally invasive tumour pre-senting with progressive pulmonary hypertension, characterized pathologically by proliferation of thin-walled capillaries throughout the lungs [183]. It is progressive and fatal unless transplantation can be carried out.

Pulmonary lymphangiectasis

Primary cystic dilatation of pulmonary lymphatics may occur in children, either as part of a generalized disease of lymphatics or as a lesion confined to the lungs [184,185]. It may occur throughout the lungs, presenting as multiple cystic shadows on chest radiography, or be localized to one or several lobes. In this latter case, it may present as a hilar or intrapulmonary solid shadow or may mimic bronchiectasis. After surgical removal it can be seen to consist of dilated very thin-walled cysts filled with lymph. The cysts are adjacent to bronchi, veins, pleura and in interlobar septa and represent grossly dilated lymphatics. The cause of this congenital abnormality is not known.

Pulmonary lymphangiomatosis

This condition, analogous to capillary haemangiomatosis but characterized by overgrowth of anastomosing lymphatic vessels throughout the lungs, presents with breath-

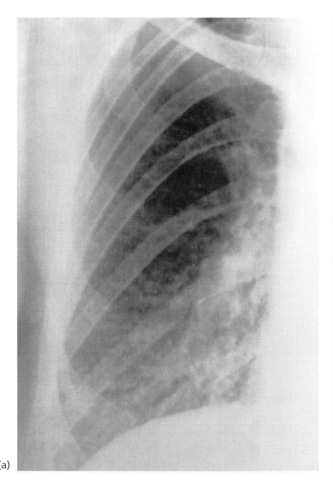
(a)

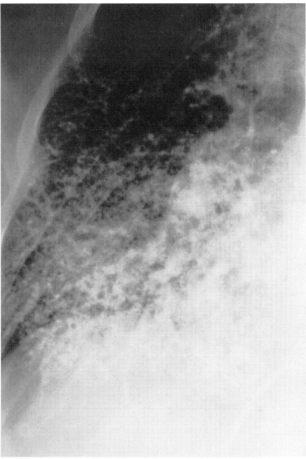
(b)

Fig. 42.16 (a) Chest film of right lower zone of cyanosed 58-year-old woman showing diffuse lower zone nodularity. (b) Angiogram of the same patient showing multiple minute arteriovenous malformations.

lessness in childhood, obstructive lung function, radiographic infiltrates and pleural effusions [186]. It runs a progressive course.

Tumours of muscle and connective tissue

Leiomyoma and leiomyosarcoma

The very rare leiomyoma originates in airway smooth muscle [187,188]. It may present as a peripheral tumour, when it has no specific features, or as a central bronchial or tracheal lesion, often polypoid or pedunculated. It tends to occur in children and young adults. Occasionally it has been removed by endoscopy [189], although surgical sleeve or wedge resection is to be preferred. Pathologically it consists of interlacing whorled smooth muscle cells and fibroblasts. On biopsy it may be difficult to distinguish from leiomyosarcoma, which is characterized by more mitotic figures and whose prognosis is related to the number of these [190]. Leiomyosarcomas present similarly

to benign leiomyomas, as incidental radiological findings when peripheral or with symptoms and signs of bronchial block when central. They may be removed surgically; in general, the larger they are at presentation, the worse the prognosis [190], although long-term cure has been reported in about 50% of cases after radical resection [187]. They appear not to be radiosensitive. Metastases occur and the prognosis is usually poor if the tumour cannot be resected. In assessing patients for surgery, care should be taken that the pulmonary tumour is not one of several metastases from a primary uterine sarcoma. Both leiomyoma and leiomyosarcoma have been reported in the trachea, presenting with signs of respiratory obstruction. They may be misdiagnosed as asthma. Resection with end-to-end tracheal anastomosis or with tracheal reconstruction with myocutaneous flaps has been associated with reported cures [191,192].

Rhabdomyosarcoma

This rare tumour has been reported in bronchi, trachea and peripheral lung [193–195]. Its apparent striated muscle origin is presumably from either primitive pluripotential mesenchymal cells or displaced teratomatous muscle cells. It presents no specific clinical features and should be removed by radical resection where possible.

Fibroma and fibrosarcoma

Benign fibroma of bronchus or lung is also an exceedingly rare tumour with no special clinical features [190,196]. Pleural fibroma, which is a benign mesothelioma, is discussed in Chapter 43. Fibrosarcoma has also been described, arising in bronchus, lung or pulmonary artery [197]. It may be difficult to distinguish pathologically from leiomyosarcoma.

Lipoma and liposarcoma

Lipomas are very rare tumours that may occur in trachea or bronchi [198,199]. They may be pedunculated and produce obstruction or arise deep in the bronchial wall and present as radiological shadows. They consist of mature lipocytes surrounded by fibrous trabeculae. Liposarcoma is a highly malignant tumour, usually derived from soft tissues, and has been reported in the mediastinum [200], pericardium [201] and trachea [199] but not so far in bronchus. It commonly metastasizes to the lung from elsewhere. It may consist of a mixture of well-differentiated fat cells and poorly differentiated lipoblasts in a myxoid stroma, or of anaplastic bizarre giant cells with some lipoblastic differentiation. It invades locally and spreads by metastasis.

Other connective tissue tumours

Other tumours have been described occasionally in the literature. These include benign chondromas [202], which may be confused with chondromatous hamartomas, chondrosarcomas [203] and myxoma [204]. Fibroma and myxoma may calcify.

Carney's triad is the name given to the coincidence of pulmonary fibromas, leiomyosarcoma of stomach and functioning paraganglionoma [205,206]. The lung lesions are benign, and may be single or multiple. If one is unaware of the syndrome, as is probably the case with most doctors, the lung lesions may be mistaken for metastases from the stomach. If the lung and stomach tumours are found, tests should be carried out for the third component, which may cause problems during anaesthesia. Removal of the stomach tumour, sometimes together with metastases, has been attended by prolonged remission so a radical surgical approach seems justified [207]. Patients have been described in whom only two of the three components of the triad have been found, and one patient where the sarcoma was in the duodenum [208]. The syndrome appears to occur predominantly in young females.

Tumours of neural tissue

Neural tumours may be classified as neurilemmoma (arising from the Schwann cell), neurofibroma (from the nerve sheath), ganglioneuroma (from the neurone) and their malignant counterparts neurosarcoma and neuroblastoma. Mixed forms occur and tumours may show transitional features between benign and malignant types; histopathological diagnosis may therefore be difficult. In addition, tumours may arise in paraganglion cells, i.e. phaeochromocytoma and chemodectoma.

Neurilemmoma, neurofibroma and neurosarcoma are exceedingly rare tumours in the trachea and bronchi [209,210], though they are the commonest tumours of the posterior mediastinum (see Chapter 49). Neurofibroma may be seen as part of von Recklinghausen's syndrome of multiple neurofibromatosis. Chemodectomas or paragangliomas occur in the posterior mediastinum and may be responsible for causing hypertension [211]. They have been described occasionally as occurring within the lung in association with the pulmonary artery [212]. Multiple minute (0.2 cm) tumours, similar on light microscopy to chemodectomas, have been seen within the lung as an incidental finding at postmortem, although their significance and histogenesis is unclear [213].

Tumours of mixed-cell origin

Teratoma

Intrathoracic teratomas are usually seen in the mediastinum (see Chapter 49). They are tumours derived from the three primitive germ layers and may contain a variety of tissues, including hair, skin, bone, muscle and teeth. Glandular tissue may actively secrete hormones. The benign type is often called a dermoid cyst. Malignant change occurs in up to 20% of teratomas, when one or more cell lines show poor differentiation and pleomorphism. Often trophoblastic tissue is predominant, the tumour taking on the characteristics of a choriocarcinoma.

Both benign and malignant teratomas have been described in the lung and, very occasionally, in the bronchus [214,215]. Their clinical characteristics are those of any slow-growing pulmonary tumour [216], with the additional possibilities of complications such as necrosis due to pancreatic hormone secretion or expectoration of components such as hair. Because of their potential for malignant change, and also because diagnosis is rarely made before excision, treatment is surgical removal. Malignant tumours in the mediastinum have also shown good response to chemotherapy in combination with surgery [217].

Hamartoma

Hamartoma has usually been regarded as a developmental anomaly [218–221]; however, recent genetic analysis of a series of such lesions has shown an abnormal karyotype, suggesting that they are neoplastic [222]. It is a lesion in which the normal components of the organ are combined in a disorganized manner. Pathologically, pulmonary hamartomas are usually small 1–3 cm lesions containing predominantly cartilage, with epithelium, fibrous tissue and fat. Calcification occurs frequently and on radiography they appear as well-demarcated, dense, round peripheral shadows often with a central dot of calcium (Fig. 42.17). Though usually single, multiple hamartomas may occur and give rise to diagnostic difficulties [223]. Multiple lesions may also be a feature of tuberous sclerosis and have been described in the trachea as an incidental finding at autopsy [224]. Cystic appearances may be due to deposits of fat within the lesion [225], and multiple cavitating tumours have been described that mimic metastases [226]. They may grow slowly and very occasionally reach a large size. They occur predominantly in the fourth decade, although they may be seen at any age, and are more common in males than females [219,227].

Less commonly, the predominant tissue in a hamartoma is smooth muscle [225,228,229]. These fibroleiomyomatous hamartomas may occur as a diffuse pulmonary infiltrate, giving the appearance of honeycomb lung, or as a localized lesion; the latter usually presents radiologically as an ill-defined subpleural shadow. The tumour may be intrabronchial, giving rise to collapse or distal infection. In contrast to the chondromatous type, fibroleiomyomatous hamartomas are more common in women [220].

If a hamartoma is diagnosed with confidence, on the basis of its presence on old radiographs, slow growth and central calcification, the patient may be spared surgery since malignant change has been described only rarely [230]. Indeed there is some doubt that it ever occurs in true hamartomas [1]. More usually, however, there is sufficient clinical doubt for surgery to be justified; the tumour has a characteristic hard feel and can often be removed without resection of lung tissue. The finding of a fibromatous hamartoma should bring to mind the possibility of Carney's triad; in one series of 65 resections this was found in two, while in eight an associated carcinoma was found [231].

Carcinosarcoma and blastoma

These tumours contain malignant cells derived from both epithelial and connective tissue [232,233]. Their histogenesis is obscure. Blastomas are regarded as tumours that contain cells of fetal type, whereas carcinosarcomas are derived from adult cells. In children the tumour is regarded as highly malignant but responsive, at least in the short term, to combination chemotherapy [234,235]. Their histological features are of interest to pathologists

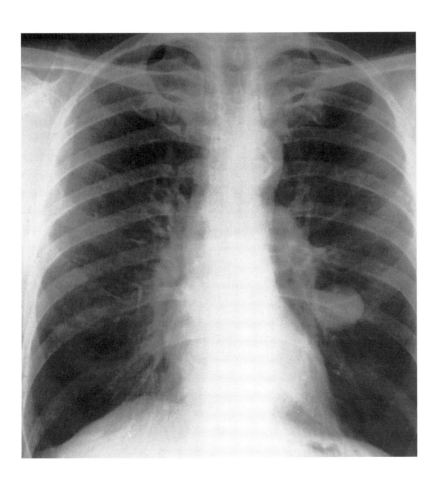

Fig. 42.17 Typical smoothly outlined, dense, spherical appearance of hamartoma.

[236], while from a clinical point of view they behave like other bronchial carcinomas; metastasis occurs and may be of single or both cell types. Treatment is by surgery if possible, usually combined with chemotherapy.

Metastatic tumours in the lung

Any malignant tumour, including bronchial carcinoma, may metastasize to the lung. Clinically, it is helpful to recognize several different patterns of metastasis, as this may be of assistance in differential diagnosis or planning treatment. These patterns include solitary metastasis, multiple cannonball lesions, diffuse nodular infiltration, lymphangitic carcinomatosis, endobronchial metastasis and carcinomatous embolization. Metastasis to hilar nodes bilaterally may also be seen.

Solitary metastasis

This lesion presents as a peripheral tumour, usually spherical and well demarcated from surrounding lung [237]. It may cavitate and clinical differentiation from primary tumour is difficult, especially as it may be the presenting feature of an occult neoplasm elsewhere. The most common sites of origin of the tumour are large bowel, breast, cervix, kidney and sarcomas. In the absence of metastases elsewhere, and if the primary tumour is resectable, there may be a case for surgical removal [237,238], although it is never certain whether reported long-term survival following this procedure owes more to the surgery or the biological nature of the tumour. Other tumours may respond to radiotherapy or chemotherapy.

Multiple cannonball tumours

Multiple spherical lesions of many different sizes are characteristic of metastatic deposits (Fig. 42.18), though similar appearances may occur occasionally in sarcoidosis, tuberculosis, hydatid and fungal disease, multiple hamartomas and Wegener's granulomatosis. Cannonball metastases originate particularly from hypernephroma, seminoma, sarcoma, colon carcinoma, choriocarcinoma and breast carcinoma. Cavitation, calcification or haemorrhage may occasionally occur in these metastases; when necrosis occurs in them adjacent to pleura, they may cause pneumothorax. It is not normally necessary to take further diagnostic steps, since the primary tumour is usually clinically evident. If it is not, care should be taken to exclude seminoma, and prostatic and breast carcinoma, which may respond to appropriate combinations of chemotherapy, hormone treatment and radiotherapy. In patients where there is no obvious primary tumour, biopsy of a lesion is justified in order to exclude rare granulomatous and infective causes.

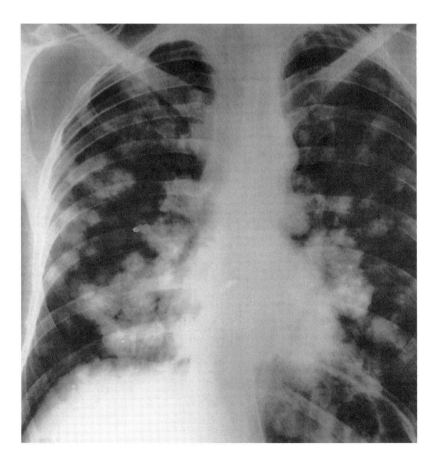

Fig. 42.18 Multiple cannonball metastases from oesophageal carcinoma. Note the oesophageal tube.

Diffuse nodular infiltration

Multiple small nodules, usually less than 5 mm in size but varying from pin-point size upwards (Fig. 42.19), occasionally occur as a manifestation of metastatic spread, particularly from breast, stomach, thyroid and colonic carcinomas. A similar appearance may occur in diffuse alveolar cell or pulmonary adenocarcinoma. The patient may present with shortness of breath, although this is initially not so severe as with lymphangitic spread. Again, it is desirable to exclude those primary sites that may be responsive to chemotherapy or hormone treatment. Spontaneous regression after removal of the primary tumour or temporary regression after corticosteroid treatment may occur very occasionally.

Lymphangitic carcinomatosis

Lymphangitic spread of carcinoma occurs particularly from breast, stomach, pancreas and prostate, as well as from bronchial carcinoma itself. The patient presents with increasingly severe dyspnoea, cough and evidence of general ill-health. Auscultation of the lungs may be normal or show repetitive inspiratory crackles. The radiograph shows multiple small nodular and linear shadows and Kerley's lines, particularly in the lower zones (Fig. 42.20). The course is usually rapidly downhill, though

remission has been described with chemosensitive or hormone-dependent tumours [239]. Partial relief of symptoms may occur on treatment with corticosteroids, diazepam or opiates.

Endobronchial metastases

Endobronchial metastasis is much less common than the patterns described above. It occurs particularly in breast, kidney, colon and cervical cancer [240]. In its mode of presentation it mimics primary bronchial carcinoma [241,242] and most cases described in the literature are of patients subjected to lobectomy or pneumonectomy on this account. The finding of clear-cell tumour on bronchial biopsy or cytology should always arouse suspicion of a renal primary. Indeed, endobronchial renal metastases may be expectorated by the patient [242]. The prognosis depends on the biological behaviour of the tumour, although long-term survival with or without resection may occasionally occur.

Carcinomatous embolization

Very rarely a patient may present with increasing dyspnoea, a clear chest radiograph and reduction in PaO_2 and diffusing capacity. In such circumstances, multiple pulmonary emboli should be considered; occasionally these

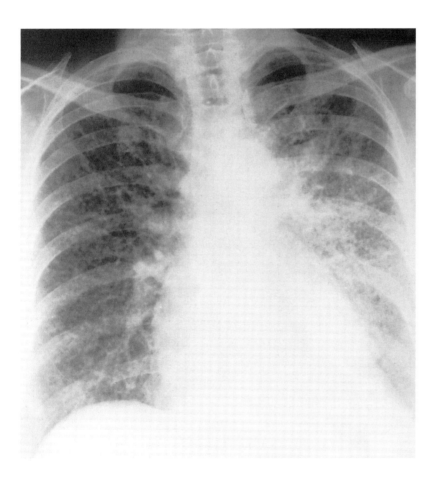

Fig. 42.19 Diffuse fine nodular infiltrate due to metastatic breast adenocarcinoma.

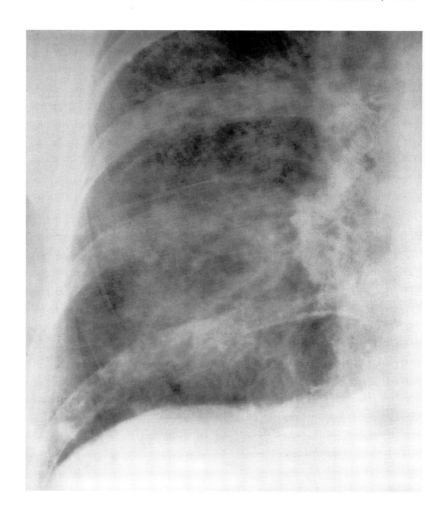

Fig. 42.20 Lymphangitic spread of breast carcinoma. Note irregular pulmonary infiltration and Kerley B lines.

are due to blood-borne tumour cells rather than thrombi. This syndrome has been described with prostatic, breast, stomach, colonic, pancreatic, hepatic and cervical cancers and with choriocarcinoma [243,244]. The lung scan shows features typical of multiple emboli. The diagnosis is usually made at postmortem, but would probably require open lung biopsy in life.

Bilateral hilar node metastasis

The common causes of bilateral hilar node enlargement are sarcoidosis, tuberculosis in Asians, and lymphoma. Oat-cell carcinoma of bronchus may metastasize bilaterally, and this may also be an occasional feature of cancers of kidney, head and neck, testicle and breast, and of malignant melanoma [245,246].

References

1 Miller DL, Allen MS. Rare pulmonary neoplasms. *Mayo Clin Proc* 1993; 68: 492.
2 Whimster WF. *Diagnostic Tumour Bibliographies. 1. Tumours of the Trachea, Bronchus and Lung.* London: Pitman Medical, 1983.
3 Carbone PB, Kaplan HS, Musshoff K *et al.* Report of the committee on Hodgkin's disease staging and classification. *Cancer Res* 1971; 31: 1860.
4 Ellman P, Bowdler AJ. Pulmonary manifestations of Hodgkin's disease. *Br J Dis Chest* 1960; 54: 59.
5 Nelson S, Prince DM, Terry P. Primary Hodgkin's disease of the lung: case report. *Thorax* 1983; 38: 310.
6 Dhingra HK, Flance JI. Cavitary primary pulmonary Hodgkin's disease presenting as pruritus. *Chest* 1970; 58: 71.
7 Macdonald JB. Lung involvement in Hodgkin's disease. *Thorax* 1977; 32: 664.

8 Wolpaw SE, Higley CS, Hauser H. Intrathoracic Hodgkin's disease. *Am J Roentgenol* 1944; 52: 374.
9 Sajjad SM, Luna MA. Primary pulmonary histiocytosis X in two patients with Hodgkin's disease. *Thorax* 1982; 37: 110.
10 Capewell SJ, Wright AJ, Ellis DA. Pulmonary venoocclusive disease in association with Hodgkin's disease. *Thorax* 1984; 39: 554.
11 Canellos GP, Anderson JR, Propert KJ *et al.* Chemotherapy of advanced Hodgkin's disease with MOPP, ABVD, or MOPP alternating with ABVD. *N Engl J Med* 1992; 327: 1478.
12 Jacquillat C, Auclert G, Weil M *et al.* Acute leukaemia, Kaposi sarcoma, epitheliomas complicating 30 observations of Hodgkin's disease. *Proc Am Assoc Cancer Res Clin Oncol* 1976; 17: 247.
13 Van Leeuwen FE, Klockman WJ, Hagenbeek

A, Noyon R *et al.* Second cancer risk following Hodgkin's disease: a 20-year follow-up study. *J Clin Oncol* 1994; 12: 312.
14 Stansfield AG, Diebold J, Kapanci Y *et al.* Updated Kiel classification for lymphomas. *Lancet* 1988; i: 292.
15 Cordier JF, Chailleux E, Lauque D, Reynaud-Gaubert M *et al.* Primary pulmonary lymphomas. A clinical study of 70 cases in non-immunocompromised patients. *Chest* 1993; 103: 201.
16 Manoharan A, Pitney WR, Schonell ME, Bader LV. Intrathoracic manifestations in non-Hodgkin's lymphoma. *Thorax* 1979; 34: 29.
17 Jenkins PF, Ward MJ, Davies P, Fletcher J. Non-Hodgkin's lymphoma, chronic lymphatic leukaemia and the lung. *Br J Dis Chest* 1981; 75: 22.
18 Jenkins BAG, Salm R. Primary lymphosarcoma of the lung. *Br J Dis Chest* 1971; 65: 225.

19 Rees GM. Primary lymphosarcoma of the lung. *Thorax* 1973; 28: 429.

20 Benfield GFA. Primary lymphosarcoma of lung associated with hypertrophic pulmonary osteoarthropathy. *Thorax* 1979; 34: 279.

21 Dalquen P, Gudat F, Ohnacker H, Perruchoud A. Immunocytoma (polymorphous subtype IgA/x) of the lung. *Thorax* 1984; 39: 208.

22 Manoharan A, Ford J, Hill J *et al.* Sputum cytology in the diagnosis of pulmonary non-Hodgkin's lymphoma. *Thorax* 1984; 39: 392.

23 Gibbs AR, Seal RME. Primary lymphoproliferative conditions of lung. *Thorax* 1978; 33: 140.

24 Weynants P, Cordier JF, Cellier CC *et al.* Primary immunocytoma of the lung: the diagnostic value of bronchoalveolar lavage. *Thorax* 1985; 40: 542.

25 Portlock CS. 'Good risk' non-Hodgkin lymphomas: approaches to management. *Semin Hematol* 1983; 20: 25.

26 Muesers P, Konig E, Brittinger G. Why not adhere to the original Kiel classification? *Lancet* 1980; ii: 1194.

27 Bodey EP, Powell RD, Hersh EM *et al.* Pulmonary complications of acute leukaemia. *Cancer* 1966; 19: 781.

28 Green RA, Nichols NJ. Pulmonary involvement in leukaemia. *Am Rev Respir Dis* 1959; 80: 833.

29 Phillips MJ, Knight RK, Green M. Fibreoptic bronchoscopy and diagnosis of pulmonary lesions in lymphoma and leukaemia. *Thorax* 1980; 35: 19.

30 Wardman AG, Cooke NJ. Pulmonary infiltrates in adult acute leukaemia: empirical treatment or lung biopsy. *Thorax* 1984; 39: 647.

31 Herskovic T, Andersen HA, Bayrd ED. Intrathoracic plasmacytomas. *Dis Chest* 1965; 47: 1.

32 Childress WG, Adie GC. Plasma cell tumours of the mediastinum and lung. *J Thorac Surg* 1950; 19: 794.

33 Kober SJ. Solitary plasmacytoma of the carina. *Thorax* 1979; 34: 567.

34 Cordier JF, Cellier CC, Vincent M *et al.* Monoclonal gammopathies in chest disease. *Thorax* 1985; 40: 629.

35 Lichtenstein L. Histiocytosis X. Integration of eosinophilic granuloma of bone, Letterer–Siwe disease and Schuller–Christian disease as related manifestations of a single nosologic entity. *Arch Pathol* 1953; 56: 84.

36 Warnke RA, Kim H, Dorfman RF. Malignant histiocytosis (histiocytic medullary reticulosis). *Cancer* 1975; 35: 215.

37 Colby TV, Carrington CB, Mark GJ. Pulmonary involvement in malignant histiocytosis. A clinicopathologic spectrum. *Am J Surg Pathol* 1981; 5: 61.

38 Stemple DA, Volberg FM, Parker BR, Lewiston NJ. Malignant histiocytosis presenting as interstitial pulmonary disease. *Am Rev Respir Dis* 1982; 126: 726.

39 Parums DV. Commentary. 'Histiocytosis X'. *Thorax* 1998; 53: 322.

40 Basset F, Corrin B, Spencer H *et al.* Pulmonary histiocytosis X. *Am Rev Respir Dis* 1976; 118: 811.

41 Basset F, Soler P, Jaurand MC, Bignon J. Ultrastructural examination of bronchoalveolar lavage for diagnosis of pulmonary histiocytosis X. *Thorax* 1977; 32: 303.

42 Avery ME, McAfee JG, Guild HG. The course and prognosis of reticuloendotheliosis (eosinophilic granuloma, Schuller–Christian disease and Letterer–Siwe disease). A study of 40 cases. *Am J Med* 1957; 22: 636.

43 Nezelof C, Frileux-Herbet F, Cronier-Sachot J. Disseminated histiocytosis X. Analysis of prognostic factors based on a retrospective study of 50 cases. *Cancer* 1979; 44: 1824.

44 Anon. Histiocytosis X. *Lancet* 1977; ii: 440.

45 Ha SY, Helms P, Fletcher M, Broadbent V, Pritchard J. Lung involvement in Langerhans cell histiocytosis: prevalence, clinical features, and outcome. *Pediatrics* 1992; 89: 466.

46 Travis WD, Borok Z, Roum JH, Zhang J *et al.* Pulmonary Langerhans cell granulomatosis (histiocytosis X). A clinico-pathologic study of 48 cases. *Am J Surg Pathol* 1993; 17: 971.

47 Friedman PJ, Liebow AA, Sokoloff J. Eosinophil granuloma of lung. Clinical aspects of primary pulmonary histiocytosis in the adult. *Medicine* 1981; 60: 385.

48 Roland AS, Merdinger WF, Froeb HF. Recurrent spontaneous pneumothorax. A clue to the diagnosis of histiocytosis X. *N Engl J Med* 1964; 270: 73.

49 Lacronique J, Roth C, Battesti J-P *et al.* Chest radiological features of pulmonary histiocytosis X: a report based on 50 adult cases. *Thorax* 1982; 37: 104.

50 Matlin AH, Young LW, Klemperer MR. Pleural effusion in two children with histiocytosis X. *Chest* 1972; 61: 33.

51 Pernod J, Kermarec J, Chambatte C. Aspects cliniques des histiocytoses X pulmonaires de l'adulte (granulomes eosinophiles du poumon). *Rev Tuberc Pneumol* 1967; 31: 591.

52 Chollet S, Dournovo P, Richard MS *et al.* Reactivity of histiocytosis X cells with monoclonal anti-T6 antibody. *N Engl J Med* 1982; 307: 685.

53 Chollet S, Soler P, Dournovo P *et al.* Diagnosis of pulmonary histiocytosis X by immunodetection of Langerhans cells in bronchoalveolar lavage fluid. *Am J Pathol* 1984; 115: 225.

54 Tazi A, Bonay M, Grandsaigne M, Battesti JP, Hance AJ, Soler P. Surface phenotype of Langerhans cells and lymphocytes in granulomatous lesions from patients with pulmonary histiocytosis X. *Am Rev Respir Dis* 1993; 147: 1531.

55 McLelland J, Broadbent V, Yeomans E, Malone M, Pritchard J. Langerhans cell histiocytosis: the case for conservative treatment. *Arch Dis Child* 1990; 65: 301.

56 Lewis JG. Eosinophilic granuloma and its variants, with special reference to lung involvement. A report of 12 patients. *Q J Med* 1964; 33: 337.

57 Jakobson AM, Kreuger A, Hagberg H, Sundström C. Treatment of Langerhans cell histiocytoma with alpha-interferon. *Lancet* 1987; ii: 1520.

58 Habib SB, Congleton J, Carr D *et al.* Recurrence of recipient Langerhans' cell granulomatosis following bilateral lung transplantation. *Thorax* 1998; 53: 323.

59 Gabbay E, Dark JH, Ashcroft T *et al.* Recurrence of Langerhans' cell histiocytosis following lung transplantation. *Thorax* 1998; 53: 326.

60 Katzenstein A-LA, Maurer JJ. Benign histiocytic tumour of lung: a light and electron microscopic study. *Am J Surg Pathol* 1979; 3: 61.

61 Bates T, Hull OH. Histiocytoma of the bronchus. Report of a case in a six year old child. *Am J Dis Child* 1958; 95: 53.

62 Kern WH, Hughes RK, Meyer BW, Harley DP. Malignant fibrous histiocytoma of the lung. *Cancer* 1979; 44: 1793.

63 Bedrossian CWM, Verani R, Unger KM, Salman J. Pulmonary malignant fibrous histiocytoma. Light and electron microscopic studies of one case. *Chest* 1979; 75: 186.

64 Gal AA, Koss MN, McCarthy WF, Hochholzer L. Prognostic factors in pulmonary fibrohistiocytic lesions. *Cancer* 1994; 73: 1817.

65 Addis BJ, Hyjek E, Isaacson PG. Primary pulmonary lymphoma: a reappraisal of its histogenesis and relationship to pseudolymphoma and lymphoid interstitial pneumonia. *Histopathology* 1988; 16: 519.

66 Saldana MJ, Mones JM. Pulmonary pathology in AIDS: atypical *Pneumocystis carinii* infection and lymphoid interstitial pneumonia. *Thorax* 1994; 49: S46.

67 Halprin GM, Ramirez RJ, Pratt PC. Lymphoid interstitial pneumonia. *Chest* 1972; 62: 418.

68 Cummings NA, Scholl GL, Asofsky R *et al.* Sjögren's syndrome: newer aspects of research, diagnosis and therapy. *Ann Intern Med* 1971; 75: 937.

69 Grieco MH, Chinoy-Acharya P. Lymphocytic interstitial pneumonia associated with the acquired immune deficiency syndrome. *Am Rev Respir Dis* 1985; 131: 952.

70 Solal-Celigny P, Couderc LJ, Herman D *et al.* Lymphoid interstitial pneumonitis in acquired immunodeficiency syndrome-related complex. *Am Rev Respir Dis* 1985; 131: 956.

71 Leblond V, Zouabi H, Sutton L, Guillon JM *et al.* Late CD8^2 lymphocytic alveolitis after allogeneic bone marrow transplantation and chronic graft-versus-host disease. *Am J Respir Crit Care Med* 1994; 150: 1056.

72 Weissman E, Becker NH. Interstitial lung disease in primary biliary cirrhosis. *Am J Med Sci* 1983; 385: 21.

73 Levinson AI, Hopewell PC, Stites DP, Spitler LE, Fudenberg HH. Coexistent lymphoid interstitial pneumonia, pernicious anemia, and agammaglobulinemia: comment on autoimmune pathogenesis. *Arch Intern Med* 1976; 136: 213.

74 Rogers BB, Browning I, Rosenblatt H, McClain K *et al.* A familial lymphoproliferative disorder presenting with primary pulmonary manifestations. *Am Rev Respir Dis* 1992; 145: 203.

75 Liebow AA, Carrington CB. Diffuse pulmonary lymphoreticular infiltrations associated with dysproteinaemia. *Med Clin North Am* 1973; 57: 809.

76 Weisbrot IM. Lymphomatoid granulomatosis of the lung associated with a long history of benign lymphoepithelial lesions of the salivary glands and lymphoid interstitial pneumonia. *Am J Clin Pathol* 1976; 66: 792.

77 Saltzstein SL. Pulmonary malignant lymphomas and pseudolymphomas: classification, therapy and prognosis. *Cancer* 1963; 16: 928.

78 Bolton-Maggs PHB, Colman A, Dixon GR *et al.* Mucosa associated lymphoma of the lung. *Thorax* 1993; 48: 670.

79 McNamara JJ, Kingsley WB, Paulson DL *et al.* Primary lymphosarcoma of the lung. *Ann Surg* 1969; 169: 133.

80 Strimlan CV, Rosenow EC, Divertie MC, Harrison EG. Pulmonary manifestations of Sjögren's syndrome. *Chest* 1976; 70: 354.

81 Bahadori M, Liebow AA. Plasma cell granulomas of the lung. *Cancer* 1973; 31: 191.

82 Hurt R, Bates M. Carcinoid tumours of the bronchus: a 33 year experience. *Thorax* 1984; 39: 617.

83 Okike N, Bernatz P, Woolner LB. Carcinoid tumours of the lung. *Ann Thorac Surg* 1976; 22: 270.

84 Blondal T, Grimelius L, Nou E *et al*. Argyrophil carcinoid tumors of the lung: incidence, clinical study and follow-up of 46 patients. *Chest* 1980; 78: 840.

85 Hasleton PS. Histopathology and prognostic factors in bronchial carcinoid tumours. *Thorax* 1994; 49: S56.

86 Mark EJ, Quay SC, Dickensin GR. Papillary carcinoid tumor of the lung. *Cancer* 1981; 48: 316.

87 Arrigoni MG, Woolner LB, Bernatz PE. Atypical carcinoid tumors of the lung. *J Thorac Cardiovasc Surg* 1972; 64: 413.

88 Skinner C, Ewen SWB. Carcinoid lung: diffuse pulmonary infiltration by a multifocal bronchial carcinoid. *Thorax* 1976; 31: 212.

89 Bertelsen S, Aasted A, Lund C *et al*. Bronchial carcinoids: review of 124 cases. *Scand J Thorac Cardiovasc Surg* 1985; 16: 105.

90 Hasleton PS, Gomm S, Blair V, Thatcher N. Pulmonary carcinoid tumours: a clinicopathological study of 35 cases. *Br J Cancer* 1986; 54: 963.

91 Overholt RH, Bougas JA, Morse DP. Bronchial adenoma: a study of 60 patients with resections. *Am Rev Tuberc* 1957; 75: 865.

92 Spitzer SA, Segal I, Lubin E *et al*. Unilateral increased transradiancy of the lung caused by bronchial carcinoid tumour. *Thorax* 1980; 35: 739.

93 Churg A, Warnock ML. Pulmonary tumorlet. A form of peripheral carcinoid. *Cancer* 1976; 37: 1469.

94 Whitwell F. Tumourlets of the lung. *J Pathol Bacteriol* 1955; 70: 529.

95 Warner RRP, Southren AL. Carcinoid syndrome produced by metastasizing bronchial adenoma. *Am J Med* 1958; 24: 903.

96 Payne WR, Fontana RS, Woolner LB. Bronchial tumors arising from mucous glands. Current classification and unusual manifestations. *Med Clin North Am* 1964; 48: 945.

97 Roberts WC, Sjoerdsma A. The cardiac disease associated with the carcinoid syndrome (carcinoid heart disease). *Am J Med* 1964; 36: 5.

98 Bernheimer H, Ehringer H, Heistracher P *et al*. Biologische actives nicht metastatsierendes Bronchuscarcinoid mit Linkshertzsyndrom. *Wien Klin Wochenschr* 1960; 72: 867.

99 Oates JA, Melmon K, Sjoerdsma A *et al*. Release of a kinin peptide in the carcinoid syndrome. *Lancet* 1964; i: 514.

100 Shalet SM, Beardwell CG, MacFarlane IA *et al*. Acromegaly due to production of a growth hormone releasing factor by a bronchial carcinoid tumour. *Clin Endocrinol* 1979; 10: 61.

101 Williams ED, Celestin LR. The association of bronchial carcinoid and pluriglandular adenomatosis. *Thorax* 1962; 17: 120.

102 Allen MB, Shamash J, Kerr KM, Leitch AG. Hypercalcaemia in atypical bronchial carcinoid tumour. *Chest* 1989; 96: 1206.

103 Allison DJ, Modlin IM, Jenkins WJ. Treatment of carcinoid liver metastases by hepatic artery embolization. *Lancet* 1977; ii: 1323.

104 Donahue JK, Weichert RF, Ochsner JL. Bronchial adenoma. *Ann Surg* 1968; 167: 873.

105 Pearson FG, Thompson DW, Weissberg D *et al*. Adenoid cystic carcinoma of trachea: experience with 16 patients managed by tracheal resection. *Ann Thorac Surg* 1974; 18: 16.

106 Conlan AA, Payne WS, Woolner LS, Sanderson DR. Adenoid cystic carcinoma (cylindroma) and mucoepidermoid carcinoma of the bronchus. *J Thorac Cardiovasc Surg* 1978; 76: 369.

107 Stalpaert G, Denette G, van Maele R. Surgical treatment of adenoid cystic carcinoma of the left main bronchus and trachea by left pneumonectomy, resection of 7.5cm of trachea, and direct reanastomosis of right lung. *Thorax* 1979; 34: 554.

108 Vieta JO, Maier HC. The treatment of adenoid cystic carcinoma (cylindroma) of the respiratory tract by surgery and radiation therapy. *Dis Chest* 1957; 31: 493.

109 Zellos S. Bronchial adenoma. *Thorax* 1962; 17: 61.

110 Enterline HT, Schoenberg HW. Carcinoma (cylindromatous type) of trachea and bronchi and bronchial adenoma: a comparative study. *Cancer* 1954; 7: 663.

111 Ozlu C, Christopherson WM, Allen JD. Mucoepidermoid tumors of the bronchus. *J Thorac Cardiovasc Surg* 1961; 42: 24.

112 Moran CA, Suster S, Askin FB, Koss MN. Benign and malignant salivary gland-type mixed tumours of the lung. Clinicopathologic and immunohistochemical study of eight cases. *Cancer* 1994; 73: 2481.

113 Payne US, Ellis FH, Woolner LB, Moersch HJ. The surgical treatment of cylindroma (adenoid cystic carcinoma) and mucoepidermoid tumors of the bronchus. *J Thorac Cardiovasc Surg* 1959; 38: 709.

114 Patel RG, Norman JR. Unilateral hyperlucency with left lower lobe mass in a patient with bronchial asthma. *Chest* 1995; 107: 569.

115 Guillou L, Luze P, Zysset F, Costa J. Papillary variant of low-grade mucoepidermoid carcinoma. *Am J Clin Pathol* 1994; 101: 269.

116 Leonardi HK, Jung-Legg Y, Legg MA, Neptune WB. Tracheobronchial mucoepidermoid carcinoma. Clinicopathological features and results of treatment. *J Thorac Cardiovasc Surg* 1978; 76: 431.

117 Salm R. A primary malignant melanoma of the bronchus. *J Pathol Bacteriol* 1963; 85: 121.

118 Robertson AJ, Sinclair DJM, Sutton PP, Guthrie W. Primary melanocarcinoma of the lower respiratory tract. *Thorax* 1980; 35: 158.

119 Reid JD, Mehta VT. Melanoma of the lower respiratory tract. *Cancer* 1966; 19: 627.

120 Jackson DA, Hatch HB. Solitary benign squamous papilloma of the bronchus. Report of two cases. *Am Rev Respir Dis* 1968; 97: 699.

121 Maxwell RJ, Gibbons JR, O'Hara MD. Solitary squamous papilloma of the bronchus. *Thorax* 1985; 40: 68.

122 Le Roux BT, Williams MA, Kallichurum S. Squamous papillomatosis of the trachea and bronchi. *Thorax* 1969; 24: 673.

123 Spencer H, Dail DH, Arneaud J. Noninvasive bronchial epithelial papillary tumours. *Cancer* 1980; 45: 1486.

124 Shale DJ, Lane DJ, Fisher CWS, Dunnill MS. Endobronchial polyp in an asthmatic subject. *Thorax* 1983; 38: 75.

125 Liebow AA, Castleman B. Benign, clear cell tumors of the lung. *Am J Pathol* 1963; 43: 13a.

126 Becker NH, Soifer I. Benign clear cell tumor (sugar tumor) of the lung. *Cancer* 1971; 27: 712.

127 Hegg CA, Flint A, Singh G. Papillary adenoma of the lung. *Am J Clin Pathol* 1992; 97: 393.

128 Edwards CW, Matthews HR. Mucous gland adenoma of the bronchus. *Thorax* 1981; 36: 147.

129 Heard BE, Dewar A, Firmin RK, Lennox SC. One very rare and one new tracheal tumour found by electron microscopy: glomus tumour and acinic cell tumour resembling carcinoid tumours by light microscopy. *Thorax* 1982; 37: 97.

130 Davis PW, Briggs JC, Seal RME, Storring FK. Benign and malignant mixed cell tumours of the lung. *Thorax* 1972; 27: 657.

131 Warter A, Walter P, Sabountchi M, Jory A. Oncocytic bronchial adenoma. Histological, histochemical and ultrastructural study. *Virchows Arch A* 1981; 392: 231.

132 Katzenstein ALA, Gmelich JT, Carrington CB. Sclerosing haemangioma of the lung. A clinicopathologic study of 51 cases. *Am J Surg Pathol* 1980; 4: 343.

133 Hirano H, Miyagawa Y, Nagata N *et al*. Transbronchial needle aspiration in the diagnosis of pulmonary sclerosing haemangioma. *Respir Med* 1993; 87: 475.

134 Chan K-W, Gibbs AR, Lo WS, Newman GR. Benign sclerosing pneumocytoma of lung (sclerosing haemangioma). *Thorax* 1982; 37: 404.

135 Magee F, Wright JL, Kay JM *et al*. Pulmonary capillary haemangiomatosis. *Am Rev Respir Dis* 1985; 132: 922.

136 Meade JB, Whitwell F, Bickford BJ, Waddington JKB. Primary haemangiopericytoma of lung. *Thorax* 1974; 29: 1.

137 Emery RW, Fox AL, Raab DE. Intravascular bronchioloalveolar tumour. *Thorax* 1982; 37: 472.

138 Marsh K, Kenyan WE, Earis JE, Pearson MG. Intravascular bronchioloalveolar tumour. *Thorax* 1982; 37: 474.

139 Yi ES, Auger WR, Friedman PJ, Morris TA, Shin SS. Intravascular bronchioloalveolar tumor of the lung presenting as pulmonary thromboembolic disease and pulmonary hypertension. *Arch Pathol Lab Med* 1995; 119: 255.

140 Corbeil J, Evans LA, Vasak E, Cooper DA, Penny R. Culture and properties of cells derived from Kaposi's sarcoma. *J Immunol* 1991; 146: 2972.

141 Chang Y, Cesarman E, Pessin MS *et al*. Identification of Herpesvirus-like DNA sequences in AIDS-associated Kaposi's sarcoma. *Science* 1994; 266: 1865.

142 Slavin G, Cameron HM, Forbes C, Mitchell RM. Kaposi's sarcoma in East African children: a report of 51 cases. *J Pathol* 1970; 100: 187.

143 Nesbitt S, Mark PF, Zimmerman HM. Disseminated visceral idiopathic hemorrhagic sarcoma (Kaposi's disease): report of a case with necropsy findings. *Ann Intern Med* 1945; 22: 601.

144 Rosen M, Tow TW, Teirstein AS *et al*. Diagnosis of pulmonary complications of the acquired immune deficiency syndrome. *Thorax* 1985; 40: 571.

145 McKenzie R, Travis WD, Dolan SA *et al*. The causes of death in patients with human immunodeficiency virus infection: a clinical and pathologic study with emphasis on the role of pulmonary diseases. *Medicine* 1991; 70: 326.

146 Misra DP, Sunderrajan EV, Hurst DJ, Maltby JD. Kaposi's sarcoma of the lung: radiology and pathology. *Thorax* 1982; 37: 155.

147 Dantzig PI, Richardson D, Rayhansadeh S *et al*. Thoracic involvement of non-African Kaposi's sarcoma. *Chest* 1971; 66: 522.

148 Gruden JF, Huang L, Webb WR, Gamsu G, Hopewell PE, Sides DM. AIDS-related Kaposi sarcoma of the lung: radiographic findings and staging system with bronchoscopic correlation. *Radiology* 1995; 195: 545.

149 Davis SD, Henschke CI, Chamides BK, Westcott JL. Intrathoracic Kaposi sarcoma in AIDS patients: radiographic–pathologic correlation. *Radiology* 1987; 163: 495.

150 Komfeld H, Axelrod JL. Pulmonary presentation of Kaposi's sarcoma in a homosexual patient. *Am Rev Respir Dis* 1983; 127: 248.

151 Volberding P, Conant MA, Stricket RB, Lewis BJ. Chemotherapy in advanced Kaposi's sarcoma: implications for current cases in homosexual men. *Am J Med* 1983; 74: 652.

152 Krown SE, Gold JW, Niedzwiecki D *et al*. Interferon-alpha with zidovudine: safety, tolerance, and clinical and virologic effects in patients with Kaposi sarcoma associated with the acquired immunodeficiency syndrome (AIDS). *Ann Intern Med* 1990; 112: 812.

153 Bogner JR, Kronawitter U, Rolinski B, Truebenbach K, Goebel FD. Liposomal doxorubicin in the treatment of advanced AIDS-related Kaposi sarcoma. *J Acquir Immun Defic Syndr* 1994; 7: 463.

154 Carrington CB, Cugell DW, Gaensler EA *et al*. Lymphangio-leiomyomatosis. Physiologic–pathologic–radiologic correlations. *Am Rev Respir Dis* 1977; 116: 977.

155 Stovin PG, Lum LC, Flower CDR *et al*. The lungs in lymphangio-myomatosis and in tuberous sclerosis. *Thorax* 1975; 30: 497.

156 Kitaichi M, Nishimura K, Itoh H, Izumi T. Pulmonary lymphangio-leiomyomatosis: a report of 46 patients including a clinico-pathologic study of prognostic factors. *Am J Respir Crit Care Med* 1995; 151: 527.

157 Sinclair W, Wright JL, Churg A. Lymphangi-oleiomyomatosis presenting in a post-menopausal woman. *Thorax* 1985; 40: 475.

158 Corrin BA, Leibow A, Friedman PJ. Pulmonary lymphangiomyomatosis: a review. *Am J Pathol* 1975; 79: 348.

159 Basset F, Soler P, Marsac J, Corrin B. Pulmonary lymphangiomyomatosis. Three new cases studied with electron microscopy. *Cancer* 1976; 38: 2357.

160 Brentani MM, Carvalho RR, Saldiva PH *et al*. Steroid receptors in pulmonary lymphangiomyomatosis. *Chest* 1984; 85: 96.

161 Logan RF, Fawcett IW. Oophorectomy for pulmonary lymphangio-leiomyomatosis: a case report. *Br J Dis Chest* 1985; 79: 98.

162 McCarty KS, Mossler JA, McClelland R, Seiker HO. Pulmonary lymphangiomyomatosis responsive to progesterone. *N Engl J Med* 1980; 303: 1461.

163 Wahedna I, Cooper S, Williams J *et al*. Relation of pulmonary lymphangio-leiomyomatosis to use of the oral contracep-tive pill and fertility in the UK: a national case-control study. *Thorax* 1994; 49: 910.

164 Dawson J. Pulmonary tuberous sclerosis and its relationship to other forms of the disease. *Q J Med* 1954; 23: 113.

165 Guinee DG, Thornberry DS, Azumi N *et al*. Unique pulmonary presentation of an angiomyolipoma. Analysis of clinical, radio-graphic, and histopathologic features. *Am J Surg Pathol* 1995; 19: 476.

166 Harris JO, Waltuck BL, Swenson EW. The pathophysiology of the lungs in tuberous sclerosis. A case report and literature review. *Am Rev Respir Dis* 1969; 100: 379.

167 Broughton RBK. Primary tuberous sclerosis presenting with pleural effusion. *Br Med J* 1970; 1: 477.

168 Castro M, Shepherd CW, Gomez MR, Lie JT, Ryu JH. Pulmonary tuberous sclerosis. *Chest* 1995; 107: 189.

169 Lindskog GE, Liebow A, Kausel H, Jansen A. Pulmonary arterio-venous aneurism. *Ann Surg* 1950; 132: 591.

170 Whitaker W. Cavernous haemangioma of lung. *Thorax* 1947; 2: 58.

171 Le Roux BT. Pulmonary 'hamartoma'. *Thorax* 1964; 19: 236.

172 White RI, Pollak JS, Wirth JA. Pulmonary arteriovenous malformations: diagnosis and transcatheter embolotherapy. *J Vasc Intervent Radiol* 1996; 7: 787.

173 Currarino G, Willis KW, Johnson AF, Miller WW. Pulmonary telangiectasia. *Am J Roentgenol* 1976; 127: 775.

174 Shuter-Eringer H, Orie NGM, Sluiter HJ. Pulmonary arteriovenous fistula: diagnosis and prognosis in noncompliant patients. *Am Rev Respir Dis* 1969; 100: 177.

175 Foley RE, Boyd DP. Pulmonary arteriove-nous aneurisms. *Surg Clin North Am* 1961; 41: 801.

176 Chandler D. Pulmonary and cerebral arteri-ovenous fistula in Osler's disease. *Arch Intern Med* 1965; 116: 277.

177 Sapru RPDC, Hall JI. Pulmonary hyperten-sion in patients with pulmonary arteriove-nous fistulae. *Br Heart J* 1969; 31: 559.

178 Genovesi MG, Tierney DF, Taplin GV, Eisenberg H. An intravenous radionuclide method to evaluate hypoxaemia caused by abnormal alveolar vessels. *Am Rev Respir Dis* 1976; 114: 59.

179 Steinberg I. Diagnosis and surgical treat-ment of pulmonary arteriovenous fistula. Report of 3 new and review of 19 consecu-tive cases. *Surg Clin North Am* 1961; 41: 523.

180 Muri JW. Artenovenous aneurism of the lung. *Am J Surg* 1955; 89: 265.

181 Armitage JM, Kurland G, Michaels M *et al*. Critical issues in pediatric lung transplanta-tion. *J Thorac Cardiovasc Surg* 1995; 109: 60.

182 Charles TJ, Davies AB. Pulmonary telang-iectasia. *Br J Dis Chest* 1979; 73: 309.

183 Eltorky MA, Headley AS, Winer-Muram H, Garrett HE, Griffin JP. Pulmonary capillary hemangiomatosis: a clinicopathologic review. *Ann Thorac Surg* 1994; 57: 772.

184 Noonan JA, Walters LR, Reeves JT. Congeni-tal pulmonary lymphangiectasis. *Am J Dis Child* 1970; 120: 314.

185 Wagenaar SS, Swierenga JA, Wagenvoort CA. Late presentation of primary pul-monary lymphangiectasis. *Thorax* 1976; 33: 791.

186 Tazelaar HD, Kerr D, Yousem SA *et al*. Diffuse pulmonary lymphangio-matosis. *Hum Pathol* 1993; 24: 1313.

187 Yellon A, Rosenman Y, Lieberman Y. Review of smooth muscle tumours of the lower res-piratory tract. *Br J Dis Chest* 1984; 78: 337.

188 White SN, Ibrahim NBW, Forrester-Wood CF, Jeyasingham K. Leiomyomas of the lower respiratory tract. *Thorax* 1985; 40: 306.

189 Shahian DM, McEnamy MT. Complete endoscopic excision of leiomyoma of the bronchus. *J Thorac Cardiovasc Surg* 1977; 77: 87.

190 Guccion JG, Rosen SH. Bronchial leiomyosarcoma and fibrosarcoma. A study of 32 cases and review of the literature. *Cancer* 1972; 30: 836.

191 Houston HE, Payne WS, Harrison EF, Olsen AM. Primary cancers of the trachea. *Arch Surg* 1969; 99: 132.

192 Frederickson JM, Jahn AF, Bryce DP. Leiomyosarcoma of the cervical trachea. Report of a case with reconstruction using a latissimus dorsi island flap. *Ann Otolaryngol* 1979; 88: 463.

193 Eriksson A, Thunell M, Lundqvist G. Pendulating endobronchial rhabdo-myosarcoma with fatal asphyxia. *Thorax* 1982; 37: 390.

194 Drennan JM, McCormack RJM. Primary rhabdomyosarcoma of lung. *J Pathol Bacteriol* 1960; 79: 147.

195 Forbes GB. Rhabdomyosarcoma of bronchus. *J Pathol Bacteriol* 1956; 70: 427.

196 Endelman RM. Pulmonary fibroma: a rare and benign tumour. *Am Rev Respir Dis* 1967; 96: 1242.

197 Elphinstone RG, Spector RG. Sarcoma of the pulmonary artery. *Thorax* 1959; 14: 333.

198 MacArthur CGC, Cheung DLC, Spiro SG. Endobronchial lipoma: a review with four cases. *Br J Dis Chest* 1977; 71: 93.

199 Van der Beukel JTI, Wagenaar SS, Vander-schuren R. Liposarcoma of the trachea. *Thorax* 1979; 34: 817.

200 Standerfer RJ, Armistead SH, Paneth M. Liposarcoma of the mediastinum: report of two cases and review of the literature. *Thorax* 1981; 36: 693.

201 Lacey CJN, Petch MC. Primary liposarcoma of the pericardium. *Thorax* 1979; 34: 120.

202 Walsh TJ, Healy TM. Chondroma of the bronchus. *Thorax* 1969; 24: 327.

203 Rees GM. Primary chondrosarcoma of lung. *Thorax* 1970; 25: 366.

204 Littlefield JB, Drash EC. Myxoma of the lung. *Thorac Surg* 1959; 37: 745.

205 Carney J, Sheps S, Go V, Gordon H. The triad of gastric leiomyosarcoma, functioning extra-adrenal paraganglioma and pul-monary chondroma. *N Engl J Med* 1977; 296: 1517.

206 Carney J. The triad of gastric epithelial leiomyosarcoma, functioning extra-adrenal paraganglioma, and pulmonary chon-droma. *Cancer* 1979; 43: 374.

207 Messina MS, Sampson MG, Chumas J, Nelson S. Carney's triad: role of transtho-racic needle biopsy. *Am Rev Respir Dis* 1983; 128: 311.

208 Ngadiman S, Horenstein MG, Campbell WG. The concurrence of duode-nal epithelioid stromal sarcoma, pulmonary chondromatous hamartoma, and non-functioning pancreatic islet cell tumor. A possible analogue of Carney's triad? *Arch Pathol Lab Med* 1994; 118: 840.

209 Crofts NF, Forbes GB. Malignant neurilem-moma of the lung metastasising to the heart. *Thorax* 1964; 19: 334.

210 Nies AT-V, van De Brekel B, Buytendijk HJ, Maesen F. Neurofibroma of the trachea: a case report. *Thorax* 1978; 33: 121.

211 Nigam BK, Hyer SL, Taylor EJ, Guha T. Intrathoracic chemodectoma with noradrenaline secretion. *Thorax* 1981; 36: 66.

212 Singh G, Lee RE, Brooks DH. Primary pulmonary paraganglioma. Report of a case and review of the literature. *Cancer* 1977; 40: 2286.

213 Churg AM, Warnock ML. So called 'minute pulmonary chemodectoma'. *Cancer* 1976; 37: 1759.

214 Prauer HW, Mack D, Babic R. Intrapulmonary teratoma 10 years after removal of a mediastinal teratoma in a young man. *Thorax* 1983; 38: 632.

215 Jamieson MPG, McGowan AR. Endobronchial teratoma. *Thorax* 1982; 37: 157.

216 Bateson EM, Hayes JA, Woo-Ming M. Endobronchial teratoma associated with bronchiectasis and bronchiolectasis. *Thorax* 1968; 23: 69.

217 Parker D, Holford CP, Begent RHJ *et al.* Effective treatment for malignant mediastinal teratoma. *Thorax* 1983; 38: 897.

218 Arrigoni MG, Woolmer LB, Bernatz PE *et al.* Benign tumors of the lung. A ten year surgical experience. *J Thorac Cardiovasc Surg* 1970; 60: 589.

219 Koutras P, Urschel HC, Paulson DL. Hamartoma of the lung. *J Thorac Cardiovasc Surg* 1971; 61: 768.

220 Petheram IS, Heard BF. Unique massive pulmonary hamartoma. Case report with review of hamartomata treated at Brompton Hospital in 27 years. *Chest* 1979; 75: 95.

221 Hansen CP, Holtveg H, Francis D, Rasch L, Bertelsen S. Pulmonary hamartoma. *J Thorac Cardiovasc Surg* 1992; 104: 674.

222 Johansson M, Dietrich C, Mandahl N *et al.* Recombinations of chromosomal bands 6p21 and 14q24 characterise pulmonary hamartomas. *Br J Cancer* 1993; 67: 1236.

223 Laroche CM, Stewart S, Wells F, Schneerson J. Multiple recurrent intrapulmonary and endobronchial mesenchymomas (hamartomas). *Thorax* 1993; 48: 572.

224 Dominguez H, Hariri J, Pless S. Multiple pulmonary chondrohamartomas in trachea, bronchi and lung parenchyma. Review of the literature. *Respir Med* 1996; 90: 111.

225 Doppman J, Wilson G. Cystic pulmonary hamartoma. *Br J Radiol* 1965; 38: 629.

226 Mushtaq M, Ward SP, Hutchison JT, Mann JS. Multiple cystic pulmonary hamartomas. *Thorax* 1992; 47: 1076.

227 Blair TC, McElvein RB. Hamartoma of the lung. A clinical study of 25 cases. *Dis Chest* 1963; 44: 296.

228 Silverman JF, Kay S. Multiple pulmonary leiomyomatous hamartomas. Report of a case with ultrastructure examination. *Cancer* 1976; 38: 1199.

229 Cruikshank DB, Harrison GK. Diffuse fibroleiomyomatous hamartomatosis of the lung. *Thorax* 1953; 8: 316.

230 Paulsen JT, Jacobsen M, Francis D. Probable malignant transformation of a pulmonary hamartoma. *Thorax* 1979; 34: 557.

231 Ribet M, Jaillard-Thery S, Nuttens MC. Pulmonary hamartoma and malignancy. *J Thorac Cardiovasc Surg* 1994; 107: 611.

232 Davis PW, Briggs JC, Seal RME, Storring FK. Benign and malignant mixed tumours of the lung. *Thorax* 1972; 27: 657.

233 Chaudhuri MR, Eastham WN, Fredriksz PA. Pulmonary blastoma with diverse mesenchymal proliferation. *Thorax* 1972; 27: 487.

234 Hachitanda Y, Aoyama C, Sato JK, Shimada H. Pleuropulmonary blastoma in childhood. A tumor of divergent differentiation. *Am J Surg Pathol* 1993; 17: 382.

235 Calabria R, Srikanth MS, Chamberlin K, Bloch J, Atkinson JB. Management of pulmonary blastoma in children. *Am Surg* 1993; 59: 192.

236 Nappi O, Wick MR. Sarcomatoid neoplasms of the respiratory tract. *Semin Diagn Pathol* 1993; 10: 137.

237 Shepherd MP. Thoracic metastases. *Thorax* 1982; 37: 366.

238 Rees GM, Cleland WP. Surgical treatment of pulmonary metastases. *Thorax* 1972; 27: 654.

239 Simpson FG, King HA, Whelan P, Cooke NJ. Prostatic carcinoma presenting with respiratory symptoms: response to orchidectomy. *Thorax* 1984; 39: 552.

240 Shepherd MP. Endobronchial metastatic disease. *Thorax* 1982; 37: 362.

241 Albertini RE, Ekberg NL. Endobronchial metastasis in breast cancer. *Thorax* 1980; 35: 435.

242 Jariwalla AG, Seaton A, McCormack RJM *et al.* Intrabronchial metastases from renal carcinoma with recurrent tumour expectoration. *Thorax* 1981; 36: 179.

243 Kane RD, Hawkins HK, Miller JA, Noce PS. Microscopic pulmonary tumor emboli associated with dyspnea. *Cancer* 1975; 36: 1473.

244 Keeping IM, Buchanan R, Dodds JH. Microscopic tumour emboli from carcinoma of the prostate. *Br J Dis Chest* 1982; 76: 298.

245 McLoud TC, Kalisher L, Stark P, Greene R. Intrathoracic lymph node metastases from extrathoracic neoplasms. *Am J Roentgenol* 1978; 131: 403.

246 King TE, Fisher J, Schwarz MI, Patzelt LH. Bilateral hilar adenopathy: an unusual presentation of renal cell carcinoma. *Thorax* 1982; 37: 317.

43

DISEASES OF THE PLEURA

ANTHONY SEATON

The two layers of the pleura (visceral and parietal) that surround the lung are described in Chapter 1. Only the parietal layer has a somatic nerve supply, derived from intercostal and diaphragmatic nerves, and is therefore sensitive to painful stimuli. In almost all instances of disease of the pleural membranes and of the potential cavity that they enclose, the cause is in the lung or elsewhere in the body, although in a few instances primary pleural disease may occur. This chapter discusses the main diseases that affect the pleura, with the exception of empyema (see Chapter 14) and pneumothorax (see Chapter 44).

Physiology of the pleura

The pleura transmits the force generated by the respiratory muscles to the lungs [1]. During normal respiration there is therefore a pressure negative to atmosphere (about −0.66 kPa at functional residual capacity) within the pleural space. This would tend to suck capillary fluid and gas from surrounding tissue into the space if it were not for other balancing factors. In the case of fluid, there is a hydrostatic pressure difference between parietal pleural capillaries, supplied by systemic arterial vessels (about 4 kPa), and visceral pleural capillaries, supplied by pulmonary arterial vessels (about 1.5 kPa). Plasma oncotic pressure is the same in both sets of capillaries (about 4.66 kPa), while pleural osmotic pressure is only about 0.8 kPa, since little protein is able to escape from the adjacent healthy capillaries. Thus there is a net force that drives fluid from parietal capillaries to pleural space (−0.66 − 4 − 0.8 + 4.66 = −0.8 kPa); similarly, a net force drives pleural fluid into visceral capillaries and lymphatics (−0.66 − 1.5 − 0.8 + 4.66 = +1.7 kPa). There is therefore a regular transfer of low-protein fluid from parietal to pleural space, although recent evidence suggests that reabsorption is not, as was thought, via the visceral pleura but through lymphatic vessels opening into the parietal pleura. In the case of gas, any that gains access to the pleural space is at atmospheric minus pleural pressure, i.e.

101.1 − 0.66 = 100.44 kPa. In contrast, the partial pressure of gas within the pleural capillary blood is some 5.3–6.6 kPa below atmospheric pressure, and thus there is a driving force of about 5.3 kPa available to resolve any pneumothorax.

The pleural fluid is in a dynamic state, 30–75% of the water being turned over every hour [2]. This is accelerated by increased lung movements, such as during exercise. Protein and particles are turned over much less rapidly, being absorbed by lymphatics only [3,4]; stomata leading into lymphatics have been demonstrated over the lower mediastinal, chest wall and diaphragmatic parietal pleura [5]. These, together with the valves of the lymphatic vessels, ensure transport of protein and particle-containing fluid from the pleural space. Any disease that causes inflammatory or neoplastic change in the parietal pleura is likely to decrease protein reabsorption and therefore alter the fluid hydrodynamics in such a way as to increase the size of the effusion.

It has generally been assumed that the pleural space is lubricated by a thin film of serous fluid, and it has been shown that a few millilitres of this fluid can be obtained from the normal space. However, it has been suggested on physical grounds that this would be unlikely to provide adequate lubrication and that a surfactant would be more efficient; such surface-active phospholipids have been identified in pleural fluid [6].

Dry or fibrinous pleurisy

Clinical features

Pleural pain is characteristically sharp and associated with inspiration, coughing and movements of the chest wall. When it is severe the patient breathes in short grunts and may attempt to splint the appropriate part of the chest by holding it or lying on it. The site of pain can usually be localized quite closely and is most frequently in the lower posterolateral parts of the chest. As the pleurisy improves, or sometimes from the beginning when the upper chest is involved, the pain may be more of an ache though still associated with movement and breathing.

The diagnostic sign of pleurisy is a rub, of a creaking superficial nature, usually localized closely to the site of the pain. At its most marked this is unmistakable and heard in inspiration and expiration; however, it may be confined to part of the inspiratory cycle and at times may be difficult to distinguish from pulmonary crackles. As the pleurisy improves, it tends to become less obvious but may persist after the pain has gone and in occasional patients a loud rub may be present indefinitely. Indeed, pleural rub may sometimes be heard in patients with no pain and pleural pain may occasionally occur without a rub.

Because of the innervation of the pleura, pleuritic pain may be referred to the shoulder tip via the phrenic nerve when the area over the central tendon of the diaphragm is involved or to the upper abdomen when the area over the peripheral diaphragm is affected. In the latter case this may cause diagnostic difficulties unless the relationship to respiration is recognized, especially as a rub is usually not audible. The pain of pleurisy is due to inflammation of the parietal pleura and is presumably provoked by stretching. The rub arises from friction between the two pleural surfaces when their normal lubricating mechanism is impaired by the inflammatory exudate.

Causes

Dry pleurisy may be due to chest trauma, usually associated with rib fracture. Apart from this, the most common cause is infection of the underlying lung; recurrent pleurisy is usually associated with recurrent infection of bronchiectatic lung. Bornholm disease, collagen diseases (especially rheumatoid and systemic lupus) and pulmonary infarction are other not infrequent causes. Tumours invading the chest usually cause a persistent, continuous pain but may occasionally present with pleurisy. Rarely dry pleurisy may be associated with asbestos exposure (see below), tuberculosis and subdiaphragmatic abscess.

Bornholm disease

Bornholm disease is named after the Danish island where an early epidemic was described and is also known as epidemic pleurodynia, epidemic myalgia or, colloquially, the devil's grip [7]. It is caused by an enterovirus, usually Coxsackie B but occasionally Coxsackie A or an echovirus [8]. In one study of an outbreak in an American football team it has been suggested that spread may have been due to contamination of a common drinking source by one of the players [9]. It has a short incubation period (3–5 days) and may occur in late summer and autumn epidemics, although sporadic cases are frequent. The disease is most common in children and young adults, usually starting with fever and upper respiratory symptoms followed by the characteristic pain. Typically this occurs in the chest or upper abdomen and may be very severe. It is worsened by movement and respiration and associated with tenderness of intercostal muscles. Pleurisy, sometimes referred to the shoulder, is common and a pleural rub is sometimes audible. Pericarditis with rub may also be present. Fever and a raised erythrocyte sedimentation rate are occasionally present at this stage but there are no characteristic haematological changes. The chest radiograph is usually normal, though a blunted costophrenic angle may be present. There may be diagnostic confusion with early herpes zoster and the eosinophilia–myalgia syndrome associated with L-tryptophan therapy.

The illness usually lasts about a week, the pain gradually subsiding. Other organs, such as the heart, central nervous system or testes, may occasionally be involved, resulting in a more prolonged course. The disease has a tendency to relapse, usually in a milder form, over several weeks. The diagnosis is made from the characteristic clinical features and may be confirmed by viral culture of stools or throat swabs and by a rise in the approriate viral antibodies. There is no specific treatment but analgesics are often needed to control the pain.

Recurrent polyserositis

This condition, also known as periodic disease or familial Mediterranean fever, is an autosomal recessive genetic disease afflicting predominantly people of Jewish, Arabic, Armenian and Turkish origins [10,11]. The genetic defect has been shown in several families to be on the short arm of chromosome 16 [12,13], although the biochemical defect remains unknown. The disease is characterized by recurrent fever and inflammation of serous membranes. Attacks occur at irregular intervals, from several days to several years. The disease almost always manifests itself in childhood and very rarely after the age of 40, and there is often a history of similar illness in other members of the family, especially siblings. It presents most commonly with peritoneal inflammation that mimics a ruptured appendix, and the patient has often been subjected to laparotomy. Pleurisy mimicking Bornholm disease is another common presentation, as is acute inflammation of one or two large joints. The pain is accompanied by fever, tachycardia and often chills, and there is often a moderate neutrophil leucocytosis during attacks. Effusions into large joints and erysipelas-like rashes on the legs may occur. A similar periodic syndrome associated with hyperimmunoglobulinaemia D has been described in European families in which prolonged myositis is more frequent and serositis and amyloidosis rarer [14]. There is no diagnostic test, though immunological changes such as circulating immune complexes and raised immunoglobulins have been described; amyloidosis of the kidneys is the most serious complication, occurring in 0–20% in different series, and may lead to renal failure. Acute attacks of the syndrome resolve spontaneously within 12–48h in almost all cases, and apart from the renal complication the condition is generally regarded as having a benign course.

Treatment of the acute attack relies on the use of analgesics. Recurrent episodes may be prevented by regular use of colchicine [15] and there is some anecdotal evidence that this may help to prevent the long-term renal complication of amyloidosis [16].

Diagnosis and management

The pain of pleurisy needs to be differentiated from that due to chest wall causes, such as rib fracture, intercostal muscle pain and Tietze's syndrome, and that due to neurogenic causes, such as herpes zoster and root compression. The presence of a pleural rub is helpful, although this may be heard sometimes following rib fractures. A chest radiograph is frequently useful in showing the primary lung condition. If this is normal, or if it only shows a small amount of fluid in the costophrenic angle, it is important to consider the possibility of pulmonary embolism, and further examination of the legs together with isotopic scanning may help in coming to a therapeutic decision (see Chapter 25). If this diagnosis is considered unlikely, it is reasonable to treat the patient with adequate analgesics and await developments; in most such cases, the pleurisy settles within a week. Paired blood samples taken in the acute and convalescent phases may be tested for viral antibodies. When the chest film is abnormal, further investigation or treatment may be necessary; for example pneumonic change would indicate bacteriological investigation and antibiotic treatment, while evidence of bronchiectasis may lead to consideration for surgery if it is giving rise to recurrent episodes of infection and pleurisy.

The pain of pleurisy is usually controlled by simple analgesia and the patient adopting a comfortable posture (often lying on the affected side). Severe pain may require opiates, although dramatic relief may often be obtained by raising intradermal wheals of local anaesthetic in four or five places around the site of maximum pain. This relief is often prolonged and the procedure, if successful, may be repeated periodically; it is particularly useful when the patient's respiratory condition makes the use of opiates inadvisable.

Pleural effusion

Clinical features

The effects of accumulation of fluid in the pleural space depend on the cause and on the amount of fluid. Small effusions are often symptomless; even very large effusions, if they accumulate slowly, may cause little or no discomfort to the patient. If the effusion is due to inflammatory disease, it often starts with pleuritic pain that may be relieved as the fluid accumulates. The usual symptom of a large effusion is shortness of breath, often accompanied by a dull ache on the affected side; this is especially likely if the effusion is due to malignant disease of the pleura. Recurrent dry cough is frequently present, especially if the fluid has accumulated quickly.

The findings on physical examination are also dependent on the size and site of the effusion. Since most effusions are in the dependent part of the pleural space, the signs of diminished movements, dull percussion note and distant or absent breath sounds are found here. Bronchial breath sounds or aegophony (a nasal or bleeting quality of transmitted voice sounds) may be heard immediately above an effusion. Large effusions displace the mediastinum to the opposite side unless there is underlying pulmonary collapse or associated pleural fibrosis. Although the signs of a large effusion are very characteristic, those of a smaller one may be mimicked by lobar collapse, pleural tumour or pleural fibrosis, and it is often difficult to assess the presence or absence of collapse or consolidation beneath an effusion. Careful clinical examination of the mediastinal position may help, as may asking the patient to change position in order to test whether the effusion moves.

Radiological features

Free pleural fluid in small amounts (about 100 mL) may be seen as blunting of the costophrenic angle on posteroanterior or lateral films. Larger effusions are most dense at the base, obscure the diaphragm and show decreasing density towards the top. As the fluid rides up around the edges of the lung, attenuation of the X-rays decreases and the radiographic appearances suggest that the effusion is higher in the axilla than anteriorly or posteriorly (Fig. 43.1). However lateral films show the level to appear higher posteriorly and anteriorly, indicating that in fact the top of the effusion is horizontal, only showing radiographically where the X-rays have to traverse sufficient depth of fluid [17]. If there is doubt about the presence of fluid radiographically, a lateral decubitus film may be taken to show the shift of the effusion to the mediastinum or lateral chest wall. This may help particularly in differentiating a small effusion from pleural thickening.

Sometimes effusions may be encysted and cause diagnostic difficulties. Interlobar effusions may mimic tumour (Fig. 43.2); they occur particularly in cardiac failure and their clearance following diuretic treatment has given rise to the term 'vanishing pulmonary tumour' [18]. Subpulmonary effusions may not appear to rise into the axilla and may look like an elevated diaphragm. On the left, the

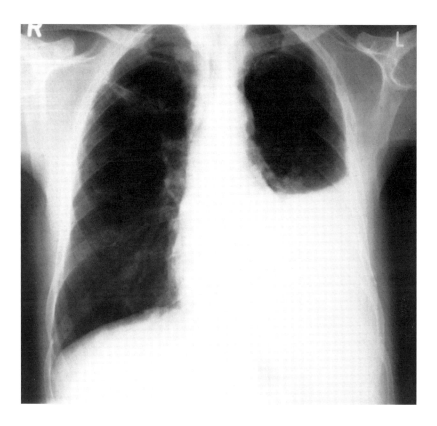

Fig. 43.1 Chest film showing left pleural effusion.

stomach air bubble allows the distinction to be made, but on the right it may be more difficult. A lateral decubitus film or ultrasound investigation may be necessary. Other encysted effusions may occur anywhere in the pleural space, especially following pleural infection or pulmonary surgery, and may look like tumours. Serial radiographs often allow the diagnosis to be made and ultrasound may be helpful [19]. Fluid together with air (hydropneumothorax) shows the characteristic fluid level (Fig. 43.3). This appearance may be mimicked by fluid in a lung cyst or bulla, especially as hydropneumothorax may often be encysted following partial resolution of the pneumothorax.

Causes

It is convenient to differentiate transudates from exudates when discussing the causes of pleural effusion.

Pleural transudates

The causes of these are given in Table 43.1. By far the most common is congestive cardiac failure [20]; this effusion is often unilateral initially, usually on the right side. In severe failure it is usually bilateral, cardiac failure being the most frequent cause of bilateral effusions. The mechanism is increased transudation of fluid from the lung, partly as a result of increased capillary pressure but also because of increased pulmonary interstitial

Table 43.1 Causes of pleural transudates.

Increased hydrostatic pressure
Congestive cardiac failure
Constrictive pericarditis
Pericardial effusion
Constrictive cardiomyopathy
Massive pulmonary embolism

Decreased capillary oncotic pressure
Cirrhosis
Nephrotic syndrome
Malnutrition
Protein-losing enteritis
Small bowel disease

Transmission from peritoneum
Any cause of ascites
Peritoneal dialysis
Liver transplantation

Increased capillary permeability
Small pulmonary emboli
Myxoedema

Obstructed lung lymphatics
Lung transplantation

pressure [21]. The diagnosis is usually obvious from associated clinical features, this being one situation when diagnostic aspiration may be avoided, at least until after a trial of diuretic treatment. An important point

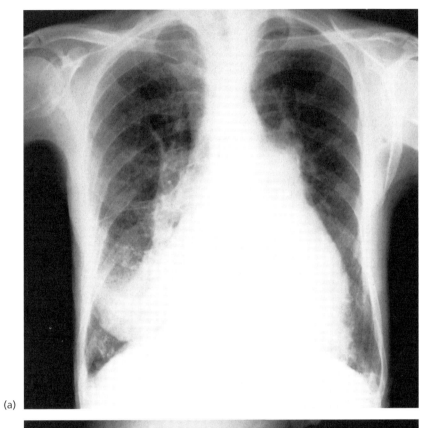

(a)

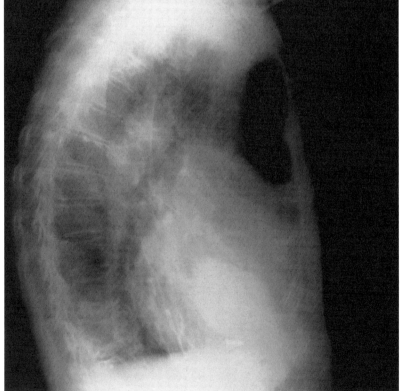

(b)

Fig. 43.2 (a) Rounded right lower zone lesion in patient with congestive heart failure. (b) Lateral view shows the lesion to be fluid in the oblique fissure.

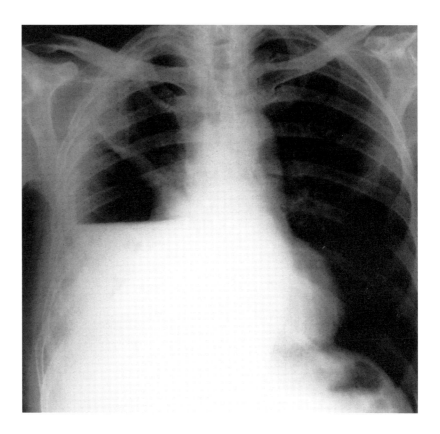

Fig. 43.3 Right hydropneumothorax in patient with mesothelioma. The tumour can be seen under the ribs above the fluid level.

in radiological diagnosis is that bilateral effusions are rarely due to cardiac failure if the cardiac size is not increased (constrictive pericarditis being an exception), in which case other causes such as pulmonary embolism, neoplasm and occasionally hypoalbuminaemia need to be considered.

Pulmonary embolism may cause pleural transudates, although blood-staining occurs in about one-quarter of cases and exudates are found in about two-thirds [22]. Again, these effusions are often bilateral but usually quite small [23]. They may be associated with typical dome-shaped or linear (not, as is commonly believed, wedge-shaped) pulmonary shadows, although the radiological appearances are often quite non-specific and further investigations are usually necessary. Transudates due to hypoproteinaemia occur in cirrhosis, nephrotic syndrome and protein malnutrition. They may be diagnosed by their associated features. Constrictive pericarditis, due to old tuberculosis, rheumatoid disease or malignant infiltration of the pericardium, and constrictive cardiomyopathies are usually also associated with ascites; often this fluid tracks up into the right pleural space through small defects in the diaphragm [24,25], producing a large unilateral effusion. Indeed, a left-sided pleural effusion in hypoproteinaemia is usually due to some other cause and should be investigated accordingly. This same mechanism is responsible for the occasional right pleural effusion occurring during peritoneal dialysis [26].

Meigs' syndrome is the rare association of a benign ovarian fibroma with ascites and accompanying, usually right-sided, pleural effusion [27]. In fact ovarian fibroma is rarely associated with serous transudates and the finding of effusions in association with ovarian disease usually leads to the realization that they are exudates and that the tumour is malignant. In Meigs' syndrome it is likely that the pleural effusion has tracked through the diaphragm from the peritoneum.

Finally, myxoedema may cause pleural effusion, either as a consequence of ascites or pericardial effusion or, very rarely, as a direct effect on pleural capillary permeability [28]. This condition responds to replacement thyroxine therapy; the metabolic basis of the alteration in permeability of the capillaries of the serous membranes is unclear.

Pleural exudates

The main causes are given in Table 43.2. Of these, the most common are metastatic tumour, infections and pulmonary embolism.

Neoplasms

A primary pleural tumour is almost always a mesothelioma. Metastasis occurs commonly from bronchial, breast, stomach and ovarian carcinoma [29]. Almost any

Table 43.2 Causes of pleural exudates.

Neoplasms
Mesothelioma, very rarely pleural sarcoma
Metastases
Lymphoma

Infections
Pneumonia, abscess
Tuberculosis
AIDS
Hantavirus syndrome
Fungal and actinomycotic disease
Subphrenic abscess
Hepatic amoebiasis

Immune disorders
Post-myocardial infarct/cardiotomy syndrome
Rheumatoid disease
Systemic lupus erythematosus
Wegener's granulomatosis
Rheumatic fever

Abdominal diseases
Pancreatitis
Uraemia
Other causes of peritoneal exudates

Pulmonary embolism and infarction

Other causes
Sarcoidosis
Drug reactions
Radiation therapy
Asbestos exposure
Recurrent polyserositis
Yellow nails syndrome
Oesophageal rupture

---

other malignant neoplasm may occasionally metastasize to pleura, while lymphoma may cause effusion without necessarily causing pleural infiltration [30]. Malignant pleural effusions are usually, though not always, blood-stained and recur after aspiration.

Infections

Bacterial pneumonia is associated with pleural effusion in about 40% of cases [31]. Initially the effusion may be amber-coloured, containing predominantly polymorphs, but may progress to increasing turbidity with a high white cell count (empyema; see Chapter 14). Viral and mycoplasmal pneumonias rarely cause effusion, although tuberculosis remains an important cause. Recently, infection with hantavirus, an often fatal syndrome occurring particularly in North American Indians, has been shown to cause non-cardiogenic pulmonary oedema and pleural effusion [32].

The effusion associated with bacterial pneumonia is initially sterile. However, it may frequently be invaded by

the causative organism, leading to empyema or eventual healing by fibrosis. For this reason, aspiration to dryness (or as near as possible) is necessary at the time of presentation; it is unwise to wait in the hope of resolution of the effusion with antibiotic treatment of the original pneumonia.

Pleural effusion may occur as a complication of tuberculosis in four situations. In all cases the disease is due to actual infection of the pleura by tubercle bacilli, though tuberculin hypersensitivity probably plays a part in potentiating the reaction.

1 Effusion may occur as part of primary tuberculosis in children, when the peripheral focus or a caseating lymph node ruptures into the pleura [33]. This disease is now relatively uncommon in developed countries but typically presented between the age of 5 and puberty and occurred in about 7% of patients with primary tuberculosis [34]. The effusion usually occurs 3–6 months after infection, and is associated with general malaise, fever and pleuritic pain [35]. In the era before chemotherapy, it would usually resolve without treatment in 3–4 months, leaving only some blunting of the costophrenic angle and evidence of the primary complex. Nowadays this syndrome is seen more frequently in middle-aged and elderly subjects who may have lost their tuberculin sensitivity. At presentation they may have negative tuberculin tests though these invariably become positive within a few weeks [36].

2 Pleural effusion may present in adolescents or young adults, often after a few weeks of malaise, with acute pleuritic pain and fever. This presentation became much less common after the introduction of bacille Calmette–Guérin (BCG) inoculation in the UK, though it is not prevented by this altogether. The illness may initially manifest with recurrent dry pleurisy and all evidence of disease may disappear without treatment over a few months. However, up to two-thirds of these patients develop active pulmonary tuberculosis within the ensuing 5 years [37,38]. Moreover, a proportion of patients in whom treatment is started late or withheld because of diagnostic uncertainty progress to pleural fibrosis, which may cause serious restrictive impairment of lung function; these individuals ultimately require surgical pleurectomy. Early diagnosis and treatment is therefore important.

3 This type of tuberculous effusion, also now seen relatively rarely in the West, occurs when a tuberculous cavity in a patient with extensive postprimary disease ruptures into the pleura. This usually causes a tuberculous pyopneumothorax, the patient becoming breathless and complaining of pleuritic pain and increased malaise and fever (Fig. 43.4). Bronchopleural fistula may result and causes considerable management problems [39]. A fatal outcome is not infrequent in these circumstances. When resolution takes place, chronic fibrothorax is almost always the result, with extensive calcification [40] (Fig. 43.5). Before the modern era of antibiotics, this was also often the

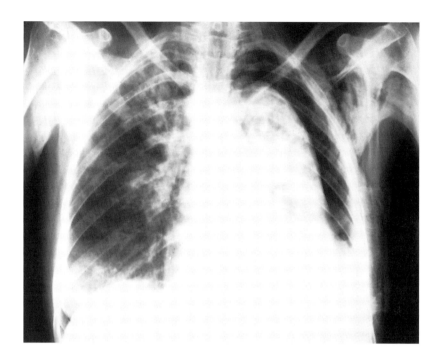

Fig. 43.4 Fatal left pyopneumothorax due to extensive pulmonary tuberculosis in an alcoholic woman.

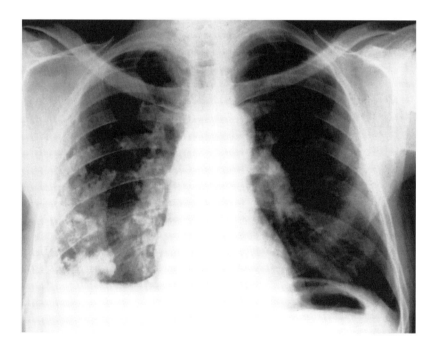

Fig. 43.5 Extensive right pleural calcification following tuberculosis effusion.

outcome of pleural effusion complicating artificial pneumothorax treatment for tuberculosis.

4 Pleural effusion as a manifestation of disseminated tuberculosis in patients with AIDS is becoming increasingly common. These patients are usually very ill and deteriorate rapidly. The effusion may contain large numbers of bacilli, although the typical granulomatous histological changes are often absent [41].

The effusion in tuberculosis is rarely massive but often occupies about one-third to half the hemithorax [34]. The fluid is usually serous and contains more than 50 g/L protein with a predominant lymphocytosis [35]. In immunocompetent people, the tuberculin test is almost always positive, save in the early stages when it may occasionally be negative; if so, it should be repeated 1 month later, when it has usually converted. The initial negativity may be due to the presence of circulating lymphocytes that suppress the activity of tuberculin-sensitized T lymphocytes [42]. Culture of pleural fluid is often negative, the chances of a positive result being increased in proportion to the amount of fluid sent to the laboratory. However, pleural biopsies show granulomas in about two-thirds of patients; repeating the biopsies and culturing them may increase the rate of diagnosis to 90% [43].

Infection with the other pathogenic mycobacteria (*Mycobacterium kansasii* and *M. avium-intracellulare*) has been recognized more frequently as the incidence of tuberculosis has declined in the West, and these organisms are a well-recognized problem in the immunosuppressed. These conditions are discussed in Chapters 20 and 52. Pleural effusion occurs in about 5% of cases, usually in association with radiological evidence of intrapulmonary disease [44]. The clinical and radiographic features of the disease in the immunocompetent are usually indistinguishable from those of tuberculosis, the diagnosis being made bacteriologically from pleural fluid and biopsies.

Fungal infections of the lung are relatively uncommon in the UK, being seen mainly in immunosuppressed patients. However they are seen more often in the USA, where they are endemic in certain areas (see Chapter 21). Pleural effusion may occur in any pulmonary fungal infection and usually mimics tuberculosis clinically, radiographically and in the features of the pleural fluid. It may occur as a self-limiting process, together with fever and malaise, in the primary infection, or as a more intractable illness in association with rupture of a lung focus in post-primary or disseminated disease. It has been described in about 7% of patients with coccidioidomycosis [45], 10% of patients with blastomycosis [46] and rarely in histoplasmosis [47], cryptococcosis [48] and other fungal infections. It is an occasional complication of invasive or disseminated aspergillosis [49] and has been described very rarely in allergic aspergillosis [50].

Actinomyces and *Nocardia* sp., filamentous branching bacteria (see Chapter 21), may infect the lung and spread to the pleura. Either parapneumonic or infected effusions may occur, almost always in association with cavitating pneumonic changes in the ipsilateral lung [51–54].

Subphrenic infection, usually due to a perforated abdominal viscus, may spread up through the diaphragm. The effusion initially contains polymorphs but no organisms; untreated it progresses to empyema [55]. Diagnosis is aided by the presence radiologically of gas under the diaphragm [56]. The usual organisms are coliforms, streptococci and clostridia.

Hepatic amoebiasis may be complicated by serous pleural effusion, usually on the right side [57]. Hepatic abscess may rupture into the pleura causing empyema; occasionally a hepatobronchial fistula forms and the so-called 'anchovy sauce' sputum is expectorated (see Chapter 22). Hydatid disease, of either liver or lung, may also rupture into the pleura, in some instances causing an anaphylactic reaction, in others leading to hepatobronchial fistula [58,59].

Immune disorders

Rheumatic fever, still quite uncommon in the West despite an apparent rise in incidence in the western USA, occurs frequently in the tropics and India, where it has an annual incidence of about 0.5 per 1000 among rural children [60]. It may be associated with pleurisy (usually accompanied by pericarditis). Pleural effusion apparently occurred in the past in about 10% of cases of acute rheumatic fever [61], although recent reviews do not mention this as a complication.

Rheumatoid arthritis may be accompanied by effusion in about 15% of males with the disease but only 2% of females. Typically the effusion occurs within about 5 years of the start of the disease, in patients with severe arthritis and subcutaneous nodules [62–64]. The effusion may be an incidental finding or may accompany worsening arthritis and increased systemic symptoms. The fluid is straw-coloured, often turbid and typically has a low glucose and pH and a high lactate dehydrogenase. Rheumatoid factor and immune complexes may be found in pleural fluid, often at higher titres than in blood [65,66]. Biopsies of pleura may show typical rheumatoid histology. Thoracoscopy shows a highly characteristic granular appearance to the parietal pleura, with some associated inflammatory changes on the visceral pleura [67]. The granular change is due to palisaded epithelioid cells and occasional giant cells, resembling an opened-out rheumatoid nodule. These nodules may be responsible for the production of the immune complexes often found in the fluid. The condition usually regresses gradually and eventually clears over several months. Corticosteroid treatment may be of value if started early but this has not been clearly established. Chronic persistence of the effusion or progressive pleural fibrosis may lead eventually to the need for pleurectomy. Occasionally the condition may be bilateral and associated with other pulmonary manifestations of rheumatoid disease. There also appears to be a risk of infection of these effusions, leading to empyema [68].

Systemic lupus erythematosus presents not infrequently with pleurisy and, in contrast to rheumatoid pleurisy, is more common in women than men [69–71]. The usual presentation is bilateral small effusions, though unilateral ones are not unusual. Some 40% of patients have pleural effusion at some stage [69,71]. Lupus cells may be demonstrated in the fluid as well as the blood and a high titre of antinuclear antibodies in the fluid is diagnostic [72]. The fluid is often blood-stained and tends to have a normal glucose and low lactate dehydrogenase. Effusions may of course occur in lupus secondary to other complications of the disease, such as uraemia or pneumonia, in which case these antibodies may be absent from the fluid. The lupoid effusion is unlikely to resolve spontaneously, but usually does so in response to corticosteroid treatment. If this fails, cyclophosphamide or azathioprine may be necessary.

Other collagen diseases seem rarely to be associated with pleural effusion unless associated with lupoid features or as a complication of renal or cardiac failure or of pulmonary infection. Wegener's granulomatosis of the lung may be complicated by pleural effusion [73,74], though this is usually small and responds to treatment with cyclophosphamide.

The post-cardiac injury syndrome, a relatively uncommon complication of myocardial infarction or cardiac surgery, is characterized by malaise, fever and pleural and pericardial pain, usually coming on about 3 weeks after the cardiac injury. Effusions may occur in pericardium and pleura, and pulmonary infiltrates may be seen; the fluid is usually bloody with high glucose and pH, and difficulty is often experienced in differentiating the condition from pulmonary infarction. It usually responds to corticosteroid treatment.

Abdominal diseases

Pleural effusion may occur as a complication of a number of non-infective abdominal conditions, apart from the infective ones mentioned above. Acute pancreatitis may lead to pleural exudate, probably by transmission of inflammation through the adjacent diaphragm and of fluid through diaphragmatic lymphatics [75]. The fluid is characterized by high amylase levels, often higher than in serum. Chronic pancreatitis may also cause pseudocyst formation, with a sinus developing between cyst and pleura [76]. Again the fluid shows high amylase levels. Pleural transudates may occur as a complication of ascites due to ovarian fibroma, Meigs' syndrome [27], but more commonly exudates are seen in relation to gastrointestinal or pelvic carcinomas. The late stages of renal failure may be accompanied by pleural and pericardial pain and effusions [77].

Pulmonary embolism and infarction

This condition is described in Chapter 25. As stated above, massive embolism may lead to right-sided heart failure and pleural transudation, although two-thirds of effusions associated with infarction are exudates, sometimes blood-stained [22,23]. The fluid may contain a high proportion of eosinophils.

Other causes

Pleural exudates are an unusual occurrence in patients with sarcoidosis, usually presenting when the disease involves the lungs and often other organs as well [78–81]. The effusions are usually small and contain lymphocytes predominantly [81]. The pleura contains sarcoid granulo-

mas that may be found on biopsy, sometimes leading to confusion with tuberculosis. Usually the tuberculin test is negative and the Kveim test or biopsy of other tissues confirms the diagnosis.

Occasional patients working with asbestos develop pleuritic pain and an effusion, which may be recurrent [82,83]. While this may be the first evidence of mesothelioma, it may be benign asbestos pleurisy. This condition is the most common asbestos-related disease during the first two decades of exposure at work, but may occur for the first time long after exposure has ceased. The effusion is sometimes blood-stained and shows no specific cytological features. It may be an incidental finding on chest radiography, and it is likely that this is the event that leads to diffuse pleural fibrotic changes in a proportion of asbestos workers (Fig. 43.6). The effusion is usually of small or moderate size and may be bilateral. It tends to recur after aspiration but eventually disappears, sometimes leading to pleural fibrosis [83,84].

The yellow nails syndrome is a condition of hypoplasia of lymphatic vessels, leading to lymphoedema of the limbs, dystrophic changes in the nails and, sometimes, intractable pleural effusions [85–87]. The nail changes, which are not always present, take the form of thickening, increased curvature in both long and transverse axes, transverse ridging and a yellow-brown pigmentation (Fig. 43.7). They also grow more slowly than normal. The condition usually presents in adult life and is distributed equally between the sexes. In some cases it appears to be inherited as a dominant characteristic [88]. The cause of the nail changes is not known but the lymphoedema and pleural effusions are related to lymphatic vessel hypoplasia, which may be demonstrated in the limbs by lymphangiography. The condition may be complicated by bronchiectasis, sinusitis or protein-losing enteropathy [89,90] and patients have an increased risk of neoplasms, especially lymphomas and sarcomas [87]. The effusions may not require treatment but can result in pleural fibrosis. If they are sufficiently large to cause symptoms, it may be necessary to carry out pleurodesis or pleuroperitoneal shunt [91]; occasionally pleurectomy has been carried out, and on one occasion the surgical specimen showed abnormal pleural lymphatic vessels [92]. It is assumed that this abnormality hinders the reabsorption of proteins in the fluid, thus leading to effusion [93]. Effusions may occasionally be chylous and have been managed by dietary reduction of fat intake [94].

Certain drugs may provoke pleural effusions as a side-effect (see also Chapter 55). Practolol and methysergide may have a direct effect on serous membranes, leading to effusion and fibrosis [95,96]. In addition, pleural effusion may be associated with eosinophilic reactions induced by such drugs as nitrofurantoin, sulphonamides, salicylates, β-blockers and para-aminosalicylic acid [97]. The eosinophilia–myalgia syndrome is associated with the use

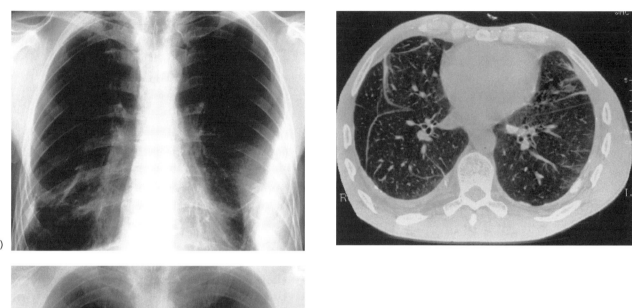

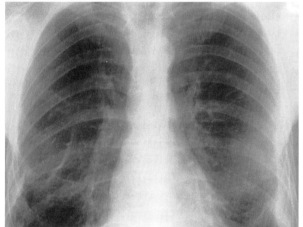

Fig. 43.6 (a) Chest film of patient who presented with pain and weight loss showing a left-sided pleural effusion. He had a 10-year history of asbestos exposure until 10 years previously, and mesothelioma was suspected. (b) Chest film 4 months later showing resolution of the effusion leaving pleural fibrosis. Pleural fibrosis is present on the right side also. (c) CT scan after resolution showing bilateral diffuse pleural fibrosis. The patient remained well 3 years later.

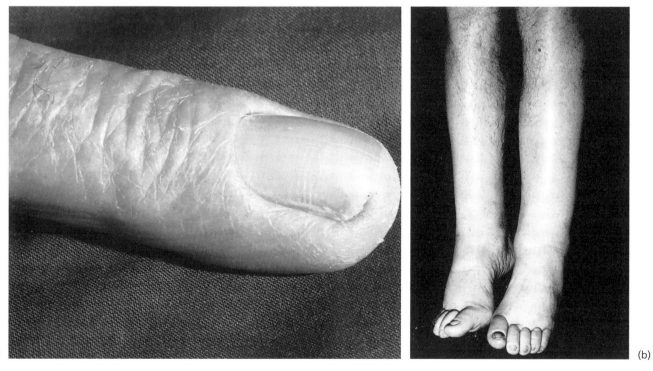

Fig. 43.7 (a) Transversely ridged curved nails of the yellow nails syndrome. (b) Chronic lymphoedema of the legs in the same patient, who presented with pleural effusion.

of L-tryptophan [98]. As mentioned above, the lupus syndrome may be associated with pleural effusion and this may also be caused by drugs such as hydralazine, procainamide, phenytoin and isoniazid [99]. Effusion occasionally follows several months after a course of radiotherapy, though this is rarely large and usually resolves after aspiration [100]. It may also occur when pericardial effusion develops as a complication of mediastinal irradiation [101,102].

The syndrome of recurrent polyserositis, discussed previously, may cause effusions as well as pleural and peritoneal pain [10,11]. Finally, oesophageal rupture leads to mediastinitis with infection of the pleura and effusions containing a high level of salivary amylase, epithelial cells and often food particles [103–105]. It may be associated with mediastinal emphysema and usually follows oesophageal instrumentation, though spontaneous rupture does occur. It is important to recognize this condition early, as it is usually fatal if surgical repair and mediastinal drainage are not instituted promptly [106].

Investigation

A pleural effusion is normally diagnosed by chest radiography, although loculated effusions may require confirmation by ultrasound. However, the radiograph does not usually provide diagnostic information on the cause of the effusion, although evidence of a proximal or pleural tumour or of tuberculosis may be seen. Similarly, the history and clinical examination may sometimes provide clues but do not often give a clear indication of the cause, except in the case of hydrothorax. When taking the history, special attention should be paid to previous illnesses, drug or radiation treatment and symptoms not directly related to the effusion. It should be apparent from the foregoing that pleural fluid often accumulates as a consequence of systemic disease.

If the history and examination indicate a clear cause, no further investigation is necessary though therapeutic aspiration may be desirable. Thus, evidence of congestive heart failure is sufficient to justify a trial of diuretic therapy prior to aspiration of a right-sided or bilateral effusion and evidence of venous thrombosis often leads to treatment with anticoagulants rather than aspiration. In most patients, however, pleural fluid needs to be aspirated.

Pleural aspiration and biopsy

Pleural aspiration should normally be combined with pleural biopsy during the one procedure. The best method is to seat the patient on a stool leaning forward over the side of the bed, with arms folded under the chin. The site is chosen carefully, taking account of the likely position of the diaphragm and the top of the effusion as judged by

percussion. Simple M-mode ultrasound may be very helpful in aspirating loculated effusion [107,108]. Local anaesthetic is infiltrated intradermally, subcutaneously and into muscle and parietal pleura, infiltration continuing until fluid is aspirated. If the pleura is felt to be much thickened, a long lumbar puncture needle may be used. Careful attention to anaesthetic technique, together with a reassuring explanation of the procedure, makes the aspiration less of an ordeal for both patient and doctor.

Care should be taken to insert all needles immediately above the lower rib in order to avoid damage to intercostal nerve and vessels, which lie immediately below each rib. After finding the fluid it is sensible to take some specimens for chemistry, cytology and culture immediately, and to follow this by pleural biopsy. If tuberculosis is suspected, as much fluid as possible should be sent to the microbiology laboratory. Biopsy is usually carried out with an Abrams punch [109], which is inserted along the anaesthetic needle track after its enlargement with a fine-pointed scalpel blade. Biopsies should be taken first laterally and the punch should then be rotated inferiorly and through 180°, avoiding the region of the intercostal bundle. Four or five bites should be taken to increase the chances of a positive finding [110].

Having collected specimens for diagnosis, it may be desirable to remove fluid in order to relieve symptoms. This should be done by aspiration into a large syringe equipped with a three-way tap rather than by insertion of a tube, although tube drainage is often necessary if the fluid is infected. The syringe may be connected to a wide-bore needle (and, after biopsy, to the Abrams needle for convenience) or to a plastic cannula introduced through a needle; the latter method is more comfortable for the patient and involves less risk of puncturing the lung. Aspiration should take place relatively slowly (hence the disadvantage of a tube) since rapid removal of fluid may result in unilateral pulmonary oedema, a complication that may be fatal and which is probably due to increased microvascular permeability in the reinflated lung [111,112]. Removal of large amounts of fluid may also cause hypoxaemia, which can be alleviated by administration of oxygen [113]. It is probable that these complications are related to the generation of excessively negative intrapleural pressures and can be prevented by careful and slow aspiration [114]. If the patient complains of shortness of breath, pain in the chest or general unease during the procedure, it is wise to stop immediately and to take a chest radiograph to exclude pneumothorax or pulmonary oedema.

A fortunately rare complication, though seen occasionally, is air embolism when air is introduced into the pulmonary venous circulation. This may be immediately fatal or attended by loss of consciousness. The patient should immediately be laid down on the left side with head below feet; if a hyperbaric chamber is available its use may be life-saving. Air embolism was a complication of the old artificial pneumothorax treatment of tuberculosis and thus was more familiar to an earlier generation of chest physicians. Pneumothorax is a more frequent complication of pleural aspiration, especially when done by the inexperienced. It is usually due to puncture of the lung, though a careless technique may allow introduction of air through needles or the chest incision. It may require tube drainage. Sometimes the introduction of a small amount of air is useful in a diagnostic sense, since it may demonstrate pleural tumour separate from the effusion. Other occasional complications attendant on careless technique include the introduction of infection and the inadvertent biopsy of lung, liver, spleen or even kidney.

Examination of the fluid

Macroscopic appearances

The fluid of a transudate is clear and pale straw-coloured. Exudates tend to be more amber-coloured and may be turbid if the cell count is high. A fresh exudate often clots on standing, while an older one has often been defibrinated and, like a transudate, remains fluid. Blood in the fluid may be due to damage to a vessel during insertion of the needle or biopsy. If this is the case, the fluid withdrawn into the local anaesthetic syringe is usually clear and later aspirates tend to be less blood-stained than the initial ones. Uniform blood-staining, of a red or brown colour, frequently indicates pleural tumour, although infarction, rheumatoid, leukaemic and tuberculous effusions may be haemorrhagic. Milky fluid is usually due to chyle (see below), though chronic effusions can mimic this appearance due to the presence of fat globules derived from degenerating cells. Purulent fluid in cases of frank empyema is easily recognized, but lesser degrees of infection give the fluid an increased turbidity indistinguishable from that due to a high cell content. A fluid with a shimmering sheen may contain high levels of cholesterol [115], another indication that the effusion is chronic but of no further significance.

Microscopic appearances

A citrated specimen of the fluid should be examined for differential cell count and for malignant cells. The polymorph is predominant when there is an infective cause in lung or pleura, other than tuberculosis, while the lymphocyte is the characteristic cell in tuberculous effusions [116,117]. It is also frequently the predominant cell in malignant effusions. An eosinophilic effusion (with >10% of white cells being eosinophils) is a non-specific finding [118,119] that occurs in association with other diseases characterized by blood eosinophilia, such as pulmonary eosinophilia, polyarteritis nodosa, tropical eosinophilia,

filariasis and Hodgkin's disease, and also in the absence of blood eosinophilia when blood has been introduced into the serous cavity [120]. It is thus seen following trauma, pulmonary infarction and infection. It is relatively unusual in carcinomatous effusions [120]. Eosinophilic effusion has also been described in response to fungal and viral infections. It may be that the common factor is the escape into the pleural fluid of eosinophil chemotactic factor derived from white cells in blood.

The examination of pleural fluid for malignant cells may lead to the diagnosis. However, caution should be exercised in interpreting positive results, since desquamated mesothelial cells may easily be mistaken for malignant cells, even by experienced pathologists [20]. Nevertheless, a high diagnostic yield following careful cytological examination has been reported from specialized laboratories [121,122], and it is likely that the use of newer cell marker techniques will improve the reliability of these diagnostic tests.

Bacteriological culture

Culture of effusions should be carried out as a routine in order to guide therapy if infection is found. If tuberculosis is thought a possibility, several large specimens of fluid should be cultured, since the chances of a positive result increase with the amount of fluid examined.

Biochemical tests

It is usual to measure the protein content of pleural fluid, 30 g/L being taken as the dividing line between transudate and exudate [20,123]. In addition the pleural fluid–serum ratios of lactate dehydrogenase and cholesterol have been found useful in differentiation. Pleural fluid cholesterol is usually less than 55 mg/dL and the fluid–blood ratio is 0.3 or below in transudates [124]. The glucose level may be helpful because it is characteristically low (<1.7 mmol/L or 30 mg/dL) in rheumatoid disease. It may also be low in infected effusions or whenever there is a high cell count [125,126]. Lactate dehydrogenase is raised in exudates above the serum level, but otherwise is a non-specific finding [127]. Amylase levels may be very high (>1000 u/L) in effusions due to pancreatitis and oesophageal rupture [126,128]. The fluid pH is reduced (acid) in pleural inflammatory disease and has been used by some as guide to the use of tube drainage in empyema [129]. In general, however, biochemical tests are not very helpful in a diagnostic sense.

Further diagnostic tests

Ultrasound and CT are now standard investigations in most centres prior to biopsy and aspiration in order to detect evidence of malignant disease, either primary or secondary [130,131]. These investigations are a particularly useful guide to the best site to biopsy, although it should be remembered that they cannot be relied on absolutely in the diagnosis of tumour and tissue diagnosis is necessary in most cases [132]. If clinical examination, aspiration and biopsy fail to give the diagnosis, further tests may be necessary. According to the surgeon's preference, thoracoscopy can be carried out using a rigid thoracoscope or video-assisted techniques with biopsy of any pleural lesions seen [133–135]. This has a high success rate in experienced hands. If it fails, a limited thoracotomy may be necessary for appropriate biopsies to be taken.

Management

The management of pleural effusion depends on the cause. In many cases aspiration is sufficient to cure the problem, although some effusions do recur, especially malignant ones. Infective effusions should be treated with the appropriate antibiotics (see Chapter 14) and tube drainage may be necessary. Tuberculous effusions require antituberculosis chemotherapy along standard lines and it is usual to add corticosteroids (prednisolone 20 mg daily for 2–3 weeks, reducing over a further 2–4 weeks) as there is evidence that this speeds reabsorption and prevents pleural fibrosis [136,137]. Corticosteroids also speed the resolution of effusions due to sarcoidosis, systemic lupus erythematosus, the post-cardiac injury syndrome and possibly rheumatoid disease.

In general, recurrent exudates eventually heal themselves by causing pleural fibrosis; however, since this may cause serious restriction of lung movements the aim of treatment is to prevent it happening by early aspiration and appropriate drugs. However, if there is no specific treatment for the underlying disease and if the effusion is large enough to cause symptoms due to lung compression, treatment may be aimed at producing pleural obliteration by fibrosis. This is the case with malignant effusions, which rarely resolve spontaneously. Several methods have been used to promote pleurodesis, including instillation of nitrogen mustard [138], radioactive colloidal gold [139], tetracycline [140], doxorubicin [141] and quinacrine [142], all of which show a success rate of up to 60%. A suspension of killed *Corynebacterium parvum* has also been used and has been shown to be more effective than nitrogen mustard in controlled trials [143–145], causing less nausea than the former and producing pleurodesis in more than 90% of subjects. There is also some evidence that it lengthens survival in some of the patients [146]. The technique is to aspirate the pleural space until no more fluid is obtained and to inject 7 mg of heat-killed, freeze-dried *C. parvum* in 20 mL saline into the pleural cavity. The patient is then tilted in the bed and placed in series of different positions for 15 min each to ensure generalized distribution of the material over the pleural surface. The usual side-effect is fever associated with malaise for 2–3 days. A brisk pleural reaction occurs that may cause widespread radiological shadowing before the space is obliterated. Reaspiration and a second instillation is sometimes necessary. The mechanism of action of *C. parvum* is not known, but it clearly excites a brisk fibrotic reaction and produces a thick rind round the lung. It may also have an indirect antitumour action, possibly by activating macrophages or natural killer cells [147].

Pleurodesis with *C. parvum* has been so successful in our hands that more aggressive treatment, with insufflation of kaolin or talc through a thoracoscope or intercostal tube or surgical pleurectomy, is now rarely necessary to prevent recurrent effusions. These techniques have been used widely, are effective [148–150] and there is still an occasional need for them, though thoracotomy should only be used as a last resort in patients with pleural tumour. In particular, when using talc for non-malignant effusions care should be taken to ensure that it is not contaminated with tremolite asbestos, the two minerals often occurring together in the same geological formations. Fortunately, one survey of patients many years after talc pleurodesis failed to show any case of mesothelioma developing to the time of the survey [151], and personal investigation of talc BP as used in the UK has shown no contamination.

Chylothorax

Anatomy and physiology

In general, the thoracic duct receives the lymph from both sides of the body below the diaphragm and from the left side above it. The lymph from the right side of the head and neck and right arm is drained into the right lymphatic duct, while that from the right hemithorax is drained into the right bronchomediastinal trunk. The thoracic duct begins in the abdomen as a dilatation called the cisterna chyli, which lies on the front of the upper two lumbar vertebrae between the aorta and the right crus of the diaphragm. The duct passes upwards through the aortic opening of the diaphragm, ascends in the posterior mediastinum behind the diaphragm and then the oesophagus, inclining to the left at the fifth thoracic vertebra to ascend in the superior mediastinum closely applied to the left side of the oesophagus. Entering the root of the neck, it turns laterally between the carotid sheath and the vertebral artery, then downwards in front of the subclavian artery and enters the venous system at the junction of the left internal jugular and subclavian veins. In rather fewer than 50% of subjects there are variations in the anatomy of the thoracic duct, two or more ducts frequently being present at some point in the course.

The right lymphatic duct is usually quite short, about 1 cm long, starting at the medial margin of the scalenus anterior muscle above the subclavian artery where it is formed by the junction of right jugular and subclavian lymph trunks. The right bronchomediastinal trunk runs up the right side of the oesophagus into the neck. Both trunks end in the innominate vein, either separately or as a common trunk. Many anastomoses occur between the bronchomediastinal trunk, thoracic duct and the azygos, intercostal and lumbar veins, so that the thoracic duct may be ligated at any point in its thoracic course without causing problems of lymph drainage [152,153]. This is important in the management of chylothorax.

The chyle that drains up the thoracic duct is an alkaline fluid which may be milky or almost serous in appearance depending on the nutritional state of the subject. On standing it separates into a creamy upper layer rich in chylomicrons, a milky middle layer and a lower layer containing lymphocytes. It has a protein content of 20–60 g/L and a fat content of up to 60 g/L. The amount of chyle produced daily may be as much as 2.5 L [154], again depending on the subject's nutritional status and especially the fat content of the food. Thus the rate of accumulation of a chylothorax may be controlled by dietary measures [94].

Clinical features and aetiology

There are no specific clinical features associated with chylothorax, which presents as does any other pleural effusion. It may be bilateral or unilateral, with a tendency to be right-sided with lesions of the thoracic duct below the fifth dorsal vertebra and left-sided with lesions above that level [155]. It is usually not associated with pleural pain, and infection does not occur because of the antibacterial properties of chyle. The diagnosis is made on aspiration of the fluid, although this is not always obviously milky; it may require biochemical analysis of triglycerides and chylomicrons to confirm the diagnosis [156]. Alternatively, detection of dye or radioactivity in pleural fluid after the patient has eaten butter containing a lipophilic dye or radioiodine-labelled triglyceride also allows confirmation [155,157].

If the effusion is milky, the only possible cause of confusion is the so-called chyliform, pseudochylous or cholesterol effusion [158]. This is usually readily distinguished because it is due to fat globules from degenerating cells in long-standing encysted effusions, usually secondary to tuberculosis or rheumatoid disease. The history and features of the primary condition should allow the distinction to be made without difficulty; if not, the presence of cholesterol crystals and negative dye or radioiodine tests settle the matter.

Chylothorax is uncommon. The most frequent cause is tumour [159], especially lymphoma and metastases from stomach and gastric carcinoma to mediastinal nodes. Occasionally radiotherapy to these tumours may provoke the chylothorax. Extensive blockage or invasion of the duct, with fistula formation, or invasion of the left subclavian vein is responsible. Some 50% of cases are due to tumour, while about 25% are due to trauma [159]. Half of these are the result of damage to the duct at surgery [160,161], especially in the region of the left subclavian vein, though many cervical and thoracic operations may cause this, from neck dissection, cervical sympathectomy and oesophagectomy to coronary bypass, high lumbar aortography and diaphragmatic hernia repair. The other half are due to knife and bullet wounds or stretching and bending injuries to the spine; sometimes these may be surprisingly minor, such as coughing, straining or vomiting [162,163]. Of the remaining 25% a few may be due to tuberculous mediastinal nodes, filariasis, left subclavian vein thrombosis, thoracic aortic aneurysm, lymphangioleiomyomatosis and thoracic duct lymphangiomatosis, sometimes associated with generalized lymphangiomatosis and lymphoedema [164,165]. Finally, a proportion of cases seem to have no obvious cause. This is particularly so with the neonatal type [166], which presents within a day or two of birth and, though rare, is the most common cause of pleural effusion at that early stage of life.

Traumatic chylothorax usually presents 2–10 days after the injury, the interval being the time taken for a mediastinal chylous cyst to rupture into the pleura [167]. Drainage is only required to relieve the symptom of increasing dyspnoea; however, since recurrent aspirations are almost always necessary, this leads to the important complication of nutritional deficiency. Thus emaciation and dehydration occur quickly without appropriate treatment, death ensuing.

Management

If the patient's nutritional status can be maintained, spontaneous or traumatic damage to the thoracic duct may heal. Thus, in such cases, a trial of conservative treatment is justified [168]. This means tube drainage of the pleural space, reduction of chyle formation by cessation of oral feeding and total parenteral nutrition. Assuming the patient's nutritional status is maintained, it is reasonable to wait about a week to see if the drainage of chyle is ceasing. If it is not, surgical treatment is indicated [169]. The surgeon usually attempts to locate the tear, using an injection of Evans blue dye into a leg as a marker, and suture the duct above and below it [155]. Alternatively, active attempts at talc, kaolin or tetracycline pleurodesis, combined with tube drainage, may be used at an early stage and have been reported to be successful [170,171].

In the case of non-traumatic chylothorax, the treatment is planned in the light of the primary disease, bearing in mind the principles of maintaining nutrition and preventing chyle leaking into the pleura. Thus, lymphoma may well respond to radiotherapy or chemotherapy, although pleurodesis and tube drainage as above may be necessary as well. Symptomatic relief in the case of metastatic carcinoma may also be provided by radiotherapy, though pleurodesis or low thoracic duct ligation may also be necessary. In some cases of terminal disease, it may be kinder to avoid all such measures and simply palliate the patient's symptoms with appropriate drugs.

Pleural plaques

Clinical features

Pleural plaques are benign fibrous lesions of the parietal pleura that occur as a result of exposure to asbestos; however, they may frequently be found at postmortem in people in whom such exposure was not known. Radiologically they present as indistinct elevations of the pleura [172], which may easily be missed unless they are large

and multiple (Fig. 43.8); indeed one autopsy series has shown only a 15% ante-mortem diagnosis rate [173]. Moreover, pleural fat pads and companion shadows may easily be mistaken for plaques, leading to a tendency to false-positive diagnoses. Thus diagnosis of fibrous plaques by routine chest radiography is unreliable. However, most long-standing plaques calcify and this leads to characteristic radiological shadows, often seen most distinctly as elongated 2–3 mm wide calcifications on the lateral chest wall, diaphragm and pericardium but also *en face* as 'holly leaf' shadows (Fig. 43.9). In cases of doubt, and where the additional radiation is considered justified, CT proves a reliable means of diagnosing and defining the extent of plaques [174]. Parietal pleural plaques would not be expected to cause any detectable lung functional impairment; studies demonstrating abnormalities in such subjects are likely due to the effects of asbestos exposure or some confounder, usually cigarette smoking, on the lungs.

Pathological features

Pathologically, pleural plaques are smooth, whitish-

Fig. 43.8 Fibrous pleural plaques (arrowed) in retired asbestos worker, best seen in left mid zone and under lateral chest wall.

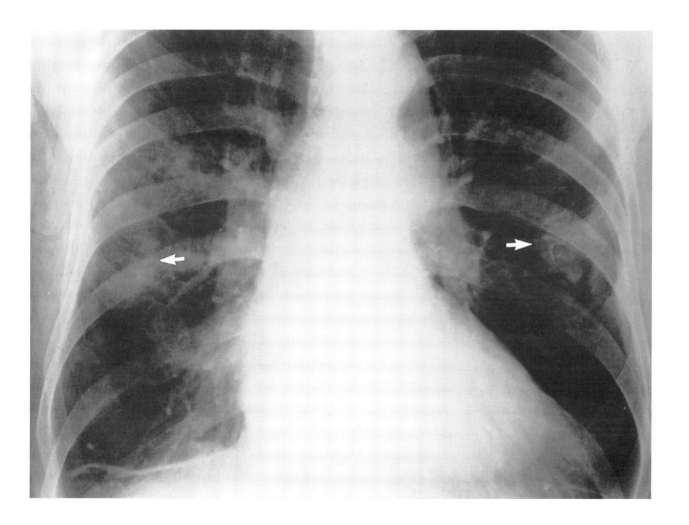

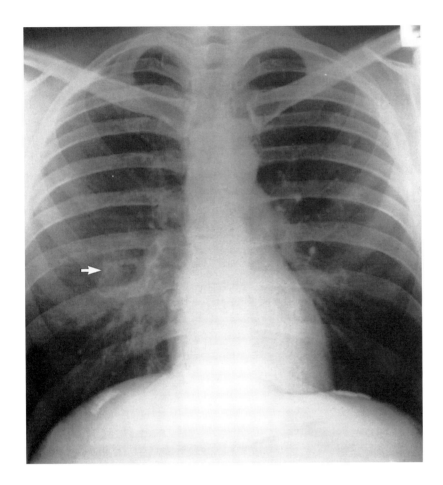

Fig. 43.9 Calcified plaques on diaphragm and, *en face*, in right mid zone (arrowed).

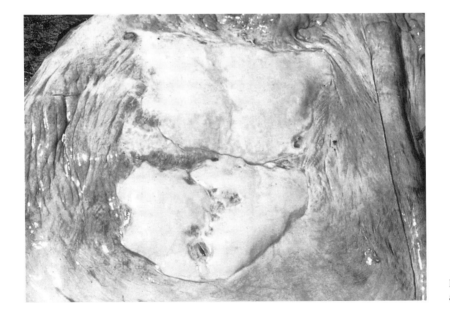

Fig. 43.10 Diaphragmatic pleural plaques as seen at necropsy.

yellow elevations of the parietal pleura, separated distinctly from surrounding mesothelium and having their centres usually over a rib or over the central tendon of the diaphragm (Fig. 43.10). They vary in size from pin-head to that of a hand and are almost always multiple. Histologically, they consist of collagen arranged in a basket-weave pattern and covered by an intact and non-metaplastic mesothelial layer [175]. In their deeper layers there may be small collections of lymphocytes and plasma cells. Asbestos fibres may be found in plaques by electron microscopy but are usually too small and sparse to be seen by light microscopy. Electron microscopy has shown these to be predominantly short chrysotile fibres [176]. Asbestos bodies are not present in plaques, although they may be found in the subject's lung.

Aetiology

It is well established that plaques occur most frequently in populations exposed industrially to asbestos, although exposure does not have to be heavy or prolonged [177]. Usually plaques only make their radiological appearance about 10 years, and calcification usually only 20 years, or more after first exposure. They have also been found in populations exposed to the non-asbestos fibrous mineral erionite present in the environment in certain parts of Turkey [178,179], and in people exposed environmentally, rather than occupationally, to naturally occurring soil or rock asbestos in parts of Finland, central Europe, Turkey and Greece [180,181].

It is likely that pleural plaques are a benign reaction to an individual fibre or a very small number of fibres that have lodged in the parietal pleura, probably being transferred via pleural lymphatics. Their site, centred over ribs and diaphragmatic tendon, suggests that the fibre's progress through the lung, as a result of forces exerted by lung movement, has been arrested by impenetrable tissue. There is no evidence that the plaque is in any way premalignant, although a subject with plaques has been exposed to asbestos and may be at increased risk of lung cancer or mesothelioma in relation to the intensity and duration of such exposure.

Management

Pleural plaques are of no account save as a marker of asbestos exposure. Since they are benign, reassurance should be given to the individual in whom they are found and he or she should not be followed up in clinic. The risk of mesothelioma in such an individual is likely to be greater than in someone without plaques, and depends upon their exposure to asbestos rather than the presence of the plaques (see Chapter 54). In any case, the risk cannot be reduced further by any action other than by ensuring no future exposure to asbestos. However, a number of people with plaques and no other disease have received compensation for having these wholly benign lesions, thus increasing anxiety and public misconceptions about their nature. The sensible physician recognizes and attempts to allay the natural anxiety of a patient in whom these plaques have been found, and is now able to provide a sensible risk estimate based on likely past exposure to asbestos (see Chapter 54).

Pleural fibrosis

Distinction should be made between pleural plaques, which are well-demarcated lesions of the parietal pleura, and pleural fibrosis, which is a diffuse process involving both layers of pleura and not infrequently extending into the surface of the lung.

Clinical features

Pleural fibrosis is usually the sequel of an unabsorbed pleural effusion, although the presence of the effusion may not have been recognized clinically (see Fig. 43.6). Thus it may present in a patient with a recent history of effusion or episode of pleural pain, or it may be found incidentally on chest radiographs. The lesion may be unilateral or bilateral. Whether it is associated with symptoms depends on its extent and on the health of the underlying lung; in general, bilateral thickening has to be quite extensive before it interferes seriously with lung expansion, while unilateral thickening is unlikely to cause symptoms unless associated with other lung disease. The physiological effects of pleural fibrosis are decreased lung volumes, without reduction in transfer coefficient, and decreased compliance. These features may be associated with exertional dyspnoea. Chest pain is not usually a feature and when it is present it should always lead the physician to suspect that the pleural thickening is due to tumour rather than fibrosis. However, it is apparent that some patients with asbestos pleural fibrosis present to their doctors with pleuritic pain or with a persistent chest wall ache [182].

The radiological features vary according to the cause. There may be localized lower zone thickening with obliteration of the costophrenic angle following an unresolved effusion, or more generalized changes. These may have the appearance of 'crow's feet', irregular streaky shadows, diffuse thickening of pleura or a combination. Calcification may be present; if this is unilateral the fibrosis is likely to be due to an old haemothorax or tuberculous effusion, but if bilateral is almost certainly due to asbestos exposure (Fig. 43.11). Grossly thickened pleura with nodular changes is unlikely to be due to fibrosis alone and usually indicates pleural infiltration by carcinoma or mesothelioma.

Occasionally, pleural thickening is responsible for distortion and atelectasis of underlying lung with infolding of pleura, causing appearances resembling tumour. This appearance is sometimes called Blesovsky's syndrome [183,184]. It should be noted that it occurs with diffuse thickening and not with pleural plaques. Some patients with this syndrome may complain of persistent non-pleuritic chest pain.

The clinical course of pleural thickening is varied. In many cases it does not progress. However, when the cause

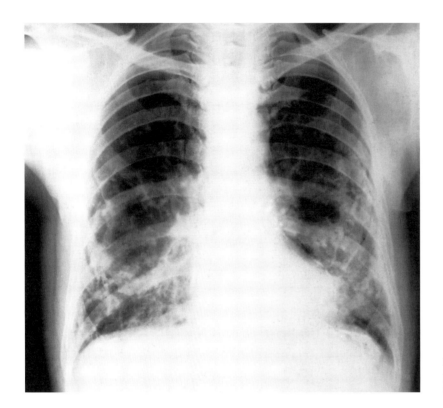

Fig. 43.11 Extensive bilateral calcified pleural fibrosis in pipe lagger exposed for many years to asbestos.

is still active, as for example with collagen disease, asbestos and drug therapy, it may progress, infiltrate the peripheral lung and cause restrictive interference with lung function. Pleural thickening is often associated with physical signs. The localized type mimics pleural effusion, with local reduction in movements, percussion note and breath sounds. The generalized type may cause marked limitation of chest wall movements, retraction of intercostal spaces and flattening of the chest wall, mimicking the features of extensive pulmonary fibrosis. As stated above, in such cases lung fibrosis is often present also by extension from the pleura. It is not uncommon to be able to hear inspiratory crackles and there is evidence that these may in some cases originate in the pleura and be distinct from those due to underlying pulmonary fibrosis; in such cases there may be a mid-expiratory component [185].

Causes

Any cause of pleural exudate may be responsible for the subsequent development of pleural fibrosis, usually of the localized type. However there are relatively few commonly recognized causes of general pleural fibrosis (Table 43.3). If it is calcified, it is likely to be due to old empyema or haemothorax, tuberculous effusion, artificial pneumothorax treatment or asbestos exposure [186]. Bilateral, diffuse, non-calcified thickening suggests a collagen disease or therapy with β-blockers or methysergide [95,96] (Fig. 43.12).

Table 43.3 Causes of generalized pleural fibrosis.

Tuberculous effusion	Unilateral	Calcified
Old artificial pneumothorax	Unilateral	Calcified
Haemothorax	Unilateral	Calcified
Multiple rib fractures	Either	Either
Old empyema	Unilateral	Either
Thoracotomy, thoracoplasty	Unilateral	Uncalcified
Radiation therapy	Unilateral	Uncalcified
Rheumatoid disease	Bilateral	Uncalcified
Systemic lupus	Bilateral	Uncalcified
Drugs (practolol, methysergide)	Bilateral	Uncalcified
Asbestos exposure	Usually bilateral	Calcified
Silicotic massive fibrosis	Overlying the PMF	Uncalcified

PMF, progressive massive fibrosis.

Investigation and management

The clinical history and chest radiograph are usually sufficient to lead to the diagnosis. Care should be taken to exclude asbestos exposure and drug therapy as causes. In the case of the former, diffuse pleural thickening should only be attributed to asbestos exposure if the patient has worked regularly with the material; occasional, incidental or non-occupational exposure to asbestos is very unlikely to cause anything other than pleural plaques. There is evidence from lung asbestos counts that diffuse pleural fibrosis occurs at exposure levels comparable to those that cause early asbestosis [187].

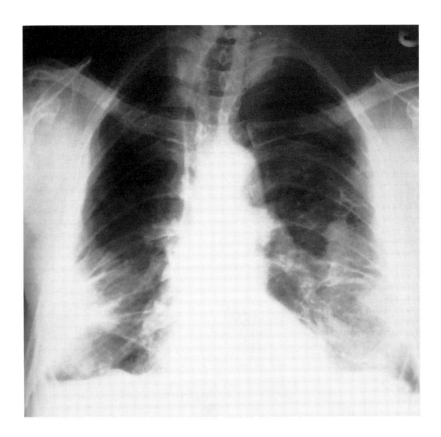

Fig. 43.12 Bilateral non-calcified pleural fibrosis in patient treated for 10 years with methysergide for migraine.

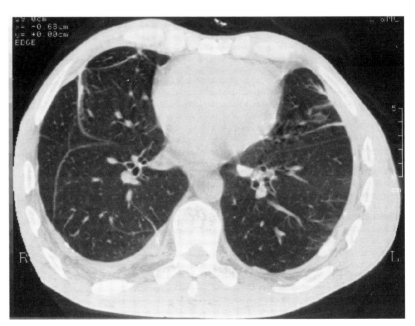

Fig. 43.13 High-resolution CT scan of asbestos worker showing diffuse pleural fibrosis with some extension into underlying lung. Calcification is visible bilaterally.

The main problem in diagnosis is differentiation of the lesion from malignant infiltration of the pleura, especially by mesothelioma. Mesothelioma is usually unilateral and associated with some nodular change. However, metastases and alveolar cell carcinoma may present with bilateral pleural involvement. If a primary tumour is not demonstrable, bronchoscopy and needle biopsy of the pleura may be necessary, though these investigations may be avoided if the appearances are shown to have been present on previous radiographs. CT may be useful in deciding whether extension of the fibrosis into lung has occurred and when surgical treatment is being contemplated [188], and is commonly used in the assessment of asbestos disease (Fig. 43.13).

Apart from the treatment of any underlying cause, such as cessation of drugs or appropriate therapy for collagen disease, there is only one therapeutic decision: whether to seek the advice of a thoracic surgeon. Pleurectomy and 'decortication', i.e. removal of the thick fibrous peel, may release the lung and chest wall and thereby relieve the restriction to ventilation. This operation has much to offer in the case of localized fibrothorax following empyema or tuberculous effusion and surgical advice should be sought early in these situations [189]. Where fibrosis is generalized and well established, the decision should be made after consideration of the patient's disability and age and in the knowledge that the procedure may be hazardous and not produce a dramatic improvement. In particular, care should be taken to assess the underlying lung for the presence of disease such as fibrosis and bronchiectasis and for the extension of pleural disease into its surface; the former prevents a good functional result while the latter causes surgical difficulties and complications. Bronchoscopy, bronchography, CT and regional lung function testing may all be of value in coming to a decision about surgery. In general, the more recent the development of the fibrothorax, the more likely is surgical success, and the more extensive the fibrosis, the better the functional result after surgery. Patients with Blesovsky's syndrome not infrequently undergo surgery in the belief that the lesion is a tumour. Long-term results are generally satisfactory in that it does not recur, although lung function may not improve and may even deteriorate [190]. Operation for asbestos pleural fibrosis is inadvisable since the underlying lung is usually involved and results are likely to be poor.

Tumours of the pleura

Secondary tumour of the pleura is quite common and is discussed briefly in Chapter 42. Primary pleural tumour is increasing in incidence. The most important and most common, occurring in over 1000 people annually in the UK, is malignant mesothelioma. Benign mesothelioma or fibroma and sarcoma are very uncommon primary pleural tumours.

Localized fibrous pleural tumour (pleural fibroma, benign mesothelioma)

Clinical features

This tumour [191–193] may present as an incidental radiological finding or on account of symptoms; when these are present they may be due to direct pressure effects of the lesion, which cause breathlessness, or to one of the recognized indirect effects: fever and chills [194,195], hypoglycaemia [196] or hypertrophic pulmonary osteoarthropathy [197]. The patient is usually over 40,

although children have been described with the disease. Clinical signs depend on the size of the tumour, which may be very large and mimic massive pleural effusion; in one case, signs suggestive of constrictive pericarditis related to gross mediastinal displacement have been reported [195].

The radiological appearance is usually that of a spherical or lobulated peripheral mass adjacent to the pleura. Occasionally it may have a broad base (Fig. 43.14a) but more usually the pleural connection is a narrow pedicle. As it may arise from parietal or visceral pleura, it may occur anywhere on the chest film in relation to chest wall, diaphragm, mediastinum or fissures. In fissures it may have an ovoid shape. It may be complicated by pleural effusion, which is sometimes blood-stained [194,198].

Pathologically, the tumour is well encapsulated, surrounded by compressed lung, from which it can be shelled out easily. The histological appearances are predominantly of interlaced fibrous tissue with few mitotic figures and areas of myxomatous degeneration (Fig. 43.14b). However, pleomorphic types are well recognized and there may be difficulty in deciding whether the tumour has undergone sarcomatous change [191,199]. While the cell of origin may be mesothelial in some cases, in others the histology suggests submesothelial mesenchymal origin [191].

Investigation and management

Localized fibrous tumour can rarely be distinguished clinically from bronchial carcinoma; in any case, because of its potential for malignant change the treatment is surgical. Sometimes the presence of hypertrophic osteoarthropathy in association with a tumour adjacent to the pleura suggests the diagnosis. The presence of a haemorrhagic effusion should not prevent surgery.

Surgical resection can usually be carried out without removing lung and is normally curative. Secondary effects of the tumour, such as fever and joint pains, disappear by the time the patient wakes from the anaesthetic, while the clubbing and swelling of the osteoarthropathy settle over a month or two. The tumour may sometimes recur and need further resection; osteoarthropathy may be the symptom that announces this. Occasionally the tumour behaves like a sarcoma and metastasizes widely.

Pleural sarcoma

This is a very rare and highly malignant tumour that occurs predominantly in young adults [191]. Although it may be confused histologically and radiologically with fibrous or malignant mesothelioma, it is distinguished by the age group of the patient and the tendency to metastasize early. The clinical course is characterized by local invasion of lung and chest wall as well as by blood-

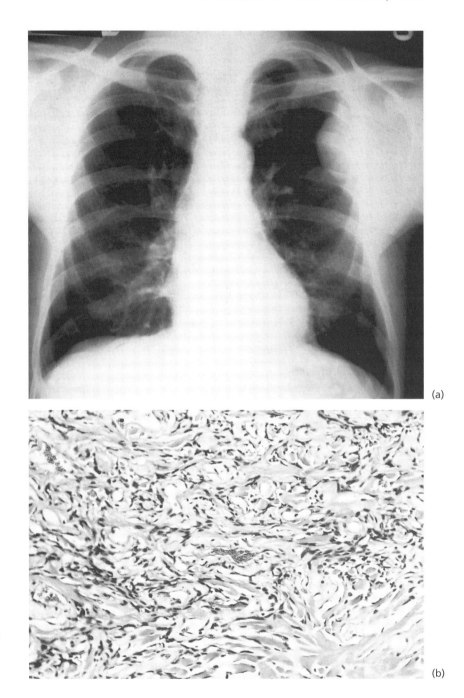

(a)

(b)

Fig. 43.14 (a) Broad-based chest wall tumour in left upper zone. At operation this proved to be a fibroma. (b) Histology of resected specimen showing admixture of spindle cells and mature collagen.

borne metastases. Histologically it has a pleomorphic appearance, with spindle and polygonal cells with many mitoses.

Malignant mesothelioma

Aetiology

Before 1960, malignant mesothelioma [200] was regarded as a very rare tumour of unknown aetiology. Several classical cases were described from Glasgow in 1945 but their histological classification was not recognized [201]. In

1960, however, Wagner and colleagues [202] described a large cluster of patients with the disease in the crocidolite asbestos mining area of the North-Western Cape in South Africa. Many further studies have now confirmed the strong association between the tumour and exposure to crocidolite, especially in asbestos product manufacture, ship-breaking and gas mask production. There has been much debate about two other important matters with respect to aetiology: whether all types of asbestos cause the disease, and how large an exposure is necessary for the risk of mesothelioma to be incurred. With respect to the former, animal studies have shown that any asbestos type, indeed many synthetic and other naturally occurring fibrous minerals, provoke mesothelioma when injected directly into the pleural or peritoneal cavity, although the frequency of this response differs with dose and with different mineral types [203]. However, studies of human populations have shown that the risks of mesothelioma are remote in people exposed only to chrysotile [204], definite in those exposed to amosite [205] and high (up to 10% after as little as a year's exposure) in those exposed to crocidolite [206]. These exposures apply to an occupational setting; para-occupational exposures, such as regular washing of a worker's overalls or close proximity to asbestos insulation work, may also involve high and prolonged dosage and may lead to mesothelioma [207]. The second, and connected, question concerns the amount of asbestos required to provoke mesothelioma. Evidence from pure exposures to crocidolite and amosite has shown that the disease may develop after exposures (almost certainly to very high fibre levels) for as little as 6 months [205,206]. However, there is no evidence associating the disease with exposures to the very low levels that may be found in buildings with undisturbed asbestos walling or insulation. Non-occupational exposures leading to mesothelioma have been described, for example children habitually playing on asbestos waste tips or people living close to a heavily polluting asbestos factory, but these levels of exposure have almost certainly been of the same order of magnitude as those of asbestos workers [207].

The apparent conflicts between the human and experimental data on aetiology are resolved by the hypothesis that chrysotile, while carcinogenic to the pleura, does not normally reach the target organ in sufficiently large doses to initiate the process. Two factors may be responsible for this: (i) its curly nature prevents sufficient being inhaled and (iii) once inhaled the fibres do not reach the pleura in sufficient numbers. Support for the hypothesis comes from the observation that in people with mixed exposures to asbestos much less chrysotile is found in the lungs at postmortem than would be expected from the exposure history, while proportionally much larger amounts of crocidolite or amosite are found [208]. It seems likely that chrysotile does not penetrate so readily into the lung because of its physical and mineralogical characteristics; once in the lung, over the years of residence it is gradually broken down into microfibrils sufficiently small to be removed by macrophages.

Thus it can be stated with reasonable confidence that mesothelioma is a disease that occurs in people who have been exposed to relatively high levels of crocidolite or amosite in the past, almost always as part of their occupation. In people with no known exposure to these minerals, the risk is about one in a million, since sporadic cases unassociated with any known aetiological agent do occur; in those with heavy past exposure, the risk may be as high as 15%. However, in terms of predicting risk in the

majority of patients presenting with fear of future disease, these figures are often unhelpful since people have usually had mixed exposures in the user industries and never know exactly what they have worked with. The matter of predicting risk is discussed in the section on management.

Mesothelioma has also been described in people living in parts of rural Turkey. Two endemic areas have been discovered, one where the use of naturally occurring tremolite asbestos as building material and whitewash is responsible [180] and another where a non-asbestos mineral, fibrous erionite, is thought to be the cause [178]. The importance of the latter observation is that erionite, though fibrous, is not related to asbestos, thus lending strong support to the hypothesis that the propensity of a mineral to cause mesothelioma is due to its physical rather than its chemical properties. This casts doubt over the safety of a number of other fibrous substitutes for asbestos, such as artificial glass and carbon fibres and naturally occurring vermiculite and wollastonite. So far no epidemiological or clinical evidence has implicated these substances in the causation of mesothelioma, although superfine glass fibres have caused the disease when injected directly into the peritoneum or pleura of rats [209]. It would therefore be prudent for industry to avoid the use of such very fine fibres and to confine commercial interest to those outside the respirable range.

One other intriguing clue to the aetiology of mesothelioma has come from a study that has shown DNA sequences resembling those of a monkey virus, SV40, in human mesothelioma tissue. This virus contaminated some of the injected Salk poliomyelitis vaccines used in the 1950s and, if these observations are confirmed, may be a factor predisposing some individuals to the disease, perhaps acting in synergy with asbestos [210,211].

Approximately 1000 people each year die of mesothelioma in the UK, this figure having risen annually since reliable records were first kept in the late 1960s. This rise has been related to the much increased importation of all forms of asbestos during and after the Second World War that continued almost exponentially until 1970. In that year, crocidolite was effectively banned and control of the use of all asbestos considerably tightened. By 1980, importation of amosite had ceased and that of chrysotile had reduced substantially (Fig. 43.15). Unfortunately, this continued extensive use of asbestos for at least 20 years after the association with mesothelioma was described, together with the fact that once in place the mineral remains a threat to those who are required to remove or otherwise work with it, means that the epidemic of mesothelioma is likely to continue rising for a further 20 years and ultimately may be responsible for some 3000 deaths in the UK each year [212]. Mesothelioma is now the most common of the serious dust-related diseases seen in the UK, as well as being the most fatal.

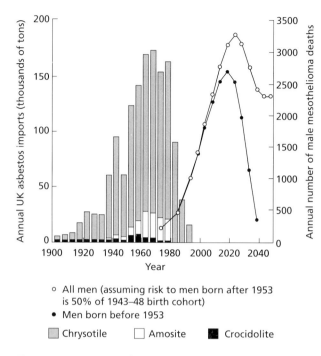

Fig. 43.15 Importation of asbestos into the UK and predicted annual deaths of British men from mesothelioma. (From Peto *et al.* [212] with permission.)

Clinical features

Mesothelioma may affect pleura, peritoneum or pericardium [213]. The last two sites are much less common than the first, and peritoneal mesothelioma seems to have occurred more frequently in the past, reflecting particularly high previous exposures. The tumour characteristically presents 20–40 years after first exposure to asbestos, and often the victim has forgotten that he or she worked with the mineral. However, it is usually possible to obtain a history of work likely to have entailed exposure; jobs in railway workshops, shipyards, ships' engine rooms, gas mask or asbestos manufacture, thermal insulation or building are those most frequently associated with the disease. The first symptoms of mesothelioma are those associated with pleural effusion, breathlessness and chest pain. Often the chest pain is a persistent dull ache, but it may be severe. As the disease progresses, the pain and breathlessness become more troublesome and the patient loses weight. Distant metastases rarely present clinical problems, although they are usually found at post-mortem. Local spread of disease, causing cardiac tamponade, superior caval or oesophageal obstruction, spinal cord and intercostal nerve involvement or chest wall infiltration, is a usual feature; tumour very frequently grows through thoracotomy scars and not uncommonly through needle tracks. Examination of the patient reveals the signs of pleural effusion, though mediastinal displacement to the opposite side is unusual; this combination of appar-

ently massive effusion without displacement of the heart should lead to suspicion of malignant pleural disease. Finger clubbing and hypertrophic osteoarthropathy are rare.

The radiographic features are usually of a large pleural effusion. If the pleura can be seen, pleural nodules may be visible (Fig. 43.16). The lesion is almost always unilateral, although spread across the mediastinum sometimes occurs. Other features of asbestos-related disease may be seen, such as pleural plaques or asbestosis in the opposite lung.

The diagnosis is made on the history and by needle biopsy of the pleura. Typically an attempt to aspirate the effusion is thwarted by encountering much-thickened pleura, and biopsy of this with a cutting needle or drill may show characteristic features. If fluid is withdrawn, it is an exudate and often haemorrhagic. Hyaluronic acid may be present in the fluid or tissue, and cytology with electron microscopy may be useful in the hands of experts [214,215]. However, often the diagnosis cannot be made on examination of the fluid. Moreover, needle biopsy specimens may provide insufficient tissue for a firm diagnosis to be made. In these circumstances, it is wise neither to repeat the procedure too frequently nor to resort to thoracotomy for diagnosis; evidence of pleural tumour, consistent with the diagnosis, is sufficient to exclude a treatable cause of the pleural disease and is also adequate evidence in the UK for industrial injuries benefit to be paid.

The only treatable condition that may mimic mesothelioma is tuberculous pleural disease, and diagnostic efforts should be directed towards excluding this. However, the usual problem in differential diagnosis is whether the condition is mesothelioma or secondary pleural carcinoma. The latter is usually bilateral, except when due to bronchial or breast carcinoma. Certain tumour markers may be helpful in differentiation if the histological appearances are equivocal. Secondary adenocarcinomas frequently stain positively for carcinoembryonic antigen or β_1 pregnancy-specific glycoprotein, whereas mesothelioma is usually negative for these [216]. However, until satisfactory treatment becomes available for these tumours, differentiation is of no value to the patient.

The clinical course of mesothelioma is one of steady deterioration to death over 1–2 years; patients are only rarely alive more than 2 years after diagnosis, although there is some evidence that those with a predominantly epithelial histological pattern have a somewhat better prognosis, a few long-term survivals in this group having been described [200]. Death usually occurs after a prolonged period of increasing chest pain and breathlessness, and may be precipitated by terminal infection or cardiac involvement. Loss of appetite and weight are constant features.

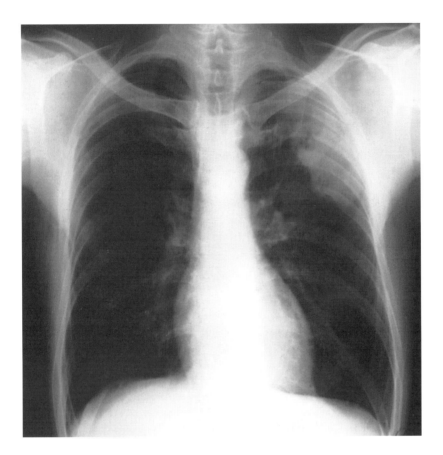

Fig. 43.16 Unusual presentation of mesothelioma without pleural effusion but with extensive tumour in left upper chest wall.

Pathology

The gross appearances are of a thick rind of white or grey-yellow tissue surrounding the lung and usually involving both pleural layers [217,218] (Fig. 43.17). The pleural space may be wholly or partly obliterated; where it persists it contains mucinous or haemorrhagic fluid. The tumour infiltrates lung, chest wall and diaphragm, and is frequently present in surgical wounds and needle tracks. Although few in number, metastases are frequently present in lung, nodes and other viscera.

The histological appearances vary, reflecting the potential of mesothelial cells to differentiate into epithelial or mesenchymal tissue. Typically there is much collagen, often containing clefts lined by tumour cells (Fig. 43.18). The predominant histological pattern may be epithelial, consisting of cuboidal or flattened cells forming tubular and papillary structures separated by a matrix that may consist of closely packed spheroidal cells, collagen or a mixture. This type may be confused with adenocarcinoma, especially with small biopsies, and it is in these circumstances that special stains may be of value in differentiation. The other main histological type consists of diffuse spindle cells, resembling sarcoma. Frequently the two types coexist in different areas of the same tumour. There is some evidence that the epithelial type has a slightly better prognosis than the mixed and sarcomatous types. Asbestos bodies are not usually seen in the tumour but may be found in the lungs of the patient. Analysis of lung tissue using phase-contrast optical microscopy for uncoated asbestos fibres usually reveals large numbers [219]. Electron microscopy is necessary to analyse the fibres, since it is not possible to differentiate asbestos from other fibres commonly found in lungs by light microscopy [220]. Electron microprobe analysis usually shows the asbestos present to be predominantly crocidolite or amosite, since over time chrysotile dissolves. It should be stressed that such expensive and time-consuming analyses are of great value in research into asbestos-related diseases but have no useful application in clinical diagnosis. However, they are used increasingly in litigation issues, since the very large numbers generated by these methods have an impressive effect on judges and juries.

Management

The prospects for curative treatment are not good. Surgery, radical radiotherapy and chemotherapy have all been tried and a number of enthusiastic reports published. However, none of these has been controlled and the few long-term survivors are matched by those from untreated series. In particular, it is wise to be sceptical of reports of improved survival rates in people treated for 'early disease'. Clearly, the earlier intervention occurs in the natural history of a disease, the longer the apparent sur-

vival unless the treatment actually reduces it, and it is therefore necessary in any such research to have controls in order to demonstrate benefit convincingly. Surgery, which is popular in the USA, has a high mortality and is attended by considerable discomfort. Radiotherapy may produce some regression and prevent reaccumulation of fluid, although the author's experience suggests that it has a useful place in palliation of tumour growing through aspiration tracks or wounds and might also have a pro-phylactic role after aspiration or pleural biopsy. Single-agent therapy with doxorubicin, cyclophosphamide, interferon γ and other drugs and multiple regimens have been tried, all with anecdotal reports of improvement. Perhaps the most promising has been interferon γ admin-istered intrapleurally, although in this study the response was seen only in very early cases who might well have been expected to live longer anyway [221]. There is clearly a need for multicentre controlled trials, and until then the management of individual patients must depend on the physician's judgement. Since the chances of achieving long-term remission seem as bad with treatment as without and the side-effects of treatment often add to the patient's misery, it is wise to confine treatment to pallia-tion of symptoms with appropriate analgesics. Radiother-apy or *C. parvum* pleurodesis may be helpful in preventing recurrent effusions and the former may be useful in the relief of local bone or nerve pain or in reducing the size of subcutaneous extensions of tumour.

An increasingly frequent aspect of management related to mesothelioma is the requirement to advise patients who have been exposed to asbestos about their risks of developing the disease. This arises particularly in relation to the finding of pleural plaques on a chest radiograph, which sometimes leads to ill-considered advice to sue an employer rather than to reassurance

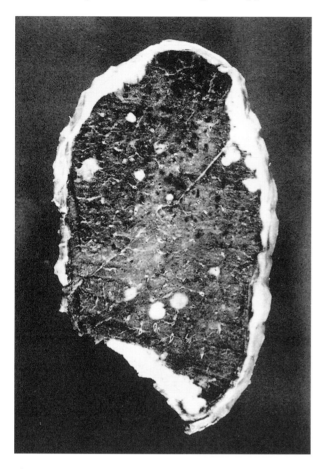

Fig. 43.17 Excised lung with surrounding mesothelioma. Some metastatic deposits are also visible in the lung.

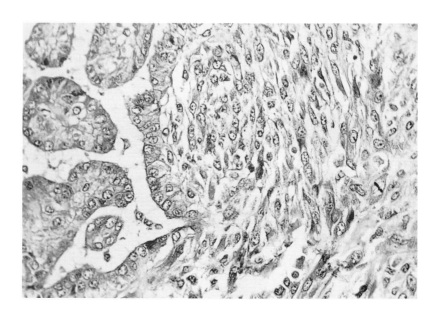

Fig. 43.18 Histological appearance of a malignant mesothelioma showing tubopapillary tumour to the left and sarcomatous cells to the right. Note the mitotic figure in the mid right (haematoxylin & eosin ×300).

about the benign nature of this condition. It is now possible to make reasonable predictions of risk from the epidemiological study of Peto and colleagues [212]. These authors have calculated lifetime probabilities of death from mesothelioma for British males by year of birth. For those born between 1933 and 1938 the risk is about 8 per 1000, rising to about 12 per 1000 in the 1943–48 birth cohort. These estimates may be multiplied by the relative risks for different trades (e.g. 7 for metal plate and shipyard workers, 4 for plumbers and 3 for electricians) to give an estimate that can be further weighted by a detailed knowledge of the individual's exposure history within the confidence intervals given in the paper. Thus a shipyard worker, such as a shipwright or boilermaker, born in 1943 might have a lifetime risk (assuming typical exposure to asbestos in that trade) of about 8%. This can be explained

to an individual in relation to risks of other diseases such as heart attack or any type of cancer in order to put matters into some sort of perspective. It has to be said that this form of prediction has become a necessary part of the business of preparing a medicolegal report and almost inevitably causes anxiety to the patient unless explained very carefully.

Other pleural lesions

Endometriosis may very rarely involve the pleura, causing haemopneumothorax associated with menstruation [222,223]. Transplantation of splenic tissue to the pleura, splenosis pleurae, has been described very rarely following abdominal injuries with rupture of the spleen [224]. They present as rounded pleural opacities.

References

1 Wiener-Kornish JP, Broaddus VC. Interrelationship of pleural and pulmonary interstitial liquid. *Annu Rev Physiol* 1993; 55: 209.
2 Claus RH, Yacoubian NH, Barker HG. Dynamics of pleural effusion. *Surg Forum* 1956; 7: 201.
3 Miserocchi G, Negrini D, Mariani E, Passafaro M. Reabsorption of a saline- or plasma-induced hydrothorax. *J Appl Physiol* 1983; 54: 1574.
4 Leckie WJH, Tothill P. Albumin turnover in pleural effusions. *Clin Sci* 1965; 29: 339.
5 Leak LV, Rahil K. Permeability of the diaphragmatic mesothelium: the ultrastructural basis for 'stomata'. *Am J Anat* 1978; 151: 557.
6 Hills BA, Butler BD, Barrow RE. Boundary lubrication imparted by pleural surfactants and their identification. *J Appl Physiol* 1982; 53: 463.
7 Gordon RB, Lennette EH, Sandrock RS. The varied clinical manifestations of Coxsackie virus infection. *Arch Intern Med* 1959; 103: 63.
8 Kantor FS, Hsiuing GD. Pleurodynia associated with Echovirus type 8. *N Engl J Med* 1962; 266: 661.
9 Ikeda RM, Kondracki SF, Drabkin PD, Birkhead GS, Morse DL. Pleurodynia among football players at a high school. An outbreak associated with coxsackievirus B1. *JAMA* 1993; 270: 2205.
10 Ehrenfeld EN, Eliakim M, Rachmilewitz M. Recurrent polyserositis (familial Mediterranean fever; periodic disease). A report of 55 cases. *Am J Med* 1961; 31: 107.
11 Sohar E, Gafni J, Pras M, Heller H. Familial Mediterranean fever. A survey of 470 cases and review of the literature. *Am J Med* 1967; 43: 227.
12 Aksentijevich I, Pras E, Gruberg L *et al.* Familial Mediterranean fever (FMF) in Moroccan Jews: demonstration of a founder effect by extended haplotype analysis. *Am J Hum Genet* 1993; 53: 644.
13 Aksentijevich I, Pras E, Gruberg L *et al.* Refined mapping of the gene causing familial Mediterranean fever, by linkage and homozygosity studies. *Am J Hum Genet* 1993; 53: 451.

14 Drenth JP, Haagsma CJ, van der Meer JW. Hyperimmunoglobulinemia D and periodic fever syndrome. The clinical spectrum in a serie of 50 patients. *Medicine* 1994; 73: 133.
15 Levy M, Eliakim M. Long-term colchicine prophylaxis in familial Mediterranean fever. *Br Med J* 1977; 2: 808.
16 Livneh A, Zemer D, Langevitz P *et al.* Colchicine in the treatment of AA and AL amyloidosis. *Semin Arthritis Rheum* 1993; 23: 206.
17 Davis S, Gardner F, Qvist G. The shape of a pleural effusion. *Br Med J* 1963; i: 436.
18 Millard CF. Vanishing or phantom tumor of the lung: localized interlobar effusion in congestive cardiac failure. *Chest* 1971; 59: 675.
19 Sandeiss DA, Hausan JC, Gosink BB, Moser KM. Ultrasound in diagnosis, localisation and treatment of loculated pleural empyema. *Ann Intern Med* 1975; 82: 50.
20 Leuallen EC, Carr DT. Pleural effusion: a statistical study of 436 patients. *N Engl J Med* 1955; 252: 79.
21 Owens MW, Milligan SA. Pleuritis and pleural effusions. *Curr Opin Pulm Med* 1995; 1: 318.
22 Bynum LJ, Wilson JE. Characteristics of pleural effusion associated with pulmonary embolism. *Arch Intern Med* 1976; 136: 159.
23 Bynum LJ, Wilson JE. Radiographic features of pleural effusions in pulmonary embolism. *Am Rev Respir Dis* 1978; 117: 829.
24 Lieberman FL, Hidemura R, Peters RL, Reynolds TB. Pathogenesis and treatment of hydrothorax complicating cirrhosis with ascites. *Ann Intern Med* 1966; 64: 341.
25 Lieberman FL, Peters RL. Cirrhotic hydrothorax: further evidence that an acquired diaphragmatic defect is at fault. *Arch Intern Med* 1970; 125: 114.
26 Rudnick MR, Coyle JF, Beck LH, McCurdy DK. Acute massive hydrothorax complicating peritoneal dialysis: report of two cases and a review of the literature. *Clin Nephrol* 1979; 12: 38.
27 Meigs JV. Fibroma of the ovary with ascites and hydrothorax: Meigs' syndrome. *Am J Obstet Gynecol* 1954; 67: 962.
28 Schneierson SJ, Katz M. Solitary pleural

effusion due to myxedema. *JAMA* 1958; 168: 1003.
29 Chernow B, Sahn SA. Carcinomatous involvement of the pleura: an analysis of 96 patients. *Am J Med* 1977; 63: 695.
30 Weick JK, Kiely JM, Harrison EG *et al.* Pleural effusion in lymphoma. *Cancer* 1973; 31: 848.
31 Light RW, Girard WM, Jenkinson SG, George RB. Parapneumonic effusions. *Am J Med* 1980; 69: 507.
32 Levy H, Simpson SQ. Hantavirus pulmonary syndrome. *Am J Respir Crit Care Med* 1994; 149: 1710.
33 Stead WW, Eichenholz A, Stauss H-K. Operative and pathological findings in twenty four patients with syndrome of idiopathic pleurisy with effusions, presumably tuberculous. *Am Rev Tuberc* 1955; 71: 473.
34 Bentley FJ, Grzybowski S. *Tuberculosis in Childhood and Adolescence.* London: National Association for the Prevention of Tuberculosis, 1954.
35 Thompson BC. Studies in primary pleurisy with effusion. *Br Med J* 1949; 2: 841.
36 Berger HW, Mejia E. Tuberculous pleurisy. *Chest* 1973; 63: 88.
37 Patiala J. Initial tuberculous pleuritis in the Finnish armed forces in 1939–45 with special reference to eventual post pleuritic tuberculosis. *Acta Tuberc Scand* 1954; Suppl 36.
38 Roper WH, Waring JJ. Primary serofibrinous pleural effusion in military personnel. *Am Rev Tuberc* 1955; 71: 616.
39 Johnson TM, McCann W, Davey WN. Tuberculous bronchopleural fistula. *Am Rev Respir Dis* 1973; 107: 30.
40 Jensen AO. Chronic calcified tuberculous empyema. *Scand J Respir Dis* 1969; 50: 19.
41 Hill AR, Premkumar S, Brustein S *et al.* Disseminated tuberculosis in the acquired immunodeficiency syndrome era. *Am Rev Respir Dis* 1991; 144: 1164.
42 Ellner JJ. Pleural fluid and peripheral blood lymphocyte function in tuberculosis. *Ann Intern Med* 1978; 89: 932.
43 Levine H, Metzger W, Lacera D, Kay L. Diagnosis of tuberculous pleurisy by culture of pleural biopsy specimen. *Arch Intern Med* 1970; 126: 269.

44 Christensen EE, Deitz GW, Ahn CH *et al.* Initial roentgenographic manifestations of pulmonary *Mycobacterium tuberculosis, M. kansasii* and *M. intracellulare* infections. *Chest* 1981; 80: 132.

45 Salkin D, Birsner TW, Tarr AD. Roentgen analysis of coccidioidomycosis. In: Ajello L, ed. *Coccidioidomycosis*. Tucson: University of Arizona Press, 1967.

46 Jay SJ, O'Neill RP, Goodman N, Penman R. Pleural effusion: a rare manifestation of pulmonary blastomycosis. *Am J Med Sci* 1977; 274: 325.

47 Goodwin RA, Loyd JE, Des Prez RM. Histoplasmosis in normal hosts. *Medicine* 1981; 60: 231.

48 Young EJ, Hirsh DD, Fainstein V, Williams TW. Pleural effusions due to *Cryptococcus neoformans*: a review of the literature and report of two cases with cryptococcal antigen determinations. *Am Rev Respir Dis* 1980; 121: 743.

49 Bertrand G, Basle M, Alquier P *et al.* Septicèmie aspergillaire et aspergillose disseminée. *Sem Hop Paris* 1972; 48: 2599.

50 Murphy D, Lane DJ. Pleural effusion in allergic bronchopulmonary aspergillosis: two case reports. *Br J Dis Chest* 1981; 75: 91.

51 Bates M, Cruikshank G. Thoracic actinomycosis. *Thorax* 1957; 12: 99.

52 Flynn MW, Felson B. The roentgen manifestations of thoracic actinomycosis. *Am J Roentgenol* 1970; 110: 707.

53 Harrison RN, Thomas DJB. Acute actinomycotic empyema. *Thorax* 1979; 34: 406.

54 Presant CA, Wiernik PH, Serpick AA. Factors affecting survival in nocardiosis. *Am Rev Respir Dis* 1974; 108: 1444.

55 Harley HRS. Subphrenic abscess. *Thorax* 1949; 4: 1.

56 Miller WT, Talman EA. Subphrenic abscess. *Am J Roentgenol* 1967; 101: 961.

57 Le Roux BT. Pleuro-pulmonary amoebiasis. *Thorax* 1969; 24: 91.

58 Borrie J, Shaw JHF. Hepatobronchial fistula caused by hydatid disease. *Thorax* 1981; 36: 25.

59 Xanthakis DS, Katsaras E, Efthimiadis M *et al.* Hydatid cyst of the liver with intrathoracic rupture. *Thorax* 1981; 36: 497.

60 Grover A, Dhawan A, Iyengar SD *et al.* Epidemiology of rheumatic fever and rheumatic heart disease in a rural community in northern India. *Bull WHO* 1993; 71: 59.

61 Paul JR. Pleural and pulmonary lesions in rheumatic fever. *Medicine* 1928; 7: 383.

62 Horler AR, Thompson M. The pleural and pulmonary complications of rheumatoid arthritis. *Ann Intern Med* 1959; 51: 1179.

63 Walker WC, Wright V. Pulmonary lesions and rheumatoid arthritis. *Medicine* 1968; 47: 501.

64 Lillington GA, Carr DT, Mayne JG. Rheumatoid pleurisy with effusion. *Arch Intern Med* 1971; 128: 764.

65 Halla JT, Schrohenloher RE, Volanakis JE. Immune complexes and other laboratory features of pleural effusions. A comparison of rheumatoid arthritis, systemic lupus erythematosus, and other diseases. *Ann Intern Med* 1980; 92: 748.

66 Andrews BS, Arora NS, Shadforth MF *et al.* The role of immune complexes in the pathogenesis of pleural effusions. *Am Rev Respir Dis* 1981; 124: 115.

67 Faurschou P, Francis D, Faarup P. Thoracoscopic, histological and clinical findings in nine cases of rheumatoid pleural effusion. *Thorax* 1985; 40: 371.

68 Jones FL, Blodgett RC. Empyema in rheumatoid pleuropulmonary disease. *Ann Intern Med* 1971; 74: 665.

69 Estes D, Christian DL. The natural history of systemic lupus erythematosus by prospective analysis. *Medicine* 1971; 50: 85.

70 Israel HC. The pulmonary manifestations of disseminated lupus erythematosus. *Am J Med Sci* 1953; 226: 387.

71 Alarcon-Segovia D, Alarcon DG. Pleuropulmonary manifestations of systemic lupus erythematosus. *Dis Chest* 1961; 39: 7.

72 Good JT, King TE, Antony VB, Sahn SA. Lupus pleuritis: clinical features and pleural fluid characteristics with special reference to pleural fluid antinuclear antibodies. *Chest* 1983; 84: 714.

73 Gonzalez L, van Ordstrand HS. Wegener's granulomatosis. *Radiology* 1973; 107: 295.

74 Carrington CB, Liebow AA. Limited forms of angiitis and granulomatosis of Wegener's type. *Am J Med* 1966; 41: 497.

75 Kaye MD. Pleuropulmonary complications of pancreatitis. *Thorax* 1968; 23: 297.

76 Tombroff M, Loicq A, de Koster J-P *et al.* Pleural effusion with pancreatico-pleural fistula. *Br Med J* 1973; i: 330.

77 Berger HW, Rammohan G, Neff MS, Buhain WJ. Uremic pleural effusion: a study of 14 patients on chronic dialysis. *Ann Intern Med* 1975; 82: 362.

78 Wilen SB, Rabinowitz JG, Ulrich S, Lyons HA. Pleural involvement in sarcoidosis. *Am J Med* 1974; 57: 200.

79 Beekman JF, Zimmet SM, Chun BK *et al.* Spectrum of pleural involvement in sarcoidosis. *Arch Intern Med* 1976; 136: 323.

80 Chusid EL, Siltzbach LE. Sarcoidosis of the pleura. *Ann Intern Med* 1974; 81: 190.

81 Nicholls AJ, Friend JAR, Legge JS. Sarcoid pleural effusions: three cases and review of the literature. *Thorax* 1980; 35: 277.

82 Martensson G, Hagberg S, Pettersson K, Thiringer G. Asbestos pleural effusion: a clinical entity. *Thorax* 1987; 42: 646.

83 Lilis R, Lerman Y, Selikoff IJ. Symptomatic benign pleural effusions among asbestos insulation workers: residual radiographic abnormalities. *Br J Ind Med* 1988; 45: 443.

84 Robinson BWS, Musk AW. Benign asbestos pleural effusion: diagnosis and course. *Thorax* 1981; 36: 896.

85 Beer DJ, Pereira W, Snider GL. Pleural effusion associated with primary lymphedema: a perspective on the yellow nail syndrome. *Am Rev Respir Dis* 1978; 117: 595.

86 Emerson PA. Yellow nails and pleural effusions. *Thorax* 1966; 21: 247.

87 Hiller E, Rosenow EC, Olsen AM. Pulmonary manifestations of the yellow nail syndrome. *Chest* 1972; 61: 452.

88 Govaert P, Leroy JG, Pauwels R *et al.* Perinatal manifestations of maternal yellow nail syndrome. *Pediatrics* 1992; 89: 1016.

89 Dilley JJ, Kierland RR, Randall RV, Schick RM. Primary lymphedema associated with yellow nails and pleural effusions. *JAMA* 1968; 204: 670.

90 Ross JD, Reid KDG, Ambujakshan VP *et al.* Recurrent pleural effusion, protein-losing enteropathy, malabsorption and mosaic warts associated with generalized lymphatic hypoplasia. *Thorax* 1971; 26: 119.

91 Brofman JD, Hall JB, Scott W, Little AG. Yellow nails, lymphedema and pleural effusion. Treatment of chronic pleural effusion with pleuroperitoneal shunting. *Chest* 1990; 97: 743.

92 Lewis M, Kallenbach J, Zaltzman M *et al.* Pleurectomy in the management of massive pleural effusion associated with primary lymphoedema: demonstration of abnormal pleural lymphatics. *Thorax* 1983; 38: 637.

93 Runyon BA, Forker EL, Sopko JA. Pleural fluid kinetics in a patient with primary lymphedema, pleural effusion and yellow nails. *Am Rev Respir Dis* 1979; 119: 821.

94 Tan WC. Dietary treatment of chylous ascites in yellow nail syndrome. *Gut* 1989; 30: 1622.

95 Hindle W, Posner E, Sweetman JT, Tan RSH. Pleural effusion and fibrosis during treatment with methysergide. *Br Med J* 1970; i: 605.

96 Hall DR, Morrison JB, Edwards FR. Pleural fibrosis after practolol therapy. *Thorax* 1978; 33: 822.

97 Israel HL, Diamond P. Recurrent pulmonary infiltration and pleural effusion due to nitrofurantoin sensitivity. *N Engl J Med* 1962; 266: 1024.

98 Williamson MR, Eidson M, Rosenberg RD, Williamson SL. Eosinophilia–myalgia syndrome: findings on chest radiographs in 18 patients. *Radiology* 1991; 180: 849.

99 Good JT, King TE, Sahn SA. Native and drug-induced lupus pleuritis: a cause of a low glucose low pH pleural effusion. *Chest* 1980; 57: 518.

100 Gross NJ. Pulmonary effects of radiation therapy. *Ann Intern Med* 1977; 86: 81.

101 Martin RG, Rukdeschel JC, Chang P *et al.* Radiation-related pericarditis. *Am J Cardiol* 1975; 35: 216.

102 Whitcomb ME, Schwarz MJ. Pleural effusion complicating intensive mediastinal radiation therapy. *Am Rev Respir Dis* 1971; 103: 100.

103 Chandrasekhara R, Levitan R. Spontaneous rupture of the esophagus. *Arch Intern Med* 1970; 126: 1008.

104 Michel L, Grillo HC, Malt RA. Operative and non-operative management of esophageal perforations. *Ann Surg* 1981; 194: 57.

105 Maulitz RM, Good JT, Kaplan RL *et al.* The pleuro-pulmonary consequences of esophageal rupture: an experimental model. *Am Rev Respir Dis* 1979; 120: 363.

106 Finley RJ, Pearson FG, Weisel RD *et al.* The management of non-malignant intrathoracic esophageal perforations. *Ann Thorac Surg* 1980; 30: 575.

107 Adams FV, Galati V. M-mode ultrasonic localization of pleural effusion. *JAMA* 1976; 239: 1761.

108 Hirsch JH, Rogers JV, Mack LA. Real-time sonography of pleural opacities. *Am J Roentgenol* 1981; 136: 297.

109 Abrams LD. A pleural biopsy punch. *Lancet* 1958; i: 30.

110 Mungal IPF, Cowan PN, Cooke NT *et al.* Multiple pleural biopsy with the Abrams needle. *Thorax* 1980; 35: 600.

111 Trapnell DH, Thurston JGB. Unilateral pulmonary oedema after pleural aspiration. *Lancet* 1970; i: 1367.

112 Wilkinson PD, Keegan J, Davies SW, Bailey J, Rudd R. Changes in microvascular permeability accompanying re-expansion oedema:

evidence from dual isotope scintigraphy. *Thorax* 1990; 45: 456.

113 Brandstetter RD, Cohen RP. Hypoxemia after thoracentesis. *JAMA* 1979; 242: 1060.

114 Light RW, Jenkinson SG, Minh V-D, George RB. Observations on pleural pressures as fluid is withdrawn during thoracentesis. *Am Rev Respir Dis* 1980; 121: 799.

115 Ferguson GC. Cholesterol pleural effusion in rheumatoid lung disease. *Thorax* 1966; 21: 577.

116 Light RW, Erozan YS, Ball WC. Cells in pleural fluid: their value in differential diagnosis. *Arch Intern Med* 1973; 132: 854.

117 Pettersson T, Riska H. Diagnostic value of total and differential leukocyte counts in pleural effusions. *Acta Med Scand* 1981; 210: 129.

118 Bower G. Eosinophilic pleural effusion. A condition with multiple causes. *Am Rev Respir Dis* 1967; 95: 746.

119 Adelman M, Abelda SM, Gottlieb J, Haponik EF. Diagnostic utility of pleural fluid eosinophilia. *Am J Med* 1984; 77: 915.

120 Chapman JS, Reynolds RC. Eosinophilic response to intraperitoneal blood. *J Lab Clin Med* 1958; 51: 516.

121 Dekker A, Bupp PA. Cytology of serous effusions: an investigation into the usefulness of cell blocks vs smears. *Am J Clin Pathol* 1978; 70: 855.

122 Dewald GW, Hicks GA, Dines DE, Gordon H. Cytogenic diagnosis of malignant pleural effusions. *Mayo Clin Proc* 1982; 57: 488.

123 Carr DT, Power MH. Clinical value of measurements of concentration of protein in pleural fluid. *N Engl J Med* 1958; 259: 926.

124 Valdes L, Pose A, Suares J et al. Cholesterol: a useful parameter for distinguishing between pleural exudates and transudates. *Chest* 1991; 99: 1097.

125 Carr DT, McGuckin WF. Pleural fluid glucose. *Am Rev Respir Dis* 1968; 97: 302.

126 Light RW, Ball WC. Glucose and amylase in pleural effusions. *JAMA* 1973; 225: 257.

127 Light RW, MacGregor MI, Luchsinger PC, Ball WC. Pleural effusions: the diagnostic separation of transudates and exudates. *Ann Intern Med* 1972; 77: 507.

128 Sherr HP, Light RW, Merson MH et al. Origin of pleural fluid amylase in esophageal rupture. *Ann Intern Med* 1972; 76: 985.

129 Potts DE, Levin DC, Sahn SA. Pleural fluid pH in parapneumonic effusions. *Chest* 1976; 70: 328.

130 Scott EM, Marshall TJ, Flower CD, Stewart S. Diffuse pleural thickening: percutaneous CT-guided cutting needle biopsy. *Radiology* 1995; 194: 867.

131 Qureshi N, Momin ZA, Brandstetter RD. Thoracentesis in clinical practice. *Heart Lung* 1994; 23: 376.

132 O'Donovan PB, Eng P. Pleural changes in malignant pleural effusions: appearance on computed tomography. *Cleve Clin J Med* 1994; 61: 127.

133 Baumgartner WA, Mark JBD. The use of thoracoscopy in the diagnosis of pleural disease. *Arch Surg* 1980; 115: 420.

134 Boutin C, Viallat JR, Cargnino P, Farisse P. Thoracoscopy in malignant pleural effusions. *Am Rev Respir Dis* 1981; 124: 588.

135 Allen MS, Trastek VF, Daly RC, Deschamps C, Pairolero PC. Equipment for thoracoscopy. *Ann Thorac Surg* 1993; 56: 620.

136 Aspin J, O'Hara H. Steroid treated tuberculous pleural effusions. *Br J Tuberc* 1958; 52: 81.

137 Menon NK. Steroid therapy in tuberculous pleural effusion. *Tubercle* 1964; 45: 17.

138 Mark JBD, Goldenberg IS, Montague ACW. Intrapleural mechlorethamine hydrochloride therapy for malignant pleural effusion. *JAMA* 1964; 187: 858.

139 Botsford TW. Experiences with radioactive colloidal gold in the treatment of pleural effusion caused by metastatic cancer of the breast. *N Engl J Med* 1964; 270: 552.

140 Wallach HW. Intrapleural tetracycline for malignant pleural effusions. *Chest* 1975; 69: 510.

141 Desai SD, Figueredo A. Intracavitary doxorubicin in malignant effusions. *Lancet* 1979; i: 872.

142 Stiksa G, Korsgaard R, Simonsson BG. Treatment of recurrent pleural effusions by pleurodesis with quinacrine. *Scand J Respir Dis* 1979; 60: 197.

143 Webbe HE, Oaten SW, Pike CP. Treatment of malignant ascitic and pleural effusions with *Corynebacterium parvum*. *Br Med J* 1978; 1: 338.

144 Millar JW, Hunter AM, Horne NW. Intrapleural immunotherapy with *Corynebacterium parvum* in recurrent malignant pleural effusions. *Thorax* 1980; 35: 856.

145 Felletti R, Ravazzoni C. Intrapleural *Corynebacterium parvum* for malignant pleural effusions. *Thorax* 1983; 38: 22.

146 McLeod DT, Calverley PMA, Millar LW, Horne NW. Further experience of *Corynebacterium parvum* in malignant pleural effusion. *Thorax* 1985; 40: 515.

147 Thatcher N, Lamb B, Swindell R, Crowther D. Effects of *Corynebacterium parvum* on cellular immunity of cancer patients, assayed sequentially over 63 days. *Cancer* 1981; 47: 285.

148 Adler RH, Rappole BW. Recurrent malignant pleural effusions and talc powder aerosol treatment. *Surgery* 1967; 62: 1000.

149 Jones GR. Treatment of recurrent malignant pleural effusions by iodised talc pleurodesis. *Thorax* 1969; 24: 69.

150 Aelony Y, King R, Boutin C. Thoracoscopic talc poudrage for chronic recurrent pleural effusions. *Ann Intern Med* 1991; 115: 778.

151 Research Committee of the British Thoracic Association and the Medical Research Council Pneumoconiosis Unit. A survey of the long-term effects of talc and kaolin pleurodesis. *Br J Dis Chest* 1979; 73: 285.

152 Lampson RS. Traumatic chylothorax. A review of the literature and report of a case treated by mediastinal ligation of the thoracic duct. *J Thorac Surg* 1948; 17: 778.

153 Bower G. Chylothorax. *Dis Chest* 1964; 46: 464.

154 Watne AL, Hatiboglu I, Moore GE. A clinical and autopsy study of tumor cells in the thoracic duct lymph. *Surg Gynecol Obstet* 1960; 110: 339.

155 Bessone LN, Ferguson TB, Burford TH. Chylothorax. *Ann Thorac Surg* 1971; 12: 527.

156 Staats BA, Ellefson RD, Budahn LL et al. The lipoprotein profile of chylous and nonchylous pleural effusions. *Mayo Clin Proc* 1980; 55: 700.

157 Woofenden JM, Struse TB. Diagnosis of chylothorax with [131]I Triolen: case report. *J Nucl Med* 1977; 18: 128.

158 Coe JE, Aikawa JK. Cholesterol pleural effusion. *Arch Intern Med* 1961; 108: 763.

159 Light RW. *Pleural Diseases*, 3rd edn. Baltimore: Williams & Wilkins, 1995.

160 Cevese PG, Vecchione R, D'Amico DF et al. Postoperative chylothorax: six cases in 2500 operations, with a survey of the world literature. *J Thorac Cardiovasc Surg* 1975; 69: 966.

161 Schmidt A. Chylothorax: review of 5 years' cases in the literature and report of a case. *Acta Chir Scand* 1959; 118: 5.

162 Herzog KA, Branscom JJ. Spontaneous chylothorax. *Chest* 1974; 65: 346.

163 Kjeldsen CS, Struve-Christensen E. Chylothorax. *Scand J Thorac Cardiovasc Surg* 1974; 8: 138.

164 Bresser P, Kromhout JG, Reekers JA, Verhage TL. Chylous pleural effusion associated with primary lymphedema and lymphangioma-like malfomations. *Chest* 1993; 103: 1916.

165 Dunkelman H, Sharief N, Berman L, Ninan T. Generalised lymphangiomatosis with chylothorax. *Arch Dis Child* 1989; 64: 1058.

166 Chernick V, Reed MH. Pneumothorax and chylothorax in the neonatal period. *J Pediatr* 1970; 76: 624.

167 Ross IK. A review of the surgery of the thoracic duct. *Thorax* 1961; 16: 12.

168 William KR, Burford TH. The management of chylothorax. *Ann Surg* 1964; 160: 131.

169 Selle JG, Snyder WH, Schreiber JT. Chylothorax: indications for surgery. *Ann Surg* 1973; 177: 245.

170 Adler RH, Levinsky L. Persistent chylothorax: treatment by talc pleurodesis. *J Thorac Cardiovasc Surg* 1970; 76: 859.

171 Gingell JC. Treatment of chylothorax by producing pleurodesis using iodised talc. *Thorax* 1965; 20: 261.

172 Hourihane DO'B, Lessof L, Richardson PC. Hyaline and calcified pleural plaques as an index of exposure to asbestos. *Br Med J* 1966; i: 1069.

173 Hillerdal G, Lindgren A. Pleural plaques: correlation of autopsy findings to radiographic findings and occupational history. *Eur J Respir Dis* 1980; 61: 315.

174 Al Jarad N, Poulakis N, Pearson MC, Rubens MB, Rudd RM. Assessment of asbestos induced pleural disease by computed tomography: correlation with chest radiograph and lung function. *Respir Med* 1991; 85: 203.

175 Roberts GH. The pathology of parietal pleural plaques. *J Clin Pathol* 1971; 24: 348.

176 Sebastien P, Janson X, Gaudichet A. Asbestos retention in human respiratory tissues: comparative measurements in lung parenchyme and in parietal pleura. In: Wagner JC, Davis JMW, eds. *Biological Effects of Mineral Fibres*, Vol 1. Lyon: IARC, 1980: 237.

177 Hillerdal G. Pleural plaques in a health survey material: frequency, development and exposure to asbestos. *Scand J Respir Dis* 1978; 59: 257.

178 Baris YI, Sahin AA, Ozesmi M et al. An outbreak of pleural mesothelioma and chronic fibrosing pleurisy in the village of Karain/Urgup in Anatolia. *Thorax* 1978; 33: 181.

179 Elmes PC. Mesotheliomas, minerals and man-made mineral fibres. *Thorax* 1980; 35: 561.

180 Yazicioglu S, Ilcayto R, Balci K et al. Pleural

calcification, pleural mesotheliomas, and bronchial cancers caused by tremolite dust. *Thorax* 1980; 35: 564.

181 Boutin G, Viallat JR, Steinbauer J, Dufour G, Gaudichet A. Bilateral pleural plaques in Corsica: a marker of non-occupational asbestos exposure. In: Bignon J, Peto J, Saracci R, eds. *Non-occupational Exposure to Mineral Fibres*. Lyon: IARC, 1989: 406.

182 Miller A. Chronic pleuritic pain in four patients with asbestos induced pleural fibrosis. *Br J Ind Med* 1990; 47: 147.

183 Payne CR, Jaques P, Kerr IH. Lung folding simulating peripheral pulmonary neoplasm (Blesovsky's syndrome). *Thorax* 1980; 35: 936.

184 Mintzer RA, Cugell DW. The association of asbestos-induced pleural disease and rounded atelectasis. *Chest* 1982; 81: 457.

185 Al Jarad N, Davies SW, Logan-Sinclair R, Rudd RM. Lung crackle characteristics in patients with asbestosis, asbestos-related pleural disease and left ventricular failure using a time expanded waveform (TEW) analysis. *Respir Dis* 1994; 88: 37.

186 Hillerdal G. Non-malignant asbestos pleural disease. *Thorax* 1981; 36: 669.

187 Gibbs AR, Stephens M, Griffiths DM, Blight BJM, Pooley FD. Fibre distribution in the lungs and pleura of subjects with asbestos related diffuse pleural fibrosis. *Br J Ind Med* 1991; 48: 762.

188 Hillerdal G. Non-malignant pleural disease related to asbestos exposure. *Clin Chest Med* 1985; 6: 141.

189 Carroll D, McClement J, Himmelstein A, Cournand A. Pulmonary function following decortication of the lung. *Am Rev Tuberc* 1951; 63: 231.

190 Dernevik L, Gatzinsky P. Long term results of operation for shrinking pleuritis. *Thorax* 1985; 40: 448.

191 Dalton WT, Zolliker AS, McCaughey W *et al.* Localised primary tumors of the pleura. *Cancer* 1979; 44: 1465.

192 Le Roux BT. Pleural tumours. *Thorax* 1962; 17: 111.

193 Briselli M, Mark EJ, Dickersin GR. Solitary tumors of the pleura: eight new cases and review of 360 cases in the literature. *Cancer* 1981; 47: 2678.

194 Clagett OT, McDonald JR, Schmidt HW. Localised benign mesothelioma of the pleura. *J Thorac Surg* 1952; 24: 213.

195 Nwafo DC, Adi FC. Giant fibromyxoma of the parietal pleura. *Thorax* 1978; 33: 520.

196 Spry CJF, Williamson DH, James ML.

Pleural mesotheliomas and hypoglycaemia. *Proc R Soc Med* 1968; 61: 1105.

197 Price-Thomas C, Drew CE. Fibroma of visceral pleura. *Thorax* 1953; 8: 180.

198 Heany JP, Overton RC, de Bakey ME. Benign localised pleural mesothelioma. Report of two cases. *J Thorac Surg* 1957; 34: 553.

199 Hernandez FJ, Femandez DB. Localised fibrous tumours of the pleura A light and electron microscopic study. *Cancer* 1974; 34: 1667.

200 Hillerdal G. Malignant mesothelioma 1982: review of 4710 published cases. *Br J Dis Chest* 1983; 77: 321.

201 Wyers H. MD thesis, University of Glasgow, quoted by Perry KMA. Diseases of the lung resulting from occupational dusts other than silica. *Thorax* 1947; 2: 91.

202 Wagner JC, Sleggs CA, Marchand P. Diffuse pleural mesothelioma and asbestos exposure in the North Western Cape Province. *Br J Ind Med* 1960; 17: 260.

203 Bolton RE, Davis JMG, Donaldson K, Wright A. Variations in the carcinogenicity of mineral fibres. In: Walton WH, ed. *Inhaled Particles V*. Oxford: Pergamon Press, 1982: 569.

204 McDonald JC, Liddell FDK. Mortality in Canadian miners and millers exposed to chrysotile. *Ann N Y Acad Sci* 1979; 330: 1.

205 Seidman H, Selikoff IJ, Hammond EC. Short-term asbestos work exposure and long-term observation. *Ann N Y Acad Sci* 1979; 330: 61 1980.

206 Jones JSP, Smith PG, Pooley FD *et al.* The consequences of exposure to asbestos dust in a war-time gas-mask factory. In: Wagner JC, Davis JMG, eds. *Biological Effects of Mineral Fibres*, Vol 1. Lyon: IARC, 1980: 637.

207 Sluis-Cremer GK, Du Toit RSJ, Asbestos-related radiological changes in residents of South African amphibole asbestos mining fields and the fibre counts to which they may have been exposed. In: Wagner JC, Davis JMG, eds. *Biological Effects of Mineral Fibres*, Vol 1. Lyon: IARC, 1980: 559.

208 Wagner JC, Pooley FD, Berry G *et al.* A pathological and mineralogical study of asbestos-related deaths in the United Kingdom in 1977. In: Walton WH, ed. *Inhaled Particles V*. Oxford: Pergamon Press, 1982: 423.

209 Stanton MF, Layard M, Tegeris A *et al.* Carcinogenicity of fibrous glass: pleural response in the rat in relation to fiber dimension. *J Natl Cancer Inst* 1977; 58: 587.

210 Carbone M, Pass HI, Rizzo P *et al.* Simian

virus 40-like DNA sequences in human pleural mesothelioma. *Oncogene* 1996 9, 781.

211 Pepper C, Jasani B, Navabi H, Wynford-Thomas D, Gibbs AR. Simian virus 40 large T antigen (SV40LTAg) primer specific DNA amplification in human pleural mesothelioma tissue. *Thorax* 1996; 51: 1074.

212 Peto J, Hodgson JT, Matthews FE, Jones JR. Continuing increase in mesothelioma mortality in Britain. *Lancet* 1995; 345: 535.

213 Elmes PC, Simpson MJC. The clinical aspects of mesothelioma. *Q J Med* 1976; 45: 427.

214 Arai H, Kang K-Y, Sato H *et al.* Significance of the quantification and demonstration of hyaluronic acid in tissue specimens for the diagnosis of pleural mesothelioma. *Am Rev Respir Dis* 1979; 120: 529 1980.

215 Butler EB, Johnson NF. The use of electron microscopy in the diagnosis of diffuse mesotheliomas using human pleural effusions. In: Wagner JC, Davis JMG, eds. *Biological Effects of Mineral Fibres*, Vol 1. Lyon: IARC, 1980: 409.

216 Gibbs AR, Harach R, Wagner JC, Jasani B. Comparison of tumour markers in malignant mesothelioma and pulmonary adenocarcinoma. *Thorax* 1985; 40: 91.

217 Churg J, Rosen SH, Moolten S. Histologic characteristics of mesothelioma associated with asbestos. *Ann N Y Acad Sci* 1965; 132: 614.

218 Hourihane D, O'B. The pathology of mesotheliomata and an analysis of their association with asbestos exposure. *Thorax* 1964; 19: 268.

219 Whitwell F, Scott J, Grimshaw M. Relationships between occupations and asbestos-fibre content of the lungs in patients with pleural mesothelioma, lung cancer and other diseases. *Thorax* 1977; 32: 377.

220 Gibbs AR, Pooley FD. Analysis and interpretation of inorganic mineral particles in 'lung' tissues. *Thorax* 1996; 51: 327.

221 Boutin C, Nussbaum E, Monnet I *et al.* Intrapleural treatment with recombinant gamma-interferon in early stage malignant pleural mesothelioma. *Cancer* 1994; 74: 2460.

222 Jelihovsky T, Grant AF. Endometriosis of the lung. A case report and a brief review of the literature. *Thorax* 1968; 23: 434.

223 Foster DC, Stern LJ, Buscema J *et al.* Pleural and parenchymal pulmonary endometriosis. *Obstet Gynecol* 1981; 58: 552.

224 Jariwalla AG, Al-Nasiri NK. Splenosis pleurae. *Thorax* 1979; 34: 123.

44

PNEUMOTHORAX

DOUGLAS SEATON

A pneumothorax is defined as the presence of air within the pleural cavity. The term was first used in the doctoral thesis of the French physician Itard in 1803 [1], although the presence of abnormal collections of air and fluid within the chest might have been inferred as early as the fifth century BC by physicians in ancient Greece who practised so-called Hippocratic succussion of the chest [2,3].

Classification and terminology

In health each lung is surrounded by two contiguous layers of pleura separated by the potential space known as the pleural cavity. The pressure in this space is negative with respect to the atmosphere and as a result the elastic structures comprising the lung are held in apposition to the chest wall. Should air gain entry to the pleural cavity by whatever means, intrapleural pressure becomes less negative with respect to atmospheric pressure and this permits the lung to move away from the chest wall by deflation until a point is reached at which the pressure remains sufficiently negative to prevent further collapse. Should the pressure in the pleural cavity reach that of the atmosphere then a complete, as opposed to a partial, pneumothorax is said to exist. Should intrapleural pressure exceed that of the atmosphere then as well as the pneumothorax being complete, the structures comprising the mediastinum are compressed and displaced to the opposite side producing a tension pneumothorax.

From the foregoing it is clear that a pneumothorax cannot occur unless the integrity of either the visceral or parietal layer of pleura, or both, is breached. Should the breach remain patent then a fistula exists and the pneumothorax may be described as open. More frequently the breach seals off, resulting in a closed pneumothorax. A tension pneumothorax arises when the defect is valve-like, permitting air to pass into the pleural cavity on inspiration but preventing its escape. A working classification of pneumothorax based on aetiology is given in Fig. 44.1.

Spontaneous pneumothorax

Any pneumothorax occurring in the absence of trauma may be described as spontaneous (syn. primary simple pneumothorax, primary pneumothorax, simple pneumothorax, pneumothorax simplex, idiopathic pneumothorax). The term 'primary spontaneous pneumothorax' is used in the absence of clinical evidence of pre-existing respiratory disease, while 'secondary spontaneous pneumothorax' denotes a clinically recognizable coexisting structural or functional abnormality in the lung. In a histopathological sense this distinction is somewhat artificial as small defects in the pleura and adjacent lung (see below) have been causally related to primary spontaneous pneumothorax. However, it should be stressed that the distinction remains clinically valid, since these defects in primary spontaneous pneumothorax are of no functional significance and usually go undetected prior to the event. Some cases of secondary spontaneous pneumothorax may at first be misclassified as primary before the underlying clinical condition evolves to the point of recognition.

Primary spontaneous pneumothorax

Spontaneous pneumothorax most commonly occurs in apparently healthy subjects with no history of pre-existing lung disease. In a series of 210 consecutive cases of spontaneous pneumothorax admitted to a teaching hospital over a 5-year period, 67% fell into this primary category [4]. Primary spontaneous pneumothorax is predominantly a disease of young adults, being rare in children [5], the peak incidence falling in the third decade [4,6,7]. One study found that spontaneous pneumothorax was primary in 81% of cases presenting at the age of 45 years or under [4]. It is also of note that the condition predominantly affects males, the male to female ratio lying somewhere between the 12:1 found in a study of 118 cases of primary spontaneous pneumothorax [8], 4:1 in a series of 400 cases [9] and 3:1 in a later Swedish community survey that included 2414 patients [10]. In a detailed community-

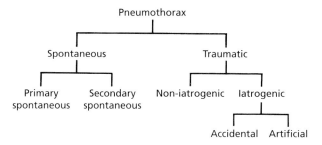

Fig. 44.1 Classification of pneumothorax.

Table 44. 1 Causes of pneumothorax.

Spontaneous pneumothorax
Primary
  apical blebs
  stature

Secondary
  chronic bronchitis and emphysema
  asthma
  suppurative pneumonia
  tuberculosis of the lungs
  cystic fibrosis
  rare causes (*see text*)

Traumatic pneumothorax
Non-iatrogenic
  open and closed chest injury
  barotrauma

Iatrogenic (accidental)
  paracentesis thoracis
  pleural biopsy
  transbronchial biopsy
  percutaneous lung biopsy/aspiration
  central venous cannulation
  barotrauma (mechanical ventilation)
  rare causes (*see text*)

Iatrogenic (deliberate)
  artificial pneumothorax

based survey carried out in Minnesota, USA, the incidence of primary spontaneous pneumothorax was found to be 7.4 per 100 000 per year for males and 1.2 per 100 000 per year for females [11]. A similar overall incidence has been reported in the UK [6]. The annual incidence in Stockholm was found to be higher at 18 per 100 000 for men and 6 per 100 000 for women [10]. The right and left lung appear to be affected with equal frequency [12].

Aetiology (Table 44.1)

In the early part of the twentieth century spontaneous pneumothorax was, in the minds of most physicians, inextricably bound up with pulmonary tuberculosis, Biach [13] having described such an association in 79% of 918 cases of pneumothorax. A gradual realization that pneumothorax could occur in the absence of underlying lung disease subsequently emerged and Kjaergaard's monograph [14] in which he reviewed 51 cases did much to cause general acceptance of the concept of primary spontaneous pneumothorax. This results from the rupture into the pleural cavity of a small air-filled space know as a pulmonary bleb (Fig. 44.2), a localized collection of air within the cellular layers of the visceral pleura that is contiguous with the lung parenchyma [15]. Blebs may arise as a result of a congenital weakness in the connective tissue of subpleural alveoli and electron microscopic studies have demonstrated that communications exist between blebs and the adjacent alveolar spaces [16]. In cases of primary spontaneous pneumothorax coming to surgery it has been shown that blebs are very common, occurring in over 90% of patients [17], are frequently multiple, occur most commonly at the lung apices and are found in the uncollapsed contralateral lung almost as frequently as in the lung where the pneumothorax has occurred [18,19]. Blebs may occur more frequently at the lung apices as a result of the regional differences in mechanical stresses known to exist within the lungs [20]. In the upright posture a gravity-dependent gradient of negative intrapleural pressure extends along the length of each lung so that distending forces are greatest over the lung apices [21], just as a loosely coiled spring, when suspended by its uppermost coil, becomes progressively more expanded by its own

weight from bottom to top (Fig. 44.3). It has also been suggested that the relative ischaemia at the apex of the lung makes this area more susceptible to infection, so that blebs may develop as a result of inflammation occurring in a zone of maximal stress [22] and there is some histological support for this view [19]. A higher incidence of primary spontaneous pneumothorax has been recorded in individuals who have a tall and thin body habitus. In a study comprising 92 patients with primary spontaneous pneumothorax, mean height was found to be 5 cm greater and mean weight 11 kg less than predicted [23]. A study in the UK recorded a similarly increased mean height in patients with primary spontaneous pneumothorax [24]. In a Japanese study that compared patients with primary spontaneous pneumothorax with controls, those in the pneumothorax group were no taller but had significantly longer lungs and were also leaner [25]. In a detailed epidemiological study in the USA it was concluded that much of the male predominance in spontaneous pneumothorax could be explained in terms of height [11].

There have been several case reports of primary spontaneous pneumothorax occurring in families [26–28]. In one such report an association between spontaneous pneumothorax and specific human leucocyte antigen (HLA) and antitrypsin phenotypes was suggested but not proved conclusively [29]. In a study of 286 Israeli military personnel, a positive family history of primary spontaneous pneumothorax was obtained in 11.5% of cases [30]. The

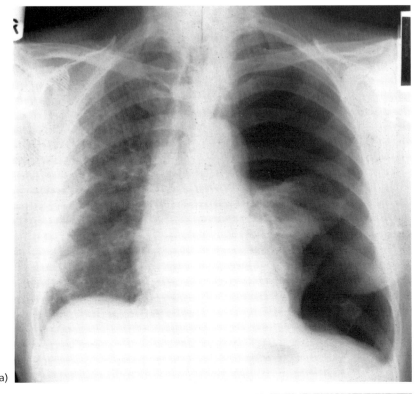

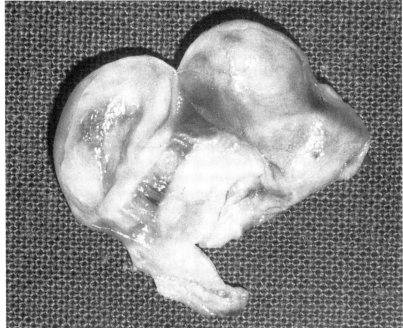

Fig. 44.2 (a) Left pneumothorax showing blebs at apex. (b) Operative specimen showing excised blebs.

lungs of some patients with spontaneous pneumothorax have been reported to contain high levels of soluble hydroxyproline. This substance is a degradation product of collagen and the finding was taken to imply an abnormality in the structure or biosynthesis of lung collagen resulting in its increased breakdown [31]. A high incidence of tobacco smoking has been reported in several series of primary spontaneous pneumothorax and this may be a

predisposing factor [7,11,32,33]. A Swedish study found that there was a significant dose–response relationship between smoking and the occurrence of primary spontaneous pneumothorax, the habit increasing the risk 22-fold among men and ninefold among women [10]. Data relating to the same group also showed that there was an apparent temporal relationship between tobacco consumption and changes in the incidence of primary sponta-

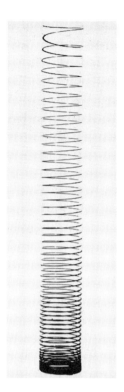

Fig. 44.3 Suspended spring showing effects of increased tension in the upper coils.

neous pneumothorax in the community, a decrease in consumption being followed by a decrease in incidence within 1–2 years [34]. It is conjectured that the repeated stress imposed upon the walls of a pulmonary bleb by a smoker's cough might make it more likely to rupture. A causal relationship between the presence of a sharp inner border to the first or second ribs and primary spontaneous pneumothorax has been proposed [35]. This finding was present at thoracotomy in 49% of a series of 57 cases compared with only 8% of control subjects coming to thoracotomy for other reasons. It has been claimed that patients presenting with primary spontaneous pneumothorax are more likely to have minor bronchial anomalies at endoscopy than controls [36] and these patients are also more likely to show localized emphysema-like changes on CT, particularly in the upper zones and towards the lung periphery [37].

Secondary spontaneous pneumothorax (Table 44.1)

Spontaneous pneumothorax that occurs as a result of disease is catergorized as secondary. Although it is less common than the primary form in developed countries, accounting for about one-third of cases [38], this may not be the case in those parts of the world where the prevalence of pulmonary tuberculosis remains high. With this possible exception, chronic bronchitis and emphysema are the most frequently associated conditions, accounting for

30–50% of cases in this group [4,33]. As these patients tend to be middle-aged or elderly, emphysema is the most common cause of pneumothorax in patient over 40 years of age [39]. Spontaneous pneumothorax has been recorded in 0.8% of a series of 1714 patients admitted to hospital with acute exacerbations of chronic bronchitis and emphysema [40]. Emphysematous bullae on the plain chest radiograph are frequently evident but this is by no means always the case [41]. In emphysema the leakage of trapped air through the weakened walls of dilated airspaces is probably assisted by the high intrabronchial pressures produced as a consequence of repeated coughing. It is also evident that pneumothorax may occur in association with large congenital bullae or cysts and in the absence of airflow limitation.

In one series, pneumothorax was reported to complicate 1.4% of cases of active tuberculosis [42]. Over 90% of these were cavitating and the pneumothoraces were thought to have resulted from the breakdown of tuberculous lesions situated close to the visceral pleura. It was observed that this might have been a more frequent complication had the overlying pleura not been thickened by fibrosis: when the pneumothorax did arise, the fibrosis caused it to be localized and limited in size. Before the advent of effective antituberculous chemotherapy, pneumothorax was frequently accompanied by a persistent bronchopleural fistula and tuberculous empyema with a mortality rate of 30–50% [43]. Pneumothorax has also been described in association with miliary tuberculosis but this is a rare complication [44].

Pneumothorax occasionally complicates asthma, having been found in 0.8% of 2000 adult asthmatics and 2.6% of 269 children admitted to hospital with severe asthma [45,46]. A more recent review of the chest radiographic findings of 1016 adult patients with asthma that was severe enough to require hospital admission in a large city in the UK found only one case (0.1%) of complicating pneumothorax [47].

Suppurative disease of the lungs and pleurae, particularly staphylococcal and *Klebsiella* pneumonia, is associated with pneumothorax. In the former, multiple lung abscesses may lead to the formation of cystic spaces or pneumatoceles that sometimes rupture into the pleural cavity, although such pneumatoceles are rare in adult compared with paediatric practice [48,49]. Prior to the availability of modern antibiotics, pneumothorax complicated approximately 5% of cases of staphylococcal pneumonia in adults and over 30% of cases in children [50,51]. Staphylococcal pneumonia continues to be the leading cause of pneumothorax in children and infants beyond the neonatal age group.

With the increasing prevalence of human immunodeficiency virus (HIV) infection, pneumothorax has become recognized as an important complication that occurs in approximately 2–4% of patients with AIDS, over 90%

of pneumothoraces in this condition being associated with active or previous episodes of *Pneumocystis carinii* pneumonia [52,53]. The chances of a patient with AIDS-associated *Pneumocystis* pneumonia developing a pneumothorax have been found to be about 6–9% [54]. One North American series of 120 patients with spontaneous pneumothorax referred to a surgical unit found that 27% of them had AIDS [55]. Patients with AIDS may be subject to bullous changes that have been termed 'premature emphysema' and *Pneumocystis* pneumonia itself has been shown to produce cystic changes on CT that persist despite clinical recovery [56]. Spontaneous pneumothoraces in AIDS are more commonly bilateral than is the case with other predisposing conditions, occurring in both lungs simultaneously in 34% according to one reported series [55]. It has been suspected that aerosolized pentamidine might predispose to spontaneous pneumothorax, although doubt remains on this score [53,57].

Patients with cystic fibrosis have a high incidence of spontaneous pneumothorax, which increases with age and which is an important cause of morbidity and mortality in this group (see Chapter 30) [58,59].

All other causes of secondary spontaneous pneumothorax may be regarded as unusual or rare. The diseases responsible include diffuse pulmonary inflammation of varying severity, which may be associated with fibrosis and cyst formation (honeycomb lung), and more localized disease processes abutting the pleural surface. Individual case reports abound and the following list is not exhaustive: cryptogenic fibrosing alveolitis [60]; occupational lung disease, particularly acute silicosis and Shaver's disease [61,62]; granulomatous disease such as sarcoidosis, usually at a late and fibrotic stage [63] but occasionally at an early stage of active inflammation [64]; Langerhans-cell histiocytosis (histiocytosis-X) [65] and Wegener's granulomatosis [66]; rheumatoid disease [67]; systemic sclerosis [68]; haemosiderosis [69]; lymphangioleiomyomatosis [70,71]; pulmonary alveolar proteinosis [72]; inherited disorders of connective tissue such as Marfan's syndrome [73], Ehlers–Danlos syndrome [74] and the marfanoid hypermobility syndrome [75]; other hereditary conditions, including neurofibromatosis [76] and tuberous sclerosis (which has been linked with lymphangioleiomyomatosis) [77,78]; coccidioidomycosis [60,79]; parasitic infections of the lung including hydatid disease [80]; intrathoracic tumours, particularly metastatic sarcomas and germ cell tumours [81,82]; primary bronchial carcinoma [83]; malignant mesothelioma of the pleura [84]; and cavitating pulmonary infarction [85]. Pneumothorax has been seen with septic pulmonary emboli occurring as a complication of staphylococcal tricuspid endocarditis in drug addicts using intravenous heroin [86]. Infection or inflammation in the gastrointestinal tract may unusually result in pneumothorax that may complicate retropharyngeal abscess formation [87]. Fistulous communications

have also been described between benign gastric ulcers and the pleural cavity across an anatomically intact diaphragm [88] and between stomach, colon and the pleural cavity in the presence of congenital diaphragmatic herniae [89,90]. Pneumothorax has also been recorded in association with hyperinflation and cystic changes occurring distal to congenital bronchial atresia [91]. Radiotherapy used to treat Hodgkin's disease above the diaphagm using a 'mantle' field may be complicated by pneumothorax [92,93].

Recurrent pneumothorax associated with menstruation was first reported by Maurer and is known as catamenial pneumothorax [94,95]. This rare condition, which is the usual way in which the thoracic endometriosis syndrome declares itself, is right-sided in about 90% of cases and is associated with multiparity, the pneumothorax occurring within 24–72 h of the onset of menstruation. Symptomatic pelvic endometriosis may be present in one-third to half of patients [96,97]. Examination of the diaphragm has occasionally revealed bluish cystic implants of endometrial tissue and there may be tiny diaphragmatic fenestrations through which it is supposed that endometrial tissue may find its way from the pelvis to the pleural cavity [98,99]. Less frequently the thoracic endometriosis syndrome presents as haemoptysis, sometimes in the presence of lung nodules consisting of islands of intrapulmonary endometrial tissue that may reach the lung by microembolization through the pelvic veins [100].

Traumatic pneumothorax

Traumatic pneumothoraces may arise from the penetration of the pleural cavity as a result of stab or gunshot wounds or from its accidental puncture by needles or cannulae. It may also occur in closed or blunt chest injury such as may result from road traffic accidents or explosions [101,102]. In this situation, rib fractures and bronchial rupture are frequent findings, as is blood loss into the pleural cavity resulting in haemopneumothorax [103,104].

Iatrogenic pneumothoraces

Iatrogenic pneumothoraces are common [105]. A 5-year study from a Veterans Administration medical centre in California found iatrogenic pneumothoraces to be slightly more common than the spontaneous variety; one-third were caused by transthoracic needle aspiration biopsy of suspected lung disease, 28% by thoracentesis and 22% by attempts to cannulate the subclavian vein [106].

About 12% of thoracenteses carried out on medical services result in pleural air leaks and pneumothoraces, although these are often shallow [107,108]. The frequency with which pneumothorax occurs may be increased further by closed needle biopsy of the pleura, although rates of 8% or less are achieved as the experience of the operator increases [108]. Pneumothorax is also a common complication of the placement of intercostal tubes intended for the drainage of malignant pleural effusions. The pneumothorax rate was found to be 31% in 88 such patients when drainage of pleural fluid was being effected by a small-bore tube [109]. None of these pneumothoraces were associated with tension or respiratory distress, the tendency being for them to either resolve spontaneously or remain stable [109].

Pneumothorax is an accepted but unwelcome complication of percutaneous lung biopsy by any form of needle or trephine (see Chapter 8), occurring in 20–45% of patients. In some but not all studies, the rate of pneumothorax has been found to be greater with increasing distance of the target lesion from the chest wall and also with smaller lesions, which may require more needle passes to locate them [110–113]. Lower complication rates have been obtained when a fine-gauge needle is employed [110,114], and lower rates may also be obtained when a modern gun-actuated cutting needle is used [115,116]. These accidental pneumothoraces are generally shallow but when they do occur chest tube placement has been recorded as necessary in 10–30% of cases [111,116]. Some investigators have found that the probability of pneumothorax is increased not only by greater depth of penetration of the needle but also by the presence of an obstructive impairment of ventilatory capacity [110,117]. Others have found that an obstructive impairment of lung function does not reliably predict complicating pneumothorax, although when pneumothorax does occur the need for tube placement clearly depends on the severity of any pre-existing pulmonary impairment [110–113]. It has been claimed that if the patient breathes pure oxygen before lung biopsy, the frequency of complicating pneumothoraces is reduced [118]. However, Poe and colleagues [117] observed an unaltered risk after breathing oxygen, although the size of the pneumothorax was reduced and the rate of its absorption increased.

Subclavian vein cannulation, with location of the vein by surface landmarks, is commonly used for measurement of central venous pressure, the administration of high-dose chemotherapy and long-term antibiotics, and total parenteral nutrition. A prospective study of 821 subclavian vein catheterizations found the overall pneumothorax rate to be 1.5% [119]. The complication rate increased with the number of passes, if body mass index was greater than 30 or less than 20 and if the patient had undergone prior surgery or radiotherapy to the ipsilateral hemithorax. The complication rate was not reduced by the use of ultrasound to help localize the vein [119]. Sometimes such pneumothoraces are 'delayed' and are not evident on the radiograph taken immediately after catheterization [120].

Pneumothorax is the most common complication of transbronchial lung biopsy, occurring in about 2–5% of cases or in a higher proportion if fluoroscopy is not used (see Chapter 8). Although pneumothorax in this situation is usually an immediate complication, it may occasionally be delayed by hours or even days [121]. The diagnostic yield of routine chest radiographs is very low in patients who have just undergone fluoroscopically guided transbronchial lung biopsy but who have no symptoms or fluoroscopic findings suggestive of pneumothorax, no unsuspected pneumothorax being found in 305 consecutive procedures in a study from the University of Virginia [122].

Pneumothorax may also complicate needle biopsy of the mediastinum, breast and liver [123–125], and may occur following tracheostomy [126].

Traumatic pneumothorax has also been described following a further miscellany of procedures, including acupuncture of the thoracic wall [127], the surgical use of a laser beam in the upper respiratory tract [128,129] and the misplacement of a small-bore nasogastric feeding tube in the respiratory tract [130]. Oesophageal rupture resulting from instrumental or other trauma may lead to pneumothorax in association with mediastinitis [131]. Pneumothorax may be self-inflicted by drug addicts who, having used all accessible veins in the arms, may resort to the practice of internal jugular or subclavian vein injection ('pocket shooting') [132,133]. The author has also seen traumatic pneumothorax occurring as a form of deliberate self-injury in a patient with psychological problems and access to hypodermic needles.

Pulmonary barotrauma

Since the volume of a given mass of gas at a constant temperature is inversely proportional to its pressure (Boyle's law), so a given volume of air, saturated at 37°C, expands to approximately 1.5 times the volume it would have occupied at sea level if it is placed at an altitude of 3050m. Should the air in question be trapped in a pleural bleb, the expansive force may cause that bleb to rupture into the pleural cavity resulting in a pneumothorax. Individuals who may be subject to such decompression occurring suddenly and by accident include aircrew, in whom radiographic screening procedures have been employed to exclude blebs prior to acceptance for flight training [134].

Considerable pressure changes may also occur underwater (see Chapter 57). The atmospheric pressure on the surface of the sea is 101 kPa (760 mmHg) but this increases linearly and doubles with every 10 m of descent. During scuba (*s*elf-*c*ontained *u*nderwater *b*reathing *a*pparatus) diving, in which compressed air is delivered to the lungs from a cylinder via a demand regulator, it is during ascent that barotrauma may occur: as ambient pressure falls rapidly, so gas contained in the lungs expands and serious damage may occur [135]. Such injury can be avoided if the diver is taught never to breath-hold and to ascend slowly,

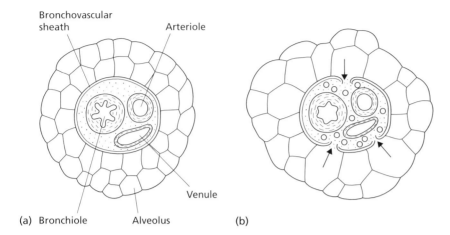

Bronchovascular sheath

Arteriole

Venule

(a) Bronchiole   Alveolus   (b)

Fig. 44.4 Barotrauma resulting in pneumomediastinum: (a) normal situation; (b) distended gas-containing spaces with air tracking from ruptured alveoli into the connective tissue plane of the bronchovascular bundle from which it may travel to the mediastinum and beyond. (After Maunder *et al.* [138].)

giving time for the expanding gas to escape by exhalation. Similarly, submariners who have to surface rapidly in submarine escape tank training must never do so with the glottis closed but must be taught to exhale continuously during ascent in order to allow the expanding intrathoracic gas to vent [136,137]. Caisson workers are at similar risk from rapid decompression.

Under all these circumstances expanding gas may break through both alveoli and subsequent anatomical barriers:
1 the visceral pleura to produce preumothorax (which may be bilateral);
2 the bronchiovascular bundle (Fig. 44.4) to produce mediastinum;
3 the connective tissue continuum leading from the mediastinum to the neck and beyond, producing subcutaneous emphysema; and
4 the diaphragmatic hiatus, entering the peritoneal carity and more rarely tracking between the diaphragm and the parietal pleura to produce encysted pockets of gas at the lung bases.

Much more seriously, rapidly expanding gas that has escaped from ruptured alveoli may track back into torn pulmonary veins, resulting in systemic arterial air embolism [139].

Pneumothorax due to barotrauma may also occur in patients who require positive-pressure mechanical ventilation, although this correlates most closely with the nature of the underlying disease. This is a particular problem in patients with adult respiratory distress syndrome (ARDS) [140,141]; 17% of 41 patients with ARDS receiving high-level (>15 cmH$_2$O) positive end-expiratory pressure ventilation developed radiographic signs of barotrauma including pneumothorax in one recent series [142]. Barotrauma may also occur as a result of attempted cardiopulmonary resuscitation [143]. Endotracheal tube misplacement, which is common, may also increase the chance of barotrauma by directing an excessive blast of air to one lung [144]. Systemic arterial air embolism has also occurred as a result of ventilator-associated barotrauma in association with ARDS and necrotizing pneumonia, but is rare [145].

There have been a number of reports of spontaneous pneumothorax occurring during the inhalation of recreational drugs, such as crystalline free base cocaine ('crack') and cannabis (marijuana, hashish, 'dope', 'pot', 'grass', 'ganja', 'hash'). The former, which looks like small crystals ('rocks'), may be smoked in a pipe or the vapour may be inhaled from a piece of heated tin foil, in contrast to cocaine powder which is taken like snuff. Cannabis is usually smoked mixed with tobacco in a rolled cigarette. Those pneumothoraces that have been described may result from a form of barotrauma, in both cases possibly being related to coughing or straining while the user is breath-holding after a deep inhalation near total lung capacity [146,147]. Pneumothorax due to presumed barotrauma has also been reported with the use of tracheo-oesophageal voice prostheses by patients who have had a total laryngectomy for carcinoma of the larynx [148].

Artificial pneumothorax

This term refers to the deliberate introduction of a measured volume of air into the pleural cavity by needle, using a device such as that illustrated in Fig. 44.5. Devised by Forlanini in the nineteenth century, this procedure became a popular method of treatment for pulmonary tuberculosis in the era before antibiotics but is now obsolete, although the technique is still employed diagnostically in order to enable the thoroscopist to visualize the surface of the lung and postoperatively in order to test whether a chemical or surgical pleurodesis has been effective [149].

Physiological disturbance

When pneumothorax occurs in a previously healthy subject, a restrictive impairment of ventilatory capacity is produced with a reduction in vital capacity, functional

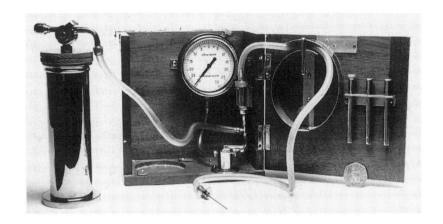

Fig. 44.5 Maxwell box used to induce artificial pneumothorax for the treatment of tuberculosis before the introduction of chemotherapy.

residual capacity and total lung capacity commensurate with the size of the pneumothorax [150]. There may also be a small reduction in diffusing capacity for carbon monoxide (D_{LCO}) and increase in the transfer coefficient (K_{CO}) [151]. If the pneumothorax is large, with greater than 20% collapse, then Pa_{O_2} falls immediately before returning to normal over the space of a few hours, despite the fact that the size of the pneumothorax may remain the same [152,153]. The initial hypoxaemia results from the shunting of blood through deaerated lung. The subsequent return to normoxaemia despite persisting lung collapse results from compensatory vasoconstriction that abolishes gross ventilation–perfusion mismatching in the affected lung [154]. Pulmonary function almost always returns to normal following re-expansion of the collapsed lung and although minor defects of gas distribution and reduced pulmonary compliance have been recorded, they appear to be of no clinical significance [155].

In tension pneumothorax the physiological disturbance may be severe and life-threatening. A valve-like tear in the visceral pleura permits air to progressively fill the pleural cavity during each inspiratory effort. As the intrapleural pressure builds up, hypoxaemia results from compression of both the ipsilateral and contralateral lung and the mediastinal structures are displaced across the midline. This mediastinal displacement and compression may cause a fall in cardiac output leading to hypotension and syncope.

Experiments with dogs have shown that the induction of pneumothorax in the conscious animal results in hyperventilation with arterial normoxaemia and hypocapnia. The belief that this behaviour is in part neuronally mediated is supported by the observation that when the same procedure is carried out in the vagotomized dog, hyperventilation does not occur and hypoxaemia ensues. General anaesthesia also impairs this adaptive response [156]. The relevance of these findings to the physiological consequences of pneumothorax in humans is unclear.

A study of regional lung function in spontaneous pneumothorax showed uniform airway closure on the affected side at low lung volumes, leading to the suggestion that this was the chief cause of ventilation–perfusion mismatch [157].

Clinical features

Symptoms

The most common mode of presentation is for a previously fit young man to develop sharp unilateral chest pain. This is frequently accompanied by shortness of breath, although pain may be the sole presenting symptom in two-thirds of patients [158]. The pain may be continuous but tends to be exacerbated by deep inspiration and postural change. It is often of moderately severe intensity but is sometimes insufficiently troublesome to cause the patient to seek medical advice for several days [159]. It is common for the pain to settle within a day or so, despite the persistence of the pneumothorax on the chest radiograph. Very occasionally a pneumothorax may be found unexpectedly on a chest film taken for routine reasons in a symptom-free individual. This suggests that spontaneous pneumothorax may occur more frequently in the population than is realized and that it may resolve unnoticed. The majority of cases of spontaneous pneumothorax are unassociated with physical exertion [33,160,161].

Extreme dyspnoea in a previously healthy subject is unusual and implies that the pneumothorax is under tension. In this situation the patient is anxious, restless and tachypnoeic, struggling for breath. Unless tension is relieved the patient may worsen, developing a rapid low-volume pulse and hypotension. Dyspnoea may be equally extreme with only a small pneumothorax; when this occurs in patients whose lung function is already impaired by underlying disease and in order that serious and unnecessary mishaps may be avoided, it is essential for clinicians to be alert to the possibility of pneumothorax when assessing a deteriorating patient with known asthma or chronic obstructive airways disease.

In the majority of patients the pneumothorax is small;

when this is the case, the presenting symptoms subside within a few hours even though there has been little or no radiographic improvement. Cough is not a prominent feature unless related to coincidental disease and when present is usually dry [17].

Spontaneous bilateral pneumothorax is rare [38,162,163], occurring in subjects who rupture bilateral apical blebs simultaneously or in patients with extensive bilateral emphysema or other cystic lung disease. It may be rapidly fatal [164].

Physical signs

A small pneumothorax may be impossible to detect on physical examination. If a sufficient volume of air enters the pleural cavity it insulates the lung from the stethoscope, producing the classical diagnostic signs described by Laënnec, comprising unilateral absent or diminished breath and voice sounds in the presence of a normal or hyperresonant percussion note [165]. Other signs are less important but complementary. Chest movement may be diminished on the affected side. When tension is present the chest may appear larger ipsilaterally and the mediastinum may be pushed to the opposite side, resulting in displacement of the trachea and apex beat. Similarly if the pneumothorax is right-sided, the liver may be displaced downwards so that the upper level of hepatic dullness moves caudally. There may be jugular venous engorgement.

A crepitous sound may be heard over the precordium and is sometimes even noticed by the patient. This noise is referred to as a 'mediastinal crunch' and may occur throughout the cardiac cycle, being influenced in its intensity by posture and the phase of respiration. It was described by Lister [166] in association with left-sided pneumothorax and later by Hamman [167], who considered it to result from free air in the mediastinum (Hamman's sign). In fact it may occur in both conditions, resulting from the close proximity of trapped air to moving heart muscle, and is not pathognomonic of pneumomediastinum. It has also given rise to the terms 'noisy' or 'clicking' pneumothorax [168,169]. Leakage of air into the mediastinum may spread to the subcutaneous tissues of the neck and beyond producing the characteristic palpable crepitus of 'surgical' emphysema, which may spread further to involve the face, anterior chest wall and beyond, sometimes alarming both onlookers and the patient who may quite suddenly come to resemble the 'Michelin man' of advertisement fame. Both may be reassured since this impressive sign is of no particular prognostic significance.

The signs of an associated pleural effusion or haemothorax are likely to be overlooked unless it is of moderate size, in which case in addition to the more usual physical signs devotees of medical history may perform Hippocratic succussion, in which a splashing sound is produced by rocking the patient to and fro [170]. The coin test is another obsolete manoeuvre, although the 'scratch sign' is sometimes usefully employed. In this test the stethoscope is placed in the mid-point of the sternum and the surface of the chest wall scratched with the finger at points equidistant to the left and right of the instrument. The sound heard is louder when the side of the pneumothorax is scratched [171].

The occurrence of pneumothorax in a mechanically ventilated patient may be suggested by (i) the sudden onset of tachycardia and hypotension, caused by a tension pneumothorax impeding venous return; (ii) an increase in peak airway pressure, resulting from external lung compression; (iii) a sudden decline in oxygen saturation; or (iv) the distressed patient appearing to 'fight the ventilator'.

Radiographic appearances

The characteristic finding is a sharply defined lung edge that is convex outwards and separated from the chest wall by a lucent zone entirely devoid of lung markings (Fig. 44.6). The thin white line representing the lung margin may be overlooked if the pneumothorax is shallow, in which case it may be hidden by bony shadows particularly if it is apical, as it may well be on an erect posteroanterior chest radiograph. If a pneumothorax is suspected clinically but cannot be detected on a standard inspiratory film, then two procedures may be used to confirm or refute the diagnosis. In the first the chest radiograph is taken in full expiration. This has the effect of reducing the volume of both the thorax and the partially deaerated lung. As the volume of gas contained within the pleural cavity is incompressible at physiological pressures, it remains the same on expiration and the pneumothorax therefore appears to enlarge in relation to the smaller thoracic volume (Fig. 44.6). In the second method the chest radiograph is taken in the lateral decubitus position with the side on which the pneumothorax is suspected uppermost [172]. Even a small pneumothorax is revealed by this technique as the air–lung interface becomes clearly visible beneath the lateral chest wall. This is also the preferred view for demonstrating pneumothorax in infants. In complete pneumothorax the lung appears as a dense globular shadow at the hilum (Figs 44.2 & 44.7). However, with lesser degrees of collapse the density of the lung may vary little from that of the fully expanded viscus. This finding is probably the result of a commensurate reduction in pulmonary blood flow [173]. Sometimes increased blood flow to the opposite lung may produce exaggerated vascular markings that may be mistaken for pneumonic shadowing.

In a tension pneumothorax the lung may be compressed into a shapeless shadow or even displaced across the

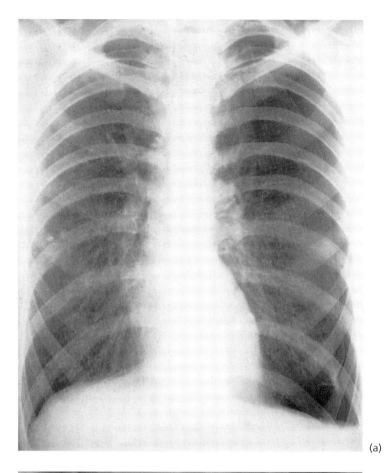

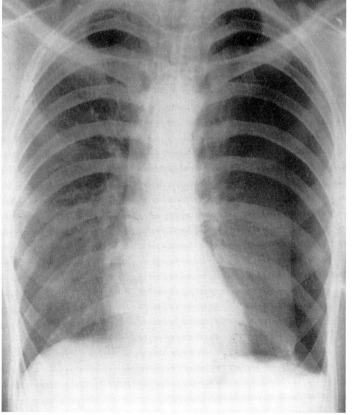

Fig. 44.6 (a) Respiratory and (b) expiratory films showing apparant enlargement of left pneumothorax on expiration.

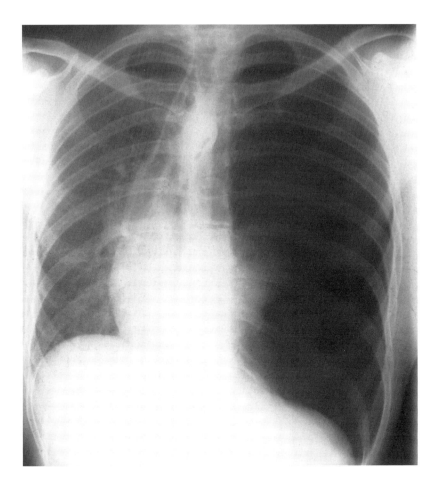

Fig. 44.7 Tension pneumothorax showing small dense shadow of collapsed left lung and deviation of mediastinum to the right. There is gross overdistension of the left thoracic cavity.

midline along with the mediastinal structures (Fig. 44.7). In addition, the diaphragm may be depressed so that its costal attachments become clearly visible. It should be noted that some degree of mediastinal displacement is to be expected on an expiratory film and that this does not indicate tension. Some mediastinal displacement is also commonly seen in large pneumothoraces in the absence of *clinical* signs of tension such as tachypnoea and hypotension. When there is also fluid as well as air in the pleural cavity it appears as a completely horizontal line with no meniscus where it abuts the lateral chest wall (Fig. 44.8) and this finding may draw the observer's attention to the presence of a small pneumothorax that might otherwise have been missed.

It has been suggested that CT may be useful in the unusual case where the distinction between a bulla and a pneumothorax cannot be easily made but in practice this is seldom necessary [102].

In patients under intensive care only supine films may be available for interpretation. In this situation a pneumothorax may be indicated by increased lucency on the ipsilateral side due to an anterior collection of gas, and by a deep lateral costophrenic angle also on the involved side. This last feature has been called the 'deep sulcus sign' and when present should lead to a request for a lateral decubitus or 'cross table lateral' view to confirm [174].

Differential diagnosis

Although the differential diagnosis includes many conditions associated with chest pain and dyspnoea, in practice few difficulties are encountered. Pain due to myocardial infarction, pleuritis associated with pulmonary infarction or pleural infection, and the pain of intra-abdominal inflammatory disease, such as a perforated peptic ulcer, may occasionally suggest pneumothorax to the clinician but any doubts should be resolved by physical examination and the chest radiograph. It should be noted that changes in the ECG typical of a transmural myocardial infarction may be produced by a left-sided pneumothorax, although these changes resolve once re-expansion has occurred [175]. A breathless patient with generalized emphysema may have physical signs that give rise to confusion with pneumothorax but again the chest film is generally diagnostic. Where a massive emphysematous bulla or congenital lung cyst occupies a large part of one hemithorax, the physical signs may be indistinguishable from pneumothorax and even the chest radiographic

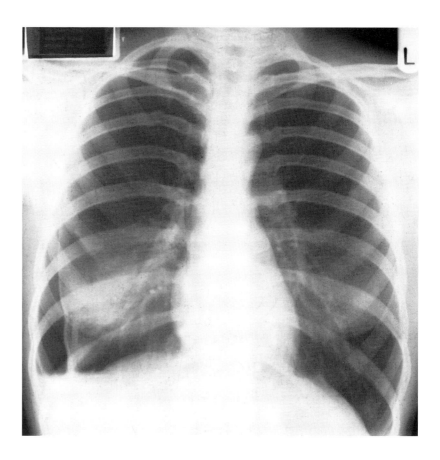

Fig. 44.8 Right hydropneumothorax showing basal fluid level.

appearances may not be dissimilar (Fig. 44.9). It is on such occasions that time taken to enquire about or to obtain previous chest radiographs is time well spent (Fig. 44.10). A lateral decubitus view is often helpful in differentiating an upper lobe bulla or cyst from a typical pneumothorax; in the first case, the gas is constrained by the anatomical boundaries of the upper lobe, whereas in pneumothorax it usually moves to lie along the lateral chest wall. The herniation of a large volume of gut through a diaphragmatic defect may also mimic the physical signs of a basal pneumothorax. Such defects may be congenital or acquired, in which case a history of recent or remote trauma to the lower chest or abdomen (e.g. road traffic accident) might be obtained. When radiographic uncertainty exists, barium contrast studies of the upper or lower bowel are diagnostic.

It is emphasized that pneumothorax should always be considered when patients with previously diagnosed lung disease, such as asthma or chronic obstructive pulmonary disease, present with an apparent deterioration.

Management of spontaneous pneumothorax

There is evidence of considerable variation in individual management of spontaneous pneumothorax, thoracic sur-geons on the whole tending to resort to more active measures than physicians [176].

Conservative management

Conservative management relies upon the natural tendency of the gases in a pneumothorax space to be reabsorbed and has the attraction of avoiding any form of invasive procedure [177,178]. This approach is indicated in an otherwise healthy adult who is not breathless and in whom the volume of the pneumothorax is judged to be small. 'Small' is widely taken to mean that the pneumothorax occupies less than 20% of the hemithoracic volume. Various methods for calculating the volume of a pneumothorax have been published [179,180] but these are rarely used in practice. Thus most clinicians leave a primary spontaneous pneumothorax that they gauge as shallow, treating those that are moderate or large [181]. As a rule of thumb, if the lateral edge of the lung is separated from the ipsilateral chest wall in the horizontal plane and at the widest point of the pneumothorax by more than one-third of the transverse diameter of the hemithorax, then the pneumothorax can be regarded as moderate to large and active treatment is reasonable. Previously healthy patients with small spontaneous pneumothoraces need not be admitted to hospital and rest in bed is not manda-

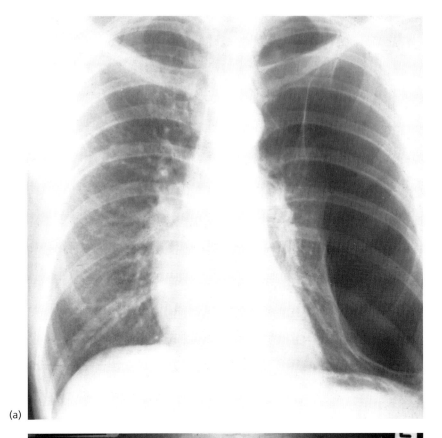

(a)

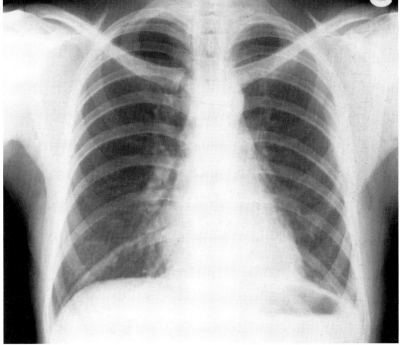

(b)

Fig. 44.9 (a) Large, presumably congenital, bulla in asymptomatic young woman mimicking pneumothorax. (b) Same patient after excision of bulla showing expansion of normal lung.

tory. Non-manual work may be continued but heavy physical exertion should be disallowed. The chest radiograph should be repeated at weekly intervals until full expansion has occurred; meanwhile the way should have been prepared for prompt admission should dyspnoea develop. If any doubt exists the safest course is to admit

and observe for 24 h in order to ensure that the pneumothorax is not enlarging. Patients with significant underlying lung disease such as emphysema should be admitted for observation even if the pneumothorax is shallow, since these patients are at risk of developing severe respiratory failure if the pneumothorax enlarges.

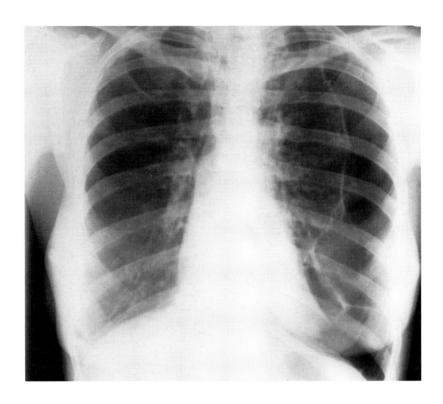

Fig. 44.10 Somewhat similar appearance to that in Fig. 44.9a but due to a tethered pneumothorax. A previous film showed no abnormality.

Provided the pneumothorax remains 'closed', the lung will re-expand slowly. This is because the rate of transfer of gases across a semi-permeable membrane is directly proportional to the difference in partial pressure of the gases on either side of the membrane. The total gas pressure of alveolar air is approximately 101 kPa (760 mmHg) at sea level, this being the same as the arterial total gas pressure; however, the venous total gas pressure is about 93.8 kPa (705 mmHg) due to the fall in P_{O_2} from approximately 13.3 kPa (100 mmHg) in the arterial system to 5.3 kPa (40 mmHg) in the venous system, the balance being due to the smaller rise in P_{CO_2} between the arterial and venous phases. Kircher and Swartzel [179] described a radiographic method to express the volume of pneumothorax as a percentage of hemithoracic volume and found an average rate of re-expansion of 1.25% hemithoracic volume per day. Thus, provided that there is no further air leak, a '10% pneumothorax' re-expands in approximately 8 days, a '20% pneumothorax' in 16 days, and so on.

Absorption of gas from a pneumothorax space may be hastened by breathing a high concentration of oxygen [180]. By breathing 100% oxygen instead of ambient air, which contains about 79% nitrogen, alveolar P_{N_2} falls and nitrogen is gradually washed out of the tissues and vascular system as oxygen is taken up, so that the end-capillary total gas tension eventually falls from approximately 93.8 kPa (705 mmHg) to around 22.6 kPa (170 mmHg). This produces a substantial gradient between the tissue capillary (low P_{N_2}) and the pneumothorax space, which is nearer atmospheric pressure (about 101 kPa, relatively high P_{N_2}), with the result that the rate of absorption of gas from the pleural space increases several fold (Fig. 44.11). Clearly, high concentrations of oxygen are contraindicated in those patients with chronic obstructive pulmonary disease whose respiratory centres may be dependent upon 'hypoxic drive'; furthermore, the potential toxicity of high concentrations of oxygen for prolonged periods in otherwise healthy individuals has to be considered [182]. However, oxygen therapy may be a useful adjunct to the conservative treatment of pneumothorax in patients who also have a bleeding diathesis in order to avoid an invasive procedure such as tube drainage with its attendant risk of haemorrhage.

Active management

Most reported hospital series show that in the majority of patients the volume of the pneumothorax exceeds 20%, fitting into the moderate or large categories mentioned above. Brooks [163], while acknowledging the difficulties in estimating size, reported 23% of patients presenting with 25% collapse, 31% with 25–50% collapse, 13% with 50–75% collapse and 33% with over 75% collapse in his series of 376 spontaneous pneumothoraces. In view of this, active treatment in hospital is employed in the vast majority of cases in order to achieve full expansion within a reasonable length of time. Hospital treatment is indicated not only for moderate or large primary spontaneous pneumothoraces but also for secondary spontaneous pneumothoraces, in which underlying lung disease is associated with a pre-existing impairment of lung function so that even a shallow pneumothorax may be serious.

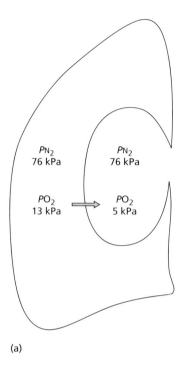 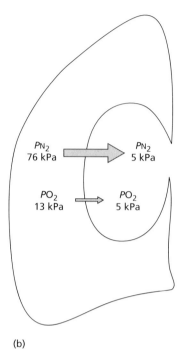

Fig. 44.11 Potential partial pressure differences for oxygen and nitrogen between a closed pneumothorax space and venous end capillaries that contribute to reabsorption of gas when the patient breaths (a) ambient air and (b) a high concentration of oxygen so that nitrogen is 'washed out'. The differences in P_{CO_2} are relatively small and are not illustrated. (a) No difference in P_{N_2}, small differences in P_{O_2}. (b) Large difference in P_{N_2}, small differences in P_{O_2}.

Aspiration

The insertion and removal of a standard intercostal drain is unpleasant for the patient and while the drain remains *in situ* regular analgesia is required. In view of this, simple manual apiration has been re-evaluated [183,184]. The technique originally employed a needle and attracted condemnation because of the risk of lacerating the lung as it expanded [162,185]; however, this complication may be avoided if a modern plastic intravenous cannula is used and various clinicians have claimed success for their techniques [186–189]. The author prefers a small (8 cm long, 10 French gauge) neonatal pneumothorax cannula with trocar and side-holes as well as an end-hole. The second intercostal space in the mid-clavicular line is conventional, although an axillary approach in the fourth, fifth or sixth space between the mid and anterior axillary lines may be used as an alternative. The cannula is inserted aseptically with local anaesthetic and air withdrawn and expelled using a large Luer–Lok syringe with a three-way tap. Placement of the exit tube underwater reduces the chance of an embarrassing mistake. Provided that the patient's condition remains stable, the procedure may be continued until no more air can be withdrawn or until 3 L has been removed, which implies that a leak is still present. Aspiration is abandoned and an intercostal drain inserted if the patient's condition deteriorates.

Simple aspiration is contraindicated if the patient is distressed as a result of a tension pneumothorax or when there is more than a little pleural fluid present. It is unnecessary if the pneumothorax is shallow. For the remainder, while aspiration may avoid the need for an intercostal drain in a significant number of patients [188], those in whom the technique fails due to reaccumulation of air require treatment by conventional means and their hospital stay is likely to be longer than would otherwise have been the case. A marker gas technique may be used in order to determine whether the pleural leak has sealed off at the time of aspiration, chest radiographs taken immediately after aspiration being unreliable in this respect. The hydrocarbon propellant gas found in metered-dose inhalers has been used in this way, being detected by a portable flame ionizer [190], the patients' breathing from a Douglas bag containing air or oxygen labelled with the tracer gas (Fig. 44.12). Those pneumothoraces that were negative for tracer gas were successfully treated by aspiration, whereas those that were positive for tracer gas frequently recollapsed over the following 12 h despite initial radiographic improvement, requiring tube placement in 60–80% of cases [191,192]. Patients negative for tracer gas may be discharged early if their general condition allows, provided that arrangements for prompt readmission have been put in place should the need arise [192].

There is evidence to suggest that patients who are treated by aspiration not only experience less pain but are also likely to spend a shorter time in hospital than those treated by intercostal tube drainage [192,193]. Manual aspiration is less likely to be successful in pneumothoraces in which the lung is completely collapsed at presentation [194]. When taking the requirement for a chest drain as the end-point, the marker gas technique has subsequently been found to have a negative predictive value of 95% and a positive predictive value of 67% when applied to 136 events.

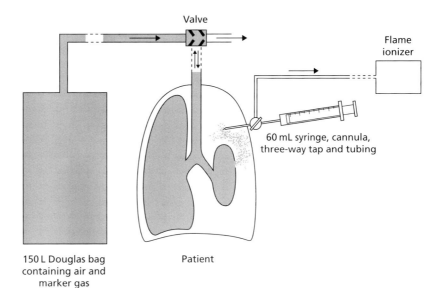

Fig. 44.12 Apparatus for detecting hydrocarbon marker gas in pleural leaks during manual aspiration of pneumothorax. (After Seaton *et al.* [191].)

Table 44.2 Indications for intercostal tube drainage in spontaneous pneumothorax.

Tension pneumothorax
Presence of dyspnoea
Intermittent positive-pressure ventilation
Previous contralateral pneumothorax
Bilateral pneumothoraces
Presence of pleural fluid
Large/complete pneumothorax
Failed manual aspiration

Intercostal tube drainage

When simple manual aspiration is contraindicated, the preferred method of treatment is intercostal tube drainage or 'tube thoracostomy', in which an intercostal drain is inserted into the pleural space and connected to an underwater seal bottle (Table 44.2).

It has been suggested that premedication with atropine 0.6 mg i.m. might reduce the chances of a vasovagal reaction. A common site for insertion is in the second intercostal space in the mid-clavicular line, thereby avoiding the internal mammary arteries (which run vertically 3–4 cm to the left and right of the sternum, posterior to the costal cartilages). The first intercostal space is immediately below the clavicle and is avoided because of the risk of major neurovascular damage; the second intercostal space is identified below the second rib, which articulates with the sternal angle of Louis.

An alternative site now commonly used and which may be preferred in women for cosmetic reasons is the fourth or fifth intercostal space between the anterior and posterior axillary lines. This site is also suitable when the pleural cavity contains fluid, because drainage is facilitated, and is also preferred in traumatic pneumothorax.

The choice of site may also be influenced by the presence of adhesions as seen on the chest radiograph. In order to avoid the upper limit of the diaphragm, it is a good rule for the physician not to insert a tube below nipple level in the male or below the sixth space in the female.

Once the entry point has been selected and the site marked with a pen, 10–15 mL of 1% lidocaine (lignocaine) is infiltrated from the skin to the parietal pleura, taking in the periosteum of the upper border of the rib at the chosen interspace and localizing the pneumothorax space by withdrawing air. This is done *before* skin preparation in order to give time for the local anaesthetic to have its effect. The needle can be left in place to mark the site of anaesthetic infiltration while aseptic skin procedures are then followed. A small (1–1.5 cm) incision is made through skin to subcutaneous fat over the body of the rib that lies below the chosen intercostal space. Two interrupted sutures, or better still a single central mattress suture, are inserted across the incision so that they can be tied later when the tube is removed. Purse-string sutures should be avoided as they may result in skin necrosis. A further silk or propylene securing suture (at least 0 gauge) is placed alongside the incision so that the drain can be tied in once inserted (Fig. 44.13). The track for the tube is made by blunt dissection with a haemostat (artery forceps). This is done by advancing the haemostat a short distance with the jaws closed, opening the jaws, withdrawing the instrument, closing the jaws and advancing it further [195]. The track is aimed obliquely upwards towards the upper border of the same rib, the objective being for the tube to follow this direction so that its tip lies at the apex of the hemithorax. The lower border of the rib above, with the neurovascular bundle lying behind its lower margin, is avoided.

The pleural cavity used to be routinely entered with a relatively short guarded steel trocar and cannula

(Fig. 44.14). Following withdrawal of the trocar, a rubber self-retaining Malecot catheter stretched on a steel introducer was passed through the cannula and the introducer and cannula then withdrawn. Nowadays Malecot catheters are virtually museum pieces and a prepacked disposable plastic tube with a long central metal trocar is usually provided instead; 18–24 French gauge is suitable for air, whereas if blood as well as air needs draining a larger tube (e.g. 28–32 French gauge) may be more successful. The central trocar on such modern tubes may have a conical point that does not cut tissues but spreads them, so that in less experienced hands and if undue pressure is applied this assembly carries the risk of causing injury to the lung or other tissues by sudden deep penetration of the

chest. This may be particularly relevant in cases of traumatic pneumothorax dealt with by accident and emergency personnel; in these patients diaphragmatic rupture may have occurred, allowing abdominal viscera such as the liver, spleen or stomach to lie within the thoracic cavity, so that various advanced life support guidelines recommend that intercostal drains should be inserted without a trocar in trauma cases (see p. 1204). A protective guard has been devised to prevent such sudden deep entry [196] (Fig. 44.14) but in truth heavy pressure should never be applied. Once the forceps have entered the pleural cavity by blunt dissection, the track may be widened with the forefinger if necessary so that the tube can then be easily introduced while being gripped firmly about 5 cm from its tip to allow for any loss of resistance when the pleural cavity is reached and to avoid sudden overpenetration. The trocar may be withdrawn a few centimetres and used to help angle the tube, which is advanced about 8 cm towards the apex. As an alternative, curved blunt plastic-coated metal introducers are also available that can be placed through a side-hole of the plastic drain in place of a trocar to enable it to be directed towards the apex of the lung. The trocar or introducer is then removed completely in order to allow the intercostal drain to be attached with a suitable untaped connection to further tubing, which joins it with an underwater seal drainage bottle. The catheter connected to the bottle passes through a double-lumen stopper or similar arrangement to rest 2.5 cm below the surface of about 0.5 L sterile water, thereby acting as a one-way low-resistance valve. Correct placement of the tube is greeted by a satisfying stream of bubbles during expiration or coughing and a rise in the level of the fluid in the underwater seal tube during inspiration.

All connections and tubing require regular inspection to avoid either leakage or blockage by kinking. So-called

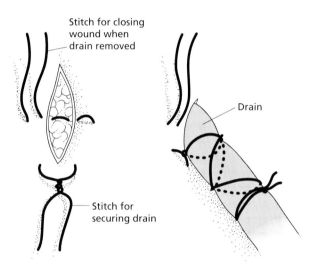

Fig. 44.13 Sutures inserted to secure the drain and for closing the wound when the drain is removed. The drain is secured to the skin by tying knots on either side of it. (After Parmar [195].)

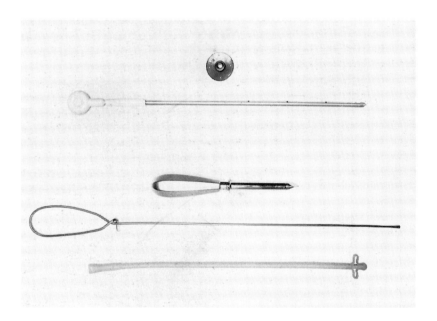

Fig. 44.14 Disposable plastic cannula, metal trocar and plastic guard (above) and early rubber Malecot catheter with steel introducer, trocar and cannula (below)

'sleek' should be avoided, and simple adhesive tape is used to cover the gauze skin dressings and may also used to fashion a supportive mesentery for the tubing but should not conceal any junctions in the drainage system. The tube itself should be attached to the skin by knotting the securing suture three or four times on each side of the drain (Fig. 44.13), which should also be looped and taped to the skin to further reduce the chance of it being accidentally pulled out.

Should the patient be in a state of cardiovascular collapse as a result of a tension pneumothorax, release of the positive pressure in the pleural cavity is a matter of urgent necessity. Provided that there is no doubt about the diagnosis, this may be quickly achieved with rapid clinical improvement by the insertion of a wide-bore hypodermic needle or preferably a plastic intravenous cannula into the pleural cavity. This allows the pressure in the pneumothorax to become atmospheric and if the diagnosis was correct results in immediate improvement in the patient's condition so that an intercostal tube can then be inserted in a more orderly manner [197].

The application of suction to the second opening of the underwater seal drain bottle has been recommended by some in order to assist expansion of the collapsed lung. This has been applied either at constant high flow using an appropriate pump (e.g. Thompson or Tubbs-Barrett rather than Roberts) or at constant pressure (e.g. 1.5–5.0 kPa, 15–50 cmH$_2$O) using wall suction with a pressure reducing valve. However, if the pneumothorax is closed this should be unnecessary as expansion will occur within 2–3 days anyway. If the pneumothorax is open then the application of suction at practicable flow rates might in theory prevent it from sealing off by drawing air through the point of leakage. This is in agreement with observations that mechanical suction does not influence the rate of re-expansion [198].

The tube is left *in situ* until the lung is fully re-expanded on the chest radiograph and the tube has not been seen to bubble for 24 h. Once this has been achieved, the tube may be removed. It is safer to remove tubes with the help of an assistant. One throw of the knot in the mattress suture is made. The patient inspires fully and is then asked to perform a Valsalva manoeuvre, thereby reducing the risk of air entering the pleura again as the drain is withdrawn. The drain is removed with one smooth quick movement while the track is compressed and the knot in the mattress suture is then completed [195]. Some practitioners prefer to clamp the tube for about 12 h once the tube has apparently stopped blowing and when no bubbles are seen on coughing, after which the intercostal tube is removed if the lung remains fully expanded. However, if the pneumothorax has reaccumulated, the clamp is removed and the air once again fully drained before the cycle is repeated. The obvious drawback of clamping is that the patient may become distressed if a substantial leak does occur and the clamp is not removed promptly because of lack of understanding by staff either at the bedside or while the patient is being transported between departments; the British Thoracic Society guidelines thus advise against this practice [181].

It is usually possible to re-expand the lung and remove the tube within 3–4 days. Intercostal tubes may occasionally kink or become blocked by blood or fibrous material before full re-expansion has taken place. The column of water in the underwater seal drainage bottle is seen to stop swinging in this situation and the intercostal tube needs to be unkinked or replaced through a second clean incision in order to achieve a satisfactory result. Sometimes several such tube changes are required and re-expansion is slow. This is particularly common in patients with diffuse emphysema, although almost always in such cases if drainage is continued the leak eventually seals. A retrospective study of 214 patients with spontaneous pneumothorax found that 51% still had a persistent leak after 2 days of tube drainage. Of those who continued to be treated medically, the median time to resolution was 7 days for those with primary spontaneous pneumothorax and 11 days for those with underlying lung disease [199]. It has been claimed that patients with uncomplicated pneumothoraces treated by intercostal catheter are usually fit to return to work within 1 week [162]. Other authors have reported an average hospital stay of 13 days for cases of pneumothorax treated with underwater seal drainage [200].

Flutter valves

Commercially available (Heimlich-type) flutter valves may be connected to the chest tube in order to avoid the encumbrance of an underwater seal drain [201,202]. This method has been used satisfactorily in battle casualties [201] and also in the civilian outpatient management of pneumothorax, sometimes by using narrow 8–14 French gauge intercostal catheters [203–207]. These valves may be more prone to blockage than standard underwater seal drainage [208] and their use in general management has not gained full acceptance. Prepacked water-free ambulatory chest drainage kits incorporating a conventional intercostal drain that connects to a plastic bag with an integral flutter valve are also available for use in trauma cases.

Chemical pleurodesis

The tendency for a pneumothorax to recur (see p. 1202) has led to the development of certain procedures intended to cause the visceral pleura to adhere to the inner surface of the chest wall. Various foreign substances may be introduced into the pleural cavity in order to produce a sterile pleurisy, with the subsequent formation of adhesions between the visceral and parietal pleural layers [209].

This method, known as chemical pleurodesis, was first described by Spengler over 80 years ago [210]. The wide variety of different substances that have been used to achieve pleural symphysis, ranging from irritants such as tetracycline, 50% glucose solution, autologous blood and iodized oil to more caustic chemicals such as silver nitrate solution to physical irritants such as iodized talc slurry or kaolin and more recently to fibrin glue sealant, implies that the search for an ideal agent continues. These substances may be injected or insufflated through an intercostal drain or in some cases may be applied to the surface of the visceral pleura under general anaesthesia using a thoracoscope.

As a rule these procedures produce pleural effusions that require drainage. Cerebral embolism has rarely been reported following the use of talc [211] and there have been fears about the possibility of subsequent mesothelioma due to potential contamination with asbestos, although this has not been borne out by experience [212,213]. Patients treated by chemical pleurodesis remain in hospital longer than those treated by intercostal tube drainage alone and the efficacy of the procedure in preventing recurrence has been questioned [214], although the balance of evidence is that it is more effective than tube thoracostomy alone but less so than surgical treatment [215,216].

Despite these disadvantages, chemical pleurodesis finds occasional application in the prevention of recurrent spontaneous pneumothorax, particularly in patients with serious respiratory impairment due to chronic lung disease, in whom more invasive surgery for pleurectomy or pleural abrasion might carry an unacceptable risk. Of the many substances that have been used, a solution of tetracycline hydrochloride (1–1.5g in 50mL of normal saline with 10mL 1% lidocaine added) is currently favoured. Lidocaine is added to the solution to diminish the considerable pain that the procedure often produces. Once the lung has almost inflated and the pleural leak sealed or become minimal, the tetracycline is injected into the chest tube and flushed through with a further 50mL saline. The tube is then clamped for the next 60–120 min while the patient is frequently repositioned (e.g. 5 min supine, prone, left and right lateral decubitus) so that the tetracycline comes into contact with all pleural surfaces, before the tube is unclamped for drainage (with or without suction) of any effusion that might have accumulated. Talc may be more effective than tetracycline, producing a vigorous granulomatous reaction but seemingly also producing greater pain and more prolonged fever [217]. Tetracycline has been claimed to be no less effective than silver nitrate, to cause less pain, diminished exudation and a shorter hospital stay [218]. Tetracycline pleurodesis has been shown to reduce ipsilateral recurrence rate significantly in a prospective controlled trial of patients with primary and secondary spontaneous pneu-

mothorax [215]. As a standard procedure for primary spontaneous pneumothorax, chemical pleurodesis does not currently find wide acceptance but continues to be used in some centres [216,218].

Parietal pleurectomy, pleural abrasion at thoracotomy and video-assisted thoracoscopic procedures

A more major operative procedure is indicated if the lung fails to expand fully with tube drainage. Most leaks close within 2–3 days of insertion of a well-placed intercostal tube [219,220], failing which is is reasonable to consider a surgical opinion provided that the patient's general condition permits thoracotomy or thoracoscopy. A further delay of a few days is not important, so that an operation can proceed if still needed after about a week has elapsed from the insertion of the drain [199]. Patients with underlying lung disease are often left longer because of the increased risks that surgical intervention carries for this group. Prior to the advent of video-assisted thoracoscopic surgery (VATS), the standard procedure was parietal pleurectomy carried out through a posterolateral thoracotomy, in which the parietal pleura is stripped off the chest wall and upper mediastinum leaving a raw area that becomes adherent to the remaining visceral pleura [211]. Some surgeons prefer to produce a similar effect less radically by either limiting the procedure to the apex of the lung (apical pleurectomy) or alternatively by scarifying the parietal pleura with a dry gauze sponge or nylon pan scourer, a procedure known as pleural abrasion [221,222]. Both types of operation may include the excision, oversewing or stapling of any visible pleural blebs or bullae and, after either of these procedures, tube drainage is maintained for a few days to allow the visceral pleura to come into close apposition with the chest wall while adhesions form. Parietal pleurectomy is almost guaranteed to prevent recurrence (0.4%) and recurrence after pleural abrasion is also unlikely (2%) [38,223,224].

Although these 'open' procedures are still carried out in many centres, increasing use is being made of VATS. The indications for this intervention are broadly similar to those for the open procedures mentioned above and the temptation to refer patients routinely after a first episode of primary spontaneous pneumothorax should be resisted as the recurrence rate is only 20% or so. VATS usually entails the surgeon making three 1–2 cm incisions to establish a port for the thoracoscopic camera and one each for the grasping forceps and stapler. This compares with a thoracotomy wound, which although sometimes limited may extend anything up to 30 cm in length and is associated with greater morbidity and a longer hospital stay. VATS lends itself to the identification of leaking apical blebs in patients with recurrent or persistent primary spontaneous pneumothorax. These blebs can often be resected after placing a row of staples across their necks

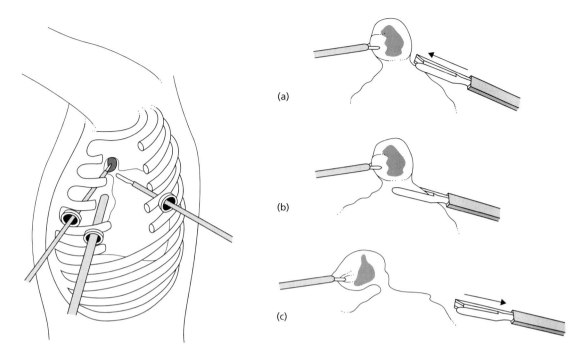

Fig. 44.15 Approximate sites of routine trocar positioning for video-assisted thoracoscopic surgery in pneumothorax, also demonstrating the stapled resection of an apical bleb. (a) The bleb is grasped; (b) the stapler is applied above a rim of normal lung tissue; (c) each staple application cuts between six rows of staples. (After Hazelrigg *et al.* [225].)

Table 44.3 Indications for parietal pleurectomy or abrasion in spontaneous pneumothorax.

Failed tube drainage (persistent pneumothorax)
Ipsilateral recurrence (First or second)
Contralateral occurrence (First)
Bilateral simultaneous pneumothorax
Persistent pleural effusion
Initial episode life-threatening
Special risk groups e.g. aircrew, divers, etc.

[225] (Fig. 44.15). The bullae in patients with emphysema tend to merge with adjacent lung and are more difficult to deal with using VATS so that leaks are more frequent and other surgical techniques may need to be used, including formal thoracotomy. In addition to dealing with the leak, VATS may be used to establish a pleural symphysis by parietal pleurectomy, pleural abrasion or chemical pleurodesis. The recurrence rate is known to be higher if no leak can be identified and dealt with at thoracoscopy, in which case VATS pleurectomy may be a surer way to proceed [226]. There are reports of thoracoscopic ablation of pulmonary blebs and bullae by laser but in the setting of pneumothorax, the recurrence rate may be too high [226].

Parietal pleurectomy or abrasion may also be recommened after the first or second ipsilateral recurrence or following the first contralateral recurrence in order to avoid the future possibility of simultaneous bilateral spontaneous pneumothoraces [227]. Pleurectomy is indicated after the initial event for categories of patient in whom a recurrence would carry a special risk, such as aircrew, divers who refuse to stop diving, seafarers or other travellers to remote parts and those in whom the first pneumothorax was a life-threatening 'near miss' (Table 44.3). Surgical treatment is also indicated when pneumothorax is complicated by a large haemothorax, pleural effusion or

empyema that cannot be satisfactorily managed by aspiration or tube drainage alone. One potential problem with pleurectomy in a patient with pneumothorax is that the symphysis is so good that were a thoracotomy to be required in the future for some other reason, it would be made technically very difficult.

Patients with spontaneous pneumothorax secondary to cystic fibrosis may be managed with aspiration or tube thoracostomy. Cases of recurrence may be treated with chemical pleurodesis or thoracoscopically with ligation of bullae and limited pleural abrasion rather than with pleurectomy, unless it is quite certain that they are not candidates for future transplantation. It is sensible to discuss the management options for those patients with cystic fibrosis who are transplant candidates with the transplant centre concerned [59].

Spontaneous pneumothorax in pregnancy has rarely been reported. It can be treated with aspiration or tube drainage. Surgical treatment during pregnancy is sometimes necessary and there is no good evidence of teratogenesis, increased risk of abortion or premature labour following general anaesthesia. However, the risks from pneumothorax in pregnancy are also small [228] and prolonged drainage with a flutter valve until after term has been reported as an alternative to surgical intervention [203,229].

Cases of catamenial pneumothorax thought to be associated with endometriosis may be treated medically by inducing a hypo-oestrogenic state with drugs such as danazol and analogues of gonadotrophin-releasing hormone, but are likely to produce improvement only while treatment is continued [230,231]. Endometriosis resolves at the menopause; however, apart from these pharmacological interventions, an earlier permanent cure requires bilateral oophorectomy, which may be appropriate (with hysterectomy) for women in their fifth decade. This may be followed with hormone replacement therapy without any recrudescence of pneumothorax since the problems in endometriosis seem to seem to depend on cyclical variation in oestrogen level [232].

Sometimes patients with barotrauma due to diving accidents, in addition to possible pneumothorax and pneumomediastinum, may develop air embolism that should be treated by transport to the nearest centre with facilities for emergency hyperbaric oxygen therapy. This has the effect of reducing the volume of the air emboli physically according to Boyle's law, as well as accelerating absorption of gas by 'washing out' nitrogen from the body, thereby increasing the gradient for diffusion of nitrogen between the trapped gas and the tissues (see Fig. 44.11). The US Navy uses a protocol of rapid recompression with air to 600 kPa for 30 min, followed by 100% oxygen at 280 kPa [135].

Complications

Failure to re-expand

Failure to re-expand the lung by tube drainage may require the insertion of a second intercostal drain [9]. A persistent air leak requiring surgical intervention is reported in 4–14% of cases in whom tube drainage has been attempted [6,8,9,162]. These failures may be caused by multiple leaks in generalized emphysema or by adhesions preventing a bronchopleural fistula from closing. In such cases the treatment of choice is a surgical procedure to produce pleurodesis (see above), provided that the patient does not have severe respiratory impairment that would make the risk of thoracotomy or thoracoscopy unacceptable. Such high-risk patients usually have severe emphysema and with prolonged tube drainage the leak frequently seals off, although this may occasionally take weeks. However, an otherwise healthy subject should be offered a surgical procedure if tube drainage remains unsuccessful after 3–7 days [199,224,225]. Occasionally re-expansion of the lung is delayed by atelectasis resulting from retained secretions. This situation is treated by chest physiotherapy with an intercostal drain in place, although

rigid bronchoscopy may be required occasionally to suck out tenacious intrabronchial material and the passage of an endotracheal tube may be required in order to achieve full reflation.

Rarely a pneumothorax becomes chronic, with the result that the lung becomes surrounded and bound down by a thickened non-expansive layer of fibrin known as a pleural rind or peel. This is more likely to occur if there is an associated pleural effusion. A chronic pneumothorax is sometimes seen in cases of inactive tuberculosis that were treated with the now obsolete technique of artificial pneumothorax; in such cases the pleural rind is frequently heavily calcified [233] (Fig. 44.16). Surgical decortication of the pleura may be required to achieve re-expansion of the trapped lung, although this is seldom technically possible because of the dense nature of the adhesions.

Recurrence

There is a tendency to overestimate the recurrence rate of spontaneous pneumothorax in the published series, many of which are retrospective and contain an unduly high proportion of patients referred to surgical units because of 'failed conservative treatment' or for the treatment of recurrence itself rather than for the primary event. In a study of 294 patients comprising all medically and surgically referred cases of spontaneous pneumothorax in a single institution, a recurrence rate of 16% was found in those treated for the first event either conservatively or with tube drainage [6]. Other series have reported a first recurrence rate of 16–50% [30,38,162,211,234,235]. At least half of those patients who experience a recurrence do so within 4 months of the initial episode [7,9,162]. Some series have recorded slightly lower recurrence rates following an intercostal tube as opposed to conservative treatment [162,236,237], although this experience is not universal [7]. After each recurrent spontaneous pneumothorax treated conservatively or by intercostal tube, the likelihood of a further episode increases; thus the chance of a third pneumothorax following the second has been found to be 40–64% [6,7,38] and the chance of a fourth pneumothorax following the third is reported to be 80% [238]. There is a risk of a subsequent contralateral spontaneous pneumothorax of 10–15% [9], although simultaneous bilateral pneumothoraces are unusual occurring in 1.3–2.5% of cases [38,162,163].

Haemopneumothorax

Significant haemorrhage in association with spontaneous pneumothorax is uncommon but potentially fatal, early reports indicating a mortality rate approaching 20% [211,239]. It was reported in 2.3% of one recent surgical series with no mortality [240]. The source of blood loss is usually the chest wall side of a vascularized adhesion that

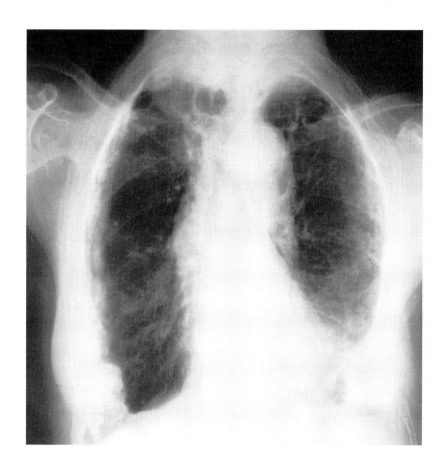

Fig. 44.16 Chronic bilateral fibrothoraces, with heavily calcified visceral pleura, in a patient previously treated for tuberculosis with artificial pneumothorax.

is torn apart as the pneumothorax develops [163]; it is of historical interest that this was also a recognized complication following the induction of artificial pneumothoraces when these were used in the treatment of pulmonary tuberculosis [241]. Blood loss may produce shock with sweating, nausea and syncope. Treatment comprises prompt replacement of blood; if blood loss is excessive, early surgical intervention to achieve haemostasis is necessary [240]. Adequate aspiration or drainage is all that is required for smaller amounts of blood. Thoracoscopy or thoracotomy may be required if the organization of substantial clot prevents expansion of the lung, although smaller amounts may gradually reabsorb without intervention.

Pyopneumothorax

Pyogenic infection of the pleural space was reported in less than 1% of cases of spontaneous pneumothorax in one early Scottish series and was also found to be surprisingly uncommon following penetrating trauma to the chest wall [104,162]. This does not apply to countries with less well-developed healthcare facilities and those with a high prevalence of tuberculosis. The infecting organisms may enter the pneumothorax space as a result of suppurative pneumonia or rupture of a lung abscess or may be introduced at pleural aspiration, during intercostal tube

drainage or at thoracotomy. Treatment comprises prompt and adequate drainage by aspiration or intercostal tube and appropriate antibiotic therapy. When these measures fail surgical intervention is indicated (see Chapter 14).

Respiratory failure

This is unlikely to occur in the absence of pre-existing respiratory disease other than when a tension pneumothorax is present. It is characterized by hypoxia, hypercapnia and respiratory acidosis and treatment involves urgent re-expansion of the deflated lung and controlled oxygen therapy according to arterial blood gas analysis.

Re-expansion pulmonary oedema

Unilateral pulmonary oedema is an unusual but well-documented complication that may follow the re-expansion of a completely collapsed lung, not only after the treatment of pneumothorax [242] but also sometimes following the aspiration of a large pleural effusion or after the relief of bronchial obstruction, as in the case of the withdrawal of a misplaced endotracheal tube. It is thought to be more likely to occur if the pneumothorax has been present for several days and if re-expansion is rapid, as may occur if suction has been applied [243,244], although it can occur when collapse of the lung has been present for only a few hours. Radiographic evidence of unilateral pulmonary oedema on the side of the treated pneumothorax was found in 0.9% of a retrospective series of 320 episodes of spontaneous pneumothorax collected over an 8-year period and treated with intercostal tube drainage [245]. The mechanisms are open to conjecture but possibilities include increased pulmonary capillary permeability resulting from raised transpulmonary negative pressures acting on lung tissue, whose elastic recoil has been increased by loss of surfactant; alternatively, there may be pulmonary microvascular injury by oxygen free radicals or other substances produced as a result of hypoxic lung injury occurring during the period of collapse [246,247]. Curiously, contralateral or bilateral pulmonary oedema has also been described on rare occasions [248,249].

This complication may be asymptomatic, being detected on a routine film, or it may result in cough and dyspnoea [245]. Although unusual, marked respiratory distress with severe hypotension and death have occasionally been reported [245,248,250]. The radiographic findings are those of unilateral pulmonary oedema and are non-specific. Treatment is by correction of hypoxaemia and hypovolaemia if present and with inotropic support where appropriate. Mechanical ventilation may sometimes be necessary [251].

Other complications of management

Some complications that may arise as a direct result of the placement of intercostal tube drains have already been mentioned. The most serious are haemorrhagic. Bleeding may occur as a result of injury to a vascular structure, usually one of the intercostal vessels, less commonly the internal mammary artery or another major vessel. Elderly patients may have more tortuous intercostal arteries than younger people and may therefore be more vulnerable [252]. Other serious structural injury is only likely to arise as a result of the misplacement or overpenetration of a trocar. Trauma cases who are dealt with as emergencies are particularly vulnerable since their thoracic cavities may contain abdominal viscera as a result of diaphragmatic rupture and the normal mediastinal structures may also be displaced. The liver, spleen, bowel, major vessels or even the heart may be inadvertently punctured during tube placement so that various advanced trauma life support guidelines recommend that intercostal drains should be inserted without a trocar in such cases [253,254]. Massive haemorrhage is best dealt with by clamping the tube in the hope that this tamponades the flow, by replacing lost volume as rapidly as possible and by requesting thoracic surgical help immediately. Smaller bleeds thought to come from intercostal vessels have been tamponaded by replacing the chest tube with a large Foley urinary catheter and applying traction to its overinflated

balloon, although experience with this technique is not widespread [255]. Misplaced tubes have been known to injure the brachial plexus and occasionally an apical drain may abut the sympathetic chain producing neuropraxia with Horner's syndrome [256]. Sometimes a track may develop between the outside of a drain and the chest wall so that the air is drawn into the pleural cavity on inspiration, thereby defeating the purpose of the exercise and necessitating removal and resiting or an alternative surgical approach, depending upon the circumstances.

Many of these problems can be prevented by scrupulous attention to detail as outlined in the section on intercostal tube drainage. It is notable that a retrospective North American study conducted to determine the complication rate of tube thoracostomy found a strikingly lower complication rate when tubes were placed by a surgeon rather than an emergency physician, implying that additional training might be important [257].

Pneumomediastinum

Air in the mediastinal tissues is referred to as pneumomediastinum or mediastinal emphysema. Although the condition of pneumomediastinum has been recognized for over a century [258], the first detailed accounts are credited to Hamman [167,259]. A working classification based on cause, similar to that applied to pneumothorax, is recommended (Fig. 44.17). Thus any pneumomediastinum occurring in the absence of trauma may be described as spontaneous. The term 'primary spontaneous pneumomediastinum' is used in the absence of any demonstrable predisposing disease and 'secondary spontaneous pneumomediastinum' where the leakage of air has arisen as a result of a recognizable coexisting structural abnormality, usually in the lungs or mediastinum; thus any of the causes of secondary spontaneous pneumothorax may also result in secondary spontaneous pneumomediastinum.

Aetiology

Pneumomediastinum may arise following alveolar rupture, in which case air tracks along interstitial and vascular supporting tissues (see Fig. 44.4) until it reaches the mediastinum [260]. Air may also be released directly into

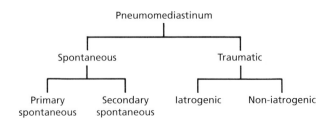

Fig. 44.17 Classification of pneumomediastinum.

the mediastinum following tracheal, bronchial or oesophageal rupture in association with chest trauma, local disease or endoscopic examination [261]. The initiating event may be a rise in intrathoracic pressure such as occurs with coughing, straining or during positive-pressure ventilation. In this regard the condition has been recorded in upper respiratory tract infection, asthma, bronchitis, whooping cough, obstructive laryngitis, choking on a foreign body and with various forms of physical exertion including childbirth [262–272]. Frequently, however, no precipitating cause is found as was emphasized in early reports [259].

Alveolar rupture may also follow the decompression of intrathoracic gas, as may occur in a surfacing diver or in aircrew subjected to sudden accidental cabin decompression at high altitude (p. 1187). The surgical dilatation of an oesophageal stricture is a frequent cause of rupture of this viscus, particularly if the lumen is blocked by carcinoma. Violent vomiting may sometimes give rise to a vertical tear in the lower 8 cm of the oesophagus postero-laterally [273]. Air is occasionally drawn into the fascial planes of the mediastinum from wounds in the neck, including tracheostomy and surgical procedures in the mouth, pharynx and upper gastrointestinal tract [274]. Gas in the mediastinum may also be introduced by high-speed air turbine dental drills [275,276] and even by attempting to uncap a carbonated beverage bottle with the teeth [277]. Strenuous physical exertion coupled with retching that may not be recalled could be the explanation for occasional reports of pneumomediastinum occurring in association with the recreational use of 3,4-methylene-dioxymethamphetamine ('ecstacy'), typically taken at discothèques and 'raves' [278]. Rarely gas may enter the thorax from a ruptured viscus in the abdomen, ascending retroperitoneally alongside the oesophagus and aorta.

Clinical features

Primary spontaneous pneumomediastinum occurs predominantly in young previously healthy males aged 15–30 years [264,279]. All grades of clinical severity exist and the condition is almost certainly underdiagnosed in milder cases. The most consistent symptom is central chest pain, produced as a result of air spreading about the mediastinal tissues [263]. It may be slight or severe, mimicking that of myocardial infarction or pericarditis and radiating to the shoulders, arms and neck. Any movement that disturbs the mediastinal structures, such as deep breathing, turning or swallowing, may aggravate the pain and the patient may obtain relief by leaning forwards in the sitting position and by breathing shallowly [280]. Pain in the neck may be accompanied by dysphagia, which may be the principal complaint [264]. There may be a change in the quality of the voice [265]. Surgical emphysema is frequently palpable in the neck and may be more

widespread, involving the face, chest or arms particularly if the channel through which air has entered the mediastinum remains patent or if the patient is being ventilated mechanically. Pulsus paradoxus has been described in the absence of asthma [264]. The normal area of cardiac dullness to percussion may be diminished and on auscultation the heart sounds may be indistinct. Hamman's sign is variously described as a crepitous, crackling or crunching sound that may be heard with the stethoscope to be synchronous with systole. It is usually maximal at the left sternal edge with the patient sitting forwards or lying in the left lateral decubitus position. This sign is present in about 50% of cases of pneumomediastinum and is occasionally noticed by the patient or even by a casual observer. It is not entirely specific for pneumomediastinum, having been described in left-sided pneumothorax [166], bullous emphysema of the lingula, distension of the lower oesophagus or stomach by air, and pneumoperitoneum with a high left hemidiaphragm [281]. On rare occasions sufficient air under tension surrounds the heart to cause cardiac tamponade, with breathlessness, cyanosis and hypotension. When secondary spontaneous or traumatic pneumomediastinum occurs, the symptoms and signs of associated disease such as pneumothorax or oesophageal rupture are frequently present. The latter condition is often indicated by the presence of fever and a pleural effusion or empyema, the source of which may be demonstrated by asking the patient to swallow dye such as methylene blue, which can then be shown to be present in an aspirate of pleural fluid. In lower oesophageal rupture the upper part of the abdomen may be rigid, suggesting a perforated gastric or duodenal ulcer. There may be the symptoms and signs of an associated pneumothorax.

Radiographic features

It is usually the chest radiograph that provides indisputable diagnostic evidence of pneumomediastinum (Fig. 44.18). Free mediastinal air is usually seen as sharp lines of increased lucency that enhance the mediastinal viscera, run along and outline one or both of the cardiac borders and extend to the superior medias-tinum, which may appear widened [172]. A continuous diaphragmatic 'shadow' has also been desribed [282]. If posteroanterior views only are taken, then about 50% of cases that would otherwise be detected with a routine lateral view may be missed [283]. This projection may show a collection of air lying between the sternum and heart. In the neck posteroanterior and lateral views may show air tracking along the fascial planes. In cases of doubt, mediastinal air may be evident using either echocardiography or CT [261,278]. A water-soluble, non-ionic (e.g. lopamidol, Gastrografin) contrast examination may be helpful where oesophageal perforation is suspected.

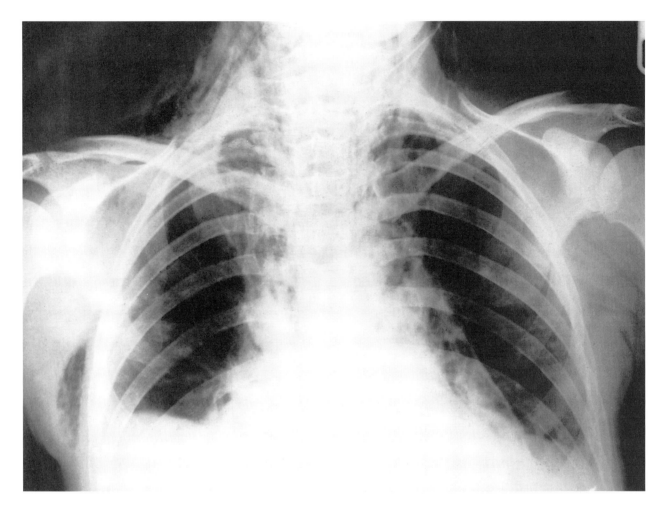

Fig. 44.18 Mediastinal and subcutaneous air due to instrumental perforation of pyriform fossa.

Diagnosis

Failure to diagnose pneumomediastinum usually results from the omission of this possibility in the differential diagnosis when a subject presents with central chest pain. Difficulty may arise when the air leak has been small, with the result that the usual physical signs are absent; in this case, free air must be assiduously sought on the radiographs. Myocardial infarction is usually easily distinguishable by serial changes on the ECG and a rise in cardiac enzyme levels. However, caution should be exercised in interpreting the ECG since ST and T wave changes have been described in both pneumothorax and pneumomediastinum [175,263,284].

Management

Primary spontaneous pneumomediastinum seldom requires any treatment other than reassurance, observation and simple analgesia should the pain require it. The

administration of high concentrations of oxygen may be beneficial in the rare situation in which trapped air in the mediastinum is limiting diastolic filling of the heart. This causes nitrogen to be washed out of the body, thereby increasing the gradient of P_{N_2} between the pneumomediastinum space and the tissues so that the trapped air is more rapidly absorbed (see Fig. 44.11) [285].

When a pneumomediastinum is secondary to another disease process or to trauma, therapeutic efforts are directed to the primary condition since it is usually of much greater clinical importance. Coexisting pneumothorax should be treated on its own merits (see above) and should be searched for, particularly when pneumomediastinum develops in patients who are being mechanically ventilated. When tracheobronchial or oesophageal ruptures are suspected, endoscopic examination or contrast swallow may be required. Major perforations, especially if they have resulted from trauma, usually require operative treatment. Minor oesophageal tears, which may have arisen from endoscopy itself, are frequently managed conservatively with antibiotics and drainage of any coexisting pleural effusion. Although air may have entered the mediastinum by purely physical means, the finding of gas in these tissues should certainly alert the physician to the possibility of mediastinitis from anaerobic organisms that may have been introduced from adjacent areas.

The majority of cases of primary spontaneous pneumo-mediastinum are absorbed within 1 week. Recurrence is unusual but has been described [260,263].

References

1 Itard JMG. *Dissertation sur le pneumo-thorax ou les congestions gazeuses qui deforment dans la poitrine.* Thesis, Paris, 1803.

2 Emerson CP. Pneumothorax: a historical, clinical and experimental study. *Johns Hopkins Hosp Rep* 1903; 11: 1.

3 Hippocrates (*c.* 5 BC) *De morbis*, Lib II.

4 Watt AG. Spontaneous pneumothorax: a review of 210 consecutive admissions to Royal Perth Hospital. *Med J Aust* 1978; 1: 186.

5 Davis AM, Wensley DF, Phelan PD. Spontaneous pneumothorax in paediatric patients. *Respir Med* 1993; 87: 531.

6 Ferguson LJ, Imrie CW, Hutchinson J. Excision of bullae without pleurectomy in patients with spontaneous pneumothorax. *Br J Surg* 1981; 68: 214.

7 Hart GJ, Stokes TC, Couch AHC. Spontaneous pneumothorax in Norfolk. *Br J Dis Chest* 1983; 77: 164.

8 Inouye WY, Berggren RB, Johnson J. Spontaneous pneumothorax: treatment and mortality. *Dis Chest* 1967; 51: 67.

9 Getz SB, Beasley WE. Spontaneous pneumothorax. *Am J Surg* 1983; 145: 823.

10 Bense L, Eklunde G, Odont D *et al.* Smoking and the increased risk of contracting spontaneous pneumothorax. *Chest* 1987; 92: 1009.

11 Melton LJ, Hepper NGG, Offord KP. Incidence of spontaneous pneumothorax in Olmsted County Minnesota: 1950–1974. *Am Rev Respir Dis* 1979; 120: 1379.

12 De Vries WC, Wolfe WG. The management of spontaneous pneumothorax and bullous emphysema. *Surg Clin North Am* 1980; 60: 851.

13 Biach A. Zur aetiologie des pneumothorax. *Wien Med Wochenschr* 1880; 30: 6.

14 Kjaergaard HPB. Spontaneous pneumothorax in the apparently healthy. *Acta Med Scand* 1932; Suppl 43: 11.

15 Thurlbeck WM. *Chronic Air Flow Obstruction in Lung Disease.* Philadelphia: WB Saunders, 1976.

16 Ohata M, Suzuki H. Pathogenesis of spontaneous pneumothorax with special reference to the ultrastructure of emphysematous bullae. *Chest* 1980; 77: 771.

17 Killen DA, Gobbel WG. *Spontaneous Pneumothorax.* Boston: Little Brown, 1968.

18 Baronofsky ID, Warden HG, Kaufman JL *et al.* Bilateral therapy for unilateral spontaneous pneumothorax. *J Thorac Surg* 1957; 34: 310.

19 Lichter I, Gwynne JF. Spontaneous pneumothorax in young subjects: a clinical and pathological study. *Thorax* 1971; 26: 409.

20 West JB. *Regional Differences in the Lung.* New York: Academic Press, 1977.

21 Glazier JB, Hughes JMB, Maloney JE *et al.* Vertical gradient of alveolar size in lungs of dogs frozen intact. *J Appl Physiol* 1967; 23: 694.

22 Ogilvie CM. Spontaneous pneumothorax and apical lung disease. *Br Med J* 1971; 4: 573.

23 Withers JN, Fishback ME, Kiehl PV *et al.* Spontaneous pneumothorax: suggested etiology and comparison of treatment methods. *Am J Surg* 1964; 108: 772.

24 Forgacs P. Stature in simple pneumothorax. *Guy's Hosp Rep* 1969; 118: 119.

25 Kawakami J, Irie T, Kamishima K. Stature, lung height and spontaneous pneumothorax. *Respiration* 1982; 43: 35.

26 Rashid A, Sendi A, Al-Kadhimi A, Donnelly RJ. Concurrent spontaneous pneumothorax in identical twins. *Thorax* 1986; 41: 971.

27 Gibson GJ. Familial pneumothoraces and bullae. *Thorax* 1977; 32: 88.

28 Nickoladze GD. Surgical management of familial spontaneous pneumothorax. *Respir Med* 1990; 84: 107.

29 Sharpe IK, Ahmad M, Braun W. Familial spontaneous pneumothorax and HLA antigens. *Chest* 1980; 78: 264.

30 Aboinik IZ, Lossos IS, Gillis D *et al.* Primary spontaneous pneumothorax in men. *Am J Med Sci* 1993; 305: 297.

31 Metivier HJ, Masse R, Vai F *et al.* Increased content of neutrosoluble collagen and dialyzable hydroxyproline in panacinar emphysema and spontaneous pneumothorax. *Exp Lung Res* 1982; 3: 129.

32 Jansveld CAF, Dijkman JH. Primary spontaneous pneumothorax and smoking. *Br Med J* 1975; 4: 559.

33 Hallgrimsson JG. Spontaneous pneumothorax in Iceland with special reference to the idiopathic type: a clinical and epidemiological investigation *Scand J Thorac Cardiovasc Surg* 1978; Suppl 21: 3.

34 Bense L, Wiman L-G. Time relation between sale of cigarettes and the incidence of spontaneous pneumothorax. *Eur J Respir Dis* 1987; 71: 362.

35 Stephenson SF. Spontaneous pneumothorax: the sharp rib syndrome. *Thorax* 1976; 31: 369.

36 Bense L, Eklund G, Wiman L-G. Bilateral bronchial anomaly. A pathogenetic factor in spontaneous pneumothorax. *Am Rev Respir Dis* 1992; 146: 513.

37 Bense L, Lewander R, Eklund G *et al.* Non-smoking, non-alpha$_1$ antitrypsin deficiency-induced emphysema in non-smokers with healed spontaneous pneumothorax, identified by computed tomography of the lungs. *Chest* 1994; 103: 433.

38 Weeden D, Smith GH. Surgical experience in the management of spontaneous pneumothorax 1972–82. *Thorax* 1983; 38: 737.

39 George RB, Herbert SJ, Shames JM *et al.* Pneumothorax complicating emphysema. *JAMA* 1975; 234: 389.

40 Cabiran LR, Ziskind MM. Spontaneous pneumothorax in pulmonary emphysema. *Dis Chest* 1964; 46: 571.

41 Brock RC. Recurrent and chronic spontaneous pneumothorax. *Thorax* 1948; 3: 88.

42 Wilder RJ, Beacham EG, Ravitch MM. Spontaneous pneumothorax complicating cavitatory tuberculosis. *J Thorac Cardiovasc Surg* 1962; 43: 561.

43 Reemtsma K, Clauss RH, Wylie RH. The management of spontaneous pneumothorax complicating pulmonary tuberculosis. *Am Rev Tuberc* 1956; 74: 351.

44 Peiken AS, Lamberta F, Seritt NS. Bilateral recurrent pneumothoraces: a rare complication of miliary tuberculosis. *Am Rev Respir Dis* 1974; 110: 512.

45 Turiaf J, Marland P, Mathieu H. Spontaneous pneumothorax, mediastinal and subcutaneous emphysema associated with asthma. *Poumon Coeur* 1955; 11: 999.

46 Jorgensen JR, Falliers CJ, Bukantz SC. Pneumothorax in mediastinal and subcutaneous emphysema in children with bronchial asthma. *Pediatrics* 1963; 31: 824.

47 Pickup CM, Nee PA, Randall PE. Radiographic features in 1016 adults admitted to hospital with acute asthma. *J Accid Emerg Med* 1994; 11: 234.

48 Lohse AW, Klein O, Hermann E *et al.* Pneumatoceles and pneumothoraces complicating staphylococcal pneumonia: treatment by synchronous independent lung ventilation. *Thorax* 1993; 48: 578.

49 Davidson AC, Creach M, Cameron I. Staphylococcal pneumonia, pneumatocele, and the toxic shock syndrome. *Thorax* 1990; 45: 639.

50 Hausmann W, Karlish AJ. Staphylococcal pneumonia in adults. *Br Med J* 1956; 2: 845.

51 Rebhan AW, Edwards ME. Staphylococcal pneumonia. *Can Med Assoc J* 1960; 82: 513.

52 Mitchell DM, Miller RF. New developments in the pulmonary diseases affecting HIV infected individuals. *Thorax* 1995; 50: 294.

53 Cocker RJ, Moss F, Peters B *et al.* Pneumothorax in patients with AIDS. *Respir Med* 1993; 87: 43.

54 McClennan MD, Miller SB, Parsons PE *et al.* Pneumothorax with *Pneumocystis carinii* pneumonia in AIDS. *Chest* 1991; 100: 1224.

55 Wait MA, Estrera A. Changing clinical spectrum of spontaneous pneumothorax. *Am J Surg* 1992; 164: 528.

56 Moskovic E, Miller R, Pearson M. High resolution computed tomography of *Pneumocystis carinii* pneumonia in AIDS. *Clin Radiol* 1990; 42: 239.

57 Renzi PM, Corbeil C, Chassé M *et al.* Bilateral pneumothoraces hasten mortality in AIDS patients receiving secondary prophylaxis with aerosolised pentamidine. *Chest* 1992; 102: 491.

58 Penketh ARL, Knight RK, Hodson ME, Batten JC. Management of pneumothorax in adults with cystic fibrosis. *Thorax* 1982; 37: 850.

59 Seddon DJ, Hodson ME. Surgical management of pneumothorax in cystic fibrosis. *Thorax* 1988; 43: 739.

60 Spencer H. *Pathology of the Lung*, 4th edn. Oxford: Pergamon Press, 1985.

61 Bailey WC, Brown M, Buechner HA *et al.* Silico-mycobacterial disease in sandblasters. *Am Rev Respir Dis* 1974; 110: 115.

62 Morgan WKC, Seaton A. *Occupational Lung Diseases*, 2nd edn. Philadelphia: WB Saunders, 1984.

63 Scadding JG. *Sarcoidosis*. London: Eyre and Spottiswood, 1967.

64 Ross RJM, Empey DW. Bilateral spontaneous pneumothorax in sarcoidosis. *Postgrad Med J* 1983; 59: 106.

65 Davidson AR. Eosinophilic granuloma of the lung. *Br J Dis Chest* 1976; 70: 125.

66 Jaspan T, Davidson AM, Walker WC. Spontaneous pneumothorax in Wegener's granulomatosis. *Thorax* 1982; 37: 774.

67 Evans WV, Stauffer JL, Carbone JE. Bilateral pneumothorax and pleural effusions in rheumatoid disease. *Thorax* 1984; 39: 213.

68 Edwards WG, Dines DE. Recurrent spontaneous pneumothorax in diffuse scleroderma. *Dis Chest* 1966; 49: 96.

69 Nickol KH. Idiopathic pulmonary haemosiderosis presenting with spontaneous pneumothorax. *Tubercle* 1960; 41: 216.

70 Berkman N, Bloom A, Cohen P *et al.* Bilateral spontaneous pneumothorax as the presenting feature in lymphangioleiomyomatosis. *Respir Med* 1995; 89: 381.

71 Tanaka H, Imada A, Morikawa T *et al.* Diagnosis of pulmonary lymphangioleiomyomatosis by HMB45 in surgically treated spontaneous pneumothorax. *Eur Respir J* 1995; 8: 1879.

72 Anton HC, Gray B. Pulmonary alveolar proteinosis presenting with pneumothorax. *Clin Radiol* 1967; 18: 428.

73 Wood JR, Bellamy D, Child AH, Citron KM. Pulmonary disease in patients with Marfan syndrome. *Thorax* 1984; 39: 780.

74 O'Neill S, Sweeney J, Walker F *et al.* Pneumothorax in the Ehlers–Danlos syndrome. *Ir J Med Sci* 1981; 150: 43.

75 Motoyoshi K, Momoi H, Mikami R *et al.* Pulmonary lesions seen in a family with marfanoid hypermobility syndrome. *Jpn J Thorac Dis* 1973; 11: 138.

76 Torrington KG, Ashbaugh DG, Stackle EG. Recklinghausen's disease. Occurrence with intrathoracic vagal neurofibroma and contralateral spontaneous pneumothorax. *Arch Intern Med* 1983; 143: 568.

77 Harris JO, Waltuck BL, Swenson EW. The pathophysiology of lungs in tuberous sclerosis. A case report and literature review. *Am Rev Respir Dis* 1969; 100: 379.

78 Sculley RE, Mark EJ, McNeely WF *et al.* Case records of the Massachusetts General Hospital. *N Engl J Med* 1994; 330: 1300.

79 Sculley RE, Mark EJ, McNeely WF *et al.* Case records of the Massachusetts General Hospital. *N Engl J Med* 1994; 330: 1516.

80 Handa AK, Eggleston FC. Pneumothorax caused by hydatid cysts. *Ind J Chest Dis Allied Sci* 1982; 24: 47.

81 Lote K, Dahl O, Vigander T. Pneumothorax during combination chemotherapy. *Cancer* 1981; 47: 1743.

82 Stein ME, Haim N, Drumea K *et al.* Spontaneous pneumothorax complicating chemotherapy for metastatic seminoma. A case report and review of the literature. *Cancer* 1995; 75: 2710.

83 Yeung K, Bonnet JD. Bronchogenic carcinoma presenting as spontaneous pneumothorax. Case report with review of the literature. *Cancer* 1976; 39: 2286.

84 Sheard JDH, Taylor W, Soorae A, Pearson MG. Pneumothorax and malignant mesothelioma in patients over the age of 40. *Thorax* 1991; 46: 584.

85 Hall FM, Salzman EW, Burton IE, Kurland GS. Pneumothorax complicating aseptic cavitating pulmonary infarction. *Chest* 1977; 72: 232.

86 Corzo JE, León FL, Gómez-Mateos J *et al.* Pneumothorax secondary to septic pulmonary emboli in tricuspid endocarditis. *Thorax* 1992; 47: 1080.

87 Lokman S, Sani A, Sidek DS. Pyopneumothorax: a rare complication of retropharyngeal abscess. *J Laryngol Otol* 1993; 107: 460.

88 Roberts CM, Gelder CM, Goldstraw P, Spiro SG. Tension pneumothorax and empyema as a consequence of gastropleural fistulae. *Respir Med* 1990; 84: 253.

89 Nayak LN, Lawrence D. Tension pneumothorax from a perforated gastric ulcer. *Br J Surg* 1976; 63: 245.

90 Sinha M, Gibbons P, Kennedy SC, Matthews HR. Colopleural fistula due to strangulated Bochdalek hernia in an adult. *Thorax* 1989; 44: 762.

91 Berkman N, Bar-Ziv J, Breuer R. Recurrent spontaneous pneumothorax associated with bronchial atresia. *Respir Med* 1996; 90: 307.

92 Penniment MG, O'Brien PC. Pneumothorax following thoracic radiation therapy for Hodgkin's disease. *Thorax* 1994; 49: 936.

93 Pezner RD, Horak DA, Sayegh HO *et al.* Spontaneous pneumothorax in patients irradiated for Hodgkin's disease and other malignant lymphomas. *Int J Radiat Oncol Biol Phys* 1990; 19: 707.

94 Maurer ER, Schaal JA, Mendez FL. Chronic recurring spontaneous pneumothorax due to endometriosis of the diaphragm. *JAMA* 1958; 168: 2013.

95 Lillington GA, Mitchell SP, Wood GA. Catamenial pneumothorax. *JAMA* 1972; 219: 1328.

96 Barrocas A. Catamenial pneumothorax: case report and a review of the literature. *Am Surg* 1979; 45: 340.

97 Foster DC, Stern JL, Buscema J *et al.* Pleural and parenchymal pulmonary endometriosis. *Obstet Gynecol* 1981; 58: 552.

98 Furman WR, Wang KP, Summer WR *et al.* Catamenial pneumothorax: evaluation by fiberoptic pleuroscopy. *Am Rev Respir Dis* 1980; 121: 137.

99 Shiraishi T. Catamenial pneumothorax: report of a case and review of the Japanese and non-Japanese literature. *Thorac Cardiovasc Surg* 1991; 39: 304.

100 Joseph J, Sahn SA. Thoracic endometriosis syndrome: new observations from an analysis of 110 cases. *Am J Med* 1996; 100: 164.

101 Sariego J, Brown JL, Matsumo T, Kerstein MD. Predictors of pulmonary complications in blunt chest trauma. *Int Surg* 1993; 78: 320.

102 Jantz MA, Pierson DJ. Pneumothorax and barotrauma. *Clin Chest Med* 1994; 15: 75.

103 Bertelsen S, Howitz P. Injuries of trachea and bronchi. *Thorax* 1972; 27: 188.

104 Muckart DJ, Luvuno FM, Baker LW. Penetrating injuries of the pleural cavity. *Thorax* 1984; 39: 789.

105 Berger R. Iatrogenous pneumothorax. *Chest* 1994; 105: 981.

106 Despars JA, Sassoon CS, Light RW. Significance of iatrogenic pneumothoraces. *Chest* 1994; 105: 1147.

107 Collins TR, Sahn SA. Thoracenteses: clinical value, complications, technical problems and patient experience. *Chest* 1987; 91: 817.

108 Ansari S, Highcock M, Parfrey H *et al.* The introduction of a pleural biopsy service improves diagnostic yield in a district general hospital. *Eur J Respir Med* 1998; 10 (Suppl 25): 325S.

109 Chang YC, Patz EF, Goodman PC. Pneumothorax after small-bore catheter placement for malignant pleural effusions. *Am J Roentgenol* 1996; 166: 1049.

110 Kazerooni EA, Lim FT, Mikhail A *et al.* Risk of pneumothorax in CT-guided transthoracic needle aspiration biopsy of the lung. *Radiology* 1996; 198: 371.

111 Hill PC, Spagnolo SV, Hockstein MJ. Pneumothorax with fine-needle aspiration of thoracic lesions. Is spirometry a predictor? *Chest* 1993; 104: 1017.

112 Anderson CLV, Crespo JCA, Lie TH. Risk of pneumothorax not increased by obstructive lung disease in percutaneous needle biopsy. *Chest* 1994; 105: 1705.

113 Vitulo P, Dore R, Cerveri I *et al.* The role of functional respiratory tests in predicting pneumothorax during lung needle biopsy. *Chest* 1996; 109: 612.

114 Kouri NF, Stitik FP, Erozan YS *et al.* Transthoracic needle biopsy of benign and malignant lesions. *Am J Roentgenol* 1985; 144: 281.

115 Zavala DC, Schoell JE. Ultrathin needle aspiration of the lung in infections and malignant disease. *Am Rev Respir Dis* 1981; 123: 125.

116 Arakawa H, Nakajima Y, Kurihara Y *et al.* CT-guided transthoracic needle biopsy: a comparison between automated biopsy gun and fine needle aspiration. *Clin Radiol* 1996; 51: 503.

117 Poe RH, Kallay MC, Wicks CM *et al.* Predicting risk of pneumothorax in needle biopsy of the lung. *Chest* 1984; 85: 232.

118 Cormier Y, Laviolette M, Tardif A. Prevention of pneumothorax in needle lung biopsy by breathing 100% oxygen. *Thorax* 1980; 35: 37.

119 Mansfield PF, Hohn DC, Fornage BD *et al.* Complications and failures of subclavian vein catheterisation. *N Engl J Med* 1994; 331: 1735.

120 Plewa MC, Ledrick D, Sferra JJ. Delayed tension pneumothorax complicating central venous catheterisation and positive pressure ventilation. *Am J Emerg Med* 1995; 13: 532.

121 Levy H, Kallenbach JM, Feldman C *et al.* Delayed pneumothorax after transbronchial lung biopsy. *Thorax* 1986; 41: 647.

122 Frazier WD, Pope TL, Findley LJ. Pneumothorax following transbronchial biopsy. Low diagnostic yield with routine chest roentgenograms. *Chest* 1990; 97: 539.

123 Morrissey B, Adams H, Gibbs AR, Crane MD. Percutaneous needle biopsy of the mediastinum: review of 94 procedures. *Thorax* 1993; 48: 632.

124 Gateley CA, Maddox PR, Mansel RE. Pneumothorax: a complication of fine needle aspiration of the breast. *Br Med J* 1991; 303: 627.

125 Kavanagh G, McNulty J, Fielding JF. Complications of liver biopsy: the incidence of pneumothorax and the role of post-biopsy chest x-ray. *Ir J Med Sci* 1991; 160: 387.

126 Barlow DW, Weymuller EA, Wood DE. Tra-

cheotomy and the role of postoperative chest radiography in adult patients. *Ann Otol Rhinol Laryngol* 1994; 103: 665.

127 Bodner G, Topilsky M, Greif J. Pneumothorax as a complication of acupuncture in the treatment of bronchial asthma. *Ann Allergy* 1983; 51: 401.

128 Ganfield RA, Chaplin JW. Pneumothorax with upper airway laser surgery. *Anesthesiology* 1982; 56: 398.

129 Shah H, Garbe L, Nussbaum E *et al*. Benign tumours of the tracheobronchial tree. Endoscopic characteristics and role of laser resection. *Chest* 1995; 107: 1744.

130 Wendell GD, Lenchner GS, Promisloff RA. Pneumothorax complicating small-bore feeding tube placement. *Arch Intern Med* 1991; 151: 599.

131 Barrett NR. *Modern Trends of Gastroenterology*, 1st edn. London: Butterworths, 1952.

132 Bell C, Borak J, Loeffler JR. Pneumothorax in drug abusers: a complication of internal jugular venous injections. *Ann Emerg Med* 1983; 12: 167.

133 Footit D. Minerva. *Br Med J* 1993; 307: 1016.

134 Fuchs HS. Incidence of spontaneous pneumothorax in apparently healthy air crew. *Riv Med Aeronaut Spaz* 1979; 42: 428.

135 Melamed Y, Shupak A, Bitterman H. Medical problems associated with underwater diving. *N Engl J Med* 1992; 326: 30.

136 Strauss RH. Diving medicine. *Am Rev Respir Dis* 1979; 119: 1001.

137 Douglas JDM. Medical problems of sport diving. *Br Med J* 1985; 291: 1224.

138 Maunder RJ, Pierson DJ, Hudson LD. Subcutaneous and mediastinal emphysema. *Arch Intern Med* 1984; 144: 1447.

139 Broome CR, Jarvis LJ, Clark J. Pulmonary barotrauma in submarine escape training. *Thorax* 1994; 49: 186.

140 Gammon RB, Shin MS, Groves RH *et al*. Clinical risk factors for pulmonary barotrauma: a multivariate analysis. *Am J Respir Crit Care Med* 1995; 152: 1235.

141 Hudson LD. Protective ventilation for patients with acute respiratory distress syndrome. *N Engl J Med* 1998; 338: 385.

142 Di Russo SM, Nelson LD, Safcsak K *et al*. Survival of patients with severe adult respiratory distress syndrome treated with high level positive end-expiratory pressure. *Crit Care Med* 1995; 23: 1485.

143 Hillman K, Albin M. Pulmonary barotrauma during cardiopulmonary resuscitation. *Crit Care Med* 1986; 14: 606.

144 Kollef MH, Legare EJ, Damiano M. Endotracheal misplacement: incidence, risk factors and impact of a quality improvement program. *South Med J* 1994; 87: 248.

145 Marini JJ, Culver BH. Systemic gas embolism complicating mechanical ventilation in the adult respiratory distress syndrome. *Ann Intern Med* 1989; 110: 699.

146 Seaman ME. Barotrauma related to inhalational drug abuse. *J Emerg Med* 1990; 8: 141.

147 Feldman AL, Sullivan JT, Passero MA *et al*. Pneumothorax in poly-substance abusing marijuana and tobacco smokers: three cases. *J Subst Abuse* 1993; 5: 183.

148 Odland R, Adams G. Pneumothorax as a complication of tracheoesophageal voice prosthesis use. *Ann Otol Rhinol Laryngol* 1988; 97: 537.

149 Hopkirk JAC, Pullen MJ, Fraser JR. Pleu-

150 Bates DV, Macklem PT, Christie RV. *Respiratory Function in Disease*. Philadelphia: WB Saunders, 1971.

151 Gilmartin JJ, Wright AJ, Gibson GJ. Effects of pneumothorax or pleural effusion on pulmonary function. *Thorax* 1985; 40: 60.

152 Richards DW, Riley CB, Niscock M. Cardiac output following artificial pneumothorax in man. *Arch Intern Med* 1932; 49: 944.

153 Guz A, Noble MIM, Eisele JH *et al*. The effect of lung deflation on breathing in man. *Clin Sci* 1971; 40: 451.

154 Norris RM, Jones JG, Bishop JM. Respiratory gas exchange in patients with spontaneous pneumothorax. *Thorax* 1968; 23: 427.

155 Williams MH, Kane C. Pulmonary function in patients who have recovered from spontaneous pneumothorax. *Dis Chest* 1965; 47: 153.

156 Kilburn KH. Cardiorespiratory effects of large pneumothorax in conscious and anaesthetised dogs. *J Appl Physiol* 1963; 18: 279.

157 Anthonisen NR. Regional lung function in spontaneous pneumothorax. *Am Rev Respir Dis* 1977; 115: 873.

158 Lidskog GE, Halasz NA. Spontaneous pneumothorax: a consideration of pathogenesis and management with review of 72 hospitalized cases. *AMA Arch Surg* 1957; 75: 693.

159 Lenox-Smith I. Spontaneous pneumothorax: a study of ninety-four cases. *Br J Dis Chest* 1962; 56: 1.

160 O'Hara VS. Spontaneous pneumothorax. *Milit Med* 1978; 143: 32.

161 Bense L, Wiman LG, Hedenstierna G. Onset of symptoms in spontaneous pneumothorax: correlations to physical activity. *Eur J Respir Dis* 1987; 71: 181.

162 Ruckley CV, McCormack RJM. The management of spontaneous pneumothorax. *Thorax* 1966; 21: 139.

163 Brooks JW. Open thoracotomy in the management of spontaneous pneumothorax. *Ann Surg* 1973; 117: 798.

164 Lenggenhager K. The blood circulation in the presence of pneumothorax. *Thorax Chirurgie* 1966; 14: 338.

165 Laënnec RTH. *A Treatise on the Diseases of the Chest and on Mediate Auscultation* (transl. Forbes J 1830). New York: Samuel Wood, 1819.

166 Lister WA. Case of pericardial knock associated with spontaneous pneumothorax. *Lancet* 1928; i: 1225.

167 Hamman L. Spontaneous interstitial emphysema of the lungs. *Trans Assoc Am Physicians* 1937; 52: 311.

168 Roelandt J, Willems J, van der Hauweart L *et al*. Clicks and sounds (whoops) in left sided pneumothorax: a clinical and phonographic study. *Dis Chest* 1969; 56: 31.

169 Desser KB, Benchimol A. Clicks secondary to pneumothorax confounding diagnosis of mitral valve prolapse. *Chest* 1977; 71: 523.

170 Klonin H, Vickery C. Insomnia as a complication of pleural aspiration. *Br Med J* 1996; 312: 1473.

171 Lawson JD. The scratch sign: a valuable aid in the diagnosis of pneumothorax. *N Engl J Med* 1961; 264: 88.

172 Felson B. *Chest Roentgenology*. Philadelphia: WB Saunders, 1973: 392.

173 Dornhorst AC, Pier JW. Pulmonary collapse and consolidation: the role of collapse in the production of lung field shadows and the significance of segments in inflammatory lung disease. *J Fac Radiol* 1954; 5: 276.

174 Gordon R. The deep sulcus sign. *Radiology* 1980; 136: 25.

175 Kaimal PK. Transient electrocardiographic Q waves in spontaneous pneumothorax: a case report. *Heart Lung* 1983; 12: 268.

176 Butland RJA, Spickett GP, Seaton D. A survey of the management of primary spontaneous pneumothorax in the UK. *Thorax* 1987; 42: 226.

177 Henderson Y, Henderson MC. The absorption of gas from any closed space within the lung. *Arch Intern Med* 1932; 49: 88.

178 Piiper J. Physiological equilibria of gas cavities in the body. In: Fenn NO, Rahn H, eds. *Handbook of Physiology, Vol 4, Respiration*. Washington, DC: American Physiological Society, 1965: 1205.

179 Kircher LT, Swartzel RL. Spontaneous pneumothorax and its treatment. *JAMA* 1954; 155: 24.

180 Chadha TS, Cohn MA. Non-invasive treatment of pneumothorax with oxygen inhalation. *Respiration* 1983; 44: 147.

181 Miller AC, Harvey JE for British Thoracic Society. Guidelines for management of spontaneous pneumothorax. *Br Med J* 1993; 307: 114.

182 Winter PM, Smith G. The toxicity of oxygen. *Anesthesiology* 1972; 37: 210.

183 Anon. Simple aspiration of pneumothorax. *Lancet* 1984; i: 434.

184 Riordan JF. Management of spontaneous pneumothorax. *Br Med J* 1984; 289: 71.

185 Klassen KP, Meckstroth CV. Treatment of spontaneous pneumothorax. *JAMA* 1962; 182: 1.

186 Raja OG, Lalor AJ. Simple aspiration of spontaneous pneumothorax. *Br J Dis Chest* 1981; 75: 207.

187 Bevalaqua FA, Aranda C. Management of spontaneous pneumothorax with small lumen catheter manual aspiration. *Chest* 1982; 81: 693.

188 Hamilton AAD, Archer GJ. Treatment of pneumothorax by simple aspiration. *Thorax* 1983; 38: 934.

189 Jones JS. A place for aspiration in the treatment of spontaneous pneumothorax. *Thorax* 1985; 40: 66.

190 Coady TJ, Seaton D, Day A *et al*. Measurement of exhaled chlorofluorocarbons. *Lancet* 1988; ii: 1286.

191 Seaton D, Yoganathan K, Coady T, Barker R. Spontaneous pneumothorax: marker gas technique for predicting outcome of manual aspiration. *Br Med J* 1991; 302: 262. (Correction *Br Med J* 1991; 302: 697.)

192 Ansari S, Highcock M, Seaton D. Spontaneous pneumothorax: predicting early safe discharge following aspiration. *Eur Respir J* 1995; 8 (Suppl 19): 536S.

193 Harvey JE, Prescott RJ for British Thoracic Society. Simple aspiration versus intercostal drainage for spontaneous pneumothorax in patients with normal lungs. *Br Med J* 1994; 309: 1338.

194 Ansari S, Seaton D. Can the chest radiograph predict early outcome of spontaneous pneumothorax? *Eur Respir J* 1996; 9 (Suppl 23): 211s.

195 Parmar JM. How to insert a chest drain. *Br J Hosp Med* 1989; 42: 231.

196 Bristol JB, Harvey JE. Safer insertion of pleural drains. *Br Med J* 1983; 286: 348.

197 Kaye W. Emergency treatment of tension pneumothorax. *Heart Lung* 1983; 12: 315.

198 So S, Yu D. Catheter drainage of spontaneous pneumothorax: suction or no suction, early or late removal? *Thorax* 1982; 37: 46.

199 Mathur R, Cullen J, Kinnear WJM, Johnston IDA. Time course of resolution of persistent air leak in spontaneous pneumothorax. *Respir Med* 1995; 89: 129.

200 Thompson HT, Bailey RR. Management of spontaneous pneumothorax. *N Z Med J* 1966; 65: 101.

201 Heimlich HJ. Valve drainage of the pleural cavity. *Dis Chest* 1968; 53: 282.

202 Samelson SL, Goldberg EM, Ferguson MK. The thoracic vent: clinical experience with a new device for treating simple pneumothorax. *Chest* 1991; 100: 880.

203 Levine AJ, Collins FJ. Treatment of pneumothorax during pregnancy. *Thorax* 1996; 51: 338.

204 Mercier C, Page A, Verdant A *et al.* Outpatient management of intercostal tube drainage in spontaneous pneumothorax. *Ann Thorac Surg* 1976; 22: 163.

205 Laub M, Milman N, Müller D *et al.* Role of small calibre chest tube drainage for iatrogenic pneumothorax. *Thorax* 1990; 45: 748.

206 Cannon WB, Mark JBD, Jamplis RW. Pneumothorax: a therapeutic update. *Am J Surg* 1981; 142: 16.

207 Kirby TJ, Ginsberg RJ. Management of the pneumothorax and barotrauma. *Clin Chest Med* 1992; 13: 97.

208 Bernstein A, Waqaruddin M, Shah M. Management of spontaneous pneumothorax using a Heimlich flutter valve. *Thorax* 1973; 28: 386.

209 Berger R. Pleurodesis for spontaneous pneumothorax. Will the procedure of choice please stand up? *Chest* 1994; 106: 992.

210 Spengler L. Zur Chirurgie des pneumothorax. *Beitr Klin Chir* 1906; 49: 68.

211 Gaensler EA. Parietal pleurectomy for recurrent spontaneous pneumothorax. *Surg Gynecol Obstet* 1956; 102: 293.

212 Research Committee of the British Thoracic Association and the Medical Research Council Pneumoconiosis Unit. The survey of long term effects of talc and kaolin pleurodesis. *Br J Dis Chest* 1979; 73: 285.

213 Lange P, Mortensen J, Groth S. Lung function 22–35 years after treatment of idiopathic spontaneous pneumothorax with talc poudrage or simple drainage. *Thorax* 1988; 43: 559.

214 Anon. Spontaneous pneumothorax. *Br Med J* 1975; 2: 526.

215 Light RW, O'Hara VS, Moritz TE *et al.* Intrapleural tetracycline for the prevention of recurrent spontaneous pneumothorax. *JAMA* 1990; 264: 2224.

216 Alfageme I, Moreno L, Huertas C *et al.* Spontaneous pneumothorax: long term results with tetracycline pleurodesis. *Chest* 1994; 106: 347.

217 Almind M, Lange P, Viskum K. Spontaneous pneumothorax: comparison of simple drainage, talc pleurodesis, and tetracycline pleurodesis. *Thorax* 1989; 44: 627.

218 Wied U, Halkier E, Hoeier-Madsen K *et al.* Tetracycline versus silver nitrate pleurodesis in spontaneous pneumothorax. *J Thorac Cardiovasc Surg* 1983; 86: 591.

219 Granke K, Fischer CR, Gogo O *et al.* The efficacy and timing of operative intervention for spontaneous pneumothorax. *Ann Thorac Surg* 1986; 42: 540.

220 Schoenenberger RA, Haefeli WE, Weiss P *et al.* Timing of invasive procedures in therapy for primary and secondary spontaneous pneumothorax. *Arch Surg* 1991; 126: 764.

221 Clagett OT. The management of spontaneous pneumothorax. *J Thorac Cardiovasc Surg* 1968; 55: 761.

222 Anon. Pot-scourer pleurodesis for pneumothorax. *Lancet* 1992; 339: 217.

223 Singh VS. The surgical treatment of spontaneous pneumothorax by parietal pleurectomy. *Scand J Thorac Cardiovasc Surg* 1982; 16: 75.

224 Nkere UU, Griffin SC, Fountain SW. Pleural abrasion: a new method of pleurodesis. *Thorax* 1991; 46: 596.

225 Hazelrigg SR, Landreneau RJ, Mack M *et al.* Thoracoscopic stapled resection for spontaneous pneumothorax. *J Thorac Cardiovasc Surg* 1993; 105: 389.

226 Berrisford RG, Page RD. Video assisted thoracic surgery for spontaneous pneumothorax. *Thorax* 1996; 51 (Suppl 2): S23.

227 Harvey JE, Jeyasingham K. The difficult pneumothorax. *Br J Dis Chest* 1987; 81: 209.

228 Terndrup TE, Bosco SF, McLean ER. Spontaneous pneumothorax complicating pregnancy: case report and review of the literature. *J Emerg Med* 1989; 7: 245.

229 van Winter JT, Nichols FC, Pairolero PC *et al.* Management of spontaneous pneumothorax during pregnancy: case report and review of the literature. *Mayo Clin Proc* 1996; 71: 249.

230 Johnson WM, Tyndal CM. Pulmonary endometriosis treated with danazol. *Obstet Gynecol* 1987; 69: 506.

231 Espaulella J, Armengol J, Bella F *et al.* Pulmonary endometriosis: conservative treatment with GnRH agonists. *Obstet Gynecol* 1991; 78: 535.

232 Edmonds DK. Commentary (on two cases). *Thorax* 1996; 51: 1064.

233 Savage T, Fleming HA. Decortication of the lung in tuberculous disease. *Thorax* 1955; 10: 293.

234 Gobbel WG, Rhea WG, Nelson IA *et al.* Spontaneous pneumothorax. *J Thorac Surg* 1963; 43: 331.

235 Clark TA, Hutchinson DE, Deaner RM *et al.* Spontaneous pneumothorax. *Am J Surg* 1972; 124: 728.

236 Reid JM, Stevenson JG, McSwan N. The management of spontaneous pneumothorax. *Scott Med J* 1963; 8: 171.

237 Seremetis MG. The management of spontaneous pneumothorax. *Chest* 1970; 57: 65.

238 Askew AR. Parietal pleurectomy for recurrent pneumothorax. *Br J Surg* 1976; 63: 203.

239 Hopkins HU. Spontaneous pneumothorax. *Am J Med Sci* 1937; 193: 763.

240 Tatebe S, Kanazawa H, Yamazaki Y *et al.* Spontaneous haemothorax. *Ann Thorac Surg* 1996; 62: 1011.

241 Ellis FJ, Carr DI. Problem of spontaneous pneumothorax. *Med Clin North Am* 1954; 38: 1065.

242 Carlson RI, Classen KI, Gollan F *et al.* Pulmonary oedema following the rapid re-expansion of a totally collapsed lung due to a pneumothorax. *Surg Forum* 1959; 9: 367.

243 Kassis E, Philipsen E, Clausen KH. Unilateral pulmonary oedema following spontaneous pneumothorax. *Eur J Respir Dis* 1981; 62: 102.

244 Henderson AF, Banham SW, Moran F. Re-expansion pulmonary oedema: a potentially serious complication of delayed diagnosis of pneumothorax. *Br Med J* 1985; 291: 593.

245 Rozenman J, Yellin A, Simansky DA, Shiner RJ. Re-expansion pulmonary oedema following spontaneous pneumothorax. *Respir Med* 1996; 90: 235.

246 Jackson RM, Veal CF, Alexander CB *et al.* Re-expansion pulmonary oedema: a potential role for free radicals in its pathogenesis. *Am Rev Respir Dis* 1988; 137: 1165.

247 Sewell RW, Fewel JG, Frederick BA *et al.* Experimental evaluation of re-expansion pulmonary oedema. *Ann Thorac Surg* 1978; 26: 126.

248 Mahfood S, Hix WR, Aaron BL *et al.* Re-expansion pulmonary oedema. *Ann Thorac Surg* 1988; 45: 340.

249 Ragozzino MW, Green R. Bilaleral re-expansion pulmonary oedema following unilateral pleurocentesis. *Chest* 1991; 99: 506.

250 Pavlin DJ, Raghu G, Rogers TR, Cheney FW. Re-expansion hypotension: a complication of prolonged pneumothorax. *Chest* 1986; 89: 70.

251 Wong CF, Cohen MAH, Chan HS. PEEP ventilation: the treatment for life-threatening re-expansion pulmonary oedema? *Respir Med* 1991; 85: 69.

252 Carney M, Ravin CE. Intercostal artery laceration during thoracentesis: increased risk in elderly patients. *Chest* 1979; 75: 520.

253 Committee on Trauma. *Advanced Trauma Life Support Student Manual.* Chicago: American College of Surgeons, 1990.

254 Haggie JA. Chest drain trochar unsafe and unnecessary. *Br Med J* 1993; 307: 443.

255 Urschel JD. Balloon tamponade for haemorrhage secondary to chest tube insertion. *Respir Med* 1994; 88: 549.

256 Campbell P, Neil T, Wake PN. Horner's syndrome caused by an intercostal drain. *Thorax* 1989; 44: 305.

257 Etoch SW, Bar Nathan MF, Miller FB *et al.* Tube thoracostomy. Factors related to complications. *Arch Surg* 1995; 130: 521.

258 Muller F. Ueber emphysem des mediastinum. *Klin Wochenschr* 1888; 25: 25.

259 Hamman L. Spontaneous mediastinal emphysema. *Bull Johns Hopkins Hosp* 1939; 64: 1.

260 Macklin MT, Macklin CC. Malignant interstitial emphysema of the lungs and mediastinum as an important occult complication of many respiratory diseases and other conditions: an interpretation of the clinical literature in the light of laboratory experiment. *Medicine* 1944; 23: 281.

261 Naughton M, Irving L, McKenzie A. Pneumomediastinum after a transbronchial lung biopsy. *Thorax* 1991; 46: 606.

262 Ramadan HH, Bu-Saba N, Baraka A *et al.* Management of an unusual presentation of foreign body aspiration. *J Laryngol Otol* 1992; 106: 751.

263 Abolnik I, Lossos IS, Breuer R. Spontaneous pneumomediastinum: a report of 25 cases. *Chest* 1991; 100: 93.

264 Yellin A, Gapany MG, Lieberman Y. Spontaneous pneumomediastinum: is it a rare cause of chest pain? *Thorax* 1983; 38: 383.

265 Sleeman D, Turner R. Spontaneous pneumomediastinum with alteration in voice. *J Laryngol Otol* 1989; 103: 1222.

266 Mitchell RE, Derbes VJ, Akenhead WR. Rupture of the oesophagus. Two instances of a hitherto undescribed complication of status asthmaticus. *Ann Allergy* 1955; 13: 15.

267 Morere P, Fleury J, Vandour P *et al.* Spontaneous microtraumatic mediastinal emphysema in children with bronchial asthma. *Presse Med* 1966; 74: 1953.

268 Griffith RS. The spontaneous rupture of the esophagus. *Penn Med J* 1932; 35: 639.

269 Spellacy WN, Prem KA. Subcutaneous emphysema and pregnancy. Report of three cases. *Obstet Gynecol* 1963; 22: 521.

270 Packham CJ, Stevenson GC, Hadley S. Pneumomediastinum during sexual intercourse. *Br Med J* 1984; 288: 1196.

271 Morgan EJ, Henderson DA. Pneumomediastinum as a complication of athletic competition. *Thorax* 1981; 36: 155.

272 Varkey B, Kory RC. Mediastinal and subcutaneous emphysema following pulmonary function tests. *Am Rev Respir Dis* 1973; 108: 1393.

273 Gray JM, Hanson GC. Mediastinal emphysema: aetiology, diagnosis and treatment. *Thorax* 1966; 21: 325.

274 Mitchell A, Steer HW. Late appearance of pneumothorax after subclavian vein catheterisation: an anaesthetic hazard. *Br Med J* 1980; 281: 1339.

275 Hunt RB, Sahler OD. Mediastinal emphysema produced by air turbine dental drills. *JAMA* 1968; 205: 241.

276 Torres-Melero J, Arias-Diaz J, Balibrea JL. Pneumomediastinum secondary to use of a high speed air turbine drill during a dental extraction. *Thorax* 1996; 51: 339.

277 Bentley TM, Asy F. Minerva. *Br Med J* 1992; 305: 724.

278 Rezvani K, Kurbaan AS, Brenton D. Ecstacy induced pneumomediastinum. *Thorax* 1996; 51: 960.

279 McMahon DJ. Spontaneous pneumothorax. *Am J Surg* 1976; 131: 550.

280 Millard CE. Pneumomediastinum. *Chest* 1969; 56: 297.

281 Sulavik S. Mediastinal crunch (Hamman's sign). *GP Kansas City* 1962; 26: 104.

282 Levin B. The continuous diaphragm sign. *Clin Radiol* 1973; 24: 337.

283 Lillard RL, Allen RP. The extra-pleural air sign in pneumomediastinum. *Radiology* 1965; 85: 1093.

284 Munsell WP. Pneumomediastinum. *JAMA* 1967; 202: 689.

285 Fine J, Hermanson L, Frehling S. Further experience with 95% oxygen for the absorption of air from the body tissues. *Ann Surg* 1938; 107: 1.

45

CHEST WALL AND NEUROMUSCULAR DISORDERS

ANTHONY SEATON

Congenital abnormalities of the chest wall

Rib abnormalities

Bifid ribs are common, particularly in the upper six ribs, and if not appreciated on the chest radiograph may give rise to confusion in interpretation [1]. Fused and absent ribs may also occur but are only of radiological interest. An asymmetrical congenital deformity has been described in adolescent patients in whom the ribs and costal cartilages on the right side are deeply depressed and the sternum rotated to the right [2]. Reconstructive surgery is possible.

Cervical ribs occur in 0.5% of the population, usually arising from the seventh cervical vertebra; they may vary greatly in size and shape, and are bilateral in 80% of cases [3,4] (Fig. 45.1). They are usually asymptomatic but may give rise to the thoracic outlet syndrome due to compression of subclavian vessels or nerves in the root of the neck. Symptoms due to compression are more prevalent in females and more common on the left [3]. The production of symptoms bears no relation to the size of the rib; a small cervical rib with a fibrous attachment may cause severe symptoms whereas a large cervical rib may be asymptomatic. The thoracic outlet syndrome has been described following correction of scoliosis in a patient with cervical ribs [5].

Neurological symptoms of cervical ribs commonly consist of pain and weakness of the arm with paraesthesiae of the fingers. Atrophy of the intrinsic muscles of the hand may occur [6,7]. Vascular symptoms may mimic Raynaud's phenomenon, and emboli from a thrombosed subclavian artery may cause fingertip gangrene [6,7]. Neurological complications need not require resection of the offending rib since the majority respond to shoulder girdle strengthening exercises and the avoidance of heavy loads. However, vascular complications may require arteriographic investigation and treatment depends on the findings, ranging from simple rib resection to arterial

reconstructive surgery plus embolectomy or thrombectomy [3,4].

Jointed xiphoid process

A jointed xiphoid process may masquerade as an upper abdominal mass but may be readily recognized on a lateral chest film or by ultrasound examination, thus preventing unnecessary operation [8].

Pectus carinatum or pigeon chest

In this condition the sternum is prominent, forming an anterior ridge like the keel of a ship with the ribs falling away steeply on either side, sometimes with a vertical groove on each side of the sternum [9,10]. It may be associated with other congenital anomalies, especially cardiac lesions and coarctation of the aorta [11].

Aetiology

Pectus carinatum may result from obliteration of all the sternal sutures at an early age, possibly due to inadequate segmentation during fetal life, with a resulting synostosis [9]. An alternative explanation, which has been confirmed at postmortem, is that the deformity results from malattachment of the anterior portion of the diaphragm to the posterior portion of the rectus sheath rather than to the xiphoid process, with consequent distorting mechanical effects [12].

Management

There is no associated functional defect and correction is not normally indicated. However, corrective procedures for both types of pectus carinatum have been described and may be required for cosmetic reasons [10,13]. Such patients are almost invariably happier with the large scar than with the deformity, though this effect of the operation

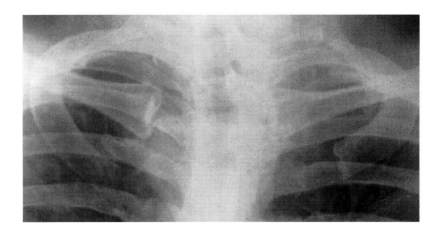

Fig. 45.1 Bilateral cervical ribs.

should be discussed with them before referral to a thoracic surgeon.

Pectus excavatum or funnel chest

In this condition the manubrium is normal but the body of the sternum is angled backwards towards the spine from the manubriosternal joint downwards with maximum recession at the xiphoid, below which the costal margin bends forwards. The condition is usually symmetrical but occasionally the sternal recession may be greater on one side than the other. As with pectus carinatum, there may be associated congenital anomalies and Marfan's syndrome may be present.

Aetiology

Pectus excavatum probably results from an imbalance of forces counteracting the inward pull of the diaphragm on the xiphisternum. Biopsies have shown that the anterior portion of the diaphragm is replaced by fibrous tissue. In the normal person the muscle in this region contracts on inspiration and its attachments to the lower chest wall on either side of the xiphisternum and lower sternum prevent these being dragged backwards as the diaphragm descends. When this muscle is lacking, the unopposed action of the posterior diaphragmatic muscle displaces the sternum and xiphisternum backwards as the diaphragm descends [12]. This movement occurs in affected newborn infants only on inspiration but after the age of 3 months the deformity progresses, with resulting secondary changes in the sternum and costal cartilages.

It has been suggested that an additional factor is a congenital laxity of the pericardium that allows the heart to fall to the left, removing its support from the sternum [14], and it has been recommended therefore that at operation the pericardial sac should be sutured into a central position. It has also been suggested that upper airway obstruction, whether due to enlarged tonsils and adenoids or segmental bronchomalacia, appears to predispose to pectus excavatum, which may resolve if the obstruction is treated early enough [15–17]. An association between pulmonary sequestration and pectus excavatum has been described [18].

There is said to be a hereditary tendency to the development of pectus excavatum but no sex linkage. The condition was reported in 2.2% of boys and 2.5% of girls in a German series [19].

Pulmonary function

Minor decreases in vital capacity (VC), total lung capacity (TLC) and maximal ventilation volume (MVV) have been reported in pectus excavatum with normal or increased residual volume (RV) and a normal forced expiratory volume in 1s (FEV_1) [20–22]. Even in the presence of normal pulmonary mechanics and lung volumes, it may be possible to demonstrate abnormal findings during exercise in symptomatic patients. Of eight such patients with exercise limitation, five demonstrated a diminished tidal volume expressed as percentage vital capacity at maximal exercise and had excessive oxygen uptake at higher loads consistent with an increased work of breathing [23].

Clinical features

In most cases the main symptom due to the deformity is the embarrassment caused to the patient by the deep furrow in the chest. In surgical series, however, where selection by degree of severity has occurred, patients are recorded with severe symptoms of dyspnoea, precordial pain, syncope on moderate exertion, palpitations and recurrent lung infections [12]. Incapacitating supraventricular tachycardia provoked by exercise and cured by surgery has been reported [24].

In children with pectus excavatum the majority have auscultatory findings suggestive of cardiac disease, with murmurs mimicking those of pulmonary stenosis or a small atrial septal defect [25]. These murmurs are presumed to be due to the resultant cardiac displacement. It has been reported that a cartilaginous horn from the inner surface of the xiphoid may impinge on the heart with resultant ECG changes and/or angina and that this may be cured by operation [26]. The ECG may show persistence of the juvenile pattern, with T inversion in the right precordial leads, incomplete right bundle branch block and right axis deviation. Because of cardiac rotation there may be P-wave inversion in V_1 and a QR pattern [27].

Radiology

On the posteroanterior chest film the heart is often displaced to the left and anterior ribs may show marked obliquity (Fig. 45.2). The depressed sternum is obvious on the lateral chest film and various indices for assessing the severity of disease and response to surgery using this film have been described [28]. Paradoxical cardiac enlargement during inspiration in children with pectus excavatum has been reported and is due to reduction of the anteroposterior diameter of the thorax caused by diaphragmatic descent [29].

Treatment

Surgery is rarely required because of cardiorespiratory symptoms, although these may occur in a minority and be disabling as described above. More often, surgical repair is sought for cosmetic reasons. It is usual to resect the deformed costal cartilages and perform an osteotomy of the anterior table of the sternum, providing internal fixation by the use of a bar that passes anterior to the rib cage but behind the sternum. Early cosmetic and functional results are usually good, and most recent reports indicate a satisfactory long-term result [30,31]. Unsatisfactory results have been recorded in patients with severe and asymmetrical deformities and with Marfan's syndrome [31]. Lung function is likely to deteriorate rather than improve shortly after surgery, thereafter sometimes recovering to its original level [22,32,33]. Nevertheless, the majority of patients are happy with the cosmetic results.

Straight back syndrome

The straight back syndrome is a presumed congenital abnormality in which there is absence of the physiological dorsal kyphosis of the spine as determined on a lateral chest radiograph.

Clinical features

Presumably because of compression of the heart and great vessels between the spine and sternum, with resultant compression of the pulmonary outflow tract, a pulmonary ejection systolic murmur is not infrequently found [34,35]. A palpable left parasternal systolic impulse may be present and exaggerated respiratory splitting of the second heart sound may be heard. An ECG may show an rSr pattern in V_1. These subjects are reported not to differ from controls in work capacity, FEV_1, diffusing capacity or arterial blood gas tensions, although total lung capacity may be reduced [36].

Radiology

The lateral chest radiograph suggests the diagnosis, showing loss of dorsal kyphosis and reduced anteroposterior diameter of the chest. On the posteroanterior film the pulmonary arteries may be prominent and the heart shadow is often displaced to the left, sometimes with a pancake configuration [36].

Poland's syndrome

Poland's syndrome consists of syndactyly plus ipsilateral absence of the pectoralis major muscle [37]. This results in hypoplasia of the ribs on the affected side and hypertranslucency of the lung on the posteroanterior chest radiograph.

Sternal abnormalities

An unusually wide sternum, with the suggested name eurysternum, and sternal foramina visible on chest radiography and bone scans have been described [38]. They are of no clinical significance

Congenital kyphoscoliosis

A minority of cases of kyphoscoliosis are congenital in origin and these are considered later in this chapter.

Acquired abnormalities of the chest wall

Fractures [39]

Traumatic fractures

Trauma to the chest wall may be inadvertent and unnoticed by the patient, particularly when under the influence of alcohol, anaesthetics or in a coma, and may sometimes give rise to problems in differential diagnosis. A rib fracture should be suspected if there is acute local rib tenderness at the site of pain of recent onset or if pain occurs on springing the ribs. Palpable or audible crepitus may be found at the site. If penetration of the parietal and visceral pleura occurs, there may be signs of pneumothorax and

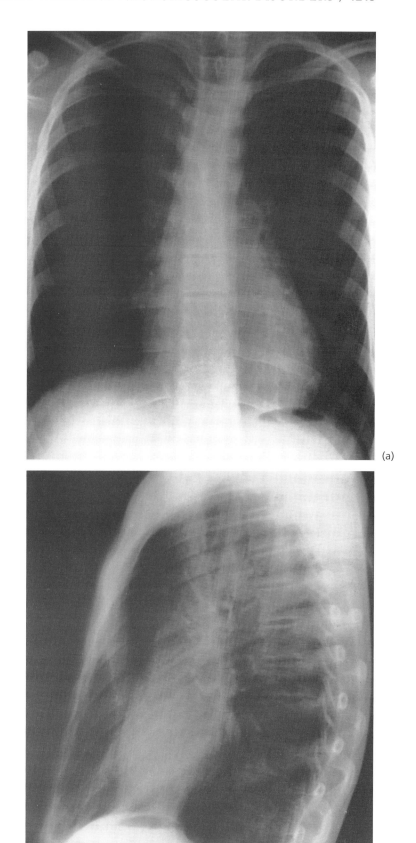

(a)

(b)

Fig. 45.2 Posteroanterior (a) and lateral (b) chest films of patient with pectus excavatum. Slight apparent enlargement at the left hilum is due to compression by the depressed sternum.

subcutaneous emphysema. The presence of multiple healed rib fractures on a chest film should call attention to the possibility of alcohol abuse.

Fatigue fractures

These may occur in the first or second ribs, most commonly in young soldiers carrying heavy rucksacks or rifles. Often there is little pain but the fracture may result in fibrous union or a residual cyst [40].

Cough fractures

Cough fractures are common and most frequently seen in patients with severe chronic airways obstruction, usually due to chronic bronchitis and emphysema, and in whooping cough. Predisposing factors include corticosteroid therapy or senile osteoporosis and osteomalacia. Cough fractures are associated with sudden onset of pain while coughing, the subsequent pain usually being worse on coughing than breathing. The local signs are as for a traumatic fracture, although pneumothorax is not usually seen. They are located most frequently in the mid-axillary line.

Pathological fractures

Pathological fractures may occur with rib metastasis or osteolytic primary tumour of rib such as myeloma.

Radiology

Unless there is displacement of a fracture it may not be visible on the radiograph even in the acute stage, and radiologically visible callus formation does not occur for several weeks. The diagnosis is therefore frequently clinical. Pneumothorax and/or subcutaneous emphysema may be seen with traumatic lesions, while the primary lesion may be visible in the case of pathological fractures. Sometimes the film may show linear shadows 2–3 cm long underlying a traumatically fractured rib, possibly due to bruising of the lung [40].

Treatment

Treatment with adequate analgesia is usually all that is required, although occasionally it may be necessary to infiltrate with local anaesthesia. Lower respiratory tract infection, particularly on the affected side, may develop in patients with chronic airways obstruction and require intervention with antibiotics. Chest wall strapping is contraindicated since it predisposes to the same complication.

Scoliosis

Scoliosis is defined as a lateral curvature of the spine and is associated with rotation of the spine and viscera adjacent to it. It may be (but is usually not) accompanied by kyphosis [41].

Aetiology

An abbreviated aetiological classification is shown in Table 45.1 [41]. Non-structural causes include the well-known sciatic scoliosis, a temporary scoliosis occasioned by irritation of sciatic nerve roots. Structural causes are identified by the persistence of fixed rotation of the spine on forward bending. The majority of cases of scoliosis nowadays are idiopathic in origin. Idiopathic scoliosis may be seen at all ages during growth and at all spinal

Table 45.1 Aetiological classification of scoliosis.

Non-structural
Postural compensatory
Sciatic
Inflammatory
Hysterical

Structural
Idiopathic
Adolescent kyphosis

Osteopathic
Congenital scoliosis
Klippel–Feil syndrome
Spondylolisthesis

Myopathic
Duchenne muscular dystrophy
Faciohumeroscapular dystrophy

Neuropathic
Poliomyelitis
Cerebral palsy
Syringomyelia
Neurofibromatosis
Friedreich's ataxia

Hereditary syndromes
Dominant
   Marfan's syndrome
   Ehlers–Danlos syndrome
Recessive
   Homocystinuria
   Morquio's syndrome
Sex-linked
   Turner's syndrome

Miscellaneous
Long-standing unilateral lung fibrosis
Burns
Irradiation
Thecoperitoneal shunts
Empyema
Thoracoplasty
Hiatus hernia

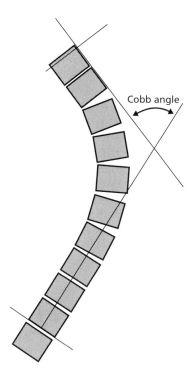

Fig. 45.3 Measurement of a thoracic scoliosis by Cobb's angle.

sites, although thoracic scoliosis to the right is the most common presentation [42,43]. The condition is more prevalent in girls. The higher in the spine the structural curve, the worse the prognosis. Prognosis is also a function of the angle of curvature, which is measured as shown in Fig. 45.3; lines are drawn parallel to the upper border of the upper vertebral body and to the lower border of the lowest vertebra of the structural curve. Perpendiculars are then erected from these lines to cross each other, the angle between the perpendiculars being the angle of curvature or Cobb's angle [44].

Neuropathic and myopathic conditions, of which poliomyelitis is the most common example, are usually associated with a worse prognosis for a given degree of curvature as a result of the associated muscle weakness and consequent ventilatory problems. Scoliosis due to poliomyelitis usually appears within 2 years of infection.

Pathology

In scoliosis the total lung volume is reduced and the lungs differ in size, with distortion of lobar shapes due to the deformity [45]. Alveolar size may vary; if scoliosis has been present from an early age, alveolar numbers per acinus may correspond to that developmental stage [46]. In severe scoliosis progressing to cor pulmonale, the pulmonary changes of marked vascular medial hypertrophy are indistinguishable from the changes seen in other causes of cor pulmonale [47].

Physiology

Because of the reduction in height occasioned by the spinal deformity, it is conventional to calculate predicted values for lung function in scoliosis on the basis of arm span measurements, arm span correlating closely with height in normal subjects [48]. Lung volumes are reduced, with a restrictive pattern even in asymptomatic adolescents with scoliosis. VC, TLC, MVV, functional residual capacity (FRC) and peak expiratory flow (PEF) and are all reduced and there is a direct relationship between the angle of curvature and the degree of reduction of these indices [49–54]. The higher the curve in the dorsal spine, the more severe its effect on function. RV may be maintained, resulting in an increased RV/TLC ratio [50]. The FEV_1/forced vital capacity (FVC) ratio is normal unless obstructive disease such as asthma supervenes [49]. Diffusing capacity for carbon monoxide (D_{LCO}) is reduced in proportion to the reduction in lung volumes, giving normal values for K_{CO} [49,52,53,55]. In paralytic scoliosis, similar changes are seen in lung volumes; however, for a given angle of curvature diminution of lung volumes is more severe [56] and the correlation of lung volume changes with Cobb's angle less clearly seen, reflecting the contribution of affected muscle to the disorder of lung function.

Lung compliance in scoliosis is commonly low, perhaps reflecting occurrence of small airway collapse due to inability to take a deep breath or a sigh [51,57,58]. This decreased compliance is also most pronounced in those with muscle weakness and can be increased by positive-pressure ventilation [59,60]. In scoliotic patients with impaired cardiorespiratory response to exercise, maximal oxygen uptake is reduced compared with age- and sex-matched normals, and ventilation at a given oxygen uptake is 20% higher than in normal subjects [61]. Exercise tolerance is thus limited in these patients by ventilatory factors.

Regional perfusion and ventilation are often normal in patients with scoliosis studied with xenon-133 techniques, although reduction in ventilation and perfusion at the lung bases does occur to a greater extent with increasing angle of curvature and age [55,62–64]. Pa_{O_2} is diminished even in asymptomatic adolescents with scoliosis, and with severe disease carbon dioxide retention occurs [64]. As a consequence of increasing hypoxia, pulmonary artery hypertension occurs, the pressure being inversely proportional to Pa_{O_2} [65,66]. In patients with severe scoliosis (with an angle ≥100°), severe desaturation may occur during sleep with episodes of central or obstructive apnoea and hypopnoea, particularly during REM sleep [67,68]. The occurrence of carbon dioxide retention raises the possibility of defective chemical control of ventilation. Diminished ventilatory responses to carbon dioxide have been demonstrated in patients with both the idiopathic and paralytic types of scoliosis, where the mechanical deformity has been the presumed explanation [51,55].

Finally, in patients with scoliosis of whatever degree, diminution in the maximum inspiratory and maximum transdiaphragmatic pressures has been recorded, suggesting that inspiratory muscle function is impaired, as a consequence of either a primary muscular problem or defective mechanical coupling between the inspiratory muscles and the rib cage [57,69].

Clinical features

It is unusual for patients with mild scoliosis to have respiratory symptoms. However, physiological studies of such patients have shown reduced muscularity and work capacity and an excessive cardiovascular response to exercise, suggesting cardiovascular unfitness [70]. Daytime somnolence may indicate the presence of nocturnal desaturation, a common occurrence as the patient's condition deteriorates. In more severe cases exertional dyspnoea may occur and is due to the restriction of lung volumes that these patients have. Airways obstruction, which is often reversible, may also develop. In patients with a mid or high thoracic curve greater than about 100°, progression to pulmonary hypertension and right ventricular failure often occurs in the fourth decade, usually presenting with increasing dyspnoea; syncope, angina or sudden death may occur. Death most commonly occurs as a result of respiratory failure or cardiac disease, and the risks are highest in juvenile scoliosis and scoliosis after polio [71]. In severe scoliosis, acute respiratory failure may be precipitated by respiratory tract infection, and deterioration in these patients may be more rapid and severe than in patients with end-stage chronic bronchitis and emphysema for example. This necessitates careful attention to antibiotics, oxygen and physiotherapy with recourse to assisted ventilation, which is employed if the future prognosis warrants such intervention.

Treatment

Surgery

Although surgical intervention, for example by spinal fusion, may ameliorate the angle of curvature and halt the progression of scoliosis, remarkably little benefit has been documented in terms of pulmonary function tests apart from an improvement in submaximal exercise ventilation [72].

Medical treatment

Following the initial episode of acute respiratory failure in severe scoliosis, the rate of deterioration of FEV_1 has been shown to be much slower than in patients with chronic

bronchitis and emphysema, and prolonged survival is possible after such an initial event [73]. Long-term domiciliary oxygen therapy may be useful as initial management of respiratory failure [74], although most patients ultimately need some form of assisted ventilation (see Chapter 58). In patients with late-onset respiratory failure in paralytic poliomyelitis, it has been shown that improvised long-term intermittent positive-pressure ventilation not only improves the patient's sense of well-being but also arterial blood gas tensions [75]. It is now apparent that home ventilation is of substantial benefit to patients with severe scoliosis. The most usual starting regimen is nasal intermittent positive-pressure ventilation, which has been shown to reduce admissions to hospital and to result in improvements in blood gases [76,77]. Alternative means of support for patients with life-threatening hypoventilation include tank respirators or cuirass shells. The latter can be individually moulded and tailored for each patient's deformity, and nocturnal ventilator support with such a system produces dramatic improvement in daytime blood gas tensions and also reduces the need for hospitalization [78–81]. Less satisfactory for the patient, but equally effective, is nocturnal ventilation via a permanent tracheostomy [82]. The effectiveness of nocturnal assisted ventilation is probably due to abolition of the more severely reduced blood gas tensions found at night [67,68]. Respiratory muscles that are rested at night and prevented from becoming fatigued are more capable of sustaining satisfactory ventilation and blood gas tensions by day.

Needless to say, appropriate diuretic therapy is indicated where right heart failure is present, and individual patients may also have superadded obstructive ventilatory defects that respond to bronchodilator therapy. Infective episodes are treated along routine lines.

Ankylosing spondylitis

Aetiology

The aetiology of ankylosing spondylitis is unknown but the strong association with HLA-B27 is now well recognized, and individuals homozygous for HLA-B27 may have more severe disease [83–88]. Blood donor studies have suggested a disease prevalence of 1–2% depending on the frequency of B27 in the population [89]. The disease is much commoner in young adult males than in females.

Pathophysiology

Fixation of the thoracic cage occurs in ankylosing spondylitis as a result of ankylosis of costotransverse and costovertebral joints. Sternomanubrial and sternoclavicular joints may also be affected [90]. In one study, 70% of patients had chest expansion of less than 5 cm when first seen [90]. In severe disease a restrictive pattern of abnormality is seen, with a reduction in VC due to reduced inspiratory capacity and a reduction in TLC [90,91]. RV and FRC are normal or slightly increased [90,92]. Gas exchange is normal [92]. As might be expected, thoracic and total respiratory compliance are decreased but lung compliance is normal [93]. Xenon-133 studies have shown normal perfusion but reduced apical ventilation in patients, although later studies suggested that apical underventilation is only seen in the presence of fibrosis [94,95].

Clinical features

Despite the functional abnormalities described, respiratory disability is uncommon in ankylosing spondylitis, although dyspnoea on exertion may occur. In most cases the diaphragm appears to compensate more than adequately for the restriction of thoracic wall movement. However, an occasional patient may develop respiratory failure due to very extensive chest wall disease. Chest pain is not uncommon and may be diffuse and prolonged or short and stabbing in character. It is usually located in the lower anterior chest and there may be an associated island of pain higher up posteriorly, suggesting that the phenomenon is one of radiating intercostal pain from posterior spinal joints [96].

In 1972, Davies [97] described seven patients with ankylosing spondylitis and apical lung fibrosis. Found late in the history of the disease, the fibrosis begins as consolidation that may extend to upper and mid zones bilaterally (Fig. 45.4) and may subsequently cavitate with bulla formation. Aspergillomas may form in the cavities or bullae with attendant symptoms of cough and/or haemoptysis (see Chapter 21). Transient pleural effusions have also been reported in ankylosing spondylitis but such pleuropulmonary manifestations are rare, occurring in only 1.3% of 2080 patients in one study [98].

Adenocarcinoma has been reported in association with the apical fibrosis of ankylosing spondylitis [99]. There has also been a further report of pathology suggestive of bronchocentric granulomatosis associated with *Aspergillus* colonization [100]. Other rare complications of ankylosing spondylitis that have been reported include acute respiratory failure from extrathoracic airway obstruction due to ankylosis of the cricoarytenoid joints [101] and amyloidosis of the lungs [102].

Treatment

Chest pain usually responds to minor analgesics. No other treatment is usually required or indicated apart from the management of mycetoma complications. In occa-

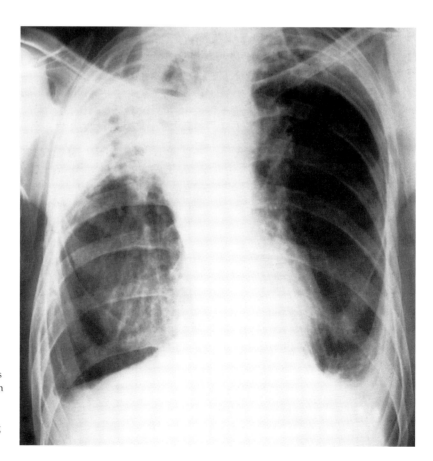

Fig. 45.4 Bilateral upper lobe fibrosis with disappearance of the main pulmonary arteries into the fibrotic lesions. There is also cavitation due to secondary bronchiectasis in the right upper lobe and bilateral basal pleural thickening. The patient had severe ankylosing spondylitis.

sional patients with severe disease, surgical attempts have been made to mobilize the chest by resection of the posterior parts of several ribs or by other procedures, some of which appear to have improved respiratory function [103].

Slipping rib syndrome

Clinical features

The slipping rib (syn. rib tip or clicking rib) syndrome [39,104,105] consists of intercostal radicular pain that may be episodic or continuous, mild or severe, and which is exacerbated by movement, as on rising from a chair. The pain is due to irritation of the intercostal nerve anteriorly by an adjacent rib or costal cartilage, and most commonly involves the eighth, ninth and tenth ribs, more frequently on the right than the left. The condition is more common in women than men, with an average age at onset of 29. The symptom may be reproduced by moving the affected rib, when a clicking or grating sound may be heard.

Treatment

The condition may respond to local injection of anaesthetics or steroids but if severe may require subperiosteal excision of the affected rib and costal cartilage. At operation the affected rib is found to be unduly mobile and to slip under the superior adjacent rib. The results of operation are good, with 82% of patients being pain-free at 7 days [106].

Sternocostoclavicular hyperostosis

Clinical features

Kohler and colleagues [107] described five patients presenting between the ages of 44 and 46 years with an 11–34 year history of a persistent pulling pain in the sternum, clavicles and upper ribs that was exacerbated by cold and dampness. Others have reported episodes of painful hot swelling at the same sites [108–110]. Club-like symmetrical enlargement of the clavicles was present, and in two patients venous congestion of the upper half of the body was seen. In these patients, atrophy of the shoulder girdle and occlusion of the subclavian vein, which was sometimes bilateral, appeared to occur for mechanical reasons [107,110]. The erythrocyte sedimentation rate (ESR) was markedly elevated.

Chest radiographs show symmetrical hyperostosis of the sternum and middle thirds of the clavicles, with synostosis of the sternoclavicular joints. The upper ribs are variably involved, with early ossification of the costochondral junctions. The disease appears to begin with an ossifying periosteitis. Biopsy of affected bones shows hyperostotic sclerosis of the spongiosa.

The aetiology is unknown, although there appears to be an association with ankylosing spondylitis and with vulgar or pustular psoriasis [108,110]. The disease is rare in the West, where it appears to be linked with HLA-B27, and is commoner in Japan where no such linkage occurs [110].

Treatment

No definitive treatment exists but symptomatic relief may be obtained with non-steroidal anti-inflammatory agents or with corticosteroids.

Tietze's syndrome or costochondritis

This condition of obscure origin results in pain, swelling and tenderness of one or more of the upper six costal cartilage, although the sternoclavicular joint was thought to be involved in one of Tietze's original four cases [111]. It has been suggested that the condition is the mechanical consequence of differences in leg length [112]. Alternatively, on the basis of an 'epidemic' of six cases occurring within 6 weeks in Zambia, a viral aetiology has been proposed [113].

Clinical features

It may occur at any age although it is commoner in young adults. There is no sex predisposition. The most common presentation is with painful swelling of one or more of the upper six costal cartilages, most commonly the second. The pain is localized and may be described as aching, gripping, sharp or dull. The intensity varies from mild to severe and may be exacerbated by coughing or deep breathing [114,115]. The onset may be sudden or gradual and the condition may persist for weeks, months or, rarely, years [116]. Biopsy shows normal cartilage [117]. The blood picture, including ESR, is normal and there are no radiological changes.

Treatment

The majority of cases respond to reassurance and the passage of time with or without the administration of a minor analgesic. Exceptionally, local injection of hydrocortisone may be required for relief of symptoms [118].

Relapsing polychondritis

This serious condition results in painful inflammation,

most commonly of the ear, nose and eyes, in association with systemic upset including fever, elevated ESR, anaemia and hyperglobulinaemia [119,120]. It is a disease of the middle decades with an equal sex distribution and is thought to be autoimmune in aetiology; antibodies to types IX and XI collagen and associations with systemic lupus and HLA-DR4 have been demonstrated [121–123]. Costochondral junction involvement is seen in about 50% of cases and laryngotracheal involvement in 70%. The disease may be rapidly fulminant, with death from pneumonia refractory to antibiotics or tracheal narrowing due to oedema, scarring and collapse of tracheal rings. Of the 49 cases reported in one series, the average lifespan of 11 who succumbed was 7 years, with a range from 10 months to 24 years [124]. The usual treatment is with systemic corticosteroids in a high initial dose (30–60 mg) followed by a maintenance dose (5–10 mg) [124]. Corticosteroids appear to suppress the fatal tracheobronchial complications of the disease. The use of stents may be necessary when tracheal or bronchial collapse is a problem [125].

Rib defects

Rib notching

Erosion of the inferior border of ribs or rib notching is most commonly seen in patients with coarctation of the aorta, when it is due to the enlarged intercostal arteries acting as collateral vessels (Fig. 45.5). It is present in 75% of adult patients but, since it is acquired, is less common in children although it has been seen in an infant [126,127]. The first two and last three ribs are never involved [126]. All other causes of this radiographic abnormality are rare, including subclavian artery obstruction after the Blalock–Taussig operation, 'pulseless disease', pulmonary arteriovenous fistula and intercostal neuroma. An idiopathic group is also recognized [126].

Superior marginal rib defects

Loss of superior marginal cortical bone in the third to sixth ribs has been reported in patients with poliomyelitis and in patients with restrictive lung disease due to connective tissue disorders, such as rheumatoid arthritis, systemic lupus erythematosus and scleroderma [128–130]. The aetiology is unknown.

Tumours of the chest wall

Tumours of the chest wall may originate in soft tissues or the bony thorax and the most common primary tumours found in these sites are shown in Table 45.2. Metastatic tumours of the chest wall are much more common than primary tumours.

Soft tissue tumours

Benign tumours

Lipoma is the most common benign soft tissue tumour of the chest wall. It is characteristically spongy, transilluminates well and is readily identified by CT. Rarely it may extend into the pleural cavity giving rise to an hourglass-shaped mass that indents the lung [131].

Chest wall haemangiomas are slow-growing tumours that arise in striated muscle. As they enlarge they may produce radiographic evidence of rib hypertrophy and notching. Phleboliths are uncommon but pathognomonic. Eventually a pulsatile mass that may have an audible bruit may form and this may be mistaken for a metastasis from thyroid or renal carcinoma.

Cystic hygroma or cavernous lymphangioma is an uncommon thin-walled multilocular tumour, usually found in the region of the neck in small children, that may extend into the mediastinum and chest wall rendering

Table 45.2 Benign and malignant tumours of the thoracic soft tissues and the bony thoracic cage.

	Benign	Malignant
Soft tissue	Lipoma	Fibrosarcoma
	Haemangioma	Liposarcoma
	Cystic hygroma	Leiomyosarcoma
	Neurofibroma	Synovioma
		Neuroectodermal tumours
Bony cage	Osteochondroma	Chondrosarcoma
	Chondroma	Ewing's tumour
	Simple cyst	Fibrosarcoma
	Osteoid osteoma	Osteogenic sarcoma
	Fibrous dysplasia	Myeloma

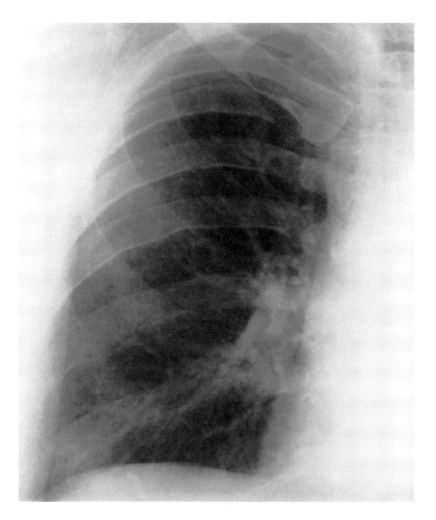

Fig. 45.5 Notching of the lower borders of upper thoracic ribs in a patient with aortic coarctation.

removal difficult. The author has seen haemorrhage into one such tumour cause acute tracheal obstruction (Fig. 45. 6).

Multiple neurofibromas, varying in size from a pea to a ping-pong ball, may be found in the intercostal spaces of the chest wall (Fig. 45.7). They are associated with neurofibromas elsewhere in the body and with the characteristic *café-au-lait* spots. Rarely malignant change may occur, with sudden acceleration in the rate of growth of a nodule.

The fibrous benign desmoid tumour, which usually arises from the fascia of the anterior abdominal wall, has also been described arising in the intercostal space [132–134].

Malignant tumours

Fibrosarcoma is the most common malignant soft tissue tumour of the chest wall and usually presents in young adults as a tumour in the region of the shoulder [133]. Haematogenous dissemination does happen but cure is possible if wide surgical excision is performed before this occurs.

Liposarcoma arises *de novo* and not from a pre-existing lipoma. It rarely metastasizes, although 50% recur after surgical resection.

Chest wall sarcomas including leiomyosarcoma have been reported in children and have proved amenable to surgical resection [135,136]. Malignant synovioma of the chest wall has also been reported [137]. A malignant chest wall tumour with features of adenocarcinoma and squamous carcinoma has been described 2 years after iodized talc pleurodesis [138]. Neuroectodermal tumours (Askin tumours) may occur in the chest wall. They are most frequent in children and may present as a large mass or with lung metastases [139].

Tumours of the bony thoracic cage

Tumours of the bony thoracic cage are most commonly found in the ribs and least commonly in the sternum, with intermediate frequencies in scapula, thoracic vertebrae and clavicle. The most common tumours are metastases from other primary tumours, most often breast, bronchial and prostatic carcinoma. Prostatic and breast metastases in particular may be osteosclerotic (Fig. 45.8). Of primary

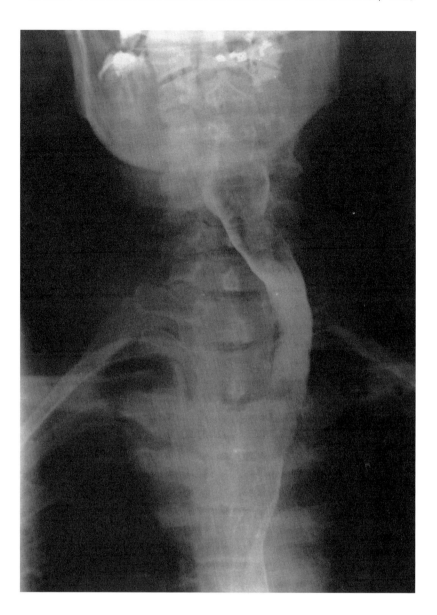

Fig. 45.6 Barium swallow in a patient who presented with stridor showing tracheal displacement to left. At surgery the lesion proved to be a cystic hygroma into which an acute bleed had occurred.

tumours of the thoracic cage, approximately 50% are benign [140–144]. Secondary tumours tend to have a short duration of symptoms, averaging 3 months in one series, whereas the mean duration of symptoms averaged 4.1 years for primary benign and 1.7 years for primary malignant tumours in the same series [141]. Patients with benign tumours are half as old on average as those with malignant tumours and about 30% of all thoracic cage tumours are discovered on routine chest radiography [141].

Patients may be asymptomatic, although the most common presentation is with local pain, which may vary from a dull ache to pain of great severity, and a mass on the chest wall. The pain of benign lesions tends not to change, whereas that of malignant lesions tends to progress and may be more readily affected by movement and coughing [140]. Where local structures are infiltrated or compressed,

pleuritic pain and referred pain, for example from intercostal nerves, may occur. It is generally agreed that it is unwise to assume that a tumour of the thoracic cage is benign, and all tumours should be treated with wide excision so that a pathological diagnosis can be obtained on the entire surgical specimen.

Benign tumours

Osteochondroma or exostosis is the most common benign tumour, often presenting as a mass arising from the scapula or a rib, most frequently near the costochondral junction, in patients in the second decade. Growth begins in childhood and is believed to stop when adult stature is achieved. There is often a bony base to the tumour with a cartilaginous cap over which a bursa may be present. These tumours may cause local pain and

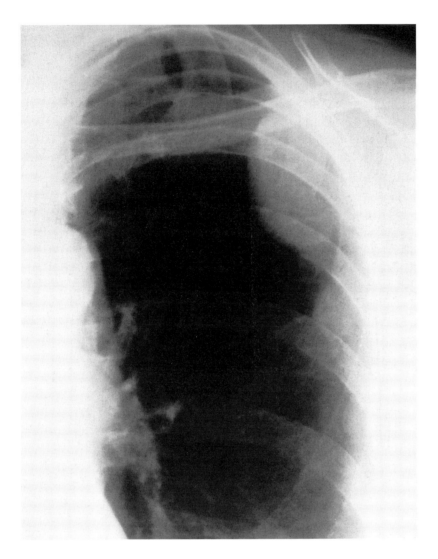

Fig. 45.7 Three neurofibromas on left lateral chest wall in patient with multiple neurofibromatosis.

should be excised since the diagnosis is never certain and chondrosarcomatous transformation of the cartilage can occur.

Chondromas appear radiologically as well-demarcated expansions of a rib near a costochondral junction. A well-defined lucent area in the rib may contain flakes of calcium. Tumours of mature cartilage, they may give rise to chondrosarcomas and the treatment of choice is wide surgical excision.

Simple (or unicameral) bone cysts are found in the anterior portion of ribs, in the clavicle or sometimes in the head of the humerus. They produce a radiolucent defect on chest radiographs that may expand and thin the cortex resulting in a pathological fracture.

Osteoid osteoma is uncommon in the thoracic skeleton but may be confused with osteomyelitis or malignancy since it causes severe progressive pain that is worse at night. The radiographic picture of a round or oval lucent area about 1 cm in diameter surrounded by sclerotic bone often assists diagnosis.

Fibrous dysplasia is the most commonly encountered rib abnormality in young adults aged 20–30 years [145, 146]. The condition is one in which primitive fibrous tissue proliferates in the medullary cavity and erodes the cortex from within, often producing expansion or distortion of the bone. The lesion is usually single and located in the posterior aspect of the ribs, although multiple lesions are found in Albright's syndrome where *café-au-lait* spots, precocious puberty or hyperthyroidism may be found [145]. Radiologically, the cortex may be thinned by a transradiant swelling that may be traversed by irregular bony trabeculae [140]. Clinically, pain is unusual but pathological fractures do occur. Excision is the treatment of choice [147].

Osteoclastoma is a rare tumour in the thorax, where it may be found in the head or tubercle of a rib; 10% are malignant and treatment is by excision.

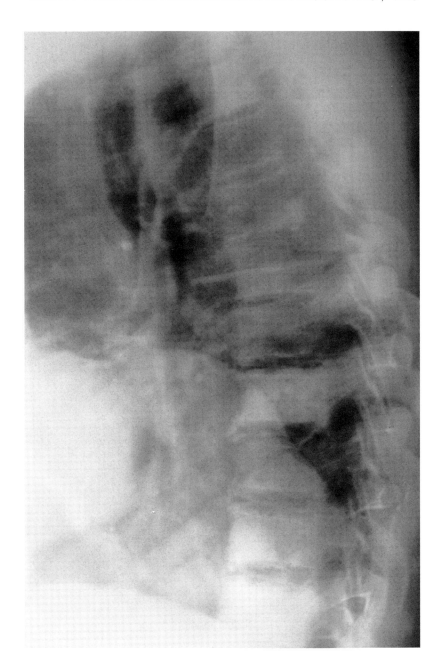

Fig. 45.8 Chest film of thoracic and upper lumbar spine showing radiodense osteosclerotic metastases from prostatic carcinoma.

Malignant tumours

Chondrosarcoma is the most common primary malignant tumour of the bony thoracic skeleton and presents usually with chest pain and swelling [140,141,148]. It has been described after radiation therapy, in Paget's disease and on one occasion following repetitive trauma from the arm of a wheelchair [149]. Most common in the upper anterior ribs, it is seen radiologically as a mass arising from the periosteum in such a way that the underlying bone shows minimal destruction (Fig. 45.9). Flakes of calcium may be seen in the tumour. It is locally invasive and may also spread via the bloodstream to the lungs in the first

instance. Treatment is by wide surgical excision and chemotherapy.

Ewing's tumour, an aggressively malignant tumour, is most common in those under 30 years of age and usually involves the ribs and less commonly the scapula or sternum [140,150]. Systemic features of fever, weight loss and malaise may occur with progressive local changes of pain, swelling and tenderness [150]. Radiographs may show progressive rib destruction with little reactive change and a soft tissue mass develops in most cases (Fig. 45.10). Multiple areas of periosteal new bone formation may produce an onion-peel appearance. The tumour metastasizes to lungs and other bones in most patients.

Treatment involves chemotherapy usually with combined radiotherapy and surgery; survival rates at 4 years of 56% have been reported after combined treatment, with no later recurrences [151].

Fibrosarcoma and osteogenic sarcoma behave like chondrosarcoma both clinically and radiologically [140].

Myeloma may present as a solitary lesion or as multiple lesions most commonly of the ribs [152,153]. The most common presenting feature is rib pain, often due to pathological fractures. Lytic lesions are seen on chest radiographs. Treatment consists of radiotherapy for local lesions and chemotherapy for multiple lesions.

Infections of the chest wall

Osteomyelitis

Osteomyelitis of ribs is relatively uncommon and is more frequent in children than adults. It often occurs after trauma and affects one of the upper three ribs, most commonly the first. The suppuration may strip the periosteum from the rib, forming a subperiosteal extrapleural abscess that may be large. Radiologically, the rib appearance may not change for 10–12 days. Initially, there is non-specific local destruction and osteolysis with reactionary sclerosis as the lesion becomes established [153].

Local osteomyelitis of a rib may be secondary to the drainage of an empyema, with infection spreading from the drainage site into the bone. Sequestra may be formed and discharge into the empyema, which persists until they are removed [154]. The most common offending microorganism is *Staphylococcus aureus*, management with appropriate antibiotics leading to resolution in most cases.

Osteomyelitis of the sternum is very uncommon [155,156]. It presents with fever and a tender swelling with radiographic evidence of bony erosion and sclerosis. *Staph. aureus* and *Pseudomonas aeruginosa* have been reported as causative organisms. Surgical drainage and curettage may be required in addition to antibiotic therapy [156].

Septic arthritis

Sternoclavicular joint infection is an unusual cause of chest pain [157]. The joint is usually swollen and tender, with fever and systemic evidence of infection. The condition is commoner in heroin users in whom infection with both *Ps. aeruginosa* and *Staph. aureus* has been reported [158]. Treatment is with antibiotics and aspiration as required.

Tuberculosis of the thoracic cage

Costal tuberculosis is rare but may give rise to local pain,

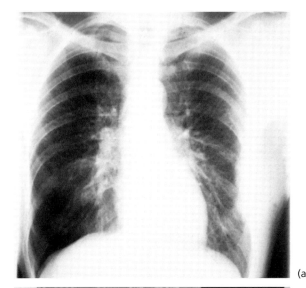
(a)

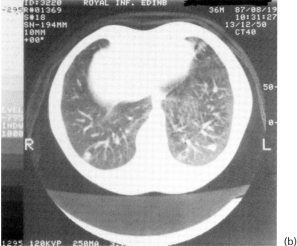
(b)

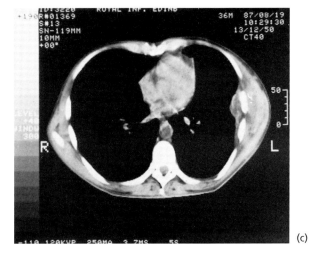
(c)

Fig. 45.9 (a) Left lateral chest wall mass that on biopsy proved to be chondrosarcoma. CT shows (b) small metastatic deposits within the lungs and (c) soft tissue expansion round enlarged rib, containing dense areas of new cartilage. (Courtesy of Dr J.R. Walsh.)

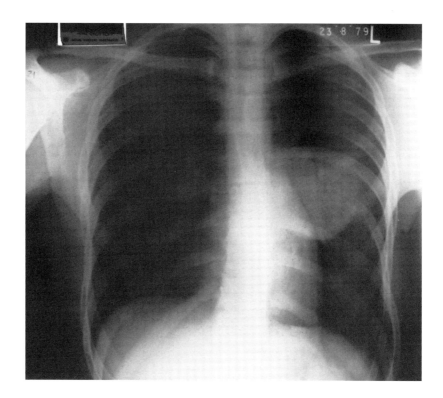

Fig. 45.10 Posterior mediastinal tumour. Destruction of the eighth rib provided the clue that this was a primary Ewing's sarcoma.

swelling and sinus formation. Radiologically there is an initial small area of bone destruction that may progress to periosteal elevation and soft tissue swelling. There is usually no evidence of pulmonary tuberculosis. Similar disease may arise in sternoclavicular or acromioclavicular joints.

Multiple lesions of the costovertebral portion of the ribs may accompany Pott's disease of the spine with paravertebral abscess formation.

Cold abscess of the chest wall

Cold abscess of the chest wall, which originates in tuberculosis of the intercostal lymph glands, can be divided into two main groups: the first lies at the angle of the ribs, from which the pus may track either backwards with the posterior primary division of the intercostal nerve, presenting near the erector spinae muscles, or forwards with the anterior division to present in the lateral chest wall; the second may arise from nodes in the region of the internal mammary artery and present near the costal cartilages. Cold abscess usually presents as a painless fluctuant swelling that may be mistaken for a lipoma. Diagnosis is made by aspiration of pus or during surgical exploration. It responds well to conventional antituberculous chemotherapy.

Syphilitic gumma of chest wall

This is now very rare and is described as arising in the anterior mediastinum and giving rise to a hard, fixed lump in the intercostal space that may later soften and form a punched-out ulcer. Radiologically, the lesion may resemble a tumour of the anterior mediastinum. The true nature may be suspected if a punched-out ulcer has developed or as a result of positive serology.

Actinomycosis

Actinomycosis may spread from the lungs into the chest wall and give rise to destructive lesions with irregularity of the rib margins caused by periosteitis. It is described in Chapter 21.

Echinococcosis

Costal echinococcosis is very rare and usually presents as a multiloculated osteolytic lesion in rib [159]. The lesions are usually posterior and may expand to transgress the bony cortex. In the costovertebral region soft tissue masses may form and neurological presentations are common in this situation. The condition is described in Chapter 22.

Fungal infections

Blastomycosis, coccidioidomycosis and cryptococcosis can cause osteolytic lesions of ribs similar to those described above for tuberculosis. These organisms are discussed in Chapter 21.

Thoracoplasty

This operation, in which a varying number of ribs was removed from one or both sides of the upper thoracic cage (Fig. 45.11), was widely practised from the 1930s until the mid-1950s as a treatment for tuberculosis [160]. In many cases it appears to have arrested previously progressive cavitating disease, one study carried out during the 1980s having shown survival of 93% at 10 years and 79% at 20 years [161]. However, the combination of the effects of the tuberculosis, the loss of the chest wall and, often, smoking has in many cases resulted ultimately in the development of respiratory failure.

Neuromuscular conditions affecting respiration

It is uncommon but not unknown for patients with neurological disease to present primarily to the chest physician. However, respiratory problems in the course of neurological disease occur frequently, and the advice of someone interested in respiratory management is often sought. These conditions may be separated into those causing acute ventilatory problems and those causing chronic failure (Table 45.3).

Acute respiratory failure

Acute problems occur most commonly as a consequence of overdose of drugs with a central nervous depressant effect, such as barbiturates and opiates, producing hypoventilation and carbon dioxide retention [162]. Management of these episodes includes a requirement for ventilatory support and, if necessary, cardiac support. Alcohol may not only cause central respiratory depression but has also been described as causing an acute rhabdomyolysis after a prolonged drinking bout [163]. A unique drug-induced cause of respiratory failure is the myasthenia syndrome that occurs as a rare side-effect of treatment with D-penicillamine, which usually resolves when the drug is discontinued [164]. Organophosphate and carbamate poisoning as a result of the widespread and careless use of insecticides is a not uncommon cause of acute respiratory failure in underdeveloped countries [165]. Similar problems occur as a result of neurological disease in acute ascending polyneuritis (Guillain–Barré syndrome), poliomyelitis, status epilepticus, tetanus and myasthenia gravis; as a result of accidents, following high spinal cord trauma and air embolism in diving; and as a consequence of lesions causing acute rises in intracranial pressure. Hypothyroidism may cause respiratory failure by a combination of central respiratory depression, upper airway

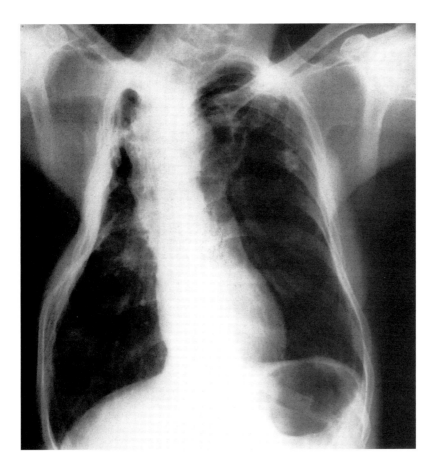

Fig. 45.11 Right-sided eight-rib thoracoplasty carried out for cavitating tuberculosis in the late 1940s. Calcified lesions of healed tuberculosis are visible in both lungs.

Table 45.3 Neuromuscular causes of ventilatory failure.

	Acute	Chronic
Neurological disease	Acute polyneuritis	Motoneurone disease
	Poliomyelitis	Poliomyelitis
	Myasthenia gravis	Cervical cord injury
	Cerebral haemorrhage	Idiopathic
	Cervical cord injury	Ondine's curse
	High intracranial pressure	Brainstem tumours
	Epilepsy	Myasthenia gravis
	Critical illness neuropathy	Eaton–Lambert syndrome
	Tetanus	Multiple sclerosis
	Air embolism	Bilateral phrenic palsy
	Hypothyroidism	Hypothyroidism
	Bilateral phrenic palsy	Parkinson's disease
Muscular disease	Acute polymyositis	Muscular dystrophies
	Dermatomyositis	Acid maltase deficiency
	Steroid myopathy	Dystrophia myotonica
	Hypokalaemia	Rigid spine syndromes
		Nemaline myopathy
Drugs' poisons	Opiates	
	Barbiturates	
	Hypnotics	
	Anaesthetics	
	Muscle relaxants	
	D-Penicillamine	
	Alcohol	
	Botulinus toxin	
	Organophosphates	
	Carbamates	

obstruction and perhaps respiratory myopathy [166,167]. Acute respiratory muscle paralysis may occur in hypokalaemia [168], most commonly of the familial type but whatever the cause, and as a result of muscular or peripheral nerve dysfunction occurring in patients acutely ill on respirators [169–171], where it may cause problems in weaning from the machine. A steroid myopathy has also been described as causing similar problems [172], and this is something to be considered especially in severe asthma attacks when a patient has required ventilation and is proving difficult to wean. Primary muscle disorders may cause acute respiratory failure, particularly those having an inflammatory basis such as polymyositis and dermatomyositis [173].

Chronic respiratory failure

Chronic ventilatory failure may be due to lesions involving the respiratory centre in the floor of the fourth ventricle, the nerves of the respiratory reflex arc or the muscles of respiration. The sleep apnoea syndromes are discussed in Chapter 47, although it should be noted that sleep hypoventilation is a usual accompaniment of all neuromuscular syndromes affecting respiration. The most common neurological causes of chronic ventilatory failure are motoneurone disease [174], poliomyelitis [175], multiple sclerosis [176] and spinal cord transection.

Chronic hypoventilation may also occur in myasthenia gravis [177], Eaton–Lambert syndrome [178] associated with bronchial carcinoma, hypothyroidism [179] and Parkinson's disease [180,181]. The drug L-dopa, used in the treatment of Parkinson's disease, may also cause respiratory muscle and respiratory centre dysfunction leading to ventilatory insufficiency [180]. Ondine's curse, a condition in which there is failure of brainstem autonomic control leading to suppression of respiratory drive when the subject is asleep, occurs as a congenital defect or may be a consequence of stroke or other pathological processes in the respiratory centre [182]. Bilateral phrenic nerve palsy has been discussed above. Muscle diseases causing chronic respiratory failure [173] include muscular dystrophies, of which the limb girdle and Duchenne types are the most common, adult acid maltase deficiency [183], dystrophia myotonica, rigid spine disorders including Emery–Dreifuss syndrome, and the autosomal dominant nemaline myopathy that sometimes presents in adult life.

Assessment of respiratory function

In neuromuscular ventilatory failure the patient may remain asymptomatic from a respiratory point of view because of the inactivity imposed by the primary disease [184]. As the condition progresses, the patient may be seen to be breathing rapidly and shallowly, except when the cause is drug overdose or brainstem disease, when the rate may be much reduced. Daytime somnolence is often present. The cause is usually obvious from the symptoms and signs of the primary disease, and treatment should be directed at its alleviation where possible. Thus it is important not to miss the less obvious causes such as hypokalaemia in, say, periodic paralysis, myxoedema or poisoning with organophosphorus insecticides. Physical signs may include the paradoxical chest wall and abdominal movements described in the section on diaphragmatic paralysis, poor cough, and difficulty with speech and swallowing. Vital capacity may be reduced but is often normal until the condition is quite advanced; nevertheless, at an earlier stage it should be possible to demonstrate reduced MVV and maximal inspiratory pressures using an oesophageal balloon. Sleep studies are essential, as the condition is usually worse during this time and in a number of conditions both central and upper airway dysfunction combine to cause the respiratory failure. In conditions with a fluctuating or progressive course, serial measurement of vital capacity is a useful means of monitoring progress and assessing the need for ventilatory assistance.

Management

Wherever possible treatment should be directed at the primary cause. General management includes assistance with coughing and treatment of any respiratory infections, although the important decision relates to the need for ventilatory assistance. This clearly depends on the primary condition and its other effects on the patient, and there is little problem in deciding to use this in acute ventilatory failure. Increasingly, however, patients with chronic neuromuscular conditions who would not have been considered suitable for long-term ventilation a decade ago are now benefiting from advances in management, which may provide fewer hospitalizations and respiratory infections and a better quality of life. Most such patients should be considered for such treatment [185]. In this chronic situation, there is time for detailed discussion of the implications of long-term support with patients and relatives, and for assessment of their suitability for domiciliary ventilation [186]. It is usually desirable to start with non-invasive measures and to delay tracheostomy until it becomes essential. Administration of low-flow oxygen to such patients without assisted ventilation is likely to give rise to carbon dioxide retention and is therefore undesirable [187]. A simple rocking bed may be suitable in some cases, where diaphragmatic weakness predominates or in relieving symptoms in terminal care [173]. The methods of ventilatory support available are described in Chapter 58. After full assessment, including polysomnography, the patient is often helped by nasal intermittent positive-pressure ventilation during the night. As the condition progresses it is often necessary to convert to intermittent positive-pressure ventilation via a permanent tracheostomy. In some cases a cuirass respirator is found to be more suitable (see Chapter 58).

All patients with chronic ventilatory failure reach a stage at which their quality of life seems not to justify initiation or continuation of ventilation, a matter that should be as fully discussed as practicable with patient and relatives. When the decision is made, some expertise in the use of drugs and ventilators is required to ensure that the gradual withdrawal of support does not cause undue distress.

References

1 Gayler BW, Donner MW. Radiographic changes of the ribs. *Am J Med Sci* 1967; 253: 586.

2 Ravitch MM. Asymmetrical congenital deformity of rib. *Ann Surg* 1980; 191: 534.

3 Dick R. Arteriography in neurovascular compression at the thoracic outlet, with special reference to embolic patterns. *Am J Roentgenol* 1970; 110: 141.

4 Scher LA, Veith FJ, Haimovici H *et al.* Staging of arterial complications of cervical rib: guidelines for surgical management. *Surgery* 1984; 95: 644.

5 Grimer RJ, Mulligan PJ, Thompson AG. Thoracic outlet syndrome following correction of scoliosis in a patient with cervical ribs. *J Bone Joint Surg* 1983; 65A: 1172.

6 Lagerquist LG, Tyler FH. Thoracic outlet syndrome with tetany of the hands. *Am J Med* 1975; 59: 281.

7 Ruckley CV. Thoracic outlet syndrome. *Br Med J* 1983; 287: 447.

8 Sanders RC, Knight RW. Radiological appearances of the xiphoid process presenting as an upper abdominal mass. *Radiology* 1981; 41: 489.

9 Currarino G, Silverman FN. Premature obliteration of the sternal sutures and pigeon-breast deformity. *Radiology* 1958; 70: 532.

10 Robicsek F, Cook JW, Daugherty HK, Selle JG. Pectus carinatum. *J Thorac Cardiovasc Surg* 1979; 78: 52.

11 Chidambaran B, Mehta AV. Currarino–Silverman syndrome (pectus carinatum type 2 deformity) and mitral valve disease. *Chest* 1992; 102: 780.

12 Chin EF. Surgery of funnel chest and congenital sternal prominence. *Br J Surg* 1956; 44: 360.

13 Fonkalsrud EW, Salman T, Guo W, Gregg JP. Repair of pectus deformities with sternal support. *J Thorac Cardiovasc Surg* 1994; 107: 37.

14 Wooler GH, Mashhour YAS, Garcia JB *et al.* Pectus excavatum. *Thorax* 1969; 24: 557.

15 Olsen KD, Kern EB, O'Connell EJ. Pectus excavatum: resolution after surgical removal of upper airway obstruction. *Laryngoscope* 1980; 90: 832.

16 Fan L, Murphy S. Pectus excavatum from chronic airway obstruction. *Am J Dis Child* 1981; 135: 550.

17 Godfrey S. Association between pectus excavatum and segmental bronchomalacia. *J Pediatr* 1980; 96: 649.

18 Iwa T, Watanabe Y. Unusual combination of pulmonary sequestration and funnel chest. *Chest* 1979; 76: 314.

19 Reusch CS. Hemodynamic studies in pectus excavatum. *Circulation* 1961; 24: 1143.

20 Fink A, Rivin A, Murray JF. Pectus excavatum. *Arch Intern Med* 1961; 108: 427.

21 Orzalesi MM, Cook CD. Pulmonary function in children with pectus excavatum. *J Pediatr* 1965; 66: 898.

22 Kaguraoka H, Ohnuki T, Itaoka T, Yokoyama M, Nitta S. Degree of severity of pectus excavatum and pulmonary function in preoperative and postoperative periods. *J Thorac Cardiovasc Surg* 1992; 104: 1483.

23 Castile RG, Staats BA, Westbrook PR.

Symptomatic pectus deformities of the chest. *Am Rev Respir Dis* 1982; 126: 564.

24 Majid PA, Zienkowicz BS, Roos JP. Pectus excavatum and cardiac dysfunction: a case report with pre- and post-operative haemodynamic studies. *Thorax* 1979; 34: 74.

25 Guller B, Hable K. Cardiac findings in pectus excavatum in children: review and differential diagnosis. *Chest* 1974; 66: 165.

26 Skinner EF. Xiphoid horn in pectus excavatum. *Thorax* 1969; 24: 750.

27 De Oliveira JM, Sambhi MP, Zimmerman HA. The electrocardiogram in pectus excavatum. *Br Heart J* 1958; 20: 495.

28 Backer OG, Brunner S, Larsen V. Radiologic evaluation of funnel chest. *Acta Radiol* 1961; 55: 249.

29 Ben-Menachem Y, O'Hara AE, Kane HA. Paradoxical cardiac enlargement during inspiration in children with pectus excavatum: a new observation. *Br J Radiol* 1973; 46: 38.

30 Actis-Dato GM, De Paulis R, Actis-Dato A *et al.* Correction of pectus excavatum with a self-retaining seagull wing prosthesis. Long-term follow-up. *Chest* 1995; 107: 303.

31 Lane-Smith DM, Gillis DA, Roy PD. Repair of pectus excavatum using a Dacron vascular graft strut. *J Pediatr Surg* 1994; 29: 1179.

32 Morshuis W, Folgering H, Barentsz J, van Lier H, Laquet L. Pulmonary function before surgery for pectus excavatum and at long-term follow-up. *Chest* 1994; 105: 1646.

33 Morshuis W, Folgering H, Barentsz J, Cox AL, van Lier H, Laquet L. Exercise cardiorespiratory function before and one year after operation for pectus excavatum. *J Thorac Cardiovasc Surg* 1994; 107: 1403.

34 Datey KK, Deshmukh MM, Engineer SD, Dalvi CP. Straight back syndrome. *Br Heart J* 1964; 26: 614.

35 De Leon AC, Perloff JK, Twigg H, Majd M. The straight back syndrome. Clinical cardiovascular manifestations. *Circulation* 1965; 32: 193.

36 Gould KG, Cooper KH, Harkleroad LE. Pulmonary function and work capacity in the absence of physiological dorsal kyphosis of the spine. *Dis Chest* 1969; 55: 405.

37 Pearl M, Chow TF, Friedman E. Poland's syndrome. *Radiology* 1971; 101: 619.

38 Park HM, Seifert MF. Eurysternum (extra-wide sternum): a rarely recognised developmental anomaly. Scintigraphic appearances. *Clin Nucl Med* 1995; 20: 306.

39 Anon. Rib pain. *Br Med J* 1976; i: 358.

40 Shanks SC, Kerley P. *A Text-book of X-ray Diagnosis by British Authors*, 4th edn. London: HK Lewis, 1973.

41 James JIP. *Scoliosis*, 2nd edn. Edinburgh: Churchill Livingstone, 1976.

42 McMaster MJ, Ohtsuka K. The natural history of congenital scoliosis. *J Bone Joint Surg* 1982; 64A: 1128.

43 McMaster MJ. Occult intraspinal anomalies and congenital scoliosis. *J Bone Joint Surg* 1984; 66A: 588.

44 Cobb JR. Outline for the study of scoliosis. *Instruct Course Lect Am Acad Orthop Surg* 1948; 5: 261.

45 Reid L. Pathological changes in the lungs in scoliosis. In: Zorab PA, ed. *Scoliosis*. London: Heinemann, 1969: 67.

46 Boffa P, Stovin P, Schneerson J. Lung developmental abnormalities in severe scoliosis. *Thorax* 1984; 39: 681.

47 Naeye RL. Kyphoscoliosis and cor pulmonale. A study of the pulmonary vascular bed. *Am J Pathol* 1961; 38: 561.

48 Hepper NGG, Black LF, Fowler WS. Relationships of lung volume to height and arm span in normal subjects and in patients with spinal deformity. *Am Rev Respir Dis* 1965; 91: 356.

49 Weber B, Smith JP, Briscoe WA *et al.* Pulmonary function in asymptomatic adolescents with scoliosis. *Am Rev Respir Dis* 1975; 111: 389.

50 Bergofsky EH, Turino GM, Fishman AP. Cardiorespiratory failure in kyphoscoliosis. *Medicine* 1959; 38: 263.

51 Kafer ER. Idiopathic scoliosis. Mechanical properties of the respiratory system and the ventilatory response to carbon dioxide. *J Clin Invest* 1975; 55: 1153.

52 Jones RS, Kennedy JD, Hasham F *et al.* Mechanical inefficiency of the thoracic cage in scoliosis. *Thorax* 1981; 36: 456.

53 Olgiati R, Levine D, Smith JP *et al.* Diffusing capacity in idiopathic scoliosis and its interpretation regarding alveolar development. *Am Rev Respir Dis* 1982; 126: 229.

54 Smyth RJ, Chapman KR, Wright TA *et al.* Pulmonary function in adolescents with mild idiopathic scoliosis. *Thorax* 1984; 39: 901.

55 Siegler D, Zorab PA. The influence of lung volume on gas transfer in scoliosis. *Br J Dis Chest* 1982; 76: 44.

56 Kafer ER. Respiratory function in paralytic scoliosis. *Am Rev Respir Dis* 1974; 110: 450.

57 Cooper DM, Rojas JV, Mellins RB *et al.* Respiratory mechanics in adolescents with idiopathic scoliosis. *Am Rev Respir Dis* 1984; 130: 16.

58 Bjure J, Grimby G, Kasalicky J *et al.* Respiratory impairment and airway closure in patients with untreated idiopathic scoliosis. *Thorax* 1970; 25: 451.

59 Anon. Respiratory function in scoliosis. *Lancet* 1985; i: 84.

60 Sinha R, Bergofsky EH. Prolonged alteration of lung mechanics in kyphoscoliosis by positive pressure hyperinflation. *Am Rev Respir Dis* 1972; 106: 47.

61 Schneerson JM. The cardiorespiratory response to exercise in thoracic scoliosis. *Thorax* 1978; 33: 457.

62 Dollery CT, Gillan PMS, Hugh-Jones P, Zorab PA. Regional lung function in kyphoscoliosis. *Thorax* 1965; 20: 175.

63 Bake B, Bjure J, Kasalicky J, Nachemson A. Regional pulmonary ventilation and perfusion distribution in patients with untreated idiopathic scoliosis. *Thorax* 1972; 27: 703.

64 Shaw DB, Read J. Hypoxia and thoracic scoliosis. *Br Med J* 1960; ii: 1486.

65 Schneerson JM, Venco A, Prime FL. A study of pulmonary artery pressure, electrocardiography and mechanocardiography in thoracic scoliosis. *Thorax* 1977; 32: 700.

66 Bruderman I, Stein M. Physiologic evaluation and treatment of kyphoscoliotic patients. *Ann Intern Med* 1961; 55: 94.

67 Mezon BL, West P, Israels J, Kryger M. Sleep breathing abnormalities in kyphoscoliosis. *Am Rev Respir Dis* 1980; 122: 617.

68 Guilleminault C, Kurland G, Winkle R, Miles LE. Severe kyphoscoliosis, breathing and sleep. The 'Quasimodo' syndrome during sleep. *Chest* 1981; 79: 626.

69 Lisboa C, Moreno R, Fava M *et al.* Inspiratory muscle function in patients with severe kyphoscoliosis. *Am Rev Respir Dis* 1985; 132: 48.

70 Kearon C, Viviani GR, Killian KJ. Factors influencing work capacity in adolescent idiopathic thoracic scoliosis. *Am Rev Respir Dis* 1993; 148: 295.

71 Pehrsson K, Larsson S, Oden A, Nachemson A. Long-term follow-up of patients with untreated scoliosis: a study of mortality, causes of death and symptoms. *Spine* 1992; 17: 1091.

72 Schneerson JM, Edgar MA. Cardiac and respiratory function before and after spinal fusion in adolescent idiopathic scoliosis. *Thorax* 1979; 34: 658.

73 Libby DM, Briscoe WA, Boyce B, Smith JP. Acute respiratory failure in scoliosis or kyphosis. Prolonged survival and treatment. *Am J Med* 1982; 73: 532.

74 Strom K, Pehrsson K, Boe J, Nachemson A. Survival of patients with severe thoracic spine deformities receiving domiciliary oxygen therapy. *Chest* 1992; 102: 164.

75 Lane DJ, Hazleman B, Nichols PJR. Late onset respiratory failure in patients with previous poliomyelitis. *Q J Med* 1974; 43: 551.

76 Leger P, Bedicam JM, Cornette A *et al.* Nasal intermittent positive pressure ventilation. Long-term follow-up in patients with severe chronic respiratory insufficiency. *Chest* 1994; 105: 100.

77 Bach JR, Robert D, Leger P, Langevin B. Sleep fragmentation in kyphoscoliotic individuals with alveolar hypoventilation treated by NIPPV. *Chest* 1995; 107: 1552.

78 Wiers PWJ, Le Coultre R, Dallinga OT *et al.* Cuirass respirator treatment of chronic respiratory failure in scoliotic patients. *Thorax* 1977; 32: 221.

79 Powner DJ, Hoffman LG. Bedside construction of a custom cuirass for respiratory failure in kyphoscoliosis. *Chest* 1978; 74: 469.

80 Fulkerson WJ, Wilkins JK, Esbenshade AM *et al.* Life threatening hypoventilation in kyphoscoliosis: successful treatment with a moulded body-brace ventilator. *Am Rev Respir Dis* 1984; 129: 185.

81 Indihar FJ, Walker NE. Experience with a prolonged respiratory care unit: revisited. *Chest* 1984; 86: 616.

82 Hoeppner VH, Cockcroft DW, Dosman JA, Cotton DJ. Night time ventilation improves respiratory function in secondary kyphoscoliosis. *Am Rev Respir Dis* 1984; 129: 240.

83 Brewerton DA, Caffrey M, Hart FD *et al.* Ankylosing spondylitis and HLA-B27. *Lancet* 1973; i: 904.

84 Danilevicius Z. HL-A system and rheumatic diseases. *JAMA* 1975; 231: 283.

85 Calin A, Fries JF. Striking prevalence of ankylosing spondylitis in healthy, W27 positive males and females. *N Engl J Med* 1975; 293: 835.

86 Luthra HS. Extra-articular manifestations of ankylosing spondylitis. *Mayo Clin Proc* 1977; 52: 655.

87 Woodrow JC, Eastmond CJ. HLA-B27 and the genetics of ankylosing spondylitis. *Ann Rheum Dis* 1978; 37: 504.

88 Khan MA, Kushner I, Braun WE *et al.* HLA-B27 homozygosity in ankylosing spondylitis: relationship to risk and severity. *Tissue Antigens* 1978; 11: 434.

89 Russell AS. The prevalence of ankylosing spondylitis. *J Rheumatol* 1979; 6: 603.

90 Dudley Hart F, Emerson PA, Gregg I. Thorax

in ankylosing spondylitis. *Ann Rheum Dis* 1963; 22: 11.

91 Renzetti AD, Nicholas W, Dutton RE, Jivoff L. Some effects of ankylosing spondylitis on gas exchange. *N Engl J Med* 1960; 262: 215.

92 Miller JM, Sproule BJ. Pulmonary function in ankylosing spondylitis. *Am Rev Respir Dis* 1964; 90: 376.

93 Sharp JT, Sweany SK, Henry JP *et al.* Lung and thoracic compliances in ankylosing spondylitis. *J Lab Clin Med* 1964; 63: 254.

94 Stewart RM, Ridyard JB, Pearson JD. Regional lung function in ankylosing spondylitis. *Thorax* 1976; 31: 433.

95 Parkin A, Robinson PJ, Hickling P. Regional lung ventilation in ankylosing spondylitis. *Br J Radiol* 1982; 55: 833.

96 Good AE. The chest pain of ankylosing spondylitis. *Ann Intern Med* 1963; 58: 926.

97 Davies D. Ankylosing spondylitis and lung fibrosis. *Q J Med* 1972; 41: 395.

98 Rosenow EC, Strimlan CV, Muhm JR, Ferguson RH. Pleuropulmonary manifestations of ankylosing spondylitis. *Mayo Clin Proc* 1977; 52: 641.

99 Ahern MJ, Maddison P, Mann S, Scott CA. Ankylosing spondylitis and adenocarcinoma of the lung. *Ann Rheum Dis* 1982; 41: 292.

100 Rohatgi P, Turrisi BC. Bronchocentric granulomatosis and ankylosing spondylitis. *Thorax* 1984; 39: 317.

101 Libby DM, Schley WS, Smith JP. Cricoarytenoid arthritis in ankylosing spondylitis. *Chest* 1981; 80: 641.

102 Blavia R, Toda MR, Vidal F, Benet A, Razquin S, Richart C. Pulmonary diffuse amyloidosis and ankylosing spondylitis. A rare association. *Chest* 1992; 102: 1608.

103 Thiranont N, Netrawichian P. Transpedicular decancellation closed wedge osteotomy for treatment of fixed flexion deformity in spine in ankylosing spondylitis. *Spine* 1993; 18: 2517.

104 Mynors JM. Clicking rib. *Lancet* 1973; i: 674.

105 McBeath AA, Keene JS. The rib-tip syndrome. *J Bone Joint Surg* 1975; 57A: 795.

106 Copeland GP, Machin DG, Shennan JM. Surgical treatment of the 'slipping rib syndrome'. *Br J Surg* 1984; 71: 522.

107 Kohler H, Neulinger E, Kutzner J, West TB. Sternocostoclavicular hyperostosis: painful swelling of the sternum, clavicles and upper ribs. *Ann Intern Med* 1977; 87: 192.

108 Resnick D. Sternocostoclavicular hyperostosis. *Am J Roentgenol* 1980; 135: 1278.

109 Resnick D, Vint V, Poteshman NL. Sternocostoclavicular hyperostosis. *J Bone Joint Surg* 1981; 63A: 1329.

110 Fallett GH, Arroyo J, Vischer TL. Sternocostoclavicular hyperostosis: case report with a 31 year follow up. *Arthritis Rheum* 1983; 26: 784.

111 Tietze A. Uber eine eigenartige Houfung von Fallen mit Dystrophie der Rippenkuorpel. *Berl Klin Wochenschr* 1921; 58: 829.

112 Dunlop RF. Tietze revisited. *Clin Orthop* 1969; 62: 223.

113 Gill GV. Epidemic of Tietze's syndrome. *Br Med J* 1977; ii: 499.

114 Kayser HL. Tietze's syndrome. *Am J Med* 1956; 21: 982.

115 Kennedy AC. Tietze's syndrome: an unusual cause of chest wall swelling. *Scott Med J* 1957; 2: 363.

116 Ausubel H, Cohen BD, Ladue JS. Tietze's disease of eight years duration. *N Engl J Med* 1959; 261: 190.

117 Carabasi RJ, Christian JJ, Brindley HH. Costosternal chondrodynia: a variant of Tietze's syndrome. *Dis Chest* 1962; 41: 559.

118 Salomon MI. Thoracochondralgia (Tietze's syndrome). Report of three cases. *N Y State J Med* 1958; 58: 530.

119 Khan AJ, Lynfield Y, Baldwin H. Relapsing polychondritis: case report and review of the literature. *Cutis* 1994; 54: 98.

120 Diebold L, Rauh G, Jager K, Lohrs U. Bone marrow pathology in relapsing polychondritis: high frequency of myelodysplastic syndromes. *Br J Haematol* 1995; 89: 820.

121 Alsalameh S, Mollenhauer J, Scheuplein F *et al.* Preferential cellular and humoral immune reactivities to native and denatured collagen types IX and XI in a patient with fatal relapsing polychondritis. *J Rheumatol* 1993; 20: 1419.

122 Lang B, Rothenfusser A, Lanchbury JS *et al.* Susceptibility to relapsing polychondritis is assocated with HLA-DR4. *Arthritis Rheum* 1993; 36: 660.

123 Harisdangkul V, Johnson WW. Association between relapsing polychondritis and systemic lupus erythematosus. *South Med J* 1994; 87: 753.

124 Dolan DL, Lemmon GB, Tietelbaum SL. Relapsing polychondritis. *Am J Med* 1966; 41: 285.

125 Tsang V, Williams AM, Goldstraw P. Sequential silastic and expandable metal stenting for tracheobronchial strictures. *Ann Thorac Surg* 1992; 53: 856.

126 Boone ML, Swenson BE, Felson B. Rib notching: its many causes. *Am J Roentgenol* 1964; 91: 1075.

127 Ferris RA, Lopresti JM. Rib notching due to coarctation of the aorta: report of a case initially observed at less than one year of age. *Br J Radiol* 1974; 47: 357.

128 Bernstein C, Loeser WD, Manning LE. Erosive rib lesions in paralytic poliomyelitis. *Radiology* 1958; 70: 368.

129 Sargent EN, Turner AF, Jacobson G. Superior marginal rib defects. An etiologic classification. *Am J Roentgenol* 1969; 106: 491.

130 Keats TE. Superior marginal rib defects in restrictive lung disease. *Am J Roentgenol* 1975; 124: 449.

131 Rosenberg RF, Rubinstein BM, Messinger NH. Intrathoracic lipomas. *Chest* 1971; 60: 507.

132 Nickel WK, Kittle CF, Boley JO. Desmoid tumour of the chest. *Thorax* 1958; 13: 218.

133 Omell GH, Anderson LS, Bramson RT. Chest wall tumours. *Radiol Clin North Am* 1973; 11: 197.

134 Jones ER, Golebiowski A. Desmoid tumour of chest wall. *Br Med J* 1960; ii: 1134.

135 Barson AJ, Ahmed A, Gibson AAM, Macdonald AM. Chest wall sarcoma of childhood with good prognosis. *Arch Dis Child* 1978; 53: 882.

136 Marshall DG, Bains M. Massive leiomyosarcoma of the chest wall in a young child. *J Pediatr Surg* 1980; 15: 666.

137 Joffe N. Malignant synovioma of the chest wall. *Br J Radiol* 1959; 32: 619.

138 Jackson JW, Bennett MH. Chest wall tumour following iodised talc pleurodesis. *Thorax* 1969; 28: 788.

139 Winer-Muram HT, Kauffman WM, Gronermeyer SA, Jennings SG. Primitive neuroectodermal tumors of the chest wall (Askin tumors): CT and MR findings. *Am J Roentgenol* 1993; 161: 265.

140 Hochberg LA. Primary tumours of the rib. *Arch Surg* 1953; 67: 566.

141 Ochsner A, Lucas JL, McFarland GB. Tumours of the thoracic skeleton. Review of 134 cases. *J Thorac Cardiovasc Surg* 1966; 52: 311.

142 Teitelbaum SL. Twenty years experience with intrinsic tumours of the bony thorax at a large institution. *J Thorac Cardiovasc Surg* 1972; 63: 776.

143 Stelzer P, Gay WA. Tumors of the chest wall. *Surg Clin North Am* 1980; 60: 779.

144 Eygelaar A, Homan van der Heide JN. Diagnosis and treatment of primary malignant costal and sternal tumours. *Dis Chest* 1967; 52: 683.

145 Buker RH, Hughes FA, Mashburn JD. Polyostotic fibrous dysplasia (Albright's syndrome). *J Thorac Cardiovasc Surg* 1965; 49: 241.

146 Anon. Fibrous dysplasia of bone. *Br Med J* 1971; i: 685.

147 Nabarro MN, Giblin PE. Monostotic fibrous dysplasia of the thoracic spine. *Spine* 1994; 19: 463.

148 Hsu JT, Finby N. Rapidly developing mass in an asymptomatic man. *Chest* 1979; 75: 703.

149 Ron IG, Amir G, Inbar MJ, Chaitchik S. Clear cell chondrosarcoma of rib following repetitive low-impact trauma. *Am J Clin Oncol* 1995; 18: 87.

150 Richardson JV, Light RW, George RB. Thoracic mass and pleuritic chest pain. *Chest* 1979; 76: 93.

151 Maygarden SJ, Askin FB, Siegal GP *et al.* Ewing sarcoma of bone in infants and toddlers. A clinicopathologic report from the Intergroup Ewing's study. *Cancer* 1993; 71: 2109.

152 Wolfel DA, Dennis JM. Multiple myeloma of the chest wall. *Am J Roentgenol* 1963; 89: 1241.

153 Subbarao K, Jacobson HG. Systemic disorders affecting the thoracic cage. *Radiol Clin North Am* 1984; 22: 497.

154 Barrett NR. The chest wall. In: Penny KMA, Sellors TH, eds. *Chest Diseases*. London: Butterworth, 1963.

155 Sant GR. Primary sternal osteomyelitis. *J R Coll Surg Edinb* 1979; 24: 368.

156 Mittapalli MR. Primary osteomyelitis of the sternum. *Thorax* 1979; 34: 680.

157 Seviour PW, Dieppe PA. Sternoclavicular joint infection as a cause of chest pain. *Br Med J* 1984; 288: 133.

158 Goldin RH, Chow AW, Edwards JE *et al.* Sternoarticular septic arthritis in heroin cases. *N Engl Med* 1973; 289: 616.

159 Bonakdarpour A, Fazl Ali Zadeh Y, Maghssoudi H *et al.* Costal echinococcosis. *Am J Roentgenol* 1973; 118: 371.

160 Keers RY. *Pulmonary Tuberculosis. A Journey Down the Centuries*. London: Baillière Tindall, 1978.

161 Phillips MS, Kinnear WJM, Schneerson JM. Late sequelae of pulmonary tuberculosis treated by thoracoplasty. *Thorax* 1987; 42: 445.

162 Parsons PE. Respiratory failure as a result of drugs, overdoses, and poisonings. *Clin Chest Med* 1994; 15: 93.

163 Hudgson P. Alcoholic myopathy. *Br Med J* 1984; 288: 584.

164 Adelman HM, Winters PR, Mahan CS, Wallach PM. D-Penicillamine-induced myasthenia gravis: diagnosis obscured by coexisting chronic obstructive pulmonary disease. *Am J Med Sci* 1995; 309: 191.

165 Goswamy R, Chaudhuri A, Mahashur AA. Study of respiratory failure in organophosphate and carbamate poisoning. *Heart Lung* 1994; 23: 466.

166 Brussel T, Matthay MA, Chernow B. Pulmonary manifestations of endocrine and metabolic disorders. *Clin Chest Med* 1989; 10: 645.

167 Weiner M, Chausow A, Szidon P. Reversible respiratory muscle weakness in hypothyroidism. *Br J Dis Chest* 1986; 80: 391.

168 Stedwell RE, Allen KM, Binder LS. Hypokalemic paralyses: a review of the etiologies, pathophysiology, presentation and therapy. *Am J Emerg Med* 1992; 10: 143.

169 Gorson KC, Ropper AH. Acute respiratory failure neuropathy: a variant of critical illness polyneuropathy. *Crit Care Med* 1993; 21: 1986.

170 Sheth RD, Pryce-Phillips WE, Riggs JE, Bodensteiner JB. Critical illness neuromuscular disease in children manifested as ventilatory dependence. *J Pediatr* 1995; 126: 259.

171 Leijten FSS, Harinck-de Weerd Poortvliet DCJ, de Weerd AW. The role of polyneuropathy in motor convalescence after prolonged mechanical ventilation. *JAMA* 1995; 274: 1221.

172 Vallet B, Fourrier F, Hurtevent JF, Parent M, Chopin C. Myasthenia gravis and steroid-induced myopathy of the respiratory muscles. *Intensive Care Med* 1992; 18: 424.

173 Howard RS, Wiles CM, Hirsch NP, Spencer GT. Respiratory involvement in primary muscle disorders: assessment and management. *Q J Med* 1993; 86: 175.

174 Howard RS, Wiles CM, Loh L. Respiratory complications and their managment in motor neurone disease. *Brain* 1989; 112: 1155.

175 Howard RS, Wiles CM, Spencer GT. The late sequelae of poliomyelitis. *Q J Med* 1988; 251: 219.

176 Howard RS, Wiles CM, Hirsch NP, Loh L, Spencer GT, Newsom Davis J. Respiratory involvement in multiple sclerosis. *Brain* 1992; 108: 845.

177 Zulueta JJ, Fanburg BL. Respiratory dysfunction in myasthenia gravis. *Clin Chest Med* 1994; 15: 683.

178 Gracey DR, Southorn PA. Respiratory failure in Lambert–Eaton syndrome. *Chest* 1987; 91: 716.

179 Marino W. Intermittent volume cycled mechanical ventilation via nasal mask in patients with respiratory failure due to COPD. *Chest* 1991; 99: 681.

180 Brown LK. Respiratory dysfunction in Parkinson's disease. *Clin Chest Med* 1994; 15: 715.

181 Vincken WG, Gauthier SG, Dollfuss RE *et al.* Involvement of upper airway muscles in extrapyramidal disorders. A cause of airflow limitation. *N Engl Med* 1986; 311: 438.

182 Vingerhoets F, Bogousslavsky J. Respiratory dysfunction in stroke. *Clin Chest Med* 1994; 15: 729.

183 Moufarrej NA, Bertorini TE. Respiratory insufficiency in adult-type acid maltase deficiency. *South Med J* 1993; 86: 560.

184 Rochester DF, Esau SA. Assessment of ventilatory function in patients with neuromuscular disease. *Clin Chest Med* 1994; 15: 751.

185 Hotes LS, Johnson JA, Sicilian L. Long-term care, rehabilitation, and legal and ethical considerations in the management of neuromuscular disease with respiratory dysfunction. *Clin Chest Med* 1994; 15: 783.

186 Sawicka EH, Loh L, Branthwaite MA. Domiciliary ventilatory support: an analysis of outcome. *Thorax* 1986; 43: 31.

187 Gay PC, Edmonds LC. Severe hypercapnia after low-flow oxygen therapy in patients with neuromuscular disease and diaphragmatic dysfunction. *Mayo Clin Proc* 1995; 70: 327.

46

ABNORMALITIES AND DISEASES OF THE DIAPHRAGM

ANTHONY SEATON

The diaphragm is the most important muscle of respiration. It is rarely affected by intrinsic disease but because of its complex embryological development is subject to a number of congenital anomalies. Primary disorders of the diaphragm may present with symptoms suggestive of intrathoracic disease. Conversely, radiographic abnormalities of the diaphragm may indicate disease in the chest or abdomen.

Embryology

The arched musculotendinous division between the thorax and the abdomen has its origin in vertebral, costal and spinal attachments from which muscular fibres curve upwards and inwards from the periphery to be inserted into the fibrous sheet called the central tendon [1]. The diaphragm derives developmentally from four sources [2].

1 The *septum transversum* is first seen at the third week of development as a mass of mesoderm situated cranial to the pericardial cavity. This structure contributes to the more ventral portions, i.e. the sternal and costal parts.

2 The second source is derived from paired dorsolateral portions, the *pleuroperitoneal membranes*, which fuse with the dorsal mesentery of the oesophagus and the dorsal portion of the septum transversum to complete the partition between the thoracic and abdominal cavities and form the primitive diaphragm at about the seventh week of development.

3 The median portion of the diaphragm is derived from an irregular medial dorsal portion of primary oesophageal mesentery that fuses with the septum transversum and pleuroperitoneal membranes. The curves of the diaphragm develop from the growth of muscle fibres into the dorsal mesentery of the oesophagus.

4 During weeks 9–12 the fourth source is contributed by marginal ingrowths of the body wall. These contributions from the thoracic myotomes also contain nerve fibres of the lower six or seven intercostal nerves that distribute sensory fibres to the peripheral parts of the diaphragm.

During the development of the diaphragm, striking positional changes of its components are seen. At the third or fourth week the septum transversum lies opposite the upper cranial somites. During the fifth week nerve fibres from the third, fourth and fifth cervical segments of the spinal cord grow into the septum transversum via the pleuropericardial membranes and together constitute the phrenic nerves, which in adult life lie within the fibrous pericardium.

A more rapid growth of the dorsal embryo results in an apparent migration of the diaphragm, which by the sixth week is at the level of the thoracic somites. The phrenic nerves are also lengthened. By the beginning of the eighth week, the diaphragm is attached to the dorsal body wall at the level of the first lumbar vertebra, giving the diaphragm the domed contour characteristic of its adult form. In the adult a threefold variation in diaphragm muscle mass has been recorded, being related to an individual's overall muscularity [3].

Radiological appearances

The right hemidiaphragm is usually higher than the left, the average level of the right dome being at the anterior end of the sixth rib [4]. The left hemidiaphragm lies half an interspace lower than the right but appreciable unilateral elevation is not uncommon [5]. In one study a raised diaphragm was seen on the left in 9% and on the right in 2% of 500 normal chest films [6]. In half the individuals with a raised diaphragm on the left the two domes were at the same level, while in the other half the left was actually higher than the right.

The normally higher position of the right hemidiaphragm is usually and illogically attributed to the bulk of the underlying liver, but the truth is that the left hemidiaphragm is depressed by the heart. In partial situs inversus with liver and heart on the same side, the diaphragm is lower on that side [7]. Inversion of the diaphragm may occur on both the right and left sides, most commonly as the result of a massive pleural effusion or a tension pneumothorax. Difficult to demonstrate on a plain chest radiograph, it is readily detected by ultrasound examination [8].

Unequal excursion of the two hemidiaphragms is normal [5]. In one series the hemidiaphragms moved asynchronously in 77%, although the difference in excursion was usually less than 1 cm [9]. The excursion in this group of normal subjects ranged from 3 to 6 cm in 75%, with 23% showing excursion of less than 3 cm and 2% more than 6 cm. Unilateral paradox on sniffing has been seen in up to 6% of normal subjects and is more common on the right [10].

Function

In normal quiet breathing the diaphragm is responsible for 75% of inspiration and the intercostal muscles for 25%. Contraction of the diaphragm leads to its descent, with a resultant rise in intra-abdominal pressure and movement of the abdominal wall outwards [11,12]. A secondary effect of diaphragmatic contraction is to elevate and push the lower ribs outwards [13]. This secondary action is a function of the costal parts of the diaphragm, for when the costal parts only are stimulated the diameter of the lower rib cage increases [14,15]. During severe hyperinflation, as seen in chronic bronchitis and emphysema, contraction of the diaphragm produces paradoxical inward movement of the lower rib cage or Hoover's sign [15].

Diaphragmatic function may be assessed clinically by checking for appropriate thoracic and abdominal wall movements during inspiration and by performing tidal percussion, although one study found poor correlation between chest radiographic and clinical measures of diaphragmatic movement and wide interobserver variation [16]. Fluoroscopy allows diaphragmatic movement to be examined and is the conventional method of screening for diaphragmatic paralysis in patients with bronchogenic carcinoma. With paralysis of the diaphragm, the affected side descends poorly on inspiration and should move paradoxically upwards during a sniff. However, contraction of abdominal muscles may confound the findings, allowing apparently normal movement of a paralysed diaphragm [13].

Phrenic nerve stimulation, with recording of the diaphragmatic action potential using either oesophageal electrodes or surface electrodes over the lateral chest wall, allows the measurement of phrenic nerve conduction time. Unfortunately, the amplitude of the action potential is not an absolute index of diaphragmatic function. The most sensitive index of function is the measurement of transdiaphragmatic pressure (Pdi) during a quiet and a maximal inspiration. Pressures are recorded from balloons in the oesophagus and the stomach; in normal subjects Pdi increases by 5–8 cmH$_2$O in a quiet inspiration and by more than 25 cmH$_2$O during a maximal inspiration. In bilateral diaphragmatic paralysis no change in pressure occurs [13]. Even this index of diaphragmatic function has been criticized because of the wide range of normal values for maximum Pdi (18–137 cmH$_2$O) occasioned by interindividual variation in utilization of accessory muscles [17]. It has been suggested that measurement of Pdi during a maximum sniff is of more value in detecting diaphragmatic weakness or paralysis (normal value 112–204 cmH$_2$O) [18].

Disorders of function

Diaphragmatic fatigue

The diaphragm shares with the myocardium continuing regular activity of varying degree throughout life. Not surprisingly the muscle fibres comprising the diaphragm show a predominance of fibre types relatively resistant to fatigue; 50% are type I or slow-twitch fibres, with a high oxidative and low glycolytic capacity, and 20% type IIA or fast-twitch fibres, with both high oxidative and glycolytic capacities. The remaining 30% are type IIB or fast-twitch fibres, with low oxidative capacity and high glycolytic activity, and are relatively susceptible to fatigue [19–22].

At its customary resting length the human diaphragm only becomes fatigued when the force of contraction during inspiration exceeds 40% of the force that it can develop in a maximal static effort. During tidal breathing it operates at only about 10% of maximal [23]. The more the respiratory force exceeds 40%, the sooner the onset of fatigue [19]. Development of fatigue can be demonstrated by stimulating the phrenic nerve and constructing Pdi–phrenic nerve stimulation frequency curves [24,25]. Fatigue produced in normal humans, for example by breathing through an inspiratory resistance for as long as possible, results in a reduction of force developed at all frequencies with a preferential reduction at low frequencies [26]. This 'low-frequency fatigue' is believed to represent a failure of excitation–contraction coupling in the muscle [13]. It has been shown to occur in normal individuals as a consequence of exhausting exercise and the exertions of the later stages of labour [27,28].

An alternative technique for detecting diaphragmatic fatigue is to record the power spectrum of the diaphragmatic electromyogram (EMG) using oesophageal or surface electrodes [13,26]. A decrease in the ratio of high-frequency to low-frequency power in the EMG indicates fatigue. Using this technique, fatigue has been detected in the normal newborn diaphragm when rib cage distortion is present [29]. The technique has also been used to detect fatigue early in neonates being weaned from a ventilator before the onset of clinical signs or carbon dioxide retention [30]. The predisposition of the neonate to diaphragmatic fatigue is presumably a reflection of the relative absence of type I muscle fibres in the infant diaphragm; premature infants have only 10% type I fibres and the full-term newborn only 25%. The adult proportion of 50% type I fibres is only achieved at 8 months [31]. In adults with chronic obstructive pulmonary disease, the force reserve of the diaphragm has been shown to be greatly reduced so that slight modifications of the pattern of breathing can bring the diaphragm above the fatigue threshold [32].

Clinical features

Two physical signs of diaphragmatic dysfunction are recognized. Prominent rib cage movement in the supine position indicates recruitment of other respiratory muscles and is a feature of any disease or condition that leads to increase in the work of breathing. More importantly, indrawing of the anterior abdominal wall during inspiration (when not due to abdominal muscle contraction) is a significant indication of diaphragmatic fatigue or paralysis [33,34]. In patients being unsuccessfully weaned from ventilators, the sequence of events that culminates in respiratory acidosis has been described [20]. Initial EMG evidence of fatigue either precedes or accompanies an increase in respiratory rate. This is followed by alternation between abdominal and rib cage breathing (respiratory alternans) and then by a paradoxical inward motion of the abdomen during inspiration (abdominal paradox). Finally, minute ventilation and respiratory rate fall with a resultant increase in $Paco_2$.

Management

The immediate management of diaphragmatic fatigue, which is probably present in all cases of life-threatening respiratory failure, involves ventilatory support with positive-pressure ventilation to allow recovery of the fatigued muscle while the precipitating factor is treated. In the longer term, in subjects predisposed to fatigue by virtue of associated disease such as chronic obstructive airways disease, quadriplegia and cystic fibrosis, ventilatory muscle training, which involves breathing against an inspiratory resistance for 30 min daily, increases both the strength and endurance of the diaphragm as well as protecting against fatigue [35–39]. Pharmacological intervention also seems possible since both aminophylline [40] and caffeine [41] have been shown to increase the contractility of the diaphragm and to increase the pressure the diaphragm develops at a constant frequency of phrenic nerve stimulation after fatigue [40].

Finally, in selected subjects, particularly quadriplegics with ventilatory failure, implanted receivers with electrodes stimulating the phrenic nerves have been used successfully in treatment. This procedure, which is restricted to a few specialist centres, involves placing a radio receiver subcutaneously with electrodes leading to the phrenic nerve usually in the neck. An external battery-powered transmitter controls the receiver and can be used to modify respiratory rate and the depth of inspiration. Each phrenic nerve is paced alternately for 8 h in order to avoid diaphragmatic fatigue [42].

Diaphragmatic paralysis

Unilateral paralysis

Aetiology

The phrenic nerve is derived from the C3–C5 nerve roots and may be affected by compression, inflammation or injury anywhere in its course from cervical spine to diaphragm. The most common cause of unilateral diaphragmatic paralysis is involvement of the phrenic nerve by bronchogenic carcinoma. Such involvement by tumour above the pulmonary hilum excludes surgical treatment, although when the lesion is below the hilum resection of the tumour, nerve and pericardium may be attempted. The causes of unilateral diaphragmatic paralysis are shown in Table 46.1 [43].

Sometimes phrenic paralysis occurs without satisfactory explanation. In the days of mass miniature radiography, it was not uncommon to recall patients in whom the film had shown an elevated hemidiaphragm and who were shown to have paralysis on screening. Such patients often gave a history of a transient febrile illness, often associated with chest or shoulder pain; no other cause was found and led to the problem being attributed to a 'viral infection'. The recent evidence that idiopathic facial nerve palsy is often caused by herpes simplex virus 1 [44] suggests that this may not have been wide of the mark. Indeed, cervical herpes zoster is a known cause of diphragmatic paralysis [45]. This appears to be analogous to the so-called neuralgic amyotrophy that affects the deltoid muscle and is attributed to inflammation of the C5–C7 nerve roots; diaphragmatic paralysis, both unilateral and bilateral, has been found in this condition [46].

The 'paralysis' seen in association with supraphrenic or subphrenic infection may be more apparent than real. In such subjects the diaphragm is often elevated and immobile but recovery occurs as the infection clears. The same is true of the elevation of the diaphragm associated with pulmonary embolism.

Clinical features

Paralysis of a hemidiaphragm alone does not usually give rise to symptoms, and where symptoms are present they usually reflect the causative disease. Altered diaphragmatic movement may be detected by careful

Table 46.1 Causes of unilateral diaphragmatic paralysis.

Surgical
Thoracic and cervical operations
Cardiac cooling during open heart surgery [47]

Tumour
Bronchogenic
Metastatic

Neurological
Cervical myelitis, neuropathy
Encephalitis
Herpes zoster [46]
Poliomyelitis
Tetanus antitoxin [48]
Diphtheria

Trauma
Thoracic cage
Cervical spine
Brachial plexus block
Birth injury
Subclavian vein puncture [49]

Mechanical
Retrosternal goitre
Aortic aneurysm
Progressive massive fibrosis (silicosis, coalworkers' pneumoconiosis)

Infection
Tuberculosis [50]
Pneumonia
? Empyema
? Subphrenic or hepatic abscess

Miscellaneous
Syphilis
Pulmonary infarction
Congenital anomalies of lung and thorax
Pott's disease

Idiopathic

percussion, although this sign requires practice to elicit and is assocated with substantial interobserver variation [16].

Radiology

The affected diaphragm may or may not be elevated and shows paradoxical movement on respiration. This is confirmed by fluoroscopy and may be accentuated by asking the patient to sniff, when the affected hemidiaphragm rises while the unaffected hemidiaphragm moves downwards. As discussed above, the diagnosis may not always be clear-cut even on screening, and ultrasonography has proved a useful means of confirming the radiological suspicions [51].

Functional effects

Unilateral paralysis of the diaphragm reduces vital capacity by 20–25% in the upright posture, with a further 10–20% reduction in the supine position [52–54]. Pao_2 may fall in the supine position due to an increase in closing volume, and compression of basal lung segments on the affected side has been demonstrated bronchographically [52,53]. A 20% reduction in ventilation and perfusion to the lung on the affected side has also been shown [52,55].

Management

In the large majority of cases, no treatment is necessary as the condition is symptomless. Occasionally, however, the development of unilateral paralysis in someone with severe pulmonary impairment precipitates ventilatory failure. This has been described particularly after lung or cardiac surgery [56–58]. In such circumstances recovery may take place with time, such as when the paralysis occurred as a consequence of phrenic stretching or hypothermia, and ventilatory support may be all that is necessary. If recovery does not occur, diaphragmatic plication has proved to be an effective method of improving lung mechanics and the patient's condition [59,60].

Bilateral paralysis

Aetiology

Paralysis or weakness of both hemidiaphragms is uncommon and may be idiopathic in origin [61], follow viral infections [62] or blunt trauma to the chest [63], or occur in association with rare neuromuscular diseases as well as the more common quadriplegia following trauma [46,64–70] (Table 46.2). A similar condition may occur in systemic lupus erythematosus [71].

Table 46.2 Causes of bilateral diaphragmatic paralysis.

Anterior horn cell disease
Poliomyelitis
Kugelberg–Welander disease
Motoneurone disease
Multiple sclerosis

Peripheral nerve disease
Guillain–Barré syndrome
Charcot–Marie–Tooth disease
Idiopathic

Muscle disease
Acid maltase deficiency
Limb girdle dystrophy
Type II atrophy
Dystrophia myotonica
Neuralgic amyotrophy

Clinical features

Dyspnoea is a usual feature of bilateral diaphragmatic paralysis as is paradoxical inward movement of the abdominal wall during inspiration, both particularly marked when the subject is in the supine position [13]. Respiratory rate is usually increased with a reduction in tidal volume. Alveolar hypoventilation may occur during sleep [63,72] with resultant carbon dioxide retention leading to disturbed sleep, morning headaches and daytime fatigue with hypersomnolence [66]. There may be associated sleep apnoea [61].

Radiology

Both diaphragms may be elevated on the chest film, move sluggishly or paradoxically with inspiration, and para-doxical movement should be (but is not always) seen during sniffing [65]. That fluoroscopy can be misleading is due to contraction of abdominal muscles during expira-tion, which pushes the diaphragm up passively and allows it to descend passively and apparently normally during inspiration [13].

Functional changes

In complete bilateral diaphragmatic paralysis, Pdi does not change during tidal breathing or a maximum inspira-tion, while reduced changes in pressure are seen in patients with bilateral weakness [13,67,68,72]. Vital capacity is reduced in the upright position and further decreased in the supine position [63,73]. Similarly, Pao_2 is reduced and falls further on lying down. Studies have shown that the ventilation–perfusion ratio is the same in both lungs in a normal subject occupying the lateral decu-bitus position, whereas it is substantially reduced in the dependent lung of patients with bilateral diaphragmatic paralysis, a phenomenon that must contribute to the postural hypoxia via shunting of blood [74]. Measurement of pressure–volume relationships in diaphragmatic paralysis has disclosed decreases in both maximal transpulmonary pressure and static compliance [75]. The reduced compliance, tentatively ascribed to microatelecta-sis, may explain the rapid respiratory rate in these patients.

Management

Although spontaneous improvement in diaphragm func-tion has been seen [68], permanent paralysis is the rule. Some patients have benefited from the use of a cuirass respirator at night to manage the associated respiratory failure [65], and it would seem reasonable to apply the principles of management, including the use of nasal con-tinuous positive airway pressure, described in Chapter 58.

The use of diaphragmatic pacing has already been men-tioned [42].

Involuntary movements of the diaphragm

Hiccup

Sudden inspiratory spasm of the diaphragm with associ-ated closure of the glottis (hiccup, or singultus for the obscurantist) is a familiar and harmless symptom in the normal subject, usually caused by gastric distension. EMG recordings have demonstrated synchronous electrical discharge in both the diaphragm and external (inspira-tory) intercostal muscles [76]. The usual cause is a reflex transmitted by vagal efferents, via vagal and respiratory nuclei in the medulla, and phrenic nerves to the diaphragm and by somatic nerves to other respiratory muscles. Occasionally the symptom becomes persistent and distressing to the patient, especially in uraemia and neurological disease [77]. The best-recognized causes of persistent hiccup are shown in Table 46.3 and reflect the reflex pathway. It has been suggested that some appar-ently idiopathic cases may be a vagal analogue of trigemi-nal neuralgia and hemifacial spasm, where the neural hyperactivity may be triggered by contact between nerve and blood vessel [78].

Treatment

Treatment depends on the cause and severity. Everyone is familiar with the various empirical homely remedies rec-ommended for transient hiccup that act via vagal stimula-

Table 46.3 Causes of hiccup.

Local causes, stimulating vagal afferents
Gastric distension or inflammation
Oesophageal reflux, achalasia
Pericarditis
Pleural effusion
Mediastinial disease
Chest and upper abdominal surgery
Diaphragmatic irritation
Subphrenic abscess
Metabolic causes
Anaesthesia
Uraemia
Addison's disease
Hypocalcaemia
Central causes, affecting brainstem
Medullary infarction, tumour
Multiple sclerosis
Viral encephalitis, including HIV
Meningitis

HIV, human immunodeficiency virus.

tion. More persistent episodes may respond to stimulation of the pharynx with a catheter introduced through the nose [79]. This intervention is believed to initiate afferent vagal impulses that inhibit the hiccup reflex. Prolonged or distressing hiccup requires investigation and removal of the cause. If this is not possible, it may respond to intravenous injection of 50 mg chlorpromazine [80]. Other drugs used have included haloperidol, metoclopramide, baclofen, antiepileptics and antidepressants [77,81]. In exceptional cases, phrenic nerve block by local anaesthetic or phrenic nerve crush has been used but is not recommended since it impairs lung function and is usually only partially successful. In one rather dramatic instance, neurosurgical separation of the vagus from contact with the posterior inferior cerebellar artery appears to have relieved the condition [78].

Tonic spasm of the diaphragm

Tonic spasm may complicate rabies, tetanus and strychnine poisoning and less commonly pregnancy toxaemia, encephalitis and epilepsy. It results in upper abdominal pain and dyspnoea, and may necessitate assisted ventilation.

Diaphragmatic tic or flutter

Diaphragmatic tic or respiratory myoclonus was first diagnosed and described by van Leeuwenhoek, the inventor of the microscope, who himself suffered from the condition [82]. It can occur at any age and in most cases the aetiology is unknown, although encephalitis and assorted causes of phrenic nerve irritation have been implicated in some [83]. The diaphragm or one hemidiaphragm contracts irregularly, with an average frequency of 150/min (range 35–480); the EMG shows bursts of electrical activity during inspiration and expiration [84,85].

Clinical features

Episodes may be precipitated by emotion, eating, exercise or assorted respiratory manoeuvres, and may last only a few seconds or persist for months. Attacks are usually associated with upper abdominal or lower chest pain that may mimic angina. Respiratory distress may occur and stridor and apneustic respiration (a prolonged breath-hold in inspiration) have been reported [86,87]. Other symptoms include belching, hiccups and retching. In some subjects epigastric pulsations may be seen, and if the stomach is full a rhythmic splashing sound may be heard [88]. Fluoroscopy demonstrates the abnormal movement of the diaphragm, which may also distort an ECG tracing [85]. The diagnosis may be confirmed if necessary by diaphragmatic EMG [89].

Treatment

Treatment with phenytoin 400 mg daily or carbamazepine has been successful in some cases [85,89], but others have required phrenic paralysis by crush or injection of local anaesthetic [86,88].

Infection

Subphrenic abscess

Clinical features

Subphrenic abscess may occur spontaneously due to perforation of a viscus, amoebic liver abscess or pancreatitis, or may follow abdominal surgery [90–94]. Such abscesses may occur on either or both sides. Features include local costal or subcostal pain and tenderness, unexplained fever, tachycardia and leucocytosis. If antibiotics have been taken, the course may be more chronic with vague pains, chronic ill-health, unexplained fever and anaemia [95]. Its importance for the chest physician lies in the associated changes that may be seen on a chest film or on fluoroscopy.

Radiology

The most common finding is an elevated hemidiaphragm on the affected side with diminished movement of the diaphragm, although it should be noted that a reduction in diaphragmatic activity is a normal finding after upper abdominal surgery [96]. Other frequent findings include blunting of the costophrenic angle, pleural effusion and pulmonary infiltrates or atelectasis. Air–fluid levels may be seen in the abscess cavity. Fixation of the diaphragm and displacement of intra-abdominal viscera may be seen. Radiologically, it may be difficult to differentiate between a subphrenic abscess and a subpulmonary collection of fluid. Multiplanar ultrasonography, especially on the right side, and CT are useful means of making the diagnosis [94,97–99]. Outlining of a hemidiaphragm by contrast medium during pulmonary angiography has been reported in subdiaphragmatic inflammation [100], although it is not recommended that such an investigation be routinely employed! Scanning techniques using gallium–technetium subtraction or following injection of gallium-labelled leucocytes have also proved useful in the localization of subphrenic abscesses [101,102].

Treatment

The management of subphrenic abscess is by surgical drainage and appropriate antibiotic therapy [103]. Percutaneous drainage under ultrasonic or fluoroscopic guidance using wide-bore catheters has been used with some success by those with special expertise [104].

Trichiniasis

One of the few primary diseases of the diaphragm is trichiniasis. When ingested in undercooked pork, or much less commonly bear meat, the larvae of the nematode *Trichinella spiralis* may be freed in the intestines where mating of male and female produces new larvae that can penetrate the intestinal wall and enter the bloodstream. Their subsequent fate is variable: some settle in organs where they die out; others reside in the muscles, including the diaphragm, where they may remain alive for years, subsequently becoming encysted.

Clinical features

The phases of intestinal invasion and encystment are usually symptomless but may be accompanied by diarrhoea and vomiting. The main symptoms usually occur 1 or 2 weeks after ingestion. These include fever, oedema that may affect the face only or be more widespread, muscle aches, skin rashes, chest pain (usually attributed to involvement of the intercostal muscles and diaphragm), hiccup, cough and haemoptysis (due probably to parasites in the lung). Respiratory failure secondary to weakness of the diaphragm and intercostal muscles has been described [105,106].

Investigations

Eosinophilia is a fairly constant and early feature and the parasite may be recovered from the blood in the early stages. Other diagnostic procedures in a suspected case are muscle biopsy (after the third week) and skin and precipitin tests with *Trichinella* antigen. In long-standing cases the calcified larvae are visible in muscles on the chest radiograph.

Treatment

The condition is usually self-limiting and no treatment is required. In severe cases treatment with corticosteroids and tiabendazole (thiabendazole) 25 mg/kg daily may be required. Prevention is the most important aspect of management of trichiniasis and the disease can be eradicated by making it known that the longer pork is cooked, the safer it is.

Tumours

Primary tumours of the diaphragm are exceedingly rare, and secondary tumours usually only occur as a direct extension from lung, liver or pleura.

Metastatic tumours

Metastatic tumours of the diaphragm are more common than primary tumours. Few are blood-borne, the majority occurring by seeding across serous membranes, infiltration from lung through pleura or direct spread, for example from the stomach [107]. The most common extrapleural primary sources are breast, ovary and stomach, while local involvement by bronchogenic carcinoma and mesothelioma is also seen. Mesothelioma is a tumour that is increasing in frequency in the UK, and it commonly involves the diaphragmatic pleura (see Chapter 43).

Benign tumours

Benign primary tumours occur more frequently than malignant ones [108]. The most common is the lipoma, which presents radiologically as a smooth rounded mass with a lower border continuous with the diaphragm [109]. The mass, which may appear less dense than would be expected on the basis of its size, usually arises from the posterolateral portion of the hemidiaphragm, more commonly on the left.

Other benign tumours include fibroma, angiofibroma, neurofibroma, neurilemmomas and haemangiopericytomas [110–113]. Angiofibromas may be calcified [111]. Mesothelial cysts may arise in relation to the pleuroperitoneal canal [112].

Malignant tumours

Most malignant tumours are of mesenchymal origin and the range of histological types is shown in Table 46.4 [111–113]; fibrosarcoma is the most common.

Clinical presentation

Malignant diaphragmatic tumours may present with severe lower chest or hypochondrial pain that radiates

Table 46.4 Some malignant tumours of the diaphragm.

Fibrosarcoma
Fibromyosarcoma
Myosarcoma
Fibroangioendothelioma
Undifferentiated sarcoma
Neurofibrosarcoma
Rhabdomyosarcoma
Sarcoma
Mixed-cell sarcoma
Haemangioendothelioma
Haemangiopericytoma
Leiomyosarcoma
Malignant synovioma

along intercostal nerves or to the shoulder [112,113]. The pain is usually exacerbated by respiration and may be associated with cough, dyspnoea or upper gastrointestinal symptoms. A haemorrhagic pleural effusion may be present. A bulging of the hypochondrium that moves with respiration may occur. A palpable mass is found in 10%. Hypertrophic pulmonary osteoarthropathy has been described in 10% of cases [112]. The tumour may metastasize or invade lung locally.

Diagnosis

On radiography a mass is seen in the lower thorax that is difficult to separate from surrounding structures. On fluoroscopy the mass is seen to move with the diaphragm. Pneumoperitoneum and pneumothorax may be needed to confirm that the mass arises from the diaphragm. CT may be helpful in diagnosis and in particular may identify lipomas by their decreased radiodensity.

Management

If possible, surgical excision is indicated, with local repair using fascia lata or prosthetic material [114].

Disorders of structure

Eventration of the diaphragm

Eventration of the diaphragm is a condition in which all or part of the diaphragm is largely composed of fibrous tissue with only a few or no interspersed muscle fibres [115,116]. It is usually congenital but may be acquired.

Complete eventration

Complete eventration almost invariably occurs on the left side and is characterized by elevation of the left hemidiaphragm (Fig. 46.1), which on screening is virtually immobile and which moves paradoxically on sniffing. The condition is usually asymptomatic in adults but occasionally upper gastrointestinal symptoms such as undue flatulence may occur and operation, with plication of the diaphragm, has occasionally been undertaken because of the severity of dyspeptic symptoms [117]. In many patients barium examination shows the stomach to be inverted beneath the hemidiaphragm.

In infants, diaphragmatic eventration may occur on either side and may give rise to severe respiratory symptoms such as cough, dyspnoea and wheeze. Recurrent bronchopneumonia with associated dyspnoea and cyanosis may be seen. Anorexia and vomiting are less common. On examination there may be bulging of the affected hemithorax and a scaphoid abdomen. Fluoroscopy may show a 'dicrotic-like' pattern of diaphragmatic movement, with the lax portion of diaphragm

Fig. 46.1 Posteroanterior (a) and lateral (b) chest films showing complete eventration of the left hemidiaphragm.

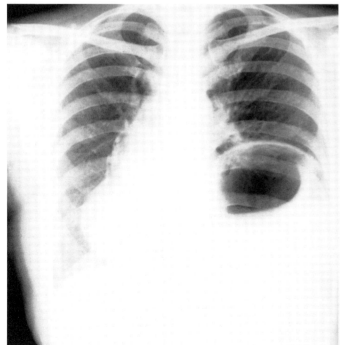

(a)

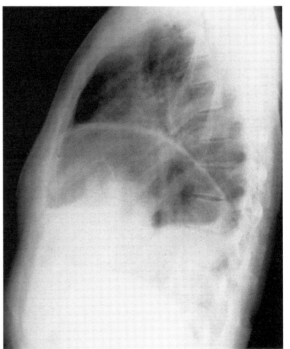

(b)

moving initially in a paradoxical manner followed by normal contraction of the periphery. Treatment by diaphragmatic plication usually gives excellent clinical and radiographic results [118,119]. However, a proportion of these patients have other congenital anomalies, including neurological and bowel disorders, that may influence their clinical outcome [120].

Partial eventration

Partial eventration of the diaphragm occurs virtually exclusively on the right side. It is detected as an antero-medial bulge of the diaphragm that moves paradoxically on respiration [121] (Fig. 46.2). There is usually a corresponding deformity of the liver or 'superior accessory lobe' that can be demonstrated by pneumoperitoneum, liver scan or ultrasound examination [122,123]. Ultrasound is particularly useful in differentiating eventration from diaphragmatic hernias and pleuropericardial cysts, both of which it may closely resemble. Liver inversion with a suprahepatic gallbladder has been reported in association with partial eventration [124].

Duplication of the diaphragm

An accessory diaphragm is a rare abnormality usually found in the oblique fissure on the right where it separates

Fig. 46.2 Posteroanterior (a) and lateral (b) chest films showing partial eventration of the right hemidiaphragm anteriorly.

all or part of the lower lobe from the rest of the lung [125–127]. It may be fibrous or muscular and contains a defect through which the normal bronchovascular supply passes to the lower lobe. Radiologically, thickening of the oblique fissure with elevation of the right hemidiaphragm may be apparent. It may be associated with neonatal respiratory distress; where the accessory diaphragm is muscular, bronchiectasis of the right lower lobe may result.

Diaphragmatic hernias

The common sites for herniation of viscera through the diaphragm are shown in Fig. 46.3.

Hiatus hernia

Herniation through the oesophageal hiatus is the most common type of diaphragmatic hernia. It is not considered in detail here but is mentioned because it may present on a chest film as a retrocardiac opacity containing a fluid level (Fig. 46.4). The uninitiated may mistakenly diagnose a lung abscess or cyst.

Bochdalek hernia

Bochdalek [128] first described the embryology and the congenital absence of the posterolateral part of the diaphragm in 1848. This is the most common site for congenital diaphragmatic hernia and an incidence of 0.8 per 1000 live births has been reported [129]. The foramen of

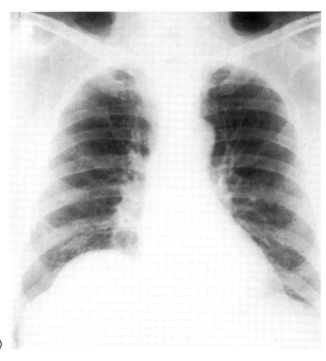

(a)

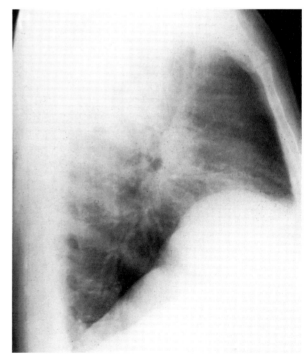

(b)

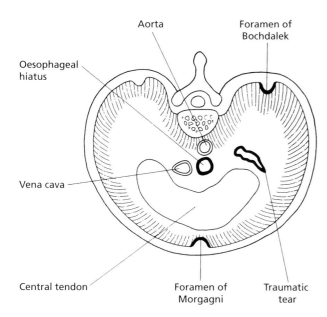

Fig. 46.3 Diaphragm viewed from above showing sites of possible herniation. Thick lines show most common sites.

Bochdalek is normally closed by the eighth week of fetal life. Failure of the pleuroperitoneal membrane to fuse with the septum transversum allows herniation of the abdominal contents into the hemithorax; 75% occur on the left and there may be other associated malformations, most commonly of the central nervous system [130]. A 13th pair of ribs is a reported association [131]. The lung on the side of hernia is usually hypoplastic with a reduction in the number of airway generations, although normal numbers of alveoli are found in the segments that are present [132,133]. The contralateral lung may also be hypoplastic and this heralds a poor prognosis [133,134]. In an extreme form, Bochdalek hernia merges with congenital diaphragmatic agenesis, a condition more readily diagnosed by antenatal ultrasound but which causes even more severe postnatal respiratory problems [135].

Clinical presentation

The majority present soon after birth with respiratory distress. A scaphoid abdomen is usually noted. Radiographically the diaphragm is not seen on the affected side and loops of intestine are found in the thorax, with displacement of the mediastinum. There is a relative absence of gas in the abdomen. Herniation on the right is less likely to be life-threatening, perhaps because the liver blocks the defect. While a right-sided hernia may occasionally present with respiratory distress, asymptomatic presentation with an intrathoracic mass of liver or bowel is more common [136,137].

Presentation in adulthood is uncommon. In a review of 50 cases in 1971, one-quarter were asymptomatic while the remainder presented with abdominal pain or vague remitting gastrointestinal symptoms with or without obstruction [138]. Delayed presentation following a previously normal chest film may occur [139].

Management and prognosis

Management of patients in respiratory distress is with ventilatory support and correction of acidosis, followed immediately by surgical repair, either by direct suture or with insertion of synthetic patches [140]. Contralateral pneumothorax may occur postoperatively due to the high inflation pressures required, and prophylactic pleural intubation has been employed by some [130,141].

Overall survival rates of 70–80% have been reported in neonates, with lower rates in those requiring operation within the first 24 h of life [142,143]. The majority of deaths are due to the presence of severely hypoplastic lungs that are incapable of sustaining life. In those with unilateral hypoplasia, compensatory emphysema may develop in the other lung [132].

Morgagni hernia

The foramen of Morgagni lies anteromedially and is bounded anteriorly by the sternum, medially by the sternal portion of the diaphragm and laterally by the costal portion of the diaphragm in the region of the attachment to the seventh costal cartilage. It is usually filled with loose connective tissue but omentum, colon, liver or other infradiaphragmatic structures, including gallbladder, may herniate through the foramen, more commonly on the right [144].

Clinical presentation

Presentation in childhood is rare, although Morgagni hernia has been reported as a cause of intermittent cyanotic attacks in an infant [145]. Where symptoms are present, feelings of pressure, tightness, fullness or pain in the right anterior chest occasionally with referral to the shoulder tip are admitted [146]. Strangulation of the bowel may occur.

The chest film shows a rounded density in the cardiophrenic angle that may or may not contain gas (Fig. 46.5). Barium studies determine the presence of intestine, and in the case of an omental hernia the transverse colon is hitched up. Pneumoperitoneum may be needed to make a definitive diagnosis.

Management

Surgical repair by suture after reduction of the hernia is normally sufficient.

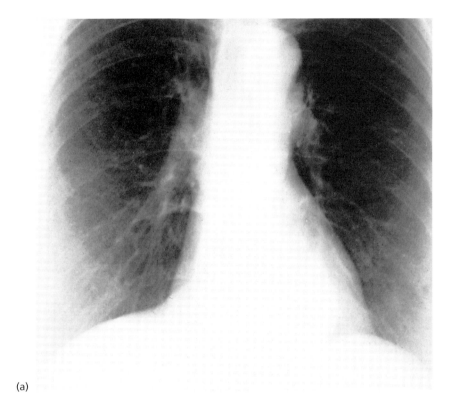

(a)

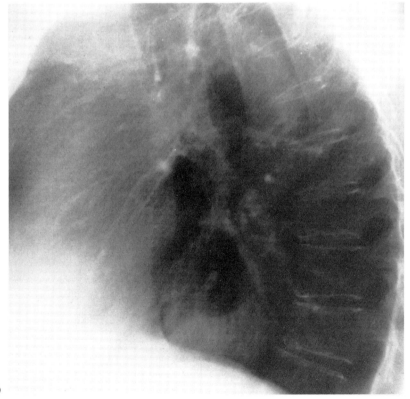

(b)

Fig. 46.4 (a) Solid lesion with indistinct air–fluid level behind heart. (b) Lateral view shows it to be a hiatus hernia.

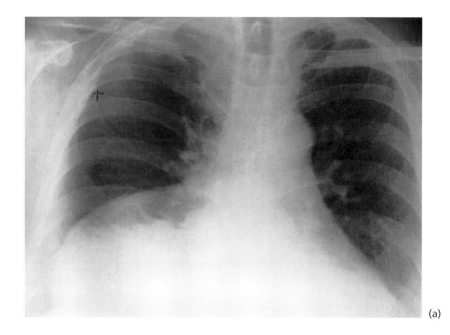

(a)

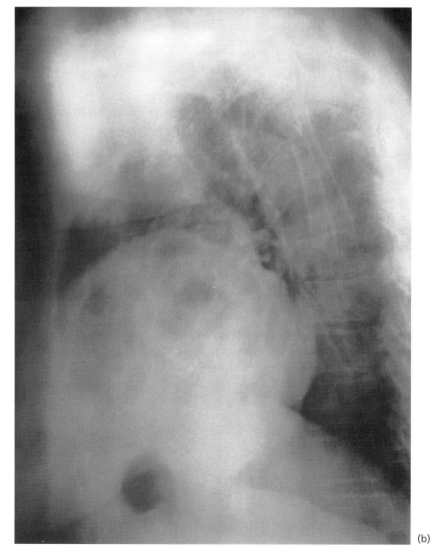

(b)

Fig. 46.5 Posteroanterior (a) and lateral (b) chest films showing Morgagni hernia. This 68-year-old patient presented with increasing dyspnoea.

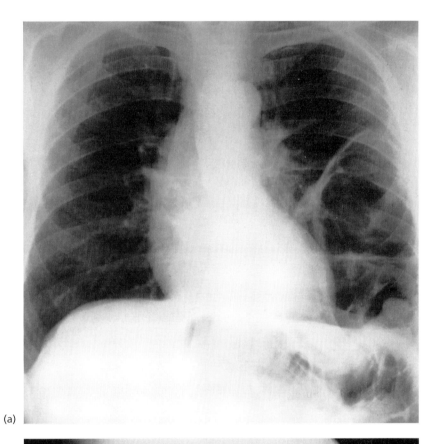

(a)

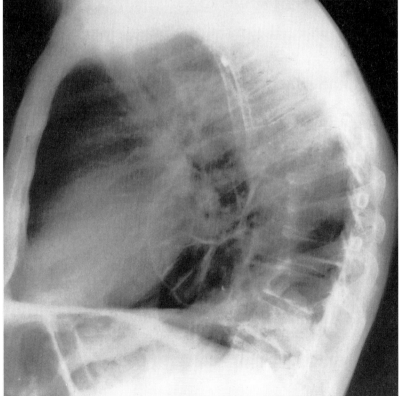

(b)

Fig. 46.6 Traumatic hernia. Posteroanterior (a) and lateral (b) chest films taken in 1987 of a 67-year-old man who suffered a shrapnel wound in Normandy in 1942 that necessitated splenectomy. No diaphragmatic lesion was noted at that time and it was not until 1958 that colon was seen in the chest on a routine chest film. No action was taken and the patient remains asymptomatic. Presumably the diaphragm was lacerated or ruptured by shrapnel in 1942.

Traumatic hernia

Traumatic diaphragmatic hernias are most commonly seen following blunt non-penetrating trauma to the chest in road traffic accidents or falls from a height. Many are detected at the time of the initial injury although a substantial number present later, even up to 15 years after the initial injury [147] (Fig. 46.6). It has been estimated that 90% of traumatic diaphragmatic hernias are overlooked at the time of injury [148].

Traumatic hernias represent only 5% of all diaphragmatic hernias, but 90% of all strangulated hernias result from trauma [149]; 90% of tears occur in the left leaf of the diaphragm, most commonly in the central and posterior portion. The most common hernial contents are omentum, stomach or colon, although any abdominal organ including kidney may be found. Rarely, herniation into the pericardium occurs [150–152].

Clinical presentation

The most common complaints are of upper abdominal or lower chest pain with dyspnoea, which may be worse after eating [147,148]. Bowel sounds may be audible in the chest. If strangulation occurs, sudden and progressive severe lower chest or upper abdominal pain is experienced, with dyspnoea, vomiting or retching. Upper abdominal guarding is found and progression to shock occurs [153,154]. On one occasion, the author has seen perforation of colon into the pleura following traumatic rupture of the diaphragm, causing pyopneumothorax. A rare complication of traumatic rupture is bronchopancreatic fistula following acute pancreatitis; this can be diagnosed by finding high levels of amylase in the profuse frothy sputum [155].

Radiology

Radiologically, the only evidence may be an elevated hemidiaphragm; at the other extreme multiple air–fluid levels may be present. Barium studies demonstrate obstruction or constriction of the stomach or colon as it passes through the tear [149]. With herniation of the liver on the right side, pneumoperitoneum (which results in pneumothorax) may be needed to confirm the diagnosis. CT may enable the discontinuity in the diaphragm to be seen [156].

Management

Surgical repair may be achieved by the abdominal, thoracic or combined routes [148]. In view of the common concurrence of injury to abdominal viscera, the abdominal route is usually preferred [157].

References

1 Leak LV. Gross and ultrastructural morphologic features of the diaphragm. *Am Rev Respir Dis* 1979; 119 (Suppl 2): 3.
2 Wells LJ. Observations on the development of the diaphragm in the human embryo. *Anat Rec* 1948; 100: 778.
3 Arora NS, Rochester DF. Effect of body weight and muscularity on human diaphragm muscle mass, thickness and area. *J Appl Physiol* 1982; 52: 64.
4 Lennon EA, Simon G. The height of the diaphragm in the chest radiograph of normal adults. *Br J Radiol* 1965; 38: 937.
5 Young DA, Simon G. Certain movements measured on inspiration–expiration chest radiographs correlated with pulmonary function studies. *Clin Radiol* 1972; 23: 37.
6 Felson B. *Chest Roentgenology*. Philadelphia: WB Saunders, 1973.
7 Wittenborg MH, Aviad I. Organ influences on the normal posture of the diaphragm: a radiological study of inversions and heterotaxies. *Br J Radiol* 1963; 36: 280.
8 Lowe SH, Cosgrove DO, Joseph AEA. Inversion of the right hemidiaphragm shown on ultrasound examination. *Br J Radiol* 1981; 54: 754.
9 Simon G, Bonnell J, Kazantzis G, Waller RE. Some radiological observations on the range of movement of the diaphragm. *Clin Radiol* 1969; 20: 231.
10 Alexander C. Diaphragm movements and the diagnosis of diaphragmatic paralysis. *Clin Radiol* 1966; 17: 79.

11 Macklem PT. Normal and abnormal function of the diaphragm. *Thorax* 1981; 36: 161.
12 Luce JM, Culver BH. Respiratory muscle function in health and disease. *Chest* 1982; 81: 82.
13 Loh L, Goldman M, Newson Davis J. The assessment of diaphragm function. *Medicine* 1977; 56: 165.
14 De Troyer A, Sampson M, Sigrist S, Macklem PT. The diaphragm: two muscles. *Science* 1981; 213: 237.
15 Roussos C, Macklem PT. The respiratory muscles. *N Engl J Med* 1982; 307: 786.
16 Williams TJ, Ahmad D, Morgan WKC. A clinical and roentgenographic correlation of diaphragm movement. *Arch Intern Med* 1981; 141: 878.
17 De Troyer A, Estenne M. Limitations of transdiaphragmatic pressure in detecting diaphragm weakness. *Thorax* 1981; 36: 169.
18 Macklem PT. Respiratory muscles: the vital pump. *Chest* 1980; 78: 753.
19 Rochester DF. Is diaphragmatic contractility important? *N Engl J Med* 1981; 305: 278.
20 Cohen CA, Zagelbaum G, Gross D *et al.* Clinical manifestations of inspiratory muscle fatigue. *Am J Med* 1982; 73: 308.
21 Grassino A, Macklem PT. Respiratory muscle fatigue and ventilatory failure. *Annu Rev Med* 1984; 35: 625.
22 Rochester DF. Respiratory muscles and ventilatory failure: 1993 perspective. *Am J Med Sci* 1993; 306: 394.
23 Seick GC. Physiological effects of

diaphragm muscle denervation and disuse. *Clin Chest Med* 1994; 15: 641.
24 Aubier M, Farkas G, De Troyer A *et al.* Detection of diaphragmatic fatigue in man by phrenic stimulation. *J Appl Physiol* 1981; 50: 538.
25 Moxham J, Morris AJR, Spiro SG *et al.* Contractile properties and fatigue of the diaphragm in man. *Thorax* 1981; 36: 164.
26 Gross D, Grassino A, Macklem PT. The EMG pattern of diaphragm fatigue. *Clin Res* 1976; 24: 690A.
27 Mador MJ, Madalang UJ, Rodis A, Kufel TJ. Diaphragmatic fatigue in healthy human subjects. *Am Rev Respir Dis* 1993; 148: 1571.
28 Nava S, Zanotti E, Ambrosino N, Fracchia C, Scarabelli C, Rampulla C. Evidence of acute diaphragmatic fatigue in a 'natural' condition. The diaphragm during labour. *Am Rev Respir Dis* 1992; 146: 1226.
29 Bryan AC. Diaphragmatic fatigue in newborns. *Am Rev Respir Dis* 1979; 119 (Suppl 2): 143.
30 Muller N, Volgyesi G, Eng P *et al.* The consequences of diaphragmatic muscle fatigue in the newborn infant. *J Pediatr* 1979; 95: 793.
31 Keens TG, Ianuzzo CD. Development of fatigue resistant muscle fibers in human ventilatory muscles. *Am Rev Respir Dis* 1979; 119 (Suppl 2): 139.
32 Bellemare F, Grassino A. Force reserve of the diaphragm in patients with chronic obstructive pulmonary disease. *J Appl Physiol* 1983; 55: 8.

33 Ashutosh K, Gilbert R, Auchincloss JH, Peppi D. Asynchronous breathing movements in patients with obstructive pulmonary disease. *Chest* 1975; 67: 553.

34 Pontoppidan H, Geffin B, Lowenstein E. Acute respiratory failure in the adult. *N Engl J Med* 1972; 287: 743.

35 Belman MJ, Mittman C. Ventilatory muscle training improves exercise capacity in chronic obstructive pulmonary disease patients. *Am Rev Respir Dis* 1980; 121: 273.

36 Gross D, Ladd HW, Riley EJ *et al.* The effect of training on strength and endurance of the diaphragm in quadriplegia. *Am J Med* 1980; 68: 27.

37 Keens TG, Krastins IRB, Wannamaker EM *et al.* Ventilatory muscle training in normal subjects and in patients with cystic fibrosis. *Am Rev Respir Dis* 1977; 116: 853.

38 Bradley ME, Leith DE. Ventilatory muscle training and the oxygen cost of sustained hyperpnea. *J Appl Physiol* 1978; 45: 885.

39 Belman MJ, Sieck GC. The ventilatory muscles. Fatigue, endurance and training. *Chest* 1982; 82: 761.

40 Aubier M, de Troyer A, Sampson M *et al.* Aminophylline improves diaphragmatic contractility. *N Engl J Med* 1981; 305: 249.

41 Supinski GS, Deal EC, Kelsen SG. The effect of caffeine and theophylline on diaphragm contractility. *Am Rev Respir Dis* 1984; 130: 429.

42 Lozewicz S, Potter DR, Costello JF *et al.* Diaphragm pacing in ventilatory failure. *Br Med J* 1981; 283: 1015.

43 Riley EA. Idiopathic diaphragmatic paralysis. *Am J Med* 1968; 32: 404.

44 Murakami S, Mizobuchi M, Nakashiso Y, Doi T, Hato N, Yanagihara N. Bell's palsy and herpes simplex virus: identification of viral DNA in endoneurial fluid and muscle. *Ann Intern Med* 1996; 124: 27.

45 Dutt AK. Diaphragmatic paralysis caused by herpes zoster. *Am Rev Respir Dis* 1970; 101: 755.

46 Mulvey DA, Aquilina RJ, Elliot MW, Moxham J, Green M. Diaphragmatic dysfunction in neuralgic amyotrophy: an electrophysiologic evaluation of 16 patients presenting with dyspnea. *Am Rev Respir Dis* 1993; 147: 66.

47 Efthimiou J, Butler J, Woodham C, Westaby S, Benson MK. Phrenic nerve and diaphragm function following open heart surgery: a prospective study with and without topical hypothermia. *Q J Med* 1992; 85: 845.

48 Smith HP, Smith HP Jr Phrenic paralysis due to serum neuritis. *Am J Med* 1955; 19: 808.

49 Epstein EJ, Quereshi MSA, Wright JS. Diaphragmatic paralysis after supraclavicular puncture of subclavian vein. *Br Med J* 1976; i: 693.

50 Gupta SK. Spontaneous paralysis of the phrenic nerve with special reference to chronic pulmonary tuberculosis. *Br J Dis Chest* 1960; 54: 283.

51 Houston JG, Fleet M, Cowan MD, McMillan NC. Comparison of ultrasound with fluoroscopy in the assessment of suspected hemidiaphragmatic movement abnormality. *Clin Radiol* 1995; 50: 95.

52 Arborelius M, Lilja B, Senyk J. Regional and total lung function studies in patients with hemidiaphragmatic paralysis. *Respiration* 1975; 32: 253.

53 Clague HW, Hall DR. Effect of posture on lung, airway closure and gas exchange in hemidiaphragmatic paralysis. *Thorax* 1979; 34: 523.

54 Svanberg L. Clinical value of analysis of lung function in some intrathoracic diseases. A spirometric, bronchospirometric and angio-pneumonographic investigation. *Acta Chir Scand* 1956; 111: 169.

55 Ridyard JB, Stewart RM. Regional lung function in unilateral diaphragmatic paralysis. *Thorax* 1976; 31: 438.

56 Diehl JL, Lofaso F, Deleuze P, Similowski T, Lemaire F, Brochard L. Clinically relevant diaphragmatic dysfunction after cardiac operations. *J Thorac Cardiovasc Surg* 1994; 107: 487.

57 Takeda S, Nakahara K, Fujii Y, Minami M, Matsuda H. Plication of paralysed hemidiaphragm after right sleeve pneumonectomy. *Ann Thorac Surg* 1994; 58: 1755.

58 Raine J, Samuels MP, Mok Q, Shinebourne EA, Southall DP. Negative extrathoracic pressure ventilation for phrenic nerve palsy after paediatric cardiac surgery. *Br Heart J* 1992; 67: 308.

59 Glassman LR, Spencer FC, Baumann FG, Adams FV, Colvin SB. Successful plication for postoperative diaphragmatic paralysis in an adult. *Ann Thorac Surg* 1994; 58: 1754.

60 Ciccolella DE, Daly BD, Celli BR. Improved diaphragmatic function after surgical plication for unilateral diaphragmatic paralysis. *Am Rev Respir Dis* 1992; 146: 797.

61 Blythe JA, Griffin JP, Gonyea EF. Bilateral diaphragmatic paralysis in association with neurogenic disease. *Arch Intern Med* 1977; 137: 1455.

62 Spitzer SA, Korczyn AD, Kalaci J. Transient bilateral diaphragmatic paralysis. *Chest* 1973; 64: 355.

63 Sandham JD, Shaw DT, Guenter CA. Acute supine respiratory failure due to bilateral diaphragmatic paralysis. *Chest* 1977; 72: 96.

64 Newsom Davis J. The diaphragm and neuromuscular diseases. *Am Rev Respir Dis* 1979; 119 (Suppl 2): 115.

65 Newsom Davis J, Goldman M, Loh L, Casson M. Diaphragm function and alveolar hypoventilation. *Q J Med* 1976; 45: 87.

66 Skatrud J, Iber C, McHugh W *et al.* Determinants of hypoventilation during wakefulness and sleep in diaphragmatic paralysis. *Am Rev Respir Dis* 1980; 121: 587.

67 Cooper CB, Trend P, StJ, Wiles CM. Severe diaphragm weakness in multiple sclerosis. *Thorax* 1985; 40: 633.

68 Graham AN, Martin PD, Haas LF. Neuralgic amyotrophy with bilateral diaphragmatic palsy. *Thorax* 1985; 40: 635.

69 Chan CK, Mohsenin V, Loke J *et al.* Diaphragmatic dysfunction in siblings with hereditary motor and sensory neuropathy (Charcot–Marie–Tooth disease). *Chest* 1987; 91: 567.

70 Patterson DL, DeRemee RA, Hunt LW. Severe asthma complicated by bilateral diaphragmatic paralysis attributed to Parsonage–Turner syndrome. *Mayo Clin Proc* 1994; 69: 774.

71 Hunninghake GW, Fauci AS. Pulmonary involvement in the collagen vascular diseases. *Am Rev Respir Dis* 1979; 119: 471.

72 Spiteri MA, Mier AK, Brophy CJ *et al.* Bilateral diaphragm weakness. *Thorax* 1985; 40: 631.

73 McCredie M, Lovejoy FW, Kaltreider NL.

Pulmonary function in diaphragmatic paralysis. *Thorax* 1962; 17: 213.

74 Loh L, Hughes JMB, Newsom Davis J. The regional distribution of ventilation and perfusion in paralysis of the diaphragm. *Am Rev Respir Dis* 1979; 119 (Suppl 2): 121.

75 Gibson GJ, Pride NB. Lung mechanics in diaphragmatic paralysis. *Am Rev Respir Dis* 1979; 119 (Suppl 2): 119.

76 Newsom Davis J. An experimental study of hiccup. *Brain* 1970; 93: 851.

77 Howard RS. Persistent hiccups. *Br Med J* 1992; 305: 1237.

78 Johnson DL. Intractable hiccups: treatment by microvascular decompression of the vagus nerve. *J Neurosurg* 1993; 78: 813.

79 Salem MR, Baraka A, Rattenborg CC, Holaday DA. Treatment of hiccups by pharyngeal stimulation in anesthetized and conscious subjects. *JAMA* 1967; 202: 32.

80 Friedgood CE, Ripstein CB. Chlorpromazine (thorazine) in the treatment of intractable hiccups. *JAMA* 1955; 157: 309.

81 Williamson BWA, McIntyre IMC. Management of intractable hiccup. *Br Med J* 1977; ii: 501.

82 van Leeuwenhoek A. De generatione animalium et de palpitatione diaphragmatis. *Philos Trans R Soc Lond* 1723; 32: 438.

83 Rigatto H, De Medeiros NP. Diaphragmatic flutter. Report of a case and review of the literature. *Am J Med* 1962; 32: 103.

84 Rigatto H, Correa CEC. Diaphragmatic flutter with an electromyographic study. *J Pediatr* 1968; 73: 757.

85 Phillips JR, Eldridge FL. Respiratory myoclonus (Leeuwenhoek's disease). *N Engl J Med* 1973; 289: 1390.

86 Ting EY, Karliner JS, Williams MH. Diaphragmatic flutter associated with apneustic respiration. *Am Rev Respir Dis* 1963; 88: 833.

87 Cvietusa PJ, Nimmagadda SR, Wood R, Liu AH. Diaphragmatic flutter presenting as inspiratory stridor. *Chest* 1995; 107: 872.

88 Corbett CL. Diaphragmatic flutter. *Postgrad Med J* 1977; 53: 399.

89 Vantrappen G, Decramer M, Harlet R. High frequency diaphragmatic flutter: symptoms and treatment by carbamazepine. *Lancet* 1992; 339: 265.

90 Miller WT, Talman EA. Sub-phrenic abscess. *Am J Roentgenol* 1967; 101: 961.

91 Johnson TH. Chest roentgen findings of subdiaphragmatic abscess with antibiotic therapy. *Am J Roentgenol* 1968; 104: 584.

92 Decosse JJ, Poulin TL, Fox PS, Condon RE. Subphrenic abscess. *Surg Gynecol Obstet* 1974; 138: 841.

93 Warracki SE, Mishad MM, Youssef HH, Fahmy AER. Sub-diaphragmatic infection. *Dis Chest* 1967; 52: 166.

94 Gupta RK, Pant CS, Prakesh R, Behl P, Swaroop K. Sonography in complicated hepatic amoebic abscess. *Clin Radiol* 1987; 38: 123.

95 Rosenberg M. Chronic subphrenic abscess. *Lancet* 1968; ii: 379.

96 Ford GT, Whitelaw WA, Rosenal TW *et al.* Diaphragm function after upper abdominal surgery in humans. *Am Rev Respir Dis* 1983; 127: 431.

97 Mueller PR. In evaluating fluid collections, how does one differentiate subpulmonic from subphrenic collections? Answer to reader's query. *Am J Roentgenol* 1994; 163: 739.

98 Carrol CL, Jeffrey RB, Federle MP, Vernacchia FS. CT evaluation in mediastinal infections. *J Comput Assist Tomogr* 1987; 11: 449.

99 Alexander ES, Proto AV, Clark RA. CT differentiation of subphrenic abscess and pleural effusion. *Am J Roentgenol* 1983; 140: 47.

100 Banham SW, Howie AD, Stevenson RD, Moran F. The pulmonary angiographic appearance of pleurisy associated with subdiaphragmatic inflammation. *Thorax* 1979; 34: 241.

101 Damron JR, Beihn RM, Selby JB, Rosenbaum HD. Gallium–technetium subtraction scanning for the localisation of sub-phrenic abscess. *Radiology* 1974; 113: 117.

102 Burleson RL, Holman BL, Tow DE. Scintigraphic demonstration of abscesses with radioactive gallium labelled leucocytes. *Surg Gynecol Obstet* 1975; 141: 379.

103 Halasz NA. Sub-phrenic abscess-myths and facts. *JAMA* 1970; 214: 724.

104 Van Gansbeke D, Matos C, Gelin M *et al*. Percutaneous drainage of subphrenic abscesses. *Br J Radiol* 1989; 62: 127.

105 Robin ED, Crump CH, Wagman RJ. Low sedimentation rate, hypofibrinogenaemia and restrictive pseudo-obstructive diseases associated with trichinosis. *N Engl J Med* 1960; 262: 758.

106 Brashear RE, Martin RR, Glover JL. Trichinosis and respiratory failure. *Am Rev Respir Dis* 1971; 104: 245.

107 Brennan JL. Metastatic tumours of the diaphragm. *Br J Surg* 1971; 58: 458.

108 Olaffson G, Rausing A, Holen O. Primary tumors of the diaphragm. *Chest* 1971; 59: 568.

109 Ferguson DD, Westcott JL. Lipoma of the diaphragm. *Radiology* 1976; 118: 527.

110 Seaton D. Primary diaphragmatic haemangiopericytoma. *Thorax* 1974; 29: 595.

111 Anderson LS, Forrest JV. Tumors of the diaphragm. *Am J Roentgenol* 1973; 119: 259.

112 Wiener MF, Chou WH. Primary tumors of the diaphragm. *Arch Surg* 1965; 90: 143.

113 Ackermann AJ. Primary tumors of the diaphragm roentgenologically considered. *Am J Roentgenol* 1942; 47: 711.

114 Tanaka F, Sawada K, Ishida I *et al*. Prosthetic replacement of entire left hemidiaphragm in malignant fibrous histiocytoma of diaphragm. *J Thorac Cardiovasc Surg* 1982; 83: 278.

115 Laxdale OE, McDougall H, Mellin GW. Congenital eventration of the diaphragm. *N Engl J Med* 1954; 250: 401.

116 Newman HW, Ellis FH, Andersen HA. Eventration of the diaphragm. *Mayo Clinic Proc* 1955; 30: 310.

117 Christensen P. Eventration of the diaphragm. *Thorax* 1959; 14: 311.

118 Paris F, Blasco E, Canto A *et al*. Diaphragmatic eventration in infants. *Thorax* 1973; 28: 66.

119 Kizilcan S, Tanyel FC, Hicsonmez A, Buyukpamukcu N. The long-term results of diaphragmatic plication. *J Pediatr Surg* 1993; 28: 42.

120 Lund DP, Mitchell J, Kharasch V, Quigley S, Kuehn M, Wilson JM. Congenital diaphragmatic hernia: the hidden morbidity. *J Pediatr Surg* 1994; 29: 258.

121 Vogl A, Small A. Partial eventration of the right diaphragm (congenital diaphragmatic herniation of the liver). *Ann Intern Med* 1955; 43: 61.

122 Spencer RP, Spackman TJ, Pearson HA. Diagnosis of right diaphragmatic eventration by means of liver scan. *Radiology* 1971; 99: 375.

123 Khan AN, Gould DA. The primary role of ultrasound in evaluating right-sided diaphragmatic humps and juxtadiaphragmatic masses: a review of 22 cases. *Clin Radiol* 1984; 35: 413.

124 Anderson RD, Connell TH, Lowman RM. Inversion of the liver and suprahepatic gall bladder associated with eventration of the diaphragm. *Radiology* 1970; 97: 87.

125 Nazarian M. Accessory diaphragm: report of a case with complete physiological evaluation and surgical correction. *J Thorac Cardiovasc Surg* 1971; 61: 293.

126 Nigogosyan G, Ozarda A. Accessory diaphragm: a case report. *Am J Roentgenol* 1961; 85: 309.

127 Hashida YM, Sherman FE. Accessory diaphragm associated with neonatal respiratory distress. *J Pediatr* 1961; 59: 529.

128 Bochdalek VA. Zinige Betrachtungen uber die Entstehung des angeborenen Zwerchfellbruches. Als Beitrag zur pathologischen Anatomie de Hernien. *Vrtljschr Prakt Heilk* 1848; 19: 89.

129 Bock HB, Zimmennann JH. Study of selected congenital abnormalities in Pennsylvania. *US Public Health Rep* 1967; 82: 446.

130 Kelvin FM, Starer F. Congenital diaphragmatic hernia and thirteen pairs of ribs. *Br J Radiol* 1975; 48: 152.

131 Bray RJ. Congenital diaphragmatic hernia. *Anaesthesia* 1979; 34: 567.

132 Reed JO, Lang EF. Diaphragmatic hernia in infancy. *Am J Roentgenol* 1959; 82: 437.

133 Berdon WE, Baker DH, Amoury R. The role of pulmonary hypoplasia in the prognosis of newborn infants with diaphragmatic hernia and eventration. *Am J Roentgenol* 1968; 103: 413.

134 Nguyen L, Guttman FM, de Chadarevian JP *et al*. The mortality of congenital diaphragmatic hernia. Is total pulmonary mass inadequate, no matter what? *Ann Surg* 1983; 198: 766.

135 Tsang TM, Tam PK, Dudley NE, Stevens J. Diaphragmatic agenesis as a distinct clinical entity. *J Pediatr Surg* 1995; 30: 16.

136 Kirchner SG, Burke HO, Neill JA,

Stahlman M. Delayed radiographic presentation of congenital right diaphragmatic hernia. *Radiology* 1975; 115: 155.

137 Campbell DN, Lilly JR. The clinical spectrum of right Bochdalek's hernia. *Arch Surg* 1982; 117: 341.

138 Ahrend TR, Thomson BW. Hernia of the foramen of Bochdalek in the adult. *Am J Surg* 1971; 122: 612.

139 Hight DW, Hixson SD, Reed JO *et al*. Intermittent diaphragmatic hernia of Bochdalek: report of a case and literature review. *Pediatrics* 1982; 69: 601.

140 Nair UR, Entress A, Walker DR. Management of neonatal posterolateral diaphragmatic hernia. *Thorax* 1983; 38: 254.

141 Young DG. Contralateral pneumothorax with congenital diaphragmatic hernia. *Br Med J* 1968; iv: 433.

142 Whittaker LD, Lynn HB, Dawson B, Chaves E. Hernias of the foramen of Bochdalek in children. *Mayo Clin Proc* 1968; 43: 580.

143 Marshall A, Sumner E. Improved prognosis in congenital diaphragmatic hernia: experience of 62 cases over a two year period. *J R Soc Med* 1982; 75: 607.

144 Fischel RE, Joel EM. Herniation of a stone-filled gall bladder through the diaphragm. *Acta Radiol (Diagn)* 1964; 2: 172.

145 Cohen MD. Intermittent cyanotic attacks in an infant: an unusual presentation of a congenital anterior diaphragmatic (Morgagni) hernia. *Br J Radiol* 1981; 54: 260.

146 Betts RA. Subcostosternal diaphragmatic hernia. *Am J Roentgenol* 1956; 75: 269.

147 Payne JH, Yellin AE. Traumatic diaphragmatic hernia. *Arch Surg* 1982; 117: 18.

148 Bernatz PE, Burnside AF, Clagett OT. Problem of the ruptured diaphragm. *JAMA* 1958; 168: 877.

149 Wiot JF. The radiologic manifestations of blunt chest trauma. *JAMA* 1975; 231: 500.

150 Lundius B. Intrathoracic kidney. *Am J Roentgenol* 1975; 125: 678.

151 Wallace DB. Intrapericardial diaphragmatic hernia. *Radiology* 1977; 122: 596.

152 Smith L, Lipperr KM. Peritoneo-pericardial diaphragmatic hernia. *Ann Surg* 1958; 148: 798.

153 Hoffman E. Strangulated diaphragmatic hernia. *Thorax* 1968; 23: 541.

154 Keshishian JM, Cox PA. Diagnosis and management of strangulated diaphragmatic hernia. *Surg Gynecol Obstet* 1962; 115: 626.

155 Cox CL, Anderson JN, Guest JL. Bronchopancreatic fistula following traumatic rupture of the diaphragm. *JAMA* 1977; 237: 1461.

156 Worthy SA, Kang EY, Hartman TE, Kwong JS, Mayo JR, Muller NL. Diaphragmatic rupture: CT findings in 11 patients. *Radiology* 1995; 194: 885.

157 Lee WC, Chen RJ, Fang JF *et al*. Rupture of the diaphragm after blunt trauma. *Eur J Surg* 1994; 160: 479.

47

SLEEP APNOEA/HYPOPNOEA SYNDROME

NEIL J. DOUGLAS

The sleep apnoea/hypopnoea syndrome is probably the most common medical disorder to be described in the second half of the twentieth century. It is not a new condition, merely a recently recognized one, as cases can be identified from manuscripts thousands of years old [1,2]. One of the earliest reports in the British medical literature was in 1829 when Wadd [3] reported a man who 'weighed 23 stone . . . and was withal so lethargic that he frequently fell asleep in company. He felt much inconvenienced and alarmed . . . and was sent to Edinburgh to consult Dr Gregory. He reduced himself to 15 stones . . . he is now well'. Joe, the fat boy in Dickens' *Posthumous Papers of the Pickwick Club* [4] made his appearance in 1837 and is testimony to Dickens' powers of observation, powers that exceeded those of most of his physician contemporaries or indeed those of physicians over the next century and a half. Joe was described as being obese, catastrophically sleepy, of ruddy complexion and having the dropsy (right heart failure).

The medical discovery of sleep apnoea occurred simultaneously in Germany and France in 1965 [5,6]. Both groups recorded physiological variables overnight and recognized the association between breathing pauses during sleep and daytime sleepiness, thus describing the condition that became known as the sleep apnoea syndrome [7]. Interest in the condition spread to North America and Australia and thereafter gradually to the rest of the world. With the identification of episodes of marked hypoventilation (hypopnoeas) during sleep not sufficiently severe to be true apnoeas but which have similar consequences [8], the condition has subsequently become known in many centres as the sleep apnoea/hypopnoea syndrome (SAHS).

Epidemiology

Over the past few years, prevalence studies have been performed in different countries and continents using different techniques. However, their conclusions have been broadly similar, namely that SAHS occurs in 2–6% of middle-aged men and 1–2% of middle-aged women [9–12].

Jennum and Sjol [12] randomly selected 2000 Danish citizens in the age group 30–60 years, of whom 1504 responded. Half the respondents were randomly selected for study of their breathing pattern overnight; 10.9% of the men and 6.3% of the women were found to have more than five apnoeas plus hypopnoeas per hour of sleep, while 1.9% of the men and 0.9% of the women had the same degree of abnormal breathing during sleep and also daytime sleepiness in socially unacceptable conditions.

Young and colleagues [9] studied a random sample of 602 employed men and women aged 30–60 years from Wisconsin using overnight polysomnography (the recording of sleep pattern from the EEG plus breathing and oxygenation patterns) in order to determine the frequency of irregular breathing during sleep; 9% of the women and 24% of the men had more than five apnoeas plus hypopnoeas per hour of sleep, whereas 2% of women and 4% of men had this degree of abnormal breathing during sleep plus daytime sleepiness. The methodology used in the study, including sampling techniques and the performance of overnight polysomnography, make this probably the most robust of the epidemiological studies, although the population studied may be more obese than is the norm in some countries.

Bearpark and colleagues [10] reported that 26% of 294 Australian men had more than five apnoeas plus hypopnoeas per hour in bed, with 3% having the same degree of breathing irregularity plus daytime sleepiness. Olson and colleagues [11], also from Australia, reported that at least 5.7% of middle-aged men and 1.2% of middle-aged women had more than 15 apnoeas plus hypopnoeas per hour of sleep but did not quote data for the coexistence of sleepiness.

With a prevalence of around 2–6% in the middle-aged, sleep apnoea thus has a similar frequency to symptomatic asthma or to diabetes in the same age group. This high prevalence, in conjunction with the significant associated morbidity, has led to the suggestion that it 'has an impact on society that rivals that of smoking' [13]. Although the epidemiology is best documented in the middle-aged, sleep apnoea also occurs in children and the elderly but the precise prevalences are not yet clear.

Mechanisms of upper airway narrowing

SAHS results from recurrent narrowing of the supraglottic airway during sleep. The patency of the pharynx depends upon a balance between transmural pressure and upper airway muscle activity (Fig. 47.1). During inspiration, the negative intraluminal pressure tends to narrow the upper airway and this is opposed by the action of upper airway dilating muscles. These muscles tense with each inspiration, thus resisting collapse of the upper airways and probably also stiffening the airway and so preventing vibration. The principal muscles involved are genioglossus, which tenses the tongue, and palatoglossus, which holds the soft palate in the downwards and forwards position thus resisting collapse of the nasopharynx (Fig. 47.2). Other palatal muscles, including palatopharyngeus, are also involved and there is some evidence to suggest that generalized tensing of palatal muscles, whatever their direction of action, results in palatal stiffening that resists upper airway collapse.

Muscle tone decreases throughout the body during sleep and the relaxation of the upper airway dilating muscles results in relative narrowing of the pharynx. In normal subjects, this narrowing results in increased airflow resistance that is of no major significance [14]. However, in about 50% of middle-aged men and 30% of middle-aged women, this upper airway narrowing is sufficient to cause marked turbulent flow with the associated vibration of snoring. In some, this tendency may progress to produce clinically significant upper airway narrowing or occlusion sufficient to cause sleep disruption and thus clinical sequelae.

The site of airway narrowing during sleep is usually at the retropalatal or retroglossal level [15,16]. In many patients, the occluded segment spans both the retropalatal and retroglossal segments and this probably explains why

surgical approaches designed to increase airway calibre in only one of these locations are frequently unsuccessful.

Upper airway

Patients with SAHS tend to have narrower upper airways when awake than either normal subjects or simple snorers; however, there is substantial overlap between the groups [17–19]. There is considerable evidence indicating that anatomical factors contribute to this upper airway narrowing. Patients with SAHS have increased deposition of adipose tissue around their upper airway, particularly lateral to the pharynx [20,21]. This increased fat deposition is found in obese patients with SAHS compared with obese controls [20] and also in non-obese patients with SAHS compared with non-obese controls [21] (Fig. 47.3).

Bony structure

Some patients with SAHS have abnormal facial bony structure [18,23,24]. The most common abnormalities are small maxillae and mandibles, with resulting retrognathia. The anteroposterior shortening of the face produces narrowing of the uppper airway [18,24,25]. These abnormalities are more common in non-obese patients with SAHS [24]. The abnormalities may be familial, although it is not yet clear whether they are inherited or environmental [25].

Physiological factors

It is difficult to test whether there are abnormalities of neuromuscular control in patients with sleep apnoea compared with normal subjects. Many studies have shown that the upper airway in patients with SAHS is more liable to collapse during both wakefulness and sleep [26–28], although this may be due to anatomical factors. Some studies [29], but not all [30], have indicated that there is

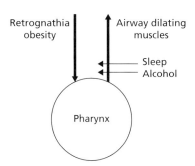

Fig. 47.1 Schematic diagram of upper airway physiology.

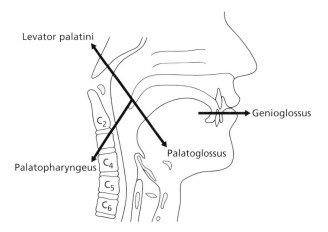

Fig. 47.2 Actions of upper airway dilator muscles.

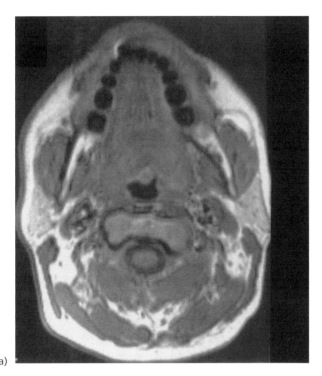

(a)

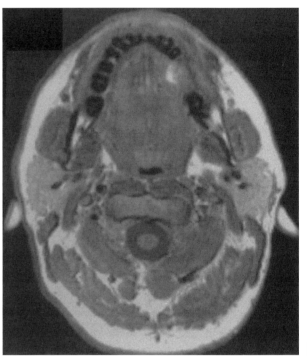

(b)

Fig. 47.3 Magnetic resonance images of a normal subject (a) and a patient of similar age and weight with the sleep apnoea/hypopnoea syndrome (b). The black area in the centre of each image is the upper airway, which is smaller in the patient with sleep apnoea compared with the normal subject even during the awake scans. The white areas lateral to the upper airway in the patient with sleep apnoea/hypopnoea syndrome represent adipose tissue. (From Douglas [22] with permission.)

increased activity of the upper airway dilating muscles in awake patients with SAHS compared with controls, suggesting that patients need to defend their upper airways to keep them patent. This might therefore be a secondary response to anatomical narrowing. Upper airway muscles tense in a reflex response to negative upper airway pressure and Mortimore and Douglas [31] have recently compared this response in normal subjects and in patients with SAHS, finding that the latter have an impaired response to negative upper airway pressure. This suggests that there may be physiological as well as anatomical abnormalities in SAHS.

Sleep induces hypotonia of the upper airway dilating muscles. This is associated with both decreased and delayed responses to negative pressure [32]. These changes thus predispose to upper airway narrowing and occlusion. However, it is not yet clear whether the decrease in upper airway muscle activity and force generation differs between patients with SAHS and normal subjects.

Consequences of upper airway narrowing

Upper airway narrowing results in a compensatory increase in respiratory effort in an attempt to maintain ventilation. This increase in respiratory effort is the under-

lying trigger that stimulates arousal from sleep [33]. It was initially thought that total airway occlusion and cessation of ventilation were required for the pathophysiological sequelae to develop; it was later realized that continued, although diminished, ventilation in the form of hypopnoeas produced identical consequences [8]. There is now evidence that increased upper airways resistance in the absence of a diminution in ventilation may also produce identical sequelae [34,35]. These arousals restore upper airway dilating muscle activity, the patient gasps, takes a few deep breaths and then falls back to sleep, at which point the upper airway dilating muscles relax again and the cycle is initiated once more. These episodes of upper airway narrowing terminated by arousal may recur many hundreds of times per night and the recurrent arousals are thought to cause the major clinical features of the condition (Fig. 47.4).

The frequency of brief arousals from sleep correlates significantly with the impairment in daytime performance found in SAHS. Specifically, arousal frequency is correlated with reaction time and with the decrease in IQ observed [37]. Further evidence that it is sleep disruption which causes symptoms in SAHS come from modelling experiments in which normal subjects have been woken very briefly repeatedly through the night without any overall change in sleep duration. In these studies, recurrent arousals produce objective and subjective daytime

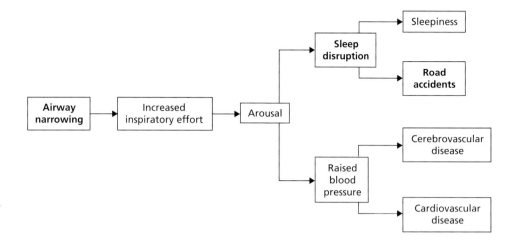

Fig. 47.4 Mechanism and consequences of arousal following airway narrowing. (From Douglas & Polo [36] with permission.)

sleepiness and impaired daytime cognitive performance of the type found in SAHS [38].

Each arousal causes a transient rise in systemic blood pressure [39], the magnitude of which may vary from a small increase to a doubling of both systolic and diastolic pressures. These blood pressure rises may occur even when there are no visually discernible features of arousal on the EEG. Such repeated elevations of blood pressure hundreds of times per night over years or decades presumably account for the reported increase in morbidity and mortality from cardiovascular and cerebrovascular disease in patients with SAHS [40].

Clinical features

Symptoms

The patient's major complaints are usually daytime sleepiness and unrefreshing nocturnal sleep (Table 47.1). Sleepiness must be differentiated from physical fatigue since both tend to be described as 'tiredness'. Many patients admit to falling asleep at least once a day when not in bed [41] and many have been troubled by sleepiness for years prior to presentation. Sleep attacks can occur at any time of day but are usually worst in the early afternoon and evening, coincident with the circadian tendencies to sleepiness in the normal population. The urge to sleep usually comes on gradually but sometimes may be rapid and is often irresistible. Initially, sleepiness tends to present only during monotonous activities, classically watching television in the evening or during unstimulating driving such as on motorways or freeways. As sleepiness becomes more severe, it intrudes progressively into daily activities until sleep intervenes during all varieties of driving, when operating machinery or during conversations and meals. Some patients deny daytime sleepiness but report that they have impaired concentration that causes significant deterioration in their work performance.

Table 47.1 Symptoms of the sleep apnoea/hypopnoea syndrome.

Reported by patient
Sleepiness
Poor concentration
Difficulty driving long distances
Unrefreshing sleep
Morning lethargy
Sleep-related choking/dyspnoea
Nocturia
Decreased sex drive

Reported by partner
Snoring: intermittent, loud
Apnoeas
Irritability

Most patients with SAHS find nocturnal sleep unsatisfying, usually waking up feeling as if they have not had a good night's sleep. However, most do not report an increased frequency of nocturnal awakenings. Approximately one-third of patients have intermittent nocturnal choking attacks related to upper airways obstruction. Usually these are occasional but often terrifying events.

Nocturia is common and often troublesome. It is due to increased salt and water excretion at night [42] and ceases with adequate therapy. Young men with SAHS may complain of loss of libido and impotence. A few patients have reported automatic behaviour and disorientation after awakening, although many more report that they have difficulty getting started in the morning. Ankle oedema is reported by a minority, most of whom have coexisting respiratory disease [43,44], presumably because they have two causes for nocturnal hypoxaemia and thus have more severe hypoxaemia and therefore more marked sequelae.

Most spouses of patients with SAHS report that the patient is a loud snorer and often that their snoring is intermittent, punctuated by multiple apnoeas. However, such a story cannot always be obtained, either because the patient does not have a bed partner or because these features have not been observed by a partner who is usually asleep. Normally, the patient has snored loudly for many years and snores in all body postures. Bed partners also report restless sleep as the patient fights for breath, the bedclothes often being rearranged. Partners may also report psychological changes, particularly irritability or depression.

Patient characteristics

Around 80% of patients with SAHS are male [41]; the reason for this is not clear, although it relates to testosterone in some way since this can induce SAHS in hypogonadal men or in women [45–47]. Males have a central pattern of obesity and this produces greater deposition of fat in the neck of men than women. This may result in greater mass loading of the upper airway on lying down. Around 50% of patients with SAHS are obese. However, an increasing number of patients with SAHS are now found to have normal body weight, with more than 50% of our new patients having a body mass index of less than $30 \, kg/m^2$ and some less than $20 \, kg/m^2$.

Most patients are middle-aged, although the reasons for this are unclear. Upper airway calibre has been found to narrow with age in awake men in some studies [48] but not all [49]. However, age has been found not to affect upper airway calibre in awake women [48].

All affected individuals should be examined for abnormalities of the nose or oropharynx. In some centres, all patients are seen by an otorhinolaryngological surgeon but in others this is reserved for selected patients with appropriate symptoms or abnormal findings on gross examination. Enlarged tonsils are a common cause of sleep apnoea in children and an occasional cause in adults and must be excluded by oropharyngeal examination. Other medical conditions that must be considered include hypothyroidism, acromegaly, Marfan's syndrome and upper airway tumours. Gross retrognathia is relatively uncommon but since it is a correctable cause it should always be sought.

Consequences of sleep apnoea

Death

Early data suggested that sleep apnoea was associated with increased mortality [40,50]. Later studies have not found any clear increase in mortality in patients with SAHS when allowance is made for coexisting risk factors such as obesity, smoking and age [51]. However, larger and better-designed studies are required before this issue can be satisfactorily resolved.

Road traffic accidents

Many patients with SAHS report falling asleep at the wheel and some have road traffic accidents as a consequence. There is convincing evidence that members of the population with irregular breathing during sleep [52] and patients with SAHS have an increased frequency of road traffic accidents [53–55]. The overall increase in frequency is around two- to four-fold, although there may be a nine-fold increase in single-vehicle accidents, i.e. the type of accident typically caused by drivers falling asleep at the wheel [55]. Not only are these accidents common but they are also dangerous. Falling asleep at the wheel accounts for 15–20% of road traffic accidents and these sleep-related accidents are associated with an increased morbidity [56]. Indeed, a recent study in Bavaria has suggested that falling asleep at the wheel is the most common cause of fatal road accidents, and specifically caused more fatal accidents than alcohol [57]. Driving simulator studies show that untreated patients with sleep apnoea drive worse than normal subjects made legally drunk [58]. Obviously, sleep apnoea is only one of several causes of sleep-related road accidents and general fatigue may be more common. Patients with SAHS often report that they have no problems driving short distances in town or on minor roads where sensory input is fairly high but have great difficulties driving on motorways or freeways where the monotonous conditions predispose to sleep. Patients with sleep apnoea also underreport the severity of their driving impairment prior to receiving treatment [59].

Hypertension

Many studies have attempted to assess whether there is an increased frequency of systemic hypertension in SAHS. Assessment of the significance of the differences observed is made difficult by the need to allow for potentially confounding factors, including obesity, age, smoking and alcohol consumption. Furthermore, some of the studies have used methods of diagnosing sleep apnoea that are not sufficiently precise by present-day criteria. Several studies have also used single measurements or even retrospective measurements of blood pressure rather than repeated measurements or 24-h recording. Others have studied patients on antihypertensive therapy, which may affect not only blood pressure but also, perhaps, nocturnal breathing pattern. Few studies stand up to rigorous review of their methodological standards.

Hla and colleagues [60] found an increased frequency of hypertension during 24-h monitoring in patients with SAHS compared with either snoring or non-snoring normal subjects. These differences persisted after controlling for age, sex and obesity. In a recent study, the same group have reported that blood pressure is correlated with frequency of apnoea/hypopnoea and that even individuals with five apnoeas plus hypopnoeas per hour have a higher blood pressure than those with none, again when controlling for other variables [61]. This strongly suggests that irregular breathing at night produces clinically important effects on blood pressure that persist even after controlling for other risk factors. Other population-based studies have also found significant relationships between SAHS and hypertension, although these were explained by associations between hypertension and sex, age, body mass and alcohol consumption [62,63]; in both these studies blood pressure was only recorded on one occasion. Whether or not the 24-h blood pressure is significantly raised in patients with SAHS, there is no doubt that patients have hundreds of transient elevations of blood pressure every night associated with each arousal from a respiratory event [39]. Recurring every night for years or even decades, these could produce significant cardiovascular and cerebrovascular sequelae even in the absence of daytime hypertension.

Cardiovascular risk

A retrospective study has shown that patients with myocardial infarction have a raised frequency of apnoeas during sleep [64]. A population-based study of 441 middle-aged subjects has indicated that patients with irregular breathing at night have a 3.5-fold increased risk of coronary artery disease; however, when adjustment was made for age, sex, body mass index, alcohol consumption and smoking, this ratio decreased to a non-significant 1.4 (95% confidence interval 0.4–3.5) [63]. Thus, the relationship between sleep apnoea and ischaemic heart disease is not yet clear.

Cerebrovascular disease

Several studies have shown associations between snoring and cerebrovascular disease [65–68] and these findings persist after correction for age, smoking and obesity, although there are no data indicating whether SAHS *per se* predisposes to cerebrovascular accidents. However, there is evidence from a retrospective study that treatment for sleep apnoea decreases 'vascular' mortality, i.e. a combination of cerebrovascular and cardiovascular death [40]. Data suggest that the severity of snoring prior to a cerebrovascular accident is a predictor of outcome [68], indicating that nocturnal breathing may be important in the pathogenesis of cerebrovascular accidents.

Right heart failure/respiratory failure

The development of chronic carbon dioxide retention, pulmonary hypertension and peripheral oedema in SAHS usually requires an additional respiratory problem, most commonly chronic airflow obstruction [43,44,69]. Occasionally, other coexisting respiratory problems, such as extreme obesity or weakness of the respiratory muscles, may also produce these complications.

Sudden infant death syndrome

There appears to be an increased frequency of sudden infant death syndrome (cot deaths) in the families of patients with SAHS [70,71]. This observation was made in the families of non-obese patients with SAHS. Families who had both SAHS and sudden infant death syndrome had retroposition of the maxilla and mandibles. A recent study indicates that victims of sudden infant death syndrome also have retroposed maxilla in comparison to age-matched control infants [72]. It is not yet clear how many, if any, cases of sudden infant death syndrome result from an SAHS-related mechanism.

Differential diagnosis

Other causes of daytime sleepiness need to be considered [73].

Narcolepsy

Narcolespy occurs in 0.05% of the population and thus has a frequency about one-hundreth that of SAHS. Narcolepsy tends to present at 10–30 years of age, whereas patients with SAHS tend to present in middle age. The four characteristic features of narcolepsy are daytime sleepiness, cataplexy, hypnagogic hallucinations and sleep paralysis.

Cataplexy is the sudden onset of muscle weakness when awake, almost always in response to amusement or some other strong emotion. It can vary between minor drooping of the head to total collapse. Hypnagogic hallucinations are vivid dreams at the onset of sleep and both these and sleep paralysis relate to the propensity for REM sleep suffered by these patients.

The diagnosis of narcolepy is easy when sleepiness is associated with one of the other features of the tetrad but it commonly is not, in which case the demonstration of sleep-onset REM during multiple sleep latency testing [74] and the demonstration of HLA-DR2, DQw1 may be helpful as may a family history, although the latter is by no means always positive. Narcolepsy is best treated by a combination of simple advice (e.g. taking postprandial naps where possible, and avoiding dangerous situations if feasible) and stimulant medication. Drugs normally used include mazindol, methylphenidate, dexamfetamine (dexamphetamine) and modafinil. Tolerance to these drugs may develop and drug holidays may be required. Cataplexy can also be difficult to treat but drugs of choice include clomipramine, imipramine, fluoxetine and phenelzine.

Idiopathic hypersomnolence

Nocturnal sleep duration tends to be longer than usual and daytime naps are also longer than those found in sleep apnoea or narcolepsy, often lasting over 1 h. The morning is often the worst time of day for patients with idiopathic hypersomnolence, with morning drunkeness as a troublesome feature for some. Like narcolepsy, this condition usually presents first at 10–30 years of age, earlier than SAHS. Treatment is the same as with narcolepsy in terms of advice and stimulant drugs.

Periodic limb movement disorder

Repetitive leg movements occur in many individuals during sleep, perhaps up to 30% by the age of 60 years. These leg movements occur around every 20 s during non-REM sleep but usually disappear totally during REM sleep. When these leg movements are followed by arousals, they may cause daytime sleepiness and treatment with either L-dopa or a benzodiazepine can be beneficial.

Post-traumatic hypersomnolence

Persisting daytime sleepiness following head injury is well documented. This may also occur following cranial surgery or a cerebrovascular accident.

Kleine–Levin syndrome

This rare syndrome causes recurrent episodes of hypersomnolence lasting several days or weeks at a time and recurring perhaps once or twice a year. The patient is often an adolescent and the episodes of prolonged sleeping may be associated with bouts of binge eating and hypersexual activity. Usually the condition gradually improves with time. Lithium therapy may be helpful.

Psychiatric illness

Severe depression and psychotic illnesses may be associated with daytime sleepiness. Psychiatric referral should be considered for not only sleepy patients with overt psychiatric illness but also those in whom no medical cause for sleepiness can be found.

Psychological sleepiness

Occasional daytime sleepiness may relate to anxiety or depression. More often these conditions are associated with insomnia rather than sleepiness.

Insufficient sleep

Patients should always be asked about their normal sleep duration. Prospective sleep diaries may be helpful in this situation.

Shift work

It can be very difficult to ascertain whether the patient's shift rota itself is causing the reported sleepiness and an accurate history is essential.

Drug abuse

Hypnotics, sedatives and alcohol in excess can all cause sleepiness. Trials of withdrawal may prove helpful.

Diagnosis

History and examination

The diagnosis of SAHS cannot be adequately made from the history alone. While questions about intensity of snoring, witnessed apnoeas and falling asleep while driving are useful for selecting patients likely to have SAHS from the general population [75], they are of less value in patients presenting to a sleep clinic, many of whom have such symptoms. Several studies have attempted to distinguish which of the patients presenting to a sleep clinic may have SAHS on history alone but the results have been disappointing. Factors increasing the likelihood of sleep apnoea are witnessed apnoeas [76–78], nocturnal choking [76,77], sleepiness [78], being male [76,77], obesity [76–78], hypertension [77] and the presence of a narrowed pharynx with a large uvula [76]. However, none of these are sufficiently specific to be diagnostically useful, the most helpful being the presence of witnessed apnoeas in 75% of patients with SAHS; however, apnoeas are also reported in around 60% of patients referred to sleep clinics who are shown not to have SAHS [76,77]. Predictive equations can be built around these observations but their value in limiting the number of sleep studies required has yet to be proved.

Sleep studies

The 'gold standard' for the diagnosis of SAHS was originally thought to be polysomnography, which involves the overnight recording of sleep, breathing patterns and oxygenation (Table 47.2). However, the need for this level of investigation in all cases and the associated expense has been questioned as a result of the limitation of healthcare budgets combined with the rapidly increasing numbers of patients being referred for investigation.

Table 47.2 Variables recorder during polysomnography.

Usual
Neurophysiology
    EEC
    Electro-oculography
    Electromyography: submental, anteriotibial

Respiratory
    Airflow
    Thoracoabdominal movement
    Oxygen saturation

General
    ECG
    Body position
    Sound

Optional
    Oesophageal pressure
    Blood pressure
    Penile tumescence
    Light intensity

The recording of sleep quality and duration appears to play little part in the routine clinical diagnosis of SAHS according to a study of 200 patients [79]. The re-examination of patients who either slept for less than 3 h per night or who had no REM sleep did not change the clinical diagnosis, and the identification of early REM sleep was also not diagnostically useful. The expense of sleep recording does not therefore appear to be justified in routine studies. However, there are occasional patients who genuinely do not sleep during either diagnostic or therapeutic sleep studies. Thus, if a technique is used that does not record sleep and the patient indicates that sleep was very poor, polysomnography should be considered to allow interpretation of the breathing pattern during sleep.

The major value of recording sleep may be to identify transient arousals; however, there is no agreement on the definition of such brief arousals [37,80]. Furthermore, even this may not be a reason for recording EEG, since arousals may be better detected by examining changes in cardio-vascular or respiratory pattern. For example, each arousal is associated with a rise in blood pressure [81] and a short-ening in pulse transit time [82] and most are associated with an increase in tidal volume and with the loss of flow limitation.

Many different respiratory sensors have been used to detect SAHS, including oximetry, airflow signals, thoracoabdominal movement, snoring detectors and oesophageal pressure. Oximetry alone can detect about two-thirds of patients with SAHS and this is best done by a trained observer examining the pattern of desaturation [79,83]. Current computerized systems designed to detect recurrent desaturations are highly specific when positive (specificity 97–100%) but are not adequately sensitive (sensitivity 30–40%). Thus, oximetry alone can be diagnos-

tic when positive although normal oximetry by no means excludes the diagnosis of sleep apnoea nor indeed can it even exclude severe sleep apnoea. It must be remembered that the magnitude of daytime impairment in patients with SAHS in terms of reaction time and driving ability relates to arousal frequency more than the degree of desaturation [37]. Thus, patients with recurrent respiratory-associated arousals who have either SAHS or the so-called upper airways resistance syndrome may show no desaturation during sleep but have severe symptoms and benefit greatly from continuous positive airway pressure (CPAP) or other treatment. These limitations of oximetry must be realized by those using this technique either on its own or as a key component in their diagnostic systems.

SAHS was initially diagnosed from recurrent episodes of flow cessation. More recently, it has been realized that events in which there is continued airflow but reduced thoracoabdominal movement (hypopnoeas) are also associated with recurrent arousals and similar clinical sequelae [8]. Indeed, even hypoventilation may not be necessary for the clinical features of the syndrome, some patients exhibiting repeated arousal following increases in upper airways resistance with no decrease in ventilation (upper airways resistance syndrome) [34,35]. There is widespread confusion about this terminology, with similar patients being diagnosed in some centres as having hypopnoeas, in others partial airways obstruction and in yet others upper airways resistance syndrome. This is of more than semantic importance since if upper airways resistance-induced arousals in the absence of any change in ventilatory pattern are common, then the diagnostic strategy must centre on proving the coincidence of an arousal with some relatively subtle respiratory change. These respiratory changes may be documented by invasive techniques such as oesophageal pressure along with EEG monitoring, or less invasively by detecting inspiratory flow limitation or changes in thoracoabdominal phase angle, or by using the static charge-sensitive bed.

There are many different techniques used to record thoracoabdominal movement, including inductance plethysmography, impedance pneumography, strain gauges, piezoelectric systems or charge-sensitive beds. Each gives different results and all users must be aware of the advantages and disadvantages of their system. Thoracoabdominal movement can be used to classify apnoeas into central or obstructive, although this may not be a useful classification since many apnoeas labelled as 'central' respond to CPAP [84]. This may be because the events are initiated with upper airway occlusion, which reflexly inhibits subsequent ventilatory efforts, or because relatively poor thoracoabdominal signals are obtained from some individuals, particularly the grossly obese. The rare true central apnoea can only be diagnosed by oesophageal manometry or respiratory muscle electromyography.

The major use of the thoracoabdominal signal is to identify hypopnoeas, which are better defined with inductance plethysmography than conventional flow sensors since temperature-based measurements do not provide a quantitative estimation of ventilation, there being little difference between the temperature of an expired volume of 100 mL and that of 1000 mL [8]. The conventionally used flow-based devices that record temperature, expired $P\text{CO}_2$ or tracheal sound are adequate to detect true apnoeas, although such apnoeas are detected adequately by inductance plethysmography and thus the need for a flow signal is unclear [85]. Flow signals based on true flow-measuring devices such as pneumotachographs or on the measurement of intranasal pressure may allow detection not only of apnoeas and hypopnoeas but also of flow limitation, thus providing a non-invasive method of diagnosing upper airways resistance syndrome [86]. This is an area of considerable research.

Many different devices have been developed to record snoring. However, the sensitivity of these for diagnosing SAHS based on snoring alone has been poor (around 27%), although specificity is high [87]. Thus, at present, these devices on their own cannot be recommended for excluding SAHS, although the addition of other monitors such as oxygen saturation greatly improves their diagnostic value [88].

There is a confusing array of limited sleep study devices that use various combinations of the above sensors. Unfortunately, most systems are poorly validated at present. It is imperative that the users of such equipment fully appreciate the potential for false-positive and false-negative results with their own system.

Ideally, all sleep studies should have the ability to detect the periodic limb movements found in at least 5% of patients referred to a respiratory sleep clinic [79]. These patients may benefit from treatment for this condition. Such limb movement can be detected either by electromyography, the classical method, or by piezoelectric, static charge bed or video techniques.

Diagnostic strategy

Many factors determine the diagnostic strategy, including the availability of resources and equipment and the distances travelled by patients. Few centres can afford the luxury of polysomnography for all patients referred; indeed, it is not required for the clinical management of most patients. The diagnostic approach depends upon the patient's presenting features and in the author's view the following approach is reasonable.

Patients highly likely to have sleep apnoea

Patients who fall asleep at least once a day when not in bed, are loud snorers with witnessed apnoeas and have no features to suggest periodic limb movement disorder or narcolepsy should have a limited sleep study performed either at home or in hospital without EEG documentation of sleep being obtained. If this overnight study is unequivocally positive, the patient may proceed to therapy but a negative study must result in further investigation.

Simple snorers with no features of sleep apnoea

Any patient who is considering dental splinting or surgery for snoring should have a limited overnight sleep study, which includes recording of snoring so that both the presence of snoring and the presence or absence of sleep apnoea can be documented. In some patients, several nights' recording of snoring may be required to establish whether there is a major problem warranting surgery, as many alleged 'habitual snorers' are found to snore rarely.

Patients with moderate likelihood of sleep apnoea

Our practice in such patients depends on their proximity to the sleep laboratory. Those living less than 80 km away have a limited sleep study performed at home. This saves time and money, although a conservative definition of abnormality has to be used since events occurring during wakefulness are included in the analysis and sensitivity and specificity may differ from that used used during polysomnography [89]. Those living more than 80 km away tend to find it inconvenient to travel to and from the sleep laboratory twice in order to collect and return the equipment and overnight sleep studies in the laboratory are more satisfactory. As the costs of a hospital bed are incurred, it is imperative that the maximal amount of diagnostic information is obtained on this night and it is the author's practice therefore to perform overnight polysomnography on all patients living more than 80 km away who give a reasonable but not totally convincing story of SAHS. This stance may change with the development of better limited sleep study equipment.

Patients who may have other diagnoses

In patients with significant daytime sleepiness without obvious drug or psychological cause and who do not have a good history of SAHS, it is reasonable to perform overnight polysomnography, perhaps combined with the daytime multiple sleep latency test both to quantify the severity of the daytime sleepiness and to help with the diagnosis of narcolepsy through the documentation of early REM sleep [74].

This scheme is just one of many and will require modification as diagnostic equipment becomes more sophisticated and better suited to home use. It supposes access to limited sleep study equipment capable of measuring breathing pattern, snoring, oxygenation and leg movement in each hospital. It is reasonable for hospitals without such facilities to use oximetry for patients with a high probability of having SAHS since it is positive in two-thirds of patients with SAHS and a positive result allows rapid initiation of CPAP. However, all patients with negative or equivocal oximetry alone need to be referred for further investigation.

Treatment

The threshold for benefit from treatment has yet to be established. Most patients with more than 15 apnoeas plus hypopnoeas per hour of sleep who are troubled by daytime sleepiness benefit from therapy [90]. However, there are a significant number of patients with fewer events who are troubled by daytime symptoms who also benefit from therapy [91]. At present, the author's policy is to offer treatment to all those with troublesome sleepiness who have more than 15 apnoeas plus hypopnoeas per hour of sleep or more than 15 respiratory-related arousals per hour in the context of the upper airways resistance syndrome.

All such patients should receive advice on weight reduction and alcohol avoidance as routine. Those with otorhinolaryngological symptoms or abnormal findings on examination should be referred in order to discover whether improvement of the nasopharyngeal airway might help. Any patients with craniofacial abnormality should be considered for surgical mandibular advancement, with or without maxillary advancement. These are highly skilled procedures that must be carried out in specialist centres.

Fig. 47.5 Mechanism of action of continuous positive airway pressure. Left-hand panel shows mechanism of airway obstruction with the throat being sucked closed by the negative intraluminal pressure. Right-hand panel shows the throat being blown open by the continuous positive airway pressure applied by nasal mask.

Continuous positive airway pressure

Those patients with severe symptoms and those not responding to the above measures require a trial of CPAP [92]. CPAP blows open the upper airway, thus preventing apnoeas, hypopnoeas, increases in upper airways resistance and snoring. CPAP is usually applied via an external nasal mask (Fig. 47.5), although some patients prefer intranasal devices. Therapy must be initiated with a careful explanation to each patient of the benefits and potential problems of CPAP. Educational videos are a useful adjunct to explanations by doctors and nurses. The patient must then be sized for an appropriate mask; each sleep centre should hold in stock at least 20 different sizes of masks from differing manufacturers so that an adequate fit can be achieved for each patient. Each patient should try CPAP for at least 30 min using the correct mask during the daytime to become accustomed to the sensation before returning for an overnight titration study. This sets the pressure required to keep the patient's airway patent and to minimize arousals: too high a pressure results in the patient being kept awake, while too low a pressure does not effect airway patency. 'Split night' studies, with the first part of the night for diagnosis and the second for CPAP titration, can be used in many patients with severe sleep apnoea but their role in milder disease is still unclear [93].

CPAP is one of the most satisfying therapies to deliver in that it can completely transform a patient's lifestyle. Patients who were unable to perform their job or drive safely because of sleepiness and who were subjected to considerable domestic strife can be returned to normality overnight, a situation rare in respiratory medicine. Randomized placebo-controlled studies have shown that CPAP improves symptoms, sleepiness, quality of life, mood, cognitive function, IQ and driving performance [90,91,94]. Uncontrolled data also suggest that CPAP may improve sleepiness [95], quality of life [96] and survival [48]. Recent evidence indicates that CPAP improves driving performance [97], decreases the rate and cost of

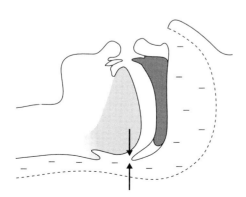
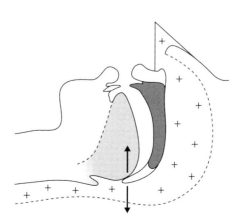

road traffic accidents [98], improves work efficiency and decreases time off work through ill-health [99].

Recently, the efficacy of CPAP has been challenged by Wright and colleagues [100]. At the time, these authors were correct in stating that there were few randomized controlled trials; however, many such studies have since been carried out and their results reviewed [101]. There is no real doubt that CPAP is effective in many patients, a conclusion shared by a recent systematic review [102], although there is a real need for further information on the cost-effectiveness and long-term use of CPAP.

Like all therapies, CPAP has side-effects. One of the major problems is the obtrusive nature of the device and careful education is the most important way of minimizing this problem. Despite careful mask fitting, local problems sometimes arise and mask sizes may need to be changed. The most common side-effects relate to nasal drying, rhinitis or dry mouth [99], all of which appear to be due to mouth leaks. Mouth leaks increase the flow of air through the nasopharynx, which may not only produce nasal drying and rhinitis but also increase airflow resistance, thus decreasing the effect of pressure delivered to the nasopharynx. Management should involve trying a chin strap but if this is not successful, then a heated humidifier may be necessary. Other problems include abnormal bloating that may be difficult to manage, although pressure reduction may prove satisfactory.

As with any other form of chronic therapy, including treatment for asthma [103], patient compliance with therapy is not as high as might be hoped. On average, patients on chronic CPAP use their machines for around 4–5h per night but there is wide variation between subjects. Short-term trials yield slightly lower compliance figures [104], probably because those who use their machines early only rarely abandon the therapy subsequently. It is not yet clear whether symptoms or initial sleep study findings can be used to predict the subsequent use of CPAP by patients, the author's own data indicating no useful relationships [104].

Follow-up of patients on CPAP must include checking for side-effects, checking the function of the mask, tubing and machine, and monitoring objective use of therapy from the time clock built into the machine, since patients are frequently inaccurate in their estimate of use [104]. Annual electrical safety checks are standard for CPAP machines.

Bilevel ventilation via a nasal mask is an acceptable form of treatment for many patients with SAHS. However, it is significantly more expensive than CPAP and there is as yet no evidence that patient compliance or outcome is improved by using this method as opposed to CPAP [105].

Those patients who do not tolerate CPAP and in whom weight reduction is either not appropriate or unachievable should be considered for either dental devices or surgery.

Oral devices

The role of dental devices in the treatment of sleep apnoea is unclear. These devices, which the subjects only use overnight, often advance the mandible and may decrease snoring and potentially also the frequency of apnoeas plus hypopnoeas [106]. Recent evidence from controlled trials suggests that oral devices may be effective in some patients with SAHS [107,108]. These data indicate that patients like oral devices and that these devices improve, but do not usually normalize, nocturnal breathing. Further studies investigating outcome measures and compliance with oral devices are awaited with interest before their role in the therapy of sleep apnoea can be stated with certainty. At present they have a role in patients who decline or do not comply with CPAP therapy, but whether they are as effective as CPAP as primary therapy remains to be seen.

Otorhinolaryngological surgery

There is considerable controversy over the role of uvulopalatopharyngoplasty, whether carried out by conventional surgical techniques or by laser. Unfortunately, there are no objective data from controlled clinical trials that indicate high success rates [109,110]. In addition, the operation tends to be painful for around 2 weeks and has been associated with significant morbidity and very occasional mortality [111,112]. Casual readers of the literature should be careful not to be confused by differing definitions of success rates between studies, few of which use definitions of cure that involve returning the frequency of apnoeas/hypopnoeas and symptoms to normal levels. Furthermore, those patients who fail to benefit from uvulopalatopharyngoplasty and who then need CPAP have difficulty with pressure leaking out through the mouth, and have more side-effects and lower use of CPAP [113].

The theoretical problem with uvulopalatopharyngoplasty is that it addresses airway occlusion only at the palatal level, whereas obstruction generally takes place at both the retropalatal and retroglossal levels [15,16]. The earlier hope that localization of the prime site of obstruction as the retropalatal level would improve the success rate of uvulopalatopharyngoplasty has not been borne out [114,115]. There is dispute whether uvulopalatopharyngoplasty improves survival in patients with SAHS [48,116]. In selected centres, this operation has been augmented by partial glossectomy and significant success rates have been claimed to ensue.

Faciomaxillary surgery

In a few centres around the world, mandibular plus maxillary advancement has been shown to benefit some patients [117]. At present, patients who may benefit from this approach should be treated by surgeons who have experience in this area. Patients who should be considered for such procedures are those with abnormal cephalometric findings and narrowed upper airway. Further factors in favour of this approach include relatively younger patients, thinner patients and those not able to tolerate CPAP.

Upper airway pacing

Pacing of the upper airway opening muscles by external or internal electrodes has been suggested as a possible treatment for SAHS [118]. Thus far, there is insufficient evidence available to recommend this approach.

Tracheostomy

This option must be remembered as a possibility in severely ill patients intolerant of CPAP, although it is rarely needed.

Central sleep apnoea

There is a small minority of patients who have true central apnoeas that do not respond to CPAP. Such patients generally have coexisting cardiovascular or cerebrovascular disease. When symptoms are troublesome, the best treatment in such cases is usually nocturnal intermittent positive-pressure ventilation via a nasal mask [41]. Acetazolamide therapy has been shown to help some patients [119].

Training

It is obviously essential that those dealing with any area of medicine are adequately trained in the clinical, diagnostic and treatment approaches relevant to that subspecialty. This is a particular problem in newly evolving areas of medicine such as the management of sleep disorders. Throughout the world, guidelines are being drawn up indicating the training requirements. The British guidelines, published by the Royal College of Physicians of London [120], indicates that trainees in respiratory medicine who wish to direct a sleep laboratory or to make sleep disorders a major component of their work should receive at least 12 months of specialist training in this area. In addition, it is recommended that all respiratory physicians in training should receive the equivalent of at least 3 months' education in a sleep laboratory during their training programme. These guidelines have yet to be rigorously enacted.

Conclusions

Our understanding of SAHS is rapidly increasing. This is a clinically rewarding area that all respiratory physicians should understand so that they may identify potential patients and refer them for appropriate investigation and treatment.

References

1 Kryger MH. Sleep apnoea: from the needles of Dionysius to continuous positive airway pressure. *Arch Intern Med* 1983; 143: 2301.

2 Lavie P. Nothing new under the moon. Historical accounts of sleep apnea syndrome. *Arch Intern Med* 1986; 144: 2025.

3 Wadd W. *Comments on Corpulency and Lineaments of Leaness and Memoirs on Diet and Dietetics.* London: John Ebers, 1829.

4 Dickens C. *The Posthumous Papers of the Pickwick Club.* London: Chapman & Hall, 1837.

5 Jung R, Kuhlo W. Neurophysiological studies of abnormal night's sleep and the Pickwickian syndrome. *Prog Brain Res* 1965; 18: 140.

6 Gastaut H, Tassinari C, Duron B. Etude polygraphic des manifestations episodiques du syndrome de Pickwick. *Rev Neurol* 1965; 112: 568.

7 Guilleminault C, Van Der Hoed J, Mitler MM. Clinical overview of the sleep apnea syndromes. In: Guilleminault C, Dement W, eds. *Sleep Apnea Syndrome.* New York: Alan R Liss, 1978: 1.

8 Gould GA, Whyte KF, Rhind GB *et al.* The sleep hypopnea syndrome. *Am Rev Respir Dis* 1988; 137: 895.

9 Young T, Palta M, Dempsey J, Skatrud J, Weber S, Badr S. The occurrence of sleep-disordered breathing among middle-aged adults. *N Engl J Med* 1993; 328: 1230.

10 Bearpark H, Elliott L, Grunstein R *et al.* Snoring and sleep apnea: a population study in Australian men. *Am J Respir Crit Care Med* 1995; 151: 1459.

11 Olson LG, King MT, Hensley MJ, Saunders NA. A community study of snoring and sleep disordered breathing: health outcomes. *Am J Respir Crit Care Med* 1995; 152: 717.

12 Jennum P, Sjol A. Epidemiology of snoring and obstructive sleep apnoea in a Danish population, age 30–60. *J Sleep Res* 1992; 1: 240.

13 Phillipson EA. Sleep apnea: a major public health problem. *N Engl J Med* 1993; 328: 1271.

14 Hudgel DW, Hendricks C. Palate and hypopharynx: sites of inspiratory narrowing of the upper airway during sleep. *Am Rev Respir Dis* 1988; 138: 1542.

15 Chaban R, Cole P, Hoffstein V. Site of upper airway obstruction in patients with idiopathic obstructive sleep apnea. *Laryngoscope* 1988; 98: 641.

16 Hudgel DW. Variable site of airway narrowing among obstructive sleep apnea patients. *J Appl Physiol* 1986; 61: 1403.

17 Bradley TD, Brown IG, Grossman RF. Pharyngeal size in snorers, non-snorers and patients with obstructive sleep apnea. *N Engl J Med* 1986; 315: 1327.

18 Shelton KE, Gay SB, Hollowell DE, Woodson H, Suratt PM. Mandible enclosure of upper airway and weight in obstructive sleep apnea. *Am Rev Respir Dis* 1993; 148: 195.

19 Martin SE, Marshall I, Douglas NJ. The effect of posture on airway caliber in the sleep apnea/hypopnea syndrome. *Am J Respir Crit Care Med* 1995; 152: 721.

20 Horner RL, Mohiaddin RH, Lowell DG. Sites and sizes of fat deposits around the pharynx in obese patients with obstructive sleep apnoea and weight matched controls. *Eur Respir J* 1989; 2: 613.

21 Mortimore IL, Marshall I, Wraith PK, Sellar RJ, Douglas NJ. Neck and total body fat deposition in nonobese and obese patients with sleep apnea compared with that in control subjects. *Am J Respir Crit Care Med* 1998; 157: 280.

22 Douglas NJ. The sleep apnoea/hypopnoea syndrome. *Eur J Clin Invest* 1995; 25: 285.

23 Partinen M, Guilleminault C, Quera-Salva M, Jamieson A. Obstructive sleep apnea and cephalometric roentgenograms: the role of anatomic upper airway abnormalities in the

definition of abnormal breathing during sleep. *Chest* 1988; 93: 1199.

24 Ferguson KA, Ono T, Lowe AA, Ryan F, Fleetham JA. The relationship between obesity and craniofacial structure in obstructive sleep apnea. *Chest* 1995; 108: 375.

25 Mathur R, Douglas NJ. Family studies in patients with the sleep apnea/hypopnea syndrome. *Ann Intern Med* 1995; 122: 174.

26 Issa FG, Sullivan CE. Upper airway closing pressures in obstructive sleep apnea. *J Appl Physiol* 1984; 57: 520.

27 Gleadhill IC, Schwartz AR, Schubert N, Wise RA, Permutt S, Smith PL. Upper airway collapsibility in snorers and in patients with obstructive hypopnea and apnea. *Am Rev Respir Dis* 1991; 143: 1300.

28 Brown IG, Bradley TD, Phillipson EA, Zamel N, Hoffstein V. Pharyngeal compliance in snoring subjects with and without obstructive sleep apnea. *Am Rev Respir Dis* 1985; 132: 211.

29 Mezzanotte WS, Tangel DJ, White DP. Waking genioglossal electromyogram in sleep apnea patients versus normal controls (a neuromuscular compensatory mechanism). *J Clin Invest* 1992; 89: 1571.

30 Douglas NJ, Jan MA, Yildirim N, Warren PM, Drummond GB. Effect of posture and breathing route on genioglossal electromyogram activity in normal subjects and in patients with the sleep apnea/hypopnea syndrome. *Am Rev Respir Dis* 1993; 148: 1341.

31 Mortimore IL, Douglas NJ. Palatal muscle EMG response to negative pressure in awake sleep apneic and control subjects. *Am J Respir Crit Care Med* 1997; 156: 867.

32 Wheatley JR, Mezzanotte WS, Tangel DJ, White DP. Influence of sleep on genioglossus muscle activation by negative pressure in normal men. *Am Rev Respir Dis* 1993; 148: 597.

33 Kimoff RJ, Cheong TH, Olha AE *et al*. Mechanisms of apnea termination in obstructive sleep apnea. *Am J Respir Crit Care Med* 1994; 149: 707.

34 Guilleminault C, Stoohs R, Duncan S. Snoring: daytime sleepiness in regular heavy snorers. *Chest* 1991; 99: 40.

35 Guilleminault C, Stoohs R, Clerk A, Cetel M, Maistros P. A cause of excessive daytime sleepiness. The upper airway resistance syndrome. *Chest* 1993; 104: 781.

36 Douglas NJ, Polo O. Pathogenesis of obstructive sleep apnoea/hypopnoea syndrome. *Lancet* 1994; 344: 653.

37 Cheshire K, Engleman H, Deary I, Douglas N. Factors impairing daytime performance in patients with the sleep apnea/hypopnea syndrome. *Arch Intern Med* 1992; 152: 538.

38 Martin SE, Engleman HM, Deary IJ, Douglas NJ. The effect of sleep fragmentation on daytime function. *Am J Respir Crit Care Med* 1996; 153: 1328.

39 Davies RJO, Vardi-Visy K, Clarke M, Stradling JR. Identification of sleep disruption and sleep disordered breathing from the systolic blood pressure profile. *Thorax* 1993; 48: 1242.

40 Partinen M, Guilleminault C. Daytime sleepiness and vascular morbidity at seven-year follow-up in obstructive sleep apnea patients. *Chest* 1990; 97: 27.

41 Whyte KF, Allen MB, Jeffrey AA, Gould GA, Douglas NJ. Clinical features of the sleep apnoea/hypopnoea syndrome. *Q J Med* 1989; 72: 659.

42 Warley AR, Stradling JR. Abnormal diurnal variation in salt and water excretion in patients with obstructive sleep apnoea. *Clin Sci* 1988; 74: 183.

43 Bradley T, Rutherford R, Grossman R. Role of daytime hypoxemia in the pathogenesis of right heart failure in obstructive sleep apnea syndrome. *Am Rev Respir Dis* 1985; 131: 835.

44 Whyte KF, Douglas NJ. Peripheral edema in the sleep apnea/hypopnea syndrome. *Sleep* 1991; 14: 354.

45 Sandblom RE, Matsumoto AM, Schoene RB. Obstructive sleep apnea syndrome induced by testosterone administration. *N Engl J Med* 1983; 308: 508.

46 Johnson MW, Anch AM, Remmers JE. Induction of the obstructive sleep apnea syndrome in a women by exogenous androgen administration. *Am Rev Respir Dis* 1984; 129: 1023.

47 Cistulli PA, Grunstein RR, Sullivan CE. Effect of testosterone administration on upper airway collapsibility during sleep. *Am J Respir Crit Care Med* 1994; 149: 530.

48 White DP, Lombard RM, Cadieux RJ, Zwillich CW. Pharyngeal resistance in normal humans: influence of age, gender and obesity. *J Appl Physiol* 1985; 58: 365.

49 Burger CD, Stanson AW, Sheedy PF, Daniels BK, Shepard JW. Fast computed tomography evaluation of age related changes in upper airway structure and function in normal men. *Am Rev Respir Dis* 1992; 145: 846.

50 HEJ, Kryger M, Zorick F, Conway W, Roth T. Mortality and apnea index in obstructive sleep apnea. Experience in 385 male patients. *Chest* 1988; 94: 9.

51 Lavie P, Herer P, Peled R *et al*. Mortality in sleep apnea patients: a multivariate analysis of risk factors. *Sleep* 1995; 18: 149.

52 Young T, Blustein J, Finn L, Palta M. Sleep-disordered breathing and motor vehicle accidents in a population-based sample of employed adults. *Sleep* 1997; 20: 608.

53 George C, Nickerson P, Millard T, Kryger M. Sleep apnea patients have more automobile accidents. *Lancet* 1987; ii: 447.

54 Findley LJ, Unverzagt ME, Suratt PM. Automobile accidents involving patients with obstructive sleep apnea. *Am Rev Respir Dis* 1988; 138: 337.

55 Haraldsson PO, Carenfelt C, Diderichsen F, Nygren A, Tingvall C. Clinical symptoms of sleep apnea syndrome and automobile accidents. *ORL J Otorhinolaryngol Relat Spec* 1990; 52: 57.

56 Horne JA, Reyner LA. Sleep related vehicle accidents. *Br Med J* 1995; 310: 565.

57 Zulley J, Cronlein T, Hell W, Langwieder K. Falling asleep at the wheel: the chief cause of severe traffic accidents. *Wien Med Wochenschr* 1995; 145: 473.

58 George CFP, Boudreau AC, Smiley A. Simulated driving performance in patients with obstructive sleep apnea. *Am J Respir Crit Care Med* 1996; 154: 175.

59 Engleman HM, Hirst WSJ, Douglas NJ. Under reporting of sleepiness and driving impairment in patients with sleep apnoea/hypopnoea syndrome. *J Sleep Res* 1997; 6: 272.

60 Hla KM, Young TB, Bidwell T, Palta M, Skatrud JB, Dempsey J. Sleep apnea and hypertension. A population-based study. *Ann Intern Med* 1994; 120: 382.

61 Young T, Peppard P, Palta M *et al*. Population-based study of sleep-disordered breathing as a risk factor for hypertension. *Arch Intern Med* 1997; 157: 1746.

62 Jennum P, Sjol A. Snoring, sleep apnea, cardiovascular risk factors: the MONICA II study. *Int J Epidemiol* 1993; 22: 439.

63 Olson LG, King MT, Hensley MJ, Saunders NA. A community study of snoring and sleep-disordered breathing. *Am J Respir Crit Care Med* 1995; 152: 711.

64 Huang J, Whitford E, Parsons R, Hillman D. Association of sleep apnea with myocardial infarction in men. *Lancet* 1990; 336: 261.

65 Norton PG, Dunn EV. Snoring as a risk factor for disease: an epidemiological survey. *Br Med J* 1985; 291: 630.

66 Partinen M, Palomaki H. Snoring and cerebral infarction. *Lancet* 1985; 2: 1325.

67 Koskenvuo M, Kaprio J, Telakivi T, Partinen M, Heikkila K, Sarna S. Snoring as a risk factor for ischaemic heart disease and stroke in men. *Br Med J* 1987; 294: 16.

68 Spriggs DA, French JM, Murdy JM, Curless RH, Bates D, James OFW. Snoring increases the risk of stroke and adversely affects prognosis. *Q J Med* 1992; 84: 555.

69 Bradley TD, Rutherford R, Lue F *et al*. Role of diffuse airway obstruction in the hypercapnia of obstructive sleep apnea. *Am Rev Respir Dis* 1986; 134: 920.

70 Mathur R, Douglas NJ. Relation between sudden infant death syndrome and adult sleep apnoea/hypopnoea syndrome. *Lancet* 1994; 344: 819.

71 Tishler PV, Redline S, Ferrette V, Hans MG, Altose MD. The association of sudden unexpected infant death with obstructive sleep apnea. *Am J Respir Crit Care Med* 1996; 153: 1857.

72 Rees K, Wright A, Keeling JW, Douglas NJ. Facial structure in the sudden infant death syndrome: case–control study. *Br Med J* 1998; 317: 179.

73 Kryger MH, Roth T, Dement WC, eds. *Principles and Practice of Sleep Medicine*, 2nd edn. Philadelphia: WB Saunders, 1994.

74 Carskadon MA, Dement WC, Mitler MM, Roth T, Westbrook PR, Keenan S. Guidelines for the multiple sleep latency test. *Sleep* 1986; 9: 519.

75 Kump K, Whalen C, Tishler P *et al*. Assessment of the validity and utility of a sleep-symptom questionnaire. *Am J Respir Crit Care Med* 1994; 150: 735.

76 Hoffstein V, Szalai J. Predictive value of clinical features in diagnosing obstructive sleep apnea. *Sleep* 1993; 16: 118.

77 Crocker BD, Olson LG, Saunders NA *et al*. Estimation of the probability of disturbed breathing during sleep before a sleep study. *Am Rev Respir Dis* 1990; 142: 14.

78 Maislin G, Pack A, Kribbs N *et al*. A survey screen for prediction of apnea. *Sleep* 1995; 18: 158.

79 Douglas NJ, Thomas S, Jan MA. Clinical value of polysomnography. *Lancet* 1992; 339: 347.

80 Atlas Taskforce of the American Sleep Disorders Association. EEG arousals: scoring, rules and examples. A preliminary report. *Sleep* 1992; 15: 174.

81 Davies RJO, Belt PJ, Roberts SJ. Arterial blood pressure responses to graded tran-

sient arousal from sleep in normal humans. *J Appl Physiol* 1993; 74: 1123.

82 Pitson D, China N, Knijn S, Herwaaden MV, Stradling J. Changes in pulse transit time and pulse rate as markers of arousal from sleep in normal subjects. *Clin Sci* 1994; 87: 269.

83 Series F, Marc I, Cormier YLA, Forge J. Utility of nocturnal home oximetry for case finding in patients with suspected sleep apnea hypopnea syndrome. *Ann Intern Med* 1993; 119: 449.

84 Issa F, Sullivan C. Reversal of central sleep apnea using nasal CPAP. *Chest* 1986; 90: 165.

85 Whyte KF, Allen MB, Fitzpatrick MF, Douglas NJ. Accuracy and significance of scoring hypopneas. *Sleep* 1992; 15: 257.

86 Condos R, Norman R, Krishnasamy I, Peduzzi N, Goldring R, Rapoport D. Flow limitation as a noninvasive assessment of residual upper-airway resistance during continuous positive airway pressure therapy of obstructive sleep apnea. *Am J Respir Crit Care Med* 1994; 150: 475.

87 Stoohs R, Guilleminault C. MESAM 4: an ambulatory device for the detection of patients at risk for obstructive sleep apnea syndrome (OSAS). *Chest* 1992; 101: 1221.

88 Issa FG, Morrison D, Hadjuk E, Iyer A, Feroah T, Remmers JE. Digital monitoring of sleep-disordered breathing using snoring sound and arterial oxygen saturation. *Am Rev Respir Dis* 1993; 148: 1023.

89 Whittle AT, Finch SP, Mortimore IL, MacKay TW, Douglas NJ. Use of home sleep studies for diagnosis of the sleep apnoea/hypopnoea syndrome. *Thorax* 1997; 52: 1068.

90 Engleman HM, Martin SE, Deary IJ, Douglas NJ. Effect of continuous positive airway pressure treatment on daytime function in sleep apnoea/hypopnoea syndrome. *Lancet* 1994; 343: 572.

91 Engleman HM, Martin SE, Deary IJ, Douglas NJ. Effect of CPAP therapy on daytime function in patients with mild sleep apnoea/hypopnoea syndrome. *Thorax* 1997; 52: 114.

92 Sullivan CE, Berthon-Jones M, Issa FG, Eves L. Reversal of obstructive sleep apnea by continuous positive airway pressure applied through the nares. *Lancet* 1981; i: 862.

93 Sanders MH, Kern NB, Constantino JP. Adequacy of prescribing positive airway pressure therapy by mask for sleep apnea on the basis of a partial-night trial. *Am Rev Respir Dis* 1993; 147: 1169.

94 Engleman HM, Martin SE, Kingshott RN, MacKay TW, Deary IJ, Douglas NJ. Randomised placebo controlled trial of daytime function after continuous positive airway pressure (CPAP) therapy for the sleep apnoea/hypopnoea syndrome. *Thorax* 1998; 53: 341.

95 Hardinge FM, Bitson DJ, Stradling JR. Use of Epworth sleepiness scale to demonstrate response treatment with nasal continuous positive airway pressure in patients with obstructive sleep apnea. *Respir Med* 1995; 89: 617.

96 Smith IE, Shneerson JM. Is the SF-36 sensitive to sleep disruption? a study in patients with sleep apnoea. *J Sleep Res* 1995; 4: 183.

97 George CFP, Boudreau AC, Smiley A. Effects of nasal CPAP on simulated driving performance in patients with obstructive sleep apnoea. *Thorax* 1997; 52: 648.

98 Krieger J, Meslier N, Lebrun T *et al.* Accidents in obstructive sleep apnea patients treated with nasal continuous positive airway pressure. *Chest* 1997; 112: 1561.

99 Engleman HM, Asgari-Jirhandeh N, McLeod AL, Ramsay CF, Deary IJ, Douglas NJ. Self-reported use of CPAP and benefits of CPAP therapy: a patient survey. *Chest* 1996; 109: 1470.

100 Wright J, Johns R, Watt I *et al.* Health effects of obstuctive sleep apnoea and effectiveness of continuous positive airway pressure: a systematic review of the research evidence. *Br Med J* 1997; 314: 851.

101 Douglas NJ. Systematic review of the efficacy of nasal CPAP. *Thorax* 1998; 53: 414.

102 Australian Health Technology Advisory Committee. *The effectiveness and cost effectiveness of nasal continuous positive airway pressure in the treatment of obstructive sleep apnoea in adults.* Canberra: Government Public Services, 1998.

103 Mawhinney H, Spector SL, Kinsman RA *et al.* Compliance in clinical trials of two nonbronchodilator, antiasthma medications. *Ann Allergy* 1991; 66: 294.

104 Engleman HM, Martin SE, Douglas NJ. Compliance with CPAP therapy in patients with the sleep apnoea/hypopnoea syndrome. *Thorax* 1994; 49: 263.

105 Reeves-Hoche MK, Hudgel DW, Meck R, Witteman R, Ross A, Zwillich CW. Continuous versus bilevel positive airway pressure for obstructive sleep apnea. *Am J Respir Crit Care Med* 1995; 151: 443.

106 Schmidt-Nowara W, Lowe A, Wiegand L, Cartwright R, Perez-Guerra F, Menn S. Oral appliances for the treatment of snoring and obstructive sleep apnea: a review. *Sleep* 1995; 18: 501.

107 Ferguson KA, Ono T, Lowe AA, Keenan SP, Fleetham JA. Randomised crossover study of oral appliances versus nasal continuous positive airway pressure therapy in the treatment of the mild-moderate obstructive sleep apnea. *Chest* 1996; 109: 1269.

108 O'Sullivan RA, Hillman DR, Mateljan R, Pantin C, Finucane KE. Mandibular advancement splint: an appliance to treat snoring in obstructive sleep apnea. *Am J Respir Crit Care Med* 1995; 151: 194.

109 Fujita S, Conway W, Zorick F, Roth T. Surgical correction of anatomic abnormalities in obstructive sleep apnea syndrome: uvulopalatopharyngoplasty. *Otolaryngol Head Neck Surg* 1981; 89: 923.

110 Gislason T, Lindholm C, Almqvist M. Uvulopalatopharyngoplasty in the sleep apnea syndrome. Predictors of results. *Arch Otolaryngol Head Neck Surg* 1988; 114: 45.

111 Larsson H, Carlsson-Nordlander B, Svanborg E. Long-time follow-up after UPPP for obstructive sleep apnea syndrome. *Acta Otolaryngol* 1991; 111: 582.

112 Conway W, Fujita S, Zorick F. Uvulopalatopharyngoplasty. One-year follow-up. *Chest* 1985; 88: 385.

113 Mortimore IL, Bradley PA, Murray JAM, Douglas NJ. Uvulopalatopharyngoplasty may compromise nasal CPAP therapy in sleep apnea syndrome. *Am J Respir Crit Care Med* 1996; 154: 1759.

114 Hudgel DW, Harasick T, Katz RL, Witt WJ, Abelson TI. Uvulopalatopharyngoplasty in obstructive apnea: value of preoperative localization of site of upper airway narrowing during sleep. *Am Rev Respir Dis* 1991; 143: 942.

115 Shepard JW, Thawley SE. Evaluation of the upper airway by computerized tomography in patients undergoing uvulopalatopharyngoplasty for obstructive sleep apnea. *Am Rev Respir Dis* 1989; 140: 711.

116 Keenan SP, Burt H, Ryan F, Fleetham JA. Long-term survival of patients with obstructive sleep apnea treated by uvulopalatopharyngoplasty or nasal CPAP. *Chest* 1994; 105: 155.

117 Riley RW, Powell NB, Guilleminault C. Maxillofacial surgery and nasal CPAP. A comparison of treatment for obstructive sleep apnea syndrome. *Chest* 1990; 98: 1421.

118 Miki H, Hida W, Chonan T, Kikuchi Y, Takishima T. Effects of submental electrical stimulation during sleep on upper airway patency in patients with obstructive sleep apnea. *Am Rev Respir Dis* 1989; 140: 1285.

119 White DP, Zwillich CW, Pickett CK, Douglas NJ, Hudgel DW, Weil JV. Central sleep apnea: improvement with acetazolamide therapy. *Arch Intern Med* 1982; 142: 1816.

120 Working Party of the Royal College of Physicians of London. *Sleep Apnoea and Related Conditions.* London: Royal College of Physicians, 1993.

48

HYPERVENTILATION SYNDROMES

ANTHONY SEATON

The symptom of breathlessness is one of the principal reasons for referral of a patient to a chest clinic and for acute admission into hospital. It is a symptom that everyone is familiar with from the effects of exertion but one that not uncommonly causes difficulties for individuals in distinguishing normal from abnormal breathlessness. The previously fit person who becomes unfit and fat from lack of exercise and overeating notices shortness of breath during activities that earlier had been carried out without difficulty, and may interpret this as indicating serious heart or lung disease. Similarly, anxious or obsessive people may seize upon an awareness of the process of respiration and interpret the pattern as abnormal. Once focused on such a symptom, it is easy to develop an obsessive interest in the suspected abnormal function of the organ, sufficient to prompt a visit to a doctor. Any subsequent indication by the doctor of uncertainty about the cause or implications of the syndrome is likely to reinforce the patient's anxiety and help perpetuate the complaint. It is therefore important that all chest physicians, to whom such patients are often referred, are aware of the syndrome of behavioural breathlessness, its causes and the methods of managing it.

The two important syndromes of behavioural breathlessness are hyperventilation, which usually occurs in attacks but rarely may become chronic, and sighing. Both types are described by patients as shortness of breath and need to be distinguished from breathlessness of organic aetiology. Hyperventilation in normal people causes a wide range of symptoms related to hypocapnia and alkalosis, vasoconstriction and stimulation of chest wall muscle receptors, and these symptoms may be interpreted by patients with hyperventilation syndrome as further evidence of organic disease.

Control of respiration

This is discussed in Chapter 2. The involuntary system is based on rhythmical discharge of neurones in the pontine and medullary respiratory nuclei that respond to stimuli from the carotid and medullary chemoreceptors; the receptors in the carotid bodies respond primarily to arterial hypoxia while those in the floor of the fourth ventricle respond to arterial and cerebrospinal fluid pH and $P\text{co}_2$. In addition, sensory stimuli from lung and airway receptors transmitted via the vagus nerve may modify the pattern of respiration. Inspiratory and expiratory neurones are found in the spinal cord, supplying the diaphragm via the phrenic nerve (C3–C5) and the intercostal, accessory respiratory and abdominal muscles through spinal nerves down to T12.

Voluntary control of respiration is possible because higher neural centres are able temporarily to override the brainstem control centres, by direct inhibition or stimulation of spinal motor nerves via corticospinal pathways or of brainstem control via corticobulbar pathways. It is with this voluntary control of respiration that this chapter is primarily concerned.

Causes

Hyperventilation may be defined as ventilation sufficient to reduce $P\text{aco}_2$ while maintaining a high $P\text{ao}_2$. This excludes breathlessness due to diseases that impair gas exchange, such as pulmonary fibroses and cardiac failure, and those with airflow obstruction such as asthma. However, it should be noted that behavioural hyperventilation can occur in these conditions as readily as it can in an otherwise healthy person. The definition also excludes breathlessness due to exercise and to hypoxia. There are organic causes of hyperventilation as well as psychogenic, and the most important are shown in Table 48.1. In any case of suspected hyperventilation it is essential to reassure oneself that there is not an organic cause. This differential diagnosis is discussed below.

Symptoms

Haldane and Poulton [1] first described the characteristic and varied symptoms associated with hyperventilation

Table 48.1 Causes of hyperventilation.

Lung disease
Asthma
Pulmonary embolism
Multiple arteriovenous fistulae

Brain disease
Midbrain tumour
Meningitis
Meningeal lymphoma
Langerhans' histiocytosis
Rett's syndrome

Metabolic acidosis
Renal failure
Renal tubular acidosis
Diabetic ketoacidosis
Lactic acidosis in shock
Gastrointestinal loss of bicarbonate
Metformin acidosis
Aspirin poisoning
Methyl alchohol poisoning
Ethylene glycol poisoning

Psychogenic
Panic attacks
Anxiety, depression
Hysteria

and hypocapnia, and generations of medical students have since experienced a selection of these symptoms in their physiology practical classes. The most common are lightheadedness, dizziness and paraesthesiae, which may lead to syncope and tetany. Other symptoms include chest pain, palpitations and a range of feelings of psychological discomfort. Symptoms occur at around an end-tidal P_{CO_2} of 2.66 kPa (20 mmHg) on average, with a threshold of no higher than 3.86 kPa (29 mmHg) [2]. Various mechanisms probably contribute to their causation, including alkalosis, cerebral and peripheral vasoconstriction, stimulation of chest wall stretch receptors and falls in blood phosphate concentrations [3–7]. The subject has been well reviewed by Gardner [8].

Behavioural breathlessness

Hyperventilation

Clinical features

Patients with psychogenic hyperventilation complain of breathlessness disproportionate to the amount of exercise taken or any cardiopulmonary impairment detected [8–10]. Indeed, they frequently complain of episodic breathlessness at rest. Their symptoms often vary substantially from day to day and, if asked, admit that breathing in is harder than breathing out. Breathlessness may be,

though not always, associated with other symptoms. These may mimic cardiac disease with chest pain or palpitations, and in some patients hyperventilation may provoke coronary artery spasm and genuine attacks of angina [11,12]. Neurological disease may be mimicked, with dizzinesss, lightheadedness, syncope, tingling in the fingers and muscle cramps. Panic attacks may be a feature [13,14], and the author has seen one patient with an epileptic tendency in whom grand mal attacks were brought on by hyperventilation. The term 'hyperventilation syndrome' was introduced in 1937 to describe this condition, in the belief that the symptoms were the result of the hyperventilation [15].

Investigation of such patients has shown that a high proportion suffer from symptoms indicating a psychiatric illness [9]. Depression, not always clinically overt, is common as is anxiety. In a relatively few cases, hysteria or motivation by the prospect of gain, for example sympathy from a spouse or in pursuit of litigation, may be important factors. A careful history often indicates that the patient has an obsessional personality and that the perceived illness was provoked by a traumatic event such as bereavement, separation or divorce. Hyperventilation does not seem to be a feature of the chronic fatigue syndrome [16], although it might be expected to occur in some cases. Bad medical management has a way of making matters much worse, and resentment at either actual or perceived medical incompetence may be detected in patients with hyperventilation. Doctors involved in examining lawyers' clients as part of civil litigation proceedings frequently see patients with disproportionate breathlessness. Not all in this situation are deliberately exaggerating (though many are); some have been made genuinely anxious by a perceived gloomy prognosis, given by rather thoughtless or stupid doctors, relating to a trivial condition such as pleural plaques or mild asthma and have developed psychogenic breathlessness.

Diagnosis

An essential step in making the diagnosis is to exclude an organic cause of the breathlessness. The syndrome is usually suspected strongly by the experienced chest physician from the history and from observation of the patient while taking it. A careful examination of lungs and heart is not only essential for diagnosis but is also of therapeutic value. It should be remembered that hyperventilation may occur in patients with organic lung or heart disease and is not uncommon in patients with asthma and other chronic airways disease [17,18]. In such subjects, a peak flow chart is of considerable value in allowing the dissociation between symptoms and flow rates to be demonstrated. Detailed lung function testing and ECG are similarly useful to reassure the patient about the absence of organic disease.

A simple exercise test, such as an 8-min run or brisk walk in or near the clinic, may be helpful as a means of indicating to the patient that exercise tolerance is unimpaired. However, many such patients complain of severe symptoms during exercise and formal testing has shown that inappropriate hyperventilation may occur on exercise as well as at rest [9].

Some physicians who have studied the syndrome find hyperventilation tests of value in diagnosis, by reproducing the patient's symptoms. Howell [9] recommended a simple test in which the patient is asked to take 20 deep breaths and to stop if he or she feels odd in any way. If this does not reproduce the patient's symptoms, the diagnosis of psychogenic breathlessness is unlikely to be correct, whereas if it does the diagnosis finds support. There is little to be gained clinically from more complex tests monitoring end-alveolar $P\text{CO}_2$. There is no clear relationship between the rate of change in $P\text{CO}_2$ and symptoms [2], and it has been shown in a controlled study that patients with hyperventilation syndrome develop symptoms similarly with hypocapnic and isocapnic hyperventilation [19]. This study also demonstrated, by using ambulatory $P\text{CO}_2$ monitoring, that symptoms did not correlate with changes in $P\text{CO}_2$. It seems therefore that hyperventilation producing hypocapnia is but one symptom of the underlying psychological illness, and not necessarily the cause of the other somatic symptoms. In support of this concept, other studies have shown symptoms to be provoked by psychological stress tests as readily as by hyperventilation [20].

Differential diagnosis

The main problem of differential diagnosis arises in patients with genuine organic disease such as asthma or other chronic heart and lung disease [21]. In lung disease, demonstration of inappropriate breathlessness on formal exercise testing or on a chart recording both symptoms and peak flow rate is necessary. In the case of chest pain, reproduction by deep breathing in the absence of ECG changes is reassuring. If ischaemic changes do occur, further investigation by angiography and hyperventilation is obviously necessary. Two respiratory diseases in particular may cause hyperventilation with no other obvious chest signs: pulmonary embolism and multiple arteriovenous fistulae [22–24]. In breathlessness due to pulmonary embolism, anxiety is often quite justifiably present and it is not uncommon for the diagnosis of psychogenic hyperventilation to be considered. $P\text{aCO}_2$ is low but $P\text{aO}_2$ is also usually reduced and the alveolar–arterial oxygen gradient is increased. Arteriovenous malformations may be multiple and not obvious on chest radiography, although finger clubbing and often a sufficiently low $P\text{aO}_2$ to cause cyanosis are present.

Hyperventilation due to acidosis may still catch the unwary [25], but in contrast to psychogenic breathlessness the patient with Kussmaul respiration may look remarkably unconcerned about what appears to be distressing breathlessness. Measurement of arterial blood gases together with blood sugar and urea quickly show the cause of the problem. The acidotic respiration of aspirin or methyl alcohol poisoning constitutes a well-known presentation in the emergency department, since these patients often look suitably anxious or depressed. Diagnostic confusion should not arise in the intensive care unit with breathlessness due to sepsis or blood loss [26]. Neurological disease is a relatively rare cause of hyperventilation, and may cause considerable diagnostic difficulties if it is not considered. A stroke in the region of the brainstem, multiple sclerosis, malignant meningeal infiltration by lymphoma, and Langerhans' cell histiocytosis (histiocytosis X) have all been described as rare causes [27–31]. In these syndromes, the hyperventilation is chronic.

Rett's syndrome is a brain disorder of young females, starting in infancy and progressing through the first two decades of life, characterized by autistic behaviour, abnormal hand movements, epilepsy, dementia, neurogenic scoliosis, and episodic hyperventilation and apnoea [32–34]. It is perhaps caused by a deficiency of dopaminergic neurotransmitters. The disordered control of breathing appears to result from higher cortical brain damage, since polysomnographic studies in such patients have shown a normal pattern during sleep [35].

Management

The first step in the management of psychogenic hyperventilation is exclusion of organic disease and reassurance of the patient that none is present. In many cases this is possible at the time of the first consultation if a few simple tests as described above prove to support the diagnosis. This reassurance should be firm, as any doubt in the doctor's mind will be readily apparent to the anxious patient. An acute attack in an anxious individual is very easily recognized, and once seen is not forgotten; it is usually managed by asking the patient to rebreathe in a paper bag, thus allowing the symptoms generated by hypocapnia to be relieved and their cause demonstrated. Subsequent steps in management are still at the stage of individual preference based on experience, experience quite likely to be of application only to the sorts of patients that one physician sees. However, in general a sensible approach would seem to be as follows.

Explain the breathlessness

Having been told that there is nothing the matter with heart and lungs, the patient, though reassured, still wishes to have an explanation of the symptoms. It is necessary therefore to explain how breathing normally occurs involuntarily but that awareness of the process can cause alterations in its pattern. A useful analogy is running downstairs, something that most people can do in a hurry but that can become awkward and even lead to a fall if too much thought is given to where one's feet should be placed on every step. It can then be explained that once one becomes aware of the process of breathing it is a small step to becoming anxious that it is not proceeding normally and this may lead to a vicious cycle of increasing anxiety and breathlessness. This explanation needs to be approached with care as some patients are quite resistant to the suggestion that their symptoms are non-organic and may interpret such an idea with denial or outright hostility. Clearly, the rapport established with the patient in the consultation is a determinant of success in managing this part of the process. The author prefers to discuss these mechanisms in a way that emphasizes their organic aspects—control by the brain, symptoms of hypocapnia (despite what was said above about this not necessarily being the cause of all the symptoms) and so on—and to explain that the syndrome is a common accompaniment of stress of one sort or another. The concept of 'stress' is now quite well appreciated by the general public and does not seem to be associated with the same amount of perceived stigma as a more psychiatric label such as depression. It is useful to point out that the syndrome is common and one with which chest physicians are quite familiar and which occurs particularly in perfectionists.

Evaluate the effectiveness of reassurance and explanation

In many less severe cases, this simple procedure is enough to give the patient sufficient insight into the condition to relieve anxiety and cure the symptoms. It is therefore sensible not to take the process any further initially but to arrange to review the patient after an interval in order to assess progress. It is apparent that overall cure depends on relief of the primary cause, and it may well be that the hyperventilation disappears but that other psychosomatic symptoms replace it. If this is the case, the psychological problem needs to be addressed, not necessarily by the chest physician.

Discuss with the patient possible causative factors

Again this requires a delicate approach and is often best done in terms of stress. The history may have revealed evidence of symptoms of depression or anxiety and of an obsessional or hysterical personality. Possible precipitating factors should be explored by asking tactfully about any events that may have occurred about the time that the symptoms started. Apart from obvious factors such as marital difficulties and bereavement, common causes nowadays include stress in the workplace, loss of employment, troublesome children and financial worries.

Treat the cause

If there is an important environmental cause, such as domestic or work-related problems, these can be addressed by appropriate agencies and this should certainly be considered before starting drug treatment. In severe cases, treatment of the symptom of hyperventilation alone is unlikely to be of benefit without additional psychological treatment. However, various forms of re-education of breathing patterns have been reported to be successful in relieving the symptom [36,37].

Take a positive attitude towards recovery

It is the author's practice, based on experience, to be optimistic about recovery. If the patient proves able to complete a simple exercise test it is often possible to demonstrate that no harm has come from that exercise and to persuade the individual to initiate a personal exercise training programme that allows confidence to increase that no serious disease is present. Since many of these patients are slightly, or indeed very, obsessional, they may take well to such advice. One of the author's patients responded to the suggestion to go swimming regularly by doing so daily in the sea off Aberdeen throughout a Scottish winter. Fortunately she did not succumb to pneumonia before being advised that the local pool was perfectly adequate.

Sighing breathlessness

Sighing breathlessness is a minor variant of the hyperventilation syndrome but one seen quite commonly in outpatient clinics [38,39]. The patient complains of the need to take a deep breath or of being unable to get a really good breath. Sometimes sighing can be observed during the consultation, occasionally to the point that one has to stifle a feeling of annoyance that one's best efforts are so boring! The symptom is usually a manifestation of mild anxiety, and reassurance that there is no abnormality of lung function (after appropriate spirometry) is all that is needed. A simple exercise test is of particular value in demonstrating to these patients that all is well with their lungs.

References

1 Haldane JS, Poulton BA. The effect of want of oxygen on respiration. *J Physiol* 1908; 37: 390.

2 Rafferty GF, Saisch SGN, Gardner WN.

Relation of hypocapnic symptoms to rate of fall of end-tidal P_{CO_2} in normal subjects. *Respir Med* 1992; 86: 335.

3 Okel BB, Hurst JW. Prolonged hyperventila-

tion in man: associated electrolyte changes and subjective symptoms. *Arch Intern Med* 1961; 108: 157.

4 Brown EB. Physiological effects of

hyperventilation. *Physiol Rev* 1953; 33: 445.

5 Mayou R. Atypical chest pain. *J Psychosom Res* 1989; 406: 393.

6 Rappoport S, Stevens CD, Engel GL, Ferris ER, Logan M. The effect of voluntary over-breathing on the electrolyte equilibrium of arterial blood in man. *J Biol Chem* 1946; 163: 411.

7 Saltzman HA, Heyman A, Sieber HO. Correlation of clinical and physiologic manifestations of hyperventilation. *N Engl J Med* 1963; 268: 1431.

8 Gardner WN. The pathophysiology of the hyperventilation disorders. *Chest* 1996; 109: 516.

9 Howell JBL. Behavioural breathlessness. *Thorax* 1990; 45: 287.

10 Gardner WN. Hyperventilation syndromes. *Respir Med* 1992; 86: 273.

11 Weiner H. Stressful experience and cardiorespiratory disorders. *Circulation* 1991; 83 (Suppl 4): 112.

12 Minoda K, Yasue H, Kugiyama K *et al.* Comparison of the distribution of myocardial blood flow between exercise-induced and hyperventilation-induced attacks of coronary spasm: a study with thallium-201 myocardial scintigraphy. *Am Heart J* 1994; 127: 1474.

13 Hoes MJ, Colla P, van Doorn P, Folgering H, de Swart J. Hyperventilation and panic attacks. *J Clin Psychol* 1987; 48: 435.

14 Cowley DS, Roy-Byrne PP. Hyperventilation and panic disorder. *Am J Med* 1987; 83: 929.

15 Kerr WJ, Dalton JW, Gliebe PA. Some physical phenomena associated with the anxiety states and their relation to hyperventilation. *Ann Intern Med* 1937; 11: 961.

16 Saisch SGN, Deale A, Gardner WN, Wessely S. Hyperventilation and chronic fatigue syndrome. *Q J Med* 1994; 87: 63.

17 McFadden ER, Lyons HA. Arterial blood gas tensions in asthma. *N Engl J Med* 1968; 278: 1027.

18 Burns BH, Howell JBL. Disproportionately severe breathlessness in chronic bronchitis. *Q J Med* 1969; 38: 277.

19 Hornsveld HK, Garssen B, Fiedeldij Dop MJC, van Spiegel PI, de Haes JCJM. Double-blind placebo-controlled study of the hyperventilation provocation test and the validity of the hyperventilation syndrome. *Lancet* 1996; 348: 154.

20 Hornsveld HK, Garssen B, Fiedeldij Dop MJC, van Spiegel PI. Symptom reporting during voluntary hyperventilation and mental load: implications for diagnosing hyperventilation syndrome. *J Psychosom Res* 1990; 34: 687.

21 Gardner WN, Bass C, Moxham J. Recurrent hyperventilation tetany due to mild asthma. *Respir Med* 1992; 86: 349.

22 Hastings GE, Seery DS, Vine DL. Recent developments in the diagnosis, treatment, and prevention of pulmonary embolism. *Arch Fam Med* 1993; 2: 655.

23 Pennington DW, Gold WM, Gordon RL, Steiger D, Ring EJ, Golden JA. Treatment of pulmonary arteriovenous malformations by therapeutic embolisation. Rest and exercise physiology in eight patients. *Am Rev Respir Dis* 1992; 145: 1047.

24 Kobayashi S, Nishimura M, Nasuhara Y, Miyamoto K, Kawayami Y. A case of pulmonary AV fistula. Possible involvement of adenosine in hyperventilation. *Am J Respir Crit Care Med* 1994; 150: 1718.

25 Treasure RA, Fowler PB, Millington HT, Wise PH. Misdiagnosis of diabetic ketoacidosis as hyperventilation syndrome. *Br Med J* 1987; 294: 630.

26 Soubani AO, Khan FA. Hyperventilation in sepsis and acidosis. What is the limit? *Chest* 1994; 105: 1632.

27 Scialdone AM. Thalamic hemorrhage imitating hyperventilation. *Ann Emerg Med* 1990; 19: 819.

28 Howard RS, Wiles CM, Hirsch NP, Loh L, Newsom Davis J. Respiratory involvement in multiple sclerosis. *Brain* 1992; 115: 479.

29 Shibata Y, Meguro K, Narushima K, Shibuya F, Doi M, Kikuchi Y. Malignant lymphoma of the central nervous system presenting with central neurogenic hyperventilation. *J Neurosurg* 1992; 76: 696.

30 Karp G, Nahum K. Hyperventilation as the initial manifestation of lymphomatous meningitis. *J Neurooncol* 1992; 13: 173.

31 Hool GJ, Marsh HM, Groover RV, Burgert EO, Simmons PS, Reese DF. Episodic central neurogenic hyperventilation in an awake child with systemic histiocytosis. *J Paediatr Child Health* 1993; 29: 154.

32 Kozinetz CA, Skender ML, MacNaughton N *et al.* Epidemiology of Rett syndrome: a population-based registry. *Pediatrics* 1993; 91: 445.

33 Migeon BR, Dunn MA, Thomas G, Schmeckpeper BJ, Naidu S. Studies of X-inactivation and isodisomy in twins provide further evidence that the X chromosome is not involved in Rett syndrome. *Am J Hum Genet* 1995; 56: 647.

34 Chiron C, Bulteau C, Loc'h C *et al.* Dopaminergic D2 receptor SPECT imaging in Rett syndrome: increase of specific binding in striatum. *J Nucl Med* 1993; 34: 1717.

35 Marcus CL, Carrol JL, McColley SA *et al.* Polysomnographic characteristics of patients with Rett syndrome. *J Pediatr* 1994; 125: 218.

36 De Guire S, Gevirtz R, Kawahara Y, Maguire W. Hyperventilation syndrome and the assessment of treatment for functional cardiac symptoms. *Am J Cardiol* 1992; 70: 673.

37 Garssen B, de Ruiter C, van Dyck R. Breathing retraining: a rational placebo? *Clin Psychol Rev* 1992; 12: 141.

38 Perin PV, Perin RJ, Rooklin AR. When a sigh is just a sigh…and not asthma. *Ann Allergy* 1993; 71: 478.

39 Aljadeff G, Molho M, Katz I, Benzaray S, Yemini Z, Shiner RJ. Pattern of lung volumes in patients with sighing breathing. *Thorax* 1993; 48: 809.

49

DISEASES OF THE MEDIASTINUM

DOUGLAS SEATON

Anatomy of the mediastinum

The mediastinum comprises those structures situated between the lungs at the centre of the thorax, the word being derived from the Latin *medius* meaning middle and *stare* to stand. It is bounded superiorly by the thoracic inlet, inferiorly by the diaphragm, posteriorly by the thoracic spine, anteriorly by the sternum and laterally by the parietal pleurae. For descriptive purposes anatomists have drawn an imaginary line on the mediastinal map from the fourth dorsal intervertebral disc (the point at which the paravertebral fascia attaches) to the sternal angle of Louis, thereby creating the superior mediastinum. The remaining inferior compartment is subdivided vertically by the heart to give anterior, middle and posterior mediastinal compartments (Fig. 49.1).

A knowledge of the normal contents of the four mediastinal compartments is helpful when considering the possible causes of a radiographic abnormality in the mediastinum or the likely consequences of its enlargement. All compartments contain vessels, lymph nodes, nerves, fat and connective tissue.

1 The superior mediastinum contains the aortic arch, its three large branches, the upper half of the superior vena cava and its two innominate tributaries. It is also traversed by the trachea, the oesophagus, the thoracic duct and the phrenic, vagus, cardiac and left recurrent laryngeal nerves.

2 The anterior mediastinum contains the thymus gland, which also extends into the superior compartment.

3 The posterior mediastinum contains the spinal nerve roots, which lie in the paravertebral gutters, the descending aorta, the oesophagus, the azygos and hemiazygos veins, the thoracic duct, the vagi and the splanchnic nerves.

4 The middle mediastinum contains the heart and pericardium, the ascending aorta, the lower half of the superior vena cava, part of the azygos vein, the pulmonary arteries and veins, the tracheal bifurcation, the phrenic nerves and inferior vena cava.

Mediastinal tumours and cysts

Predictably, the reported series of mediastinal masses appear in the surgical literature and generally include those tumours and cysts requiring an invasive procedure for diagnosis. For detailed descriptive purposes, many lesions are conventionally omitted from such series although they remain important in the differential diagnosis of a mediastinal lesion. These include the following:

1 diaphragmatic lesions, including eventrations and herniae (commonly oesophageal hiatus, occasionally foramina of Morgagni, Bockdalek or post-traumatic), as discussed in Chapter 46;

2 oesophageal tumours and megaoesophagus due to achalasia of the cardia;

3 mediastinal metastases and direct invasion of the mediastinum by tumour from other anatomical areas;

4 mediastinal lymph node enlargment as a manifestation of systemic disease, including lymphoma (see Chapter 42) and non-neoplastic granulomatous disease;

5 retrosternal extension of a thyroid goitre in the neck, except for a minority that cannot be removed by a cervical approach;

6 aneurysms of the aorta and its major branches;

7 ventricular aneurysms;

8 a minority of rare conditions, including tumours of the trachea and heart, skeletal lesions and paravertebral abscess.

Incidence

The overall incidence of mediastinal cysts and tumours is not known. A series of 105 patients collected over a 10-year period in Edinburgh resulted in an estimated incidence of 1 per 100000 per year. These lesions were seen approximately three times more commonly than bronchial adenomas over the same period. Conversely, for every case of primary mediastinal cyst or tumour, 30 cases of bronchial carcinoma and seven cases of oesophageal carcinoma were seen [1]. North American estimates for

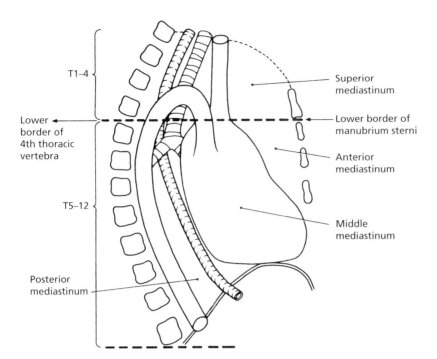

Fig. 49.1 Subdivisions of the mediastinum.

mediastinal lesions have ranged from 1 per 2500 to 1 per 3400 admissions to large medical centres [2,3].

The relative proportion of different mediastinal lesions varies according to individual series and must reflect both local patterns of referral and surgical practice. Four large series containing 974, 251, 209 and 202 cases all found that neural tumours were the most common mediastinal lesion, accounting for 20–27% of cases [4–7]. The two largest series placed thymic lesions a close second (19 and 26% respectively), with developmental cysts a close third (18 and 21% respectively) [4,5]. Thus for practical purposes, neural tumours, thymic lesions and developmental cysts can each be regarded as having a similar incidence of about 20%.

If the foregoing three groups of tumours vie for first place, then mediastinal teratomas and lymphomas compete for fourth. One series did not include cases of extrathymic mediastinal lymphoma (regarded as a mediastinal manifestation of a systemic disease) [5], but those that included this pathological group found that it accounted for approximately 12% of cases compared with about 11% for teratomas and other germ-cell tumours [4–7].

Neural tumours, thymic lesions, developmental cysts, teratomas/germ-cell tumours and lymphoma together account for approximately 88% of primary mediastinal masses, those lesions that remain being rare (Table 49.1). These frequencies are in broad agreement with the earlier calculations of Silverman and Sabiston [8].

The relative frequencies of primary mediastinal lesions differ in children in that neural tumours are more common, accounting for 40% of the total compared with

20% in adults. Conversely, thymic cysts and tumours, which make up 20% of adult lesions, are extremely rare in childhood. Most series place lymphoma as the second most common mediastinal lesion in children (20%), with teratomas and developmental cysts accounting for about 10–15%.

Clinical features

About one-third to half of patients in whom mediastinal cysts or tumours are found are asymptomatic at the time of diagnosis [2,5,8–10]. These figures also apply to children [8,11]. If the practice of performing routine chest radiographs on apparently healthy subjects were to become more widespread, then this proportion would increase. This is illustrated by one series in which 72% of military personnel found to have mediastinal tumours on routine radiographic screening were symptom-free [12].

The absence of symptoms at the time of diagnosis is a good prognostic sign as about 90% of these patients have a benign lesion [1,10,12], whereas in patients who are symptomatic about half have benign and half malignant lesions. It follows that although malignant lesions are more likely to produce symptoms than benign ones, the presence of symptoms need not imply malignancy.

The symptoms most frequently encountered are cough, breathlessness and chest pain [1,2,8–10,13]. These are usually a consequence of compression or invasion of mediastinal structures. Malaise, anorexia, weight loss, weakness and fever may occur as the non-specific features of any malignant process. When cough is present it is often recurrent and the patient may receive repeated courses of

Table 49.1 Classification of principal mediastinal tumours and cysts (see text).

Neural
Nerve sheath tumours
   Schwannoma*
   Neurofibroma*
   Malignant peripheral nerve sheath tumour*†

Autonomic nervous system tumours
   Ganglioneuroma
   Ganglioneuroblastoma*†
   Neuroblastoma†
   Paraganglioma†
      Aorticopulmonary*
      Aorticosympathetic*

Thymic
Thymic hyperplasia
Thymoma†
Thymic cyst

Thyroid
Retrosternal goitre

Germ-cell tumours
Benign
   Mature cystic teratoma*
Malignant
   Seminoma*†
   Non-seminomatous
      Teratocarcinoma*†
      Choriocarcinoma*†
      Endodermal sinus tumour*†
      Embryonal carcinoma†
      Mixed varieties†

Lymphoma†

*Foregut duplications or cysts**
Bronchogenic*
Gastroenteric*
Neurenteric

*Pleuropericardial cyst**

*Synonymous terms indicated in the text.
†Malignant neoplasm.
Note: other lesions, many of them rare, are dicussed in the text.

Table 49.2 Some systemic and endocrine syndromes associated with mediastinal tumours (see text).

Syndrome	Tumour
Myasthenia gravis	Thymoma; thymic hyperplasia
Gynaecomastia, Klinefelter's syndrome	Non-seminomatous germ-cell tumour
Hyperparathyroidism	Parathyroid adenoma
von Recklinghausen's disease	Neurofibromas
Diarrhoea, sweating, tachycardia, headache, hypertension	Functioning autonomic nervous system tumours
Spinal cord compression	Neural (dumb-bell) tumours
Hypoglycaemia	Sarcomas, benign teratomas
Hypogammaglobulinaemia, hypoplastic bone marrow, connective tissue diseases, Whipple's disease	Thymoma
Haematological malignancies	Thymoma, non-seminomatous germ-cell tumours
Malaise, weight loss, pyrexia	Lymphomas, sarcomas, any malignant tumour
Cushing's syndrome	Thymic carcinoid tumour
Multiple endocrine neoplasia syndromes	Parathyroid adenomas

or compression produces neurological impairment less frequently, but may result in hoarseness due to left recurrent laryngeal nerve palsy, hemidiaphragmatic elevation due to phrenic nerve palsy, or incomplete ptosis and a constricted pupil due to involvement of the upper thoracic sympathetic nerves. Spinal cord compression may result from the dumb-bell type of neural tumour (see Fig. 49.3c, p. 1275). Anterior or middle mediastinal tumours may rarely result in pericarditis and cardiac tamponade or heart failure due to obstruction of the right ventricular outflow tract [10]. Pleural effusion is occasionally present and may be chylous because of involvement of the thoracic duct or as a consequence of lymphangiomas [15,16].

In infants and small children compression of the upper airways, superior vena cava and oesophagus may develop with great rapidity as a result of the rapid expansion of a foregut cyst or other lesion in the close confinement of the superior mediastinum. In adults a similar life-threatening situation may rarely arise from the sudden expansion of a retrosternal goitre as a result of haemorrhage into its substance.

Apart from symptoms and signs arising as a result of the compression or invasion of adjacent mediastinal structures, there are several systemic or endocrine syndromes associated with mediastinal tumours. These are listed in Table 49.2 and discussed individually under the appropri-

antibiotic for supposed respiratory tract infection before referral to hospital. Haemoptysis may occur and sometimes the contents of a ruptured cyst are expectorated. Dyspnoea may be associated with wheeze and may lead to inappropriate treatment for asthma. Proximal airway compression is usually accompanied by stridor, which need not always imply a neoplastic cause [14]. Chest pain may be caused by either thoracic wall invasion or intercostal neuralgia and need not indicate inoperability.

Oesophageal compression results in dysphagia, while compression of the superior vena cava causes neck vein engorgement and facial swelling, a syndrome more often associated with malignancy than not. Mechanical traction

ate pathological headings that follow. All of them are rare, with the exception of myasthenia gravis occurring in association with thymic lesions.

Mediastinal neural tumours

Mediastinal neural tumours (Table 49.3) are usually but not exclusively found in the posterior mediastinum in both adults and children and comprise the largest single group of tumours in this compartment. They account for about 20% of mediastinal lesions in adults [17]. Over three-quarters of neural tumours in adults are benign, whereas about half are malignant in children [18]. The terminology surrounding these tumours may confuse as the literature is stiff with synonyms. The embryogenesis of the cell types from which neural tumours are derived is a controversial field. However, it has been claimed that during the folding of the primitive dorsal neural plate, certain ectodermal cells separate from it and migrate so that they come to lie apart from the developing neural tube in the embryo. These have been called neural crest cells and it is supposed that they subsequently differentiate via primitive blast cells into different types of mature neural cell, including peripheral nerve cells (or neurocytes) and peripheral nerve sheath (or Schwann) cells.

Peripheral nerve cells (neurocytes) are those from which sympathetic ganglia, including the spinal sympathetic ganglia, are formed. It is from these cells or from more primitive neuroblasts that mediastinal nerve cell, neurocytic or autonomic tumours develop. Benign mediastinal

neurocytic tumours arising from the sympathetic ganglia in the thorax are called ganglioneuromas. The malignant counterparts of these tumours are ganglioneuroblastomas, in which histological ganglionic differentiation remains strong, and the more aggressive neuroblastomas, which are in fact undifferentiated ganglioneuroblastomas in which ganglion cells are no longer an easily recognizable feature. Some earlier authors referred to neuroblastomas as sympatheticoblastomas [19], while others regarded this as a histological subtype [10]. All tumours belonging to this group may produce catecholamines and they are more common in children.

Mediastinal paragangliomas are very rare neurogenic tumours that arise, as the name implies, from the paraganglia, the cellular precursors of which are likely to have migrated from the embryonic neural crest to their final destination juxtaposed to the ganglia of the autonomic nervous system. They are found in the posterior mediastinum in the costovertebral sulcus and also in the region of the aortic arch. These tumours, which tend to occur in adults, may also be hormonally active, producing catecholamines. Hormonally inactive paragangliomas of the chemoreceptor system have been called chemodectomas, while those near the aortic arch have been called aortic body tumours. Hormonally active mediastinal paragangliomas have previously been classified as phaeochromocytomas because they may be morphologically indistinguishable from the adrenal paraganglioma of that name. Indeed all these mediastinal tumours are paragangliomas, so it is best to drop the terms 'chemodectoma' and 'aortic body tumour' and reserve the term 'phaeochromocytoma' for paragangliomas occurring in the adrenal medulla. The anatomical site of mediastinal paragangliomas can be described as aorticopulmonary for those found in the region of the aortic arch and aorticosympathetic for those found in the costovertebral sulcus of the posterior mediastinum [20]. It used to be thought that the presence or absence of chromaffin substance in paragangliomas correlated closely with hormonal activity, those that were chromaffin-positive being active (e.g. phaeochromocytoma) and those that were chromaffin-negative being inactive. However, it is now appreciated that the chromaffin reaction may be capricious [20] and that some chromaffin-negative paragangliomas may be hormonally active [21] and vice versa [22,23]; thus paragangliomas should be described as 'hormonally active/functioning' or 'hormonally inactive/non-functioning', without attaching complete reliance to their chromaffin status.

Nerve sheath cells give rise to both the Schwann cells and the perineural and endoneural fibrous tissue. Schwannomas (syn. neurilemmoma) are tumours that arise from Schwann cells, previously known as lemmocytes. It was thought that neurofibromas arose from perineural or endoneural fibrous tissue but it now appears

Table 49.3 Mediastinal neural tumours (see text).

Currently favoured term	Synonyms
Benign peripheral nerve sheath tumours	
Schwannoma*	Neurilemmoma
Neurofibroma*	
Malignant peripheral nerve sheath tumour	Neurosarcoma, neurofibrosarcoma, neurogenic sarcoma, malignant schwannoma, malignant neurinoma
Granular cell tumour	Granular cell myoblastoma
Automonic nervous system tumours	Nerve cell or neurocytic tumours
Ganglioneuroma*	
Ganglioneuroblastoma	
Neuroblastoma	Sympatheticoblastoma,
Paraganglioma	
Aorticopulmonary	Chemodectoma
Aorticosympathetic	aortic body tumour
	Mediastinal phaeochromocytoma, chromaffinoma

*Benign neoplasm.

that they too arise predominantly from Schwann cells, although they contain all elements of the nerve. The fact that both these neoplasms may occur in the same patient and sometimes even within the same tumour mass lends further credence to a common cell of origin. Both schwannomas and neurofibromas were referred to collectively in the older literature as neurofibromas. They may be regarded as benign although neurofibromas and rarely schwannomas have potential for undergoing change to their malignant counterpart, the malignant peripheral nerve sheath tumour (MPNST). Earlier authorities used the terms 'malignant neurilemmoma' or 'malignant schwannoma' synonymously with MPNST [24]. A third and extremely rare type of nerve sheath tumour thought to be derived from either Schwann cells or their precursors is the granular cell tumour, originally thought to be of muscle cell origin and called granular cell myoblastoma [25,26].

Peripheral nerve sheath tumours

There are three major neoplasms in this category, the benign schwannoma and neurofibroma and MPNST.

Benign: schwannoma and neurofibroma

Relative frequency and pathological features

In adult series, benign nerve sheath tumours constitute the largest single group of neural neoplasms in the mediastinum [4,5], although in children they are much less common than autonomic nervous system (syn. nerve cell or neurocytic) tumours [11]. Several authors have reported that neurofibroma is the more common tumour [2,5,13,27–29]. However, the majority of workers find that schwannoma is by far the most common and review of 10 different series reporting 398 cases of these two tumour types finds that 70% of them were schwannomas [2,4,6,9,13,27,28,30–32]. Histologically mixed forms have been reported in which the pattern varies between sections in the same tumour [28] and this may account for some differences in histopathological reporting. Most neural tissue in the mediastinum is situated posteriorly in the paravertebral gutters and for this reason benign nerve sheath tumours in common with other neurogenic tumours are often found in this location, although they may also arise from other intrathoracic nerves.

Schwannomas are rounded tumours that are well encapsulated and easily removed surgically [28]. They arise from the lateral aspect of their parent nerve, which is usually spinal although occasionally the sympathetic chain or rarely the vagus, phrenic or recurrent laryngeal nerves may be involved [32–34]. They have an organized architecture that may assume a pallisaded or reticular pattern of growth, referred to as Antoris types A and B respectively

[8,35]. Neurofibromas are also nearly always rounded with a similar gross appearance and although usually unencapsulated are generally easily removed [28]. They tend to expand from within the parent nerve, which is usually spinal [31], and present a different histological picture of a less orderly arrangement of tangled and reticular fibrous tissue in which all elements of the nerve trunk may be represented [9]. Both benign nerve sheath tumours enlarge slowly [32,36]; during this process cellular degenerative changes may occur in schwannomas but not neurofibromas [6]. Neurofibromas may be multiple and rarely take on a plexiform configuration in which the tumour assumes a serpentine shape, insinuating itself around the various mediastinal structures so that complete excision may be impossible [5,28,36]. In such cases, the patient is likely to have von Recklinghausen's disease (neurofibromatosis) type 1, and plexiform neurofibromatous proliferation in a limb or elsewhere may produce massive enlargement (elephantiasis neuromatosa). The reported frequency of type 1 (or peripheral) von Recklinghausen's disease in patients from whom neurofibromas are resected varies widely between series but approaches 30% on average [4,6,28,30,31]. Patients with this type of neurofibromatosis, which is inherited as an autosomal dominant, may have neurofibromas at every conceivable site, usually presenting with cutaneous lumps and multiple *café-au-lait* spots plus the common finding of a thoracolumbar scoliosis. Such patients may also have some schwannomas.

Clinical features

Schwannoma and neurofibroma are approximately equally distributed between the sexes. They may both occur at any age but are usually diagnosed between the ages of 30 and 60 years [4,32,36]. The majority are asymptomatic and are discovered following a routine chest radiograph (Fig. 49.2). When symptoms do occur they fall into the general pattern produced by any benign lesion that occupies space in the mediastinum (see above). Spinal cord compression as a result of a dumb-bell or hourglass tumour straddling the intervertebral foramen is a rare but well-recognized complication of both schwannomas and neurofibromas. Segmental pain may be caused by spinal nerve involvement. The radiographic appearances are of a solitary, sharply defined, rounded mass, usually occupying a paravertebral sulcus (Fig. 49.3a,b). The ribs may sometimes be splayed by lesions of sufficient size and the adjacent intervertebral foramen may be enlarged, particularly in the case of a dumb-bell tumour, the presence of which may be confirmed by spinal magnetic resonance imaging (MRI) (Fig. 49.3c). Posterior mediastinal opacities in patients with von Recklinghausen's disease are very occasionally caused by an intrathoracic meningocele, which may easily be mistaken for a neurofibroma on a chest radiograph. In this case the dura may herniate through an intervertebral foramen, the meningeal sac coming to lie in the paravertebral gutter. Associated scalloping of the posterior margins of two or three adjacent vertebral bodies with splaying of the overlying ribs are characteristic findings, as is widening of the corresponding intervertebral foramen. The nature of this problem may be shown by MRI. If intervention is required, the sac may be excised and its neck closed at thoracotomy [37].

Both schwannomas and neurofibromas may very rarely occur intratracheally, in which case they may be treated by either endoscopic or laser resection [38,39]. Two cases of mediastinal schwannoma apparently occurring in association with nephrotic syndrome have been described in the literature [40]. Sudden, presumed dysrhythmic death has been reported in a young man with type 1 von Recklinghausen's disease, who was found at postmortem to have a massive neurofibroma involving the vagus nerve [33]. Uncomplicated benign neural tumours in the posterior mediastinum are conventionally removed by posterolateral thoracotomy, although more recently 'three-hole' thoracoscopic removal has been used. The latter procedure takes longer and may be difficult with large tumours but patients tend to have a shorter hospital stay and may return to work sooner [41]. Dumb-bell tumours are dealt with by a joint neurosurgical and thoracic approach (see below).

Malignant: MPNST

Although MPNST is now the usual term, there are the inevitable synonyms including neurosarcoma, neurofibrosarcoma, neurogenic sarcoma, malignant schwannoma and malignant neurinoma. About half of all cases are thought to occur *de novo*, the remainder developing in a neurofibroma or rarely in a schwannoma. They are more

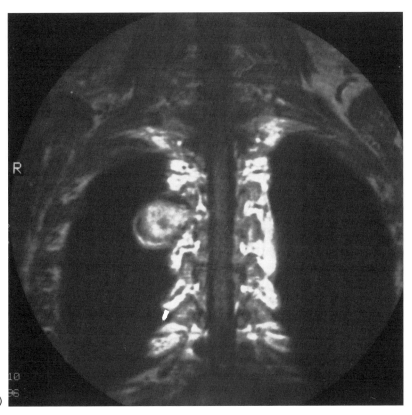

(a)

(b)

Fig. 49.2 (a) Asymptomatic right upper mediastinal tumour that on excision proved to be a neurofibroma. (b) MRI of the neurofibroma showing no evidence of spinal cord compression or displacement.

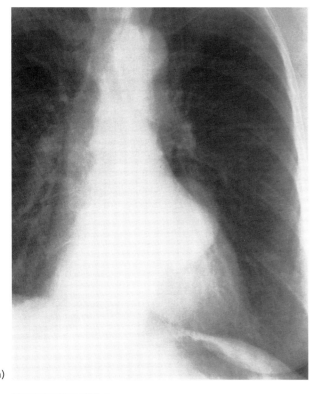

(a)

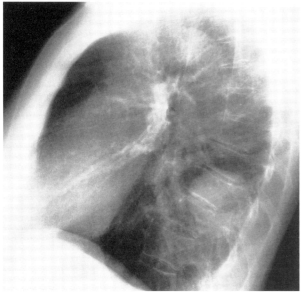

(b)

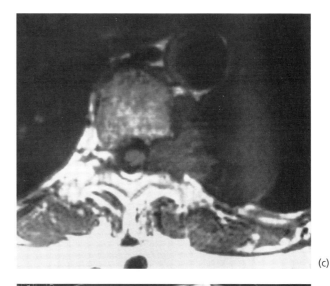

(c)

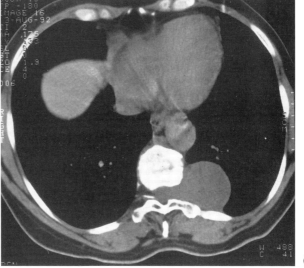

(d)

Fig. 49.3 (a,b) Asymptomatic tumour situated in the posterior mediastinum and on excision found to be a neurofibroma. (c) MRI of the lesion shows a dumb-bell tumour at the T9/T10 level extending through the intervertebral foramen and reaching the spinal cord without deforming or displacing it. (d) CT of the lesion shows the neurofibroma at the T9/T10 level widening the intervertebral foramen.

likely to occur in patients with type 1 von Recklinghausen's disease and it has been estimated that 10–15% of these individuals harbour tumours that undergo malignant transformation. When this transformation occurs in this group of patients, the site is usually a large nerve trunk in the neck or an extremity, whereas mediastinal or superficial neurofibromas in the periphery rarely become malignant [5,29,42]. MPNST is rare at any age and in nine combined series containing about 400 nerve sheath tumours accounted for 5% [2,6,9,13,27,28,30–32]. In a

small paediatric series of eight nerve sheath tumours only one was an MPNST [11]. As with other neurogenic tumours, the majority are situated in the posterior mediastinum. In addition to the usual symptoms of space occupation in the mediastinum (see p. 1270), MPNST may also produce the general systemic and metastatic features of any malignancy. Nausea and vomiting have been recorded in nerve sheath tumours of the vagus [34,43], and as with other sarcomatous tumours hypoglycaemia may occur. There may be extrathoracic evidence of neurofibromatosis, such as cutaneous *café-au-lait* patches. The prognosis with MPNST is poor because of its tendency to both invade locally and metastasize.

Some MPNSTs of the mediastinum display metaplastic changes and those that contain well-developed skeletal muscle are sometimes referred to as malignant triton tumours [44].

Autonomic nervous system tumours

These arise from autonomic nerve cells, prinicipally the ganglia of the sympathetic chain. They span a spectrum of gradual histopathological change, from the benign ganglioneuroma to the highly malignant neuroblastoma, with ganglioneuroblastoma occupying an intermediate histopathological stage. These mediastinal sympathetic nervous system tumours tend to show greater differentiation than their retroperitoneal counterparts and as a group carry a better prognosis. The benign lesions tend to be seen in older children and adolescents, whereas the malignant lesions tend to occur in younger children. Paragangliomas, as the name suggests, arise from autonomic paraganglionic tissue.

Ganglioneuroma

This is the most common of the three mediastinal sympathetic tumours in both adults and older children but occurs in a younger age group than nerve sheath tumours, most patients being less than 20 years of age [4]. Ganglioneuromas may be found on a chest radiograph taken for some other reason and are usually large before they cause symptoms. They contain nerve fibres and varying numbers of large mature ganglion cells. They are nearly all situated in the posterior mediastinum and in common with other neural tumours occasionally straddle the intervertebral foramen in dumb-bell fashion (see p. 1278), having similar radiographic features to the nerve sheath tumours described above (see Figs 49.2 & 49.3). Their sex incidence is equal and they are benign, encapsulated and slow-growing, lending themselves to curative surgical removal, which is indicated both for diagnostic purposes and because they may have malignant potential [2]. Although von Recklinghausen's disease is typified by the presence of neurofibromas, ganglioneuromas, like schwannomas, may also occasionally occur in this condition [2]. As with all automonic nervous system tumours, ganglioneuromas may be metabolically active, producing catecholamines, although these hormones are less likely to produce symptoms than is the case with neuroblastoma.

Treatment is by surgical removal. Uncomplicated benign neural tumours in the posterior mediastinum are conventionally removed by posterolateral thoracotomy, although more recently 'three-hole' thoracoscopic removal has been used. The latter procedure takes longer and may be difficult with large tumours but patients tend to have a shorter hospital stay and may return to work sooner [41].

Ganglioneuroblastoma

Mediastinal ganglioneuroblastomas are rare tumours in adults. A review of 80 cases found that 50% occurred in the first 3 years of life, while only three were found in patients aged over 20 years [45]. Their sex incidence is equal. As with neuroblastoma, the overall majority occur primarily in the adrenal medulla. Half of all mediastinal cases are diagnosed following a routine chest radiograph and the most common symptoms in the remainder are respiratory. They show histological features intermediate between ganglioneuroma and neuroblastoma, being characterized by ganglion cells with immature forms in a background of differentiating neuroblasts. Their intermediate position may result in some being classified as 'malignant ganglioneuromas' or 'differentiating neuroblastomas'. The vast majority of those occurring in the thorax arise posteriorly from the sympathetic chain. Insinuation into the intervertebral foramina in dumb-bell fashion has been described as with other neurogenic tumours (see Fig. 49.3c). They are often large pear-shaped or lobulated tumours and although the majority are encapsulated they must be regarded as malignant, with a propensity to invade locally more often than spreading by metastasis. Despite this, cure by excision is often possible and this approach, combined in some cases with radiotherapy, has achieved a 5-year survival rate of almost 90% [36]. The outlook is therefore much better than for its more malignant cousin the neuroblastoma, ganglioneuroblastoma being similar in its clincal behaviour to ganglioneuroma. Diagnosis at a young age (<3 years), a localized situation and a high degree of histological differentiation are all good predictive factors. The prognosis of mediastinal ganglioneuroblastoma is better than for abdominal forms, and if bony metastases are found a primary adrenal sympathetic tumour should be suspected.

The tumour is biochemically active in about 10% of cases, producing catecholamines whose metabolites, vanillylmandelic acid, homovanillic acid or cystathionine, may be detected in the urine. These findings may be helpful in a diagnostic sense and are also useful tumour markers, a failure of the levels to fall or a subsequent rise indicating persistent or recurrent tumour. Biochemical activity may account for the symptom of chronic diarrhoea that occurs in some cases.

Neuroblastoma

Neuroblastomas are the third most common tumour in children after acute leukaemia and intracranial neoplasms [46]. They occur only rarely in adults, 50% presenting within the first 2 years of life [47,48]. The sex incidence is equal [48]. Most neuroblastomas are retroperitoneal, usually occurring in the adrenal medulla, although 20% are found in the thorax and nearly all of these arise in the posterior mediastinum from sympathetic neural cells. This malignant autonomic tumour tends to be less well radiographically defined than its more benign counterparts, although in other respects its appearance is similar. In contrast with the preceding two members of this group, patients are usually unwell with anorexia, fever and cough. They occasionally display symptoms such as flushing, sweating, tachycardia, hypertension and diarrhoea that result from catecholamine synthesis, as may occur less frequently with the other members of this group of tumours [11,49]. Spinal cord compression due to dumbbell forms may occur in common with other neural tumours and paraplegia may result [11]. Horner's syndrome, dyspnoea and dysphagia may also occur [17].

Histology shows small round immature cells that may be arranged in rosettes and there may be a variable degree of differentiation within the same neoplasm [8,48]. These tumours are highly malignant and form fleshy masses with ill-defined margins that may attain a large size. They are both locally invasive and prone to metastasize but are notable for their infrequent but well-documented propensity either to regress spontaneously or to mature into benign ganglioneuroma forms [50]. Tumour regression may even occur in the presence of metastases and probably accounts for some 'cures' [51–54]. This behaviour may be due to a phenomemon known as immunological coercion [55].

In those rare cases that occur in adulthood, the natural history of neuroblastomas is rapid in comparison with other malignancies so that survival for 2 years after diagnosis and treatment is an accepted definition of cure, provided there is no evidence of persistent or recurrent disease at that point [48]. Treatment is by surgery, to remove the tumour if possible (if not, to relieve pressure symptoms by debulking) and to obtain histological confirmation [48,56]. Radiotherapy and chemotherapy may provide additional benefit [57]. The main prognostic determinant is the age of the patient at diagnosis; a cure rate of 87% in patients aged under 2 years compared with 34% for those aged 2–12 years has been reported [48]. Localized disease carries a better prognosis, although cures may be achieved with metastatic disease provided there is no radiographic evidence of bony destruction.

Paraganglioma

These tumours are very rare, accounting for 1–5% of neural tumours in the mediastinum [4,30,31]. They arise from autonomic paraganglionic tissue in two principal sites.

1 Most arise in the chemoreceptor tissue around the aortic arch and pulmonary artery, which gives rise to so-called aorticopulmonary paragangliomas. These are the mediastinal counterpart of the carotid body and glomus jugulare tumour. Generally, they are hormonally non-functioning and chromaffin-negative, and in the literature are also referred to as chemodectomas, non-functional non-chromaffin paragangliomas and aortic body tumours [58]. They tend to occur in young adults with an equal sex distribution.

2 The second important site is close to the ganglia of the sympathetic chains in the paravertebral gutters, in which case they are referred to as aorticosympathetic paragangliomas [59]. These tend to be hormonally functioning and chromaffin-positive, producing catecholamines in about 50% of cases. They are sometimes referred to in the literature as chromaffinomas, functional chromaffin paragangliomas or mediastinal phaeochromocytomas, although it is now usual to reserve the term 'phaeochromocytoma' for the corresponding paraganglioma arising in the adrenal medulla [58,60].

There are a few reports of both functioning and nonfunctioning paragangliomas arising in relation to the heart, presumably from the cardiac plexus [61–63]. They may also very rarely occur as a primary intratracheal tumour [64]. The heart and great vessels may both be invaded and obstruction of the superior vena cava has been described [65].

Mediastinal paragangliomas have been recorded in both adults and children and in both sexes, the aorticosympathetic paraganglioma being more common in males, usually occurring in the third to fifth decades [29,66,67].

Paragangliomas are usually encapsulated, yellowish in colour and haemorrhagic; multiple tumours have been described [22,68]. Paragangliomas are highly vascular and the cellular characteristics of those occurring in the usual mediastinal sites are similar [8,22]; furthermore, the usual histological criteria for determining malignant potential cannot be readily applied to them [8,10,31] since they may recur locally or metastasize despite a benign appearance [69].

Aorticopulmonary paragangliomas rarely metastasize but tend to cause significant morbidity and mortality as a result of local spread and recurrence despite the fact that they grow only slowly [8,60]. Although they are traditionally regarded as chromaffin-negative and hormonally inactive, evidence exists to show that they may produce catecholamines in about 3% of cases [21,70].

Aorticosympathetic paragangliomas are usually hormonally active and account for about 2% of catecholamine-producing tumours, the vast majority of which are intra-abdominal, about 80% arising in the adrenal medulla [66]. Very few of these mediastinal tumours are malignant as evidenced by distant metastases [8,10,71]. They may present with episodic hypertension, palpitations, sweating and headache, or they may not produce catecholamines in sufficient quantities to produce symptoms and are discovered as a posterior mediastinal opacity on a routine radiograph. Any suspicion that hypertension is secondary to a catecholamine-producing tumour can be substantiated by assay of blood or urine for catecholamines or their metabolites (vanillylmandelic acid, homovanillic acid or cystathionine) and by performing a phentolamine test if these other tests are equivocal [21,72]. Localization of the tumour first involves abdominal CT to exclude a primary adrenal site followed by a combination of thoracic CT and radioactive isotope scanning using a labelled norepinephrine (noradrenaline) analogue, such as ^{131}I-metaiodobenzylguanidine [66]. Thoracic aortography has also been found useful in localizing mediastinal paragangliomas because of their vascularity [36,73].

The treatment for paragangliomas is surgical and they are relatively radioresistant. Less than half of those in the aorticopulmonary area can be completely resected because of their close association with great vessels; thus they are ultimately fatal, although prolonged survival is still possible as these tumours are usually slow-growing [4,18]. The assay of catecholamine metabolites may prove a useful monitor of disease activity postoperatively in functioning tumours [71].

Clinical problem of dumb-bell tumours

As implied above, the term 'dumb-bell' refers to the shape of neural tumours of various histological types, about 10% of which may straddle an intravertebral foramen and have both intrathoracic and intraspinal components (see Fig. 49.3c) [74]. These tumours are usually but not invariably of nerve sheath origin and are also sometimes referred to as hourglass tumours. They are important to recognize since their removal may be beyond the competence of either a thoracic surgeon or a neurosurgeon alone, the expertise of both being necessary. These tumours should be suspected preoperatively if any long tract signs are present or if the radiographs show either a widened intervertebral foramen or erosion of vertebral pedicles or lamellae. The lesions may be well shown by CT (see Fig. 49.3d), although MRI produces better images with regard to spinal cord displacement. Spinal aortography to identify the artery of Adamkiewicz (which arises from a posterior intercostal artery to supply the inferior portion of the anterior spinal artery) is recommended if the tumour is situated in the lower thoracic region in order that this vessel is not compromised during surgery.

There are considerable advantages in removing the tumour at a single combined neurosurgical/thoracic operation, with a posterior hemilaminectomy to free tumour within the spinal canal and a posterolateral thoracotomy [30,74–76]. This reduces the possibility of cord damage caused by undue traction at the intervertebral foramen or of uncontrolled haemorrhage in the same area.

Other mediastinal tumours of possible neural progenitor cell origin

Some migrating neural crest progenitor cells may differentiate into so-called APUD cells capable of *a*mine *p*recursor *u*ptake and *d*ecarboxylation; tumours that may have arisen from APUD cells have been functionally grouped as APUDomas or neuroendocrine tumours. These include carcinoid tumours (of both 'typical' and 'atypical' histological types), small-cell carcinomas and large-cell neuroendocrine carcinomas. These tumours are found in the lung, where large-cell neuroendocrine carcinoma is often classified as large-cell undifferentiated carcinoma. Carcinoids may occur as primary thymic tumours, as may small-cell carcinoma, although it may be difficult to exclude spread from the lung in the latter case. Atypical carcinoid tumours are more aggressive and may themselves be mistaken for small-cell carcinoma on small biopsies due to sampling error. The capacity for these precursor cells to be chemically active accounts for the propensity of some APUDomas to be hormonally active. Melanocytes are also thought to originate from the neural crest. However, the malignant melanomas that arise from these cells are nearly always cutaneous. Although primary visceral melanomas may occur, they have not been described in the mediastinum other than in the oesophagus [77], those melanomas found in the vicinity of the mediastinum being secondary; two-thirds of patients dying of disseminated melanoma are found to have cardiac metastases [77,78].

Disorders of the thymus

Thymic lesions comprise the largest group of anterior mediastinal masses [2,4,36] (Table 49.4). The thymus gland is a lymphoreticular organ that develops as a pair of solid buds arising predominantly from the third branchial pouch at about the sixth week of embryonic life. It migrates caudally during intrauterine development to lie

Table 49.4 Disorders of the thymus.

Thymic hyperplasia
Thymic cysts
Thymoma
Thymic carcinoma
Thymic carcinoid tumour
Thymolipoma
Germ-cell tumours
Ectopic parathyroid adenomas
Lymphoma
Secondary neoplastic disease

retrosternally in the upper part of the anterior mediastinum. Sometimes this migration is incomplete or bizarre so that it occupies a cervical or some other ectopic site [79]. The thymus has two lobes bound together by fatty tissue and contained in a capsule of loose connective tissue, from which septa arise dividing the gland into lobules. Each lobule has a cortex packed with small lymphocytes and a medulla comprising reticular cells and Hassall's corpuscles, which are zones of squamous cells surrounded by epithelial cells.

In infancy, the thymus gland is large relative to the size of the mediastinum, weighing perhaps 15 g. It doubles in size by puberty and thereafter gradually involutes, returning to its original infantile weight.

Thymic hyperplasia

It is difficult to decide whether a thymus gland that appears to be enlarged on a chest radiograph in early childhood represents one extreme of a wide range of normal variation or whether it contains tumour (Fig. 49.4). In a number of cases coming to surgery with a preoperative diagnosis of thymoma no tumour is present but the gland is grossly hyperplastic and these patients are nearly always infants or small children [4,80]. Thymic hyperplasia may also sometimes occur in adults after successful treatment of malignant disease elsewhere with chemotherapy [81].

The histological criterion of lymphoid follicular hyperplasia of the thymus is the presence of germinal centres in the medulla [5,82]. This may occur without the gland increasing in size, whereas for true thymic hyperplasia to be present the gland itself must increase beyond the upper limits of normal for age. Thymic hyperplasia is not usually associated with symptoms [11] but when symptoms do occur they are seen in small children and are nearly always respiratory [5,6]. The thymus may involute in childhood during any form of stress, including illness and injury, and upon recovery the phenomenon of 'rebound hyperplasia' may occur with resultant pressure symptoms [83]. Thymic involution has also been noted to be pronounced in human immunodeficiency virus infection [84]. Both thymic hyperplasia and thymoma may occur in patients with myasthenia gravis, the former accounting for 50% of thymic abnormalities found after thymectomy in one series of 10 myasthenics [85]. Thymic hyperplasia may also occur in other autoimmune disorders, such as systemic lupus erythematosus and thyrotoxicosis [80]. Thymic hyperplasia cannot normally be differentiated from an intrinsic thymic tumour by radiography, including CT [86].

When an enlarged thymus is found in infancy, steroids have been given as a diagnostic test since they may reduce the size of the hyperplastic gland. Lymphoma, which might also regress with the same therapy, is unusual before the age of 18 months [87]. When surgery has to be undertaken to relieve pressure symptoms, the histological nature of the disorder should be confirmed at operation; resection should be subtotal and confined to that part of the hyperplastic gland causing compression [5].

Thymoma

Pathology

Thymoma is used to refer to tumours of epithelial origin arising in the thymus gland and containing a non-

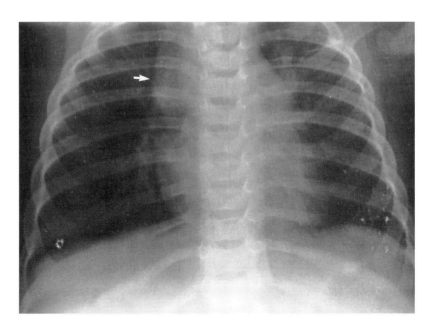

Fig. 49.4 Chest film of infant showing normal thymus as a right upper mediastinal mass (arrowed).

neoplastic lymphocytic component, representing functioning thymic tissue. They comprise about 20% of all mediastinal tumours and cysts and are the most common anterior mediastinal tumours [8]. Three principal histological groups were described in early classifications [88–90]: (i) the epithelial type, in which up to 80% of cells are epithelially derived (subgroups of this class are sometimes referred to as spindle cell, oval cell or epidermoid); (ii) the lymphocytic type, in which up to 80% of cells are lymphocytically derived; and (iii) the mixed or lymphoepithelial type, in which neither cell type predominates. However, these cellular characteristics do not appear to influence prognosis and although more recent histological classifications have related aggressiveness to the appearance of the neoplastic epithelial cell component and their numerical predominance over lymphocytes [91], this remains a controversial area. Prognosis appears to be mainly governed by clinical stage. Thymomas in which the capsule is intact, with no gross or microscopic evidence of invasion, tend to behave in a benign fashion and this is the case in two-thirds to three-quarters of cases [92], whereas those with gross or microscopic invasion through the capsule are regarded as malignant. These have a tendency to invade local structures and also to metastasize [93–95]. Clinical staging is therefore important and all thymomas should be regarded as potentially malignant [96–99].

Clinical features and diagnosis

Thymomas may occur at any age but nearly all present in adult life and are rare before the age of 20 years. There is probably a slight overall male predominance [83,85,96]. Symptoms are present at the time of diagnosis in about 60% of patients, chest pain, dyspnoea, dysphagia and other mediastinal pressure effects having been described. There is in addition a large number of associated immune-mediated systemic syndromes, the most common of which is myasthenia gravis [92,100–103]. Pure red cell hypoplasia is unusual, occurring in about 5% of cases of thymoma [104,105]. Hypogammaglobulinaemia may also occur as may a number of other conditions, the majority of which are rare associations [92,106–108] (see Table 49.2).

The usual chest radiographic features are those of an anterosuperior mediastinal mass (Fig. 49.5) and this impression may be confirmed by CT (Fig. 49.6) [86,109]. Thymomas may rarely occur ectopically in the neck or lung or as a pleural tumour [110]. It is impossible to reliably discriminate between thymic tumour and hyperplasia by imaging techniques. Cystic changes may sometimes occur. The diagnosis of thymoma may be confirmed preoperatively by fine-needle biopsy [96], although this is not usually necessary and should be avoided if surgery is to be undertaken in any case as it runs the risk of tumour implantation [111].

Treatment

The treatment of choice is surgical removal of both the tumour and the entire surrounding gland [96,112,113]. Every effort should be made to keep the capsule intact, although this may not be possible with large tumours such as that illustrated in Fig. 49.6. Surgery is by median sternotomy or thoracotomy or by a transcervical approach. Fortunately, most patients present with localized disease and routine postoperative irradiation following surgery for thymomas with an intact capsule does not improve survival, which is already good [113]. Radiotherapy is usually reserved for cases in which excision has been incomplete, and it may be a useful adjunct for these locally invasive thymomas [112,114,115]. In cases where local invasion prevents complete excision, more extensive surgical debulking procedures, as opposed to simple biopsy, appear to confer no advantage in terms of survival when both are followed by radiotherapy [116,117]. When thymoma does behave in malignant fashion it is usually by local invasion, sometimes with pleural seeding, or by local recurrence. Distant metastases, although less common, are well described and may occur as a late phenomenon, so that long-term follow up is advisable [100,118–120]. The role of chemotherapy in the management of invasive or recurrent thymoma is more controversial and has yet to be properly determined. Suffice to say that thymoma is chemosensitive and remissions have been obtained in small series with combinations of cisplatin, doxorubicin, vincristine and cyclophosphamide, sometimes as an adjunct to surgery and/or radiotherapy, although prospective randomized controlled trials are lacking [112,121,122].

Prognosis

The most important factor contributing to long-term survival is complete surgical resection of tumour with an intact capsule, and when this is achieved the prognosis is excellent. An early large North American surgical series reported the survival rate for patients with non-invasive tumours to be not much dissimilar to that of the general population, whereas more invasive tumours produced a 15-year survival rate of 12.5% [123]. Series where the extent of tumour has been staged report a 5–10-year survival of over 80% for thymomas without evidence of extracapsular invasion, falling to a 10-year survival of 23% where such invasion was evident [124,125].

Myasthenia gravis and thymic disease

Myasthenia gravis is an autoimmune disease, as indicated in nearly all cases by the presence of circulating autoantibodies that bind to acetylcholine receptors in the motor end-plates [126]. It is thought that T lymphocytes

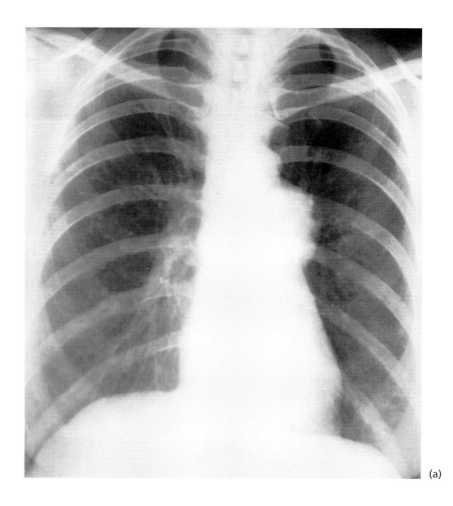

(a)

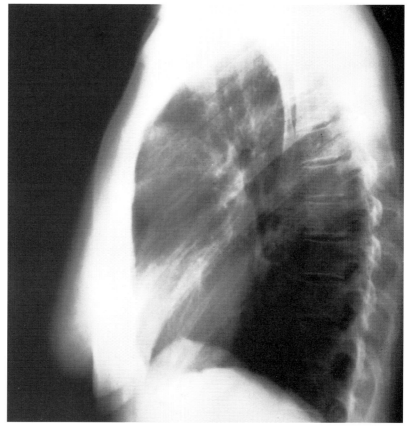

Fig. 49.5 (a) Posteroanterior film showing enlargement over left hilum. (b) Left lateral film showing lesion occupying the anterior mediastinum. On excision it proved to be a thymoma.

(b)

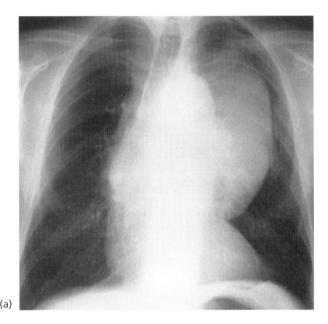

(a)

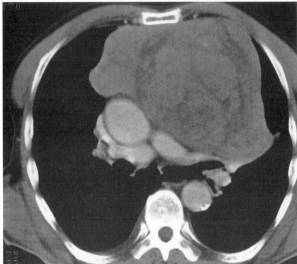

(b)

Fig. 49.6 (a,b) A large anterior mediastinal mass that did not enhance with contrast on CT in a 77-year-old man. It was removed at thoracotomy and found to be a thymoma.

elaborated by the thymus interact with B lymphocytes in order to produce these antibodies, which then result in the depletion of functioning acetylcholine receptor sites at the postsynaptic membranes.

An association between myasthenia gravis and thymic tumours was recorded in 1901 [127]. The reported frequency of thymoma in patients with myasthenia gravis is variable, approximately 10–20% [5,128]. Conversely, 35–40% of patients with thymoma develop myasthenia gravis, sometimes after the tumour has been removed [98,129]. In patients with myasthenia gravis in whom the thymus is removed, the gland is seldom found to be histologically normal and thymic hyperplasia is common, particularly in younger patients, occurring in about 65% of

cases [91]. A thymoma is more likely when a patient with myasthenia gravis is older than 50 years, and this is particularly true in males [130]. A thymoma may therefore be diagnosed before, at the time of or after the onset of myasthenic symptoms. Myasthenia gravis may occur in association with any histological type of thymoma. It remains unclear if or how the pathogenesis of myasthenia gravis is related to the presence of thymomas [92]. It has been shown that the presence of striated muscle antibodies in patients with myasthenia gravis correlates with the presence of a thymoma; these antibodies were absent in over 90% of myasthenic patients without a tumour [86,131].

Thymectomy has an important role in the treatment of myasthenic patients whether a thymoma is present or not [126,132]; indeed symptomatic response may be better when the gland is found to contain follicular hyperplasia rather than thymoma or normal tissue. The results are best in younger patients with a short history of severe myasthenia, although thymectomy may be employed in any patient with deteriorating myasthenia gravis of sufficient severity despite optimal medical treatment [133,134]. Thymectomy in such patients requires close cooperation between the thoracic surgeon, neurologist and anaesthetist. The operation may be carried out successfully using a suprasternal approach, although a sternotomy is often preferred [135]. Preoperatively the dose of anticholinesterase is reduced to a minimum before complete omission in the postoperative period, when the patient is ventilated mechanically and narcotic analgesics need to be administered. Weaning from the ventilator is controlled by blood gas analyses and measurements of ventilatory capacity. Difficulties may arise in distinguishing between weakness as a result of a stress-related myasthenic crisis and a cholinergic crisis due to overdosage with anticholinesterases, the distinction being made by using the edrophonium test. Some work has indicated that high-dose corticosteroid therapy postoperatively may assist in the weaning process [136].

The standards of postoperative care of these patients have improved to such an extent that the presence of myasthenia gravis no longer adversely influences the prognosis of thymoma [96,137]; indeed, paradoxically, patients with thymomas and myasthenia gravis may survive better because their neurological symptoms result in the early detection of the tumour. Although the results from thymectomy are best in young females without tumour, those who do have thymomas may also benefit from an improvement in their myasthenic symptoms, although continued anticholinesterase therapy is the rule in this group.

Thymic cysts

Unilocular or multilocular cystic spaces containing clear fluid or pasty material may occur in otherwise normal thymic tissue. These thymic cysts occur with equal frequency in adults and children [138]. Some are likely to be congenital and these tend to be unilocular, being found anywhere along a line running from the angle of the mandible to the manubrium sterni. Others may be acquired, probably as a result of an inflammatory reaction in thymic tissue; these tend to be multilocular and fibrotic. Although the presence of cysts may be predicted by CT, certain differentiation from thymoma can only follow histological examination, particularly as thymic tumours of various types may cavitate [92]. Cysts are usually asymptomatic but occasionally become very large (Fig. 49.7), in which case they may produce symptoms due to mediastinal compression, including in extreme cases cardiac tamponade [139]. They are otherwise benign but because of the inevitable preoperative diagnostic uncertainty, treatment is by surgical excision. Thymic cysts in association with Hodgkin's disease are rare but well descibed and also tend to cause diagnostic difficulties (see p. 1290) [140,141]. It has been suggested that they may form as a result of the degeneration of treated lymphomatous tissue within the thymus but this is seemingly not always the case and their pathogenesis is uncertain.

Other thymic tumours

The thymus gland may be the site of other tumours, although these are all encountered less frequently than thymoma. Thymic carcinoma is a rare group of tumours distict from thymomas and seemingly unassociated with myasthenia gravis or the other immune-mediated disorders listed in Table 49.2. Various cell types have been described, including squamous, small-cell and undifferentiated carcinomas [142]. Care should be taken to ensure that these are not secondaries from lung as these and other primary tumours elsewhere may occasionally metastasize to the thymus.

Lymphomas of both Hodgkin and non-Hodgkin type may involve the thymus (see p. 1290) and are occasionally confined to it. The diagnosis can reliably be made by open or excision biopsy and treatment depends upon the extent of disease as determined by formal staging.

Carcinoid tumours may rarely arise in thymic neuroendocrine cells and the morphology of most of them is similar to that of the 'atypical' type of bronchial carcinoid tumour. They appear to be more frequent in males, are unassociated with myasthenia gravis and behave in a much more aggressive manner than thymomas, with a tendency to both recur locally and to metastasise [143,144]. A minority of them are associated with endocrine abnormalities, such as Cushing's syndrome and multiple endocrine neoplasia types 1 or 2a [145–147].

Thymolipoma (syn. lipothymoma) is a rare, benign, slowly growing tumour that has the gross appearance of a lipoma but which contains both thymic and fatty elements [148–150]. This tumour may become enormous and is sometimes mistaken for cardiomegaly on plain films because of its propensity to mould itself about the mediastinal structures in a plastic fashion. The use of CT shows it to have the density of fat and may help to make the proper distinction.

Germ-cell tumours, both benign and malignant, may arise in the thymus gland and these are discussed in the following section. Secondary neoplastic disease in the thymus is not uncommon and may sometimes respond to surgery [151]. Occasionally ectopic parathyroid adenomas may be found embedded in the substance of the thymus (see p. 1298).

Miscellaneous thymic disease

Thymic masses have been reported in children with Langerhans' cell histiocytosis (histiocytosis X) [152], in patients with Churg–Strauss syndrome [153] and in giant lymph node hyperplasia (Castleman's syndrome), a condition of uncertain pathogenesis that some regard as hamartomatous, the diagnosis being made after excision biopsy [154,155].

Mediastinal germ-cell tumours

The histogenesis of mediastinal germ-cell tumours remains controversial but it seems probable that these tumours arise as a result of the proliferation of primitive extragonadal germ cells that have the potential to differentiate into various cell types of ectodermal, mesodermal and endodermal origin [36,156,157]. The anterior mediastinum is the most common adult extragonadal site for these tumours, which for some undetermined reason arise in relation to the thymus gland but which are histologically entirely distinct from thymomas. In children, extragonadal germ-cell tumours occur with greater frequency in the sacrococcygeal area [36]. Mediastinal germ-cell tumours may be benign or malignant. The terminology of germ-cell tumours is confusing because of uncertainties surrounding their pathogenesis and because of the wide histological variety that may be encountered. A plethora of synonymous terms have been used and are found scattered in the literature, nomenclature inevitably changing as wise men ponder and as the years go by (Table 49.5).

The most common mediastinal germ-cell neoplasm is mature cystic teratoma (syn. teratoma, benign or mature teratoma, dermoid cyst or tumour, teratodermoid). This tumour is benign and accounts for approximately 80% of germ-cell neoplasms, affecting both sexes equally. The term 'teratoma' was defined by Willis [158] as 'a true tumour comprised of multiple tissues foreign to the part in which the tumour is found'. This term is well entrenched in medical literature and its use will continue but is best

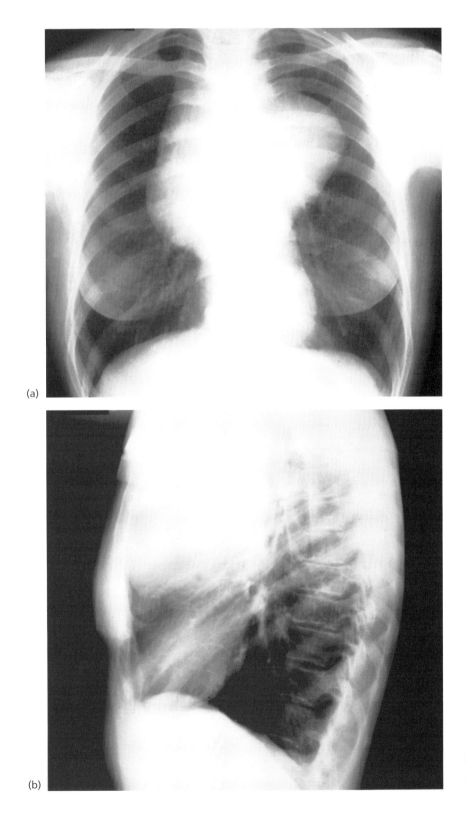

(a)

(b)

Fig. 49.7 Posteroanterior (a) and left lateral (b) chest films of asymptomatic patient with huge thymic cyst.

reserved for benign tumours, the term 'teratocarcinoma' being applied to a malignant counterpart containing a combination of benign teratomatous components and embryonal carcinoma (see below and Table 49.5).

Five distinct subtypes of malignant germ-cell tumour are described: seminoma (affecting males exclusively), teratocarcinoma, embryonal carcinoma, choriocarcinoma and endodermal sinus (or yolk sac) tumour, all of which have a strong male predilection, although rare cases have been reported in females. It is important to realize that the

Table 49.5 Germ-cell tumours of the mediastinum (see text).

Currently favoured terms	Synonyms
Benign germ cell tumour	
Mature cystic teratoma*	Teratoma,
	benign teratoma,
	mature teratoma,
	dermoid cyst,
	dermoid tumour,
	teratodermoid
Malignant germ-cell tumour	
1 Seminoma†	Germinoma,
	dysgerminoma
2 Choriocarcinoma†	Trophoblastic teratoma
3 Endodermal sinus tumour†	Yolk-sac tumour
4 Embryonal carcinoma†	
5 Mixed germ-cell tumour†	
(of types **1–4**)	
6 Teratocarcinoma*	Malignant teratoma
7 Immature teratoma* (age-dependent	
malignant potential)	

* Tissue non-specific.
† Tissue specific.

histological boundaries between these tumours may be indistinct and that they may occur both in mixed and pure form. The reader should be aware that some authors have used the term 'malignant teratoma' subgenerically to include all the above malignant germ-cell tumours, although this practice is not recommended.

Both mature cystic teratomas (benign teratomas) and teratocarcinomas, in common with all germ-cell tumours, arise from immature or primordial germ cells during development. However, in the case of benign teratomas and teratocarcinomas these immature germ cells are pluripotential and still capable of producing a regionally diverse cellular output that results in different lines of embryonal tissue (epithelial, mesenchymal and neural), whereas the remaining pure histological types of germ-cell tumour (seminoma, embryonal carcinoma, choriocarcinoma and endodermal sinus tumours) possess tissue specificity [5,159]. These tissue-specific germ-cell tumours arise in an organ-formative field or 'blastoma' in which the immature germ cells are restricted to single regionally determined patterns of cellular output. Tissue-specific germ-cell tumours are all malignant and although their response to treatment is variable some are curable. The management of these neoplasms has altered significantly in the last 20 years, especially with the introduction of cisplatin-based combination chemotherapy which been found capable of curing advanced disease [160].

The histogenesis of mediastinal germ-cell tumours is controversial. Some investigators have claimed that the tissue-specific germ-cell tumours found in this site represent metastases from occult primary gonadal tumours

[161]. This is improbable for various reasons. Firstly, several studies have excluded a gonadal primary by multiple testicular sectioning [162–164]; secondly, in the case of mediastinal seminoma the disease can be cured by local therapy to the chest [165]. Furthermore, mediastinal metastases from known testicular primary seminomas are rare [166]. Extragonadal germ-cell tumours are all found near the midline and it has been suggested that they arise from primordial germ cells that fail to migrate from the urogenital ridge to the gonads during embryogenesis [162].

Benign germ cell tumours

Mature cystic teratoma

Mature cystic teratomas account for approximately 80% of all mediastinal germ-cell tumours and about 8% of mediastinal tumours of all types [4,5,36]. With very few exceptions indeed they are situated in the anterior or anterosuperior mediastinum, although they are less common anterior mediastinal masses than thymomas and lymphomas [167]. Rare cases have been described in the posterior mediastinum and at more than one intrathoracic site [168–170].

Pathology

Macroscopically, benign germ-cell tumours of the mediastinum are rounded or lobulated and well-encapsulated tumours. They vary very widely in size, the average diameter in a large North American series being about 8 cm [167]. As the name suggests, they are often cystic or loculated and are commonly found at operation to be closely associated with the thymus and adherent to surrounding tissues.

Microscopically, mature tissue from all three germ layers is represented. Ectodermal elements predominate and of these the most common is skin, the cysts being lined by stratified squamous epithelium, hence the old term 'dermoid'. The other common ectodermal elements are hair and sebaceous glands (pilosebaceous units). The most common mesodermal element is smooth muscle followed by fat, cartilage and less frequently bone. Respiratory epithelium is the endodermal component most often found, followed by gut epithelium [167]. Pancreatic tissue may be found and can be enzymatically active, leading to the suggestion that digestive enzyme activity may account for the dense adhesions with surrounding tissues that characterize this tumour [171]. Islet of Langerhans components may also occur, giving mature cystic teratomas the potential to produce hypoglycaemia. A wide variety of other tissues are identifiable, including neural components and occasionally formed teeth. Calcification may also occur in the wall of this tumour (Fig. 49.8), which is

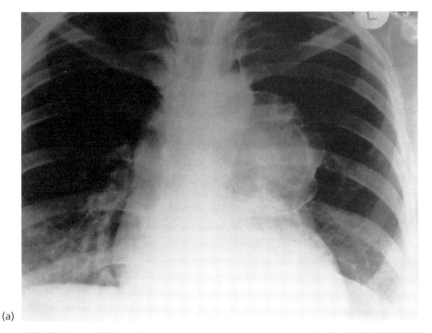

(a)

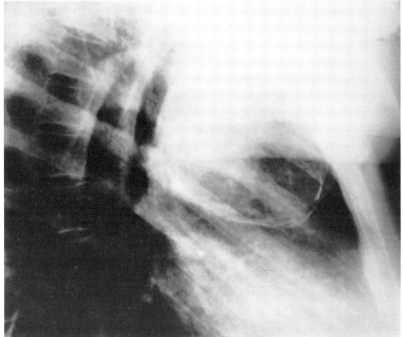

(b)

Fig. 49.8 Posteroanterior (a) and right lateral (b) chest films of asymptomatic patient with calcified anterior mediastinal teratoma. The tumour was found to contain hair.

histologically similar to the more common mature cystic teratoma of the ovary.

Benign mediastinal teratomas may be found at any age but most series show a diagnostic peak in early adulthood [167]. They affect both sexes more or less equally [4,167,172,173], in contrast with malignant germ-cell tumours of the mediastinum that affect males almost exclusively. They are usually a chance radiographic findings in a subject with no respiratory symptoms and there is evidence that asymptomatic diagnosis has become more common [167,172]. Symptoms are more often present in children than adults, pain in the sternal region, back or shoulder and dyspnoea with cough being usual [4,5,167,172]. Uncommonly, symptoms may occur as the result of the erosion of a teratoma into surrounding structures. Bronchial erosion may lead to haemoptysis, with the expectoration of sebaceous material or even hair (trichoptysis). The release of fatty material into the bronchial tree may cause lipoid pneumonia and its spillage into the mediastinum may incite a granulomatous reaction. Rupture into the pericardium may cause pericarditis or tamponade and rupture through the chest wall or into the pleura, aorta and superior vena cava have been recorded [174–176], although all these complications are becoming increasingly uncommon [167]. In subjects with large tumours, evidence of obstruction of the superior vena cava, splaying of ribs, dullness to percussion, wheeze or a pulmonary systolic murmur may sometimes be found, but more commonly physical examination reveals no localizing signs.

Investigations

Chest radiography characteristically shows a well-circumscribed or lobulated anterior mediastinal mass that may extend into one or other lung field (see Fig. 49.8). Flecks of calcification in the wall or substance of the mass and sometimes bone or tooth may be found in 15–40% of cases [167,172,177]. The presence of an air–fluid level may indicate a bronchial communication. Ultrasound examination or CT may show cystic changes with areas of fat density [178], although the diagnosis can only be established with certainty by pathological examination after surgical removal.

Treatment

The treatment of choice is total excision via either thoracotomy or sternotomy. This operation is advisable because of the diagnostic uncertainty that would otherwise exist and also because of the possibility of complications, including very rare malignant change [179,180]. Although these benign germ-cell tumours may be 'shelled out' easily [5], removal is often difficult because of dense adhesions between the lesion and surrounding structures, such as the pericardium, lung, great vessels, thymus and chest wall [172]. Lobectomy may be necessary when a teratobronchial fistula is present. Surgical removal achieves total cure even if excision has been incomplete because of adherence to mediastinal structures [172].

Immature teratoma

Immature teratoma of the mediastinum may be regarded as the potentially malignant counterpart of mature cystic teratoma. It contains immature elements of the three germ layers but unlike teratocarcinoma (see below) contains no component of embryonal carcinoma. The behaviour of this tumour is age-dependent (parallels with neuroblastoma) so that in infancy and early childhood it acts mainly as a space-occupying lesion, whereas after the age of about 14 years it behaves as a malignant tumour invading adjacent structures and metastasizing widely [159].

Malignant germ cell tumours

Approximately 20% of germ-cell tumours of the medi-astinum are malignant [5]. Therapeutically and prognostically it is very important to distinguish between those malignant germ-cell tumours that are pure seminomas and those that contain any non-seminomatous elements [165]. Seminomas and non-seminomatous germ-cell tumours are therefore considered separately.

Non-seminomatous tumours

Classification

Immature teratoma, which straddles both groups, has already been discussed above and this section therefore includes (i) teratocarcinoma (syn. malignant teratoma), which comprises embryonal carcinoma surrounding foci of benign teratoma with elements of immature teratoma, and (ii) three other tumours of more specific cellularity: choriocarcinoma (syn. trophoblastic teratoma), endodermal sinus (or yolk-sac) tumour and embryonal carcinoma, the latter being the least differentiated of this group but having the potential to transform into the other non-seminomatous cell types. Many malignant germ-cell tumours contain mixtures of the specific cell types within this group and one or more of the non-seminomatous tumour cell types may also occur in combination with seminomatous elements, so-called mixed germ-cell tumours in which all individual cell types should be specified. Occasionally, sarcomatous elements may occur in malignant mediastinal germ-cell tumours, a finding that worsens the prognosis as these components are less susceptible to chemotherapeutic agents [181].

Clinical features

Non-seminomatous germ-cell tumours of the mediastinum occur most commonly in the third decade of life and are extremely rare in females [5,165]. With the exception of immature teratoma in infancy and early childhood, they behave in a highly malignant fashion, with local invasion and a tendency to metastasize, and are usually associated with symptoms at the time of diagnosis. Chest pain, cough and dyspnoea are common and may be accompanied by systemic symptoms [5,165]. Obstruction of the superior vena cava may occur. Gynaecomastia is commonly present in these patients, especially in those with choriocarcinoma, presumably due to the elaboration of human chorionic gonadotrophin (hCG) from trophoblastic elements of the tumour [182,183]. There is also a well-recognized association between the development of malignant non-seminomatous germ-cell tumours and the presence of Klinefelter's syndrome; indeed germ-cell tumours may be 30–40% more common in this group of patients than in the population as a whole [184–188]. There is also an association between non-seminomatous mediastinal germ-cell tumours, particularly those with a yolk-sac component, and various haematological malignancies including acute leukaemias and malignant histiocytosis [189,190].

Investigation

Chest radiography shows an anterior mediastinal mass that may cause mediastinal displacement and there may be evidence of metastatic intrathoracic spread. A more accurate disposition of the tumour is demonstrated by CT, which shows the neoplasm to be more solid than mature cystic teratoma but with areas of heterogeneity, corresponding to haemorrhage and necrosis. The tumour is also less likely to contain areas of fat density than benign teratoma [191]. An accurate diagnosis may be obtained by the submission of a generous surgical biopsy in order to facilitate identification of the tumour type and to enable immunohistochemical and genetic studies to be carried out. Occasionally such genetic studies reveal a chromosome marker that confirms the germ-cell origin in a tumour of otherwise uncertain histology, a finding that may be therapeutically important in terms of indicating appropriate cisplatin-based chemotherapy [192]. CT- or ultrasound-guided percutaneous needle biopsy may result in an inaccurate diagnosis in these tumours.

Diagnosis is also assisted by the detection of two protein tumour markers in the patient's serum [193]:

1 the β subunit of hCG may be detectable at any surgical stage and in 40–60% of patients with metastatic non-seminomatous malignant tumours but only 15–20% of metastatic seminomas;

2 α-fetoprotein (AFP) may also be present at any surgical stage and in 40–60% of non-seminomatous metastatic malignant tumours [160,183,194,195].

AFP has never been detected in pure seminomas and its presence in a patient with a germ-cell tumour is always taken to indicate a non-seminomatous element, a finding of crucial therapeutic and prognostic importance. Of the non-seminomatous germ-cell tumour components, AFP is specifically produced by embryonal carcinoma and endodermal sinus (yolk-sac) tumours. AFP concentrations may also be raised in inflammatory or toxic liver damage, hepatomas and other gastrointestinal tract tumours [196]. hCG is not as specific but high levels are suggestive and one or other, or both, of these two markers is present in about 90% of malignant non-seminomatous germ-cell tumours. Serum lactate dehydrogenase may also be raised in both seminomatous and non-seminomatous germ-cell tumours [160].

Treatment and prognosis

The extent of disease is determined as for seminoma. The possibility of spread from an occult testicular tumour is considered in all extragonadal presentations of malignant germ-cell tumour since a testicular primary may be very small even though metastases have occurred (see section on seminoma). Unfortunately, invasion of adjacent mediastinal structures or metastases are usually present at the time of diagnosis in non-seminomatous germ-cell cancers and surgery has ceased to be a primary treatment, complete removal having been found to be most unusual though not unheard of [165]. Patients with mediastinal non-seminomatous germ-cell cancer are considered 'poor-risk', with a low likelihood of cure, and are usually relatively insensitive to radiotherapy, the mainstay of treatment being chemotherapy [160]. The management of non-seminomatous germ-cell tumours, as with seminomas, has been the subject of much research and collaborative effort and is a matter for the expert.

Trials to improve the effectiveness of treatment in poor-risk germ-cell cancer are ongoing, one current approach comprising four cycles of conventional-dose bleomycin, etoposide and cisplatin. Some patients die within a year, although success has been achieved using cisplatin-based chemotherapy as primary treatment [197,198]. One early study achieved a median survival time of 14 months using this approach provided that cisplatin and bleomycin were included in the regimens [165]; more recent series have reported a 2-year survival of 53% (median 28 months) in 64 patients [197] and a median survival of 55 months in a small group of 11 patients [198]. Surgery may have a role in debulking residual disease after chemotherapy, once normal levels of tumour markers have been achieved. Although these tumours still carry a poor prognosis compared with their testicular counterparts, about half should be cured with modern chemotherapy [199].

The serum levels of tumour markers are used as an essential tool in monitoring the response of disease to treatment, AFP and hCG being measured and monitored before, during and after treatment. A sustained rise or increasing levels of either AFP or hCG or both may be taken to indicate active disease, even in the absence of symptoms, signs or radiographic change, and may lead to therapeutic intervention. The levels decline after treatment and a failure to do so is indicative of residual active disease [200]. Furthermore, there is evidence to suggest that a bulky tumour need not indicate a poor prognosis in the absence of high tumour marker levels [201].

Seminoma

Clinical features

Seminoma (syn. germinoma, dysgerminoma) is the most common single malignant mediastinal germ-cell tumour, accounting for approximately half of all these neoplasms [165]. They affect young men, 95% occurring between the ages of 20 and 40 years [202], so that sperm banking should be considered prior to chemotherapy. Mediastinal seminomas almost always arise within the thymus gland. They are histologically indistinguishable from testicular seminomas. Only one-third of patients are asymptomatic, in contrast with benign mediastinal germ-cell tumours, the most common symptom being chest pain [165,202]. Dyspnoea and obstruction of the superior vena cava sometimes occur. It is not unusual for these tumours to metastasize.

Investigation

The chest radiograph shows a lobulated, usually non-calcified anterior mediastinal mass (Fig. 49.9). More accurate disposition of the tumour is confirmed by CT, which often shows the neoplasm to be large, lobulated, more solid and less likely to contain fat than benign mature teratomas [191]. Diagnosis is established by the removal of a generous piece of tumour in order to identify the tumour type and to enable immunohistochemical and genetic studies to be carried out. CT- or ultrasound-guided percutaneous needle biopsy may result in an inaccurate diagnosis in these tumours. Further evidence that the tumour is free of non-seminomatous germ-cell tumour elements, whose presence would alter management, is provided by a normal serum level of AFP. hCG is also usually absent, occurring in only 7–10% of pure seminomas and 15–20% of patients with metastatic seminoma [160,165]. Other tumour markers for seminoma, such as serum lactate dehydrogenase, are being evaluated but are less specific, also being found in non-seminomatous germ-cell tumours. For practical purposes, a seminoma is only diagnosed if the histology shows pure seminoma and if the serum level of AFP is not raised [203].

The possibility of metastasis from a testicular tumour should always be considered in any malignant germ-cell tumour, although primary mediastinal seminoma is a sufficiently well-recognized entity for surgical exploration of the testis to be unnecessary provided that (i) physical examination provides no evidence of testicular swelling or atrophy, (ii) ultrasound examination of the testes is normal and (iii) no evidence of retroperitoneal lymph node involvement is found by CT of the abdomen and pelvis [163,164,166].

The ultrasonographic findings of testicular germ-cell tumour include one or more discrete hypoechoic masses or more diffuse abnormalities with microcalcifications.

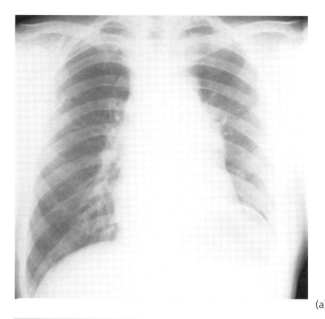

(a)

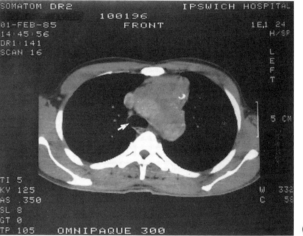

(b)

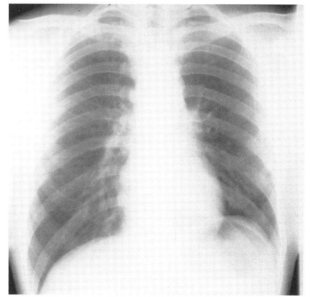

(c)

Fig. 49.9 (*Right.*) (a) Posteroanterior film of young man with seminoma in anterior mediastinum. (b) CT shows irregular mass of tissue displacing trachea (arrowed) to right. (c) Posteroanterior film after radiotherapy showing regression of tumour.

Treatment and prognosis

Seminomas carry a better prognosis than non-seminomatous germ-cell tumours and it is important to make the diagnosis accurately. As with germ-cell tumours in general, the management of seminomas has been the subject of national and international collaborative research and is a matter for the expert. Although seminomas are highly radiosensitive (and indeed complete cure may be obtained by radiotherapy) [165,166], the treatment of choice for seminoma has shifted from radiotherapy to chemotherapy, irradiation tending to be reserved for bulky tumours. Although cure has been achieved in the past when all gross evidence of tumour has been removed by surgery [5], operative attempts to remove tumour other than for histological diagnosis have generally been incomplete and are usually no longer indicated. Currently, chemotherapy takes the form of four cycles of standard etoposide and cisplatin or three cycles of bleomycin, standard etoposide and cisplatin [160]. Patients with an incomplete remission and those who relapse may be given second- and third-line 'salvage' chemotherapy, from which a significant number of cures have been obtained [160]. Such treatment may include high-dose chemotherapy with autologous bone marrow (stem cell) rescue [204]. A 2-year survival rate of 86% was reported in a series of 23 patients with pure mediastinal seminomas, most of whom were treated (between 1983 and 1990) with cisplatin-based chemotherapy, although some had been primarily treated with radiotherapy [197]. In a small series of seven patients with pure mediastinal seminomas treated with cisplatin-based combination chemotherapy and in some cases additional radiotherapy, 100% disease-free survival was reported at a median follow-up time of 41 months [198]. With modern cisplatin-based chemotherapy and radiotherapy, long-term survival or cure can be expected in around 80% of this group [199].

Other mediastinal tumours and tumour-like conditions

Mediastinal lymphoma

Any type of lymphoma can involve any lymph node, including those in the mediastinum as well as those radiographically more obvious nodes in the hila. The thymus gland may also be the seat of a lymphoma, although whether the disease originates in this site is not clear. Lymphomatous involvement of the lungs is described in Chapter 42. The mediastinum is involved in over 50% of patients with Hodgkin's disease [205]. Mediastinal Hodgkin's disease is considered 'massive' if the ratio of the maximal horizontal width of the mediastinal mass to the maximum intrathoracic diameter on a standard chest radiograph exceeds one-third [205]. Most cases of Hodgkin's disease found in the mediastinum are of the nodular sclerosing type. The correct diagnosis (as with other mediastinal tumours) is clearly important since lymphomas are eminently treatable and in many cases curable. The temptation to establish the diagnosis of a mediastinal tumour by CT- or ultrasound-guided percutaneous needle biopsy, although attractive in avoiding a more invasive surgical biopsy, runs the risk of misdiagnosis in cases of lymphoma, for which the pathologist requires a block of tissue so that a full morphological and immunohistochemical analysis can be carried out (as is the case with germ-cell tumours, see above). Failure to do this may result in some treatable non-Hodgkin lymphomas being mistakenly labelled as anaplastic carcinomas [206,207], with prognostic consequences.

Treatment may be with intensive chemotherapy regimens or primary radiotherapy or both, depending on the type, stage and bulk of the disease [205,206,208,209], and is a matter for experts in this field. Management dilemmas may sometimes be created by the persistence of cysts in the substance of the thymus following the treatment of thymic lymphoma, as there may be uncertainty about whether such cysts represent residual or recurrent disease or indeed whether they are benign. In such cases it is probably best to withhold further treatment unless pathological confirmation of active disease is obtained [141]. Similar dilemmas arise when imaging shows residual opacities in lymph node areas following treatment; indeed these are found in over 60% of patients with mediastinal disease, particularly when the original lymph node mass was large [205]. Persistent gallium isotope uptake or positron emission tomography may be helpful in distinguishing disease activity from non-malignant tissue in doubtful cases and may lead to further biopsy [205,206,209].

Patients with stage II massive mediastinal Hodgkin's disease have relapse rates of 50–74% when treated with nodal radiotherapy alone, while chemotherapy alone has been found to have relapse rates of 33–50% [205]. Improved survival may be obtained by using a combined approach, and some workers have favoured chlormethine (mustine)/vincristine/procarbazine/prednisolone (so-called 'MOPP') or doxorubicin/bleomycin/vinblastine/dacarbazine (DBVD) followed by radiotherapy [205]. The prognosis for non-Hodgkin's lymphoma varies according to the histology and stage. For well-localized high-grade tumours, disease-free survival rates of 60–80% may be achieved at 5 years. Where disease is widespread and treated with chemotherapy, the rates are 30–40%. Low-grade non-Hodgkin lymphoma runs a more indolent course, with a median survival of 7–8 years [210]. The freedom-from-relapse rate at 5 years for primary mediastinal large-cell and immunoblastic lymphoma was found to be 45% in a study of 57 patients, and the presence of pleural effusion at presentation was associated with an extremely poor outcome [209].

Mediastinal amlyoid

Amyloidosis is the term used for a group of diseases characterized by the extracellular deposition of fibrillar proteins consisting of fragments of immunoglobulin light chains. There have been a number of case reports of tumorous or lymph node deposits of amyloid in the mediastinum. The diagnosis of this very rare condition can only be made by histological examination of biopsy material, which shows a characteristic amorphous eosinophilic substance that stains positive with Congo red and which shows characteristic apple-green birefringence under polarized light microscopy [211,212]. An aspirate of subcutaneous abdominal fat may also stain similarly if other involved tissue is inaccessible. Monoclonal proteins are usually detected on electrophoresis of serum or urine. The prognosis depends upon the type and extent of disease, length of survival varying from months to years. Treatment is generally supportive but experience is accumulating with the use of colchicine, melphalan and, in certain cases, organ transplantation [213].

Mediastinal mesenchymal tumours and tumour-like lesions

Mediastinal mesenchymal (connective tissue) tumours form a diverse group of rare neoplasms that account for only about 6% of mediastinal tumours [18]. They arise from mesenchymal or connective tissue elements, including lymphatic tissue, blood vessels, fat, smooth and skeletal muscle [92]. Some are regarded as hamartomatous malformations, others as true neoplasms, either benign or their malignant (sarcomatous) counterpart. Their morphology may be heterogeneous, depending on the differentiation of the primitive mesenchymal cell, so that different cell lines are sometimes found in the same tumour. The precise diagnosis depends upon histological examination following surgical biopsy or excision, only fatty tumours lending themselves to more confident preoperative dignosis because of their characteristically low attenuation values on CT.

Benign tumours such as lipomas are usually asymptomatic findings but may produce compressive sypmtoms and signs if they attain a large size. Their malignant counterpart, the liposarcoma, is more likely to produce dyspnoea and chest pain but may also be asymptomatic at the time of diagnosis [214]. This may arise in any mediastinal compartment but possibly favours the anterior mediastinum, where it may also arise within the thymus [215]. Surgical excision may be curative but these tumours have a tendency to run an aggressive course with local recurrence, although distant metastases are not a common feature.

A series of 10 surgically resected malignant smooth muscle tumours (leiomyosarcomas) reported seven in the posterior and three in the anterior mediastinum. Most of those patients with posterior lesions were asymptomatic, whereas the anterior ones tended to produce compressive symptoms. Survival was related to histological grade and surgical staging [216]. Malignant skeletal muscle tumours (rhabdomyosarcomas) may arise in the anterior mediastinum of younger adults and behave in a highly aggressive manner [217]. Rhabdomyosarcomatous elements may also occur focally within non-seminomatous germ-cell tumours [199].

Benign tumours of blood vessels (haemangiomas) tend to be diagnosed in children and young adults but may occur at any age. They favour the anterior mediastinal compartment and range in size from small to very large. Two types are described: one is more solid and lobular, the so-called capillary haemangioma; the other, known as cavernous haemangioma, has larger dilated vascular spaces. The most common presenting symptoms in a series of 18 cases were dyspnoea, cough and chest pain [218]. These tumours tend to enhance on CT [219]. Haemangiosarcoma is an even rarer tumour in this location and has been treated by radical excision and postoperative radiotherapy [220].

Mediastinal lymphangiomas are probably hamartomatous malformations rather than true neoplasms and may result from a localized failure of the developing lymphatic system to communicate with its venous counterpart. Cystic forms of lymphangioma (so-called cystic hygroma, see below) most commonly arise in the neck of infants and sometimes extend into the superior mediastinum [221]. Solitary lymphangiomas arising exclusively in the mediastinum rather than extending from the neck are most commonly found in adults [221]. They are benign localized lesions up to several centimetres in diameter, comprising endothelial-lined spaces with a supporting connective tissue stroma that may contain smooth muscle. They are morphologically similar to haemangiomas but may contain straw-coloured fluid or chyle rather than blood [221]. They may occur anywhere in the mediastinum and although benign can infiltrate along tissue planes in a serpiginous fashion, proving difficult to remove completely at surgery. They may produce symptoms as a result of pressure on surrounding structures and are sometimes complicated by chylous pleural effusions but are often completely asymptomatic [16,221]. Lymphangiomas sometimes occur in multiple form as part of a generalized maldevelopment of the lymphatic system, so-called lymphangiomatosis, in which the tumours may be found in the mediastinum and the lungs as well as in abdominal viscera and the retroperitoneal space [222–225]. Lymphangiomatosis may also involve bones, producing cystic endothelium-lined spaces [222].

Mediastinal lymphangiomas should not be confused with lymphangiomyomas (previously called lymphangiopericytomas), which are true neoplasms seen only in females, the tumour consisting of intimately mingled lymph vessels and smooth muscle elements with particular immunohistochemical characteristics [92]. Lymphangiomyomas may occur in localized form, often in association with the thoracic duct or its tributaries in the mediastinum or retroperitoneal space and sometimes result in chylothorax. There is a generalized or systemic form of this condition known as lymphangiomyomatosis (or lymphangioleiomyomatosis) that occurs in postpubertal women. This condition is characterized by a proliferation of immature smooth muscle derived from associated lymphatics [226,227]. This smooth muscle infiltrates the walls of alveoli and bronchi with resultant air trapping and impaired gas transfer that may mimic emphysema. These women tend to present in their thirties with slowly progressive breathlessness and radiographic and CT changes that alter from a reticular infiltrate to 'honeycombing' with diffuse cystic change, so that pneumothoraces are a common feature [228]. The myoproliferative process may involve pulmonary blood vessels and lymphatics, resulting in haemoptysis and chylothorax respectively (see Chapter 42). There are close histological parallels between lymphangioleiomyomatosis and the

pulmonary manifestations of tuberous sclerosis, although this hereditary condition affects both sexes and also has cutaneous and cerebral manifestations. The pathogenesis of lymphangioleiomyomatosis remains obscure but the condition is probably a hamartomatous malformation of smooth muscle [229].

Cystic hygromas rarely develop in the superior mediastinum but more usually present as a poorly defined swelling in the neck, usually posterior to the sternomastoid muscle. However, these may extend into the mediastinum in about 10% of cases [221,230,231]. Even in this situation they are rare in adults, the vast majority being diagnosed within the first 2 years of life. They are thin-walled endothelially lined cystic tumours that contain lymph and are usually multilocular. The term 'cystic hygroma' is used synonymously with 'cystic lymphangioma' [232] and they are regarded as congenital hamartomatous malformations that may arise as a result of a bud of lymphatic tissue becoming pinched off during early development [233]. They are soft and yielding structures and although they may increase in size in adults as a result of the accumulation of lymph and the enlargement of their spaces, they do not usually produce pressure symptoms unless distended by haemorrhage into the cyst (Fig. 49.10)

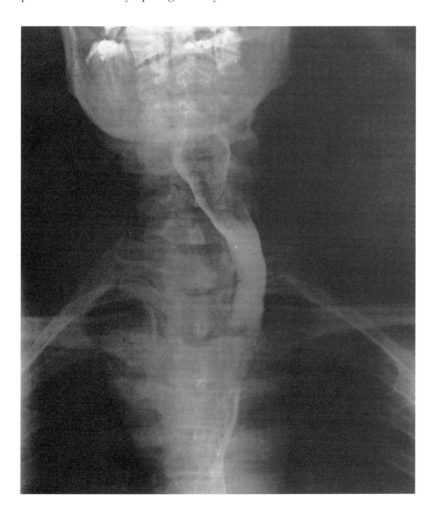

Fig. 49.10 Barium swallow in patient who presented with stridor showing mediastinal displacement to left. At operation, the tumour proved to be a cystic hygroma into which an acute bleed had occurred.

or by infection [234]. The diagnosis in adults usually follows the finding on the chest radiograph of a well-defined, rounded, homogeneous density with a sharp border in the superior mediastinum. CT shows the lesion to be cystic and of low density [234]. Treatment is by surgical excision, which may be difficult as cystic hygromas tend to mould themselves to the contours of the mediastinal contents so that a plane of cleavage may not be easy to establish [5,235].

Developmental mediastinal cysts

Congenital cysts of the mediastinum account for an average of 16% of all mediastinal cysts and tumours [2–4,6,10,30,36]. Foregut duplications are the largest group followed by pleuropericardial cysts. Congenital cysts may also occur in the thymus as described above (see Fig. 49.7) and also in relation to the thoracic duct and occasionally in ectopic thyroid or parathyroid tissue (see below).

Foregut cyst or duplication

Classification

The term 'foregut duplication' (or reduplication) may be applied to cysts, diverticula and fistulae that have resulted from developmental malformations of the primitive foregut in the embryo. Such cysts therefore contain tissues derived from primitive endoderm and mesoderm. The term 'bronchogenic cyst' is often used synonymously with 'bronchial cyst' for foregut duplications that are clearly related to the airways, especially the trachea and main bronchi, a common site being posterior to the carina. Those closely related to the gut are variously referred to as gastric, enteric or gastroenteric cysts, depending on their principal histological constituents; those where there is an associated vertebral abnormality are often called neurenteric cysts.

Pathogenesis

The pathogenesis of foregut duplications is incompletely understood, although several different mechanisms are likely to be operative [236].
1 One possible mechanism is the defective separation of the tracheobronchial bud from the foregut proper so that a bud or diverticulum becomes pinched off, creating a cystic space that may be found between the trachea or a major bronchus and the oesophagus or stomach. Such a cyst may be connected by a fibrous strand to the gut, the tracheobronchial tree or both and may be referred to as a tracheobronchial foregut duplication. When one of the connecting strands remains patent, then the 'cyst' is in fact a diverticulum of either the gut or the tracheobronchial tree; if both

connections are patent, then a tracheobronchial fistula results.
2 A second mechanism may involve the defective coalescence of chains of vacuoles that form during epithelial proliferation within the developing tracheobronchial tree, giving rise to solitary or multiple intralobar bronchogenic cysts or oesophageal cysts embedded in the oesophageal wall.
3 A third mechanism may give rise to so-called neurenteric cysts, in which a tract of abnormal development runs between a part of the upper gastrointestinal tract and the skin surface, usually over the upper thoracic spine. This anomaly is presumably initiated at an embryonic stage when the cellular precursors of the spine and the upper gastrointestinal tract are still contiguous, the neural tube and foregut being connected by the primitive neurenteric canal [237]. The persistence of this may result in a fistulous tract running from the alimentary canal to the surface of the skin [238]. This canal or its remnants may divide both the spinal cord and a corresponding vertebral body and has therefore been referred to as the split notochord syndrome [239]. Reabsorption of parts of this fistula may give rise to incomplete forms of the split notochord syndrome but upper thoracic spine anomalies are a common feature.

Intrathoracic foregut duplications may be intrapulmonary or extrapulmonary and, as suggested above, usually occur in relation to the oesophagus, the trachea or a major bronchus. They are reportedly more common in the right hemithorax than the left [5,236,238,240]. They are more likely to be diagnosed in infancy rather than adult life because their expansion in a limited space exerts pressure effects on surrounding structures [36,241].

Pathology

Macroscopically, foregut duplications appear as rounded or oval saccular structures. Bronchogenic cysts are usually spherical and thin-walled, containing gelatenous mucoid green/blue material with an average diameter of about 4cm [92]. Their wall may be lined by ciliated columnar epithelium or pseudostratified epithelium of respiratory type and may contain bronchial glandular elements as well as cartilage and neural tissue. These walls may undergo calcification. Oesophageal cysts may be found in the wall of that viscus and characteristically contain a double layer of smooth muscle in their own wall. They are occasionally tubular, traversing the long axis of the entire thorax and may contain thick mucus [238]. Rarely there may be a communication with the parent organ and exceptionally they may be multiple [5,238,242]. Gastroenteric and neurenteric cysts usually occur in the posterior mediastinum paravertebrally and are associated with vertebral, spinal cord and skin abnormalities, the cysts sometimes communicating with the skin surface through a spina bifida [238,239,243]. Microscopically, gastroenteric and neurenteric cysts have walls simulating stomach or intestine. Those with gastric features may contain parietal cells and the latter may form peptic ulcers [241]. Some cysts contain ectopic pancreatic tissue [244]. The histological findings are not always specific enough to allow differentiation between these various foregut duplications and overlap may occur.

Clinical features

The majority of children with intrathoracic foregut cysts are symptomatic, with dyspnoea, stridor or persistent cough; one-third of those with neurenteric cysts may present with a motor or sensory neurological deficit, back pain or an abnormality of gait resulting from spinal cord involvement [241,245]. In adults the majority of foregut cysts are asymptomatic and are chance radiographic findings on a routine chest film [246]. Large cysts may cause cough, stridor or dysphagia. Complications include recurrent lower respiratory tract infection due to pressure, and perforation due to either infection of the cyst itself or peptic ulceration in the case of gastric or gastroenteric cysts. Perforation may occur into the lung, pleural or pericardial cavities, causing haemoptysis, empyema or septic pericarditis [247,248]. Adenocarcinoma has been reported in a foregut cyst but is an exceptional complication [249,250].

Chest radiography

The chest radiograph may show a rounded opacity sometimes with a hair-line margin (Fig. 49.11). The majority exceed 5 cm along their longest axis [5]. The cyst occasionally contains a fluid level, indicating communication with the respiratory or gastrointestinal tract [251]. Calcification is sometimes seen in the wall of the cyst, if not with plain radiography then with CT. The presence of spinal abnormalities, such as fused vertebral bodies or a dorsal scoliosis, implies that the cyst is neurenteric and is an indication for spinal MRI, which may reveal an intraspinal cystic abnormality even in the absence of neurological symptoms or signs [241,243,252]. Radioactive technetium-99m scanning may be positive in cysts lined by gastric mucosa [253].

Treatment

Treatment is by surgical excision, which both establishes the diagnosis and avoids the possibility of future complications. In an acutely breathless child, emergency needle aspiration of a tense cyst offers temporary relief. When a coincidental intraspinal cystic component is discovered, neurosurgical removal is recommended because of the possible subsequent development of a neurological deficit [241]. Ulceration of a mediastinal cyst into the lung may necessitate both excision of the cyst and lobectomy. The

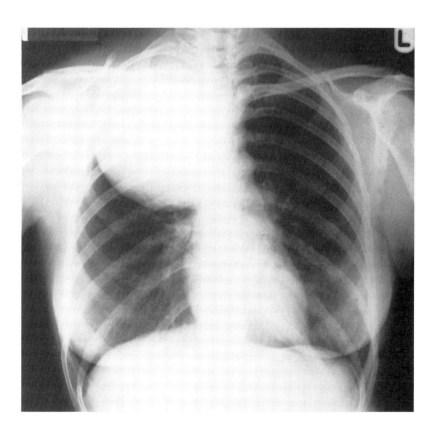

Fig. 49.11 Large right-sided foregut cyst that caused tracheal compression and stridor.

prognosis for these cytic malformations is generally excellent, although incompletely resected foregut duplications may recur.

Pleuropericardial cyst

Synonyms for pleuropericardial cysts abound and include pericardial cyst, coelomic cyst, springwater cyst, serosal cyst, mesothelial cyst, parapericardial cyst, simple cyst and hydrocele of the mediastinum! They are usually reported in surgical series as the second most common form of mediastinal cyst after foregut duplications, although it is possible that they may be seen more commonly in a physician's practice. Le Roux [254] estimated that one pericardial cyst was diagnosed per year for every 100 000 of the population studied.

Pathology

Pleuropericardial cysts are usually considered to be developmental anomalies whose origin is uncertain. It has been suggested that they arise as a result of the persistence of the ventral parietal recess of the primitive intraembryonic coelomic cavity, from which the pericardial, pleural and peritoneal cavities develop [255,256]. The coelomic cavity itself may be formed by the fusion of multiple disconnected lacunae in the primitive mesenchyme and a failure of one of these lacunae to fuse with the continuum may result in the formation of a pleuropericardial cyst [257].

Of these cysts, 70% occur in the right cardiophrenic angle and are usually situated anteriorly, tending to be loosely adherent to the pericardium and diaphragm [258,259]. Most of the remainder occur in the left cardiophrenic angle but are occasionally found in unusual locations such as the superior or posterior mediastinal compartments [260–262].

The sex incidence is approximately equal and they may occur from infancy to old age [255]. They may vary widely in size, from 5 to 25 cm in diameter [263]. They are soft and are usually unilocular, their walls being thin, consisting of a single layer of flattened mesothelial cells supported by a connective tissue stroma [255,258]. They characteristically contain crystal-clear 'springwater', although this is occasionally a more brackish yellow. The fluid is acellular and contains little protein, having the features of a transudate. They are usually truly cystic, although a small proportion communicate with the pericardial or pleural cavities via a tubular connection and in such cases are therefore diverticula [5,255].

Clinical features

Between 60 and 80% of pleuropericardial cysts are asymp-
tomatic, presenting as a chance chest radiographic finding [5,255,258]. When symptoms are a feature, chest pain is most common, occurring in about 20% of cases. Pericardial cysts may compress the right middle lobe bronchus, causing cough and dyspnoea but this is unusual as they are under low pressure.

Diagnosis and treatment

The provisional diagnosis is usually made following posteroanterior and lateral chest radiographs on the basis of a sharply demarcated, smooth-edged, rounded 'mass' shadow of uniform density situated anteriorly in the right, or less commonly the left, cardiophrenic angle and abutting the heart, diaphragm and anterior chest wall (Fig. 49.12a). Pericardial cysts have been observed to increase in size over a number of years on serial radiographs and a previously normal chest film does not exclude the diagnosis [255,258,264]. It is unusual for the rim of the cyst, which is very thin, to calcify. The absence of pulsation may be noted at fluoroscopy, as may the propensity of the cyst to alter shape during respiration and with postural change [257]. Echocardiography confirms the cystic nature of the lesion by showing a typical echolucent area that is anatomically distinct from the cardiac cavities [264]. CT shows a mass of fluid density that does not enhance following intravenous contrast [265–267] (Fig. 49.12b). The presence of a fluid-containing cyst may be confirmed by fine-needle thoracentesis of the lesion under ultrasound or CT control [268].

The most usual differential diagnoses are a prominent pericardial fat pad, an anterior diaphragmatic eventration and a diaphragmatic hernia through the foramen of Morgagni, which may contain gut or extraperitoneal fat. Less commonly, a pericardial cyst may be mimicked by a ventricular aneurysm and rarely by a rounded tumour of the middle lobe, pleura or diaphragm, or by a hydatid cyst, all of which may abut the heart or occupy the cardiophrenic angle. The differential diagnosis is much wider where a pericardial cyst is atypically situated elsewhere in the mediastinum or hilar regions.

The diagnosis may be confirmed and treated in symptomatic patients at thoracotomy or video thoracoscopy, in which case the pericardial cyst is excised [5,255,269,270]. This course of action removes doubt about the validity of the preoperative diagnosis, which has been shown to have been misplaced in earlier literature in up to 50% of cases [258]. Nowadays the diagnosis is more usually made using non-invasive imaging techniques and asymptomatic patients are managed conservatively [257,258,271,272]. CT may not always reliably differentiate between pericardial cysts and other cystic or low-density lesions, so that the uncertainty and anxiety of extended follow-up may be best removed by active surgical inter-

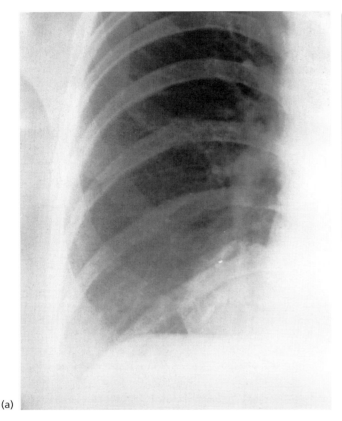

(a)

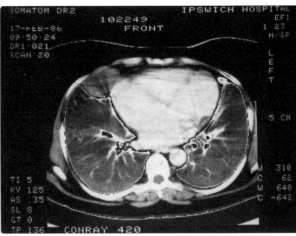

(b)

Fig. 49.12 (a) Characteristic appearance of pericardial cyst in right cardiophrenic angle. (b) CT shows pericardial cyst at right cardiac border anteriorly.

vention [255,272,273]. Aspiration, although usually safe, carries a small risk of dissemination of disease or anaphylaxis in the rare case of hydatid cyst, which should be serologically excluded prior to needling if this is a concern. When aspiration is used the fluid often reaccumulates [258].

The prognosis following surgical excision is excellent and there have been no reported cases of malignant change [255]. Symptoms are not always relieved by cyst excision, implying that they are often coincidental [5].

Thoracic duct cyst

These solitary cysts are a very rare intrathoracic finding and probably arise as a result of a developmental defect or weakness in the wall of the thoracic duct, of which they are really diverticula. They may be found accidently on a routine chest radiograph that reveals a posterior mediastinal mass shadow, although symptoms of oesophageal or tracheal compression may sometimes be produced [274–276]. Ascending lymphangiography may be diagnostic if the condition is considered preoperatively [275]. Treatment is by surgical excision, which confirms the diagnosis and which should be curative. At operation a thin-walled, unilocular 'cyst' that contains chyle and which communicates with the thoracic duct is found. Chylothorax is a potential complication of operative treatment, although it should be possible for the surgeon to avoid this

by identifying and ligating the neck of the diverticulum as it arises from the thoracic duct [276].

Retrosternal goitre and associated lesions

An extension of a cervical goitre into the thorax is probably the most common mediastinal tumour [5]. However, its true proportion is unknown as it is often managed by general rather than thoracic surgeons and its frequency therefore tends to be underestimated in surveys of mediastinal masses that appear in the thoracic literature. It is reported in one large series that 6% of cervical goitres have a retrosternal extension [277], whereas the finding of a retrosternal goitre in the absence of a goitre in the neck is rare.

Developmental features

Enlarging cervical goitres may expand into the thorax as a result of the anatomical restraints imposed by the cervical musculature and fascia, and also as a consequence of the effects of gravity and negative intrathoracic pressure. The usual pathological change in such intrathoracic extensions is nodular hyperplasia. Less commonly, thyroid tissue may find its way into the mediastinum during embryological development. A hollow diverticulum arises from the floor of the primitive pharynx in the fourth week of life at a site marked in the adult by the foramen caecum of the tongue. The thyroid rudiment is formed in this process and it migrates caudally on a tube that becomes the thyroglossal duct. During the unfolding of the embryo, this rudiment may be dragged caudally in relation to the primitive aorta so that truly ectopic thyroid tissue may be found anywhere along a track extending from the tongue through the superior and anterior mediastinal compartments to the pericardium and heart [278,279].

Pathology

Macroscopically, intrathoracic goitres nearly always extend from the lower pole of a lateral lobe, anterior to the trachea and immediately behind the sternum, although about 10% are situated posterior to the trachea and oesophagus. The histological features are no different from those of a cervical goitre and they are usually non-toxic.

Clinical features

Retrosternal goitre occurs more commonly in females and in the middle-aged and elderly [277]. An Australian epidemidological study carried out during a mass radiography campaign found the incidence to be 1 in 2000 in females over the age of 45 years compared with 1 in 5000 for the whole of the population that was screened [280]. When symptoms occur, they usually come on insidiously as growth is generally slow. Dyspnoea is the most common symptom and may be accompanied by cough and stridor due to tracheal compression. Other symptoms are less frequently encountered and include dysphagia, hoarseness due to recurrent laryngeal nerve palsy and,

occasionally, those of thyrotoxicosis. Obstruction of the superior vena cava may occur [277]. A goitre is usually palpable in the neck but this sign may be easily missed in an obese patient. A retrosternal extension should always be suspected in a breathless patient with a cervical goitre or a thyroidectomy scar. Patients with ectopic thyroid tissue in the absence of a goitre in the neck are usually free of symptoms, the diagnosis being made at thoracotomy following the finding of an anterior mediastinal mass shadow on a routine chest radiograph taken for some other purpose.

Intrathoracic goitres may be complicated by haemorrhage into the substance of the gland, which can produce sudden severe dyspnoea that constitutes a surgical emergency. Malignant change was found in 16% of one surgical series of retrosternal goitres and is no less likely if the goitre is long-standing [277].

Investigation and diagnosis

Posteroanterior and lateral chest radiographs show a rounded opacity occupying the anterior and superior mediastinal compartments. The upper border is usually indefinable because of extension into the neck. The shadow is often more prominent on the right and may displace the trachea (Fig. 49.13). Calcification is occasionally visible.

A positive radioactive iodine isotope scan is diagnostic of the presence of functioning thyroid tissue in the neck and mediastinum and is found in over half of all cases of retrosternal goitre. However, a negative scan does not exclude goitre since the thyroid tissue may be non-functioning [281]. Technetium-99m is sometimes used but

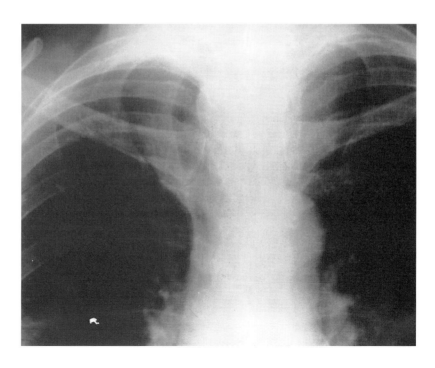

Fig. 49.13 Retrosternal goitre showing marked displacement of trachea to the right.

although more convenient is less reliable, occasionally giving negative results where iodine-131 uptake is positive.

CT is capable of demonstrating the anatomical continuity of a retrosternal goitre with the lower pole of cervical thyroid; where there is no such continuity, the presence of ectopic thyroid may be suspected [282]. The iodine content of thyroid tissue may give higher attenuation values than would be expected from a soft tissue mass of non-thyroid origin. A barium swallow may be carried out when dysphagia is present and thyroid function is assessed biochemically.

The differential diagnosis includes any superior or anterior mediastinal tumour, particularly thymic masses and germ-cell tumours. Sometimes an aortic aneurysm may be suspected, in which case MRI, CT with contrast or aortography may be used.

Treatment

It is a general rule that intrathoracic goitres should be surgically removed provided that the patient is fit enough to undergo the operation. The reasons for this are obvious in a symptomatic patient, although removal is still justified in symptom-free subjects in order to avoid the development of rare potentially life-threatening complications, such as haemorrhage into the substance of the gland [277]. The vast majority of thoracic extensions are removed using a cervical approach. Where an anterior mediastinal component is very large, the collar incision may need to be extended by a sternotomy [4].

Parathyroid adenomas and cysts

Mediastinal parathyroid adenomas are sometimes found when surgical exploration of the neck in a patient with hyperparathyroidism fails to reveal a tumour in the usual location. The occasional ectopic position of these adenomas is explicable in terms of the common embryological development of the inferior parathyroid gland and the thymus, both of which arise from the third branchial pouch, so that ectopic parathyroid lesions may be found embedded in the thymus gland. One series found 7% of parathyroid adenomas to be situated in the mediastinum [283]. In another series of 400 patients with hyperparathyroidism, 21% had mediastinal adenomas [284]. The majority of these could be removed via a cervical incision and only 19 required a sternotomy. About 65% of mediastinal parathyroid adenomas are situated in the anterior part of the superior mediastinum and the remainder in the posterior part [285]. They often go unnoticed preoperatively because they are often small and nodular, although they may grow larger than their counterparts in the neck without exciting attention. Attempts may be made to identify small tumours by CT, MRI, radioisotope scintigraphy,

selective arteriography and venous sampling with parathormone assay [286–289]. Hormonally inactive mediastinal parathyroid cysts occasionally occur and may be large enough to manifest themselves on plain chest radiographs [290]. They have been known to cause symptoms of tracheal compression and recurrent laryngeal nerve palsy [291].

Aortic aneurysm

Aortic aneurysms enter the differential diagnosis when a widened mediastinum is found on the chest radiograph. They have been defined as a permanent localized dilatation of the aorta that results in a diameter at least 50% greater than normal [292]. The possible causes range from degenerative change associated with cystic medial degeneration and atherosclerosis, to congenital disorders such as Marfan's syndrome and Ehlers–Danlos sydrome to connective tissue disorders, trauma and infection [293]; the most important single risk factor for dissection is hypertension.

Clinical features

Frequently, thoracic aortic aneurysms are asymptomatic at the time of detection. However, pressure on adjacent structures may occur during the course of enlargement, with dysphagia, stridor or dysphonia due to compression of the oesophagus, trachea and left recurrent laryngeal nerve. Compression of the superior vena cava may also occur. Aneurysms of the aortic arch may cause pain referred to the neck and jaw, and those involving the descending thoracic aorta may cause interscapular or left chest pain. The sudden onset of such pain may indicate an acute aortic dissection or intramural bleed [293]. Other symptoms may result from heart failure in connection with associated aortic regurgitation or may be the result of the occlusion of aortic branches. Aneurysms of the brachiocephalic (innominate) and left common carotid arteries may also produce superior mediastinal 'mass lesions' on the chest radiograph and symptoms of tracheal compression [294].

Investigation

Although often first suspected following chest radiography, plain chest films may miss significant retrosternal aneurysmal dilatation and cannot always differentiate a vascular opacity from other mediastinal masses [295]; indeed thoracic aortic aneurysms have sometimes been unwittingly subjected to percutaneous needle biopsy with alarming results for all concerned. MRI provides the best images of thoracic aortic disease, particularly dissections, and does not require contrast; however, it is difficult to perform on iller patients who may be attached to monitoring devices and CT is still widely used [294] (Fig. 49.14). CT or MRI may be carried out serially in order to monitor the size of aneurysms so that decisions can be made about when to intervene surgically, although aortography is still usually required before elective surgical intervention.

Treatment

Surgical treatment is intended to reduce complications and in particular to prevent death from rupture. Series of patients with thoracic aortic aneurysms who did not undergo surgery showed that rupture of the aneurysm

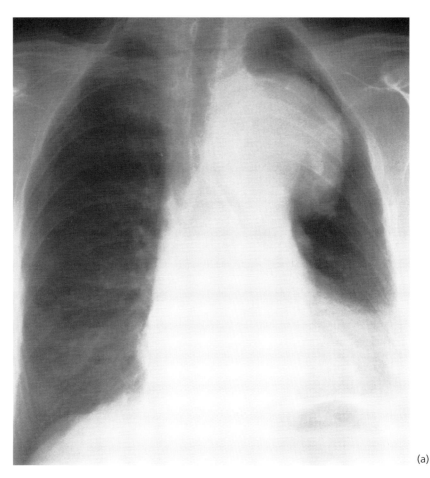

(a)

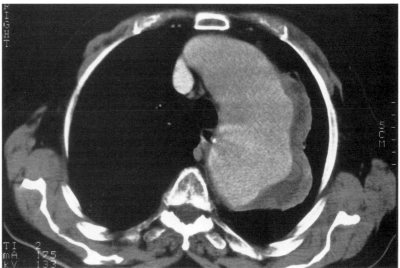

Fig. 49.14 (a) Chest radiograph showing a large suprahilar mass, which CT contrast imaging (b) showed to be a hugely dilated aneurysmal aortic arch containing mural thrombus in its lateral aspect.

(b)

was the most common cause of death, rates ranging from 42 to 70% [293,296]. The risk of rupture is increased for dissecting aneurysms and is also much greater for aneurysms exceeding 6 cm in diameter [296]. The earliest successful cardiothoracic surgical replacements of the ascending aorta and aortic arch were carried out over 40 years ago, since when there have been considerable improvements in both surgical and cardiopulmonary bypass techniques. At present, in asymptomatic patients consideration is given to replacing thoracic aortic aneurysms with grafts when the diameter of the aneurysm exceeds 5–6 cm, although these figures may well be reviewed as experience accrues. All patients with acute dissections of the ascending aorta should be considered for surgery, without which about 90% die within 3 months. A mechanical aortic valve prosthesis may be incorporated into the ascending aortic graft if this is necessary and the coronary arteries are implanted into the graft. The aortic arch may also be replaced with a graft where necessary and this may be indicated in acute dissection where an intimal tear has occurred in the arch. Most acute aortic dissections affecting the descending aorta may be managed medically at first, blood pressure being controlled with drugs such as nitroprusside.

Diaphragmatic herniae

Hiatus herniae are a common cause of a double retrocardiac 'shadow' that often contains a fluid level, the lateral radiographic projection confirming the physician's suspicion. These are often incidental findings on a radiograph taken for some other reason and patients with suprisingly large hiatus herniae may have no symptoms referable to them, in which case surgical intervention is seldom justified. Symptoms of oesophageal reflux may occur and can usually be dealt with medically. There is a small risk of paraoesophageal herniae becoming incarcerated and strangulating and when this does happen it creates an acute surgical emergency. Surgical intervention may also be needed to dilate oesophageal strictures should these arise. Diaphragmatic herniae may also occur posteriorly through the foramen of Bochdalek or anteriorly through the foramen of Morgagni. Bowel or omentum or both may be contained in the hernial sac. These and other diaphragmatic lesions that may sometimes abut the mediastinum are described more fully in Chapter 46.

Mediastinitis

Acute mediastinitis

Causes

The commonest cause of acute mediastinitis is oesophageal perforation [297]. This may occur as the result of a difficult endoscopy. Attempts to dilate a stric-

ture or to insert a tube or stent for palliative purposes in carcinoma may have the same effect and a carcinoma may itself perforate spontaneously. Other causes of oesophageal perforation include accidental blunt or penetrating injury of the chest, surgery to the oesophagus or adjacent structures and ingestion of a foreign body. Forceful vomiting commonly causes a Mallory–Weiss mucosal tear but it is unusual for the entire wall of the oesophagus to rupture (Boerhaave's syndrome).

Infection may also track down to the mediastinum from higher levels, particularly along the so-called 'danger space', a potential cavity created by a fascial plane that runs from the upper cervical level as far caudally as the diaphragm [298]. Infection from the mouth, neck or retropharyngeal space may extend into this space, between the prevertebral fascia posteriorly and the alar fascia anteriorly, and result in acute mediastinitis. The portal of entry is occasionally a small oropharyngeal mucosal tear resulting from a difficult endotracheal intubation. Other less common causes include the extension of infection from the lung, pleural or pericardial cavities, with or without abscess formation. The spread of such infection may be direct or it may be carried by lymphatic drainage, with subsequent suppuration of mediastinal nodes. Osteomyelitis of the cervical or dorsal spine, ribs or sternum may also spread directly to the mediastinum. Surgical incisions in the neck and thorax may become infected with subsequent mediastinitis, particularly following tracheostomy and sternotomy. Infection may also reach the mediastinum from central venous cannulation sites in the neck. Tuberculous mediastinitis is now rare as is haematogenous spread of infection from remote sites.

Clinical features

The patient usually feels ill and is febrile. There may be rigors. Swallowing often produces pain so that food is refused. Movements of the neck may produce discomfort if infection has tracked down from this area, so that the anxious patient may look fixedly to the front. A cough may indicate tracheal involvement. Mediastinal and subcutaneous emphysema may occur, particularly if the oesophagus is perforated, and a pleural effusion, empyema or pyopneumothorax may sometimes be produced. Retrosternal pain may be present and sternal tenderness may be elicited.

Investigation

The chest radiograph may be normal or if fluid or pus are collecting in the mediastinum, a smooth-walled convex opacity may be seen bulging laterally beyond the mediastinal boundaries with displacement of the trachea and oesophagus (Fig. 49.15). Gas may be seen in the

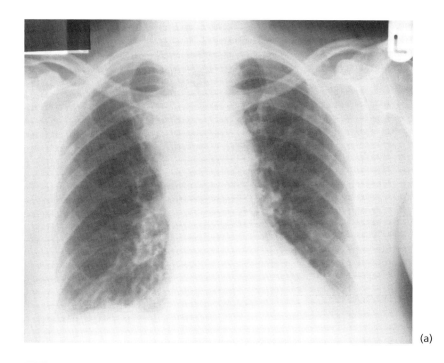

(a)

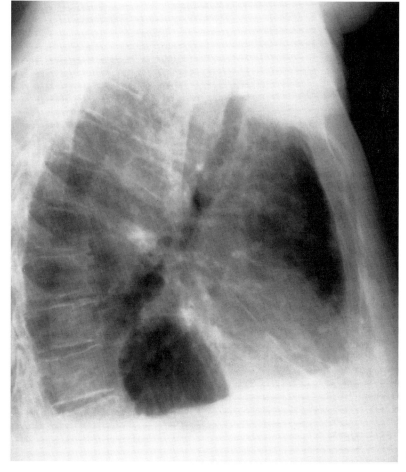

Fig. 49.15 (a) Posteroanterior film of patient with mediastinal abscess following faulty placement of central venous canula showing mass to right of upper mediastinum. (b) Right lateral view showing opacity surrounding trachea and displacing it forwards.

(b)

mediastinum or fascial planes of the neck, this being a feature of a mixed anaerobic infection in which organisms have gained entry from the oropharynx. There may be evidence of a pleural effusion or pyopneumothorax. Lateral soft tissue radiographs of the neck may show an increase in width of the retropharyngeal soft tissue. CT may show retropharyngeal inflammatory changes and gas, with possible extension to the mediastinum. This examination should be performed early as it may well show abnormalities at a time when plain radiographs are normal or show only subtle changes. The presence of a mediastinal abscess may also be shown by CT. Leakage through an oesophageal or pharyngeal tear may sometimes be demonstrated if a water-soluble non-ionic contrast (e.g. lopamidol, Gastromiro) examination of the oesophagus is undertaken. High-osmolality contrast media such as Gastrografin tend to be avoided as any 'spillover' into the lung in the presence of dysphagia may result in pulmonary oedema.

Treatment

The patient should be monitored closely as acute mediastinitis is potentially fatal. Treatment consists of a broad spectrum of parenteral antibiotics, including cover for anaerobic bacteria [299]. Initial combinations might include penicillin and metronidazole plus an aminoglycoside, or clindamycin also with an aminoglycoside. Surgical drainage is essential where there is radiographic evidence of an accumulation of pus in the neck and/or mediastinum, in which case early thoracic and otorhinolaryngological opinions are necessary. Both these territories may require separate drainage and a thoracotomy may be required to achieve adequate mediastinal drainage [298]. Any pleural collections that may be present also require adequate drainage. The degree of intervention depends upon the nature and extent of the underlying disease process, so that a foreign body may be removed endoscopically, a postemetic oesophageal rupture repaired, and an advanced and inoperable oesophageal carcinoma managed conservatively. A literature review of necrotizing mediastinitis found a mortality rate of 31%, despite the availability of antibiotics [298].

Chronic mediastinitis

Chronic mediastinitis may be caused by low-grade infection and in such cases the responsible organisms may be fungal or mycobacterial. It is possible that John Hunter's mid-eighteenth century description of mediastinal fibrosis (see below) may have been caused by tuberculosis or even syphilis [300]. More recent series from North America have implicated *Histoplasma capsulatum*, this organism having been found to be responsible for 26 cases of mediastinal granuloma or fibrosis in the series of Goodwin, the remaining 12 cases being thought to have been caused by *Mycobacterium tuberculosis* [301]. The condition may also sometimes occur with nocardiosis [302], actinomycosis [303], blastomycosis [304], coccidioidomycosis [304] and aspergillosis [305]. Patients may be asymptomatic, coming to attention following the finding of mediastinal widening on a chest radiograph taken for some unrelated reason. They may also present with symptoms of cryptogenic mediastinal fibrosis, into which chronic mediastinitis imperceptibly merges. Where an infecting agent is identified, appropriate antimicrobial therapy can be tried but usually fibrotic change predominates so that any therapeutic distinction from cryptogenic mediastinal fibrosis is problematical. Antifungal agents have been tried when histoplasmosis was suspected as the cause but evidence of benefit is somewhat anecdotal and no controlled trials have been carried out [306].

Cryptogenic mediastinal fibrosis

The different names that have been attached to this condition are a reflection of both its rarity and a general sense of ignorance about its cause. These names include fibrosing mediastinitis, sclerosing mediastinitis, chronic fibrous mediastinitis, chronic mediastinal fibrosis and idiopathic fibrosis of the mediastinum. All these terms are intended to convey the slowly progressive envelopment of mediastinal structures in fibrotic tissue.

Possible causes

The first description has been attributed to John Hunter in 1757 [300]. Although such early reports may well have included cases due to tuberculosis or even syphilis, which were highly prevalent at the time, more recent descriptions have failed to identify a cause in over 80% of cases, hence the use of the term 'cryptogenic'. Those few cases where the aetiology is known should be referred to as chronic mediastinitis or mediastinal fibrosis due to whatever causal agent has been identified (as above). Infection with *H. capsulatum* is a recurrent theme in North American reports of fibrosing mediastinitis [307,308]. This infection is highly endemic in parts of the central USA, where residence produces almost invariable infection that is of no clinical consequence in the vast majority [309]. It has been proposed that immune stimulation may result from the seepage of material from infected lymph nodes; however, cultures and silver stains are usually negative in these cases and although there is a strong suspicion of an association between *Histoplasma* infection and consequent mediastinal fibrosis, clear proof is often lacking. It has also been suggested that the mediastinal fibrosis in these cases results from a delayed hypersensitivity reaction to mycobacterial, fungal or other unidentified antigens [301]. It is notable that histological reports where histoplasmosis is the supposed cause refer to the presence of granuloma formation and caseation, hence the term 'mediastinal granuloma', whereas these are not regarded as typical features in European reports of the cryptogenic form [310,311].

A retrospective series of 18 patients collected at one British centre over the space of 23 years obtained a history of previous pulmonary tuberculosis in half of them but with no evidence of active infection at the time of diagnosis [311]. Cryptogenic fibrosing mediastinitis is occasionally associated with retroperitoneal fibrosis and both these conditions may sometimes coexist with Riedel's thyroiditis, sclerosing cholangitis, orbital pseudotumour and sclerosing mesenteritis. The histological similarities between all these conditions have been noted and have given rise to the term 'multifocal fibrosclerosis', which implies a systemic disorder with a possible common aetiology [310]. There have been reports of hypergammaglobulinaemia and hypercomplementaemia, as well as a prominent plasma cell infiltration, in patients with cryptogenic fibrosing mediastinitis and this has stimulated speculation that there may be an immune basis for the disorder [312]. Practolol and methysergide have been associated with peritoneal and retroperitoneal fibrosis. The former, a β-blocker, has been withdrawn from use and neither of these drugs, the second of which is used as prophylactic treatment for severe migraine, has been shown to cause mediastinal fibrosis, although pleural effusions, pleural friction rubs and microscopic evidence of pulmonary fibrosis have been described in a few patients receiving methysergide therapy [313].

Pathology

Masses of ill-defined sclerotic tissue encase and may compress the mediastinal structures. Any part of the mediastinum may be involved and tissue planes are not respected. Histology shows that the predominant feature is the presence of bundles of intertwining hypocellular collagenous tissue containing an infiltrate of mainly plasma cells with some lymphocytes, polymorphs and fibroblasts, the process extending into surrounding connective tissue and fat [310,312].

Clinical features

The diagnosis is most commonly made in the fourth decade of life, although the condition may occur at any age. It is found with equal frequency in men and women. It may be identified following the finding of mediastinal widening on the chest radiograph of an asymptomatic individual or it may present with the insidious onset of symptoms of obstruction of the superior vena cava, so that the patient may notice swelling of the face, neck and arms, particularly in the mornings, at which time there may be

headache and difficulty in buttoning the shirt collar [314]. Conjunctival oedema and anterior chest wall and neck vein engorgement may become evident and the patient may have a suffused complexion. These symptoms do not inevitably progress, presumably due to either the cessation of the fibrotic process or the opening up of collateral vessels [304]. Other symptoms may include dyspnoea and dysphagia, since both tracheobronchial and oesophageal compression may occur.

In some cases the fibrotic process may be limited to one or both hilar regions, with possible narrowing of the hilar vasculature and bronchi [315]. Bronchial compression may cause cough, breathlessness and recurrent lower respiratory tract infection. Pulmonary arterial hypertension may be produced if compression is bilateral. Haemoptysis may be produced by infection, bronchial invasion or as a result of pulmonary venous hypertension. It has been suggested that this distribution of fibrosis is more likely to be found in younger age groups but this may be an oversimplification [315,316].

Radiographic features

These are non-specific. There may be widening of the mediastinal shadow and the mediastinum may be displaced towards the side of the most dense fibrosis. Either hilar shadow may be prominent. Calcification within the fibrotic mass may sometimes be seen. An affected pulmonary artery may be small. There may be cardiomegaly and compressed pulmonary veins may produce Kerley's B lines. A barium swallow or bronchoscopy may demonstrate areas of compression or distortion. There may be confusion with chronic thrombotic pulmonary arterial occlusion in those cases with pulmonary arterial hypertension, and this may be compounded by similar appearances on ventilation–perfusion lung scanning and pulmonary arteriography [317]. CT and MRI of the mediastinum may help to delineate the extent of the disease process [318,319], although biopsy is necessary to provide a tissue diagnosis and to exclude a neoplastic process, particularly as a fibrotic reaction may be associated with some tumours including lymphoma. This is best done surgically, usually by mediastinoscopy or anterior mediastinotomy provided that the patient is fit enough, and several blocks of tissue should be obtained. It is important that the diagnosis is confirmed histologically, since in the days before CT 'blind treatment' with radiotherapy on the assumption that a carcinoma was responsible for obstruction of the superior vena cava has been known to produce a later myelopathy with a tragic and permanent neurological deficit.

Treatment

Medical treatment has nothing to offer, corticosteroids

having proved ineffectual and penicillamine having been of no demonstrable benefit [320]. Occasionally, fibrotic tissue may be localized and is surgically removable but usually it is diffuse and cannot be cleared. A bypass graft may relieve obstruction of the superior vena cava in severe cases that do not develop an adequate collateral drainage [311,321]. Oesophageal strictures may require dilatation. Attempts to dilate bronchial strictures have been known to cause severe bleeding.

References

1 Le Roux BT, Dodds TC. *A Portfolio of Chest Radiographs*. Edinburgh: E & S Livingstone, 1964.

2 Rubush JL, Gardner IR, Boyd WL *et al*. Mediastinal tumors, review of 186 cases. *J Thorac Cardiovasc Surg* 1973; 65: 216.

3 Sabiston DC, Scott HW. Primary neoplasm and cysts of mediastinum. *Ann Surg* 1952; 136: 777.

4 Wychulis AR, Payne WS, Clagett OT *et al*. Surgical treatment of mediastinal tumors. *J Thorac Cardiovasc Surg* 1971; 62: 379.

5 Le Roux BT, Kallichurum S, Shama DM. Mediastinal cysts and tumors. *Curr Probl Surg* 1984; 21: 5.

6 Benjamin SP, McCormack LJ, Effler RB *et al*. Primary tumors of the mediastinum. *Chest* 1972; 62: 297.

7 Lvosto R, Koikkalainen K, Jyr AA *et al*. Mediastinal tumours: a follow-up study of 208 patients. *Scand J Thorac Cardiovasc Surg* 1978; 12: 253.

8 Silverman NA, Sabiston DC. Primary tumors and cysts of the mediastinum. *Curr Probl Cancer* 1977; 2: 3.

9 Ovrum E, Birkeland S. Mediastinal tumours and cysts. A review of 91 cases. *Scand J Thorac Cardiovasc Surg* 1979; 13: 161.

10 Oldham HN. Mediastinal tumors and cysts. *Ann Thorac Surg* 1971; 11: 246.

11 Whittaker LD, Lynn HB. Mediastinal tumors and cysts in the pediatric patient. *Surg Clin North Am* 1973; 53: 893.

12 Fontenelle LJ, Armstrong RG, Stanford W *et al*. The asymptomatic mediastinal mass. *Arch Surg* 1971; 102: 98.

13 Boyd DP, Midell AI. Mediastinal cysts and tumors. An analysis of 96 cases. *Surg Clin North Am* 1968; 48: 493.

14 Morrow A, Coady TJ, Seaton D. Tracheal compression relieved by cardiomyotomy. *Thorax* 1982; 37: 776.

15 Dische MR. Mediastinal lymphangioma with chylothorax in infancy. *Am J Clin Pathol* 1968; 49: 392.

16 Teglbjherg PS, Svendsen V. Lymphangioma of the thoracic duct with previously undescribed epithelial tubules. *Tumori* 1978; 64: 63.

17 Shields TW, Reynolds M. Neurogenic tumours of the thorax. *Surg Clin North Am* 1988; 68: 645.

18 Hofmann OA, Gillespie DJ, Aughenbaugh GL, Brown LR. Primary mediastinal neoplasms (other than thymoma). *Mayo Clin Proc* 1993; 68: 880.

19 Buthker W, Feltkamp-Vroom T, Groen AS *et al*. Sympatheticoblastoma in the anterior mediastinum. *Dis Chest* 1964; 46: 531.

20 Glenner GG, Grimley PM. *Tumors of the Extra-adrenal Paraganglion System (Including Chemoreceptors)*, 2nd series, fasc 9. Washington, DC: Armed Forces Institute of Pathology, 1974.

21 Molinatti GM, Camanni F, Pizzini A. Malignant hypertension in a case of non-chromaf-

fin paraganglioma with a high concentration of catecholamine. *Cancer* 1959; 12: 878.

22 Abell MR, Hart WR, Olson JR. Tumors of the peripheral nervous system. *Hum Pathol* 1970; 1: 503.

23 Brantigan CO, Katase RY. Clinical and pathological features of paraganglioma of the organ of Zuckerkandl. *Surgery* 1969; 65: 898.

24 Enzinger F, ed. *Histologic Typing of Soft Tissue Tumours*. Geneva: WHO, 1969.

25 Pearse AGE, Polak JM. Endocrine tumours of neural crest origin: neurolophomas, APU-Domas and the APUD concept. *Med Biol* 1974; 52: 3.

26 Sobel HJ, Marquet E, Schwarz R. Is schwannoma related to granular cell myoblastoma? *Arch Pathol* 1973; 95: 396.

27 Parish C. Complications of mediastinal neural tumours. *Thorax* 1971; 26: 392.

28 Davidson KG, Walbaum PR, McCormack RJM. Intrathoracic neural tumours. *Thorax* 1978; 33: 359.

29 Smith LH. Thoracic neurolophomomas. *Ann Thorac Surg* 1977; 23: 586.

30 Morrison IM. Tumours and cysts of the mediastinum. *Thorax* 1958; 13: 294.

31 Reed JC, Hallet KK, Feigin DS. Neural tumours of the thorax: subject review from the Armed Forces Institute of Pathology. *Diagn Radiol* 1978; 126: 9.

32 Gale AW, Jelihovsky T, Grant AF *et al*. Neurogenic tumours of the mediastinum. *Ann Thorac Surg* 1974; 17: 434.

33 Chow LT-C, Shum BS-F, Chow W-H. Intrathoracic vagus nerve neurofibroma and sudden death in a patient with neurofibromatosis. *Thorax* 1993; 48: 298.

34 Gayola G, Weil PH, Janis M *et al*. Intrathoracic nerve sheath tumour of the vagus. *J Thorac Cardiovasc Surg* 1965; 49: 412.

35 Stout AP. Peripheral manifestations of specific nerve sheath tumors (neurilemmoma). *Am J Cancer* 1946; 24: 751.

36 Silverman NA, Sabiston DC. Mediastinal masses. *Surg Clin North Am* 1980; 60: 757.

37 Sarkar PK, Fagan AM. Intrathoracic meningocele in a patient with neurofibromatosis. *Respir Med* 1991; 85: 163.

38 Davies MJ, Hall DR, Ross BA. Rare tracheal tumours: two case reports of primary neurogenic tumours occurring in the trachea. *Respir Med* 1993; 87: 145.

39 Rusch VW, Schmidt RA. Tracheal schwannoma: management by endoscopic laser resection. *Thorax* 1994; 49: 85.

40 Sood AK, Dua A, Mahajan A *et al*. Minimal change nephrotic syndrome associated with extrarenal neurilemoma. *Nephron* 1997; 75: 230.

41 Bousamra M, Haasler GB, Patterson GA *et al*. A comparative study of thoracoscopic versus open removal of benign neurogenic tumours. *Chest* 1996; 109: 1461.

42 Sorensen SA, Mulvihill JJ, Nielsen A. Long term follow up of von Recklinghausen neu-

rofibromatosis. Survival and malignant neoplasms. *N Engl J Med* 1986; 314: 1010.

43 Gilbertsen VA, Lillehei CW. Bilateral intrathoracic neurofibroma of vagus nerves with note on physiologic effects of cervico-thoracic vagectomy in man: case report. *J Thorac Surg* 1954; 28: 78.

44 Otani Y, Morishita Y, Yoshida I *et al*. A malignant triton tumour in the anterior mediastinum requiring emergency surgery: report of a case. *Surg Today* 1996; 26: 834.

45 Adam A, Hochholzer L. Ganglioneuroblastoma of the posterior mediastinum. A clinico-pathologic review of 80 cases. *Cancer* 1981; 47: 373.

46 Swank RL, Fetterman GH, Sieber WK *et al*. Prognostic factors in neuroblastoma. *Ann Surg* 1971; 14: 428.

47 Salter JE, Gibson D, Ordóñez NG *et al*. Neuroblastoma of the anterior mediastinum in an 80 year old woman. *Ultrastruct Pathol* 1995; 19: 305.

48 Catalano PW, Newton WA, Williams TE *et al*. Reasonable surgery for thoracic neuroblastoma in infants and children. *J Thorac Cardiovasc Surg* 1978; 76: 459.

49 Gitlow SE, Dziedzic LB, Strauss L *et al*. Biochemical and histologic determinants in the prognosis of neuroblastoma. *Cancer* 1973; 32: 898.

50 Ambros IM, Zellner A, Roald B *et al*. Role of ploidy, chromosome 1p and schwann cells in the maturation of neuroblastoma. *N Engl J Med* 1996; 334: 1505.

51 Donohue JP, Garrett RA, Baehner RL *et al*. The multiple manifestations of neuroblastoma. *J Urol* 1974; 111: 260.

52 Priebe CJ, Clatworthy HW. Neuroblastoma. Evaluation of the treatment of 90 children. *Arch Surg* 1967; 95: 538.

53 Cushing H, Wohlback SB. The transformation of a malignant paravertebral sympathetico-blastoma into a benign ganglioneuroma. *Am J Pathol* 1927; 3: 203.

54 Fox F, Davidson J, Thomas LB. Maturation of sympathetico-blastoma into ganglioneuroma. *Cancer* 1959; 12: 108.

55 Kinnier-Wilson LM, Draper GJ. Neuroblastoma, its natural history and progress. A study of 487 cases. *Br Med J* 1974; 3: 301.

56 Adams GA, Shochat SJ, Smith EI *et al*. Thoracic neuroblastoma: a pediatric oncology group study. *J Pediatr Surg* 1993; 28: 372.

57 Kushner BH, LaQuaglia MP, Bonilla MA *et al*. Highly effective induction therapy for stage 4 neuroblastoma in children over one year of age. *J Clin Oncol* 1994; 12: 2607.

58 Ogana J, Inoue H, Koide S. Functioning paraganglioma in the posterior mediastinum. *Ann Thorac Surg* 1981; 33: 507.

59 Glenner GG, Crout JR, Roberts WC. A functional carotid-body-like tumor. *Arch Pathol* 1962; 73: 230.

60 Oslon JL, Salyer WR. Mediastinal paragangliomas (aortic body tumor): a report of four

cases and a review of the literature. *Cancer* 1978; 41: 2405.

61 Hodgson SF, Sheps SG, Subramanian R *et al.* Catecholamine-secreting paraganglioma of the interatrial septum. *Am J Med* 1984; 77: 157.

62 Besterman E, Bromley LL, Peart WS. An intrapericardial phaeochromocytoma. *Br Heart J* 1974; 36: 318.

63 Del Fante FM, Watkins E. Chemodectomas of the heart in a patient with multiple chemodectomas and familial history. *Lahey Clin Found Bull* 1967; 16: 224.

64 Gallimore AP, Goldstraw P. Tracheal paraganglioma. *Thorax* 1993; 48: 866.

65 Sharma SK, Sharma S, Mukhopadhyay S. mediastinal paraganglioma presenting as an intracardiac mass with superior vena caval obstruction. *Thorax* 1993; 48: 1181.

66 Sheps SG, Brown ML. Localisation of mediastinal paragangliomas (pheochromocytoma). *Chest* 1985; 87: 807.

67 Surakiatchanukul S, Goodsitt E, Storer J. Chemodectoma of the aortic body. *Chest* 1971; 60: 464.

68 Karasov RS, Sheps SG, Carney JA *et al.* Paragangliomatosis with numerous catecholamine-producing tumors. *Mayo Clin Proc* 1982; 57: 590.

69 Odze R, Bégin LR. Malignant paraganglioma of the posterior mediastinum. A case report and review of the literature. *Cancer* 1990; 65: 564.

70 Pryse-Davies J, Dawson IMP, Westbury J. Some morphologic, histochemical and chemical observations on chemodectomas and the normal carotid body, including a study of the chromaffin reaction and possible ganglion cell elements. *Cancer* 1964; 17: 185.

71 McNeill AD, Groden BM, Neville AM. Intrathoracic phaeochromocytoma. *Br J Surg* 1970; 57: 457.

72 Bravo EL, Gifford RW. Phaeochromocytoma. Diagnosis, localisation and management. *N Engl J Med* 1984; 311: 1298.

73 Phillips LA. Mediastinal chemodectoma and thoracic aortography. *Clin Radiol* 1963; 14: 119.

74 Akwari OE, Payne WS, Onofriol BM. Dumbbell neurogenic tumors of the mediastinum. *Mayo Clin Proc* 1978; 53: 353.

75 Grillo HC, Ojemann RG, Scannell JG. Combined approach to 'dumb-bell' intrathoracic and intraspinal neurogenic tumors. *Ann Thorac Surg* 1983; 36: 402.

76 Yuksel M, Pamir N, Ozer F *et al.* The principles of surgical management in dumb-bell tumours. *Eur J Cardiothorac Surg* 1996; 10: 569.

77 Hendricks GL, Barnes WT, Suter HJ. Primary malignant melanoma of the esophagus: a case report. *Am Surg* 1974; 40: 468.

78 Glancy DL, Roberts WL. The heart in malignant melanoma. *Am J Cardiol* 1968; 21: 555.

79 Cohen MD, Weber TR, Sequeira FW *et al.* The diagnostic dilemma of the posterior mediastinal thymus: CT manifestations. *Radiology* 1983; 146: 691.

80 Linegar AG, Odell JA, Fennell WM *et al.* Massive thymic hyperplasia. *Ann Thorac Surg* 1993; 55: 1197.

81 Pendlebury SC, Boyages S, Koutts J, Boyages J. Thymic hyperplasia associated with Hodgkin disease and thyrotoxicosis. *Cancer* 1992; 70: 1985.

82 Rosai J, Levine GD. *Tumor of the Thymus:*

Atlas of Tumor Pathology, 2nd series, fasc 13. Washington, DC: Armed Forces Institute of Pathology, 1979.

83 Cohen M, Hill CA, Cangir A *et al.* Thymic rebound after treatment of childhood tumors. *Am J Radiol* 1980; 135: 151.

84 Joshi VV, Oleske JM, Saad S *et al.* Thymus biopsy in children with acquired immunodeficiency syndrome. *Arch Pathol Lab Med* 1986; 110: 837.

85 Large SR, Shneerson JM, Stovin PGI *et al.* Surgical pathology of the thymus: 20 years' experience. *Thorax* 1986; 41: 51.

86 Keesey J, Bein M, Mink J *et al.* Detection of thymoma in myasthenia gravis. *Neurology* 1980; 30: 233.

87 Filler RM, Simpson JS, Ein SH. Mediastinal masses in infants and children. *Pediatr Clin North Am* 1979; 26: 677.

88 Castleman B. *Tumors of the Thymus Gland: Atlas of Tumor Pathology*, section V, fasc 19. Washington, DC: Armed Forces Institute of Pathology, 1955.

89 Bernatz PE, Harrison EG, Glagett OT. Thymoma: a clinico-pathologic study. *J Thorac Cardiovasc Surg* 1961; 42: 424.

90 Lattes R, Jonas S. The pathological and clinical features in eighty cases of thymoma. *Bull N Y Acad Med* 1957; 33: 145.

91 Ho FC, Fu KH, Lam SY *et al.* Evaluation of a histogenetic classification for thymic epithelial tumours. *Histopathology* 1994; 25: 21.

92 Rosai J. *Akerman's Surgical Pathology*. St Louis: Mosby, 1996.

93 Cohen DJ, Ronnigen LD, Graleber GM *et al.* Management of patients with malignant thymoma. *J Thorac Cardiovasc Surg* 1984; 87: 301.

94 Salyer WR, Eggleston JC. Thymoma: a clinical and pathological study of 65 cases. *Cancer* 1976; 37: 229.

95 Moran CA, Suster S. Current status of the histologic classification of thymoma. *Int J Surg Pathol* 1995; 31: 67.

96 Shamji F, Pearson FG, Todd TRJ. Results of surgical treatment for thymoma. *J Thorac Cardiovasc Surg* 1984; 87: 43.

97 Bergh NP, Gatzinsky P, Larsson S *et al.* Tumors of the thymus and thymic region. I. Clinicopathological studies on thymomas. *Ann Thorac Surg* 1978; 25: 91.

98 Lewis JE, Wick MR, Sheithauer BW *et al.* Thymoma. A clinicopathological review. *Cancer* 1987; 60: 2727.

99 Yamakawa Y, Masaoka A, Hashimoto T *et al.* A tentative tumour–node–metastasis classification of thymoma. *Cancer* 1991; 68: 1984.

100 Guillan RA, Kelman S, Smalley RL *et al.* Malignant thymoma associated with myasthenia gravis and evidence of extrathoracic metastases. *Cancer* 1971; 27: 823.

101 Castleman B. The pathology of the thymus gland in myasthenia gravis. *Ann N Y Acad Sci* 1966; 135: 496.

102 Friedman NB. Tumors of the thymus. *J Thorac Cardiovasc Surg* 1967; 53: 163.

103 Katz JH. Malignant thymoma in myasthenia gravis; report of an unusual case with a brief discussion of the role of the thymus in disease. *N Engl J Med* 1953; 248: 1059.

104 Zeok JV, Todd EP, Dillon M *et al.* The role of thymectomy in red cell aplasia. *Ann Thorac Surg* 1979; 28: 257.

105 De Sevilla E, Forrest JV, Zivnuska FR *et al.* Metastatic thymoma with myasthenia gravis and pure red cell aplasia. *Cancer* 1975; 36: 1154.

106 Goldstein G, Mackay IR. Thymic tumours and systemic disease associated with thymoma. In: Warren H, Green I, eds. *The Human Thymus*. St Louis: Mosby, 1969.

107 Rubin M, Straus B, Allen L. Clinical disorders associated with thymic tumors. *Arch Intern Med* 1964; 114: 389.

108 Burrows S, Carroll R. Thymoma associated with pancytopenia. *Arch Pathol* 1971; 92: 465.

109 Keen SJ, Libshitz HI. Thymic lesions. Experience with computed tomography in 24 patients. *Cancer* 1987; 59: 1520.

110 Moran CA, Travis WD, Rosado de Christenson M *et al.* Thymomas presenting as pleural tumours. Report of eight cases. *Am J Surg Pathol* 1992; 16: 138.

111 Nagasaka T, Nakashima N, Nunome H. Needle tract implantation of thymoma after transthoracic needle biopsy. *J Clin Pathol* 1993; 46: 278.

112 Loehrer PJ. Thymomas: current experience and future directions in therapy. *Drugs* 1993; 45: 477.

113 Maggi G, Casadio C, Cavallo A *et al.* Thymoma: results of 241 operated cases. *Ann Thorac Surg* 1991; 52: 175.

114 Haniuda M, Morimoto M, Nishimura H *et al.* Adjuvant radiotherapy after complete resection of thymoma. *Ann Thorac Surg* 1992; 54: 311.

115 Curran WJ, Kornstein MJ, Brooks JJ *et al.* Invasive thymoma: the role of mediastinal irradiation following complete or incomplete surgical resection. *J Clin Oncol* 1988; 6: 1722.

116 Marks RD, Wallace KM, Pettit HS. Radiation therapy control of nine patients with malignant thymoma. *Cancer* 1978; 41: 117.

117 Penn CRH, Hope-Stone HF. The role of radiotherapy in the management of malignant thymoma. *Br J Surg* 1972; 59: 533.

118 Ibrahim NBN, Briggs JC, Jeyasingham K, Owen JR. Metastasising thymoma. *Thorax* 1982; 37: 771.

119 Gravanis MB. Metastasizing thymoma. Report of a case and review of the literature. *Am J Clin Pathol* 1968; 49: 690.

120 Ruffini E, Mancuso M, Oliaro A *et al.* Recurrence of thymoma: analysis of clinicopathologic features, treatment and outcome. *J Thorac Cardiovasc Surg* 1997; 113: 55.

121 Lara PN, Bonomi PD, Faber LP. Retreatment of recurrent invasive thymoma with platinum, doxorubicin and cyclophosphamide. *Chest* 1996; 110: 1115.

122 Rea F, Sartori F, Loy M *et al.* Chemotherapy and operation for invasive thymoma. *J Thorac Cardiovasc Surg* 1993; 106: 543.

123 Bernatz PE, Khonsari S, Harrison EG *et al.* Thymoma: factors influencing prognosis. *Surg Clin North Am* 1973; 53: 885.

124 Masaoka A, Monden Y, Nakahara K *et al.* Follow up study of thymomas with special reference to their clinical stages. *Cancer* 1981; 48: 2485.

125 Wilkins EW, Castleman B. Thymoma: a continuing survey at the Massachusetts General Hospital. *Ann Thorac Surg* 1979; 28: 252.

126 Drachman DB, McIntosh KR, Reim J *et al.* Strategies for treatment of myasthenia gravis. *Ann N Y Acad Sci* 1993; 681: 515.

127 Weigerlt C. Pathologisch-anatomischer Beitrag zur Krankheit (Myasthenia Gravis) Erb'schen. *Neurol Zbl* 1901; 20: 597.

128 Wilkins EW, Edmunds LH, Castleman B. Cases of thymoma at the Massachusetts

General Hospital. *J Thorac Cardiovasc Surg* 1966; 52: 322.

129 Namba T, Brunner NG. Myasthenia gravis in patients with thymoma, with particular reference to onset after thymectomy. *Medicine* 1978; 57: 411.

130 Monden Y, Nakahara K, Kagotani F *et al.* Myasthenia gravis with thymoma. Analysis of postoperative prognosis for 65 patients with thymomatous myasthenia gravis. *Ann Thorac Surg* 1984; 38: 46.

131 Aarli JA, Thunold S. Serological detection of thymoma in myasthenia gravis. *Eur Neurol* 1981; 20: 380.

132 Masaoka A, Yamakawa Y, Niwa H *et al.* Extended thymectomy for myasthenia gravis patients: a 20 year review. *Ann Thorac Surg* 1996; 62: 853.

133 Scadding GK, Havard CWH, Lange MJ, Domb I. The long term experience of thymectomy for myasthenia gravis. *J Neurol Neurosurg Psychiatry* 1985; 48: 401.

134 Maggi G, Casadio C, Cavallo A *et al.* Thymectomy in myasthenia gravis. Results of 662 cases operated upon in 15 years. *Eur J Cardiothorac Surg* 1989; 3: 504.

135 Ferguson MK. Transcervical thymectomy. *Chest Surg Clin North Am* 1996; 6: 105.

136 Bolooki H, Schwartzman RJ. High-dose steroids for perioperative management of patients with myasthenia gravis undergoing thymectomy. *J Thorac Cardiovasc Surg* 1978; 75: 754.

137 Wilkins EW, Castleman B. Thymoma: a continuing survey at the Massachusetts General Hospital. *Ann Thorac Surg* 1979; 28: 252.

138 Welch KJ, Tapper D, Vawter GP. Surgical treatment: thymic cysts and neoplasms in children. *J Pediatr Surg* 1979; 14: 691.

139 McCafferty MH, Bahnson HT. Thymic cyst extending into the pericardium. *Ann Thorac Surg* 1982; 33: 503.

140 Lewis CR, Manoharan A. Benign thymic cysts in Hodgkin's disease: report of a case and review of published cases. *Thorax* 1987; 42: 633.

141 El-Sharkawi AMM, Patel B. Management of residual thymic cysts in patients treated for mediastinal Hodgkin's disease. *Thorax* 1994; 50: 1118.

142 Kuo T-T, Chang J-P, Lin F-J *et al.* Thymic carcinomas: histopathological varieties and immunohistochemical study. *Am J Surg Pathol* 1990; 14: 24.

143 Wick MR, Carney JA, Bernatz PE, Brown LR. Primary mediastinal carcinoid tumours. *Am J Surg Pathol* 1982; 6: 195.

144 Wang D-Y, Chang D-B, Kuo S-H *et al.* Carcinoid tumours of the thymus. *Thorax* 1994; 49: 357.

145 Salyer WR, Salyer DC, Eggleston JLC. Carcinoid tumors of the thymus. *Cancer* 1976; 37: 958.

146 Rao U, Takita H. Carcinoid tumour of possible thymic origin: case report. *Thorax* 1977; 32: 771.

147 Gartner L, Voorhess M. Adrenocorticotrophic hormone-producing thymic carcinoid in a teenager. *Cancer* 1993; 71: 106.

148 Ringe B, Dragojevic D, Frank G *et al.* Thymolipoma: a rare benign tumor of the thymus gland. *Thorac Cardiovasc Surg* 1979; 27: 369.

149 Mok CK, Ho FCS, Nandi P *et al.* Lipothymoma. *Med J Aust* 1980; 1: 272.

150 Moran CA, Rosado de Christenson M, Suster S. Thymolipoma. Clinicopathological review of 33 cases. *Mod Pathol* 1995; 8: 71.

151 Middleton G. Involvement of the thymus by metastatic neoplasms. *Br J Cancer* 1966; 20: 41.

152 Siegal GP, Dehner LP, Rosai J. Histiocytosis X (Langerhans' cell granulomatosis) of the thymus. A clinicopathologic study of four childhood cases. *Am J Surg Pathol* 1985; 9: 117.

153 Jessurun J, Azevedo M, Saldana M. Allergic angiitis and granulomatosis (Churg–Strauss syndrome). A report of a case with massive thymic enlargement in a non-asthmatic patient. *Hum Pathol* 1986; 17: 637.

154 Karcher DS, Pearson CE, Butler WM *et al.* Giant lymph node hyperplasia involving the thymus with associated nephrotic syndrome and myelofibrosis. *Am J Clin Pathol* 1982; 77: 100.

155 Serour F, Lieberman Y, Rosenman J *et al.* Castleman's disease of the mediastinum: misleading clinical and radiological characteristics. *Respir Med* 1989; 83: 509.

156 Rosai J, Parkash V, Reuter VE. The origin of mediastinal germ cell tumours in men. *Int J Surg Pathol* 1994; 2: 73.

157 Hailemariam S, Engeler DS, Bannwart F *et al.* Primary mediastinal germ cell tumour with intratubular germ cell neoplasia of the testis; further support for germ cell origin of these tumours. *Cancer* 1997; 79: 1031.

158 Willis RA. *Borderland of Embryology and Pathology.* London: Butterworth, 1958.

159 Carter D, Bibro MC, Touloukian RJ. Benign clinical behaviour of immature mediastinal teratoma in infancy and childhood. *Cancer* 1982; 49: 398.

160 Bosl GJ, Motzer RJ. Testicular germ-cell cancer. *N Engl J Med* 1997; 337: 242.

161 Chaganti RS, Rodriguez E, Mathew S. Origin of adult male mediastinal germ cell tumours. *Lancet* 1994; 343: 1130.

162 Luna MA, Valenzuela-Tamariz J. Germ-cell tumors of the mediastinum. Postmortem findings. *Am J Clin Pathol* 1976; 65: 450.

163 Burt ME, Javadpour N. Germ-cell tumors in patients with apparently normal testes. *Cancer* 1981; 47: 1911.

164 Daugaard G, Rrth M, von der Maase H *et al.* Management of extragonadal tumours and the significance of bilateral testicular biopsies. *Ann Oncol* 1992; 4: 283.

165 Economou JS, Trump DL, Holmes EC *et al.* Management of primary germ cell tumors of the mediastinum. *J Thorac Cardiovasc Surg* 1982; 83: 643.

166 Clamon GH. Management of primary mediastinal seminoma. *Chest* 1983; 83: 263.

167 Lewis BD, Hurt RD, Payne WS *et al.* Benign teratoma of the mediastinum. *J Thorac Cardiovasc Surg* 1983; 86: 727.

168 Philip WP, Harrison K, Cruikshank DB. A posterior mediastinal dermoid tumour with marked anatomical differentiation. *Thorax* 1954; 9: 245.

169 Weinberg B, Rose JS, Efremidis SC *et al.* Posterior mediastinal teratoma (cystic dermoid): diagnosis by computerised tomography. *Chest* 1980; 77: 694.

170 Prauer HW, Mack D, Babic R. Intrapulmonary teratoma 10 years after removal of a mediastinal teratoma in a young man. *Thorax* 1983; 38: 632.

171 Southgate J, Slade PR. Teratodermoid cyst of the mediastinum with pancreatic enzyme secretion. *Thorax* 1982; 37: 476.

172 Le Roux BT. Mediastinal teratoma. *Thorax* 1960; 15: 333.

173 Pachter MR, Lattes R. 'Germinal' tumors of the mediastinum. A clinicopathologic study of adult teratomas, teratocarcinomas, choriocarcinomas and seminomas. *Chest* 1964; 45: 301.

174 Paterson IM, Cockburn JS. Acute pericarditis due to perforation of a benign mediastinal teratodermoid into the pericardial sac. *Thorax* 1982; 37: 863.

175 Rusby NL. Dermoid cysts and teratoma of the mediastinum: a review. *J Thorac Surg* 1944; 13: 169.

176 Ashour M, El-Din Hawass Adam KAR *et al.* Spontaneous intrapleural rupture of mediastinal teratoma. *Respir Med* 1993; 87: 69.

177 Pantoja E, Wendth AJ, Cross VF. Radiographic manifestations of teratoma. *N Y State J Med* 1975; 75: 2353.

178 Brown LR, Muhm JR, Aughenbaugh GL *et al.* Computed tomography of benign mature teratomas of the mediastinum. *J Thorac Imaging* 1987; 2: 66.

179 Canty TG, Siemens R. Malignant mediastinal teratoma in a 15 year old girl. *Cancer* 1978; 41: 1623.

180 Morinaga S, Nomori H, Kobayashi R *et al.* Well-differentiated adenocarcinoma arising from mature cystic teratoma of the mediastinum (teratoma with malignant transformation). Report of a surgical case. *Am J Clin Pathol* 1994; 101: 531.

181 Gonzalez-Vela JL, Savage PD, Manivel JC *et al.* Poor prognosis of mediastinal germ cell cancers containing sarcomatous components. *Cancer* 1990; 66: 1114.

182 Wenger ME, Dines DE, Ahmann DL *et al.* Primary mediastinal choriocarcinoma. *Mayo Clin Proc* 1968; 43: 570.

183 Stepanas AV, Samaan NA, Schultz PN *et al.* Endocrine studies in testicular tumor patients with and without gynecomastia. A report of 45 cases. *Cancer* 1978; 41: 369.

184 Sogge MR, McDonald SD, Cofold PB. The malignant potential of the dysgenetic germ cell in Klinefelter's syndrome. *Am J Med* 1979; 66: 515.

185 McNeil MM, Leong AS-Y, Sage RE. Primary mediastinal embryonal carcinoma in association with Klinefelter's syndrome. *Cancer* 1981; 47: 343.

186 Lachman MF, Kim K, Koo B-C. Mediastinal teratoma associated with Klinefelter's syndrome. *Arch Pathol Lab Med* 1986; 110: 1067.

187 Nichols CR, Heerema NA, Palmer C *et al.* Klinefelter's syndrome associated with mediastinal germ cell neoplasms. *J Clin Oncol* 1987; 5: 1290.

188 Traveline JM, Criner GJ, Ming P-MI *et al.* Anterior mediastinal mass in a young man. *Thorax* 1994; 49: 283.

189 Nichols CR, Roth BJ, Heerema N *et al.* Hematologic neoplasia associated with primary mediastinal germ-cell tumours. *N Engl J Med* 1990; 322: 1425.

190 Orazi A, Neiman RS, Ulbright TM *et al.* Haemopoietic cells within the yolk sac tumour component are the source of secondary haemopoietic malignancies in patients with mediastinal germ cell tumours. *Cancer* 1993; 71: 3873.

191 Quillan SP, Siegel MJ. CT features of benign and malignant teratomas in children. *J Comput Assist Tomogr* 1992; 16: 722.

192 Motzer RJ, Rodriguez E, Reuter VE *et al.* Molecular and cytogenetic studies in the

diagnosis of patients with poorly differentiated carcinomas of unknown primary site. *J Clin Oncol* 1995; 13: 274.

193 Rustin GJS. Tumour markers in germ cell tumours. *Br Med J* 1986; 292: 713.

194 Javadpour N. The value of biologic markers in diagnosis and treatment of testicular cancer. *Semin Oncol* 1979; 6: 37.

195 Grigor KM, Detre SI, Kone J *et al.* Serum alpha-fetoprotein levels in 153 male patients with germ cell tumours. *Br J Cancer* 1977; 35: 52.

196 Pandha HS, Wasan HS, Harrington K *et al.* Failure of normalisation of alpha-fetoprotein concentration after successful treatment of teratoma. *Br Med J* 1995; 311: 434.

197 Lemarie E, Assouline PS, Diot P *et al.* Primary mediastinal germ cell tumours. Results of a French retrospective study. *Chest* 1992; 102: 1477.

198 Childs WJ, Goldstraw P, Nicholls JE *et al.* Primary malignant mediastinal germ cell tumours: improved prognosis with platinum-based chemotherapy and surgery. *Br J Cancer* 1993; 67: 1098.

199 Nichols CR. Mediastinal germ cell tumours. *Semin Thorac Cardiovasc Surg* 1992; 4: 45.

200 Toner GC, Geller NL, Tan C *et al.* Serum tumour marker half-life during chemotherapy allows early prediction of complete response and survival in non-seminomatous germ cell tumours. *Cancer Res* 1990; 50: 5904.

201 Newlands ES, Begent RHJ, Rustin GJS. Further advances in the management of malignant teratomas of the testis and other sites. *Cancer* 1983; 1: 948.

202 Polansky SM, Barwik KW, Ravin CE. Primary mediastinal seminoma. *Am J Roentgenol* 1979; 132: 17.

203 Mencel PJ, Motzer RJ, Mazumdar M *et al.* Advanced seminoma: treatment results, survival and prognostic factors in 142 patients. *J Clin Oncol* 1994; 12: 120.

204 Motzer RJ, Bosl GJ. High dose chemotherapy for resistant germ cell tumours: recent advances and future directions. *J Natl Cancer Inst* 1990; 84: 1703.

205 Urba WJ, Longo DL. Hodgkin's disease. *N Engl J Med* 1992; 326: 678.

206 Ledermann JA. Lymphoma involving the mediastinum: challenges in diagnosis and management. *Thorax* 1995; 50: 1121.

207 Gatter KC, Alcock C, Heryet A *et al.* Clinical importance of analysing malignant tumours of uncertain origin with immunohistochemical techniques. *Lancet* 1985; i: 1302.

208 Gaynor ER, Fisher RI. Chemotherapy and combined modality treatment in Hodgkin's disease. *Curr Opin Oncol* 1991; 3: 822.

209 Kirn D, Mauch P, Shaffer K *et al.* Large cell and immunoblastic lymphoma of the mediastinum: prognostic features and outcome in 57 patients. *J Clin Oncol* 1993; 11: 1336.

210 Hancock BW. Non-Hodgkin's lymphoma. *J R Coll Physicians Lond* 1995; 29: 340.

211 Hiller N, Fisher D, Shmesh O *et al.* Primary amyloidosis presenting as an isolated mediastinal mass: diagnosis by fine needle biopsy. *Thorax* 1994; 50: 908.

212 Jenkins MCF, Potter M. Calcified pseudotumoural mediastinal amyloidosis. *Thorax* 1991; 46: 686.

213 Falk RH, Comenzo RL, Skinner M. The systemic amyloidoses. *N Engl J Med* 1997; 337: 898.

214 Grewal RG, Prager K, Austin JHM *et al.* Long term survival in non-encapsulated primary liposarcoma of the mediastinum. *Thorax* 1993; 48: 1276.

215 Klimstra DS, Moran CA, Perino G *et al.* Liposarcoma of the anterior mediastinum and thymus. A clinicopathological study of 28 cases. *Am J Surg Pathol* 1995; 19: 782.

216 Moran CA, Suster S, Perino G *et al.* Malignant smooth muscle tumours presenting as mediastinal soft tissue masses. A clinicopathological study of 10 cases. *Cancer* 1994; 74: 2251.

217 Suster S, Moran CA, Koss MN. Rhabdomyosarcomas of the anterior mediastinum: report of four cases unassociated with germ cell, teratomatous or thymic carcinomatous components. *Hum Pathol* 1994; 25: 349.

218 Moran CA, Suster S. Mediastinal haemangiomas: a study of 18 cases with emphasis on the spectrum of morphological features. *Hum Pathol* 1995; 26: 416.

219 Eline TH, Gross BH, Francis IR. CT and MR imaging of mediastinal haemangiomas. *J Comput Assist Tomogr* 1990; 14: 766.

220 Kardamakis D, Bouboulis N, Ravazoula P *et al.* Primary haemangiosarcoma of the mediastinum. *Lung Cancer* 1996; 16: 81.

221 Brown LR, Reiman HM, Rosenow EC *et al.* Intrathoracic lymphangioma. *Mayo Clin Proc* 1986; 61: 882.

222 Ramani P, Shah A. Lymphangiomatosis. Histologic and immunohistochemical analysis of four cases. *Am J Surg Pathol* 1993; 17: 329.

223 Leeds SE, Benioff MA, Ortega P. Pulmonary lymphangiomyoma with renal angiomyolipomas. *Calif Med* 1973; 119: 74.

224 Watts MA, Gibbons JA, Aaron BL. Mediastinal and osseous lymphangiomatosis. *Ann Thorac Surg* 1982; 34: 324.

225 Fukuda S, Hossain Z. Cystic lymphangioma of the mediastinum and the small bowel. *Del Med J* 1977; 49: 575.

226 Shuman RL, Engelman R, Kittle CFL. Pulmonary lymphangiomyomatosis. *Ann Thorac Surg* 1979; 27: 70.

227 Sinclair W, Wright JL, Churg A. Lymphangioleiomyomatosis presenting in a postmenopausal woman. *Thorax* 1985; 40: 475.

228 Taylor JR, Ryu J, Colby TV *et al.* Lymphangioleiomyomatosis: clinical course in 32 patients. *N Engl J Med* 1990; 323: 1254.

229 Chan JK, Tsang WY, Pau MY *et al.* Lymphangiomyomatosis and angiomyolipoma. Closely related entities characterised by hamartomatous proliferation of HMB-45-positive smooth muscle. *Histopathology* 1993; 22: 445.

230 Rasaretnam R, Chanmugam D, Sabanathan K *et al.* Cervico-mediastinal lymphangioma. *Aust N Z J Surg* 1976; 46: 378.

231 Feutz EP, Yune HY, Mandelbaum I *et al.* Intrathoracic cystic hygroma: a report of three cases. *Radiology* 1973; 108: 61.

232 Bill AH, Sumner DS. A unified concept of lymphangioma and cystic hygroma. *Surg Gynecol Obstet* 1965; 120: 79.

233 Godart S. Embryological significance of lymphangioma. *Arch Dis Child* 1966; 4: 204.

234 Shin MS, Berland LL, Ho K-L. Mediastinal cystic hygromas: CT characteristics and pathogenetic considerations. *J Comput Assist Tomogr* 1985; 9: 297.

235 Grosfield JL, Weber TR, Vane DW. One-stage resection for massive cervicomediastinal hygroma. *Surgery* 1982; 92: 693.

236 Vaage S, Knutrud O. Congenital duplications of the alimentary tract with special regard to their embryogenesis. A follow up study of 16 surgically corrected cases. *Prog Pediatr Surg* 1974; 7: 103.

237 McLetchie NGB, Purves JK, Saunders RL. The genesis of gastric and certain intestinal diverticula and enterogenous cysts. *Surg Gynecol Obstet* 1954; 99: 135.

238 Tarnay TJ, Chang CH, Nugent RG *et al.* Esophageal duplication (foregut cyst) with spinal malformation. *J Thorac Cardiovasc Surg* 1970; 59: 293.

239 Bentley JFR, Smith JR. Developmental posterior enteric remnants and spinal malformations. The split notochord synrome. *Arch Dis Child* 1960; 35: 76.

240 Smith JR. Accessory enteric formations. A classification and nomenclature. *Arch Dis Child* 1960; 35: 87.

241 Superina RA, Ein SH, Humphreys RP. Cystic duplications of the esophagus and neurenteric cysts. *J Pediatr Surg* 1984; 19: 527.

242 Agha FP, Master K, Kaplan S *et al.* Multiple bronchogenic cysts in the mediastinum. *Br J Radiol* 1975; 48: 54.

243 Beardmore HE, Wiglesworth FW. Vertebral anomalies and alimentary duplications. Clinical and embryological aspects. *Pediatr Clin North Am* 1958; 5: 457.

244 Carr MJT, Deiraniya AK, Judd PA. Mediastinal cyst containing mural pancreatic tissue. *Thorax* 1977; 32: 512.

245 Eraklis AJ, Griscrom NT, McGovern JB. Bronchogenic cysts of the mediastinum in infancy. *N Engl J Med* 1969; 281: 1150.

246 Le Roux BT. Intrathoracic duplication of the foregut. *Thorax* 1962; 17: 357.

247 Kirwan WO, Walbaum PR, McCormack RJM. Cystic intrathoracic deviations of the foregut and their complications. *Thorax* 1973; 28: 424.

248 Owen SF, Fitzgerald FT. Acute infection of a mediastinal cyst. *Respiration* 1982; 43: 150.

249 Chuang MT, Barba FA, Kaneko M *et al.* Adenocarcinoma arising in an intrathoracic duplication cyst of foregut origin. *Cancer* 1981; 47: 1887.

250 Olsen JB, Clemmensen O, Andersen K. Adenocarcinoma arising in a foregut cyst of the mediastinum. *Ann Thorac Surg* 1991; 51: 497.

251 Mindelzun R, Long P. Mediastinal bronchogenic cyst with esophageal communication. *Radiology* 1978; 126: 28.

252 Gleeson JA, Stovin PGI. Mediastinal enterogenous cysts associated with vertebral anomalies. *Clin Radiol* 1961; 21: 41.

253 Kamoi I, Nishitani H, Oshiumi Y. Intrathoracic gastric cyst demonstrated by 99m-Tc pertechnetate scintigraphy. *Am J Radiol* 1980; 134: 1080.

254 Le Roux BT. Pericardial coelomic cysts. *Thorax* 1959; 14: 27.

255 Feigin DS, Fenoglio JJL, McAllister HA *et al.* Pericardial cysts. A radiologic–pathologic correlation and review. *Radiology* 1977; 125: 15.

256 Lillie WI, McDonald JR, Clagett OT. Pericardial celomic cysts and pericardial diverticula. A concept of etiology and report of cases. *J Thorac Surg* 1950; 20: 494.

257 Klatte EC, Yune HY. Diagnosis and treatment of pericardial cysts. *Radiology* 1972; 104: 541.

258 Unverferth DV, Wooley CF. The differential

diagnosis of paracardiac lesions: pericardial cysts. *Cathet Cardiovasc Diagn* 1979; 5: 31.

259 Wick MR. Mediastinal cysts and intrathoracic thyroid tumours. *Semin Diagn Pathol* 1990; 7: 285.

260 Mills NL. Pericardial cyst in the superior mediastinum. *Br J Radiol* 1959; 32: 554.

261 Sarin CL. Pericardial cyst in the superior mediastinum treated by mediastinoscopy. *Br J Surg* 1970; 57: 232.

262 Slasky BS, Hardesty RL. Midline pericardial cyst in the posterior mediastinum. *J Comput Assist Tomogr* 1982; 6: 171.

263 Kisner WH, Reganis JC. Pericardial celomic cyst with symptoms. *J Thorac Surg* 1950; 19: 779.

264 Hynes JK, Tajik AJ, Osborn MJ *et al.* Two dimensional echocardiographic diagnosis of pericardial cysts. *Mayo Clin Proc* 1983; 58: 60.

265 Modic MT, Janicki PC. Computed tomography of mass lesions of the right cardiophrenic angle. *J Comput Assist Tomogr* 1980; 4: 521.

266 Moncada R, Baker M, Salinas M *et al.* Diagnostic role of computed tomography in pericardial heart disease: congenital defects, thickening, neoplasms and effusions. *Am Heart J* 1982; 103: 263.

267 Daniel WG, Dohring W, Frank G *et al.* Non-invasive diagnosis of a pericardial cyst. Combined use of M-mode echocardiography and computed tomography. *Eur Heart J* 1980; 1: 201.

268 Friday RO. Paracardiac cyst: diagnosis by ultrasound and puncture. *JAMA* 1973; 226: 82.

269 De Roover PH, Maisin J, Lacquet A. Congenital pleuro-pericardial cysts. *Thorax* 1963; 18: 146.

270 Mouroux J, Pandovani B, Maalouf J *et al.* Pleuropericardial cysts: treatment by videothoracoscopy. *Surg Laparosc Endosc* 1996; 6: 403.

271 Lippert KM, Potozky H, Furman IK. Clinical significance of pleuropericardial cyst. *Arch Intern Med* 1951; 88: 378.

272 Kaimal KP. Computed tomography in the diagnosis of pericardial cyst. *Am Heart J* 1982; 103: 566.

273 Cardello FP, McQuown DS, Dollinger M. Ultrasound in diagnosis of paracardiac masses. *JAMA* 1974; 227: 1124.

274 Fromang DR, Seltzer MB, Tobias JA. Thoracic duct cyst causing mediastinal compression and acute respiratory insufficiency. *Chest* 1975; 67: 725.

275 Tsuchiya R, Sugiura Y, Ogata LT *et al.* Thoracic duct cyst of the mediastinum. *J Thorac Cardiovasc Surg* 1980; 79: 856.

276 Mori M, Kidogawa H, Isoshima K. Thoracic duct cyst in the mediastinum. *Thorax* 1992; 47: 325.

277 Allo MD, Thompson NW. Rationale for the operative management of substernal goitre. *Surgery* 1983; 94: 969.

278 Larochelle D, Arcand P, Belzile M *et al.* Ectopic thyroid tissue: a review of the literature. *J Otolaryngol* 1979; 8: 523.

279 Richmond I, Whittaker JS, Deiraniya AK *et al.* Intracardiac ectopic thyroid: a case report and review of published cases. *Thorax* 1990; 45: 293.

280 Reeve TS. Intrathoracic goitre: investigation and management. In: *Proceedings of the First Asian Congress on Thoracic and Cardiovascular Surgery.* Manila, 1972: 78.

281 Shih W-J, Cho S-R, Purcell M *et al.* Diagnostic imaging in mediastinal thyroid tumour. *Clin Nucl Med* 1984; 12: 702.

282 Bashist B, Ellis K, Gold RP. Computed tomography of intrathoracic goitres. *Am J Radiol* 1983; 140: 455.

283 Schlinkert RT, Whitaker MD, Argueta R. Resection of select mediastinal adenomas through an anterior mediastinotomy. *Mayo Clin Proc* 1991; 66: 1110.

284 Nathaniels EK, Nathaniels AM, Wang C-A. Mediastinal parathyroid tumours: a clinical and pathological study of 84 cases. *Ann Surg* 1970; 171: 165.

285 Scholz DA, Purnell DC, Woolner LB *et al.* Mediastinal hyperfunctioning parathyroid tumors: review of 14 cases. *Ann Surg* 1972; 178: 173.

286 Doppman JL. Parathyroid localization: arteriography and venous sampling. *Radiol Clin North Am* 1976; 14: 163.

287 Ubhi CS, Hardy JG, Pegg CAS. Mediastinal parathyroid adenoma: a new method of localization. *Br J Surg* 1984; 71: 859.

288 Krudy AG, Doppman JL, Brennan MF *et al.* The detection of mediastinal parathyroid glands by computed tomography, selective arteriography and venous sampling. *Radiology* 1981; 140: 739.

289 Shimada T, Higashi K, Kimura K *et al.* Magnetic resonance imaging as an effective tool for successful localization of superior mediastinal parathyroid adenoma. *Jpn J Med* 1990; 29: 647.

290 Thacker WC, Wells VH, Hall ER. Parathyroid cyst of the mediastinum. *Ann Surg* 1971; 174: 969.

291 Landau O, Chamberlain DW, Kennedy RS *et al.* Mediastinal parathyroid cysts. *Ann Thorac Surg* 1997; 63: 951.

292 Johnston KW, Rutherford RB, Tilson MD *et al.* Suggested standards for reporting on arterial aneurysms. *J Vasc Surg* 1991; 13: 452.

293 Kouchoukos NT, Dougenis D. Surgery of the thoracic aorta. *N Engl J Med* 1997; 336: 1876.

294 Munro NC, Soppitt D, Brewis RAL. Tracheal stenosis due to bilateral arterial aneurysms. *Thorax* 1994; 49: 183.

295 Chen JT. Plain radiographic evaluation of the aorta. *J Thorac Imaging* 1990; 5: 1.

296 Perko MJ, Norgaard M, Herzog TM *et al.* Unoperated aortic aneurysms: a survey of 170 patients. *Ann Thorac Surg* 1995; 59: 1204.

297 Payne WS, Larson RH. Acute mediastinitis. *Surg Clin North Am* 1969; 49: 999.

298 Corsten MJ, Shamji FM, Odell PF *et al.* Optimum treatment of descending necrotising mediastinitis. *Thorax* 1997; 52: 702.

299 Murray PM, Finegold SM. Anaerobic mediastinitis. *Rev Infect Dis* 1984; 6: S123.

300 Barrett NR. Idiopathic mediastinal fibrosis. *Br J Surg* 1958; 46: 207.

301 Goodwin RA, Nickell JA, des Prez RM. Mediastinal fibrosis complicating healed primary histoplasmosis and tuberculosis. *Medicine* 1972; 51: 227.

302 Poland GA, Jorgensen CR, Sarosi GA. *Nocardia asteroides* pericarditis: report of a case and review of the literature. *Mayo Clin Proc* 1990; 65: 819.

303 Bennhoff DF. Actinomycosis: diagnostic and therapeutic considerations and a review of 32 cases. *Laryngoscope* 1984; 94: 1198.

304 Dunn EJ, Ulicny KS, Wright CB *et al.* Surgical implications of sclerosing mediastinitis. *Chest* 1990; 97: 338.

305 Ahmad M, Weinstein AJ, Hughes JA *et al.* Granulomatous mediastinitis due to *Aspergillus flavus* in a non-immunocompromised patient. *Am J Med* 1981; 70: 887.

306 Urscel HC, Razzuk MA, Netto GL *et al.* Sclerosing mediastinitis: improved management with histoplasmosis titre and ketoconazole. *Ann Thorac Surg* 1990; 50: 215.

307 Dines DE, Payne LWS, Bernatz PE *et al.* Mediastinal granuloma and fibrosing mediastinitis. *Chest* 1979; 75: 320.

308 Sculley RE, Mark EJ, McNeely WF *et al.* Case records of the Massachusetts General Hospital. *N Engl J Med* 1989; 320: 380.

309 Goodwin RA, Loyd JE, Des Prez RM. Histoplasmosis in normal hosts. *Medicine* 1981; 60: 231.

310 Light AM. Idiopathic fibrosis of mediastinum: a discussion of three cases and review of the literature. *J Clin Pathol* 1978; 31: 78.

311 Mole TM, Glover J, Sheppard MN. Sclerosing mediastinitis: a report on 18 cases. *Thorax* 1995; 50: 280.

312 Sobrinho-Simoes MA, Vaz Saliero J, Wagenvoort CA. Mediastinal and hilar fibrosis. *Histopathology* 1981; 5: 53.

313 Graham JR, Suby HI, Leclompte PR *et al.* Fibrotic disorders associated with methysergide therapy for headache. *N Engl J Med* 1966; 274: 359.

314 Loeb JM, Lombard CM. Ideopathic mediastinitis with superior vena cava obstruction, cardiac tamponade and cutaneous vasculitis. *West J Med* 1991; 155: 296.

315 Yacoub MH, Thompson VC. Chronic idiopathic pulmonary hilar fibrosis: a clinico-pathological entity. *Thorax* 1971; 26: 365.

316 Anon. Mediastinal and hilar fibrosis. *Br Med J* 1971; 4: 639.

317 Berry DF, Buccigrossi D, Peabody J *et al.* Pulmonary vascular occlusion and fibrosing mediastinitis. *Chest* 1986; 89: 296.

318 Weinstein JBL, Aronberg DJ, Sagel SS. CT of fibrosing mediastinitis: findings and their utility. *Am J Radiol* 1983; 141: 247.

319 Rholl KS, Levitt RG, Glaser HS. Magnetic resonance imaging of fibrosing mediastinitis. *Am J Roentgenol* 1985; 145: 255.

320 Cardasco EM, Ahmad M, Mehta A *et al.* The effects of steroid therapy on pulmonary hypertension secondary to fibrosing mediastinitis. *Cleve Clin J Med* 1990; 57: 647.

321 Mitchell IM, Saunders NR, Maher O *et al.* Surgical treatment of idiopathic mediastinal fibrosis: report of five cases. *Thorax* 1986; 41: 210.

50

DEVELOPMENTAL DISORDERS OF THE LUNGS

DOUGLAS SEATON AND ANTHONY SEATON

Developmental disorders of the lungs are for the most part congenital, i.e. they exist from birth, being the consequence of disordered organogenesis following conception. As the development of the respiratory tract occurs according to a strict timetable (see Chapter 1), abnormalities present at birth may be accurately dated to disturbances of intercellular relationships that have occurred at fixed points in intrauterine life. Although major structural abnormalities of the respiratory tract and its adnexae are usually fatal, such effects are now frequently diagnosed before birth or early in postnatal life so that corrective surgery may be applied in certain cases. Other developmental anomalies may not manifest themselves until much later in life and although rare are of considerable interest to the practising physician.

A number of genetically based and ultrastructural disorders, including ciliary abnormalities, cystic fibrosis, α_1-antitrypsin deficiency and skeletal dysplastic syndromes or chondrodystrophies, are considered elsewhere in this book. Hamartomas of the lung (mesenchymomas) are considered as benign neoplasms in Chapter 42.

Tracheobronchial anomalies

The lower respiratory tract shares its embryological origin with the primitive foregut, arising from its ventral surface in the fourth week of intrauterine life as an epithelial laryngotracheal bud or 'respiratory primordial pouch' [1–3]. The subsequent development of the tracheobronchial tree and oesophagus proceeds concurrently, with the result that congenital abnormalities of one frequently involve the other, over 50 such anomalies having been recorded [4]. Respiratory tissues comprising airways and spaces distal to the terminal bronchioles are derived from mesoderm and are developmentally connected to epithelially derived proximal conducting airways in order to form a normal gas-exchanging pathway. Developmental errors of the tracheobronchial tree cannot arise after the 16th week of intrauterine life, since by this time its formation is complete [5].

Tracheal agenesis

Tracheal agenesis or aplasia refers to the absence of growth in the trachea or in part of it. It has a male to female preponderance of 2:1 and is often incompatible with life [6,7]. Three main anatomical patterns are recognized [8].

Type 1, in which there is agenesis of the proximal trachea, accounts for 20% of cases. The distal trachea is present and is often connected to the oesophagus by a fistulous communication.

Type 2, in which the main bronchi join in the midline and communicate with the oesophagus by a single fistula, is the most common variety accounting for 60% of cases.

Type 3, in which the left and right main bronchi join the oesophagus independently, accounts for the remaining 20% of cases.

Occasionally, the coexistence of a tracheo-oesophageal fistula permits air to enter the lungs so that the infant may survive for a period. In these circumstances, early diagnosis may allow temporary measures to sustain respiration and later reconstructive surgery to be undertaken [9–11].

Sometimes the trachea, though patent, is shortened owing to the absence of a number of cartilaginous rings, as in congenital brevicollis or the 'short neck syndrome', most commonly associated with Klippel–Feil syndrome, and characterized by a triad of short neck, decreased neck mobility and low occipital hairline [8,12].

Tracheo-oesophageal fistula

The H-type tracheo-oesophageal fistula (Fig. 50.1), in which both the trachea and oesophagus remain patent, may be sufficiently small to go undetected until adult life, despite the presence of recurrent symptoms from infancy [13,14]. Aspiration of oesophageal contents into the airways may cause choking, with cough and cyanotic episodes after feeding. The passage of air through the fistula and into the oesophagus in the reverse direction

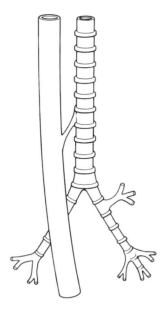

Fig. 50.1 H-type tracheo-oesophageal fistula.

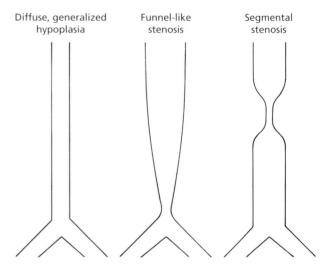

Fig. 50.2 Three types of tracheal stenosis.

may cause abdominal distension. Recurrent pneumonia is common [15]. Tracheo-oesophageal fistula may occur in partial tracheal agenesis [8] and also in oesophageal atresia, typified by a blind proximal pouch and distal fistulous communication between the lower oesophagus and trachea [16]. Tracheo-oesophageal fistula may also occur familially [17].

Tracheal stenosis

Tracheal stenosis (Fig. 50.2) is diffuse in 30% of cases, the pars membranacea being absent so that the trachea is encircled by 'napkin-ring' cartilages, the total number of which may exceed the usual complement of 22. More commonly (50% of cases) the stenoses are segmental and may occur with equal frequency in the upper, middle and lower parts of the trachea. In 20% of cases the stenosis is carrot or funnel-like and this is associated with the 'sling' left pulmonary artery syndrome, described below [18,19]. Tracheal stenoses are associated with tracheo-oesophageal fistulae, and accessory bronchi arising from the trachea may also be found [20]. An association with Down's syndrome has been reported [21]. The condition usually presents in infancy with stridor and respiratory insufficiency. Surgical treatment may be necessary, and various plastic tracheal reconstruction procedures have been described [22–24].

Tracheal narrowing due to extrinsic pressure

Congenital tracheal narrowing due to extrinsic pressure generally results from the close proximity of unusually large or abnormally placed vessels that have arisen as the result of faulty development of the primitive system of branchial arches (see Chapter 1). These anomalies are, in order of frequency, double aortic arch (47%), right aortic arch with left ligamentum arteriosum (20%), retro-oesophageal right subclavian artery (14%), anomalous innominate artery (11%), anomalous left carotid artery (4%), retrotracheal or 'sling' left pulmonary artery (3%) and right aortic arch with aberrant left subclavian artery (1%) [8,25]. Occasionally, the combination of anomalous vessels with congenital tracheal stenosis requires surgical repair [26].

Tracheomalacia

This term is used to indicate excessive weakness and collapsibility of the tracheal walls as a result of abnormally soft or pliable cartilages. It may occur in localized form as the result of a deficiency of cartilage in a short segment of trachea [27]. This condition may be mistakenly diagnosed in the presence of obstructive airways disease in which high intrathoracic pressures are produced during expiration, with resultant compression of even the normal upper respiratory tract. It should be noted that acquired forms of tracheomalacia occur as a result of prolonged endotracheal intubation and in the rare systemic disorder of cartilage known as relapsing polychondritis (see Chapter 45). Tracheomalacia may be associated with other tracheo-oesophageal anomalies and presents in childhood with expiratory airflow obstruction and apnoeic episodes. In severe cases surgical intervention with aortopexy and various tracheal splinting procedures may be necessary [28,29].

Tracheobronchomegaly

Tracheobronchomegaly [30–33] is a rare disease characterized by unusual width of the trachea and main bronchi and, because of the ineffectiveness of cough, often complicated by lower respiratory infection and bronchiectasis [34]. The cough may have a loud booming quality. The disease is probably congenital and may be inherited as an autosomal recessive; it has been recorded in association with Ehlers–Danlos syndrome. Most reported cases have been in young adults but it has been found in children. There is an atrophic or congenital defect of the connective tissues of the trachea and main bronchi. The condition may be missed on the plain chest film but is obvious on the tracheo-bronchogram and on CT or magnetic resonance imaging [35]. There is gross variation in diameter of the trachea with respiration and there may be other distortions and irregularities.

Those of the foregoing conditions that cause either a structural or functional narrowing of the trachea may produce clinical features, including wheezy dyspnoea, respiratory distress during feeding, recurrent lower respiratory tract infection, stridor, tugging inspiratory effort with intercostal muscle retraction, cyanosis and apnoeic episodes.

Abnormal patterns of bronchial branching

These are usually found at bronchoscopy and are seldom of clinical significance, other than when resective surgery is being undertaken for some other reason. The abnormalities are more often additive than subtractive and, as might be anticipated, more variability is found at segmental level than in larger proximal bronchi. The most common major anomaly is a supernumerary right upper lobe bronchus [36], which may arise anywhere from the trachea or right main bronchus (Fig. 50.3). The frequency of tracheal origin is estimated at 0.9% and of double origin from the right upper lobe bronchus at 0.4% [37]. Sometimes the origin of an upper lobe bronchus may be displaced so that it arises only from the trachea with no separate main bronchial origin. Absence of an upper lobe bronchus is the most common of the major subtractive abnormalities (0.3%). The most common segmental anomaly is a double-stem apical lower lobe segmental bronchus that occurred in 7% of one series [37], the incidence being slightly higher on the right than on the left. Unusually, an apical upper lobe segmental bronchus may arise from the trachea in either displaced or supernumerary fashion.

Bronchial isomerism is a term applied to a rare group of developmentally anomalous syndromes in which the normal pattern of bronchial branching in either the left or the right lung is mirrored in the contralateral lung, resulting in a so-called bilateral left or right lung. Developmen-

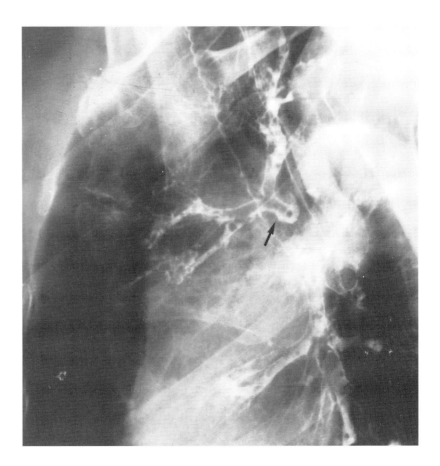

Fig. 50.3 Supernumerary right upper lobe bronchus arising from trachea shown at bronchography.

tal abnormalities of the heart, great vessels, liver, spleen and gut frequently coexist [38].

Bronchial atresia

This rare condition has been reviewed by Meng and colleagues [39]. It probably arises as a result of a developmental interruption of normal bronchial continuity in which a length of bronchus, usually the apicoposterior segmental bronchus of the left upper lobe [40], becomes sealed off from the larger proximal airways to which it may remain connected by thin, uncanalized, fibrous, vestigial strands. This sealed-off or atretic bronchus becomes distended by bronchial secretions, resulting in the formation of a cystic space or mucocele. Some degree of collateral ventilation to lung subtended by the atresia is maintained via the interalveolar pores of Kohn, although normal postnatal alveolar development to this part of the lung is retarded, with a reduced alveolar count. The pattern of bronchial branching distal to the atretic segment, having developed antenatally, remains intact [41]. Abnormalities of the vascular supply of the affected lungs have been recorded and may be causally related to bronchial atresia, as may a described association with pectus excavatum [42].

The majority of patients are asymptomatic and the diagnosis of bronchial atresia is made in young adult life following a chest radiograph that has been requested for some other reason. Less than one-third of patients present with symptoms due to lower respiratory tract infection. The chest radiograph shows the mucocele as a coin lesion and part of the lung distal to it appears hyperlucent as a result of collateral air trapping. Bronchography showed non-filling of the affected bronchus, and the surrounding bronchi may appear to be displaced by the peripheral zone of hyperlucency [5]. CT allows the diagnosis to be made with some confidence [43]. Although the risk of infection in untreated bronchial atresia is estimated to be low, in most reported cases the diagnosis has been made following surgical excision of the atretic segment by lobectomy or segmentectomy [39].

Bronchogenic cysts (syn. bronchial cysts)

Bronchogenic cysts arise as a result of abnormal budding of the tracheobronchial tree during the course of its development between the 26th day and 16th week of intrauterine life [1,44], in which a tracheal or bronchial bud becomes detached from its parent, thereafter developing separately to produce a cystic structure. Bronchogenic cysts are more common in males and apparently in Yemenite Jews [45,46]. They may be classified according to their situation as either central (syn. mediastinal) or peripheral (syn. intraparenchymal, intralobar). Central bronchogenic cysts presumably arise earlier in the developmental process, detaching themselves from major airways and occupying a position alongside the trachea, at the level of the carina or close to a main or lobar bronchus, or juxtaposed to the oesophagus [47,48]. If the developmental anomaly arises at a later stage, then the cyst or cysts are situated towards the periphery of the lung. In several reported series the peripheral situation is at least as common as the central one [49–52], and two-thirds of peripheral cysts occur in the lower lobes [36,52]. Bronchogenic cysts are usually single but are occasionally multiple and may sometimes arise in both lungs [36,52]; unusually they may occur in ectopic situations in relation to the pericardium [53], diaphragm [54], vertebral column [55] and skin [56].

Pathological features

Bronchogenic cysts vary in size and may reach 10 cm in diameter [48,52]. Their walls may be thin but increase in thickness following infection. They are usually lined by ciliated respiratory epithelium and contain smooth muscle, elastic tissue, cartilaginous trabeculations and mucous glands. The presence of cartilage in their walls serves to distinguish them from cysts of different origin. A fistulous communication with an adjacent airway may be present, and in these circumstances the cyst may be filled with air. A ball-valve mechanism may cause it to enlarge and present in infancy or exceedingly rarely in young adult life by causing displacement of normal lung [57]. Intact and uninfected cysts contain clear fluid. The presence of infection tends to destroy the characteristic histological features so that it may become extremely difficult to distinguish between a chronically infected bronchogenic cyst and an acquired lung abscess [58]. Complication by development of rhabdomyosarcoma has been described [59].

Clinical features

Bronchogenic cysts are frequently asymptomatic and may come to light as an abnormal shadow on a chest radiograph that has been requested for some unrelated reason. When symptoms do occur, they result from either a mass effect on adjacent structures or more frequently infection. Pressure on the trachea or a proximal bronchus may produce dyspnoea, cough and stridor, and on the heart may cause dysrhythmias. Oesophageal compression may result in dysphagia. Repeated lower respiratory tract infection or atelectasis may be caused by bronchial compression. Should the contents of the cyst become infected, it may enlarge and rupture into either the mediastinum or an adjacent airway, resulting in a cough productive of mucopurulent material or haemoptysis.

Radiographic features

The diagnosis is suspected following the radiographic finding of a well-circumscribed, rounded, homogeneous opacity situated either in the mediastinum close to a major airway or in the lung periphery (Fig. 50.4). If a fistulous communication is present, an air–fluid level may be visible and rarely it may mimic a large emphysematous bulla. The presence of calcification in the wall of the cyst is a variable and uncertain feature. If the cyst is centrally situated, a barium swallow may demonstrate oesophageal compression.

Treatment

Elective surgical resection of the lesion is generally advised because it is often impossible to make a firm diagnosis preoperatively, and a neoplastic condition cannot be excluded with certainty. Furthermore, there is a tendency for bronchogenic cysts to undergo serious or even lethal complications [60–62]. Only with small asymptomatic cysts or in patients in whom surgery is contraindicated is there a case for their being left *in situ*, and then only after needle aspiration [63].

Congenital adenomatoid malformation of the lung

This condition is synonymous with congenital cystic adenomatoid malformation of the lung and in older literature was probably called congenital bronchiectasis or pulmonary cystic disease [8]. It may involve either a part or the whole of a lobe or rarely an entire lung. The affected lobe or lung derives its blood supply from the pulmonary circulation and comprises a firm and airless mass of disorganized pulmonary tissue that lacks a properly defined bronchial system but contains an excess of air passages resembling terminal bronchioles and often includes mucous cysts of varying sizes [64]. Occasionally, the congenital adenomatoid malformation may consist of a separate mass connected by an extra bronchus to the normal bronchial tree, in which case it can be regarded as a form of accessory lung. Stocker and colleagues [65] described 38 cases that they classified into three types.

Type I, characterized by single or multiple large cysts, was the most common form, accounting for 50% and carrying a good prognosis.

Type II, consisting of multiple small cysts of less than 1 cm in diameter, accounted for 40% of cases and carried a poor prognosis.

Type III carried a very poor prognosis and consisted of a solid airless mass of tissue.

It has been suggested that adenomatoid malformation of the lung results from a developmental failure of the proximal bronchial system, arising from the epithelial laryngotracheal bud, to unite in a normal manner with mesodermally derived distal alveolated tissue [58]. To this extent it may be regarded as a developmental anomaly of both the tracheobronchial tree and the lung parenchyma.

About 50% of cases are born prematurely and 25% are stillborn [8]. Many of those born alive die within a few hours, often with anasarca caused by vena caval compression due to the space-occupying effect of the abnormal tissue mass. Infection of the cysts commonly occurs if the infant survives beyond the neonatal period, although the onset of symptoms may be delayed for 2 or 3 years [66]. The condition may be complicated by pneumothorax that occurs as a result of air trapping in the cystic spaces [67]. The condition may now be diagnosed antenatally by ultrasound examination, and in some cases treatment by surgical resection of the affected parts of the lung is practicable [68].

Anomalies involving the lung parenchyma

Agenesis and hypoplasia of the lung

Inconsistencies in the use of the terms 'agenesis' and 'hypoplasia' may be found in the literature [8,36]. In this book the term 'agenesis' is taken to mean absence or almost complete absence of growth in the lung [58], while the term 'hypoplasia' indicates underdevelopment but not non-development of the lung. Thus the hypoplastic lung contains a normal number of lobes but is diminished in size, with fewer bronchial branchings and reduced numbers of alveoli.

Complete bilateral agenesis of the lungs is extremely rare [69]. Needless to say, it is incompatible with life. Unilateral agenesis of the lung is much less rare and may be present to varying degrees of severity [8,70]. The left lung is affected more frequently than the right and the majority of cases exhibit other congenital abnormalities, one of the most common being patent ductus arteriosus [71–73]. In the most common form of unilateral agenesis there is a rudimentary bronchus but complete absence of lung tissue. In a second form there is a total absence of both the lung and bronchial system, and in a third, the least common, there is a rudimentary bronchial system attached to a reduced amount of alveolated tissue, this form being more properly regarded as an example of lung hypoplasia.

In many patients the aetiology is unknown. However, conditions that decrease intrathoracic space, especially congenital diaphragmatic herniae, may cause unilateral lung hypoplasia [74–76] and this may also be associated with ipsilateral congenital vascular anomalies [77]. Bilateral pulmonary hypoplasia is associated with the presence

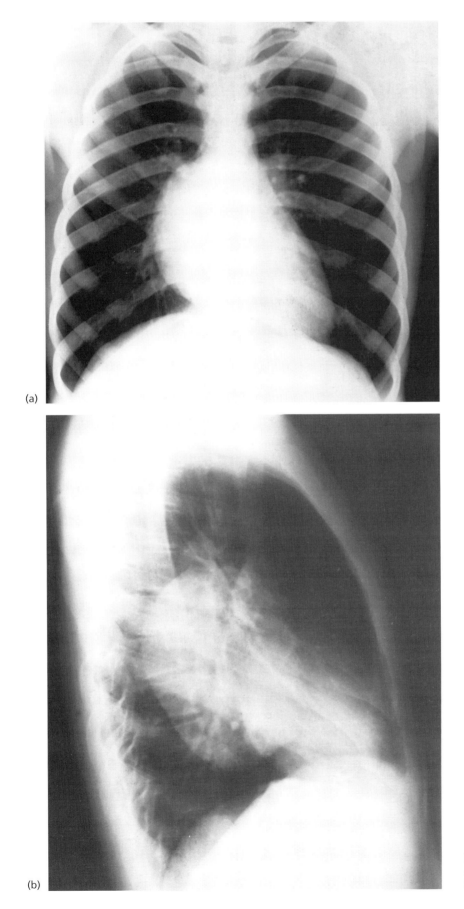

(a)

(b)

Fig. 50.4 Posteroanterior (a) and lateral (b) chest radiographs of a 24-year-old man with large right-sided bronchogenic cyst.

of oligohydramnios caused variously by renal tract disorders or by amniotic fluid leak [78,79]. An important cause is premature rupture of the membranes, and impaired lung development is detectable antenatally by ultrasonographic measurement of chest wall diameter [75,80,81]. It has also been shown that maternal treatment with angiotensin-converting enzyme inhibitors during pregnancy may be associated with lung hypoplasia [82].

Clinical features and diagnosis

Agenesis or hypoplasia of the lung is frequently associated with major extrapulmonary developmental abnormalities, and when this is the case death frequently occurs in infancy. When the anomaly is confined to a lung or part of it, prolonged survival may be possible but is likely to be accompanied by recurrent episodes of lower respiratory tract infection. This may result from imperfect drainage of lung secretions or from the spillover of pooled secretions from a blind bronchial stump into initially normal lung tissue [83].

The chest radiograph in agenesis or hypoplasia of the lung shows a hemithorax of diminished volume with crowded ribs, elevated hemidiaphragm and mediastinal displacement to the affected side. The contralateral lung tends to overinflate and may expand across

Fig. 50.5 (a) Posteroanterior chest film showing a hypoplastic right lung. (b) Tomogram of same patient showing anomalous veins draining a hypoplastic lung.

the midline [84] (Fig. 50.5). These appearances resemble atelectasis, and bronchoscopy, CT and occasionally pulmonary angiography may be required to make the distinction.

Congenital abnormalities of lobulation

Whereas complete agenesis of a lobe of the lung is rare [85], congenital anomalies of lobulation are much more common and one of those most frequently encountered is the so-called azygos lobe. An azygos lobe is really the medial portion of a bifurcated right upper lobe and in humans may be regarded as an anatomical variation, although students of comparative anatomy are aware that it is said to be a constant feature in the porpoise. It is formed during lung development if the apex of the right lung, as it enlarges, encounters the azygos vein as this vessel arches over the root of the right lung to join the superior vena cava. Whereas in normal circumstances the entire right upper lobe lies lateral to the azygos vein, in the case of this anomaly the right upper lobe assumes a bifid configuration so that a portion of lung lies on either side of the venous arch formed by the azygos vein [86]. The invagination that the azygos vein produces in the right upper lobe is in effect a supernumerary fissure and is bounded on each side by a layer of visceral and parietal pleura (Fig. 50.6). This fissure shows characteristically on chest radiographs as a thin outwardly convex line ending in a small triangular shadow at its lower end (Fig. 50.7).

The bronchial anatomy remains intact and the presence

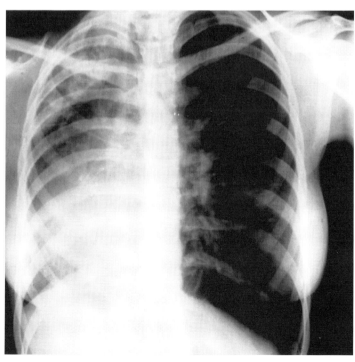
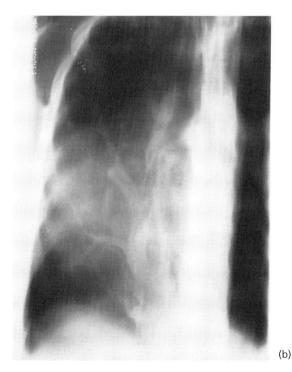

(a)
(b)

of an azygos lobe carries no morbidity. It is important only in that its features, which are present in about 0.25% of chest radiographs, require correct interpretation. A similar anomaly may very rarely occur in the left upper lobe [87].

Lung sequestration

This term covers a spectrum of related developmental pulmonary anomalies generally characterized by the forma-

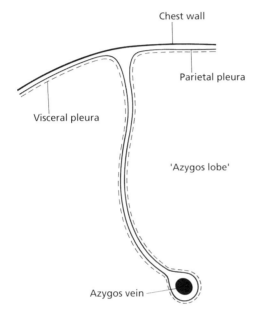

Fig. 50.6 Pleural infolding of an azygos lobe.

tion of an island of abnormal unventilated lung tissue that has no normal communication with the bronchial system and derives its arterial supply from the systemic rather than the pulmonary circulation.

Two principal types are defined for clinical convenience, namely intralobar and extralobar sequestration [88], although numerous variants have been described and much overlap may occur between these types [58,89]. The abnormal lung tissue in intralobar sequestration, which is the more common of the two types, is contained within the substance of normal lung tissue that completely surrounds it. In the rarer extralobar form the abnormal lung tissue, although lying close to normal lung, is situated outside the pleural coverings of the lung and is indeed invested by its own separate pleural membranes (Fig. 50.8). Since the latter form is entirely disconnected from normal lung, some authors refer to an extralobar sequestration as an 'accessory lung without a bronchial connection' [8,58]. The gender incidence is said to be equal for intralobar sequestration, while the extralobar form occurs four times more commonly in males than females [91]. Both forms occur more commonly in the left hemithorax; however, whereas the intralobar variety occurs on this side in 60% of cases, in the extralobular variety over 90% are left-sided [8,58,71,92]. The reasons for this left-sided propensity are unclear but may be connected with the observation that in normal development the primitive pleuroperitoneal canal closes on the left side later than on the right. Furthermore the absence of hepatic tissue on the left provides additional space in which abnormal tissue may develop. An ipsilateral diaphragmatic defect is

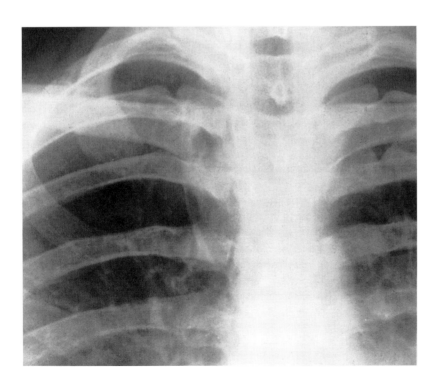

Fig. 50.7 Normal chest film showing typical appearance of an azygos lobe in the right upper zone medially.

common in extralobar sequestration, occurring in 60% of cases, but is rare in intralobar forms [8].

The posterior basal segment of either lower lobe is the most common site for intralobar sequestration. An upper lobe may be involved but this is rare [8,93]. Very occasionally an entire lung may be sequestrated [94,95]. The majority of extralobar sequestrations are sandwiched between

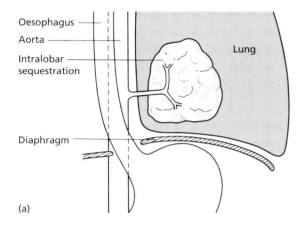

(a)

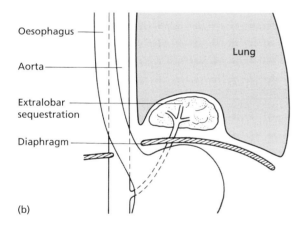

(b)

Fig. 50.8 Intralobar (a) and extralobar (b) sequestration. (After Gerle *et al.* [90].)

the left lower lobe and the diaphragm but may also occur below the diaphragm, within the diaphragmatic substance itself, within the mediastinum or even as far cephalad as the neck [58,96].

The various ways in which sequestrated lung may receive its vascular supply have been reviewed by Thilenius and colleagues [97]. Both intralobar and extralobar sequestrations usually receive their arterial supply from the descending aorta or one of its branches, either above or below the diaphragm. Subdiaphragmatic supply is reportedly more common in extralobar sequestration [98], in which case the vessel passes through the aortic or oesophageal hiatus or through a separate diaphragmatic defect. Arteries that supply the intralobar variety tend to be disproportionately large with respect to the volume of tissue supplied [58]; in both the intralobar and extralobar types the supplying arteries may be multiple. The veins draining intralobar sequestrations usually empty into the pulmonary venous circulation, whereas it is more usual for extralobar sequestrations to be drained by the azygos system of veins. Considerable shunts may sometimes result, so that the patient may present in early life with heart failure [99,100].

About half of all patients with extralobar sequestration have other congenital abnormalities of sufficient severity to bring them to medical attention, so that the sequestration is diagnosed in the first year of life in up to 60% of patients. On the other hand, widespread congenital abnormalities in intralobar sequestration are rare [8,58,71] so that the diagnosis is seldom made in neonatal life and, in over 50% of cases, not before the age of 20. Table 50.1 compares some of the features of intralobar and extralobar sequestration.

Aetiology

Pulmonary sequestration comprises a variety of congenital anomalies for which there is no hereditary basis, and none of the many theories of causation is entirely acceptable unless it has sufficient flexibility to explain the

Table 50.1 Points of comparison between intralobar and extralobar pulmonary sequestration.

Feature	Intralobar	Extralobar
Frequency	More common	Less common
Sex incidence (male : female)	1 : 1	4 : 1
Most common site	Within posterior basal segment	Between lower lobe and diaphragm
Side of thorax	*c.*60% left	*c.*90% left
Arterial supply	*c.*70% thoracic aorta	*c.*45% thoracic aorta
Venous drainage	Usually pulmonary veins	Often systemic veins
Diagnosed in neonates	Rarely	Commonly
Other congenital defects	Uncommon	Frequent

development of both intralobar and extralobar sequestration as well as more complex variants [58,89,101–103]. Occasional reports of the occurrence of both intralobar and extralobar sequestration in the same patient provide some evidence in support of a unitary theory [104,105]. One such proposition is that pulmonary sequestration develops as a result of the formation of an accessory lung bud distal to the normal laryngotracheal bud on the ventral aspect of the primitive foregut [103]. As this anomalous bronchial tissue grows, it becomes invested by primitive respiratory mesenchyme. The amount of mesenchyme determines the size of the sequestration and results in the development of its respiratory bronchioles and alveolar tissue [106]. The original foregut connection may involve and disappear, possibly as a result of outgrowth of its blood supply, although occasionally a foregut communication persists, particularly in the case of extralobar forms. Those accessory buds that arise in close proximity to the laryngotracheal bud may become incorporated into it during its development to become intralobar sequestrations, whereas those that arise from the foregut more distally either from the oesophagus or from the proximal part of the stomach escape envelopment and become extralobar sequestrations [102]. Each type of sequestration usually retains its primitive systemic arterial supply; venous drainage may be either into the pulmonary system if the sequestration developed in close proximity to the normal laryngotracheal bud, or to the systemic system if it arose more distally [100].

Pathology

Intralobar pulmonary sequestration appears macroscopically as a well-circumscribed reddish-grey area that may be clearly differentiated from healthy lung but which is intimately related to it, being usually situated within the substance of the posterior basal segment of either lower lobe. An extralobar sequestration is separated from normal lung and the surface is shiny and homogeneous, being covered by its own pleural investment. Both forms typically receive a systemic arterial supply and although this is usually derived from the aorta, the vessels tend to have the elastic structure of a pulmonary artery rather than the muscular structure found in a normal aortic branch. Histologically both intralobar and extralobar sequestrations typically contain dilated ciliated bronchi together with focal development of alveolated tissue. Bronchial dilatation by retained secretions and oedema may result in the formation of cysts visible to the naked eye. The usual histological features may be lost in cases where the sequestration has become infected.

Clinical features

Those sequestrations diagnosed in the first year of life are frequently brought to light in the course of the investigation of multiple congenital abnormalities and are usually extralobar in type. Some of those that escape detection in this manner are found in adult life in asymptomatic individuals following a routine chest radiograph. Others may present with non-specific symptoms of lower respiratory tract infection or with recurrent pneumonic episodes, characterized by cough, sputum production and occasionally haemoptysis, which may be massive. These complications may arise because there is a tendency for a sequestrated segment to become distended by mucous secretions which, in the absence of a foregut communication, are unable to drain away so that surrounding normal lung tissue becomes compressed and liable to infection. Once infection is established in adjacent lung, a fistula between the sequestrated segment and surrounding lung may develop and the infection tends to persist as a result of inadequate drainage.

Extralobar sequestrations may be less liable to infection as they are entirely separate from the normal lung [105]. Signs of pneumonic consolidation may be present but features of pleurisy and pleural effusion are said to be unusual [92]. Finger clubbing has been described, as have associated bony deformities of the ribs and chest wall.

Radiology and treatment

The radiographic features are variable. The diagnosis of intralobar sequestration should be suspected in the presence of a persistent opacity situated in either of the posterior basal segments (Fig. 50.9). The non-aerated tissue contained in the sequestration may produce a homogeneous shadow, the margins of which are not always well defined but which may have the appearance of a solitary pulmonary nodule. Cystic change may be visible radiographically and the 'cysts' may contain air–fluid levels, implying the presence of either a fistulous bronchial communication resulting from infection or some degree of collateral ventilation occurring at alveolar level (Fig. 50.10). Extralobar sequestration is less easily seen and may produce a small opacity contiguous with the left hemidiaphragmatic shadow. Both types of sequestration occasionally have persistent foregut connections and these are sometimes demonstrable by barium swallow [102,107].

Bronchography showed non-opacification of the sequestration, which was seen to be surrounded by displaced but normally ramifying bronchial branches. The diagnosis is now confirmed by CT and if necessary by retrograde thoracic aortography, which demonstrates one or more feeding arteries that usually arise from the descending aorta just above or below the diaphragm (see Fig. 1.2). These investigations are desirable because by identifying aberrant arteries they exclude other possibilities such as pneumonia, bronchiectasis, lung abscess and tumour, and also forewarn the thoracic surgeon of the existence and

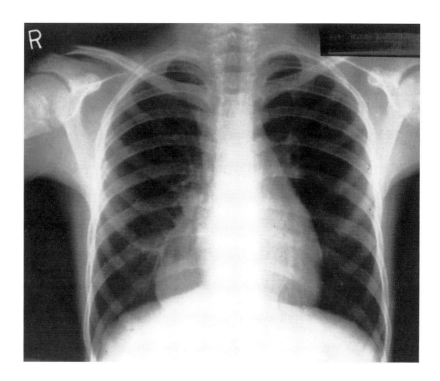

Fig. 50.9 Sequestrated segment in right lower lobe posterior to right cardiac border.

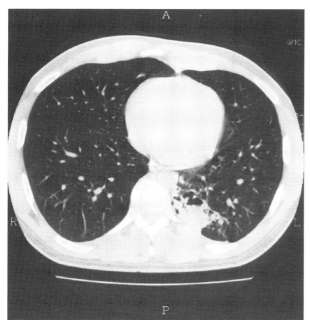

Fig. 50.10 CT scan of man showing extralobar sequestration posteriorly in the left lung. Note cavitation with fluid level following infection.

distribution of the vessels that require identification and ligation at thoracotomy.

Resection of a symptomatic pulmonary sequestration is indicated. Any infection that might be present is first treated with appropriate antibiotics. Intralobar sequestrations usually require segmental resection or lobectomy [100]. Extralobar sequestration may be resected without disturbing normal lung. Disastrous bleeding may occur as a result of failure to identify properly the aberrant vascular supply [100] but has also been described as a complication of unresected sequestration [108].

Anomalies of the pulmonary vasculature

The embryology of the pulmonary vasculature is relevant to the description of the developmental anomalies that follows (see Chapter 1). The intrapulmonary vasculature is derived from the mesenchymal investment of the primitive lung bud. The pulmonary vascular plexus so formed receives its initial arterial supply from paired segmental arteries arising from the aorta. Later the vascular plexus is joined by ramifications of the pulmonary arteries that are themselves derived from the sixth branchial arch. Once this connection is established, and as the aorta migrates caudally, the segmental aortic arteries normally involute and are lost, being replaced by the bronchial arteries that grow out of the aorta at what ultimately will be thoracic level.

The venous side of the pulmonary vascular plexus at first drains into the primitive anterior and posterior cardinal veins, although this route is later replaced when the pulmonary veins from each lung grow out to fuse with a single large pulmonary vein that in turn develops from the sinus venosus. Ultimately this structure is completely absorbed into the atrium to such an extent that the four pulmonary veins normally enter the left atrium separately.

The pulmonary vasculature is well developed by the 16th week of intrauterine life but clearly growth continues *in utero*, as does vascular remodelling at a microscopic level. Disturbances of this remodelling may result in the excessive muscularization of the intra-acinar arteries found in the condition referred to as persistent pulmonary hypertension of the newborn [5,109]. One such case has been described following maternal aspirin ingestion during pregnancy, and it was postulated that pulmonary hypertension in this patient arose as a consequence of premature closure of the ductus arteriosus that had in turn resulted from the prostaglandin-inhibiting effects of this drug [110].

Absent pulmonary artery trunk

The pulmonary artery trunk may be completely absent as a result of agenesis of the primitive sixth branchial arch or of developmental failure of the septum that normally divides the truncus arteriosus into aorta and pulmonary artery trunk. A left-to-right shunt exists in such cases, the lungs being supplied by bronchial or other aberrant systemic vessels; prolonged survival is impossible unless major corrective surgery proves feasible [58,111].

Absent unilateral pulmonary artery

Absence of one or other main pulmonary artery is rare and is a consequence of the failure of either the left or right side of the primitive sixth branchial arch to develop in the embryo. No connection exists between the main pulmonary artery trunk and the lung parenchymal vasculature on the affected side, which receives its blood supply systemically, most frequently from enlarged bronchial vessels but occasionally from aberrant arteries that usually arise from the descending aorta or less frequently from the ascending aorta, the arch, the left innominate artery, the left subclavian artery, their immediate branches or from a persistent right-sided ductus arteriosus.

The left and right pulmonary arteries are affected with equal frequency [112,113] but the right-sided lesion is more common in adult life because absence of the left pulmonary artery is strongly associated with congenital heart disease and therefore with increased early mortality [114]. In one series, 40% of cases of absent left pulmonary artery also had Fallot's tetralogy (ventricular septal defect, pulmonary outflow tract obstruction, overriding aorta and right ventricular hypertrophy) [113]. Absence of the right pulmonary artery carries no strong association with congenital heart disease and hence the tendency for patients with this anomaly to survive. The lung that receives the abnormal blood supply is frequently hypoplastic and may contain cystic and bronchiectatic changes [58]; 20% of patients with a right-sided absent pulmonary artery have been found to have pulmonary hypertension [115]. Whereas patients who present in infancy usually do so as a result of associated cardiac disease, adults with unilateral absence of a pulmonary artery may be asymptomatic, the diagnosis being made following a chest radiograph requested for some other reason [36]. The affected lung receives its blood supply from systemic vessels and occasionally patients present with haemoptysis. The chest radiograph shows a small hilar shadow and a small hyperlucent lung on the involved side. The diagnosis may be confirmed and differentiated from Macleod's syndrome by a perfusion lung scan or pulmonary angiogram, both of which show complete lack of perfusion on the affected side. Treatment is not usually possible, although reconstructive anastomotic surgery and recanalization procedures may be practicable in some cases [116]. Rarely pneumonectomy has been required to control haemoptysis, in which case thoracic aortography to demonstrate the collateral circulation is desirable [36].

Pulmonary artery stenosis

Postvalvular pulmonary artery stenosis (syn. pulmonary artery coarctation) is rare and may occur at any level from above the valve to the segmental arteries and beyond [117]. Centrally placed stenoses involving the pulmonary artery trunk or left or right main pulmonary artery branches are less common than multiple peripheral lesions, which are sometimes accompanied by pulmonary hypertension. Although pulmonary stenosis may occur in isolated form, this condition is more commonly detected in the course of the investigation of associated congenital heart disease. Postvalvular pulmonary artery stenosis has been described as part of the rubella syndrome [118] and in idiopathic hypercalcaemia. Chest radiography may show poststenotic dilatations that produce a beaded appearance contiguous with the lung vascular markings. Occasionally the poststenotic dilatations may reach aneurysmal proportions and may rupture causing haemoptysis. The diagnosis is confirmed by pulmonary angiography.

Large centrally placed lesions may be amenable to corrective surgery but this carries the risk of massive intrapulmonary bleeding due to the rupture of more distally placed pulmonary vessels as these are frequently hypoplastic [58].

Anomalous origin of the left pulmonary artery

The failure of the pulmonary arterial plexus of the left lung and the left part of the sixth primitive branchial arch to connect in the normal way may result in the left pulmonary artery arising in anomalous fashion from the right pulmonary artery. In order to reach the left lung, this aberrant left pulmonary artery loops around the right main bronchus like a sling and runs a peculiar course between the lower end of the trachea anteriorly and the oesophagus posteriorly, thereby crossing the midline to enter the left hilum [119] (Fig. 50.11). A condition known as 'sling' pulmonary artery syndrome may result, in which pressure from the aberrant left pulmonary artery may cause varying degrees of obstruction to the left main bronchus, trachea and oesophagus with consequent dyspnoea and dysphagia. Further tracheal obstruction may be produced in this developmental anomaly by an associated intrinsic tracheal defect, in which the pars membranacea is absent and the lumen of the trachea is completely encircled by so-called 'napkin-ring' cartilages [8]. The aberrant pulmonary sling vessel may be seen on a lateral chest radiograph as a rounded opacity between the air-filled trachea and oesophagus at the level of the carina. A barium swallow may provide supportive evidence and the diagnosis is confirmed by pulmonary angiography [115,120].

Anomalous systemic pulmonary perfusion

Dysplastic lung tissue may sometimes receive a blood supply from systemic vessels other than the normal bronchial arteries, as has been described in pulmonary sequestration above. Other examples of abnormal systemic arterial supply may be found in the absence of sequestration and where the lung tissue supplied is apparently normal [121,122]. Such arteries usually arise from the descending thoracic aorta but may also originate from the ascending aorta, the arch, the innominate, subclavian, internal mammary and intercostal arteries or below the diaphragm from the abdominal aorta or the coeliac artery [115] (Fig. 50.11). These vessels usually have the characteristic elastic structure of a pulmonary artery, rather than the

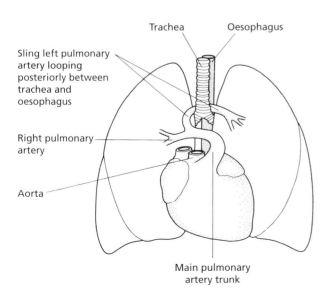

Sling left pulmonary artery looping posteriorly between trachea and oesophagus

Trachea   Oesophagus

Right pulmonary artery

Aorta

Main pulmonary artery trunk

Fig. 50.11 'Sling' left pulmonary artery. (After Kale *et al.* [120].)

muscular form of an aortic branch, and may communicate with the pulmonary circulation or drain systemically, creating a left-to-right shunt. The patient is frequently asymptomatic but may come to medical attention through recurrent haemoptysis. A systolic or a continous bruit with systolic accentuation may be heard over the involved area of the chest. The chest radiograph may be normal or show increased irregular vascular markings in the vicinity of the anomalous vessels. Pulmonary angiography shows no abnormality, while aortography is diagnostic. Surgical ligation or clipping of anomalous vessels, therapeutic embolism or even resection of lung may occasionally be indicated to control haemoptysis. These anomalies may be classified as a rare form of pulmonary arteriovenous malformation (see below).

Anomalous pulmonary venous drainage

Anomalous venous drainage of a lung arises as a result of persistent communications between the embryonic system of cardinal veins and the pulmonary venous plexus. These communications develop into aberrant pulmonary veins that drain systemically, usually into the inferior vena cava, rather than returning oxygenated blood into the left atrium in the manner of normal pulmonary veins. This anomalous drainage, which is usually partial rather than total, creates a left-to-right shunt and as with other developmental abnormalities of the lungs may be associated with congenital heart disease, the extent of which may govern the prognosis [123,124].

Scimitar syndrome

The scimitar syndrome is synonymous with congenital pulmonary venolobar syndrome and vena cava bronchovascular syndrome [123–125]. The most consistent feature of the syndrome is drainage of part of the right lung by an anomalous scimitar-shaped pulmonary vein that passes through the lung running parallel to, but separate from, the mediastinal structures before joining the inferior vena cava, usually below the diaphragm. Other variable features that may be present include:

1 an anomalous systemic arterial supply to the territory drained by the scimitar vein, taking the form of multiple small arteries arising from the descending aorta, often below the diaphragm and entering the base of the right lung, the right main pulmonary artery being frequently small or even absent;

2 hypoplasia of the right lung itself, which is small and contains fewer airways that may show bronchial isomerism [125];

3 cardiac dextroposition, which is a consequence of the small right lung;

4 diaphragmatic abnormalities in which the right hemidiaphragm may have an accessory leaf, being fused anteriorly but separated posteriorly and containing lung between its layers [126,127].

The scimitar syndrome may occur familially with an autosomal dominant pattern of inheritance [128]. The left-to-right shunt in these patients is usually of insufficient magnitude to produce ill-effects and the condition is most frequently diagnosed in adult life in asymptomatic subjects following a routine chest radiograph [124]. The chest radiograph shows a characteristic curvilinear vascular density in the right lower lung (from which the syndrome derives its name), with features of ipsilateral loss of lung volume as evidenced by mediastinal shift to the right and an elevated diaphragm (see Fig. 50.5). The abnormalities may be demonstrated in detail by CT and pulmonary angiography, although plain radiographs are usually adequate for diagnostic purposes and surgical intervention is in any case rarely necessary [126,129,130].

Other variant syndromes

Further examples of anomalous pulmonary venous drainage that have been described include the following.
1 Drainage of the right lung into the superior vena cava, azygos vein or right innominate vein.
2 Drainage of the left lung into a left-sided superior vena cava or vertical vein, representing a persistence of the embryonic left anterior cardinal vein. This vessel may drain in a cephalic direction to join the left innominate vein or caudally to join the coronary sinus.
3 Drainage of the pulmonary veins into the coronary sinus attached to the right atrium.
4 Drainage of a common single pulmonary vein into the right atrium by way of an additional atrium-like chamber, an anomaly referred to as a cor triatriatum deformity [58,131].

Pulmonary arteriovenous malformations and telangiectasia (see also Chapter 42)

Several terms used synonymously with pulmonary arteriovenous malformation are found in the literature, including pulmonary arteriovenous fistula, pulmonary arteriovenous aneurysm, pulmonary angioma, pulmonary haemangioma and pulmonary cavernous angioma.

Definition and pathology

These lesions, although sometimes categorized as tumours, contain no neoplastic cells and are in fact developmental anomalies in which there are persistent vascular communications between arteries and veins within the lung that effectively bypass parts of the normal pulmonary capillary bed. Arteriovenous malformations are rare, approximately three per year having been recorded

at a major North American centre of referral over a 20-year period [132]. Le Roux [133] reported less than one case per year in a European thoracic surgical centre compared with approximately 300 cases of bronchial carcinoma and 13 bronchial adenomas seen in the same period. The majority of arteriovenous malformations probably originate during the development of the primitive pulmonary vascular plexus, when an anastomotic vessel arises which presents a significantly lower resistance to flow than that provided by the surrounding pulmonary vascular bed [58] (Fig. 50.12). Physical principles dictate that arterial blood is diverted through this passage of least resistance, and with increasing flow there is a gradual dilatation and enlargement both of the anastomotic vessel and of the arteries and the tributaries that feed it. Those veins draining the fistulous communication also distend and become varicose. The ultimate size of the lesion depends upon haemodynamic factors and ranges from the very small to a large labyrinthine mass of dilated interconnecting thin-walled vascular spaces of lobar proportions [135].

About 95% of arteriovenous malformations derive their blood supply from branches of the pulmonary artery and drain into the pulmonary venous circulation [132]. In the few remaining cases, the supplying vessels originate systemically from the aorta and innominate, subclavian, internal mammary, bronchial and intercostal arteries and drainage may be via systemic or pulmonary veins [136].

Pulmonary telangiectasis results if there is a fistulous communication between a small peripheral arteriole and venule. If large numbers of these defects are present and if they are diffusely distributed, then the condition may be referred to as pulmonary telangiectasia [137,138].

There is a close association between pulmonary arteriovenous malformations and hereditary haemorrhagic telangiectasia (Osler–Rendu–Weber syndrome), an autosomal dominant condition present in 50–60% of cases [132,139,140]. Conversely, only 5–15% of patients with hereditary haemorrhagic telangiectasia develop pulmonary arteriovenous malformations [141]. It has been shown that a gene located on chromosome 9q3 is strongly associated with the presence of the two conditions, whereas those subjects with Osler–Rendu–Weber disease without pulmonary telangiectasia do not have this abnormal gene [142–144].

Arteriovenous malformations are slightly more common in women than men [108,115]. The majority occur as single lesions, multiple malformations being found in 20–30% of cases, occurring more frequently in patients with hereditary haemorrhagic telangiectasia [108,109]. Approximately 10% of lesions occur bilaterally [132,133]. Arteriovenous malformations are usually closely related to the visceral pleura and 70% occur in the lower lobes [132]. Associated vascular anomalies have been recorded in other organs [140].

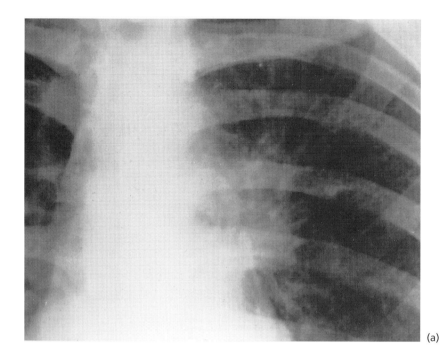

(a)

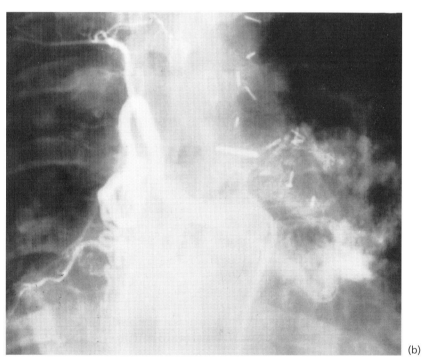

(b)

Fig. 50.12 (a) Chest film shows abnormal vascularity in left upper zone. (b) Retrograde aortic catheter shows the aberrant artery supplying lung directly from the aorta.

Clinical features

It is unusual for discrete arteriovenous malformations to be diagnosed before the third decade of life; hereditary haemorrhagic telangiectasia also usually manifests itself at puberty or later. In a series of 101 cases of all types of pulmonary arteriovenous malformation, the mean age at diagnosis was 40 years [132,145]. However, occasionally the condition is detected in infancy, especially in patients with hereditary telangiectasia, and in some such cases treatment becomes necessary [146,147]. More than half of all patients have no symptoms referable to the malformations at the time of diagnosis, which is frequently made following a routine chest radiograph or during the investigation of hereditary haemorrhagic telangiectasia. This condition is characterized by the presence of small, raised, red telangiectatic lesions of 2–3 mm diameter that blanch on pressure and are found on the skin and mucosal

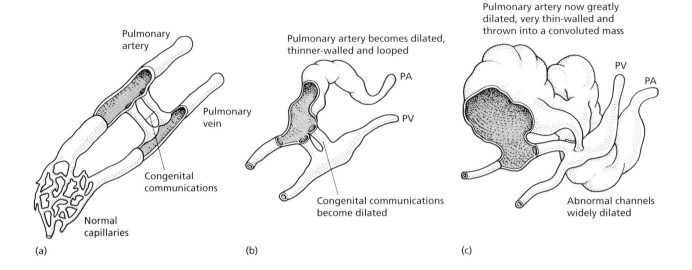

Fig. 50.13 (a–c) Evolution of a convoluted vascular malformation from congenital precapillary arteriovenous malformations. (After Cope [134].)

surfaces, particularly about the face, lips, mouth and nasopharynx (Fig. 50.13). The mucosal lesions tend to bleed and the patient may present with epistaxis, an acute gastrointestinal bleed or symptoms of anaemia as a consequence of occult bleeding into the gut.

The respiratory symptom most commonly present at the time of diagnosis is dyspnoea, haemoptysis being less frequent [132,148]. A bruit is audible in over half of all patients with arteriovenous malformations [132,149]. This is typically heard over the site of the lesion and is systolic or continuous with systolic and inspiratory accentuation. Cyanosis may be present as a result of right-to-left shunting and, when this is present, finger clubbing is a frequent accompaniment [132,150]. Symptoms are unlikely to occur in the case of single discrete lesions provided that the radiographic diameter of the malformation is less than 2 cm. The frequency of symptoms need not be greater in the presence of multiple lesions with the exception of the numerous tiny lesions found in the syndrome of pulmonary telangiectasia, in which symptoms and signs are usually evident from childhood [137,138].

Complications

The most common complication is haemorrhage, either into the bronchial tree producing haemoptysis or rarely into the pleural cavity producing a haemothorax [151–155]. Exceptionally pneumothorax may occur. Transient cerebral ischaemic attacks or cerebral infarction may be produced by a combination of systemic arterial hypoxaemia and secondary polycythaemia, while in some series as many as 50% of patients have had episodes suggestive of paradoxical embolization [132,156,157]. Less frequently, cerebrovascular accidents may result from the rupture of an associated intracranial arteriovenous malformation or from an embolus arising within a pulmonary arteriovenous malformation or passing through it in paradoxical fashion [157]. Bacterial endangiitis may occur with a pulmonary arteriovenous malformation, giving rise to metastatic abscesses in the brain or at other sites [156]. Cerebral abscesses may also occur if infected material passes straight through an arteriovenous malformation rather than being filtered by the pulmonary capillaries.

Radiographic features

Arteriovenous malformations may be seen on the chest radiograph as one or more rounded lobulated or tortuous opacities, frequently occupying the periphery of the lower lung fields [133]. Feeding or draining vessels that link the malformation with the hilum are sometimes visible on either plain films or tomograms [158]. CT is a useful method for identification and delineation of lesions [159]. Vascular calcification is uncommon [145]. Serial radiographs may show gradual enlargement of the malformations with the passage of time. The shadows are often well defined and the radiograph may be misinterpreted as indicating metastatic tumour [145]. The radiographic size of the discrete lesion may be shown to vary according to intrathoracic pressure, increasing in size during a Müller manoeuvre and becoming smaller with a Valsalva manoeuvre [160]. Bilateral pulmonary angiography confirms the diagnosis in all but a few cases [158] (Fig. 50.14). This investigation, together with CT, should always be undertaken if surgical treatment is being

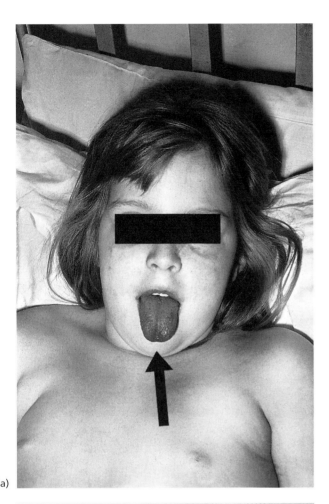

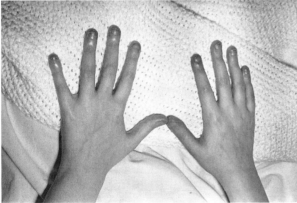

Fig. 50.14 (a) Facial appearance of 10-year-old girl, cyanosed from birth, with Osler–Rendu–Weber syndrome showing cyanosed lips and an angioma on her tongue (arrowed). (b) Finger clubbing in the same patient.

considered since they may demonstrate small lesions not detectable on plain radiographs. In the few malformations that derive their arterial supply from systemic vessels, aortography is required in order to demonstrate them adequately.

The radiographic appearance of pulmonary telangiectasia differs in that the salient feature is diffuse nodularity, particularly in the lower zones, which may be mistaken for pulmonary fibrosis and which may increase as time passes. As the vascular lesions in pulmonary telangiectasia are small, they are not usually demonstrable by pulmonary angiography.

Functional abnormalities

The majority of pulmonary arteriovenous malformations produce a right-to-left shunt, an exception being those lesions with a systemic arterial supply. If the shunt is of sufficient size, arterial hypoxaemia results. However, this is usually mild and is associated with a normal or reduced $P\text{co}_2$. In such cases, Sao_2 is reduced and is not entirely correctable by the administration of pure oxygen. The size of the intrapulmonary shunt, expressed as a percentage of cardiac output, may be obtained from measurements of mixed venous and arterial oxygen content while the patient is breathing 100% oxygen for 20 min [161]. Dye dilution curves are of little value in the quantification of shunt in pulmonary arteriovenous malformations because the fistulae are so close to capillary level that two separate peaks of dye are not seen at the arterial sampling site [145]. The former technique may also be inaccurate in the case of pulmonary telangiectasia, in which the proximity of the abnormal vessels to the alveoli and their small size (relative to larger discrete arteriovenous malformations) permits them to take up significant quantities of oxygen when this is being breathed in pure form. An alternative method of determining shunt has been developed in order to overcome this difficulty, by means of radioactively labelled albumin macroaggregates injected into a peripheral vein. Normally almost all of these particles would be arrested in the pulmonary capillaries, but in pulmonary telangiectasia a significant quantity pass straight through the telangiectatic vessels. Since the proportion of cardiac output normally received by the cranial and renal circulations is known, the size of the shunt may be estimated by counting radioactivity over the lungs, brain and kidneys [137,162].

Secondary polycythaemia was present in 23% of a combined series of 101 patients with arteriovenous malformation, anaemia due to hereditary haemorrhagic telangiectasia being present in 19% [132,145]. Right heart and pulmonary artery pressures were recorded in 22 patients in this series and the values obtained were normal in all cases. However, pulmonary hypertension, the mechanism of which is uncertain, has been reported in a few cases [163].

Measurements of diffusing capacity using carbon monoxide ($D\text{lco}$) require correction for haemoglobin level if polycythaemia or anaemia is present [164]. $D\text{lco}$ may be reduced in pulmonary telangiectasia, presumably as a result of a diminished pulmonary capillary blood volume [136].

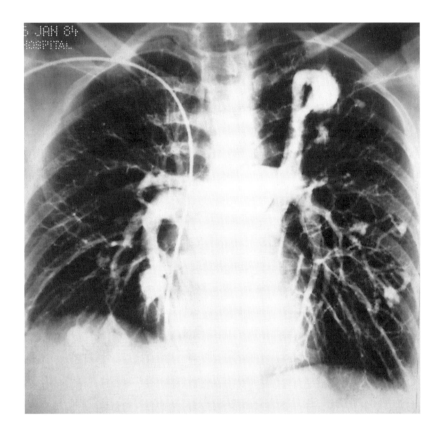

Fig. 50.15 Pulmonary arteriogram in patient with multiple arteriovenous malformations.

Treatment

The more widespread availability of embolization techniques and studies of their success rates and complications has led to a reappraisal of management of arteriovenous malformations, and it is now generally agreed that active treatment is desirable for lesions with feeding vessels greater than 3 mm in diameter [165–168]. Indeed, the relatively high rate of complications in untreated malformations is regarded by some as a reason for screening of relatives of patients with hereditary haemorrhagic telangiectasia in order to detect and treat asymptomatic lung lesions. Surgical treatment should be considered following full evaluation of a solitary pulmonary arteriovenous malformation. Discrete peripheral arteriovenous malformations may be removed by local resection with ligation of the afferent and efferent vessels. Deeper and more extensive lesions may be removed by wedge resection, segmental resection or lobectomy with the general aim of conserving as much lung tissue as possible [145,160]. When the arteriovenous malformations are multiple or bilateral, selective treatment is indicated and embolization or occlusion techniques, using balloons or steel coils, have been used with success. The occluding devices are lodged in a distal part of the feeding vessels. These methods have become the treatment of choice in patients with multiple or bilateral arteriovenous malformations in order to avoid the need for extensive or repeated surgery [165–168]. Complications occur in around 10% of embolizations, including systemic displacement of the embolus and puncture of the myocardium. Nevertheless, these forms of therapy result in increased Pao_2 and improved exercise tolerance, and recanalization is relatively infrequent.

Finally, in some cases of multiple lesions and telangiectasia with cyanosis, lung transplantation becomes an option [169].

References

1 Boyden EA. Development and growth of the airways. In: Hodson WA, ed. *Lung Biology in Health and Disease*, Vol 6. New York: Marcel Decker, 1977.

2 O'Rahilly R, Boyden EA. The timing and sequence of events in the development of the human respiratory system during the embryonic period proper. *Z Anat Entwickl* 1973; 141: 237.

3 Zaw-Tun HA. The tracheo-esophageal septum: fact or fantasy? Origin and development of the respiratory primordium and esophagus. *Acta Anat* 1982; 114: 1.

4 Kluth D. Atlas of esophageal atresia. *J Pediatr Surg* 1976; 11: 901.

5 Reid LM. Lung growth in health and disease. *Br J Dis Chest* 1984; 78: 113.

6 Altman RP, Randolph JG, Shearin RB. Tracheal agenesis: recognition and management. *J Pediatr Surg* 1972; 7: 112.

7 Hopkinson JM. Congenital absence of the trachea. *J Pathol* 1972; 107: 63.

8 Landing BH, Dixon LG. Congenital malformations and genetic disorders of the respiratory tract (larynx, trachea, bronchi and lungs). *Am Rev Respir Dis* 1979; 120: 151.

9 Fonkalsrud EW, Martelle RR, Maloney JV. Surgical treatment of tracheal agenesis. *J Thorac Cardiovasc Surg* 1963; 45: 520.

10 Hiyama E, Yokoyama T, Ichikawa T, Matsuura Y. Surgical management of tracheal agenesis. *J Thorac Cardiovasc Surg* 1994; 108: 830.

11 Koltai PJ, Quiney R. Tracheal agenesis. *Ann Otol Rhinol Laryngol* 1992; 101: 560.

12 Morrison SG, Perry LW, Scott LP. Congenital brevicollis (Klippel–Feil syndrome). *Am J Dis Child* 1968; 115: 614.

13 Mullard KS. Congenital tracheo-oesophageal fistula without atresia of the oesophagus. *J Thorac Surg* 1954; 28: 39.

14 Stephens RW, Lingeman RE, Lawson JL. Congenital tracheo-oesophageal fistulas in adults. *Ann Otol Rhinol Laryngol* 1976; 85: 613.

15 Schneider KM, Becker JM. The 'H type' tracheo-esophageal fistula in infants and children. *Surgery* 1962; 51: 677.

16 Engel PMA, Vos LJM, de Vries JA *et al.* Esophageal atresia with tracheoesophageal fistula in mother and child. *J Pediatr Surg* 1970; 5: 564.

17 Van Staey M, de Bie S, Matton MT *et al.* Familial congenital esophageal atresia. Personal case report and review of the literature. *Hum Genet* 1984; 66: 260.

18 Cantrell JR, Guild HG. Congenital stenosis of the trachea. *Am J Surg* 1964; 108: 297.

19 Cohen SR, Landing BH. Tracheostenosis and bronchial abnormalities associated with pulmonary artery sling. *Ann Otol Rhinol Laryngol* 1976; 85: 582.

20 Holinger PH. Congenital abnormalities of the tracheobronchial tree. *Postgrad Med* 1964; 36: 454.

21 Wells TR, Landing BH, Shamszadeh M, Thompson JW, Bove KE, Caron KH. Association of Down syndrome and segmental tracheal stenosis with ring tracheal cartilages: a review of nine cases. *Pediatr Pathol* 1992; 12: 673.

22 Johnson DG. Tracheal reconstruction. *Semin Pediatr Surg* 1994; 3: 244.

23 Andrews TM, Cotton RT, Bailey WW, Myer CM, Vester SR. Tracheoplasty for congenital complete tracheal rings. *Arch Otolaryngol Head Neck Surg* 1994; 120: 1363.

24 Grillo HC. Slide tracheoplasty for long-segment congenital tracheal stenosis. *Ann Thorac Surg* 1994; 58: 613.

25 Lincoln JCR, Deverall PB, Stark J *et al.* Vascular anomalies compressing the oesophagus and trachea. *Thorax* 1969; 24: 295.

26 Ziemer G, Heinemann M, Kaulitz R, Freihorst J, Seidenberg J, Wilken M. Pulmonary artery sling with tracheal stenosis: primary one-stage repair in infancy. *Ann Thorac Surg* 1992; 54: 971.

27 Landing BH. Syndromes of congenital heart disease with tracheobronchial anomalies. *Am J Roentgenol* 1975; 123: 679.

28 Messineo A, Filler RM. Tracheomalacia. *Semin Pediatr Surg* 1994; 3: 253.

29 Filler RM, Messineo A, Vinograd I. Severe tracheomalacia associated with esophageal atresia: results of surgical treatment. *J Pediatr Surg* 1992; 27: 1136.

30 Al-Mallah Z, Quantock OP. Tracheobronchomegaly. *Thorax* 1968; 23: 320.

31 Himalstein MR, Gallagher JC. Tracheobronchomegaly. *Ann Otol* 1973; 82: 223.

32 Katz I, LeVine M, Herman P. Tracheobronchomegaly. *Am J Roentgenol* 1962; 88: 1084.

33 Rahbar M, Tabatabai D. Tracheobronchomegaly. *Br J Dis Chest* 1971; 65: 65.

34 Guest JL, Anderson JN. Tracheobronchomegaly (Mounier–Kuhn syndrome). *JAMA* 1977; 238: 1754.

35 Smith DL, Withers N, Holloway B, Collins JV. Tracheobronchomegaly: an unusual presentation of a rare condition. *Thorax* 1994; 49: 840.

36 Mehta AC, Muzaffar A, Golish JA *et al.* Congenital anomalies of the lung in the adult. *Clev Clin Q* 1983; 50: 401.

37 Atwell SW. Major anomalies of the tracheobronchial tree with a list of the minor anomalies. *Dis Chest* 1967; 52: 611.

38 Landing BH, Lawrence T-YK, Payne VC *et al.* Bronchial anatomy in syndromes with abnormal visceral situs, abnormal spleen and congenital heart disease. *Am J Cardiol* 1971; 28: 456.

39 Meng RL, Jensik RJ, Faber LP *et al.* Bronchial atresia. *Ann Thorac Surg* 1978; 25: 184.

40 Warner JO, Rubin S, Heard BE. Congenital lobar emphysema, a case with bronchial atresia and abnormal bronchial cartilages. *Br J Dis Chest* 1982; 76: 177.

41 Williams AJ, Schuster SR. Bronchial atresia associated with a bronchogenic cyst. Evidence of early appearance of atretic segments. *Chest* 1985; 87: 396.

42 van Klaveren RJ, Morshuis WJ, Lacquet LK, Cox AL, Festen J, Heystraten FM. Congenital atresia with regional emphysema associated with pectus excavatum. *Thorax* 1992; 47: 1082.

43 Jederlinic PJ, Sicilian IS, Baigelman W, Gaensler EA. Congenital bronchial atresia. A report of 4 cases and a review of the literature. *Medicine* 1987; 66: 73.

44 Bucher U, Reid L. Development of the intrasegmental bronchial tree: the pattern of branching and development of cartilage at various stages of intrauterine life. *Thorax* 1961; 16: 207.

45 Racz I, Baum GL. The relationship of ethnic origin to prevalence of cystic lung disease in Israel: a preliminary report. *Am Rev Respir Dis* 1965; 91: 552.

46 Baum GL, Racz I, Bubis JJ *et al.* Cystic disease of the lung: report of eighty-eight cases with an ethnologic relationship. *Am J Med* 1966; 40: 578.

47 Maier HC. Bronchiogenic cysts of the mediastinum. *Ann Surg* 1948; 127: 476.

48 Editorial. Bronchial cysts. *Br Med J* 1973; ii: 501.

49 Rogers LF, Osmer JG. Bronchogenic cyst: a review of 46 cases. *Am J Roentgenol* 1964; 91: 273.

50 Hutchin P. Congenital cystic disease of the lung. *Rev Surg* 1971; 28: 79.

51 Ramenofsky ML, Leape LL, McCaulay RG. Bronchogenic cyst. *J Pediatr Surg* 1979; 14: 219.

52 Mayo P, Saha SP, Long GA *et al.* Surgical management of congenital lung cysts: a sixteen year review. *J Ky Med Assoc* 1984; 82: 327.

53 Kwak D, Stork WJ, Greenberg SD. Partial defect of the pericardium associated with a bronchogenic cyst. *Radiology* 1971; 101: 287.

54 Buddington WT. Intradiaphragmatic cyst: 9th reported case. *N Engl J Med* 1957; 257: 613.

55 Yamashita J, Maloney AF, Harris P. Intradural spinal bronchogenic cyst. *J Neurosurg* 1973; 39: 240.

56 Fraga S, Helwig EB, Rosen SH. Bronchogenic cysts in the skin and subcutaneous tissue. *Am J Clin Pathol* 1971; 56: 230.

57 Tarpy SP, Kornfeld H, Moroz K, Lazar HL. Unusual presentation of a large tension bronchogenic cyst in an adult. *Thorax* 1993; 48: 951.

58 Spencer H. *Pathology of the Lung.* Oxford: Pergamon Press, 1985.

59 Murphy JJ, Blair GK, Fraser GC *et al.* Rhabdomyosarcoma arising within congenital pulmonary cysts: report of three cases. *J Pediatr Surg* 1992; 27: 1364.

60 Kirwan WO, Walbaum PR, McCormack RJM. Cystic intrathoracic derivatives of the foregut and their complications. *Thorax* 1973; 28: 424.

61 Patel SR, Meeker DP, Biscotti CV, Kirby TJ, Rice TW. Presentation and management of bronchogenic cysts in the adult. *Chest* 1994; 106: 79.

62 Suen H-C, Mathisen DJ, Grillo HC *et al.* Surgical management and radiological characteristics of bronchogenic cysts. *Ann Thorac Surg* 1993; 55: 476.

63 Bolton JWR, Shahian DM. Asymptomatic bronchogenic cysts: what is the best management? *Ann Thorac Surg* 1992; 53: 1134.

64 Parodi-Hueck L, Densler JF, Reed RC *et al.* Congenital cystic adenomatoid malformation of the lung. *Clin Pediatr* 1969; 8: 327.

65 Stocker JT, Drake RM, Madwell JE. Cystic and congenital lung disease in the newborn. In: Rosenberg H, Blonde R, eds. *Prospectives in Pediatric Pathology* Vol 4. Chicago: Year Book Medical, 1978. Publishers.

66 Wexler HA, Valdes-Dapena M. Congenital cystic adenomatoid malformation: a report of three unusual cases. *Radiology* 1978; 126: 737.

67 Spector RG, Claireaux AE, Williams ER. Congenital adenomatoid malformation of the lung with pneumothorax. *Arch Dis Child* 1960; 35: 475.

68 Ng KJ, Hasan N, Gray ES, Jeffrey RR, Youngson GG. Intralobar bronchopulmonary sequestration: antenatal diagnosis. *Thorax* 1994; 49: 379.

69 DeBuse PJ, Morris G. Bilateral pulmonary agenesis, oesophageal atresia and the first arch syndrome. *Thorax* 1973; 28: 526.

70 Wexels P. Agenesis of the lung. *Thorax* 1951; 6: 171.

71 Wier JA. Congenital anomalies of the lung. *Ann Intern Med* 1960; 52: 330.

72 Booth JB, Berry CL. Unilateral pulmonary agenesis. *Arch Dis Child* 1967; 42: 361.

73 Jimenez-Martinez M, Perez-Alvarez JJ, Perez-Trevino C *et al.* Agenesis of the lung with patent ductus arteriosus treated surgically. *J Thorac Cardiovasc Surg* 1965; 50: 59.

74 DeLorimier AA, Tierney DF, Parker HR. Hypoplastic lungs in fetal lambs with surgically produced congenital diaphragmatic hernia. *Surgery* 1967; 62: 12.

75 Wigglesworth JS, Desai R, Guerrini P. Fetal lung hypoplasia: biochemical and structural variations and their possible significance. *Arch Dis Child* 1981; 56: 606.

76 Nakamura Y, Harada K, Yamamoto I *et al.* Human pulmonary hypoplasia. Statistical, morphological, morphometric, and biochemical study. *Arch Pathol Lab Med* 1992; 116: 635.

77 Mendelsohn G, Hutchins GM. Primary pulmonary hypoplasia. *Am J Dis Child* 1977; 131: 1220.

78 Carroll SG, Blott M, Nicolaides KH. Preterm prelabor amniorrhexis: outcome of live births. *Obstet Gynecol* 1995; 86: 18.

79 Husain AN, Hessel RG. Neonatal pulmonary hypoplasia: an autopsy study of 25 cases. *Pediatr Pathol* 1993; 13: 475.

80 Perlman M, Williams J, Hirsch M. Neonatal pulmonary hypoplasia after prolonged leakage of amniotic fluid. *Arch Dis Child* 1976; 51: 349.

81 Ohlsson A, Fong K, Rose T *et al.* Prenatal ultrasonic prediction of autopsy-proven pulmonary hypoplasia. *Am J Perinatol* 1992; 9: 334.

82 Shotan A, Widerhorn J, Hurst A, Elkayam U. Risks of angiotensin-converting enzyme inhibition during pregnancy: experimental and clinical evidence, potential mechanisms, and recommendations for use. *Am J Med* 1994; 96: 451.

83 Borja AR, Ransdell HT, Villa S. Congenital developmental arrest of the lung. *Ann Thorac Surg* 1970; 10: 317.

84 Daves ML, Walsh JA. Minihemithorax. *Am J Roentgenol* 1970; 109: 528.

85 Storey CF, Marrangoni AG. Lobar agenesis of the lung. *J Thorac Surg* 1954; 28: 536.

86 Grant JCB. *An Atlas of Anatomy.* Baltimore: Williams & Wilkins, 1962.

87 Lesser MB. Left azygos lobe: report of a case. *Dis Chest* 1964; 46: 95.

88 Abbey Smith R. Theory of origin of intralobar sequestration of lung. *Thorax* 1956; 11: 10.

89 Clements BS, Warner JO. Pulmonary sequestration and related congenital bronchopulmonary-vascular malformations: nomenclature and classification based on anatomical and embryological considerations. *Thorax* 1987; 42: 401.

90 Gerle RD, Jaretksi A, Ashley CA, Berne AS. Congenital bronchopulmonary-foregut malformation. Pulmonary sequestration communicating with the gastrointestinal tract. *N Engl J Med* 1968; 278: 1413.

91 DeParedes CG, Pierce WS, Johnson DG. Pulmonary sequestration in infants and children: a 20 year experience and review of the literature. *J Pediatr Surg* 1970; 5: 136.

92 Savic B, Birtel FJ, Tholen W *et al.* Lung sequestration: report of seven cases and review of 540 published cases. *Thorax* 1979; 34: 96.

93 Marks C, Wiener SN, Reydman M. Pulmonary sequestration. *Chest* 1972; 61: 253.

94 Halasz NA, Lindskog GE, Liebow AA. Esophagobronchial fistula and bronchopulmonary sequestration: report of a case and review of the literature. *Ann Surg* 1962; 155: 215.

95 Bates M. Total unilateral pulmonary sequestration. *Thorax* 1968; 23: 311.

96 Williams AO, Enumah FI. Extralobar pulmonary sequestration. *Thorax* 1968; 23: 200.

97 Thilenius OG, Ruschhaupt DG, Replogle RL *et al.* Spectrum of pulmonary sequestration: association with anomalous pulmonary venous drainage in infants. *Pediatr Cardiol* 1983; 4: 97.

98 Khalil KG, Kilman JW. Pulmonary sequestration. *J Thorac Cardiovasc Surg* 1975; 70: 928.

99 Levine MM, Nudel DB, Gootman N *et al.* Pulmonary sequestration causing congestive heart failure in infancy: a report of two cases and review of the literature. *Ann Thorac Surg* 1982; 34: 581.

100 Haller JA, Golladay ES, Pickard LR *et al.* Surgical management of lung bud anomalies: lobar emphysema, bronchogenic cyst, cystic adenomatoid malformation and intralobar pulmonary sequestration. *Ann Thorac Surg* 1979; 28: 33.

101 Blesovsky A. Pulmonary sequestration: a report of an unusual case and a review of the literature. *Thorax* 1967; 22: 351.

102 Flye MW, Izant RJ. Extralobar pulmonary sequestration with esophageal communication and complete duplication of the colon. *Surgery* 1972; 71: 744.

103 Nicolette LA, Kosloske AM, Bartow SA, Murphy S. Intralobar pulmonary sequestration: a clinical and pathological spectrum. *J Pediatr Surg* 1993; 28: 802.

104 Kafka V, Beco V. Simultaneous intra- and extrapulmonary sequestration. *Arch Dis Child* 1960; 35: 51.

105 Iwai K, Shindo G, Hajikano H *et al.* Intralobar pulmonary sequestration with special reference to developmental pathology. *Am Rev Respir Dis* 1973; 107: 911.

106 Stovin PGI. Early lung development. *Thorax* 1985; 40: 401.

107 Heithoff KB, Sane SM, Williams HJ *et al.* Bronchopulmonary foregut malformations: a unifying etiological concept. *Am J Roentgenol* 1976; 126: 46.

108 Rubin EM, Garcia H, Horowitz MD, Guerra JJ. Fatal massive hemoptysis secondary to intralobar sequestration. *Chest* 1994; 106: 954.

109 Murphy JD, Rabinovitch M, Goldstein JD *et al.* The structural basis of persistent pulmonary hypertension of the newborn infant. *J Pediatr* 1981; 98: 962.

110 Levin DL, Fixler DE, Morriss FC *et al.* Morphologic analysis of the pulmonary vascular bed in infants exposed *in utero* to prostaglandin synthetase inhibitors. *J Pediatr* 1978; 92: 478.

111 Manhoff LJ, Howe JS. Absence of the pulmonary artery: a classification for pulmonary arteries of anomalous origin. *Arch Pathol* 1949; 48: 155.

112 Steinberg I. Congenital absence of a main branch of the pulmonary artery. Report of three new cases associated respectively with bronchiectasis, atrial septal defect and Eisenmenger's complex. *Am J Med* 1958; 24: 559.

113 Pool PE, Vogel JHK, Blount SG. Congenital unilateral absence of a pulmonary artery. *Am J Cardiol* 1962; 10: 706.

114 Shenick DW, Kincaid OW, DuShane JW. Agenesis of a main branch of the pulmonary artery. *Am J Roentgenol* 1962; 87: 917.

115 Ellis K, Seaman WB, Griffiths SP *et al.* Some congenital abnormalities of the pulmonary arteries. *Semin Roentgenol* 1967; 2: 325.

116 Kieffer SA, Amplatz K, Anderson RC *et al.* Proximal interruption of a pulmonary artery. *Am J Roentgenol* 1965; 95: 592.

117 Franch RH, Gay BB. Congenital stenosis of the pulmonary artery branches: a classification with postmortem findings in two cases. *Am J Med* 1963; 35: 512.

118 Liggins GC, Phillips LI. Rubella embryopathy: an interim report on a New Zealand epidemic. *Br Med J* 1963; i: 711.

119 Philp T, Sumerling MD, Fleming J *et al.* Aberrant left pulmonary artery. *Clin Radiol* 1972; 23: 153.

120 Kale MK, Rafferty RE, Carton RW. Aberrant left pulmonary artery presenting as a mediastinal mass: report of a case in an adult. *Arch Intern Med* 1970; 125: 121.

121 Campbell DC, Murney JA, Dominy DE. Systemic arterial blood supply to a normal lung. *JAMA* 1962; 182: 497.

122 Ernst SMPG, Bruschke AVG. An aberrant systemic artery to the right lung with normal pulmonary tissue. *Chest* 1971; 60: 606.

123 Farnsworth AE, Ankeney JL. The spectrum of the scimitar syndrome. *J Thorac Cardiovasc Surg* 1974; 68: 37.

124 Kiely B, Filler J, Stone S *et al.* Syndrome of anomalous venous drainage of the right lung to the inferior vena cava: a review of 67 reported cases and three new cases in children. *Am J Cardiol* 1967; 20: 102.

125 Mathey J, Galey JJ, Logeais Y *et al.* Anomalous pulmonary venous return into inferior vena cava and associated bronchovascular anomalies (the scimitar syndrome): report of three cases and review of the literature. *Thorax* 1968; 23: 398.

126 Roehm JOF, Jue KL, Amplatz K. Radiographic features of the scimitar syndrome. *Radiology* 1966; 86: 856.

127 Davis WS, Allen RP. Accessory diaphragm: duplication of the diaphragm. *Radiol Clin North Am* 1968; 6: 253.

128 Tomsick TA, Moesner SE, Smith WL. The congenital pulmonary venolobar syndrome in three successive generations. *J Can Assoc Radiol* 1976; 27: 196.

129 Dalith F, Neufeld H. Radiological diagnosis of anomalous pulmonary venous connection: a tomographic study. *Radiology* 1960; 74: 1.

130 McKusick VA, Cooley RN. Drainage of right pulmonary vein into inferior vena cava: report of a case, with a radiologic analysis of the principal types of anomalous venous return from the lung. *N Engl J Med* 1955; 252: 291.

131 Burroughs JT, Edwards JE. Total anomalous pulmonary venous connection. *Am Heart J* 1960; 59: 913.

132 Dines DE, Arms RA, Bernatz PE *et al.* Pulmonary arteriovenous fistulas. *Mayo Clin Proc* 1974; 49: 460.

133 Le Roux BT. Pulmonary 'hamartoma'. *Thorax* 1964; 19: 236.

134 Cope GC. The development of arteriovenous aneurisms in the lung. *Br J Tuberc* 1952; 47: 166.

135 Lindskog GE, Liebow A, Kausel H *et al.* Pulmonary arteriovenous aneurysm. *Ann Surg* 1950; 132: 591.

136 Grishman A, Poppel MH, Simpson RS *et al.* The roentgenographic and angiocardiographic aspects of (1) aberrant insertion of pulmonary veins and (2) congenital arteriovenous aneurysm of the lung. *Am J Roentgenol* 1949; 62: 500.

137 Currarino G, Willis KW, Johnson AF *et al.* Pulmonary telangiectasia. *Am J Roentgenol* 1976; 127: 775.

138 Charles TJ, Davies AB. Pulmonary telangiectasia. *Br J Dis Chest* 1979; 73: 309.

139 Chandler D. Pulmonary and cerebral arteriovenous fistula with Osler's disease. *Arch Intern Med* 1965; 116: 277.

140 Gomes MR, Bernatz PE, Dines DE. Pulmonary arteriovenous fistulas. *Ann Thorac Surg* 1969; 7: 582.

141 Hodgson CH, Burchell HB, Good CA *et al.*

Hereditary haemorrhagic telangiectasia and pulmonary arteriovenous fistula. *N Engl J Med* 1959; 261: 625.

142 McAllister KA, Lennon F, Bowles-Biesecker B *et al.* Genetic heterogeneity in hereditary haemorrhagic telangiectasia: possible correlation with clinical phenotype. *J Med Genet* 1994; 31: 927.

143 Heutink P, Haitjema T, Breedveld GJ *et al.* Linkage of hereditary haemorrhagic telangiectasia to chromosome 9q3 and evidence for locus heterogeneity. *J Med Genet* 1994; 31: 933.

144 Porteous ME, Curtis A, Williams O, Marchuk D, Bhattacharya SS, Burn J. Genetic heterogeneity in hereditary haemorrhagic telangiectasia. *J Med Genet* 1994; 31: 925.

145 Dines DE, Seward JB, Bernatz PE. Pulmonary arteriovenous fistulas. *Mayo Clin Proc* 1983; 58: 176.

146 Mitchell RO, Austin EH. Pulmonary arteriovenous malformation in the neonate. *J Pediatr Surg* 1993; 28: 1536.

147 Grady RM, Sharkey AM, Bridges ND. Transcatheter coil embolisation of a pulmonary arteriovenous malformation in a neonate. *Br Heart J* 1994; 71: 370.

148 Shumacker HB, Waldhausen JA. Pulmonary arteriovenous fistulas in children. *Ann Surg* 1963; 158: 713.

149 Foley RE, Boyd DP. Pulmonary arteriovenous aneurysms. *Surg Clin North Am* 1961; 41: 801.

150 Moyer JH, Glantz G, Brest AN. Pulmonary arteriovenous fistulas: physiologic and clinical considerations. *Am J Med* 1962; 32: 417.

151 Hodgson CH, Kaye RL. Pulmonary arteriovenous fistula and hereditary hemorrhagic telangiectasia: a review and report of 35 cases of fistula. *Dis Chest* 1963; 43: 449.

152 Dalton ML, Goodwin FC, Bronwell AW *et al.* Intrapleural rupture of pulmonary arteriovenous aneurysm: report of a case. *Dis Chest* 1967; 52: 97.

153 Moore BP. Pulmonary arteriovenous fistula. *Thorax* 1969; 24: 381.

154 Livingston SO, Carr RE. Hereditary hemorrhagic telangiectasia: report of a case with haemothorax. *J Thorac Cardiovasc Surg* 1956; 31: 497.

155 Ference BA, Shannon TM, White RI, Zawin M, Burdge CM. Life-threatening pulmonary hemorrhage with pulmonary arteriovenous malformations and hereditary hemorrhagic telangiectasia. *Chest* 1994; 106: 1387.

156 Maier HC, Himmelstein A, Riley RL *et al.* Arteriovenous fistula of the lung. *J Thorac Surg* 1948; 17: 13.

157 Roman G, Fisher M, Perl DP, Poser CM. Neurological manifestations of hereditary hemorrhagic telangiectasia (Rendu–Osler–Weber disease): report of two cases and review of the literature. *Ann Neurol* 1978; 4: 130.

158 Flower CDR. Imaging pulmonary arteriovenous malformations. *Br Med J* 1987; 294: 1633.

159 Remy J, Remy-Jardin M, Wattinne L, Deffontaines C. Pulmonary arteriovenous malformations: evaluation with CT of the chest before and after treatment. *Radiology* 1992; 182: 809.

160 Steinberg I. Diagnosis and surgical treatment of pulmonary arteriovenous fistula. Report of three new and review of nineteen consecutive cases. *Surg Clin North Am* 1961; 41: 523.

161 Comroe JH, Forster RE, DuBois AB *et al. The Lung.* Chicago: Year Book Medical Publishers, 1962.

162 Genovesi MG, Tierney DF, Taplin GV *et al.* An intravenous radionuclide method to evaluate hypoxemia caused by abnormal alveolar vessels. Limitation of conventional techniques. *Am Rev Respir Dis* 1976; 114: 59.

163 Sapru RP, Hutchison DC, Hall JI. Pulmonary hypertension in patients with pulmonary arteriovenous fistulae. *Br Heart J* 1969; 31: 559.

164 Cotes JE. *Lung Function. Assessment and Application in Medicine.* Oxford: Blackwell Scientific Publications, 1979.

165 White RI, Lynch-Nyhan A, Terry PI *et al.* Pulmonary arteriovenous malformations: techniques and long-term outcome of embolotherapy. *Radiology* 1988; 169: 663.

166 Haitjema TJ, Overtoom TTC, Westermann CJJ, Lammers JWJ. Embolization of pulmonary arteriovenous malformations: results and follow up in 32 patients. *Thorax* 1995; 50: 719.

167 White RI, Pollak JS, Wirth JA. Pulmonary arteriovenous malformations: diagnosis and transcatheter embolotherapy. *J Vasc Intervent Radiol* 1996; 7: 787.

168 Dutton JA, Jackson JE, Hughes JMB *et al.* Pulmonary arteriovenous malformations: results of treatment with coil embolization in 53 patients. *Am J Roentgenol* 1995; 165: 1119.

169 Armitage JM, Fricker FJ, Kurland G *et al.* Pediatric lung transplantation. The years 1985 to 1992 and the clinical trial of FK 506. *J Thorac Cardiovasc Surg* 1993; 105: 337.

51

SOME LESS COMMON PULMONARY DISEASES

ANTHONY SEATON

Alveolar haemorrhage

Intrapulmonary bleeding occurs in many lung disorders. In general, two patterns are discernible: bleeding from the main conducting airways, as in carcinoma, may be distributed to peripheral areas of the lung but most of the bleeding becomes evident as haemoptysis; in contrast, when bleeding occurs distal to the mucociliary transport system, much or even all of the blood may remain in the lung. This form of alveolar haemorrhage may cause haemoptysis but is also associated with breathlessness, anaemia, hypoxaemia and diffuse pulmonary shadowing.

Causes

The common causes of alveolar haemorrhage are shown in Table 51.1. Goodpasture's syndrome consists of alveolar haemorrhage/haemoptysis and nephritis [1], and is now further classified into four main conditions: antiglomerular basement membrane antibody disease [2–7], the vasculitides and collagen vascular disorders (although not all cases are associated with nephritis) [8–18], idiopathic rapidly progressive glomerulonephritis [4,12,19,20], and D-penicillamine-induced disease [21,22].

Alveolar haemorrhage may also result from chemical insults such as exposure to trimellitic anhydride [23] and as a consequence of lymphangiography [24], and has been described with azathioprine sensitivity [25] and following exposure to hard metal (tungsten carbide) [26]. Finally, idiopathic pulmonary haemosiderosis is a syndrome of alveolar haemorrhage of unknown cause without involvement of other organ systems. In most series of Goodpasture's syndrome, the vasculitides account for 40–60% of cases of alveolar haemorrhage, idiopathic rapidly progressive glomerulonephritis for 15–30% and antibasement membrane antibody disease for 20–40% [4,7,12]. This section is principally concerned with antibasement membrane antibody disease as a cause of Goodpasture's syndrome and with idiopathic pulmonary haemosiderosis. The other causes of Goodpasture's syn-

drome and alveolar haemorrhage are discussed in the chapters indicated in Table 51.1.

Antiglomerular basement membrane antibody disease

Definition

This disease is characterized by alveolar haemorrhage and glomerulonephritis with linear deposition of IgG on the basement membranes of glomeruli and alveoli. Circulating antibodies to glomerular basement membrane can be detected in the blood [3,5–7].

Aetiology and prevalence

Between 1980 and 1984, 71 patients with this condition were reported in the British Isles [6], although this is certainly an underestimate, and the disease is now thought to occur in rather fewer than 1 per million of the population annually [6]. The peak incidence is seen between 20 and 30 years of age with a 4:1 male predominance. A second peak is seen in middle age where women in their sixties may present with glomerulonephritis alone [6].

The precipitating factor for the disease is unknown, although some cases have followed exposure to hydrocarbon vapour [27] and study of workers exposed to petroleum mineral oils have shown an excess of antibasement membrane antibodies [28]. In other cases, including the original description by Goodpasture, the illness has been preceded by a viral infection. The distinguishing feature of the disease is the presence of circulating antibody to glomerular basement membranes, with linear deposition of this antibody on alveolar and glomerular basement membranes [29]. The antigen to which the antibody is directed is located in the C-terminal domain of type IV collagen from glomerular and alveolar basement membrane and has a molecular mass of 26 000 kDa [30–33]. It has been shown that the antigen is the non-collagenous part of the α_3 chain of type IV collagen, expressed by a gene in the

Table 51.1 Causes of alveolar haemorrhage and references to the literature.

Goodpasture's syndrome (alveolar haemorrhage plus nephritis)
Antibasement membrane antibody disease [2–7]
Vasculitides and collagen vascular diseases (Chapters 40 & 53)
    Systemic lupus erythematosus [8–10]
    Wegener's granulomatosis [4,11]
    Non-specific systemic necrotizing vasculitis [4,12]
    Rheumatoid arthritis [13,14]
    Progressive systemic sclerosis [15]
    Mixed connective tissue disease [16]
    Polyarteritis nodosa [13]
    Behçet's disease [17]
    Essential mixed cryoglobulinaemia [18]
    Tumour-related vasculitis [12]
    Endocarditis-related vasculitis [12]
Idiopathic rapidly progressive glomerulonephritis [4,12,19,20]
D-Penicillamine induced [21,22]

Chemical related
    Trimellitic anhydride [23]
    Lymphangiography [24]

Idiopathic pulmonary haemosiderosis

---

q35–37 region of chromosome 2 [34,35]. The pathogenesis is believed to involve a cytotoxic type II hypersensitivity reaction consequent on antibody binding to this antigen. Certainly the disease can be passively transferred to monkeys by administration of human antiglomerular basement membrane antibody and the severity of the disease is proportional to the titre of circulating antibodies [36]. Savage and colleagues [6] reported a peak incidence of the disease in spring and early summer, which might be consistent with a viral trigger factor. Genetic factors would also appear to have some importance; cases have been reported in identical twin sisters living together and in two brothers who lived apart [37,38]. In addition, there is a strong association with HLA-DR2, which is present in 60–70% of cases [39–41]. It is tempting to speculate that, in those genetically predisposed, infection with a virus that shares a similar antigen to the Goodpasture antigen may precipitate disease. Such an association with influenza A2 virus infection has been described [42].

It thus seems likely that pulmonary haemorrhage occurs as a result of damage to type IV collagen in alveolar basement membrane and that, particularly in the genetically predisposed, this may occur as a consequence of a number of trigger factors, which may include viral infection and inhaled or ingested toxic substances. Type IV collagen is important in protecting the pulmonary capillaries from physical stress, and when weakened allows leakage of blood [43]. Other factors may damage collagen in the lung, perhaps explaining why cigarette smokers are at greater risk of Goodpasture's syndrome [44]. In most cases the renal lesion is presumably a consequence of the anti-

collagen IV antibodies also attacking the collagen of the glomerular basement membrane.

Pathology

Renal biopsy shows a diffuse crescentic or focal glomerulonephritis or even, rarely, normal glomeruli [2,45]. Linear deposits of IgG can be detected on the glomerular basement membrane using immunofluorescence techniques . Occasionally, immunofluorescent stains for IgA, IgM, the C3 component of complement and fibrinogen are positive [46]. Similar techniques can be applied to lung tissue obtained by open, needle or transbronchial biopsy in order to demonstrate linear deposition of IgG on alveolar basement membranes [47,48]. Light microscopy of lung biopsies shows active intra-alveolar haemorrhage with collections of haemosiderin-laden macrophages [46].

Functional abnormality

Where measured, a restrictive pattern of lung volumes is usually found. The diffusing capacity for carbon monoxide ($D_{L}CO$) is increased during episodes of haemorrhage as a result of sequestration of blood within the alveoli. The single-breath diffusion coefficient for carbon monoxide (K_{CO}) is considered abnormal if raised by more than 30% and serial measurements are of considerable value in monitoring the progress of alveolar haemorrhage [49–52]. Although K_{CO} frequently parallels the extent of airspace shadowing on the chest radiograph, it may also increase in the presence of a persistently normal film or alternatively precede the development of shadowing by up to 48 h [53].

Clinical and radiological features

There is often a preceding upper respiratory tract infection [2,3,5,6,12,54–58]. Haemoptysis is found in 80–90% of presentations and is more common in smokers. In one series of 51 patients, 100% of smokers with this disease developed pulmonary haemorrhage while only 20% of nonsmokers did so [44]. Cough, dyspnoea, weakness and fatigue are common complaints. Fever and chills may occur. Pallor is common and hypertension is found in a minority of cases. Auscultation of the chest frequently reveals inspiratory crepitations. The chest radiograph is abnormal in over 80% of cases and most commonly shows diffuse bilateral patchy consolidation in the mid and lower zones with relative sparing of the apices and costophrenic angles (Fig. 51.1). Air bronchograms may be seen. Urinalysis is abnormal in over 90% of patients, with microscopic haematuria, proteinuria, granular casts and occasionally frank haematuria. An iron-deficiency anaemia is usual and uraemia is found in over 70% of cases. Examination of sputum or bronchoalveolar washings reveals the presence of blood

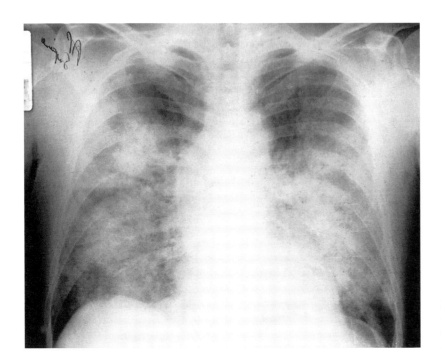

Fig. 51.1 Radiograph of patient acutely dyspnoeic with Goodpasture's syndrome showing extensive bilateral consolidation and air bronchograms.

and/or haemosiderin-containing alveolar macrophages. Occasionally renal involvement without pulmonary haemorrhage or pulmonary involvement without obvious renal disease may occur [3,6,45].

Differential diagnosis

The differential diagnosis includes the disorders listed in Table 51.1. Drug or chemical-related disease is readily identified by taking a history. The vasculitides and collagen vascular diseases frequently have other systemic manifestations (see Chapters 40 & 53) that assist in diagnosis. Idiopathic rapidly progressive glomerulonephritis is diagnosed when a renal biopsy shows crescentic glomerulonephritis without arteritis or linear immunofluorescence in the absence of any other features of a multisystem disorder. Nevertheless, it is managed in the same way as the vasculitides. It has been suggested that it is a variant of Wegener's disease, with antineutrophil cytoplasmic antibodies [59]. The definitive diagnosis of antiglomerular basement membrane disease is made by demonstrating linear immunofluorescence (usually to IgG) on the glomerular basement membrane (less commonly the alveolar basement membrane) and by detecting an elevated titre of antiglomerular basement membrane antibodies in the serum using radioimmunoassay or enzyme-linked immunosorbent assay [60].

Treatment and progress

The condition often presents to the chest physician as rapidly increasing haemoptysis with progressive renal failure, although there is frequently a history of previous smaller haemoptyses. While spontaneous remission may occur, the course is usually progressive and fatal unless treated [61–63]. The renal manifestations require treatment with high-dose prednisolone (60 mg daily reducing to 20 mg over 4 weeks) and cyclophosphamide (2–3 mg/kg daily). As the patient responds, the cyclophosphamide may be stopped after about 2–3 months and the predisolone tailed off and stopped within about 6 months.

The addition of plasmapheresis to immunosuppression has improved the speed of response and effectiveness of the above regimen and in general a good response can be expected if the patient is not already oliguric at the time of presentation [64]. Usually this is associated with resolution of the pulmonary haemorrhage within a few days and recovery of renal function. The plasma exchange is usually continued for about 2 weeks until the antibasement membrane antibodies are reduced to baseline levels. There has been one report of successful treatment of a patient unresponsive to plasmapheresis by immunoadsorption of IgG to staphylococcal protein A [65]. In patients with severe renal failure, dialysis may be necessary and ultimately transplantation if recovery does not occur. In this case, the operation should be delayed until antiglomerular basement membrane antibodies have fallen to low levels [3]. In exceptional cases bilateral nephrectomy has been necessary to control alveolar haemorrhage when all else has failed [3,66].

Relapse of disease may occur during treatment, when it is more often due to an intercurrent infection than to a rise in antibody titres [67]. Once successfully treated, recurrence is rare but has been reported, on one occasion following exposure to hydrocarbon solvents [68–70]. Lung function often shows permanently reduced gas transfer [71] and sometimes there is a slow decline in renal function. If relapse does occur, it is likely to respond to the same regimen as described above.

Idiopathic pulmonary haemosiderosis

Idiopathic pulmonary haemosiderosis is a condition of uncertain cause characterized by recurrent episodes of alveolar haemorrhage, haemoptysis and secondary iron-deficiency anaemia. Most cases begin in childhood but some start in adult life. The disease is often fatal though apparently complete recovery can occur.

Aetiology and prevalence

This is a rare disease but in 1962 Soergel and Sommers [72] were able to review 132 cases from the literature and from personal experience. Most were aged 1–7 years at onset but about 15% were aged 16 or over when symptoms began. The sex distribution was equal in childhood but in adult life the disease was twice as common in men. The disease is not familial and from the number of different associations recorded in the literature it seems likely that its aetiology is multifactorial.

The accompanying iron-deficiency anaemia is certainly due to loss of iron into the lung through haemorrhage, as has been shown by iron turnover studies, although the cause of the haemorrhage is uncertain [73]. Epidemiological observations in northern Greece have shown an excess of cases in poor rural areas where toxic insecticides were often applied to cereals stored within or close to the dwelling place [74]. A reduction in case numbers was seen when these conditions were improved, possibly implicating insecticides in the pathogenesis.

Immunological causes are fashionable and might be supported by the presence of eosinophilia in one-eighth of cases, the aggregation of mast cells in the lung, an increase in plasma cells in the reticuloendothelial system and the presence of cold agglutinins in some cases [75,76]. Immunological diseases that have been associated with pulmonary haemosiderosis include rheumatoid arthritis, autoimmune haemolytic anaemia, dermatitis herpetiformis, thyrotoxicosis and coeliac disease [77–82]. In addition, children and adults have been described with idiopathic pulmonary haemosiderosis secondary to gluten enteropathy and cows' milk allergy who responded clinically to withdrawal of gluten and cows' milk respectively [75,83–85]. Nevertheless, the aetiology in the majority of cases remains unknown.

Pathology

Histologically, there is degeneration, shedding and hyperplasia of alveolar epithelial cells with marked localized alveolar capillary dilatation [72]. Haemosiderin-containing macrophages are plentiful in the alveolar spaces and interstitium [86,87]. Depending on the chronicity of the condition there may be varying degrees of interstitial fibrosis, degeneration of the alveolar, interstitial and vascular elastic fibres, dilatation and moderate subendothelial sclerosis of pulmonary arteries and veins, and slight muscular hypertrophy of the bronchial arteries. These changes are secondary to the recurrent bleeding [72]. Electron microscopic examination has shown widespread capillary endothelial and basement membrane damage [88,89]. Deposits of protein, in one case characterized as IgA, have occasionally been observed on the alveolar basement membrane [79,88].

Functional abnormality

In acute incidents of alveolar haemorrhage $K\text{CO}$ is elevated, values of greater than 130% predicted being considered abnormal [49,50]. In chronic cases, where interstitial fibrosis has developed, a restrictive pattern of lung volumes and reduced $D\text{LCO}$ is usual, although a pattern of airways obstruction is also seen in some patients [82,87].

Clinical and radiological features

The intensity and duration of the pulmonary haemorrhages determine the clinical course, which may be very variable [72,79,86,90,91]. Commonly, continuous mild intrapulmonary bleeding results in a chronic non-productive cough with tiredness, pallor and failure to thrive in children. The sputum may be intermittently blood-stained or the child may vomit swallowed blood. An iron-deficiency anaemia is usual and the faecal occult blood test may be positive. A minority of patients may have generalized lymphadenopathy or hepatosplenomegaly. The chest radiograph may show transient blotchy shadows. With a severe bleed, cough and haemoptysis worsen and dyspnoea, chest pain or tightness and pyrexia may develop. The anaemia worsens and the chest radiograph is likely to show more extensive, bilateral, patchy shadows particularly in the middle and lower zones. Crepitations may be audible in the chest.

Bleeding episodes continue for years and eventually chronic dyspnoea becomes a feature in addition to the anaemia. Finger clubbing develops in 25%. The chest film may show reticulonodular infiltrates, fine stippling or a ground-glass appearance in the perihilar or lower lung zones due to pulmonary fibrosis. The apices and costophrenic angles are often spared. Hilar lymphadenopathy is occasionally seen. Cor pulmonale secondary to pulmonary fibrosis and hypoxaemia develop in a minority [92]. Massive pulmonary haemorrhage may occur at any time and most patients die in a severe bleeding episode.

Investigations

Haemosiderin-laden macrophages are found in sputum or bronchial washings. A hypochromic microcytic anaemia is usual and a minority of blood films show an eosinophilia [72]. Idiopathic pulmonary haemosiderosis is a diagnosis of exclusion and no evidence of other organ involvement is found, although confusion with Goodpasture's syndrome before renal disease presents may lead to diagnostic problems. Diagnosis depends on excluding other causes of pulmonary haemorrhage, especially those such as Wegener's syndrome, Goodpasture's disease and microscopic polyarteritis that may require immunosuppressive treatment.

Treatment

Patients with cows' milk allergy or gluten enteropathy have responded to withdrawal of the offending substance [83–85]; unfortunately, these patients are a small minority. Iron-deficiency anaemia responds to replacement therapy and occasionally blood transfusion is required during severe bleeding episodes. Corticosteroid and immunosuppressive drugs do not appear to affect the long-term prognosis but either may be of value during acute episodes of alveolar haemorrhage, as in Goodpasture's syndrome [93]. Anecdotal reports of therapeutic success with assorted agents such as sodium cromoglicate (cromoglycate) [76] and budesonide [94] abound. However, the disease may remit spontaneously and these reports should be viewed with caution.

Prognosis

The course of the disease is very variable. Although it is often fatal, a number of patients appear to recover and remain symptom-free for long periods. Soergel and Sommers [72] found that 20 of 68 patients were dead after an average duration of disease of 3.3 years; 17 still had active disease after an average duration of 5.5 years; 12 had relatively inactive disease but still with chronic symptoms, such as exertional dyspnoea and anaemia, after an average duration of 5.4 years; and 19 were apparently completely free of the disease and symptoms after an average duration of 4.5 years. These authors contrast a 28-year-old woman who died after an illness of only 9 days and a boy aged 6 years at onset who died of cor pulmonale 20 years later.

Pulmonary alveolar proteinosis

First described in 1958 by Rosen and colleagues [95], pulmonary alveolar proteinosis is a rare disease of unknown origin characterized by progressive dyspnoea, febrile episodes and a cough that is usually unproductive. The radiological appearances are often similar to those of pulmonary oedema. Histologically, the alveoli contain a granular eosinophilic material strongly positive to periodic acid–Schiff (PAS) stain.

Aetiology

The disease is three times as common in men as in women and usually occurs in young adults, although it has been described in the neonatal period, in children and in old age [96,97]. Primary alveolar proteinosis is characterized by uniform immunoperoxidase staining of the specific surfactant apoprotein in alveoli [98,99]. Two surfactant proteins, Sp-A and Sp-D, have been described in alveolar fluid from such patients [100,101]. Secondary alveolar proteinosis, which is found in association with immunosuppression due to haematological malignancy [102–106], myeloma [107], hypogammaglobulinaemia [108] or, more recently, human immunodeficiency virus (HIV) infection [109,110], shows only focal immunoperoxidase staining of the specific apoprotein [98]. Congenital alveolar proteinosis was first described in four siblings [111] and appears to be associated with an inherited deficiency of Sp-B [112]. The syndrome has also been described in children with a recessive amino acid transport disease, lysinuric protein intolerance [113]. Opportunistic infections, especially *Nocardia*, *Aspergillus*, *Mycobacterium* and *Cryptococcus* spp., are common in secondary alveolar proteinosis but rare in the primary condition [105,114]. Exposure to aluminium or silica dust has been associated with alveolar proteinosis and the condition can be produced in experimental animals by inhalation of large doses of finely divided mineral dust [106,115].

Pulmonary alveolar proteinosis is believed to be due to a failure of reprocessing of surfactant by type II alveolar cells, with resultant accumulation of phospholipid and glycoprotein-rich material in the alveolar spaces [116]. Electron microscopy of the alveolar material shows myelin-like multilamellated structures, which represent phospholipid bilayers separated from each other by amorphous proteinaceous material [117]. The glycoprotein has been isolated and characterized and appears to be a monomeric and dimeric form of the surfactant glycoprotein found in normal alveolar lining fluid [118,119]. Macrophage numbers are diminished in bronchoalveolar lavage fluid from patients with alveolar proteinosis and the cells may be increased in size [120,121]. The macrophages also have diminished phagocytic capacity, with decreased phagolysosome fusion [121,122]. These phagocytic defects can be induced in mouse peritoneal or human macrophages on exposure to cell-free fractions of the alveolar material, suggesting that the macrophage defect is secondary and not primary [121,122]. Leukotriene (LT)C_4-like substances and LTB_4 have been found in significant quantities in alveolar proteinosis lavage fluid, although the source and their contribution to the pathogenesis of the disease are not clear [123].

Pathology

Macroscopically, the lungs contain firm, grey-white, nodular or diffuse masses, which microscopically consist of alveoli, bronchioles and bronchi stuffed with eosinophilic granular material staining with PAS (Fig. 51.2). Bronchial and alveolar walls may be infiltrated by lymphocytes. The alveoli are often lined by flattened epithelial cells and occasional foamy mononuclear cells containing lipoid. In frozen sections, long, thin, birefringent crystals may be present. A few cases may have some interstitial fibrosis.

Functional abnormality

The extent of the abnormality depends on the amount of lung involved. A restrictive pattern of lung volumes with reduced $D\text{LCO}$ is usual and hypoxaemia, which may be extreme, occurs. The ratio of forced expiratory volume in 1 s to forced vital capacity is usually normal.

Clinical features

The usual presentation is with progressive dyspnoea on exertion with or without a dry unproductive cough [116,120,124,125]. Weight loss, chest pain and fever may also occur. The initial presentation is often wrongly diagnosed as pneumonia, sarcoidosis, allergic alveolitis or tuberculosis; in one series the median interval between onset of symptoms and diagnosis was 2 years, with a range of 6 weeks to 6 years [124]. Fine inspiratory crackles may be audible in the chest and finger clubbing develops in a minority.

Radiology

The chest film most often shows diffuse perihilar shadows resembling pulmonary oedema (Fig. 51.3). Peripheral nodular and lobar consolidation may also occur [126,127]. There may be numerous cyst-like translucencies possibly due to pneumatoceles from bronchial obstruction. Occasionally, shifting densities may suggest pulmonary eosinophilia. Changes in the radiological appearances are not always related to changes in the patient's symptoms, and clinical improvement may coincide with radiological deterioration and vice versa. Sometimes the initial radiographic appearances may suggest interstitial fibrosis [128,129]. In children, the radiographic appearance may differ from the classical adult picture; reticulonodular and miliary nodular patterns have been recorded as well as focal consolidation [97].

Investigations

Sputum or bronchial washings contain PAS-positive, alcian blue-negative staining material. Lamellar bodies may be seen on electron microscopy [130]. Serum lactate dehydrogenase levels may be elevated [131].

Treatment

A number of patients with this condition (25% in one series [120]) improve spontaneously and do not require treatment. Spontaneous remission for 18 years has been reported [132]. However, the majority require treatment for progressive symptomatology and deteriorating pulmonary function. The treatment of choice is unilateral lung lavage while the contralateral lung is isolated and ventilated by using a double-lumen endobronchial tube [116,124,133]. The lavage lung is filled with saline buffered

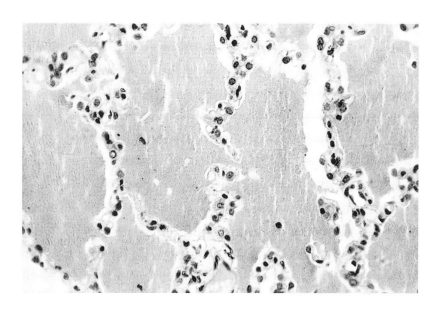

Fig. 51.2 Open lung biopsy from patient with alveolar proteinosis showing typical granular exudate, strongly eosinophilic (and also PAS-positive) (haematoxylin & eosin × 300).

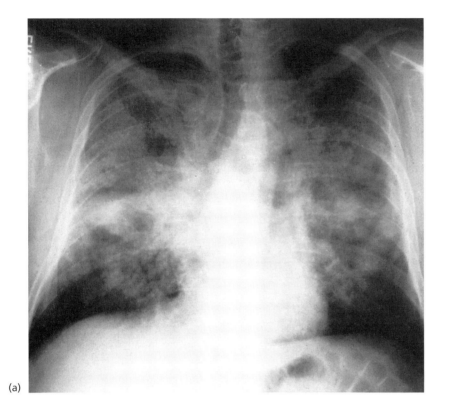

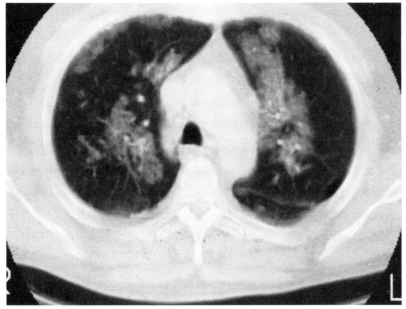

Fig. 51.3 (a) Radiograph of a patient with alveolar proteinosis showing diffuse patchy shadows, more dense round the hila. (b) CT of another patient with alveolar proteinosis shows the patchy distribution of alveolar filling. (Courtesy of Dr N. LeRoy Lapp.)

to pH 7.4 at a temperature of 37°C and volumes of 500–1000 mL are washed in and out until a total of 40–50 L has been exchanged or the effluent has become clear. At the conclusion of the procedure, vigorous suction and manual ventilation are followed by a short period of assisted ventilation. The second lung can be lavaged at a later date. Not surprisingly, chest radiographs taken during the lavage procedure show worsening of the pulmonary shadowing; within a few hours the chest film may have deteriorated further or improved but thereafter there is a gradual improvement at 1 week and marked to moderate improvement at 6 weeks [134]. Lavage may need to be repeated at intervals, the frequency varying between individual patients. Lavage via the fibreoptic bronchoscope is less satisfactory than the above but has been successfully employed to treat the right middle and upper lobes in a patient with only one lung [135].

In patients who are too hypoxic to undergo lung lavage,

various forms of support, including hyperbaric oxygen [136], use of a membrane oxygenator [137] and partial cardiopulmonary bypass [138], have been employed to maintain Pao_2 during the procedure. In one patient who refused bronchopulmonary lavage a satisfactory response was obtained to treatment with ambroxol, a surfactant activator [139].

Prognosis

The prognosis of primary alveolar proteinosis in adults has been much improved by bronchopulmonary lavage, which helps in 80% of those who require it although it may have to be repeated at intervals to maintain this improvement [120]. Death is more likely to occur in children and in those with secondary alveolar proteinosis, where opportunistic infection and the underlying disease are the main causes.

Amyloidosis

Amyloidosis is usually secondary to one of the well-recognized causes, although primary amyloidosis of unknown cause may occur. Amyloid consists of protein that shows a characteristic fibrillar pattern on electron microscopy. The amyloid in primary amyloidosis (AL) is formed from the light chains or part of the light chains of immunoglobulin [140]. In secondary amyloidosis the protein differs from that found in primary amyloidosis and is designated AA. Additional amyloid types such as AEt, found with endocrine neoplasms and which is related to calcitonin, have also been described [140]. Both primary and secondary amyloidosis may be generalized or localized to the lung. A convenient classification is shown in Table 51.2.

In generalized amyloidosis, whether primary or secondary, amyloid infiltrates are commonly found in alveolar septa and pulmonary arteries though these lesions seldom give rise to important symptoms, which are more commonly due to amyloid infiltration at other sites, particularly the heart.

Localized primary or secondary amyloidosis may affect the tracheobronchial tree or the pulmonary parenchyma. The most common form of tracheobronchial involvement is with multifocal submucosal plaques, often with diffuse infiltration of the entire airway wall leading to stenosis [141–144] (Fig. 51.4). The less common form of tracheobronchial involvement is with single or multiple amyloid tumour-like masses that are sometimes discovered incidentally at bronchoscopy. Parenchymal involvement is most frequently in the form of single or multiple nodules of 1–15 cm in diameter [145–150] with or without hilar or mediastinal node involvement [151–154]. One case of an isolated mediastinal amyloid mass has been reported [155]. Diffuse alveolar septal involvement with amyloid

Table 51.2 Classification of lower respiratory tract amyloidosis.

Generalized (systemic) amyloidosis*
Primary
Secondary
Localized amyloidosis*
Primary
Tracheobronchial
Multifocal submucosal plaques
Tumour-like mass
Pulmonary
Nodular: multiple (parenchymal) or solitary
Diffuse alveolar septal
Secondary
Tracheobronchial
Multifocal submucosal plaques
Tumour-like mass
Pulmonary
Nodular: multiple (parenchymal) or solitary
Diffuse alveolar septal.

* Including hilar lymph node involvement.

[156] is probably more common than is reported, although only 4 of 157 cases reviewed by Thomson and Citron [141] were in this category.

Clinical and radiological features

Patients with tracheobronchial involvement are usually in their fifties, on average 10 years younger than those with pulmonary parenchymal involvement [142]. Tracheobronchial lesions come to notice by causing symptoms of obstruction, such as cough, wheeze and dyspnoea, which may be slowly progressive over the years. Parenchymal lesions are often detected on routine radiography when they are usually thought to be carcinoma or, if multiple, metastases [157]. The diagnosis of airway lesions can be established by endoscopic biopsy; pulmonary lesions can also be diagnosed by transbronchial biopsy [158], although this may not be without risk [159]. In secondary cases there is evidence of the primary cause. In some cases this causes diagnostic difficulties, for example when it is confused with rheumatoid, Sjögren's or ankylosing spondylitis lung or the lung disease associated with inflammatory bowel disease [160–163].

Rarely amyloidosis can cause respiratory failure by infiltration of the diaphragm or other respiratory muscles [164,165]. Sleep apnoea due to amyloid macroglossia has also been reported [166].

Functional abnormality

With extensive nodular or diffuse disease of the pulmonary parenchyma, a restrictive pattern of lung volumes with reduced gas transfer may be seen.

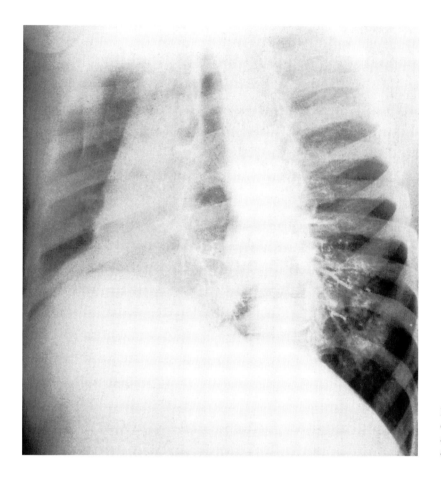

Fig. 51.4 Left anterior oblique bronchogram of patient with diffuse tracheobronchial amyloidosis showing multiple areas of airway narrowing.

Tracheobronchial involvement may result in an obstructive pattern of lung volumes and sometimes the typical findings of large airway obstruction on flow–volume loops (Fig. 51.5).

Treatment

The only possible treatment is surgical. Isolated pulmonary nodules are usually removed (and cured) under suspicion of carcinoma. No treatment is available for multiple pulmonary nodules. Tracheobronchial amyloid may be successfully controlled by endoscopic removal or by laser photoresection [167]. Untreated lesions progress slowly over the years and long survivals have been documented [153]. One patient with primary tracheobronchial amyloidosis treated personally for over 10 years responded clinically to the combination of prednisolone and melphalan. The melphalan was subsequently discontinued but deterioration in symptoms and lung function always followed attempts to stop the steroids.

Tracheopathia and bronchopathia osteoplastica

The term 'tracheopathia osteoplastica' was first used by Aschoff [168], although Wilks in 1857 [169] was the first to

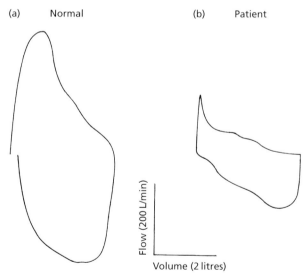

Fig. 51.5 Flow–volume loops of (a) normal subject and (b) patient with tracheobronchial amyloid, which shows the severe inspiratory and expiratory obstruction.

report the presence of large numbers of bony plates protruding into the lumen of the larynx, trachea and bronchi of a 38-year-old man dying of pulmonary tuberculosis. The term 'tracheobronchopathia osteoplastica' has been coined to embrace all the possible sites of the disease process [170].

Prevalence, aetiology and pathology

Some 245 cases had been reported in the world literature up to 1974, mostly in middle-aged and elderly men but occasionally in women [171]. Since then there have been regular isolated case reports. The bony or cartilaginous bosses or plaques arise over the cartilages and are continuous with the perichondrium. Histologically, the lesions are of bone, cartilage or calcified acellular protein matrix. The mucosa overlying the protrusions is usually intact and histologically normal, although squamous metaplasia has been reported [171–173]. The lesions may be localized or diffuse and are usually only diagnosed at autopsy, although occasionally they may be diagnosed because they cause bronchial obstruction. While the aetiology is unknown, it has been suggested that metaplastic changes occur in elastic tissue with conversion to elastic cartilage that may then ossify [174]. A simpler explanation is that the protrusions simply represent exostoses and ecchondroses from tracheal cartilage rings [175]. Finally, it has been suggested that the condition may be a late development in tracheobronchial amyloidosis [176].

Clinical features

Most cases have only been diagnosed at autopsy in patients dying of other diseases, although a few have been diagnosed by the characteristic bronchoscopic appearances [177]. Recurrent pneumonia may occur distal to obstruction and lead to a bronchoscopic diagnosis [178]. Minor symptoms may include cough, dry throat, voice change, dyspnoea and haemoptysis. The complaint of haemoptysis frequently leads to diagnosis at bronchoscopy [177].

Radiology

Bronchial obstruction may cause collapse and pneumonia. The condition cannot be recognized on routine radiography, although tomography of the trachea or main bronchi may reveal the characteristic projecting nodules [177,179].

Treatment

Treatment is only necessary for complications such as infection or collapse. If the collapsed lung is not severely damaged, endoscopic removal or sleeve resection of the blocked bronchus might be justified. When the larynx is affected, laser treatment has been used to remove protrusions [180].

Alveolar microlithiasis

Pulmonary alveolar microlithiasis is a disease that is often familial and characterized by a radiographic appearance of very fine, sand-like mottling uniformly distributed through both lungs. This mottling represents an extensive intra-alveolar deposit of calcium-containing bodies. Despite extensive radiographic changes, symptoms at the time of discovery are often minimal or absent, but later there is gradual progression to respiratory failure and cor pulmonale.

Aetiology

The cause of the disease is quite unknown. It may occur at any age between infancy and 80 years but the majority are diagnosed between the ages of 30 and 50 years. The sex distribution is equal. A familial incidence, particularly in siblings, is common, leading to the suggestion that a local defect of calcium metabolism may be responsible [181]. A report from Turkey indicates that the condition seems to be more frequent than would be expected on the basis of reports from elsewhere in the world, 52 cases having been described over 30 years; several of these were also familial [182].

Pathology

The lungs are solid and may sink in water [181], and throughout there are sand-like grains diffusely distributed but maximal at the bases. At necropsy, a saw may be required to cut the lung. Microscopically, there are 'onion-skin' bodies, resembling corpora amylacea, in 30–80% of alveoli and these bodies are usually densely calcified. There may or may not be interstitial fibrosis and inflammatory cell infiltration. Emphysematous blebs may be found at the apices or anterior margins of the lungs. There are usually no changes in other organs, although deposits in the lumbar sympathetic chain and probably in the testes have been reported in one patient [183].

Clinical and radiological features

These patients are often discovered by routine radiography at an asymptomatic stage when they may have no complaints despite dramatic changes on the chest film. Over a period of years there is progression of disease, with the development of increasing dyspnoea, cough and, later still, cyanosis, polycythaemia and cor pulmonale. Haemoptysis occasionally occurs [184] and clubbing may be seen [185]. The patient may occasionally cough up calcified bodies. Recurrent pneumothoraces may occur [186]. There are often no physical signs in the chest even when the radiograph is grossly abnormal. Later there may be inspiratory crepitations and, ultimately, the signs of cor pulmonale. Death usually results from respiratory or cardiac failure.

Functional abnormality

Respiratory function tests are often normal or near normal even with extensive radiographic changes. However, with progression of disease, a restrictive pattern of lung volumes develops and impairment of gas transfer with disturbed ventilation–perfusion ratios have been reported [185,187].

Treatment and prognosis

Therapeutic bronchoalveolar lavage has been shown to be ineffective in one case [185], and it is apparent that in progressive cases the only management course may be lung transplantation. This has been carried out successfully in at least one patient, a 32-year-old man who developed severe pulmonary hypertension [188]. Prior to this extreme measure, there is one report of nasal continuous positive pressure ventilatory support being used to improve gas exchange in a patient with respiratory failure [189].

The disease is probably slowly progressive, although occasionally it appears to arrest. One reported patient was followed for 22 years from diagnosis to death [185].

Idiopathic pulmonary hilar fibrosis

Chronic idiopathic pulmonary hilar fibrosis is a fibrosing condition restricted to the pulmonary hila that appears to have many similarities to idiopathic mediastinal fibrosis and retroperitoneal fibrosis [190–192]. The aetiology is unknown.

Pathology

Hilar fibrosis has been classified into two types depending on the relative involvement of the pulmonary artery or vein [190]. In type I disease, the pulmonary artery is narrowed or occluded by the fibrotic hilar mass, with the resultant development of exuberant bronchopulmonary anastomoses. Loss of lung volume is seen on the affected side and pleural thickening occurs due to repeated chest infections and the development of collateral vessels between the lung and chest wall. Narrowing of one of the main bronchi by the fibrotic process is often seen. In type II disease, the main pulmonary veins are occluded by fibrous tissue, with resultant pulmonary capillary hypertension in the affected lung. Loss of lung volume, pleural thickening and narrowing of main bronchi due to the fibrotic process are again seen. The fibrous tissue may extend through the bronchial cartilage. Histologically, the fibrous mass is composed of relatively acellular fibrous

tissue comprising intertwining collagen fibres. The interstices contain a few fibroblasts and lymphocytes with more plasma cells and occasional foci of polymorphonuclear leucocytes. Various degrees of hyalinization, calcification and ossification may be present.

Clinical and radiological features

Patients commonly present in young adult life with repeated haemoptyses and dyspnoea and there may be clinical signs of pulmonary hypertension. Radiographically, there may be pleural thickening and diminution of the size of the affected lung, and segmental narrowing of one or more major bronchi may be demonstrated at bronchoscopy or with bronchography (Fig. 51.6). The pulmonary artery shadow may be diminished in type I disease and pulmonary angiography shows absent or diminished pulmonary blood flow. In type II disease, an ill-defined hilar shadow may be seen with radiographic evidence of pulmonary venous distension.

Treatment and prognosis

No form of medical treatment is available. Most patients are subjected to thoracotomy, and resection of the 'tumour' and affected lung is carried out in the belief that the process is malignant. Treatment by simple ligation of bronchial arteries on the affected side also appears to have been effective in one case [190]. Where the condition is unilateral the prognosis, given surgical intervention, appears to be relatively good [190]. Bilateral hilar fibrosis has a poor prognosis when bilateral pulmonary venous obstruction occurs [193,194].

Pulmonary hyalinizing granuloma

Pulmonary hyalinizing granuloma is a condition of unknown aetiology, usually diagnosed by pathological examination of nodules resected following their discovery on routine chest radiography.

Pathology

Macroscopically, the waxy white lesions are found in the pulmonary parenchyma or just below the pleural surface [195]. Microscopically, they are seen to be composed of homogeneous pink hyaline lamellae surrounded by plasma cells, lymphocytes and histiocytes, which may also be found locally in a perivascular distribution. Occasional eosinophils and foci of ischaemic necrosis may be seen and foreign body giant cells may be present at the periphery of the lesion. In many of the 20 patients reported by Engleman and colleagues [195] the hyaline material stained with Congo red and had the characteristics of amyloid.

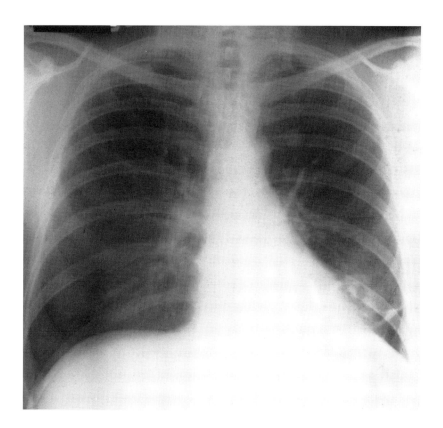

Fig. 51.6 Chest film of patient with left-sided idiopathic hilar fibrosis who presented with left lower lobe bronchial obstruction and secondary lung abscesses in posterior basal segment.

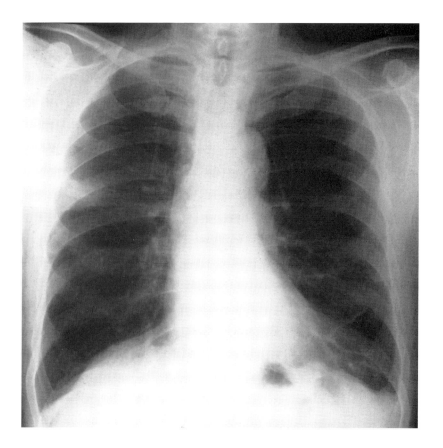

Fig. 51.7 Peripheral lesion in right mid zone that on excision proved to be a hyalinizing granuloma.

Clinical and radiological features

The average age of patients reported by Engleman and colleagues [195] was 45 years, with a range of 27–66 years. The majority were asymptomatic or had only mild symptoms, including cough, haemoptysis, fever, fatigue and pleuritic chest pain. The abnormality was commonly detected on routine chest radiography, which usually showed multiple, frequently bilateral, nodules with no predilection for any particular lung zone. Single lesions also occur (Fig. 51.7). The lesions were usually well defined and round, although irregular ill-defined nodules and cavitation were also seen. Calcification was not present. Lesions tended to grow very slowly, in one case with a doubling time of 2.5 years. The behaviour of the lesions was reminiscent of nodular pulmonary amyloid.

Treatment and prognosis

Isolated lesions are often resected as suspected carcinomas with resultant cure. No treatment is available for multiple lesions but the prognosis appears to be good, with no significant impact on longevity [195]. Four patients have been reported as developing sclerosing mediastinitis and two retroperitoneal fibrosis [195,196], an association that must be considered significant even though the aetiology of all these conditions is unknown.

Castleman's disease

Two subtypes of the very rare Castleman's disease, angiofollicular hyperplasia, have been described [197,198]. The more common presents as a mediastinal or hilar lymph node mass, usually asymptomatic or with cough or wheeze due to local compression. Occasionally there are febrile symptoms and a raised erythrocyte sedimentation rate. Biopsy at mediastinoscopy shows follicles of pericapillary lymphocytes, with proliferation of the plump and eosinophilic capillary endothelial cells. Patients with this condition generally do not seem to show a progressive illness and symptoms may be relieved by removal of the nodes.

A more aggressive variant, with prominent plasma cell infiltration, may be associated with other systemic manifestations, including generalized lymph node enlargement, hepatosplenomegaly, paraproteinaemia and skin rash. It may require treatment with corticosteroids and sometimes chemotherapy as for lymphoma, though it is thought not to be truly neoplastic but associated with overproduction of interleukin 6. There seems to be some evidence of an association with HIV infection and Kaposi's sarcoma.

References

1 Goodpasture EW. The significance of certain pulmonary lesions in relation to the etiology of influenza. *Am J Med Sci* 1919; 158: 863.

2 Teague CA, Doak PB, Simpson IJ *et al.* Goodpasture's syndrome: an analysis of 29 cases. *Kidney Int* 1978; 13: 492.

3 Wilson CB, Dixon FJ. Antiglomerular basement membrane antibody-induced glomerulonephritis. *Kidney Int* 1973; 3: 74.

4 Leatherman JW, Davies SF, Hoidal JR. Alveolar hemorrhage syndromes: diffuse microvascular lung hemorrhage in immune and idiopathic disorders. *Medicine* 1984; 63: 343.

5 Walker RG, Scheinkestel C, Becker GJ *et al.* Clinical and morphological aspects of the management of crescentic anti-glomerular basement membrane antibody (anti-GBM nephritis) Goodpasture's syndrome. *Q J Med* 1985; 54: 75.

6 Savage COS, Pusey CD, Bowman C *et al.* Antiglomerular basement antibody mediated disease in the British Isles 1980–1984. *Br Med J* 1986; 292: 301.

7 Leatherman JW. Immune alveolar hemorrhage. *Chest* 1987; 91: 891.

8 Mintz G, Galindo LF, Fernandez-Diez J *et al.* Acute massive pulmonary hemorrhage in systemic lupus erythematosus *J Rheumatol* 1978; 5: 39.

9 Eagen JW, Memoli VA, Roberts JL *et al.* Pulmonary hemorrhage in systemic lupus erythematosus. *Medicine* 1978; 57: 545.

10 Abud-Mendoza C, Diaz-Jouanen E, Alarcon-Segovia D. Fatal pulmonary hemorrhage in systemic lupus erythematosus: occurrence without hemoptysis. *J Rheumatol* 1985; 12: 558.

11 Haworth SJ, Savage COS, Carr DE *et al.* Pulmonary haemorrhage complicating Wegener's granulomatosis and microscopic polyarteritis. *Br Med J* 1985; 290: 1775.

12 Holdsworth S, Boyce N, Thomson NM, Atkins RC. The clinical spectrum of acute glomerulonephritis and lung haemorrhage (Goodpasture's syndrome). *Q J Med* 1985; 55: 75.

13 Leatherman JW, Sibley RK, Davies SF. Diffuse intrapulmonary hemorrhage and glomerulonephritis unrelated to antiglomerular basement membrane antibody. *Am J Med* 1982; 72: 401.

14 Smith BS. Idiopathic pulmonary haemosiderosis and rheumatoid arthritis. *Br Med J* 1966; i: 1403.

15 Kallenbach J, Prinsloo I, Zwi S. Progressive systemic sclerosis complicated by diffuse pulmonary haemorrhage. *Thorax* 1977; 32: 767.

16 Germain MJ, Davidman M. Pulmonary hemorrhage and acute renal failure in a patient with mixed connective tissue disease. *Am J Kidney Dis* 1984; 3: 420.

17 Cadman EC, Lundberg WB, Mitchell MS. Pulmonary manifestations in Behcet's syndrome. *Arch Intern Med* 1976; 136: 944.

18 Martinez JS, Kohler PF. Variant 'Goodpasture's syndrome'? *Ann Intern Med* 1971; 75: 67.

19 Loughlin GM, Taussig LM, Murphy SA *et al.* Immune-complex mediated glomerulonephritis and pulmonary hemorrhage simulating Goodpasture's syndrome. *J Pediatr* 1978; 93: 181.

20 Beirne GJ, Wagnild JP, Zimmerman SW *et al.* Idiopathic crescentic glomerulonephritis. *Medicine* 1977; 56: 349.

21 Sternlieb I, Bennet B, Scheinberg IW. D-Penicillamine-induced Goodpasture's syndrome in Wilson's disease. *Ann Intern Med* 1975; 82: 673,.

22 Matloff DS, Kaplan MM. D-Penicillamine-induced Goodpasture's syndrome in primary biliary cirrhosis: successful treatment with plasmapheresis and immunosuppressives. *Gastroenterology* 1980; 78: 1046.

23 Herbert FA, Orford R. Pulmonary hemorrhage and edema due to inhalation of resins containing trimellitic anhydride. *Chest* 1979; 76: 546.

24 Marglin SI, Castellino RA. Severe pulmonary hemorrhage following lymphography. *Cancer* 1979; 43: 482.

25 Stetter M, Schmidl M, Krapf R. Azathioprine hypersensitivity mimicking Goodpasture's syndrome. *Am J Kidney Dis* 1994; 23: 874.

26 Lechleitner P, Defregger M, Lhotta K, Totsch M, Fend F. Goodpasture's syndrome. Unusual presentation after exposure to hard metal dust. *Chest* 1993; 103: 956.

27 Keogh AM, Ibels LS, Allen DH *et al.* Exacerbation of Goodpasture's syndrome after inadvertent exposure to hydrocarbon fumes. *Br Med J* 1984; 288: 188.

28 Stevenson A, Yaqoob M, Mason H, Pai P,

Bell GM. Biochemical markers of basement membrane disturbances and occupational exposure to hydrocarbons and mixed solvents. *Q J Med* 1995; 88: 23.

29 Markowitz AS, Battifora HA, Schwartz F, Aseron C. Immunological aspects of Goodpasture's syndrome. *Clin Exp Immunol* 1968; 3: 585.

30 Wieslander J, Heinegard D. The involvement of type IV collagen in Goodpasture's syndrome. *Ann N Y Acad Sci* 1985; 460: 363.

31 Wieslander J, Bygren P, Heinegard D. Isolation of the specific glomerular basement membrane antigen involved in Goodpasture's syndrome. *Proc Natl Acad Sci USA* 1984; 81: 1544.

32 Pusey CD, Dash A, Kershaw MJ et al. A single autoantigen in Goodpasture's syndrome identified by a monoclonal antibody to human glomerular basement membrane. *Lab Invest* 1987; 56: 23.

33 Weber M, Kohler H, Manns M et al. Identification of Goodpasture target antigens in basement membranes of human glomeruli, lung and placenta. *Clin Exp Immunol* 1987; 67: 262.

34 Turner N, Mason PJG, Brown R et al. Molecular cloning of the human Goodpasture antigen demonstrates it to be the alpha 3 chain of type IV collagen. *J Clin Invest* 1992; 89: 592.

35 Hudson BG, Kalluri R, Gunwar S, Noelken ME, Mariyama M, Reeders ST. Molecular characteristics of the Goodpasture autoantigen. *Kidney Int* 1993; 43: 135.

36 Kefalides NA. The Goodpasture antigen and basement membranes: the search must go on. *Lab Invest* 1987; 56: 1.

37 Gossain VV, Gerstein AR, Janes AW. Goodpasture's syndrome: a familial occurrence. *Am Rev Respir Dis* 1972; 105: 621.

38 Simonsen H, Brun C, Frokjaer Thomson O et al. Goodpasture's syndrome in twins. *Acta Med Scand* 1982; 212: 425.

39 Rees AJ, Peters DK, Compston DAS, Batchelor JR. Strong association between HLA-DRW2 and antibody-mediated Goodpasture's syndrome. *Lancet* 1978; i: 966.

40 Burns AP, Fisher M, Li P, Pusey CD, Rees AJ. Molecular analysis of HLA class II genes in Goodpasture's disease. *Q J Med* 1995; 88: 93.

41 Perl SI, Pussell BA, Charlesworth JA, Macdonald GJ, Wolnizer M. Goodpasture's (antiGBM) disease and HLA Drw2. *N Engl J Med* 1981; 305: 463.

42 Wilson CB, Smith RC. Goodpasture's syndrome associated with influenza A2 virus infection. *Ann Intern Med* 1972; 76: 91.

43 West JB, Mathieu-Costello O. Stress failure of pulmonary capillaries: role in lung and heart disease. *Lancet* 1992; 340: 762.

44 Donaghy M, Rees AJ. Cigarette smoking and lung haemorrhage in glomerulonephritis caused by antibodies to glomerular basement membrane. *Lancet* 1983; ii: 1390.

45 Zimmerman SW, Varanasi UR, Hoff B. Goodpasture's syndrome with normal renal function. *Am J Med* 1979; 66: 163.

46 Donald KJ, Edwards RL, McEvoy JDS. Alveolar capillary basement membrane lesions in Goodpasture's syndrome and idiopathic pulmonary hemosiderosis. *Am J Med* 1975; 59: 642.

47 Abboud RT, Chase WH, Ballon HS et al. Goodpasture's syndrome: diagnosis by transbronchial biopsy. *Ann Intern Med* 1978; 89: 635.

48 Hogan PG, Donald KJ, McEvoy JDS. Immunofluorescence studies of lung biopsy tissue. *Am Rev Respir Dis* 1978; 118: 537.

49 Ewan PW, Jones HA, Rhodes CG, Hughes JMB. Detection of intrapulmonary haemorrhage with carbon monoxide uptake. *N Engl J Med* 1976; 295: 1391.

50 Greening AP, Hughes JMB. Serial estimations of carbon monoxide diffusing capacity in intrapulmonary haemorrhage. *Clin Sci* 1981; 60: 507.

51 Anon. Alveolar haemorrhage. *Lancet* 1985; i: 853.

52 Addelman M, Logan AS, Grossman RF. Monitoring intrapulmonary hemorrhage in Goodpasture's syndrome. *Chest* 1985; 87: 119.

53 Bowley NB, Hughes JMB, Steiner RE. The chest X-ray in pulmonary capillary haemorrhage: correlation with carbon monoxide uptake. *Clin Radiol* 1979; 30: 413.

54 Benoit FL, Rulon DB, Theil GB et al. Goodpasture's syndrome. *Am J Med* 1964; 37: 424.

55 Proskey AJ, Weatherbee L, Easterling RE et al. Goodpasture's syndrome. *Am J Med* 1970; 48: 162.

56 Nilssen DE, Talseth T, Brodwall EK. The many faces of Goodpasture's syndrome. *Acta Med Scand* 1986; 220: 489.

57 Bowley NB, Steiner RE, Chin WS. The chest X-ray in antiglomerular basement membrane antibody disease (Goodpasture's syndrome). *Clin Radiol* 1979; 30: 419.

58 Kelly PT, Haponik EF. Goodpasture syndrome: molecular and clinical advances. *Medicine* 1994; 73: 171.

59 Falk R, Jennette JC. Antineutrophil cytoplasmic antibodies with specificity for myeloperoxidase in patients with systemic vasculitis and idiopathic necrotising and crescentic glomerulonephritis. *N Engl J Med* 1988; 318: 1651.

60 Fish AJ, Kleppel M, Jeraj K, Michael AF. Enzyme immunoassay of antiglomerular basement membrane antibodies. *J Lab Clin Med* 1985; 105: 700.

61 Walker RG, Scheinkestel C, Becker GJ, Owen JE, Dowling JP, Kincaid-Smith P. Clinical and morphological aspects of the management of crescentic anti-glomerular basement membrane antibody (anti-GBM) nephritis/Goodpasture's syndrome. *Q J Med* 1985; 54: 75.

62 Johnson JP, Moore J, Austin HA, Balow JE, Antonovych TT, Wilson CB. Therapy of antiglomerular basement membrane antibody disease: analysis of prognostic significance of clinical, pathologic and treatment factors. *Medicine* 1985; 64: 219.

63 Seaton A, Meland JM, Lapp NL. Remission in Goodpasture's syndrome: report of two patients treated by immunosuppression and review of the literature. *Thorax* 1971; 26: 683.

64 Peters DK, Rees AJ, Lockwood CM, Pusey CD. Treatment and prognosis in anti-basement membrane mediated nephritis. *Transplant Proc* 1982; 14: 513.

65 Bygren P, Freiburghaus C, Lindholm T. Goodpasture's syndrome treated with staphylococcal protein A immunoadsorption. *Lancet* 1985; ii: 1275.

66 Nowakowski A, Grove RB, King LH et al. Goodpasture's syndrome: recovery from severe pulmonary hemorrhage after bilateral nephrectomy. *Ann Intern Med* 1971; 75: 243.

67 Rees AJ, Lockwood CM, Peters DK. Enhanced allergic tissue injury in Goodpasture's syndrome by intercurrent bacterial infection. *Br Med J* 1977; ii: 723.

68 Burke BR, Bear RA. Recurrent Goodpasture's syndrome. *Can Med Assoc J* 1983; 129: 978.

69 Keller F, Nekarda H. Fatal relapse in Goodpasture's syndrome 3 years after plasma exchange. *Respiration* 1985; 48: 62.

70 Mehler PS, Brunvand MW, Hutt MP, Anderson RJ. Chronic recurrent Goodpasture's syndrome. *Am J Med* 1987; 82: 833.

71 Conlon PJ, Walshe JJ, Daly C et al. Antiglomerular basement membrane disease: the long-term pulmonary outcome. *Am J Kidney Dis* 1994; 23: 794.

72 Soergel KH, Sommers SC. Idiopathic pulmonary hemosiderosis and related syndromes. *Am J Med* 1962; 32: 499.

73 Kennedy WPU, Shearman DJC, Delamore IW et al. Idiopathic pulmonary haemosiderosis with myocarditis. *Thorax* 1966; 21: 220.

74 Cassimos CD, Chryssanthopoulos C, Panagiotidou C. Epidemiologic observations in idiopathic pulmonary hemosiderosis. *J Pediatr* 1983; 102: 698.

75 Anon. Idiopathic pulmonary haemosiderosis. *Lancet* 1963; i: 979.

76 Dolan J, McGuire S, Sweeney E et al. Mast cells in pulmonary haemosiderosis. *Arch Dis Child* 1984; 59: 276.

77 Lemley DE, Katz P. Rheumatoid-like arthritis presenting as idiopathic pulmonary hemosiderosis. *J Rheumatol* 1986; 13: 954.

78 Rafferty JR, Cook MK. Idiopathic pulmonary haemosiderosis with auto-immune haemolytic anaemia. *Br J Dis Chest* 1984; 78: 282.

79 Nomura S, Kanoh T. Association of idiopathic pulmonary haemosiderosis with IgA monoclonal gammopathy. *Thorax* 1987; 42: 696.

80 Bain SC, Bryan RL, Hawkins JB. Idiopathic pulmonary haemosiderosis and autoimmune thyrotoxicosis. *Respir Med* 1989; 83: 447.

81 Wright PH, Menzies IS, Pounder RE, Keeling PWN. Adult idiopathic pulmonary haemosiderosis and coeliac disease. *Q J Med* 1981; 50: 95.

82 Wright PH, Buxton-Thomas M, Keeling PWN, Kreel L. Adult idiopathic pulmonary haemosiderosis: a comparison of lung function changes and the distribution of disease in patients with and without coeliac disease. *Br J Dis Chest* 1983; 77: 282.

83 Reading R, Watson JG, Platt JW, Bird AG. Pulmonary hemosiderosis and gluten. *Arch Dis Child* 1987; 62: 513.

84 Pacheco A, Casanova C, Fogue L, Sueiro A. Long-term clinical follow-up of adult idiopathic pulmonary hemosiderosis and celiac disease. *Chest* 1991; 99: 1525.

85 Heiner DC, Sears JW, Kniker WT. Multiple precipitins to cow's milk in chronic respiratory disease. *Am J Dis Child* 1962; 103: 634.

86 Morgan PGM, Turner-Warwick M. Pulmonary haemosiderosis and pulmonary haemorrhage. *Br J Dis Chest* 1981; 75: 225.

87 Turner-Warwick M, Dewar A. Pulmonary haemorrhage and pulmonary haemosiderosis. *Clin Radiol* 1982; 33: 361.

88 Elliot ML, Kohn C. Idiopathic pulmonary hemosiderosis. Ultrastructural abnormalities in the capillary walls. *Am Rev Respir Dis* 1970; 102: 895.

89 Corrin B, Jagusch M, Dewar A et al. Fine

structural changes in idiopathic pulmonary haemosiderosis. *J Pathol* 1987; 153: 249.

90 Ellman P. Pulmonary haemosiderosis. *Proc R Soc Med* 1960; 53: 333.

91 Bronson SM. Idiopathic pulmonary hemosiderosis in adults. Report of a case and review of the literature. *Am J Roentgenol* 1960; 83: 260.

92 Frankel LR, Smith DW, Pearl RG, Lewiston NJ. Nitroglycerin-responsive pulmonary hypertension in idiopathic pulmonary hemosiderosis. *Am Rev Respir Dis* 1986; 133: 170.

93 Colombo JL, Stoltz SM. Treatment of life-threatening pulmonary hemosiderosis with cyclophosphamide. *Chest* 1992; 102: 959.

94 Elinder G. Budesonide inhalation to treat idiopathic pulmonary haemosiderosis. *Lancet* 1985; i: 981.

95 Rosen JH, Castleman B, Liebow AA. Pulmonary alveolar proteinosis. *N Engl J Med* 1958; 258: 1123.

96 Coleman M, Dehner LP, Sibley RK *et al.* Pulmonary alveolar proteinosis: an uncommon cause of chronic neonatal respiratory distress. *Am Rev Respir Dis* 1980; 121: 583.

97 McCook TA, Kirks DR, Merten DF *et al.* Pulmonary alveolar proteinosis in children. *Am J Roentgenol* 1981; 137: 1023.

98 Singh G, Katyal S, Bedrossian CWM, Rogers RM. Pulmonary alveolar proteinosis. Staining for surfactant apoprotein in alveolar proteinosis and in conditions simulating it. *Chest* 1983; 83: 82.

99 Harris JO. Pulmonary alveolar proteinosis. Specific or non-specific response? *Chest* 1983; 84: 1.

100 Honda Y, Takahashi H, Shijubo N, Kuroki Y, Akino T. Surfactant protein-A concentration in bronchoalveolar lavage fluids of patients with pulmonary alveolar proteinosis. *Chest* 1993; 103: 496.

101 Crouch E, Persson A, Chang D. Accumulation of surfactant protein D in human pulmonary alveolar proteinosis. *Am J Pathol* 1993; 142: 241.

102 Eldar M, Shoenfeld Y, Zaizov R *et al.* Pulmonary alveolar proteinosis associated with Fanconi's anaemia. *Respiration* 1979; 38: 177.

103 Steens RD, Summers QA, Tarala RA. Pulmonary alveolar proteinosis in association with Fanconi's anaemia and psoriasis. A possible common pathogenetic mechanism. *Chest* 1992; 102: 637.

104 Cordonnier C, Fleury-Feith J, Escudier E, Atassi K, Bernaudin JF. Secondary alveolar proteinosis is a reversible cause of respiratory failure in leukemic patients. *Am J Respir Crit Care Med* 1994; 149: 788.

105 Bedrossian CWM, Luna MA, Conklin RH, Miller WC. Alveolar proteinosis as a consequence of immunosuppression. *Hum Pathol* 1980; 11: 527.

106 Rubin E, Weisbrod GL, Sanders DE. Pulmonary alveolar proteinosis. Relationship to silicosis and pulmonary infection. *Radiology* 1980; 135: 35.

107 Meijer WG, van Marwijk-Kooy M, Ladde BE. A patient with multiple myeloma and respiratory insufficiency due to accumulation of paraprotein in the alveolar space. *Br J Haematol* 1994; 87: 663.

108 Webster JR, Battifora H, Furey C *et al.* Pulmonary alveolar proteinosis in two siblings with decreased immunoglobulin A. *Am J Med* 1980; 69: 786.

109 Case records of the Massachusetts General Hospital. Case 14–1984. *N Engl J Med* 1984; 310: 906.

110 Ruben FL, Talamo TS. Secondary pulmonary alveolar proteinosis occurring in two patients with the acquired immunodeficiency syndrome. *Am J Med* 1986; 80: 1187.

111 Teja K, Cooper PH, Squires JE, Schnatterly PT. Pulmonary alveolar proteinosis in four siblings. *N Engl J Med* 1981; 305: 1390.

112 DeMello DE, Nogee LM, Heyman S *et al.* Molecular and phenotypic variability in the congenital alveolar proteinosis syndrome associated with inherited surfactant protein B deficiency. *J Pediatr* 1994; 125: 43.

113 Parto K, Kallajoki M, Aho H, Simell O. Pulmonary alveolar proteinosis and glomerulonephritis in lysinuric protein intolerance: case reports and autopsy findings in four pediatric patients. *Hum Pathol* 1994; 25: 400.

114 Witty LA, Tapson VF, Piantadosi CA. Isolation of mycobacteria in patients with pulmonary alveolar proteinosis. *Medicine* 1994; 73: 103.

115 Miller RR, Churg AM, Hutcheon M, Lam S. Pulmonary alveolar proteinosis and aluminium dust exposure. *Am Rev Respir Dis* 1984; 130: 312.

116 Claypool WD, Rogers RM, Matuschak GM. Update on the clinical diagnosis, management and pathogenesis of pulmonary alveolar proteinosis (phospholiposis). *Chest* 1984; 85: 550.

117 Hook GER, Gilmore LB, Talley FA. Dissolution and reassembly of tubular myelin-like multilamellated structures from the lungs of patients with pulmonary alveolar proteinosis. *Lab Invest* 1986; 55: 194.

118 Glen RH, Balis JU, Shelley S *et al.* Isolation, characterization and localization of a 45,000 molecular weight, soluble glycoprotein from the lung in pulmonary alveolar proteinosis. *Biochim Biophys Acta* 1981; 670: 101.

119 Ross GF, Ohning BL, Tannenbaum D, Whitsett JA. Structural relationships of the major glycoproteins from human alveolar proteinosis surfactant. *Biochim Biophys Acta* 1987; 911: 294.

120 Kariman K, Kylstra JA, Spock A. Pulmonary alveolar proteinosis: prospective clinical experience in 23 patients for 15 years. *Lung* 1984; 162: 223.

121 Nugent KM, Pesanti EL. Macrophage function in pulmonary alveolar proteinosis. *Am Rev Respir Dis* 1983; 127: 780.

122 Gonzaleth-Rothi RJ, Harris JO. Pulmonary alveolar proteinosis. Further evaluation of abnormal alveolar macrophages. *Chest* 1986; 90: 656.

123 Zijlstra FJ, Vincent JE, van den Berg B *et al.* Pulmonary alveolar proteinosis: determination of prostaglandins and leukotrienes in lavage fluid. *Lung* 1987; 165: 79.

124 Dubois RM, McAllister WAC, Branthwaite MA. Alveolar proteinosis: diagnosis and treatment over a 10-year period. *Thorax* 1983; 38: 360.

125 Case records of the Massachusetts General Hospital. *N Engl J Med* 1983; 308: 1147.

126 Anton HC. Pulmonary alveolar proteinosis. *Br Med J* 1972; i: 626.

127 Preger L. Pulmonary alveolar proteinosis. *Radiology* 1969; 92: 1291.

128 Miller PA, Ravin CE, Walker Smith GJ, Osborne DRS. Pulmonary alveolar proteinosis with interstitial involvement. *Am J Roentgenol* 1981; 137: 1069.

129 Clague HW, Wallace AC, Morgan WKC. Pulmonary interstitial fibrosis associated with alveolar proteinosis. *Thorax* 1983; 38: 865.

130 Costello JF, Moriarty DC, Branthwaite MA *et al.* Diagnosis and management of alveolar proteinosis: the role of electron microscopy. *Thorax* 1975; 30: 121.

131 Martin RJ, Rogers RM, Myers NM. Pulmonary alveolar proteinosis: shunt fraction and lactic acid dehydrogenase concentrations as aids to diagnosis. *Am Rev Respir Dis* 1978; 117: 1059.

132 Wilson DO, Rogers RM. Prolonged spontaneous remission in a patient with untreated pulmonary alveolar proteinosis. *Am J Med* 1987; 82: 1014.

133 Smith LJ, Katzenstein A-L, Ankin MG, Shapiro BA. Management of pulmonary alveolar proteinosis. *Chest* 1980; 78: 765.

134 Gale ME, Karlinsky JB, Robins AG. Bronchopulmonary lavage in pulmonary alveolar proteinosis: chest radiograph observations. *Am J Roentgenol* 1986; 146: 981.

135 Heymach GJ, Shaw RC, McDonald JA, Vest JV. Fibreoptic bronchopulmonary lavage for alveolar proteinosis in a patient with only one lung. *Chest* 1982; 81: 508.

136 Jansen HM, Zuurmond WWA, Roos CM *et al.* Whole lung lavage under hyperbaric oxygen conditions for alveolar proteinosis with respiratory failure. *Chest* 1987; 91: 829.

137 Hiratzka LF, Swan DM, Rose EF, Ahrens RC. Bilateral simultaneous lung lavage utilising membrane oxygenator for pulmonary alveolar proteinosis in an 8 month old infant. *Ann Thorac Surg* 1983; 35: 313.

138 Freedman AP, Pelias A, Johnston RF *et al.* Alveolar proteinosis lung lavage using partial cardiopulmonary bypass. *Thorax* 1981; 36: 543.

139 Diaz JP, Manresa Presas F, Benasco C *et al.* Response to surfactant activator (ambroxol) in alveolar proteinosis. *Lancet* 1984; i: 1023.

140 Glenner GG. Amyloid deposits and amyloidosis. *N Engl J Med* 1980; 302: 1283.

141 Thompson PJ, Citron KM. Amyloid and the lower respiratory tract. *Thorax* 1983; 38: 84.

142 Rubinow A, Celli BR, Cohen AS *et al.* Localised amyloidosis of the lower respiratory tract. *Am Rev Respir Dis* 1978; 118: 603.

143 Cordier JF, Loire R, Brune J. Amyloidosis of the lower respiratory tract. Clinical and pathological features in a series of 21 patients. *Chest* 1986; 90: 827.

144 Gertz MA, Greipp PR. Clinical aspects of pulmonary amyloidosis. *Chest* 1986; 90: 790.

145 Polansky SM, Ravin CE. Nodular pulmonary infiltrate in a patient with Sjögren's syndrome. *Chest* 1980; 77: 411.

146 Bignold LP, Martyn M, Basten A. Nodular pulmonary amyloidosis associated with benign hypergammaglobulinemic purpura. *Chest* 1980; 78: 334.

147 Lee AB, Bogaars HA, Passero MA. Nodular pulmonary amyloidosis. A cause of bronchiectasis and fatal pulmonary hemorrhage. *Arch Intern Med* 1983; 143: 603.

148 Shaw P, Grossman R, Fernandes BJ. Nodular mediastinal amyloidosis. *Hum Pathol* 1984; 15: 1183.

149 Laden SA, Cohen ML, Harley RA. Nodular pulmonary amyloidosis with extrapulmonary involvement. *Hum Pathol* 1984; 15: 594.

150 Pinto A, Rasmussen SL, Campbell TM, Lester WM. Nodular pulmonary amyloidosis. *Can Med Assoc J* 1984; 131: 215.

151 Thompson PJ, Jewkes J, Corrin B, Citron KM. Primary bronchopulmonary amyloid tumour with massive hilar lymphadenopathy. *Thorax* 1983; 38: 153.

152 Melato M, Antonutto G, Falconieri G, Manconi R. Massive amyloidosis of mediastinal lymph nodes in a patient with multiple myeloma. *Thorax* 1983; 38: 151.

153 Eisenberg R, Sharma OP. Primary pulmonary amyloidosis. An unusual case with 14 years survival. *Chest* 1986; 89: 889.

154 Naschitz JE, Yeshurun D, Pick AI. Intrathoracic amyloid lymphadenopathy. *Respiration* 1986; 49: 73.

155 Osnoss KL, Harrell DD. Isolated mediastinal mass in primary amyloidosis. *Chest* 1980; 78: 786.

156 Road JD, Jacques J, Sparling JR. Diffuse alveolar septal amyloidosis presenting with recurrent hemoptysis and medial dissection of pulmonary arteries. *Am Rev Respir Dis* 1985; 132: 1368.

157 Liaw YS, Kuo SH, Yang PC, Chen CL, Luh KT. Nodular amyloidosis of the lung and breast mimicking breast carcinoma with pulmonary metastasis. *Eur Respir J* 1995; 8: 871.

158 Kline LR, Dise CA, Ferro TJ, Hansen-Flaschen JH. Diagnosis of pulmonary amyloidosis by transbronchial biopsy. *Am Rev Respir Dis* 1985; 132: 191.

159 Strange C, Heffner JE, Collins BS *et al.* Pulmonary hemorrhage and air embolism complicating transbronchial biopsy in pulmonary amyloidosis. *Chest* 1987; 92: 367.

160 Sumiya M, Ohya N, Shinoura H *et al.* Diffuse interstitial pulmonary amyloidosis in rheumatoid arthritis. *J Rheumatol* 1996; 23: 933.

161 Wong BC, Wong KL, Ip MS, Wang EP, Chan KW, Cheng LC. Sjörgren's syndrome with amyloid A presenting as multiple pulmonary nodules. *J Rheumatol* 1994; 21: 165.

162 Blavia R, Toda MR, Vidal F, Benet A, Razquin S, Richart C. Pulmonary diffuse amyloidosis and ankylosing spondylitis. A rare association. *Chest* 1992; 102: 1608.

163 Beer TW, Edwards CW. Pulmonary nodules due to reactive systemic amyloidosis (AA) in Crohn's disease. *Thorax* 1993; 48: 1287.

164 Streeten EA, De La Monte SM, Kennedy TP. Amyloid infiltration of the diaphragm as a cause of respiratory failure. *Chest* 1986; 89: 760.

165 Santiago RM, Scharnhorst D, Ratkin G, Crouch EC. Respiratory muscle weakness and ventilatory failure in AL amyloidosis with muscular pseudohypertrophy. *Am J Med* 1987; 83: 175.

166 Carbone JE, Barker D, Stauffer JL. Sleep apnea in amyloidosis. *Chest* 1985; 87: 401.

167 Breuer R, Simpson GT, Rubinow A *et al.* Tracheobronchial amyloidosis: treatment by carbon dioxide laser photoresection. *Thorax* 1985; 40: 870.

168 Aschoff L. Uber Tracheopathia osteoplastica. *Verh Dtsch Pathol Ges* 1910; 14: 125.

169 Wilks S. Ossific deposits on larynx, trachea and bronchi. *Trans Pathol Soc Lond* 1857; 8: 88.

170 Secrest PG, Kendig TA, Beland AJ. Tracheobronchopathia osteoplastica. *Am J Med* 1964; 36: 815.

171 Martin CJ. Tracheobronchopathia osteochondroplastica. *Arch Otolaryngol* 1974; 100: 290.

172 Jepsen O, Sorensen H. Tracheopathia osteoplastica and ozaena. *Acta Otolaryngol* 1960; 51: 79.

173 Smith CC, Dixon MF. Tracheopathia osteoplastica with pulmonary thrombo-embolic disease. *Br J Dis Chest* 1972; 66: 192.

174 Dalgaard JB. Tracheopathia chondro-osteoplastica. A case elucidating the problems concerning development and ossification of elastic cartilage. *Acta Pathol Microbiol Scand* 1947; 24: 118.

175 Virchow R. *Die Krankhaften Geschwalsten*, Vol 1. Berlin: Hirschwala, 1863: 443. Cited by Sakula [176].

176 Sakula A. Tracheobronchopathia osteoplastica. *Thorax* 1968; 23: 105.

177 Clee MD, Anderson JM, Johnston RN. Clinical aspects of tracheobronchopathia osteochondroplastica. *Br J Dis Chest* 1983; 77: 308.

178 Carr DT, Olsen AM. Tracheopathia osteoplastica. *JAMA* 1954; 155: 1563.

179 Baird RB, Macartney JN. Tracheopathia osteoplastica. *Thorax* 1966; 21: 321.

180 Birzgalis AR, Farrington WT, O'Keefe L, Shaw J. Localised tracheopathia osteoplastica of the subglottis. *J Laryngol Otol* 1993; 107: 352.

181 Sosman MC, Dodd GD, Jones WD, Pillmore GU. The familial occurrence of pulmonary alveolar microlithiasis. *Am J Roentgenol* 1957; 77: 947.

182 Ucan ES, Keyf AI, Aydilek R *et al.* Pulmonary alveolar microlithiasis: review of Turkish reports. *Thorax* 1993; 48: 171.

183 Coetzee T. Pulmonary alveolar microlithiasis with involvement of the sympathetic nervous system and gonads. *Thorax* 1970; 25: 637.

184 Thind GS, Bhatia JL. Pulmonary alveolar microlithiasis. *Br J Dis Chest* 1978; 72: 151.

185 Mascie-Taylor BH, Wardman AG, Madden CA, Page RL. A case of alveolar microlithiasis: observation over 22 years and recovery of material by lavage. *Thorax* 1985; 40: 952.

186 Sears MR, Chang AR, Taylor AJ. Pulmonary alveolar microlithiasis. *Thorax* 1971; 26: 704.

187 Fuliehan FJD, Abboud RT, Balikian JP, Nucho CKN. Pulmonary alveolar microlithiasis: lung function in five cases. *Thorax* 1969; 24: 84.

188 Stamatis G, Zerkowski HR, Doetsch N, Greschuchna D, Konietzko N, Reidermeister JC. Sequential bilateral lung transplantation for pulmonary alveolar microlithiasis. *Ann Thorac Surg* 1993; 56: 972.

189 Freiberg DB, Young IH, Laks L, Regnis JA, Lehrhaft B, Sullivan CE. Improvement in gas exchange with nasal continuous positive airway pressure in pulmonary alveolar microlithiasis. *Am Rev Respir Dis* 1992; 145: 1215.

190 Yacoub MH, Thompson VC. Chronic idiopathic pulmonary hilar fibrosis. *Thorax* 1971; 26: 365.

191 Bradfield EO. Bilateral ureteric obstruction due to envelopment and compression by an inflammatory retroperitoneal process. *J Urol* 1953; 69: 769.

192 Cameron DG, Ing ST, Boyle M, Matthews WH. Idiopathic mediastinal and retroperitoneal fibrosis. *Can Med Assoc J* 1961; 85: 227.

193 Bindelglass IL, Trubowitz S. Pulmonary vein obstruction: an uncommon sequel to chronic fibrous mediastinitis. *Ann Intern Med* 1958; 48: 876.

194 Espinosa RE, Edwards WD, Rosenow EC, Schaff HV. Idiopathic pulmonary hilar fibrosis: an unusual cause of pulmonary hypertension. *Mayo Clin Proc* 1993; 68: 778.

195 Engleman P, Liebow AA, Gmelich J, Friedman PJ. Pulmonary hyalinising granuloma. *Am Rev Respir Dis* 1977; 115: 997.

196 Dent RG, Godden DJ, Stovin PGI, Stark JE. Pulmonary hyalinising granuloma in association with retroperitoneal fibrosis. *Thorax* 1983; 38: 955.

197 Shahidi H, Myers JL, Kvale PA. Castleman's disease. *Mayo Clin Proc* 1995; 70: 969.

198 Blankenship ME, Rowlett J, Timby JW, Roth RS, Jones RE. Giant lymph node hyperplasia (Castleman's disease) presenting with chylous pleural effusion. *Chest* 1997; 112: 1132.

52

RESPIRATORY INFECTION IN THE IMMUNOSUPPRESSED

R. ANDREW SEATON, JULIAN M. HOPKIN AND DOUGLAS SEATON

Respiratory infection in the immunosuppressed has become a major clinical issue with the advance of human immunodeficiency virus (HIV) and with progress in transplant and oncology programmes. Defence of the lungs against infection is complex, comprising laryngeal and cough reflexes, the mucociliary escalator, the scavenging macrophages of the alveolar spaces, a range of innate immune factors (e.g. mannose-binding protein, surfactant proteins A and D) and acquired T-cell immunoglobulin immunity.

Defects in these defences are various and can produce characteristic syndromes of infection. The first part of this chapter focuses on the general principles of respiratory infection complicating severe deficiency of acquired immunity, most commonly seen among patients on cancer chemotherapy and organ transplantation programmes, in those with AIDS and in those receiving immunosuppressive agents for inflammatory disorders, for example vasculitis. Among these patients, pneumonia is a leading cause of disease and death. The second part of the chapter deals specifically with an important opportunistic lung infection, *Pneumocystis carinii* pneumonia (PCP). Actinomycotic and fungal pneumonias are covered in Chapter 21, tuberculosis and opportunistic mycobacterial disease in Chapters 17–20 and bacterial and viral pneumonias in Chapter 13. Diseases that may mimic infection in the immunosuppressed are dealt with elsewhere: radiation pneumonitis in Chapter 13, cytotoxic and other drug-induced lung disease in Chapters 9 and 55, and lymphomas and Kaposi's sarcoma in Chapter 42. The minimally invasive procedures used in diagnosing lung disease in immunosuppressed patients are described in Chapter 8.

Pulmonary complications in the immunosuppressed may be due to infection with pathogenic organisms and opportunistic organisms of medium to low pathogenicity (Table 52.1) or to various non-infective complications (Table 52.2). These often have overlapping clinical and radiographic features, and pose diagnostic and therapeutic difficulties. Establishing a diagnosis, often by invasive investigation, allows the use of specific and effective treatment, with the minimum of side-effects. This significantly improves survival [1].

An effective diagnostic approach requires knowledge of the potential pulmonary complications, a thorough approach to clinical assessment and a strategy for further investigation.

Patterns of pulmonary complication

The type of immune disruption provides useful clues to the likely causes of infection (Table 52.1). However, the immunosuppression can be mixed in type in any patient and may vary with the stage of the underlying disease and treatment.

Cancer chemotherapy programmes

Patients receiving vigorous cytotoxic chemotherapy for leukaemia and lymphoma have a high risk of fatal respiratory infection that threatens their survival, despite control of the malignancy.

Profound neutropenia during the early phases of treatment and consequent Gram-negative pneumonia is a special risk; fungal pneumonia (see Chapter 21), particularly that caused by *Aspergillus fumigatus*, is also possible if the neutropenia is severe and prolonged. Later in the course of the illness, T-lymphocyte immune deficiency develops and with it the special risk of PCP; before the introduction of specific chemoprophylaxis, this produced an attack rate of 18% annually in the childhood leukaemia population.

Non-infectious complications are various and include diffuse pneumonitis as a reaction to cytotoxic agents and the rare leucagglutinin reaction of the lung, in which diffuse radiographic change and hypoxaemia may follow white cell transfusion.

Table 52.1 Opportunistic respiratory infection in the immunosuppressed.

Defect	Infections
Neutropenia, e.g. treated leukaemia	Bacteria: Gram-negatives, *Staphylococcus aureus* Fungi: *Aspergillus fumigatus*, *Mucor* spp.
Immunoglobulin deficiency, e.g. multiple myeloma, inherited defects	Encapsulated bacteria: *Streptococcus pneumoniae*, *Haemophilus influenzae*
T-lymphocyte deficiency e.g. AIDS organ transplant recipients, treated malignancy	Fungi: *Pneumocystis carinii*, *Cryptococcus neoformans* Cytomegalovirus Mycobacteria: tuberculous and atypical Bacteria including *Legionella pneumophila*, *Nocardia asteroides*

Table 52.2 Non-infectious complications in the immunosuppressed.

Pulmonary oedema
Pulmonary haemorrhage
Pulmonary embolism
Tumour (solid tumour, lymphoma/leukaemia, Kaposi's sarcoma)
Drug-induced pneumonitis
Radiation pneumonitis
Alveolar proteinosis
Leucagglutinin reaction

Organ transplantation

Renal

Bacterial pneumonias, particularly due to Gram-negative organisms including *Legionella* spp., may occur at any stage after transplantation [2,3]. Mycobacterial disease, especially tuberculosis, is a high risk for individuals with a past history of tuberculosis or likely exposure due to their country of origin. The disease often takes a rapid and disseminated pulmonary form.

Cytomegalovirus (CMV) pneumonia usually presents as a diffuse pneumonitis of mild to moderate severity at 4–6 weeks after transplantation. The most severe form occurs in patients with negative serology for CMV who receive a CMV-positive donor kidney [4].

Fungal infections are significant, particularly *P. carinii*; without chemoprophylaxis the attack rate for *Pneumocystis* in most centres is 10–12% annually [3]. The disease occurs typically from the onset of the second to the sixth month after transplantation, when immunosuppression is at its greatest, and presents with a rapidly progressive diffuse pneumonitis that is fatal unless specific treatment is initiated quickly. Other fungal pneumonias can be caused by *A. fumigatus*, *Mucor*, *Fusarium* and *Trichosporon* spp. and, in some parts of the world, by *Coccidioides* and *Histoplasma*.

Non-infectious complications are frequent and include pulmonary oedema (the result of impaired renal salt and water excretion, cardiac dysfunction or fluid overload) and thromboembolism. Recurrence in the lung of the original renal-destroying disease may occur, as in Wegener's granulomatosis or Goodpasture's syndrome.

Liver

The infective risks are similar to those for renal transplantation. Non-infectious complications include postoperative collapse and effusion, particularly at the right base, and also postoperative adult respiratory distress syndrome (ARDS).

Heart/lung

The infective complications are similar to those listed for renal transplantation but there are also risks of disease due to *Nocardia asteroides* and the protozoan *Toxoplasma gondii*, both of which may be transmitted with the donor heart.

Non-infectious complications include collapse of the left lower lobe and paralysis of the left diaphragm, often due to cold injury of the phrenic nerve. Pulmonary oedema, due to heart failure or ARDS (post-pump syndrome), is not rare. A common late complication after lung transplantation is the development of obliterative bronchiolitis as a manifestation of organ rejection.

Bone marrow transplantation

Profound neutropenia makes Gram-negative pneumonia a special risk [5]. CMV pneumonia, occurring at 6–12 weeks, is especially common; it is often progressive in this patient group and carries a high mortality despite initiation of treatment.

Non-infectious complications include early pulmonary oedema due to large-volume donations of intravenous fluid or to the cardiotoxicity of cytotoxic drugs. Common and important is an often fatal interstitial pneumonitis likely to be due to the direct pulmonary toxicity of the preparative irradiation and methotrexate therapy.

AIDS

The current AIDS pandemic has had a major impact on respiratory medicine. The many pulmonary manifestations of HIV infection are discussed later in this chapter.

Hypogammaglobulinaemia

Hypogammaglobulinaemia may be due to a variety of congenital and acquired causes and may be global or confined to subclass deficiency of IgA or IgG. Pulmonary complications can take the form of recurring bronchial infection, the development of bronchiectasis or bacterial pneumonias due to encapsulated *Streptococcus pneumoniae* or *Haemophilus influenzae*. Pneumococcal disease is especially common in the marked hypogammaglobulinaemia that accompanies multiple myeloma.

Clinical features of lung disease

Thorough clinical and radiographic review is essential, and needs to take account of the various potential infectious and non-infectious pulmonary problems and the clues that arise from the history, examination, review of fluid charts, drug schedules and chest radiology. In many instances, the respiratory illness may simply be an episode of acute bronchitis; cough and purulent sputum follow a coryzal illness and there is little constitutional disturbance and no clinical or radiographic signs of pulmonary consolidation. The more important clinical problem is the patient with breathlessness or radiographic consolidation accompanied by fever, for whom the differential diagnosis is broad and includes non-infectious disease. Fever itself, particularly when it is high and associated with chills, suggests infection though some non-infectious conditions such as drug reactions may also cause this.

The patient's background provides useful pointers in the differential diagnosis. Gram-negative sepsis and fungal disease are particular risks in the profound neutropenia seen in the early vigorous treatment of leukaemias and lymphomas, while PCP is a possibility at a later stage; CMV complicates organ transplantation usually at about 2 months and may be severe and fatal in bone marrow transplantation, whereas it is relatively milder after renal transplantation. Geographical factors may be relevant: infection with fungal disease such as coccidioidomycosis or histoplasmosis occurs in the Americas, while disseminated strongyloidiasis is seen in patients particularly from the West Indies and Far East. Tuberculosis may be reactivated in patients from developing countries but especially the Indian subcontinent and South-East Asia. The disease may disseminate and progress more rapidly in the immunosuppressed.

Physical examination needs to be comprehensive and should include a search for tumour or bleeding at extra-pulmonary sites. Skin disease may be present in graft-versus-host disease and cutaneous lesions may provide diagnostic clues of systemic vasculitis. Signs of intracerebral infection are a principal feature of cryptococcal disease and may complicate aspergillar and nocardial infections. Arthropathy and biochemical evidence of hepatitis occur frequently in CMV disease. Haemoptysis may be part of an infective syndrome but raises the possibility of pulmonary embolism or haemorrhage. Pleurisy with pleural pain and pleural rub is neither a feature of infection with *Pneumocystis* nor of cardiogenic pulmonary oedema or alveolar haemorrhage. In PCP, fever and breathlessness may precede definite radiographic changes; absence of auscultatory physical signs in the chest is characteristic.

Radiology and lung sampling

The plain chest radiograph usually provides definitive evidence of the presence, extent, distribution and character of pulmonary consolidation, and the presence or absence of other features including those of cardiac failure (cardiomegaly, pulmonary venous congestion and Kerley B lines) or pleural disease. The lateral chest radiograph is valuable in localizing lesions for further investigation by bronchoscopy. Focal radiographic abnormalities are more likely to be infective than non-infective and are also more likely to be due to bacterial than opportunistic organisms. A retrospective review of the aetiology of episodes of pulmonary infiltration in 139 patients with leukaemia showed that in those with focal radiographic abnormalities, 74% of infiltrates were infective and, of these, 87% were bacterial and only 13% opportunistic [6]. On the other hand, 65% of diffuse infiltrates were non-infective but of the remaining 45% that were infective, the great majority (93%) were opportunistic.

CT may provide more detailed information, including anatomical information for targeting of sampling procedures. However, there are few microbe-specific radiographic changes, for instance the radiographic features of *Pneumocystis*, mycobacterial and CMV infection can be very similar. However, confluent segmental or lobar consolidation accompanying an acute clinical illness (<48 h) strongly suggests bacterial pneumonia.

Sputum, if expectorated, provides a valuable sample for preliminary microbiological assessment by Gram staining and culture. Sputum may be induced by the inhalation of nebulized hypertonic (2.7%) saline [7]; such samples have proved useful in the diagnosis of PCP (see below) in AIDS subjects, although precautions are needed to protect other patients from the dissemination of microorganisms in this process.

Blood cultures should be taken in all patients in whom sepsis is a possibility and may give a positive yield in up to one-third of such cases [8], although it is probable that appropriate antimicrobial therapy has been initiated on empirical grounds in advance of the result.

Open lung biopsy (see Chapter 8) provides the best sample of pulmonary tissue but may precipitate the need for assisted ventilation or be complicated by pneumothorax or wound sepsis. Percutaneous lung biopsy or fine-needle aspiration (see Chapter 8) carries risks of bleeding or pneumothorax (proportional to the calibre of the needle) but is very useful in sampling peripheral nodules. Fibreoptic bronchoscopy (see Chapter 8), with bronchoalveolar lavage (BAL) and with or without transbronchial biopsy, is now widely used for investigating pneumonitis in the immunosuppressed and can produce diagnostic rates of 50–80% [9–12]. BAL provides a good specimen for microbiological assessment using staining, monoclonal antibodies and DNA probes, and culture; cytological examination of the fluid may diagnose pulmonary haemorrhage and malignant infiltrates. BAL rarely produces bleeding or pneumothorax. It does not provide definitive information on drug-induced lung disease or other non-infective alveolitis, which need biopsy of tissue for histology.

In all these samplings, the application of molecular techniques such as DNA amplification is improving the rapidity and sensitivity of screening for organisms such as *P. carinii* and *Mycobacterium tuberculosis* [13,14].

Practical approach to diagnosis

Episodes of bronchitis are typified by prominent cough producing purulent sputum but no clinical or radiographic evidence of consolidation. After sputum has been obtained for study, these episodes should be treated with an antibiotic effective against the likely pathogens, *H. influenzae* and *Strep. pneumoniae*. There are β-lactamase-producing strains of *H. influenzae* (20% of isolates in the UK currently), although treatment with oral co-amoxiclav or doxycycline is usually effective.

A pneumonia of abrupt onset and progress, with accompanying segmental or lobar radiographic shadowing, strongly suggests bacterial infection. Antibiotic treatment should be started promptly after swift and simple microbiological investigation based on blood, urine, natural or induced sputum and, if available, pleural fluid samplings. A regimen that provides broad antibacterial activity, i.e. covering *Strep. pneumoniae*, *H. influenzae*, *Staphylococcus aureus* and many Gram-negative organisms, should be given intravenously. One suitable combination is an antipseudomonal penicillin with a β-lactamase inhibitor and gentamicin. The possibility of infection by *Legionella* spp. (see Chapter 13) should be considered and may be covered with a macrolide [15].

When the pace of the illness is less acute or when the chest radiograph shows more diffuse or scattered change, the differential diagnosis enlarges. First, sputum or induced sputum should be examined by microscopy using both Gram stain and appropriate techniques for *P. carinii* (see below) and mycobacteria; the sample should also be cultured. If this does not provide a prompt diagnosis, a decision needs to be made about further diagnostic techniques. Percutaneous fine-needle aspiration for cytology and microbiology is most applicable in the case of peripherally placed nodules. For infiltrative or pneumonic radiographic changes when infection is primarily suspected, fibreoptic bronchoscopy with BAL is appropriate. If there is suspicion of autoimmune or drug-induced alveolitis, transbronchial lung biopsies can also be taken at bronchoscopy (see Chapter 8). The procedure can be completed in 15 min and be performed in hypoxaemic patients using local anaesthesia with concurrent oxygen supplementation. Chest radiographs allow localization of the pneumonia and the accurate direction of the flexible bronchoscope to a bronchus subtending the site. In diffuse disease, the middle lobe may be chosen and the bronchoscope is impacted firmly there. Three or four 50-mL aliquots of sterile saline are instilled singly and 30–60% of the fluid recovered by suction into a trap. Some of this sample is centrifuged and slides made from the deposit for diagnostic microscopy. The remainder is used for culture. Semi-quantitative techniques improve accuracy in diagnosing bacterial disease. The use of monoclonal antibodies facilitates the counting of CMV-'positive' alveolar macrophages. Immunofluorescent staining with conjugated *P. carinii* monoclonal antibodies also demonstrates brightly stained cysts and is a very useful microbiological search technique. Grocott–Gomori methenamine silver staining of BAL fluid for *P. carinii* has been shown on correlative postmortem studies to have sensitivity and specificity approaching 100%. Mycobacteria are more efficiently screened using fluorescent microscopy with auramine stains rather than by the Ziehl–Nielsen method. Giemsa stains are used to assess haemorrhage or malignant infiltration. *Legionella* may be identified in secretions by direct immunofluorescent antibody testing. Many of these foregoing results should be available within 4 h and simple cultures within 36 h.

If the procedure provides no diagnosis in a patient who is in a declining state, then open lung biopsy offers definitive sampling. Open lung biopsy is the only technique that gives totally reliable information on alveolitis of non-infective origin. Pulmonary capillary wedge pressure measurements, pulmonary angiography and ventilation–perfusion lung scanning may be required to establish the diagnosis of pulmonary oedema or embolism. A diagnostic algorithm is presented in Fig. 52.1.

Treatment

With the exception of acute-onset lobar pneumonia, antimicrobial therapy is best started when a specific diag-

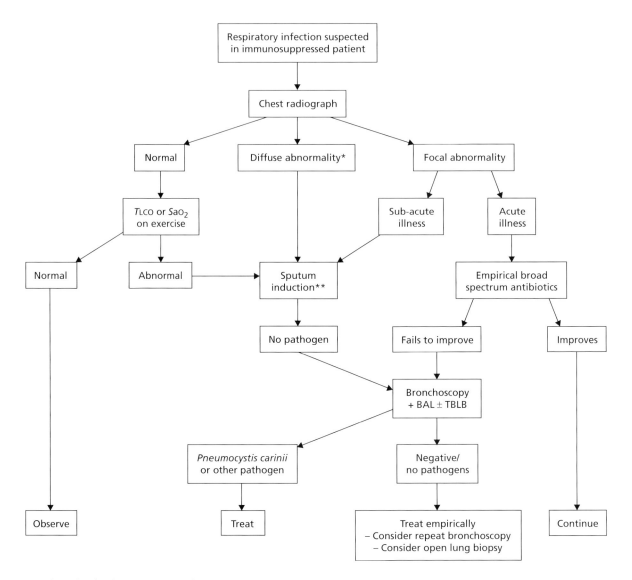

Fig. 52.1 Algorithm for the management of an immunosuppressed patient in whom respiratory infection is suspected. *, If suspicion of *Pneumocystis* pneumonia is high, start treatment at this point. **, If mycobacterial or *Pneumocystis* pneumonia is suspected and patient is unable to expectorate. BAL, bronchoalveolar lavage; TBLB, transbronchial lung biopsies.

nosis has been made. In PCP, the first-line treatment is still high-dose co-trimoxazole or pentamidine [16] as described later in this chapter. In the AIDS population, the rate of side-effects of these agents is high and reactions that include fever, rash and renal impairment often demand change of therapy to the alternative agent or to other agents, including trimetrexate-folinate or dapsone-trimethoprim, in order to allow the necessary 3 weeks of treatment to be completed. There is little evidence that changing regimens because of failure of the pneumonia to respond is useful, although there are data supporting the

coadministration of corticosteroids particularly in AIDS (see below).

Despite the severity of the disease, recovery is frequently seen in aspergillar pneumonia treated vigorously with amphotericin [17,18]; the side-effects of this agent may be limited by formulation of the drug with liposomes or lipid emulsion (see Chapter 9).

The standard chemotherapeutic regimens should be used for tuberculosis, though increasing rates of drug resistance to agents that include isoniazid and rifampicin are being documented in cities in the USA [19].

CMV pneumonia is most effectively treated with the guanine analogue ganciclovir (see Chapter 9); the addition of intravenous immunoglobulin should be considered in severe disease [20,21].

Often the severe hypoxaemia accompanying many of these pneumonias may demand a period of mechanical ventilation, high concentrations of inspired oxygen and the use of positive end-expiratory pressure. Previously, the outlook for AIDS patients with disease of such severity was grim so in appropriate circumstances humane terminal care was often more appropriate for this group [22]. In recent years, with the advent of highly active antiretroviral therapy, patients can attain sustained good health even after such a life-threatening illness.

In transplant patients and oncology patients still receiving immunosuppressive chemotherapy, there may be need to taper the dosage of such agents to allow recovery from pneumonia. Neutropenic patients (including those with HIV infection) benefit from adjuvant treatment with granulocyte colony-stimulating factor.

Prevention

Prevention of PCP depends upon chemoprophylaxis with either thrice-weekly oral co-trimoxazole or monthly inhaled pentamidine [16,23]. Such prophylaxis is a routine part of leukaemia chemotherapy in childhood, organ transplantation schedules and the management of AIDS patients, provided the agent can be tolerated (see below).

Chemoprophylaxis is also important in the prevention of tuberculosis. Daily oral isoniazid over 1 year can be used at the initiation of immunosuppressive chemotherapy, for example in the transplant group, if there is a past history of tuberculosis or if the patient is from a geographical location where the disease is prevalent. CMV disease is most severe in transplant patients who are seronegative and who receive seropositive blood products or transplant. Avoidance of a positive organ is advised if possible, although many centres now administer live attenuated CMV vaccine to CMV-seronegative potential transplant recipients since it offers protection against disease of moderate to high severity [24].

The risk of any opportunistic pneumonia is increased by the number and dosage of immunosuppressant agents. Clinicians and investigators should try to define the lowest dosages of such agents that achieve the goals of suppressing inflammatory vasculitis, maintaining an organ transplant or eradicating treatable tumour.

HIV and AIDS

AIDS was first recognized in 1981 following clusters of PCP in young gay and drug-using men in California and New York [25,26]. Since that time pulmonary infections have accounted for much of the morbidity and mortality related to this infection. About 70% of patients with HIV infection experience a pulmonary complication during life [27], and additional pulmonary pathology (particularly pneumonia, tuberculosis and pulmonary embolism) is an often unexpected finding at autopsy [28]. Worldwide, it is estimated that 30.6 million patients are living with HIV and 90% of these are in developing countries [29]. The burden of HIV-related pulmonary disease in developing countries is therefore immense.

The nature of the pulmonary complications of HIV reflect level of immunodeficiency, socioeconomic status, lifestyle, country of residence and access to prophylactic and HIV disease-modifying therapies. For the fortunate few in developed countries, HIV disease-modifying drugs dramatically alter the natural history and hence pulmonary complications of the disease (see below). The great cost of antiretroviral therapy (estimated at $US12 000 per person per annum) makes therapy unfeasible for those dependent on state healthcare in developing countries.

The three most important and common pulmonary complications of HIV are tuberculosis, PCP and bacterial pneumonia, these comprise greater than 90% of pulmonary complications worldwide. The incidence of PCP in developed countries has markedly declined since the introduction of effective prophylaxis with co-trimoxazole and HIV disease-modifying therapy. In developing countries, bacterial infections (including *M. tuberculosis and Strep. pneumoniae*) are of much greater importance, perhaps because these virulent infections occur at an earlier stage in the disease before the profound immunosuppression required for PCP.

Although most of the pulmonary complications of HIV infection are not unique to the disease, the variability and non-specificity of clinical and radiological findings in these patients frequently complicate their diagnosis.

HIV and lung defences

HIV-infected patients with respiratory symptoms frequently have detectable HIV in BAL fluid, even in the absence of opportunistic infections or tumours [30]. The lung may become diseased via pro-monocytes infected in the bone marrow that subsequently migrate and then mature into alveolar macrophages. Alternatively, free virus may be transported to the lungs via the pulmonary circulation [31]. The nature of the deficiencies in pulmonary host defences to infection in patients infected with HIV is complex and largely extrapolated from studies of circulating immune cells. HIV infection is characterized by an acquired depletion of circulating CD4+ lymphocytes whose primary role is in the regulation of cell-mediated immunity. CD4+ lymphocytes recognize antigens presented by accessory cells, regulate the expansion and differentiation of antibodies (B lymphocytes) and regulate the development of macrophages and other cytotoxic cells. HIV is directly cytopathic to CD4+ lymphocytes but also leads to qualitative defects in surviving cells, including functional defects in response to soluble mitogens, reduced recall proliferation to previously encountered antigens, defective interleukin 2 production and reduced production of interferon γ in response to antigen. Such defects in cell-mediated immunity lead to increased susceptibility to viral, fungal and protozoal infections.

Antibody production is also critically dependent on activation of B lymphocytes by CD4+ lymphocytes, so humoral defects in immunity such as recurrent serious bacterial infections are common. Natural killer cells, which are important in host defence against infection and tumour surveillance, may be non-functional in HIV infection as they require signals from CD4+ lymphocytes for optimal function. BAL fluid in patients with AIDS generally shows increased numbers of lymphocytes in comparison with HIV-negative patients; however, the numbers of CD4+ cells are markedly reduced and CD8+ lymphocytes (which are cytotoxic to HIV-infected cells) are increased. Non-specific interstitial pneumonitis (found in about half of asymptomatic HIV-infected adults) and lymphocytic interstitial pneumonitis (found in about half of HIV-infected children with pulmonary disease) are characterized by pulmonary infiltration with CD8+ lymphocytes (see later). The conditions differ histologically but it is thought that they both occur as a result of an immunological response of CD8+ cells to HIV-infected cells in the lungs.

In addition to the changes described in T-cell lymphocytes, there are also disturbances in the numbers and function of a wide variety of other cell types. In particular, alveolar macrophages (which express the CD4 receptor and are directly infected by HIV) show decreased chemotaxis, which may account for the reduced granulomatous reaction seen in mycobacterial disease. Defects in phagocytosis, intracellular killing and antigen presentation have also been described.

Differential diagnosis in HIV-infected patients with pulmonary disease

The pulmonary complications of HIV infection can be broadly classified as infectious or non-infectious (Table 52.3). For the physician presented with an HIV-infected patient with respiratory symptoms, the clinical history can give important clues as to the nature of the pulmonary disease (Table 52.4). Respiratory symptoms and signs may be less rewarding in determining the aetiology of pulmonary involvement, although general physical examination is more helpful. Radiological signs are highly variable and may mask dual pathology (Table 52.5).

Formal staging of HIV infection is of some help in guiding a differential diagnosis and is also an important epidemiological tool. The Centers for Disease Control and Prevention in the USA published a revised classification system for HIV infection in 1993 (Table 52.6), which takes into account the CD4+ lymphocyte count as well as the occurrence of opportunistic infections; this system is now widely adopted and more usefully reflects disease progression than previous definitions [32]. In developing countries, where radiological and laboratory facilities may be limited, these definitions can be adapted [33].

Table 52.3 Infectious and non-infectious respiratory tract complications of patients with HIV infection.

Infectious
Upper respiratory tract infections
Acute bronchitis
Acute sinusitis (viral, bacterial, fungal)
Bacterial pneumonia
   Streptococcus pneumoniae
   Haemophilus influenzae
   Staphylococcus aureus
   Moraxella catarrhalis
   Rhodococcus equi
Fungal pneumonia
   Pneumocystis carinii
   Cryptococcus neoformans
   Histoplasma capsulatum
   Aspergillus fumigatus
   Coccidioides immitis
Mycobacterium tuberculosis
Mycobacterium avium-intracellulare
Other mycobacteria
Protozoal infections
   Strongyloides stercoralis
   Toxoplasma gondii
   Cryptosporidium parvum
Viral pneumonitis
   Cytomegalovirus
   Herpes simplex
   Varicella zoster

Non-infectious complications*
Malignancies
   Kaposi's sarcoma
   Non-Hodgkin's lymphoma
   Hodgkin's lymphoma
   Adenocarcinoma lung

Others
   Lymphocytic interstitial pneumonitis
   Non-specific interstitial pneumonitis
   Bronchiolitis obliterans organizing pneumonia
   Primary pulmonary hypertension
   Pulmonary embolism

* Some 'non-infectious' complications are associated with infectious agents (see text).

Patients with primary HIV infection

An acute seroconversion illness occurs in upwards of half of those infected with HIV within the first few weeks of exposure (sexual or parenteral). This is manifested by a mononucleosis-type syndrome, with fever, rash, myalgia, lymphadenopathy and sore throat. It may be associated with high circulating levels of virus and can lead to a precipitous but short-lived depression of cell-mediated immunity, manifested by a low CD4+ lymphocyte count. At this time a minority of patients may develop PCP or bacterial pneumonia as well as a variety of neurological conditions and oesophageal candidiasis.

Table 52.4 Clinical evaluation of a patient with HIV infection and respiratory disease.

Risk factor	Pulmonary disease
Nationality and travel history	Tuberculosis, endemic mycoses
Use of prophylaxis for PCP, MAI	Reduce risk of PCP, MAI and other bacteria
Past and present antiretroviral use and compliance	Reduces risk of opportunistic infections and Kaposi's sarcoma
Intravenous drug misuse	Bacterial infection, *Rhodococcus*, tuberculosis, pulmonary embolic and granulomatous disease
Sexuality	Kaposi's sarcoma, cytomegalovirus in gay men
Smoking history	Bacterial infection, *Legionella*
Social deprivation	Tuberculosis
Prior respiratory disease	Consider in differential diagnosis
Occupation	Exposure to airborne particles/agents Farms (*Rhodococcus*)
Pets	Cats (toxoplasmosis) Pigeons (cryptococcosis)
Undercooked meat	Toxoplasmosis
CD4+ T-lymphocyte count* $<0.5 \times 10^9/L$ $<0.2 \times 10^9/L$ $<0.1 \times 10^9/L$	 Tuberculosis in selected groups (above), bacterial infection PCP Kaposi's sarcoma, MAI, cytomegalovirus, non-Hodgkin's lymphoma
HIV RNA viral load > 30 000/mL	Increased risk of progression to opportunistic infections
Low neutrophil count	Aspergillosis, candidosis, Gram-negatives

* These CD4+ counts are offered as a guide only. Opportunistic infections may occur outwith these ranges.
PCP, *Pneumocystis carinii* pneumonia; MAI, *Mycobacterium avium-intracellulare*.

Table 52.5 Chest radiograph findings in patients with HIV infection.

Chest radiograph	Diagnosis
Normal	No pulmonary disease Bronchitis *Pneumocystis carinii* pneumonia
Focal infiltrate(s) (may cavitate)	Bacterial pneumonia Tuberculosis and other mycobacteria *Pneumocystis carinii* pneumonia Cryptococcosis and other mycoses Adenocarcinoma Kaposi's sarcoma
Pleural effusion	Bacterial pneumonia Tuberculosis and other mycobacteria Kaposi's sarcoma Adenocarcinoma
Mediastinal adenopathy	Tuberculosis and other mycobacteria Non-Hodgkin's lymphoma Kaposi's sarcoma
Interstitial infiltrate (may have focal nodularity)	*Pneumocystis carinii* pneumonia Bacterial pneumonia Tuberculosis and other mycobacteria Lymphocytic interstitial pneumonitis Non-specific pneumonitis Cytomegalovirus pneumonitis

Progressive immunosuppression

The spectrum of respiratory disease changes as immunodeficiency develops. In the patient with a normal CD4+ lymphocyte count and undetectable or low HIV RNA in blood (<10 000 copies/mL), the risks of opportunistic infection are low. Lower respiratory tract infections are no more common than in the normal population at this early stage, although there is increased reporting of upper respiratory tract infections. This may simply reflect increased surveillance in the HIV-infected population. Intravenous drug misusers who are infected with HIV run the risk of endocarditis, septic pulmonary emboli and talc (magnesium trisilicate) embolism with subsequent granulomatous reactions [34].

As one might expect, more virulent organisms cause problems earlier in the natural history of HIV infection. Bacterial pathogens such as *Strep. pneumoniae* and *H. influenzae* are important at CD4+ counts of less than $0.5 \times 10^9/L$ in both developing [35] and developed [36] worlds. In areas of endemicity, tuberculosis also occurs at relatively preserved CD4+ counts and tends to dominate the burden of HIV-related ill-health [37,38]. Such high-virulence infections, when occurring early in the course of HIV infection, present in a similar fashion to disease

Table 52.6 Revised classification system for HIV infection and expanded AIDS surveillance case definition for adolescents and adults, 1993.

	Clinical categories		
CD4+ T-cell count	A: asymptomatic, acute (primary) HIV or PGL	B: symptomatic, not A or C conditions	C: AIDS-indicator conditions*
1 $\geq 0.5 \times 10^9/\text{L}$	A1	B1	C1
2 $0.2–0.499 \times 10^9/\text{L}$	A2	B2	C2
3 $< 0.2 \times 10^9/\text{L}$ AIDS-indicator T-cell count	A3	B3	C3

* AIDS-defining conditions are shown in Table 52.7.
PGL, persistent generalized lymphadenopathy.
Categories A3, B3 and C1–C3 are included in the AIDS case definition.

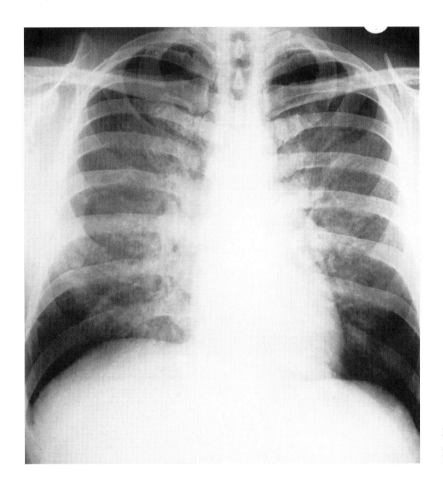

Fig. 52.2 Miliary tuberculosis in young African woman with AIDS. (Courtesy of Dr Dwight McLeod.)

in immunocompetent HIV-negative patients. Tuberculosis presenting in advanced immunosuppression can be more cryptic and is more frequently extrapulmonary than in HIV-negative patients (Figs 52.2–52.4). Although PCP does occur in developing countries it is infrequently isolated (when facilities for its detection are available), presumably because it is a true opportunist and does not occur at the level of immunosuppression that predisposes patients to bacterial and tuberculous infections [39].

Opportunistic infections that occur later in HIV infection depend on the endemic infections of the patient's country of past and present residence, for example cryptococcosis is rare in cold climates, tuberculosis is common in developing countries and deprived social groups, histoplasmosis is common in the Americas and toxoplasmosis is more common in Africa. Pulmonary complications may also be suggested by other systemic features of the disease (Table 52.7). Examples include characteristic skin and mucosal lesions in Kaposi's sarcoma, meningoencephalitis in cryptococcosis, cerebral mass lesions in toxoplasmosis, oral/pharyngeal thrush in patients with pulmonary candidiasis, and retinitis with CMV pneumonitis. In such

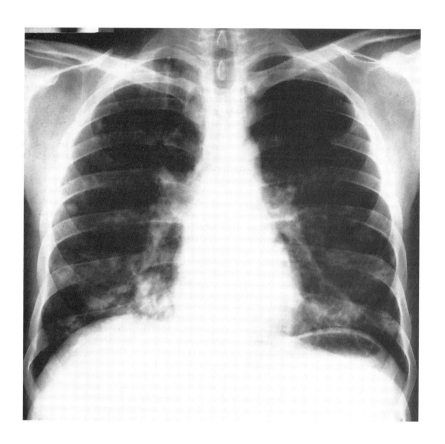

Fig. 52.8 Chest film of AIDS patient showing multiple nodules of Kaposi's sarcoma. (Courtesy of Dr Diana Buchanan.)

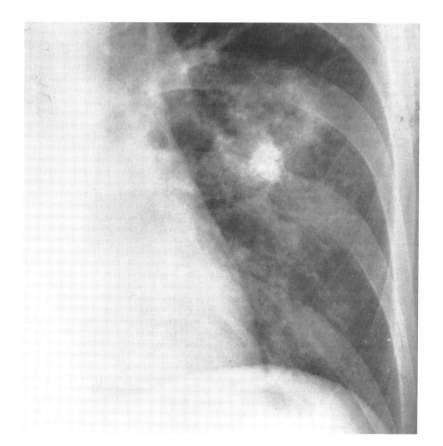

Fig. 52.9 Cavitating consolidation in left mid zone of AIDS patient with intrapulmonary Kaposi's sarcoma. (Courtesy of Dr Diana Buchanan.)

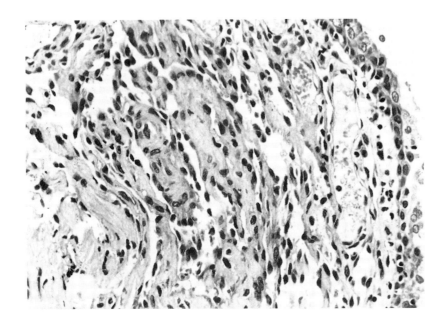

Fig. 52.10 Kaposi's sarcoma of bronchus showing epithelium to right with underlying slit-like vascular spaces lined by prominent endothelial cells (haematoxylin & eosin×250). (Courtesy of Dr Nick Francis.)

night sweats, fever and weight loss, usually when CD4+ counts are less than 0.1×10^9/L. Disease is often extranodal and although patients may have an enlarging mass on a chest radiograph, many other radiographic signs may be present. Transbronchial biopsies are often not successful in obtaining diagnostic tissue, which usually requires more invasive measures. Prognosis following a diagnosis of non-Hodgkin's lymphoma is extremely poor.

Interstitial pneumonitis

This is a group of histologically well-defined pulmonary complications whose aetiology and clinical significance is currently uncertain [45–47]. Lymphocytic interstitial pneumonitis occurs frequently in children infected with HIV but is only occasionally seen in adults (usually Afro-Caribbeans). It is also associated with other autoimmune disorders such as Sjögren's syndrome and chronic active hepatitis. Lymphocytic interstitial pneumonitis is thought to occur as a result of an immunological reaction to HIV or Epstein–Barr virus within the lung and is classified as a lymphoproliferative disorder by some. Symptoms and signs are non-specific in HIV infection but patients usually develop progressive dyspnoea. Symptoms may resolve spontaneously or progress to respiratory failure. Diagnosis depends on histology and exclusion of opportunistic infections. Lung biopsy reveals firm grey nodules characterized by a lymphocytic infiltrate. Although granulomas are not present, the infiltrate can take on a follicular appearance with germinal centres. Antiretroviral therapy may help and corticosteroids have been used in patients without HIV infection.

Non-specific interstitial pneumonitis is well described in adults with HIV infection and is characterized by an interstitial inflammatory infiltrate with a predominance of lymphocytes and plasma cells. In contrast to lymphocytic interstitial pneumonitis, a follicular pattern with germinal centres is not seen. The aetiology is not known but it may occur as a result of previous opportunistic infections or, like lymphocytic interstitial pneumonitis, as an immune response to HIV in the lung. There are no specific clinical features that distinguish non-specific interstitial pneumonitis from other more common pulmonary disorders, although symptoms are usually mild and the condition may resolve or stabilize spontaneously.

Bronchiolitis obliterans organizing pneumonia has been described in patients infected with HIV. Its mode of presentation is similar to the condition in HIV-negative patients and there is no evidence to suggest that it occurs more frequently in the HIV-infected population [48].

Pulmonary hypertension

Pulmonary hypertension is estimated to occur in 1 in 200 patients with HIV infection. It does not correlate with the stage of HIV infection or with the occurrence of opportunistic infections. Compared to patients with primary pulmonary hypertension, patients with HIV-related pulmonary hypertension are younger, less dyspnoeic and have lower peak pulmonary artery pressures. The pathological findings are usually of plexogenic pulmonary arteriopathy, although less frequently the thrombotic–fibrotic variant occurs. It is believed that HIV infection is the cause, perhaps through release of epidermal growth factors, induction of nitric oxide synthase and subsequent increased vessel tone and endothelial proliferation [49]. Secondary causes of pulmonary hypertension in patients with HIV include obstructive talc granulomas within small pulmonary arteries in intravenous drug users and pulmonary hypertension associated with chronic liver disease and portal hypertension (e.g. induced by hepatitis C virus). In addition, pulmonary thromboembolic disease is often an unexpected finding in autopsies in patients with HIV infection.

Primary lung tumours

Primary lung tumours are weakly associated with HIV infection. A recent large-scale survey of 98 336 patients with HIV infection and a large cancer register in the USA estimated a relative risk of lung adenocarcinoma of 2.5 (95% confidence interval 1–5.1). Other tumours, such as Kaposi's sarcoma, non-Hodgkin's lymphoma, Hodgkin's lymphoma, multiple myeloma, brain tumours and seminomas, were unequivocally associated with HIV infection [50].

Prevention of HIV-related pulmonary disease

The 1990s has seen an explosion in the development of new antiretroviral agents that have revolutionized the management of HIV infection. Initial pessimism following the poor success of monotherapy with the nucleoside analogue zidovudine [51] has been replaced with optimism as dual and triple drug regimens have shown at least short-term promise [52]. Highly active antiretroviral therapy is a combination of an HIV-protease inhibitor and two nucleoside reverse transcriptase inhibitors and is the standard care for many patients in developed countries. The nucleoside reverse transcriptase inhibitors (zidovudine, lamivudine, didanosine, zalcitabine, stavudine) are phosphorylated by thymidine kinase and then bind preferentially to retroviral reverse transcriptase. Proviral DNA formation is blocked because the drug is incorporated into the viral DNA with resultant 'misreading' and chain termination. The protease inhibitors inhibit post-translational processing of the polyprotein products of *gag* and *gag-pol* genes into the functional core proteins and viral enzymes, leading to release of immature non-infectious virus [53].

Outside clinical trials in countries where such therapy is freely available, AIDS-related mortality has dramatically declined [54]. In addition, the rate of progression to an AIDS diagnosis (particularly PCP) has been reduced [55]. Guidelines in HIV therapy are evolving as trial data emerge and experience with newer agents such as the non-nucleoside reverse transcriptase inhibitors improves [56].

Long-term compliance with complex drug regimens with large side-effect profiles may be difficult for many patients. The protease inhibitors are associated with a growing number of metabolic disturbances, including renal stones, diabetes mellitus, body fat redistribution and abnormalities in lipid metabolism [57]. In addition, cryptic mycobacterial and CMV infection may flare up during ini-

tiation of highly active antiretroviral therapy, presumably due to immune reconstitution. There is good evidence that viral resistance, leading to renewed risk of opportunistic infections, rapidly emerges with suboptimal therapy (potentially through non-compliance) and this has tempered enthusiasm for the long-term efficacy of current antiretroviral combinations. Guidelines for prophylaxis of opportunistic infections are still based on lowest measured CD4+ count, symptoms and prior opportunistic infections [58]. However, recent evidence suggests that primary prophylaxis against PCP may be discontinued when there is virological and immunological response to HIV therapy. HIV RNA viral load tests are useful in guiding the initiation and monitoring of therapy, but their usefulness in guiding prophylaxis has not yet been fully evaluated.

Prophylaxis against PCP with co-trimoxazole (described later) is also effective prophylactic therapy for toxoplasmosis and gives some protection against bacterial pathogens. Primary prophylaxis against *M. avium-intracellulare* infection is usually initiated when the CD4+ count is less than 0.1×10^9/L. Clarithromycin or azithromycin (in combination with rifabutin) not only protects against *M. avium-intracellulare* but also reduces the incidence of, and hospital admissions due to, other bacterial infections [59,60]. Currently, prophylaxis against community-acquired respiratory tract infection is not recommended except in unusual circumstances such as recurrent serious bacterial infections. However, pneumococcal vaccine is recommended, preferably when the CD4+ count is greater than 0.2×10^9/L [58], and probably should be repeated at 5-yearly intervals. In the USA it is also recommended that patients are immunized against influenza annually [58], although there is little evidence to justify this.

Prophylaxis against tuberculosis with isoniazid (300 mg daily) in African HIV-infected patients has been shown to be efficacious in purified protein derivative (PPD)-positive patients [61] and probably is also indicated in high-risk PPD-negative patients as this may reflect anergy due to immunosuppression. In the USA, where bacille Calmette–Guérin (BCG) is not available, a positive PPD skin reaction or contact with a case of active tuberculosis is an indication for prophylaxis, assuming there is no evidence of active disease [58]. Primary prophylaxis against endemic mycoses depends on place of residence and relative risk. There is evidence in appropriate settings for the efficacy of fluconazole against cryptococcosis [62]. The risks of primary prophylaxis include the emergence of drug-resistant organisms (particularly *Candida* spp.).

Pneumocystis carinii pneumonia

On the basis of various microbiological characteristics, *P. carinii* is classed as a eukaryote as are protozoa, algae and fungi. It used to be regarded as a protozoon on the basis of its morphology, and this supposition was supported by the responsiveness of the pneumonia that it causes to antiprotozoal antibiotics. However, ultrastructural findings, DNA sequencing and other molecular data have now led taxonomists to classify it as an atypical fungus [63,64]. Such considerations have been of no practical consequence to clinicians who are well aware that, unlike fungi, *P. carinii* cannot be cultured on cell-free media nor is it susceptible to treatment with any antifungal agents that target the usual fungal pathway of sterol synthesis (see Chapter 9).

P. carinii exists extracellularly in the form of tiny unicellular trophozoites. These form cysts, each cyst containing up to eight sporozoites or 'intracystic bodies'. Once mature, the cyst ruptures and the released sporozoites complete the life cycle as new trophozoites.

P. carinii is not a recent discovery. The organism was first described over 80 years ago in guinea-pig and rat lung and was mistakenly thought to be trypanosomal by Carini, after whom it was later named [65]. Infection of the lungs of mammals by strains of *P. carinii* appears to be species specific, with no good evidence of transmission from animal to humans and no known animal reservoirs. It is of low pathogenicity and was first associated with pneumonia in malnourished and debilitated institutionalized children on the European mainland during the Second World War, subsequently being identified as a cause of pneumonia in premature infants in the 1950s [65,66]. By the 1970s *P. carinii* had become a fairly well-recognized but somewhat infrequently diagnosed opportunistic cause of pneumonia in immunocompromised patients, particularly those receiving chemotherapy for leukaemia and other forms of cancer [67]. Reports of outbreaks of PCP in 1981 in previously healthy homosexual men and intravenous drug abusers led to the recognition and description of AIDS [25,26]. The incidence of PCP increased dramatically in the early 1980s in parallel with the AIDS pandemic.

Epidemiology

Although *P. carinii* only causes disease in susceptible individuals who are significantly immunocompromised, harmless infection by this organism appears to be common and antibodies to *P. carinii* have been found to develop in the majority of non-immunosuppressed persons before the age of 13 years [68,69]. This has led to the suggestion that PCP is caused by a reactivation of latent infection that occurs once the patient's resistance has become sufficiently impaired. Opposing this hypothesis have been the negative findings of absent *P. carinii* DNA when lung tissue from immunocompetent patients has been examined using sensitive DNA amplification polymerase chain reaction (PCR) techniques [70]. Although no environmental reservoir of human pathogenic *P. carinii* has been identified, the organism has never-

theless been detected in outdoor air samples [71]. Furthermore, cluster cases have been described in groups of immunodeficient patients, implying that case-to-case transmission may occur [72], and *P. carinii* DNA has also been detected in air filters serving the rooms of units in which patients with PCP have been managed, supporting the hypothesis of airborne transmission [73]. The chance of such transmission is evidently low, so that it is not general practice to isolate patients with PCP. It seems probable that (i) the population in general encounters environmental *P. carinii* [71] and develops immunity against it [68,69], (ii) patients whose cell-mediated immunity becomes sufficiently impaired are susceptible to reinfection and colonization with the subsequent development of PCP [74,75] and (iii) airborne spread of the organism may occur between susceptible individuals who come into close contact with one another [72]. The reported incidence of PCP in sub-Saharan Africa in patients with HIV infection has been much lower than found in Europe and North America, probably as a result of earlier deaths from bacterial infection including tuberculosis, which is much more prevalent in the countries of these regions [76].

Susceptibility

PCP occurs almost exclusively in the immunocompromised host. The chief characteristic of conditions that predispose to PCP is impaired cell-mediated immunity, as may be found in patients with HIV infection, those receiving chemotherapy for haematological and solid malignant lesions, those receiving immunosuppressive drugs following organ transplantation or for other inflammatory conditions, and premature infants and those suffering from protein malnutrition and primary immunodeficiency disorders. Highly unusual cases have been reported in elderly adults without apparent predisposing causes [77], although it is possible to speculate that these patients may have had subtle immune defects that went undetected. Although cell-mediated immunity is the primary defence against *P. carinii*, it is possible that defects of humoral immunity may play a role since PCP has exceptionally occurred in patients in whom only B-cell defects have been detectable [78].

HIV-seropositive patients are at greatest risk of PCP, although this risk has been substantially reduced by chemoprophylaxis. Without chemoprophylaxis, PCP was the AIDS-defining diagnosis in about 47% of HIV-seropositive patients in Europe and North America, this figure having fallen progressively to about 15% following the gradual uptake of chemoprophylaxis [79–82]. Despite this reduced incidence, PCP remains the most common opportunistic lung infection in HIV-infected patients in the western world; in one North American cohort, 28% of patients developed PCP at some point in their illness despite chemoprophylaxis, this intervention delaying the onset of the first AIDS-defining illness by 6–12 months, by which time the CD4+ count was lower [79]. The risk of developing PCP in HIV-infected patients correlates with the number of circulating CD4+ lymphocytes, patients with counts of less than 0.2×10^9/L being at considerably greater risk than those with counts above this level [83,84]. It is also recognized that there may be a transient but quite profound fall in the CD4+ count in patients at the initial or 'primary' stage of their infection, at which time they are in the process of seroconversion, and that this early fall may also result in PCP [85].

Patients receiving chemotherapy for malignant disease are at risk, particularly those with haematological neoplasms that may themselves impair cellular immunity. Acute lymphocytic leukaemia was the prominent disorder reported as predisposing to PCP before 1970 [67], although the disease also arises during the course of chemotherapy for lymphomas as well as other neoplastic diseases. The infection is unlikely to occur until 1 month of chemotherapy has elapsed. Treatment with fludarabine is thought to carry a particular risk of PCP [86].

PCP following organ transplantation is most likely from the onset of the second to the sixth month following the procedure, during which time immunosuppression is usually at its highest, although the infection may occur beyond these boundaries if immunosuppression is also required preoperatively or if it has been intensified at a later stage because of rejection [2]. In most centres, the incidence of PCP in those transplant patients who do not take prophylaxis is reportedly 10–12%, whereas in those who do the risk is largely eliminated [2].

Of the group receiving immunosuppressive therapy for other conditions, patients with Wegener's granulomatosis appear to be at particular risk of PCP, an incidence of 6% having been reported in one large retrospective group who did not receive prophylaxis [87]. All these patients were receiving a corticosteroid as well as another immunosuppressive agent. Further groups at risk include those receiving potent immunosuppressive treatment for other antineutrophil cytoplasmic antibody-positive vasculitis, connective tissue disorders such as systemic lupus erythematosus, polymyositis/dermatomyositis, rheumatoid arthritis and severe skin diseases [88].

A review from a single large North American centre of 116 cases of PCP occurring in patients who were not infected with HIV found that the first episode of PCP was associated with haematological malignancy in 30% of cases, organ transplantation in 25%, inflammatory disorders in 22%, solid tumours in 13% and other miscellaneous conditions in 10%. Over 90% of patients had been treated with systemic steroids, the median daily dose being up to 30 mg, although one-quarter of patients had received about half this dose [89]. The incidence of PCP in such susceptible groups may be reduced by the use of chemoprophylaxis and also by control of the retroviral load in patients with HIV infection.

Pathophysiology

P. carinii is an obligate extracellular pathogen. The trophozoite is believed to become attached to alveolar epithelial cells (principally type I pneumocytes) by mechanisms that include the formation of fibronectin bridges, following which the cell membrane of the invading organism interdigitates with the surface epithelium of the host cell to form a more intimate attachment, a process which may take 2 days. In the immunocompetent host, the invading organisms are phagocytosed by alveolar macrophages, although there are also humoral responses with the production of IgG and IgM antibodies against various *P. carinii* antigens. Experimental studies using immunosuppressed rodents imply that, given favourable circumstances, the organism enters a slow proliferative reproductive phase, so that it may take several weeks before large numbers of organisms have been produced. These developments result in cellular damage to the alveoli, with destruction of type I and subsequent proliferation of type II pneumocytes. Disruption of the epithelial barrier causes increased alveolar–capillary membrane permeability so that the alveolar spaces tend to fill with a foamy, vacuolated, proteinaceous, eosinophilic exudate (Fig. 52.11) containing cellular debris, surfactant and the cysts of *P. carinii*, which are up to 7 μm in diameter.

As with yeasts, the cyst walls of *P. carinii* contain β-1,3-glucan that allows them to take up fungal stains such as Grocott–Gomori methenamine silver nitrate, which marks the cyst walls black and is the most valuable histological *P. carinii* 'search stain' (Fig. 52.12). The alveolar exudate also contains numerous trophozoites. Although these do not take up the foregoing stain and are less easily seen with light microscopy, they may be shown as minute dots in the alveolar spaces with polychromatic stains such as Giemsa or the rapid modified Wright–Giemsa (Diff Quik), as may the intracystic sporozoites. Immunofluorescent staining with conjugated anti-*P. carinii* monoclonal antibodies also demonstrates brightly stained cysts and is a very useful microbiological search technique (see p. 1368).

The foregoing alveolar changes are associated with a patchy inflammatory interstitial infiltrate, which may become more chronic with interstitial and intraluminal fibrosis. Increased phospholipase activity may result in the degradation of surfactant with subsequent microatelectases, which are likely to contribute to physiological shunting, reduced lung compliance and hypoxaemia [70,78]. Atypical histological findings in PCP may occur and include modular forms with granuloma formation, cavitation, local consolidation, hilar lymphadenopathy, interstitial microcalcification and vascular infiltration [64,90]. Small pleural effusions are sometimes found. The

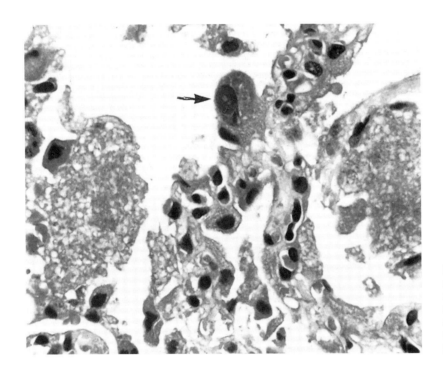

Fig. 52.11 Section of lung from AIDS patient showing alveoli containing granular material of *Pneumocystis* pneumonia and some larger cells (one arrowed) with inclusions typical of cytomegalovirus (haematoxylin & eosin × 460). (Courtesy of Dr Nick Francis.)

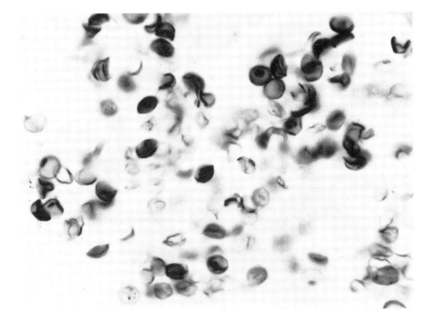

Fig. 52.12 Higher power view of the granular material in Fig. 52.11 showing the cysts (Grocott methenamine silver × 1040). (Courtesy of Dr Nick Francis.)

pneumonic process more usually arises multifocally and is diffuse, although a predominantly upper lobe distribution may be encountered in patients who develop PCP despite prophylaxis with nebulized pentamidine [91–94], an observation explained by the relative alveolar hypoventilation that occurs in the uppermost parts of the lungs in the upright posture in humans [95]. Unusually, *P. carinii* infection may become disseminated in an extrapulmonary fashion to lymph nodes, bone marrow, spleen, liver, etc., so that virtually any organ system may become involved [96].

Clinical features

Most patients have a low-grade fever, a dry cough and dyspnoea that progresses from mild breathlessness on physical exertion to tachypnoea at rest [64,97]. Less than one-third of patients produce sputum without induction (see below) and less than one-quarter experience chest pain [97]. The duration of symptoms from onset to diagnosis is highly variable, as some cases may be fulminant whereas others may be quite insidious. In general, PCP complicating HIV infection is more insidious, with a median time from onset of mild symptoms to diagnosis of 4 weeks, whereas the same condition complicating other disease states tends to be more acute in its onset and development [98]. Patients with initially mild and insidious symptoms may postpone a visit to the physician until later in their illness but nevertheless present in a sick and uncomfortable state. On physical examination the patient may be febrile and tachypnoeic. Added sounds such as scattered crackles or, less commonly, wheezes may be heard but are absent in over half of cases. Patients may present with spontaneous pneumothorax and this occurrence in HIV-positive patients is highly suggestive of underlying PCP with subpleural cyst formation Patients with HIV infection usually have noticed moderate to severe weight loss and oropharyngeal thrush may be present with other stigmata of HIV infection. In patients with typical clinical features of PCP but in whom HIV status is not known, a careful assessment of risk factors for HIV infection should be made. However, a lack of risk factors does not exclude a diagnosis of PCP and therefore the possibility of this treatable condition should not be neglected in 'low-risk patients'.

Investigation and diagnosis

Whether it is desirable to investigate all patients with suspected PCP to a definite microbiological conclusion is somewhat controversial. On the one hand, there is the desire to be sure of the diagnosis before submitting the patient to a potentially toxic antimicrobial regimen, on the other the wish to initiate treatment as speedily as possible while sparing the patient uncomfortable and potentially hazardous tests. Very often some sort of compromise has to be reached depending on the individual circumstances of the case and the facilities available in the institution. Sometimes the diagnosis of PCP seems so probable that treatment may be started without confirmation. Such a situation is illustrated by the patient known to be HIV-positive and who presents with a typical history of exertional dyspnoea, a non-productive cough, arterial hypoxaemia and whose chest radiograph shows diffuse bilateral hazy interstitial infiltrates, with no features to suggest bacterial pneumonia [99]. There is evidence that such an empirical approach is not associated with any worse outcome [100], although it should be realized that the diagnostic yield from BAL, should this subsequently become necessary, may decline within a few days of treatment [101].

Diagnostic imaging

Patients with early PCP may sometimes develop mild symptoms before the appearance of any definite chest radiographic abnormality. This is more frequently found in HIV-positive than HIV-negative patients so that a normal chest film does not rule out the diagnosis of PCP [93]. The most typical early abnormality in PCP is that of bilateral, hazy, ground-glass, perihilar infiltrates with sparing of the lung peripheries (Figs 52.13 & 52.14). As the disease progresses, more homogeneous consolidation with air bronchograms may develop. These typical appearances may occur in up to 80% of all cases [93]. Ultimately the lungs may become massively consolidated and seemingly airless (Figs 52.15 & 52.16). The radiographic

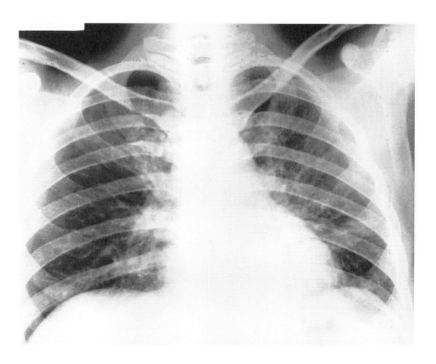

Fig. 52.13 Early *Pneumocystis* pneumonia showing perihilar infiltrates and loss of vascular definition. (Courtesy of Dr Diana Buchanan.)

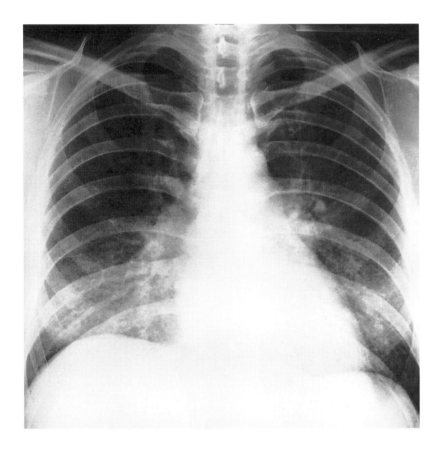

Fig. 52.14 Bilateral reticulonodular infiltrates in *Pneumocystis* pneumonia. (Courtesy of Dr Diana Buchanan.)

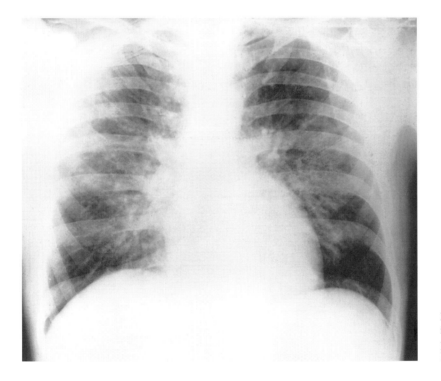

Fig. 52.15 More extensive bilateral infiltrates in *Pneumocystis* pneumonia with apparent peripheral sparing. (Courtesy of Dr Diana Buchanan.)

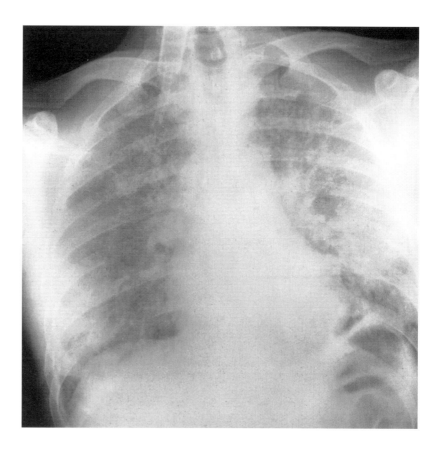

Fig. 52.16 Extensive infiltration in severe *Pneumocystis* pneumonia. (Courtesy of Dr Diana Buchanan.)

changes in PCP have been reviewed and less common appearances include (i) more focal infiltrates; (ii) nodular appearances, sometimes with cavitation (coarse multiple nodules in the HIV patient usually indicate disseminated Kaposi's sarcoma and sometimes fungal disease); (iii) selective upper lobe involvement that may mimic mycobacterial disease, this sometimes occurring in patients who have developed PCP despite nebulized pentamidine prophylaxis; (iv) subpleural cyst formation (also associated with pentamidine prophylaxis) and sometimes leading to secondary spontaneous pneumothorax; (v) hilar lymphadenopathy; and (vi) small pleural effusions and changes consistent with bronchiectasis [90,93,94]. With successful treatment there is gradual clearing of the diffuse infiltrates over a period of weeks or even months as the patient improves, radiographic resolution commonly lagging behind clinical improvement.

High-resolution CT may be useful in excluding *Pneumocystis* pneumonia when the history is suspicious but the chest radiograph remains normal, in which case an incidence of PCP of 12% has been reported [102]. Such scans may show bilateral ground-glass opacification, sometimes with sparing of the subpleural lung tissue. Less commonly, there may be some lobular inhomogeneity that can result in a mosaic pattern in which ground-glass involvement is interspersed with normal lung appearances. However, CT need not be carried out as a matter of routine in more typical cases as the images may not add clinically

useful information to that obtained from plain radiographs. Subpleural cysts may sometimes be clearly shown. Nuclear medicine scans using gallium-67 or indium-111 have also been used in the investigation of PCP in some centres, although the uptake of these investigations, which lack specificity and are both expensive and cumbersome, has not been widespread [64,103].

Non-microbiological investigations

The $CD4^+$ count is a very useful predictor of the likelihood of PCP in patients with HIV infection; it has been found that PCP is unlikely to develop in HIV-infected patients with $CD4^+$ counts above 0.2×10^9/L, whereas patients with counts below this level have a greatly enhanced risk [84]. A number of other tests have been found to have a helpful negative predictive value despite a low specificity, so that a normal result makes PCP unlikely but an abnormal result could be due to a number of different conditions and does not rule it out.

Serum lactate dehydrogenase levels are usually raised in PCP [104], although it has been suggested that this non-specific finding may simply correlate with the degree of radiographic abnormality irrespective of the pathogen [105].

Similarly, the finding of a normal diffusing capacity (D_{LCO}) for carbon monoxide in a patient at risk of PCP who has mild symptoms and a chest radiograph that looks normal makes this diagnosis highly improbable, whereas the finding of a reduced D_LCO or one that shows a downward trend in such a patient is suspicious enough to lead to further investigation for PCP [106].

An exercise test with simple monitoring of oxygen saturation by pulse oximetry may also be useful for excluding PCP in doubtful cases, since treadmill testing in 85 HIV-positive patients suspected of having PCP found that a 3% fall in saturation with exercise was 100% sensitive with a specificity of 70% [107]. Once again this test may be used to screen outpatients with normal or minimally abnormal chest radiographs and normal resting saturations, in which case a failure to desaturate with exercise effectively rules out PCP [64].

Arterial blood gas analysis is an essential assessment of severity, as with any pneumonia, although in the early stages of PCP is likely to be normal. Patients with PCP are commonly anaemic as a result of their underlying disease or its treatment. The total white cell count is more often normal or low rather than raised. Hypoalbuminaemia is not uncommon.

Microbiological investigations

Induced sputum analysis

Most patients with PCP do not produce sputum. In those few that do, a good specimen should be submitted to the microbiology department and the physician should make sure that the laboratory staff are aware of the nature of the clinical problem in order that the material be dealt with quickly and to best effect.

Sputum production may be induced in the majority of patients whose coughs are dry [7]. The specimen is obtained by having the patient breathe a mist of nebulized saline, which causes coughing. A hypertonic (2.7–5%) saline solution is conventionally used, a jet nebulizer being driven at a flow rate of at least 6 L/min and being applied to the face with a mask. Ultrasonic nebulization may be used as an alternative. The mouth should first be prepared by teeth cleaning, mouth rinsing and gargling in order to reduce any proteinaceous debris to a minimum, as this might otherwise obscure the organism. The procedure is at best unenjoyable and some patients find it distinctly unpleasant, so that it needs to be supervised by motivated staff, ideally an experienced physiotherapist, in order that an adequate specimen is obtained [108]. Sensible precautions should be taken to protect other patients from the dissemination of microorganisms during this process. Since the differential diagnosis often includes infection with *M. tuberculosis*, it is advisable to perform the investigation in a negative air flow room with attention paid to the safety of staff and visitors. A small percentage of patients may develop nausea, vomiting or wheeze and some may develop arterial desaturation [109]. It is never-

theless usually possible to obtain a satisfactory sample, although sputum induction is poorly tolerated by the more breathless subject and may prove impossible in up to 20% of patients. Although the test has been claimed to be very sensitive (up to 92%) by some groups [110], its usefulness is highly dependent on procedures being meticulously followed from the bedside to the laboratory. A sensitivity for PCP in HIV-positive patients of 28% was found on adequate samples by an experienced group in 1991, compared with 73% for BAL (see Chapter 8) [108]. Many centres now report higher sensitivities for both tests [110] so that the more invasive BAL may be avoided in a significant number of patients. A high sensitivity (63%) for induced sputum analysis has also been reported in patients with PCP due to disease other than HIV infection [111], although it might be expected that the yield in this group would be lower, as the alveolar burden of *P. carinii* is not usually as high in the absence of HIV infection [112].

Many laboratories now examine sputum for *P. carinii* using a direct immunofluorescent test (DIFT), which employs anti-*P. carinii* monoclonal antibodies and which demonstrates brightly stained cysts and results in significantly improved sensitivity compared with standard staining methods [113]. However, a negative induced sputum analysis by no means excludes PCP and it is usual for BAL to be carried out in such patients.

More invasive sampling techniques

Bronchoscopic sampling is appropriate for cases of suspected PCP in whom induced sputum analysis has been negative or as the initial investigation in centres where the positive yield from induced sputum is too low to make the test worth while. One retrospective review of all cases of suspected PCP in a large North American centre over a 4-year period found that a positive diagnosis was made bronchoscopically in 50% of patients in whom induced sputum had been negative, PCP being confirmed in over half of these, other common diagnoses including tracheo-bronchial Kaposi's sarcoma (diagnosed by its visual appearance), tuberculosis and cryptococcal pneumonia [114]. There have been reports of diagnostic sensitivities of over 90% for PCP using both BAL and transbronchial lung biopsy, although these high success rates have generally been achieved in populations with a high prevalence of HIV-positivity. Some centres add transbronchial lung biopsy to BAL as a matter of routine, in the belief that it increases the likelihood of reaching a positive diagnosis, particularly as a significant number of patients may turn out to have diagnoses other than PCP; thus a retrospective European study involving 142 immunocompromised patients found that the *overall* diagnostic yield was 68% for transbronchial lung biopsy compared with 36% for BAL [115]. However, the same authors found that when the diagnosis was found to be PCP, there was little difference in yield between transbronchial lung biopsy and BAL [115]. Many centres therefore use BAL without biopsy as the initial invasive diagnostic procedure of choice when the chance of PCP seems high, and use transbronchial biopsies only in selected cases. Thus a retrospective study covering a 3-year period in a large North American centre investigated the bronchoscopic results in patients with suspected PCP. Paired samples of both BAL fluid (examined using monoclonal antibody DIFT) and transbronchial lung biopsies (examined using conventional silver staining) showed that the one-fifth of patients in whom samples were adequate had PCP and that the sensitivity for DIFT on BAL fluid was 95% compared with 43% for silver staining on biopsies [116]. These and other seemingly conflicting results reported in the literature may result from methodological variables as well as from differences in the patient populations studied, so that individual clinicians may wish to modify their own approach according to the results of local audit. A decision to obtain histology for transbronchial biopsy may become necessary if less invasive methods have not produced a definitive diagnosis or if the patient is failing to respond to empirical antimicrobial therapy. It carries an increased risk of pneumothorax and haemorrhage. Brush biopsy does not increase the yield. It may occasionally be necessary to obtain a larger block of tissue by thorascopic or open lung biopsy (see Chapter 8).

Although the diagnostic yield may be increased by the use of PCR to detect *P. carinii* DNA in specimens such as induced sputum or BAL fluid [117,118], this costly investigation, which is not routinely available, may mislead as positive results may be obtained in the presence of residual non-viable organisms that may persist for some weeks after successful treatment of PCP.

Supportive treatment

Patients who die as a result of PCP do so because of worsening tissue hypoxia, so that immediate steps should be taken to assess the level of hypoxaemia and to correct it appropriately. This basic respiratory support is provided by high-flow oxygen administered using standard face masks. If Pa_{O_2} cannot be adequately maintained using high-flow oxygen via a mask with a reservoir bag, then the addition of continuous positive airway pressure by mask should be considered, provided that a pneumothorax has been excluded [119]. This may be well tolerated since sputum production is often minimal and it presumably improves oxygenation by splinting open small airways. Nasal positive-pressure ventilation may also improve gas exchange and avoid intubation. Patients who continue to deteriorate despite these measures remain tachypnoeic and become increasingly exhausted with worsening hypoxaemia (Pa_{O_2} <6.7 kPa, 50 mmHg) and eventually become hypercarbic. An individual decision has to be made in this situation about whether to intubate and mechanically ventilate the patient [120]. Ideally, this should be based on a knowledge of the patient's underlying disease and its prognosis, the patient's quality of life and any wishes that he or she might have expressed. Suffice to say that although the mortality is high in patients with PCP who require ventilation, particularly those with HIV infection [121], the authors have nevertheless seen successful outcomes, particularly in patients whose predisposing disease was controlled and whose performance was not significantly reduced before the onset of the pneumonic symptoms.

Antimicrobial treatment

Pentamidine isethionate (see Chapter 9) is an antiparasitic agent that has been used for over 50 years in the treatment of African trypanosomiasis (sleeping sickness) and leishmaniasis (kala-azar). It was found to be effective against *P. carinii* in the 1950s, and PCP is the only respiratory application for this drug. The use of pentamidine increased both as a result of the AIDS pandemic and the increasing use of immunosuppressant therapy in medicine. In the 1970s, co-trimoxazole, a combination of trimethoprim and sulfamethoxazole (sulphamethoxazole) (see Chapter 9), emerged as an alternative drug for treating PCP, having been found to be as effective as pentamidine but with fewer side-effects when used in children [122]. Although there have been no large comparative trials of the two, there is evidence that both response time and survival are better with co-trimoxazole [123], which has subsequently been adopted as the treatment of choice for PCP both in HIV infection and other disease [124]. Adverse effects with co-trimoxazole remain a major problem in view of the high doses that have to be used. This is particularly so in those patients with AIDS, in whom side-effects are reported in 50–80% of cases leading to discontinuation of the drug in as many as 57% [97,125], whereas the adverse side-effect rate is lower (10–20%) in other immunosuppressed patients [97].

It is accepted practice to treat the iller, more hypoxic patient intravenously, the drug of choice being co-trimoxazole, with pentamidine as a second-line agent if co-trimoxazole cannot be tolerated. Intravenous/trexate trimetrexate/folinic acid (see Chapter 9) may be used as a third-line agent for patients who are intolerant of, or unresponsive to, co-trimoxazole and pentamidine [97].

The patient with mild disease (Pa_{O_2} >10 kPa, 75 mmHg) may be treated with oral therapy, co-trimoxazole being the drug of choice. Orally administered alternatives for the intolerant patient are dapsone–trimethoprim, atovaquone or clindamycin–primaquine. The main drug regimens are illustrated in Table 52.8. Treatment of PCP in patients with HIV infection should be followed by lifelong prophylaxis.

Drugs	Dosage	Route
First line		
Co-trimoxazole	90–120 mg/kg daily in three to four divided doses	Oral or i.v.
Second line		
Pentamidine	3–4 mg/kg daily over 1–2 h once daily	i.v.
Alternatives		
Trimetrexate	45 mg/m² trimetrexate once daily	i.v.
	20 mg/m² calcium folinate four times daily	i.v. or oral
Dapsone–trimethoprim	100 mg dapsone once daily	Oral
	15 mg/kg daily trimethoprim in two to four divided doses	Oral
Atovaquone	750 mg two to three times daily	Oral
Clindamycin–primaquine	See text	i.v. and oral or oral

Table 52.8 Antimicrobial treatment for *Pneumocystis carinii* pneumonia (see text for details).

First-line treatment with co-trimoxazole

The conventional dose of co-trimoxazole required to treat PCP is 20 mg/kg daily of trimethoprim and 100 mg/kg daily of sulfamethoxazole, usually expressed as 120 mg/kg daily of the combined preparation. It is usual to administer co-trimoxazole as three to four divided doses and to treat for at least 2 weeks in the case of non-AIDS-associated PCP and for 3 weeks in the presence of HIV infection, provided that the therapy is tolerated and that a clinical response is taking place. In all but the milder case of PCP ($Pa_{O_2} > 10$ kPa, 75 mmHg), the course of co-trimoxazole is usually given intravenously for the first 10 days or so, using the same 120 mg/kg daily schedule. The manufacturer's recommendation is that the intravenous fixed combination preparation should be diluted 1/25 in 0.9% saline or 5% dextrose solution, i.e. 125 mL to one 480-mg co-trimoxazole ampoule (5 mL), and infused over 90–120 min. Despite this recommendation, it is probably safe to reduce the volume to 75 mL 5% dextrose per 480-mg ampoule if volume overload is likely to be a problem [126]. Patients with PCP receiving intravenous co-trimoxazole may deteriorate before they start to improve (see p. 1372) and a significant improvement in oxygenation may not be seen for 4–9 days. Patients with HIV-associated disease tend to respond more slowly than those without, so that it should not be assumed that therapy with co-trimoxazole has failed in such cases until about a week has passed [127]. Before switching treatment, it also has to be borne in mind that apparent deterioration may be caused by superadded pulmonary infection with bacteria or other pathogens, by coexisting disease such as Kaposi's sarcoma or lymphoma, or by complications such as pneumothorax or pulmonary oedema due to fluid overload. Once clear clinical improvement occurs, the course may be com-

pleted orally as the drug combination is well absorbed in the absence of gastrointestinal disease [125].

Milder cases may be treated orally from the start [64] provided that they have no problems with absorption, and this may be done under outpatient supervision. It is common practice to achieve this by prescribing 1920 mg (as two double-strength 960-mg tablets) three or four times daily. In patients who are finding it difficult to tolerate the drug, it may prove possible to reduce the total daily dose by 25%, from the usual 120 mg/kg daily to 90 mg/kg daily, without losing efficacy [128]. Dosage reductions are also made in renal insufficiency. The full dose may be given if the estimated creatinine clearance (see Chapter 9) is greater than 30 mL/min, the dose being halved in the range 15–30 mL/min and omitted completely if less than 15 mL/min. It is possible to assay drug levels of trimethoprim and sulfamethoxazole in such situations in order to attempt to maintain the trimethoprim level in the range 5–8 µg/mL and the sulfamethoxazole level in the range 100–150 µg/mL.

The necessity for 3-week courses has been questioned and it may be possible to conclude treatment after 2 weeks in the face of adverse effects if the patient has apparently responded and provided that secondary prophylaxis is started at the conclusion of the course [129]. It is advisable during treatment to check urea/creatinine and electrolytes, blood count and liver function tests at least twice weekly because of the likelihood of adverse effects.

Adverse effects (see Chapter 9) are common when high-dose co-trimoxazole is used in the above fashion to treat PCP, particularly when the patient has AIDS, in which case the drug may need to be discontinued in about 30% of cases [130]. Side-effects usually become evident after 1–2 weeks of treatment and include nausea and vomiting (25%), anaemia and neutropenia (40%), thrombocytopenia

(5%), abnormalities of liver function (10%), rashes (20%) and fever (25%) [123,124]. The drug need not be discontinued for mild rashes, which may be managed with antihistamines without progression [131]. Patients who have had co-trimoxazole rashes in the past have been successfully rechallenged on subsequent occasions, although severe systemic reactions may occur so caution should be exercised [131]. Rashes with involvement of the mucous membranes or those associated with the formation of bullae are reasons for discontinuance, as is intractable pruritus. The potential for marrow depression may be increased by other drugs such as zidovudine and ganciclovir, which should be stopped while treatment with high-dose co-trimoxazole is in progress. Trimethoprim has a mild potassium-sparing diuretic effect that may produce hyperkalaemia. Uraemia, hypocalcaemia and hyponatraemia sometimes occur. As with other antibiotics, *Clostridium difficile* colitis may occur. Patients with a previous history of a rash and fever in relation to co-trimoxazole have been given 8-day courses of desensitization, involving three or four times daily oral dosing with initially tiny concentrations of co-trimoxazole in solution prepared by diluting the standard oral suspension (240 mg/5 mL) [127]. One practical method is to start with a $1/10^6$ dilution on day 1, giving 1, 2, 4 and 8 mL doses at 6-h intervals, then continuing with the same volumes at 6-h intervals but reducing the dilution by a tenth power each day until day 7 when a 1/1 dilution of 20 mg sulfamethoxazole and 4 mg trimethoprim is reached. On day 8 the standard oral suspension is given as 1, 2 and 4 mL for the first three doses, culminating in one double-strength tablet for the fourth dose. Such desensitization should not be attempted in patients who have previously experienced a serious skin reaction such as Stevens–Johnson syndrome or toxic epidermal necrolysis [132]. The overall rate of intolerance to co-trimoxazole is reduced in patients ill enough to require adjuvant corticosteroids (see below) [133].

Second-line intravenous treatment with pentamidine

Intravenous pentamidine (see Chapter 9) may be used as an alternative treatment in patients who are intolerant or unresponsive to co-trimoxazole. It is probably as effective as co-trimoxazole but is more toxic [123]. It is given as a single daily dose of 3–4 mg/kg diluted in 250 mL of 5% dextrose solution (infused slowly over 1–2 h to prevent hypotension) and continued for 3 weeks in patients with AIDS; those with non-HIV-related PCP are sometimes treated for 2 weeks. Adverse effects from pentamidine are sometimes avoided by switching therapy after about 10 days to a less toxic oral regimen, such as trimethoprim in combination with dapsone or atovaquone singly, in order to complete 3 weeks of treatment. Nebulized pentamidine in doses of up to 8 mg/kg daily has been used to treat less

severe PCP but patients respond more slowly, the mortality rate is significantly higher and relapse is more common; thus this route of administration is rarely used other than for prophylaxis [127,134].

As with co-trimoxazole, adverse effects are frequent and include renal impairment (60%), leucopenia (45%), nausea and vomiting (25%), hypotension (25%) and hypoglycaemia/hypocalcaemia (20%) [123]. Fewer side-effects are encountered if 3 mg/kg daily is used. Hypotension is avoided by the slow infusion rate and blood pressure should be monitored as should serum urea/creatinine, electrolytes, glucose and calcium. Other side-effects are described in Chapter 9.

Alternative intravenous treatment with trimetrexate–folinate

Trimetrexate (an analogue of methotrexate) may be used as third-line treatment in hospitalized patients who are intolerant of both co-trimoxazole and pentamidine or in whom these drugs have failed. However, some experts use trimetrexate–folinate alone or in combination with dapsone as a second-line treatment, in preference to the more toxic pentamidine, in patients intolerant of co-trimoxazole or in whom this drug has failed [125]. Trimetrexate has its effect by preventing *P. carinii* from synthesizing folate. The folinate component of the regimen prevents or reduces myelosuppression, the microbe itself being unable to take up this supplement as it lacks a folate transport system.

The dose of trimetrexate is 45 mg/m² once daily intravenously for 21 days and that of calcium folinate (leucovorin) 20 mg/m² daily intravenously (at a separate site) or orally as four divided doses for 24 days [135]. Neutropenia is the main adverse effect, this being attenuated by folinate. Other possible adverse effects include oral and gastrointestinal mucosal ulceration, hepatic and renal dysfunction and peripheral neuropathy. However, the combination may be better tolerated than co-trimoxazole [136]. In one trial, trimetrexate–folinate proved less effective than co-trimoxazole, with a 69% survival compared with an 84% survival for co-trimoxazole at 7 weeks [135]. It is possible that the efficacy of trimetrexate–folinate may be improved by the addition of oral dapsone and this approach is being investigated.

Alternative oral treatment using dapsone–trimethoprim

This orally administered combination may be used in patients with mild to moderate PCP (Pa_{O_2} >9.3 kPa, 70 mmHg) who are intolerant of co-trimoxazole or in those cases with more severe intolerance to co-trimoxazole once the condition has been brought under control with pentamidine. The regimen is dapsone 100 mg daily as one dose, trimethoprim 15 mg/kg daily in two to four divided doses for 21 days [127,137]. The response rate appears to be similar to that achieved with co-trimoxazole with fewer side-effects.

Adverse effects include rashes, nausea and vomiting, haemolytic anaemia, methaemoglobinaemia, neutropenia, thrombocytopenia and disturbances of liver function, hyponatraemia and mild hyperkalaemia. Dapsone results in the production of hydrogen peroxide that may reduce haemoglobin to methaemoglobin, a useless molecule that cannot carry oxygen and which may result in cyanosis. This process is accelerated in subjects who have glucose 6-phosphate dehydrogenase (G6PD) deficiency, so that dapsone should not be used in patients with this condition; patients who are not G6PD deficient are unlikely to become symptomatic from any associated methaemoglobinaemia. There are reliable screening tests that demonstrate decreased red cell G6PD activity in the blood of such patients. Although used in co-trimoxazole-intolerant patients, dapsone–trimethoprim should not be tried in those who have developed a serious skin rash or type I hypersensitivity reaction to co-trimoxazole.

Alternative treatment using clindamycin–primaquine

This combination (unlicensed for PCP in the UK) is an alternative in patients with mild to moderate PCP (Pa_{O_2} > 9.3 kPa, 70 mmHg) who are intolerant of co-trimoxazole and dapsone–trimethoprim; clindamycin is administered first intravenously and then orally and primaquine orally. It is also being increasingly used in the sicker patient as an alternative to intravenous pentamidine. Clindamycin may be given at a dose of 600 mg (450 mg if body weight < 60 kg) intravenously every 6 h for 10 days, then 450 mg orally four times daily for 11 days, primaquine being given at a single dose of 15 mg (30 mg base) for the whole 21-day course. A trial comparing this regimen with co-trimoxazole in patients with HIV-associated PCP of this severity showed similar rates for response, adverse effects and survival following completion of treatment for both groups [138]. Clindamycin–primaquine is probably of similar efficacy to dapsone–trimethoprim [139].

Adverse effects with clindamycin–primaquine are generally mild. They include nausea, vomiting, abdominal discomfort, diarrhoea (including *C. difficile* diarrhoea), disturbances of liver function, methaemoglobinaemia (primaquine especially in G6PD-deficient subjects, who may develop haemolytic anaemia and who should be screened out) [125] and fever. Rashes may occur in about 20% of recipients and neutropenia or other haematological toxicity in about 25% of patients with AIDS treated for PCP [124,130].

Alternative oral treatment using atovaquone

This orally administered compound is probably best reserved for patients with mild PCP (Pa_{O_2} > 10 kPa, 75 mmHg) who are intolerant of co-trimoxazole and second-line oral regimens such as dapsone–trimethoprim or clindamycin–primaquine. It has good activity against *P. carinii* but its efficacy in clinical practice is impaired by relatively poor absorption, although this may be improved if the drug is taken with fatty food. It has a higher failure rate than co-trimoxazole [140]. It is best avoided in patients with malabsorptive problems, including those with diarrhoea [140]. The dose is 750 mg in tablet form taken with food three times daily, or 750 mg twice daily as a suspension, for 3 weeks. Side-effects are infrequent, possibly reflecting its poor absorption, although rashes (often transient), nausea, vomiting, disturbances of liver function and diarrhoea may occur, the latter further impairing absorption.

Adjunctive corticosteroids

It was found by serendipity that a patient with PCP recovered after receiving oral corticosteroids [141]. There followed a small trial that showed improvement when patients with respiratory failure received methylprednisolone as an adjunct to conventional therapy for PCP [142]. After this, a double-blind placebo-controlled trial was carried out that also used early adjunctive high-dose methylprednisolone in a similar group of ill, hypoxic and tachypnoeic patients with PCP. It had to be discontinued when it became statistically obvious that the group receiving placebo and co-trimoxazole were more likely to develop worsening respiratory failure and less likely to survive than the group receiving steroids. Similar improvements were then found in a further double-blind placebo-controlled trial when high-dose prednisolone rather than methylprednisolone was used, except that in this study patients who deteriorated initially on placebo improved when switched to steroids [143]. The accumulation of this and other evidence showed that early high-dose corticosteroids given as an adjunct to conventional antimicrobial treatment in patients with moderate to severe PCP can be expected to significantly reduce the chances of deterioration and death [127]. Patients with mild disease at presentation (Pa_{O_2} > 10 kPa, 75 mmHg) probably do *not* benefit from this intervention [144].

The mechanism by which corticosteroids produce these benefits is unknown but it has been suggested that they blunt the early inflammatory response associated with drug-induced death of *P. carinii* that might otherwise lead to deterioration before improvement sets in. A consensus view is that steroids should be used in patients with a Pa_{O_2} of less than 9.3 kPa (70 mmHg) at the onset of treatment and that this intervention is probably of no value if delayed for more than 72 h. An appropriate regimen is prednisolone 40 mg twice daily for 5 days, 20 mg twice daily for 5 days, followed by 20 mg daily until completion of the course of antimicrobial. Methylprednisolone may be used at 75% of the dose of prednisolone in patients who cannot take oral medication [127]. Whether or not a similar approach is applicable to patients who have PCP in the absence of AIDS is unknown, as most of the published work refers to HIV-positive patients. There is evidence to suggest that the early use of steroids has reduced the incidence of acute respiratory failure and the need for mechanical ventilation in patients with PCP, whereas those who progressed to respiratory failure requiring mechanical ventilation despite receiving steroids seem to fare worse as a group than those who had ventilation for PCP in the years prior to the introduction and general use of steroids in this situation [145].

One concern about adjuvant corticosteroids is that they could make matters worse if used inappropriately, for example in the presence of mycobacterial or CMV infection in the severely immunosuppressed patient [146].

Prophylaxis

Patients belonging to the 'at-risk' categories described above should receive PCP prophylaxis. This may take the form of primary prophylaxis, intended to prevent the initial attack of pneumonia in a predisposed individual, or secondary prophylaxis, intended to prevent relapse after the successful treatment of a first episode. In the case of HIV infection this should be for life, since prior to the introduction of prophylaxis 60% of patients would experience a relapse within a year [147] and the median survival after the first attack of PCP was only 11 months [148]. There are now convincing data to indicate that PCP prophylaxis has had a significantly beneficial effect on the morbidity, mortality and healthcare costs of HIV [149–151]. It is currently recommended that prophylaxis in HIV infection should be given to patients in whom:

1 the CD4+ count falls below 0.2×10^9/L;

2 the CD4+/total lymphocyte ratio is less than 1 : 5;

3 there is oropharyngeal thrush or an unexplained fever for two or more weeks even if the cell counts exceed the values given above;

4 there is another AIDS-defining diagnosis, such as Kaposi's sarcoma, cerebral toxoplasmosis or cryptococcal meningitis;

5 there has been recovery from a previous episode of PCP [64,152].

The prophylactic agent of choice is oral co-trimoxazole. Alternative regimens use dapsone or nebulized pentamidine (Table 52.9). In practice it is common for a patient with HIV infection to start with one drug regimen and to switch to another because of poor tolerance or interaction with other drugs.

Pregnancy is not a contraindication to PCP prophylaxis. Co-trimoxazole remains the drug of choice and may be used in pregnancy, although some physicians prefer to

Table 52.9 Antimicrobial prophylaxis for *Pneumocystis carinii* pneumonia.

Drugs	Doses
Co-trimoxazole	960 mg once daily* *or* 480 mg once daily* *or* 960 mg three times a week
Dapsone	100 mg once daily *or* 50 mg twice daily
Dapsone–pyrimethamine	Dapsone 50 mg once daily Pyrimethamine 50 mg once a week Calcium folinate 25 mg once a week *or* Dapsone 200 mg once a week Pyrimethamine 75 mg once a week Calcium folinate 25 mg once a week
Pentamidine (nebulized)	300 mg once monthly (appropriate nebulizer, see text)

* Regimens of first choice.
Routes of administration oral except for pentamidine.

withhold systemic treatment in the first trimester because of theoretical concerns about teratogenicity, in which case they may opt for nebulized pentamidine in these first 12 weeks because little of it is systemically absorbed.

Co-trimoxazole

Co-trimoxazole is the most effective form of primary prophylaxis for PCP in HIV infection and is taken as one double-strength tablet (960 mg) once daily, this being the regimen of first choice [152]. This results in a low attack rate of PCP of about 0.5% per year in patients with HIV infection [153]. Three-times weekly dosing with one double-strength tablet may bring the attack rate up to about 1.8% per year but produces almost a 50% reduction in toxicity and thus is an acceptable alternative regimen if higher doses cannot be tolerated [153]. However, there is the risk that intermittent dosing may produce difficulties with compliance and therefore loss of efficacy. There is also strong evidence for the efficacy and substantial clinical benefit of one single-strength tablet (480 mg) daily and this is the preferred regimen if daily double-strength tablets cannot be tolerated [152]. When side-effects have not been severe an alternative is to attempt desensitization (p. 1371), this having been successful in over 70% of patients with some regimens [132]. The efficacy of co-trimoxazole may be better maintained in the face of a falling CD4+ count in HIV infection than is the case with other prophylactic drugs. Resistance of *P. carinii* to co-trimoxazole has so far not been a problem. It also provides protection against toxoplasmosis, as well as bacterial upper and lower respiratory tract infections [152,153]. Its main drawback is its propensity to produce adverse effects such as rash (20%), fever, nausea and vomiting, neutropenia, anaemia or abnormalities of liver function, all leading to reduced compliance so that between one-fifth and half of patients may need to switch therapy [127]. It is nevertheless still reasonable to persist with or resume co-trimoxazole prophylaxis in a patient who has previously experienced mild intolerance to this compound, although not if a skin reaction has been associated with mucositis, the formation of bullae or exfoliation [70]. It has not yet been shown whether it is best to reintroduce co-trimoxazole that has been discontinued at the same dose, at a lower dose, at a gradually increasing dose or whether desensitization should be tried. Co-trimoxazole has been found to provide more effective primary and secondary prophylaxis than nebulized pentamidine [154,155], although it is possible that this difference may only become evident once the CD4+ count has dropped below $0.1 \times 10^9/L$ [156]. Trimethoprim alone is not an effective prophylactic agent. Co-trimoxazole is also regarded as the most effective prophylactic therapy against PCP in other immunosuppressed groups, for example in transplant recipients one single-strength 480-mg tablet is prescribed for up to 12 months after transplantation. This has reduced the incidence of PCP following transplant from 10–12% to virtually zero, while also reducing the risk of infection by other pathogens, including *Listeria monocytogenes*, *Nocardia asteroides* and *Toxoplasma gondii* [2]. This dose may also be prescribed in other categories of non-HIV-infected immunosuppressed patients.

Dapsone

Dapsone 100 mg daily (as a single dose or as 50 mg twice daily) may also be used as prophylaxis in patients who are intolerant of co-trimoxazole (and who may fail desensitization to it). Some studies have found dapsone to be as effective as co-trimoxazole [156,157]; however, its efficacy appears to diminish as disease advances so that the attack rate of PCP is about 7% per year once the CD4+ count has fallen to less than $0.1 \times 10^9/L$ [127,156]. Dapsone 50 mg daily is sometimes combined with pyrimethamine 50 mg per week and with calcium folinate (leucovorin) 25 mg per week, this combination having been found to be of similar efficacy to nebulized pentamidine in primary PCP prophylaxis but with more adverse effects [152]. An alternative is dapsone 200 mg, pyrimethamine 75 mg and calcium folinate 25 mg, all once weekly. Combinations that contain both dapsone and pyrimethamine are also protective against cerebral toxoplasmosis but not against bacterial infections. The incidence of adverse effects is broadly similar to that encountered with co-trimoxazole [157]. Although some data suggest a low incidence of side-effects in patients switched to dapsone after intolerance to co-trimoxazole [158], other data have shown that a high proportion of dapsone-treated patients become intolerant to it [156]. Nausea, rashes, fever, pancreatitis, liver enzyme disturbances, leucopenia, methaemoglobinaemia and haemolytic anaemia in patients with G6PD deficiency may occur. Twice-weekly dosing produces fewer side-effects but carries a higher failure rate, as does a reduction in the dose to 50 mg daily [153,156]. Dapsone has been found to provide more effective primary prophylaxis than nebulized pentamidine, although it is possible that this difference may only become evidence once the CD4+ count has dropped below $0.1 \times 10^9/L$ [156]. There are concerns about the possible teratogenicity of pyrimethamine, which should be avoided in pregnancy.

Aerosolized pentamidine

Aerosolized pentamidine was the first form of PCP prophylaxis to be used in HIV-infected patients and was shown to be effective in a placebo-controlled trial [159]. It is conventionally used at a single dose of 300 mg monthly. The type of jet nebulizer and the flow rate used are important in achieving adequate lung deposition, as the optimal particle size for alveolar deposition is 1–2 μm. The production of this size of particle diminishes deposition in the more proximal respiratory tract and therefore reduces adverse effects. The system with which there is the most experience is the Respirgard II jet nebulizer (Marquest). This should be driven by air or oxygen at a flow rate of 6–8 L/min [160,161]. The System 22 Mizer (Medic-Aid) was also validated for use with pentamidine but is no longer available. Although other systems may be effective, this has yet to be clearly shown in published work. The principal advantage of nebulized pentamidine as prophylaxis is the relatively low incidence of adverse effects compared with other options such as co-trimoxazole or dapsone [154,156]. The main disadvantage is reduced efficacy compared with standard doses of co-trimoxazole or dapsone, this becoming particularly evident in AIDS when the CD4+ count falls below $0.1 \times 10^9/L$ [154–156]. Other disadvantages include the inability of topical pentamidine to prevent bacterial infection, cerebral toxoplasmosis or extrapulmonary *Pneumocystis* that arises as a result of haematogenous dissemination [147,152,155]. The inhalation of a nebulized solution is less convenient than swallowing a tablet and is five to ten times more expensive. It is best administered in a small room or booth with extraction to the exterior of the building because of the potential risk of the dissemination of tuberculosis [161]. Nebulized pentamidine is usually well tolerated. Cough is common and wheeze may occur in about 10% of recipients [162], although these may be prevented or diminished by first giving a dose of β agonist such as 200 μg salbutamol from a standard metered-dose inhaler or 2.5 mg from a nebulizer. The patient may complain of an unpleasant metallic taste or nausea, as indeed may also be the case with parenteral administration, although nebulized pentamidine is usually free from the systemic side-effects seen when the parenteral route is used (see above and Chapter 9) as little of it is absorbed [147]. It remains an important form of prophylaxis for patients who are intolerant of co-trimoxazole and dapsone and who are at low risk of cerebral toxoplasmosis [155,163], although nowadays most patients manage one of the oral regimens satisfactorily.

Complications

Patients who develop frank respiratory failure as a consequence of PCP commonly display the clinical features of ARDS, with a virtual radiographic 'white-out' and severe hypoxaemia resulting from the shunting of blood through areas of unventilated lung [164,165]. A few of these patients recover if mechanically ventilated [120,121]. Pneumothoraces may occur in patients with PCP, presumably as a result of the rupture of necrotic subpleural blebs; indeed PCP has become a leading cause of spontaneous pneumothorax in populations with a high prevalence of AIDS [90,166,167]. Small pleural effusions may also occur in association with PCP but are unusual [90, 166]. Haemoptysis and hypertrophic pulmonary osteoarthropathy are unusual associations that have been described in association with atypical histological patterns such as nodular forms with granuloma formation, cavitation, local consolidation and vascular infiltration [64,90,168,169]. Hyponatraemia as part of the syndrome of inappropriate secretion of antidiuretic hormone has been described with PCP, as indeed it has with other pneumonias [170]. Haematogenous extrapulmonary spread of *Pneumocystis* is uncommon but can occur in virtually any organ system [171]. It was found to have occurred in approximately 3% of patients with AIDS coming to necropsy at one North American centre [172].

Outcome

Widely varying mortality rates for PCP of 5–43% have been reported in patients with AIDS [97]. Assuming a reasonable level of competence in the management of patients with PCP, mortality is chiefly influenced by the severity of the infection at presentation. This is reflected by the duration of symptoms prior to presentation (>4 weeks), the presence of tachypnoea (>30/min), the level of hypoxaemia (Pa_{O_2} <6.7 kPa, 50 mmHg) and the extent of chest radiographic change [134,173]. Haematological and biochemical parameters that have been shown to predict poor outcome include a leucocytosis (>10.8×10⁹/L), hypoalbuminaemia (<35 g/L) or a raised serum lactate dehydrogenase (>300 iu/mL) [134,173]. Mortality does not necessarily increase between the first and recurrent episodes of PCP, one cohort study of over 200 patients reporting mortality rates of 14%, 16% and 12% for the first, second and third episodes of PCP respectively [174]. Mortality is also greater in older age groups and in patients in whom pulmonary copathogens, such as bacteria, mycobacteria, *Cryptococcus* or *Toxoplasma*, are found [70,173]. The same may be true in patients receiving adjunctive steroids and from whom CMV is recovered from BAL fluid [146]. Patients who worsen after 5 days or who fail to improve after 7–10 days of treatment with appropriate medication may require treatment with an alternative drug regimen but in this group the mortality rate rises to 75–100% [97]. A prospective study of the first episode of PCP in 102 patients with AIDS found the mortality rate to be 28%, rising to 79% in those who required mechanical ventilation [173]. A relatively high mortality rate of 34% was reported in a recent retrospective survey of 116 non-HIV-infected patients with underlying diseases complicated by PCP [89]. A survival rate of 52% has been reported in a group of 29 patients who had extrapulmonary PCP [175].

References

1 Hopkin JM. Respiratory infection in the immunocompromised patient. In: Sheppard MC, ed. *Advanced Medicine*. London: Baillière Tindall, 1988.

2 Ettinger NA, Trulock EP. Pulmonary considerations of organ transplantation. *Am Rev Respir Dis* 1991; 143: 1382 and 144: 213, 433.

3 Fishman JA, Rubin RH. Infection in organ-transplant recipients. *N Engl J Med* 1998; 338: 1741.

4 Smiley MC, Wlodavier CG, Grossman RA *et al*. The role of pretransplant immunity in protection from CMV disease following renal transplantation. *Transplantation* 1985; 41: 157.

5 Hamilton PJ, Pearson ADJ. Bone marrow transplantation and the lung. *Thorax* 1986; 41: 497.

6 Tenholder MF, Hooper RG. Pulmonary infiltrates in leukaemia. *Chest* 1980; 78: 468.

7 Bigby TD, Margolskee D, Curtis JL *et al*. The usefulness of induced sputum in the diagnosis of *Pneumocystis carinii* pneumonia in patients with the acquired immunodeficiency syndrome. *Am Rev Respir Dis* 1986; 133: 515.

8 Valdivieso M, Gil-Extremera B, Zornoza J *et al*. Gram-negative bacillary pneumonia in the compromised host. *Medicine* 1977; 56: 241.

9 Hopkin JM, Turney JH, Young JA *et al*. Rapid diagnosis of obscure pneumonia in immunosuppressed renal patients by cytology of alveolar lavage fluid. *Lancet* 1983; ii: 299.

10 Young JA, Hopkin JM, Cuthbertson WP. Pulmonary infiltrates in immunocompro-mised patients: diagnosis by cytological examination of bronchoalveolar lavage fluid. *J Clin Pathol* 1984; 37: 390.

11 Broaddus C, Dake MD, Stulbarg MS *et al*. Bronchoalveolar lavage and transbronchial biopsy for the diagnosis of pulmonary infections in the acquired immunodeficiency syndrome. *Ann Intern Med* 1985; 102: 747.

12 Thorpe JE, Baughman RP, Frame PT. Alveolar lavage for diagnosis of acute bacterial pneumonia. *J Infect Dis* 1987; 155: 855.

13 Wakefield AE, Millar RM, Guiver L, Hopkin JM. DNA amplification for the diagnosis of *Pneumocystis* pneumonia from induced sputum. *Lancet* 1991; 337: 1378.

14 Carpentier E, Drouillard B, Dailloux M *et al*. Diagnosis of tuberculosis by Amplicor *Mycobacterium tuberculosis* test: a multicenter study. *J Clin Microbiol* 1995; 33: 3106.

15 Skogberg K, Ruutu P, Koivula I. Effect of immunosuppressive therapy on the clinical presentation of legionellosis. *Eur J Clin Microbiol Infect Dis* 1994; 13: 535.

16 Masur H. Prevention and treatment of *Pneumocystis* pneumonia. *N Engl J Med* 1992; 327: 1853.

17 Bowden RA, Cays M, Gooley T *et al.* Phase I study of amphotericin B colloidal dispersion for the treatment of invasive fungal infections after marrow transplant. *J Infect Dis* 1996; 173: 1208.

18 Warnock DW. Fungal complications of transplantation: diagnosis, treatment and prevention. *J Antimicrob Chemother* 1995; 36 (Suppl B): 73.

19 Grosset JH. Treatment of tuberculosis in HIV infection. *Tuberc Lung Dis* 1992; 73: 378.

20 Ljungman P. Cytomegalovirus pneumonia: presentation, diagnosis and treatment. *Semin Respir Infect* 1995; 10: 209.

21 Reed EC. Treatment of cytomegalovirus pneumonia in transplant patients. *Transplant Proc* 1991; 23 (Suppl 1): 8.

22 Maxfield RA, Sorkin IB, Fazzini EP *et al.* Respiratory failure in patients with the acquired immunodeficiency syndrome and *Pneumocystis carinii* pneumonia. *Crit Care Med* 1986; 14: 443.

23 McIvor RA, Berger P, Pack LL *et al.* An effectiveness community-based clinical trial of Respirgard II and Fisoneb nebulizers for *Pneumocystis carinii* prophylaxis with aerosol pentamidine in HIV-infected individuals. Toronto Aerosol Pentamidine Study (TAPS) group. *Chest* 1996; 110: 141.

24 Winston DJ, Ho WG, Lin CH. Intravenous immunoglobulin for prevention of cytomegalovirus infection and interstitial pneumonia after bone marrow transplantation. *Ann Intern Med* 1987; 106: 12.

25 Gottlieb MS, Schroff R, Schanker HM *et al.* *Pneumocystis carinii* pneumonia and mucosal candidiasis in previously healthy homosexual men. *N Engl J Med* 1981; 305: 1425.

26 Masur H, Michelis MA, Greene JB *et al.* An outbreak of community-acquired *Pneumocystis carinii* pneumonia: initial manifestation of cellular immune dysfunction. *N Engl J Med* 1981; 305: 1431.

27 Miller R. HIV-associated respiratory disease. *Lancet* 1996; 348: 307.

28 Wilkes MS, Fortin AH, Felix JC, Godwin TA, Thompson WG. Value of necropsy in acquired immunodeficiency syndrome. *Lancet* 1988; 332: 85.

29 Mann JM. Leadership is a global issue. *Lancet* 1997; 350 (Suppl 111): 23.

30 Davis L, Beck JM, Shellito J. Update: HIV infection and pulmonary host defenses. *Semin Respir Infect* 1993; 8: 75.

31 Clarke JR, Mitchell D. Evidence for human immunodeficiency virus infection of the lung. *Monaldi Arch Chest Dis* 1993; 48: 360.

32 Centers for Disease Control and Prevention. Revised classification system for HIV infection and expanded surveillance case definition for AIDS among adolescents and adults. *MMWR* 1993; 41 (RR-17): 1.

33 World Health Organization. *Global Programme on AIDS. Guidelines for the Clinical Management of HIV Infection in Adults.* Geneva: WHO.

34 O'Donnell AE. HIV in illicit drug users. *Clin Chest Med* 1996; 17: 797.

35 Gilks CF, Brindle RJ, Otieno LS *et al.* Life-threatening bacteraemia in HIV-1 seropositive adults admitted to hospital in Nairobi, Kenya. *Lancet* 1990; 336: 545.

36 Selwyn PA, Feingold AR, Hartel D *et al.* Increased risk of bacterial pneumonia in HIV-infected intravenous drug users without AIDS. *AIDS* 1988; 2: 267.

37 Egboga A, Corrah T, Todd J *et al.* Immunological findings in African patients with pulmonary tuberculosis and asymptomatic HIV infection. *AIDS* 1992; 6: 1045.

38 Seaton RA, Wembri JP, Armstrong P *et al.* Symptomatic human immunodeficiency virus infection in Papua New Guinea. *Aust N Z J Med* 1997; 26: 783.

39 Atzori C, Bruno A, Chichino G, Gatti S, Scaglia M. *Pneumocystis carinii* pneumonia and tuberculosis in Tanzanian patients infected with HIV. *Trans R Soc Trop Med Hyg* 1993; 87: 55.

40 Hocqueloux L, Lesprit P, Hermann J-L *et al.* Pulmonary *Mycobacterium avium* complex disease without dissemination in HIV-infected patients. *Chest* 1998; 113: 542.

41 Fiaccadori F, Elia GF, Calzetti C, Antoni AD, Magnani C. *Rhodococcus equi* infection in HIV-positive patients: report of 5 cases and literature overview. *Monaldi Arch Chest Dis* 1994; 49: 380.

42 Wallace JM. Pulmonary complications of HIV infection. Viruses and other miscellaneous organisms. *Clin Chest Med* 1996; 17: 745.

43 Huang YQ, Li JJ, Kaplan MH *et al.* Human herpes-like nucleic acid in various forms of Kaposi's sarcoma. *Lancet* 1995; 345: 759.

44 Aboulafia DM. Regression of acquired immunodeficiency syndrome-related pulmonary Kaposi's sarcoma after highly active antiretroviral therapy. *Mayo Clin Proc* 1998; 73: 439.

45 Fishback N, Koss M. Update on lymphoid interstitial pneumonitis. *Curr Opin Pulm Med* 1996; 2: 429.

46 De Leon FC, Britt EJ. The noninfectious respiratory complications of infection with HIV. *Curr Opin Pulm Med* 1995; 1: 223.

47 White DA, Matthay RA. Noninfectious pulmonary complications of infection with the human immunodeficiency virus. *Am Rev Respir Dis* 1989; 140: 1763.

48 Sanito NJ, Morley TF, Condoluci DV. Bronchiolitis obliterans organising pneumonia in an AIDS patient. *Eur Respir J* 1995; 8: 1021.

49 Mesa RA, Edell ES, Dunn WF, Edwards EW. Human immunodeficiency virus infection and pulmonary hypertension: two new cases and a review of 86 reported cases. *Mayo Clin Proc* 1998; 73: 37.

50 Goedert JJ, Cote TR, Virgo P *et al.* Spectrum of AIDS-associated malignant disorders. *Lancet* 1998; 351: 1833.

51 Concord Coordinating Committee. Concord: MRC/ANRS randomised double-blind controlled trial in immediate and deferred zidovudine in symptom-free HIV infection. *Lancet* 1994; 343: 871.

52 Delta Coordinating Committee. Delta: a randomised double-blind controlled trial comparing combinations of zidovudine plus didanosine or zalcitabine with zidovudine alone in HIV-infected individuals. *Lancet* 1996; 348: 283.

53 Moyle GJ, Barton SE. HIV-proteinase inhibitors in the management of HIV-infection. *J Antimicrob Chemother* 1996; 38: 921.

54 Hogg R, O'Shaughnessy MV, Gataric *et al.* Decline in death from AIDS due to new antiretrovirals. *Lancet* 1997; 349: 1294.

55 Egger M, Hirschel B, Francioli P *et al.* Impact of new antiretroviral combination therapies in HIV infected patients in Switzerland: prospective multicentre study. *Br Med J* 1997; 315: 1194.

56 Gazzard B, Moyle G on behalf of the BHIVA Guidelines Writing Committee. 1998 revision to the British HIV association guidelines for antiretroviral treatment of HIV seropositive individuals. *Lancet* 1998; 352: 314.

57 Carr A, Samaras K, Chisholm DJ, Cooper M. Pathogenesis of HIV-1-protease inhibitor-associated peripheral lipodystrophy, hyperlipidaemia, and insulin resistance. *Lancet* 1998; 351: 1881.

58 Kaplan JE, Masur H, Holmes KK. Prevention of opportunistic infections in persons infected with human immunodeficiency virus. *Clin Infect Dis* 1997; 25: S299.

59 Pierce M, Crampton S, Henry D *et al.* A randomized trial of clarithromycin as prophylaxis against *Mycobacterium avium* complex infection in patients with advanced acquired immunodeficiency syndrome. *N Engl J Med* 1996; 335: 384.

60 Havlir DV, Dube MP, Sattler FR *et al.* Prophylaxis against disseminated *Mycobacterium avium* complex with weekly azithromycin, daily rifabutin, or both. *N Engl J Med* 1996; 335: 392.

61 Pape JW, Jean SS, Ho JL, Hafner A, Johnson WD. Effect of isoniazid prophylaxis on incidence of active tuberculosis and progression of HIV infection. *Lancet* 1993; 342: 268.

62 Quagliarello VJ, Viscoli C, Horwitz RI. Primary prevention of cryptococcal meningitis by fluconazole in HIV infected patients. *Lancet* 1995; 345: 548.

63 Stringer JR. *Pneumocystis carinii*: what is it, exactly? *Clin Microbiol Rev* 1996; 9: 489.

64 Miller RF, Mitchell DM. *Pneumocystis carinii* pneumonia. *Thorax* 1995; 50: 191.

65 Armengol CE. A historical review of *Pneumocystis carinii*. *JAMA* 1995; 273: 747.

66 Gajdusek DC. *Pneumocystis carinii*: etiologic agent of interstitial plasma cell pneumonia of premature and young infants. *Pediatrics* 1957; 19: 543.

67 Walzer PD, Perl DP, Krogstadt DJ *et al.* *Pneumocystis carinii* pneumonia in the United States. *Ann Intern Med* 1974; 80: 83.

68 Peglow SL, Smulian AG, Linke MJ *et al.* Serologic responses to *Pneumocystis carinii* antigens in health and disease. *J Infect Dis* 1990; 161: 296.

69 Lundgren B, Lundgren JD, Nielsen T *et al.* Antibody response to a major human *Pneumocystis carinii* surface antigen in patients without evidence of immunosuppression and in patients with suspected atypical pneumonia. *Eur J Clin Microbiol Infect Dis* 1993; 12: 105.

70 Levine SJ. *Pneumocystis carinii*. *Clin Chest Med* 1996; 17: 665.

71 Cushion MT. Transmission and epidemiology. In: Walzer PD, ed. Pneumocystis carinii *Pneumonia*. New York: Marcel Dekker, 1994.

72 Chave JP, David S, Wauters JP *et al.* Transmission of *Pneumocystis carinii* from AIDS patients to other immunosuppressed patients: a cluster of *Pneumocystis carinii* pneumonia in renal transplant patients. *AIDS* 1991; 5: 927.

73 Lundgren B, Elvin K, Rothman LP *et al.*

Transmission of *Pneumocystis carinii* from patients to hospital staff. *Thorax* 1997; 52: 422.

74 Lipschik GY, Gill VJ, Lundgren JD *et al.* Improved diagnosis of *Pneumocystis carinii* infection by polymerase chain reaction on induced sputum and blood. *Lancet* 1992; 340: 203.

75 Leigh TR, Kangro HO, Gazzard BG *et al.* DNA amplification by the polymerase chain reaction to detect sub-clinical *Pneumocystis carinii* colonisation in HIV-positive and HIV-negative male homosexuals with and without respiratory symptoms. *Respir Med* 1993; 87: 525.

76 Abouya YL, Beaumel A, Lucas S *et al. Pneumocystis carinii* pneumonia. An unusual cause of death in African patients with acquired immune deficiency syndrome. *Am Rev Respir Dis* 1992; 145: 617.

77 Jacobs JL, Libby DM, Winters RA *et al.* A cluster of *Pneumocystis carinii* pneumonia in adults without predisposing illness. *N Engl J Med* 1991; 324: 246.

78 Waltzer PD. Pathogenic mechanisms. In: Walzer PD, ed. Pneumocystis carinii *Pneumonia.* New York: Marcel Dekker, 1994.

79 Hoover DR, Saah AJ, Bacellar H *et al.* Clinical manifestations of AIDS in the era of *Pneumocystis* prophylaxis. *N Engl J Med* 1993; 329: 1922.

80 Chien SM, Rawji M, Mintz S *et al.* Changes in hospital admissions pattern in patients with human immunodeficiency virus infection in the era of *Pneumocystis carinii* prophylaxis. *Chest* 1992; 102: 1035.

81 Wall PG, Porter K, Noone A *et al.* Changing incidence of *Pneumocystis carinii* pneumonia as initial AIDS-defining disease in the United Kingdom. *AIDS* 1993; 7: 1523.

82 Morlat P, Hubert JB, Chene G *et al.* Effect of primary prevention of *Pneumocystis carinii* pneumonia on the inaugural presentation of AIDS: 624 cases. *Rev Med Interne* 1995; 16: 815.

83 Masur H, Ognibene FP, Yarchoan R *et al.* CD4 counts as predictors of opportunistic pneumonias in human immunodeficiency virus (HIV) infection. *Ann Intern Med* 1989; 111: 223.

84 Phair J, Munoz A, Detels R *et al.* The risk of *Pneumocystis carinii* pneumonia among men infected with human immunodeficiency virus type I. *N Engl J Med* 1990; 322: 161.

85 Vento S, Di Perri G, Garofano T *et al. Pneumocystis carinii* pneumonia during primary HIV-1 infection. *Lancet* 1993; 342: 24.

86 Byrd JC, Hargis JB, Kester KE *et al.* Opportunistic pulmonary infections with fludarabine in previously treated patients with low-grade lymphoid malignancies: a role for *Pneumocystis carinii* pneumonia prophylaxis. *Am J Hematol* 1995; 49: 135.

87 Ognibene FP, Shelhamer JH, Hoffman GS *et al. Pneumocystis carinii* pneumonia: a major complication of immunosuppressive therapy in patients with Wegener's granulomatosis. *Am J Respir Crit Care Med* 1995; 151: 795.

88 Santamauro JT, White DA. Respiratory infections in HIV-negative immunocompromised patients. *Curr Opin Pulm Med* 1996; 2: 253.

89 Yale SH, Limper AH. *Pneumocystis carinii* pneumonia in patients without acquired immunodeficiency syndrome: associated illnesses and prior corticosteroid therapy. *Mayo Clin Proc* 1996; 71: 5.

90 Sculley RE, Mark EJ, McNeely WF *et al.* Case records of the Massachusetts General Hospital: case 27. *N Engl J Med* 1997; 337: 619.

91 Bradburne RM, Bettensohn DB, Opal SM *et al.* Relapse of *Pneumocystis carinii* pneumonia in the upper lobes during aerosol pentamidine prophylaxis. *Thorax* 1989; 44: 591.

92 Jules-Elysee KM, Stover DE, Zaman MB *et al.* Aerosolised pentamidine: effect on diagnosis and presentation of *Pneumocystis carinii* pneumonia. *Ann Intern Med* 1990; 112: 750.

93 Kennedy JW, Goetz MB. Atypical roentgenographic manifestations of *Pneumocystis carinii* pneumonia. *Arch Intern Med* 1992; 152: 1390.

94 Kuhlman JE. *Pneumocystis* infections: the radiologist's perspective. *Radiology* 1996; 198: 623.

95 West JB, ed. *Regional Differences in the Lung.* New York: Academic Press, 1977.

96 Cocker RJ, Clark D, Clayton EL *et al.* Disseminated *Pneumocystis carinii* infection in AIDS. *J Clin Pathol* 1991; 44: 820.

97 Santamauro JT, Stover DE. *Pneumocystis carinii* pneumonia. *Med Clin North Am* 1997; 81: 229.

98 Kovacs JA, Hiemenz JW, Macher AM *et al. Pneumocystis carinii* pneumonia: a comparison between patients with the acquired immunodeficiency syndrome and patients with other immunodeficiencies. *Ann Intern Med* 1984; 100: 663.

99 Miller RF, Millar AB, Weller IVD *et al.* Empirical treatment without bronchoscopy for *Pneumocystis carinii* pneumonia in the acquired immunodeficiency syndrome. *Thorax* 1989; 44: 559.

100 Tu JV, Biem HJ, Detsky AS. Bronchoscopy versus empirical therapy in HIV infected patients with presumptive *Pneumocystis carinii* pneumonia: a decision analysis. *Am Rev Respir Dis* 1993; 148: 370.

101 Gracia JD, Miravitlles M, Mayordomo C *et al.* Empiric treatments impair the diagnostic yield of BAL in HIV-positive patients. *Chest* 1997; 111: 1180.

102 Gruden JF, Huang L, Turner J *et al.* High-resolution CT in the evaluation of clinically suspected *Pneumocystis carinii* pneumonia in AIDS patients with normal, equivocal, or nonspecific radiographic findings. *Am J Roentgenol* 1997; 169: 967.

103 Fineman DS, Palestro CJ, Kim CK *et al.* Detection of abnormalities in febrile AIDS patients with In-111-labelled leukocyte and Ga-67 scintigraphy. *Radiology* 1989; 170: 677.

104 Zaman MK, White DA. Serum lactic dehydrogenase levels and *Pneumocystis carinii* pneumonia. *Am Rev Respir Dis* 1988; 137: 796.

105 Boldt MJ, Bai TR. Utility of lactate dehydrogenase vs radiographic severity in the differential diagnosis of *Pneumocystis carinii* pneumonia. *Chest* 1997; 111: 1187.

106 Stansell JD, Osmond DH, Charlebois E. Predictors of *Pneumocystis carinii* pneumonia in HIV-infected persons. Pulmonary Complications of HIV Infection Study Group. *Am J Respir Crit Care Med* 1997; 155: 60.

107 Chouaid C, Maillard D, Housset B *et al.* Cost effectiveness of noninvasive oxygen saturation measurement during exercise for the diagnosis of *Pneumocystis carinii* pneumonia. *Am Rev Respir Dis* 1993; 147: 1360.

108 Miller RF, Kocjan G, Buckland J *et al.* Sputum induction for the diagnosis of pulmonary disease in HIV positive patients. *J Infect* 1991; 23: 5.

109 Miller RF, Buckland J, Semple SJG. Arterial desaturation in HIV positive patients undergoing sputum induction. *Thorax* 1991; 46: 449.

110 Limper AH. Diagnosis of *Pneumocystis carinii* pneumonia: does only bronchoalveolar lavage suffice? *Mayo Clin Proc* 1996; 71: 1121.

111 Masur H, Gill VJ, Ognibene FP *et al.* Diagnosis of *Pneumocystis carinii* pneumonia by induced sputum technique in patients without the acquired immunodeficiency syndrome. *Ann Intern Med* 1988; 109: 755.

112 Limper AH, Offord KP, Smith TF *et al. Pneumocystis carinii* pneumonia: differences in lung parasite number and inflammation in patients with and without AIDS. *Am Rev Respir Dis* 1989; 140: 1204.

113 Kroe DM, Kirsch CM, Jensen WA. Diagnostic strategies for *Pneumocystis carinii* pneumonia. *Semin Respir Infect* 1997; 12: 70.

114 Huang L, Hecht FM, Stansell JD *et al.* Suspected *Pneumocystis carinii* pneumonia with a negative induced sputum examination. Is early bronchoscopy useful? *Am J Respir Crit Care Med* 1995; 151: 1866.

115 Cazzadori A, di Perri G, Todeschini G *et al.* Transbronchial biopsy in the diagnosis of pulmonary infiltrates in immunocompromised patients. *Chest* 1996; 107: 101.

116 Fraser JL, Lilly C, Israel E *et al.* Diagnostic yield of bronchoalveolar lavage and bronchoscopic lung biopsy for detection of *Pneumocystis carinii*. *Mayo Clin Proc* 1996; 71: 1121.

117 Chouaid C, Roux P, Lavard I *et al.* Use of the polymerase chain reaction technique on induced sputum samples for the diagnosis of *Pneumocystis carinii* pneumonia in HIV-infected patients. *Am J Clin Pathol* 1995; 104: 72.

118 Ribes JA, Limper AH, Espy MJ *et al.* PCR detection of *Pneumocystis carinii* in bronchoalveolar lavage specimens: analysis of sensitivity and specificity. *J Clin Microbiol* 1997; 35: 830.

119 DeVita MA, Friedman Y, Patrella V. Mask continuous positive airway pressure in AIDS. *Crit Care Clin* 1993; 9: 137.

120 Cowan MJ, Shelhamer JH, Levine SJ. Acute respiratory failure in the HIV-seropositive patient. *Crit Care Clin* 1997; 13: 523.

121 Rosen MJ, Clayton K, Schneider RF *et al.* Intensive care of patients with HIV infection: utilization, critical illnesses, and outcomes. Pulmonary Complications of HIV Infection Study Group. *Am J Respir Crit Care Med* 1997; 155: 67.

122 Hughes WT, Feldman S, Chaudhary SC *et al.* Comparison of pentamidine isoethonate and trimethoprim–sulfamethoxazole in the treatment of *Pneumocystis carinii* pneumonia. *J Pediatr* 1978; 92: 285.

123 Sattler FR, Cowan R, Nielsen DM *et al.* Trimethoprim–sulfamethoxazole compared with pentamidine for the treatment of *Pneumocystis carinii* pneumonia in the acquired immunodeficiency syndrome. *Ann Intern Med* 1988; 109: 280.

124 Morris-Jones SD, Easterbrook PJ. Current issues in the treatment and prophylaxis of *Pneumocystis carinii* pneumonia. *J Antimicrob Chemother* 1997; 40: 315.

125 Deresinski SC. Tretment of *Pneumocystis carinii* pneumonia in adults with AIDS. *Semin Respir Infect* 1997; 12: 79.

126 Gleckman R, Gantz NM, Joubert DW. Intravenous sulfamethoxazole–trimethoprim: pharmacokinetics, therapeutic indications, and adverse reactions. *Pharmacotherapy* 1981; 1: 206.

127 Warren E, George S et al. Advances in the treatment and prophylaxis of *Pneumocystis carinii* pneumonia. *Pharmacotherapy* 1997; 17: 900.

128 Sattler FR, Feinberg J. New developments in the treatment of *Pneumocystis carinii* pneumonia. *Chest* 1992; 101: 451.

129 Schattenkerk EJ, Lange JM, van Steenwijk RP et al. Can the course of high dose co-trimoxazole for *Pneumocystis carinii* pneumonia in AIDS be shorter? A possible solution to the problem of co-trimoxazole toxicity. *J Intern Med* 1990; 227: 359.

130 Safrin S, Finkelstein DM, Feinberg J et al. Comparison of three regimens for treating mild to moderate *Pneumocystis carinii* pneumonia in patients with AIDS. *Ann Intern Med* 1996; 124: 792.

131 Jung AC, Paauw DS. Management of adverse reactions to trimethoprim–sulfamethoxazole in human immunodeficiency virus-infected patients. *Arch Intern Med* 1994; 154: 2402.

132 Gluckstein D, Ruskin J. Rapid oral desensitisation to trimethoprim–sulfamethoxazole (TPM-SMZ): use in prophylaxis for *Pneumocystis carinii* pneumonia in patients with AIDS who were previously intolerant to TPM-SMZ. *Clin Infect Dis* 1995; 20: 849.

133 Caumes E, Roudier C, Rogeaux O et al. Effect of corticosteroids on the adverse cutaneous reactions to trimethoprin–sulfamethoxazole during treatment of AIDS-associated *Pneumocystis carinii* pneumonia. *Clin Infect Dis* 1994; 18: 319.

134 Miller RF, Le Noury J, Corbett EL et al. *Pneumocystis carinii* infection: current treatment and prevention. *J Antimicrob Chemother* 1996; 37 (Suppl B): 33.

135 Sattler FR, Allegra CJ, Verdegem TD et al. Trimetrexate–leucorvin dosage evaluation study for treatment of *Pneumocystis carinii* pneumonia. *J Infect Dis* 1990; 161: 91.

136 Sattler FR, Frame P, Davis R et al. Trimetrexate with leucovorin versus trimethoprim–sulfamethoxazole for moderate to severe episodes of *Pneumocystis carinii* pneumonia in patients with AIDS: a prospective, controlled multicenter investigation of the AIDS Clinical Trials Group Protocol 029/031. *J Infect Dis* 1994; 170: 165.

137 Medina I, Mills J, Leoung GS et al. Oral therapy for *Pneumocystis carinii* pneumonia in the acquired immunodeficiency syndrome: a controlled trial of trimethoprim–sulfamethoxazole versus trimethoprim–dapsone. *N Engl J Med* 1990; 323: 776.

138 Toma E, Fournier S, Dumont M et al. Clindamycin/primaquine versus trimethoprim/sulfamethoxazole as primary therapy for *Pneumocystis carinii* pneumonia in AIDS: a randomized, double-blind pilot trial. *Clin Infect Dis* 1993; 17: 178.

139 Safrin S, Finkelstein DM, Dumont M et al. Comparison of three regimens for treatment of mild to moderate *Pneumocystis carinii* pneumonia in patients with AIDS. *Ann Intern Med* 1996; 124: 792.

140 Hughes W, Leoung G, Kramer F et al. Comparison of atovaquone (566C80) with trimethoprim–sulfamethoxazole to treat *Pneumocystis carinii* pneumonia in patients with AIDS. *N Engl J Med* 1993; 328: 1521.

141 MacFadden DK, Edelson JD, Rebuck AS. *Pneumocystis carinii* pneumonia in the acquired immune deficiency syndrome: response to inadvertant steroid therapy. *Can Med Assoc J* 1985; 132: 1161.

142 MacFadden DK, Hyland RH, Inouye T et al. Corticosteroids as adjunctive therapy in *Pneumocystis carinii* pneumonia in patients with acquired immunodeficiency syndrome. *Lancet* 1987; i: 1477.

143 Montaner JSG, Lawson LM, Levitt N et al. Corticosteroids prevent early deterioration in patients with moderately severe *Pneumocystis carinii* pneumonia and the acquired immunodeficiency syndrome (AIDS). *Ann Intern Med* 1990; 113: 14.

144 Bozette SA, Sattler FR, Chiu J et al. A controlled trial of early adjunctive treatment with corticosteroids for *Pneumocystis carinii* pneumonia in the acquired immunodeficiency syndrome. *N Engl J Med* 1990; 323: 1451.

145 Hawley PH, Ronco JJ, Guillemi SA et al. Decreasing frequency but worsening mortality of acute respiratory failure secondary to AIDS-related *Pneumocystis carinii* pneumonia. *Chest* 1994; 106: 1456.

146 Jensen AMB, Lundgren JD, Benfield T et al. Does cytomegalovirus predict a poor prognosis in *Pneumocystis carinii* pneumonia treated with corticosteroids? *Chest* 1995; 108: 411.

147 Held M, Goebel F-D. Primary and secondary prophylaxis for *Pneumocystis carinii* related complications in HIV patients. *Eur Respir J* 1996; 9: 868.

148 Bacchetti P, Osmond D, Chaisson RE et al. Survival patterns of the first 500 patients with AIDS in San Francisco. *J Infect Dis* 1988; 157: 1044.

149 Gallant JE, McAvinue SM, Moore RD et al. The impact of prophylaxis on outcome and resource utilization in *Pneumocystis carinii* pneumonia. *Chest* 1995; 107: 1018.

150 Pitkin AD, Grant AD, Foley NM et al. Changing patterns of respiratory disease in HIV-positive patients in a referral centre in the United Kingdom between 1986–7 and 1990–1. *Thorax* 1993; 48: 204.

151 Chein S-M, Rawji M, Mintz S et al. Changes in hospital admission pattern in patients with human immunodeficiency virus infection in the era of *Pneumocystis carinii* prophylaxis. *Chest* 1992; 102: 1035.

152 Centers for Disease Control. USPHS/IDSA guidelines for the prevention of opportunistic infections in persons infected with human immunodeficiency virus: a summary. *Ann Intern Med* 1997; 127: 922.

153 Ioannidis JP, Cappelleri JC, Skolnik PR et al. A meta-analysis of the relative efficacy and toxicity of *Pneumocystis carinii* prophylactic regimens. *Arch Intern Med* 1996; 156: 177.

154 Schneider MME, Moepelman AIM, Eeftink Schattenkerk JKM et al. A controlled trial of aerosolized pentamidine or trimethoprim–sulfamethoxazole as primary prophylaxis against *Pneumocystis carinii* pneumonia in patients with human immunodeficiency virus infection. *N Engl J Med* 1992; 372: 1836.

155 Hardy WD, Feinberg J, Finkelstein DM et al. A controlled trial of trimethoprim–sulfamethoxazole or aerosolized pentamidine for secondary prophylaxis of *Pneumocystis carinii* pneumonia in patients with the acquired immunodeficiency syndrome. AIDS Clinical Trials Group Protocol 021. *N Engl J Med* 1992; 327: 1842.

156 Bozzette SA, Finkelstein DM, Spector SA et al. A randomized trial of three antipneumocystis agents in patients with advanced human immunodeficiency virus infection. *N Engl J Med* 1995; 332: 693.

157 Blum RN, Miller LA, Gaggini LC et al. Comparative trials of dapsone versus trimethoprim/sulfamethoxazole for primary prophylaxis of *Pneumocystis carinii* pneumonia. *J AIDS* 1992; 5: 341.

158 Beumont MG, Graziani A, Ubel PA et al. Safety of dapsone as *Pneumocystis carinii* pneumonia prophylaxis in human immunodeficiency virus-infected patients with allergy to trimethoprim/sulfamethoxazole. *Am J Med* 1996; 100: 611.

159 Hirschel B, Lazzarin A, Chopard P et al. A controlled study of inhaled pentamidine for primary prevention of *Pneumocystis carinii* pneumonia. *N Engl J Med* 1991; 324: 1079.

160 O'Doherty MO, Thomas S, Page C et al. Pulmonary deposition of nebulised pentamidine isethionate: effect of nebuliser type, dose and volume of fill. *Thorax* 1990; 45: 460.

161 Miller RF, Mitchell DM. Nebulisers for patients with HIV infection and AIDS. *Thorax* 1995; 52 (Suppl 2): S60.

162 Leoung GS, Feigal DW, Montgomery AB et al. Aerosolised pentamidine for prophylaxis against *Pneumocystis carinii* pneumonia. The San Francisco community prophylaxis trial. *N Engl J Med* 1990; 324: 696.

163 Simonds RJ, Hughes WT, Feinberg J et al. Preventing *Pneumocystis carinii* pneumonia in persons infected with human immunodeficiency virus. *Clin Infect Dis* 1995; 21 (Suppl 1): S44.

164 Maxfield R, Sorkin B, Fazzini E et al. Respiratory failure in patients with acquired immunodeficiency syndrome and *Pneumocystis carinii* pneumonia. *Crit Care Med* 1986; 14: 443.

165 Hopewell PC, Masur H. *Pneumocystis carinii* pneumonia: current concepts. In: Sande MA, Volberding MD, eds. *The Medical Management of AIDS*. Philadelphia: WB Saunders, 1995.

166 Light RW, Hamm H. Pleural disease and acquired immune deficiency syndrome. *Eur Respir J* 1997; 10: 2638.

167 Sassoon CS. The etiology and treatment of spontaneous pneumothorax. *Curr Opin Pulm Med* 1995; 1: 331.

168 Mascarehnas DAN, Vasudevan VP, Vaidya KP. *Pneumocystis carinii* pneumonia. Rare cause of haemoptysis. *Chest* 1991; 99: 251.

169 May T, Rabaud C, Amiel C et al. Hypertrophic pulmonary osteoarthropathy associated with granulomatous *Pneumocystis carinii* pneumonia in AIDS. *Scand J Infect Dis* 1993; 25: 771.

170 Tang WW, Kaptein EM, Feinstein EI et al. Hyponatremia in hospitalized patients with the acquired immunodeficiency syndrome and AIDS-related complex. *Am J Med* 1993; 94: 169.

171 Ng VL, Yajko DM, Hadley WK. Extrapulmonary pneumocystosis. *Clin Microbiol Rev* 1997; 10: 401.

172 Telzak EE, Armstrong D. Extrapulmonary infection and other unusual manifestations of *Pneumocystis carinii*. In: Walzer PD, ed. Pneumocystis carinii *Pneumonia*, 2nd edn. New York: Marcel Dekker, 1994.

173 Fernandez P, Torres A, Miro JM *et al*. Prognostic factors influencing the outcome in *Pneumocystis carinii* pneumonia in patients with AIDS. *Thorax* 1995; 50: 668.

174 Dohn MN, Bauhman RP, Vigdorth EM *et al*. Equal survival rates for first, second and third episodes of *Pneumocystis carinii* pneumonia in patients with acquired immunodeficiency syndrome. *Arch Intern Med* 1992; 152: 2465.

175 Raviglione MC. Extrapulmonary pneumocystosis: the first 50 cases. *Rev Infect Dis* 1990; 12: 1127.

53

PULMONARY MANIFESTATIONS OF SYSTEMIC DISEASE

ANTHONY SEATON

Many of the diseases discussed in this book have systemic manifestations or may demonstrate a major pulmonary component of a primarily systemic disease. This chapter considers diseases primarily of other organs in which lung manifestations may occur and, in some cases, may be an important or presenting feature. For convenience, they are divided into inherited and acquired diseases, although it is clear that many in the latter category may manifest because of an inherited susceptibility, while those in the former category may also be influenced by environmental factors.

Inherited disorders

The most important of these is cystic fibrosis, dealt with separately in Chapter 30. Less common, occurring as a potentially clinically important genotype in about 1 per 1000 Europeans, is α_1-antitrypsin deficiency. Other inherited disorders are sickle cell disease (common in certain racial groups), neurofibromatosis, tuberous sclerosis, Ehlers–Danlos, Marfan and cutis laxa syndromes, Shwachman's disease and Hermansky–Pudlak syndrome.

α_1-Antitrypsin deficiency

The relatively short glycoprotein α_1-antitrypsin is synthesized in the liver hepatocytes [1]. The molecule is shaped like a shepherd's crook, with a reactive methionine group on an exposed part of the handle of the crook [2]. This amino acid binds tightly to protease, inactivating it. However, the methionine can be readily oxidized and inactivated itself, a mechanism that fits well with the concept that, in defending itself against attack, the lung may need to produce oxidases and also allow elastase activity to continue. However, marked overproduction of oxidases (e.g. from leucocytes stimulated by cigarette smoke or in Gram-negative septicaemia) can result in inactivation of α_1-antitrypsin and other closely related enzymes such as antithrombin and complement

inhibitors, thus contributing to the severity of the disease process.

Many genotypes of α_1-antitrypsin deficiency have been described but the clinically important ones in terms of lung disease are PiZZ and PiSZ [3–6]. The former results from homozygous inheritance of a gene causing substitution of a single glutamic acid responsible for the primary bend in the crook. This alters the shape of the molecule, preventing hepatocytes from transporting it into the blood. Thus α_1-antitrypsin accumulates in these cells, where it may be visible as inclusion bodies and where it is probably responsible for the other serious manifestations of the disease, namely neonatal jaundice, infantile cirrhosis and a usually mild adult portal cirrhosis. The PiZZ genotype results in levels of α_1-antitrypsin in the blood of about 15% of normal. The homozygote PiSS results in levels of about 60% of normal and is not usually associated with clinical disease; neither are the heterozygotes PiMZ and PiMS, which are associated with levels 60 and 80% of normal respectively. The PiS variant results from inheritance of a gene that codes for replacement of a different glutamic acid in the α_1-antitrypsin molecule that acts as a signal for splicing; this substitution causes decreased synthesis of a normally functioning molecule. The PiSZ genotype is associated with levels of α_1-antitrypsin of about 40% of normal and may be associated with clinical lung disease.

Details of the clinical features of α_1-antitrypsin deficiency are given in Chapter 23. It is worth pointing out here that study of the biochemistry and genetics of this relatively rare lung disease has given rise to the most plausible theory of the causation of emphysema and is now leading to prospects of treatment with genetically engineered substitute antitrypsin. For the moment, however, the mainstay of management is encouragement to stop smoking.

Neurofibromatosis

Two types of this condition are recognized, both inherited

as an autosomal dominant [7]. It occurs in about 1 in 2500 births. Perhaps half of all cases are the results of new mutations, a fact that is very important in genetic counselling. If a family have a child with evidence of the condition, they will wish to know the risks associated with a future pregnancy. If there is no evidence of the condition in other family members (and careful examination for minimal evidence is necessary), a new mutation in the child is likely. On the other hand, if other family members have evidence of the disease, there is an evens chance of a further child having it. Two types are now recognized, either of which may cause thoracic spinal nerve manifestations. Type 1 is von Recklinghausen's disease and is caused by a mutation on the long arm of chromosome 17q that codes for a GTPase-activating protein known as neurofibromin [8,9]. This condition may be complicated by kyphoscoliosis, phaeochromocytoma, malignant change in fibromas, pathological bone fractures and mental retardation. The type 2 disease causes mainly bilateral acoustic neuromas and other intracranial lesions such as gliomas and meningiomas, cataracts and retinal abnormalities but may involve spinal nerves. It is caused by a mutation on chromosome 22q coding for a protein called schwannomin [10].

Since incomplete penetrance is common, the type 1 gene may be expressed by a range of clinical manifestations, from a few *café-au-lait* patches (six is regarded as the minimum for diagnosis), through multiple small subcutaneous nodules, to a serious crippling condition with multiple plexiform skin tumours with gross skin thickening and involvement of the spinal canal and central nervous system. Unfortunately, the severity of manifestations in the parent is no indicator of the abnormalities to be expected in the offspring, 50% of whom are likely to show some features of the disease. Similarly, type 2 disease may present with multiple tumours early in life or in much more benign form with few lesions later in life; there is some evidence that the severity of manifestations depends on the type of mutation [10,11].

Thoracic manifestations are usually confined to chest wall neurofibromas associated with intercostal nerves and which sometimes show the dumb-bell appearance, with enlarged intervertebral foramen associated with an extension into the spinal canal (see Chapter 45). Occasionally, however, the condition is associated with diffuse pulmonary fibrosis and bullous emphysema [12], and may present as pneumothorax.

Tuberous sclerosis

This condition occurs in about 1 per 10 000 births in the UK and is also inherited as an autosomal dominant, although many cases occur as a new mutation and severe disease may be transmitted by someone with minimal evidence [13,14]. Two mutations have been identified: on chromo-

some 9q encoding a protein called hamartin; and on chromosome 16p encoding tuberin, a GTPase-activating protein [15,16]. The clinical manifestations vary considerably and are due to the presence throughout the body of abnormal hamartomatous malformations. Skin lesions (ranging from irregular depigmentation to multiple warty nodules), central nervous nodules (causing epilepsy and mental retardation) and hamartomas of kidney, heart, bone and other organs may be present. Lung lesions include multiple nodular hamartomas and a patchy fibrosis that pathologically shows associated muscle hyperplasia as well [17]. Carney's triad, i.e. pulmonary hamartomas, gastric leiomyosarcoma and paraganglionoma, is mentioned in Chapter 42 [18]. Patients with diffuse pulmonary disease often present with pneumothorax. Pleural effusion has been described [19].

The diagnosis is made from the presence of typical associated lesions, especially mental retardation, the warty facial adenoma sebaceum, the yellowish rough 'shagreen patch' over the lower spine, subungual fibromas, retinal fibromas, and bone lesions showing increased radiographic density. In patients with diffuse lung disease, the prognosis is poor once symptoms are present. However, one patient has been described in whom mild stigmata of tuberous sclerosis were associated with diffuse lymphangioleiomyomatosis and who responded partially to treatment with tamoxifen [20]. Two others with a similar syndrome seem not to have responded [21]. Such treatment would be justified on a trial basis in such patients in the absence of any more promising therapy. If it were to be used, it would be of interest to look for oestrogen receptors in the lung biopsy.

Marfan's syndrome

This condition is characterized by excessive height and disproportionately long limbs and digits, dislocation of the lens and cardiovascular abnormalities including aortic regurgitation, dissecting aneurysm due to medial degeneration of aorta, and mitral valve prolapse [22]. Joint dislocations may also occur in relation to lax ligaments. Like the above two conditions, it is inherited as an autosomal dominant, in this case due to a mutation on chromosome 15 that encodes the protein fibrillin, important in elastin-containing tissues [23,24]. The presentation is variable in severity but many patients die in early middle age of cardiovascular problems [25]. The manifestations of the disease result from reduced tensile strength of connective tissues in the suspensory ligament of the lens and major blood vessels.

Apart from aortic dissection and regurgitation, the thoracic manifestations are not usually very important. Scoliosis of mild degree is common but pulmonary function is generally normal when allowance is made for any spinal deformity [26]. However, pneumothorax is more common in such patients than in the general population and both upper lobe bullae and upper lobe fibrosis have been described in patients with the syndrome. Aspergillomas may complicate bullae.

Ehlers–Danlos syndrome

This is a name given to what is now known to be a group of at least nine separate inherited disorders of collagen characterized by abnormal skin, lax ligaments and hyper-extensible joints. Different types are inherited differently, although most are transmitted as autosomal dominants. It is not certain how commonly thoracic problems occur in this syndrome but haemoptysis, recurrent sinusitis and pneumonia, pneumothorax, tracheomegaly and pectus excavatum have been described more frequently than might be expected [27–29].

Cutis laxa syndrome

This syndrome includes a number of inherited abnormalities of elastic tissue, characterized clinically by the development in childhood of abnormally lax and inelastic skin. The patient has characteristically loose skin around the eyes and on the ear lobes, and biopsy may show short fragmented elastic fibres with normal collagen in the skin. At least three types are recognized. The most severe is transmitted as an autosomal recessive and the skin lesion is present at birth. Severe emphysema leading to death may occur in infancy. Autosomal dominant inheritance is associated with a milder condition without pulmonary disease, while X-linked inheritance is associated with urinary tract, skeletal and joint abnormalities. Although the recessive type usually appears to be fatal in early childhood, some patients with what seems to be this variant have survived to adolescence. Severe emphysema in a child should always raise the suspicion of this condition [30–33].

Hermansky–Pudlak syndrome

This is a rare condition in which albinism, a platelet aggregation defect and chromolipid inclusions in bone marrow macrophages are found [34–36]. It is inherited as an autosomal recessive. The gene has been identified on chromosome 10q and encodes a transmembrane polypeptide that is probably a component of many cytoplasmic organelles [37,38]. The patients complain of bruising, menorrhagia and bleeding after dental extraction. In a few instances, the condition has been accompanied by evidence of interstitial lung fibrosis. Accumulations of chromolipid have been demonstrated in lung macrophages, and it has been suggested that these or chronic lung haemorrhage and haemosiderosis may cause the fibrosis [39,40]. However, it seems more likely that growth factors released in the lung may be responsible, and platelet-derived growth factor, produced by lung macrophages, has been found in raised concentrations in lavage fluid from patients with the syndrome [41].

Sickle cell disease

In contrast to the other conditions in this section, sickle cell disease is very common, occurring in about 1 in 200 births in affected racial groups from West and Central Africa, Greece, Turkey, the Middle East and India. Homozygotes (sickle cell disease) inherit haemoglobin S from both parents and exhibit the disease, while heterozygotes (sickle cell trait) have a mixture of haemoglobins S and A and only show evidence of sickling when stressed by hypoxia. The full syndrome also occurs in heterozygotes having haemoglobin S combined with other variant β-globin haemoglobins, such as haemoglobin C or β thalassaemia. Haemoglobin S has a valine substituted for glutamic acid in the β chain due to a mutation on chromosome 11.

The homozygous disease varies in its manifestations and tends to be milder in people of the Indian races than in Africans. It is characterized by sickling crises, in which vascular occlusion, bone marrow aplasia or sequestration of blood in liver and spleen occur as a result of the deformation of red cells, and which usually present with bone or abdominal pain. Relatively frequently (in up to 20% of crises) the disease presents as an acute chest syndrome [42,43]. This typically starts with bone pain in the thoracic cage, often accompanied by pleurisy, tachycardia and tachypnoea. Inspiratory crackles and signs of consolidation tend to occur later; radiographic shadowing usually appears first at the bases and in severe cases spreads throughout the lungs. The episode is accompanied by fever and falls in haemoglobin and, in severe cases, platelet count. Pains in the abdomen and other bones may be a feature. The episode may be fatal, and pathologically the lungs show evidence of alveolar wall necrosis with obstruction of capillaries by sickled red cells [44,45]. Bone marrow and fat emboli may also be found in the pulmonary vessels.

Apart from the acute chest syndrome, patients with sickle cell disease may be at increased risk of infections [42], including pneumonia, though this diagnosis may often be made in error when infarction occurs [46]. There may also be a greater risk of pulmonary embolism in pregnancy. Heterozygotes rarely develop symptoms unless exposed to hypoxic conditions, such as in unpressurized aircraft or under unwary anaesthesia. The author has seen one such patient from the Middle East whose first crisis, induced by climbing in the Himalayas, caused ischaemic necrosis of the hips and whose second crisis occurred during surgery for that condition, resulting in pulmonary infarction (Fig. 53.1).

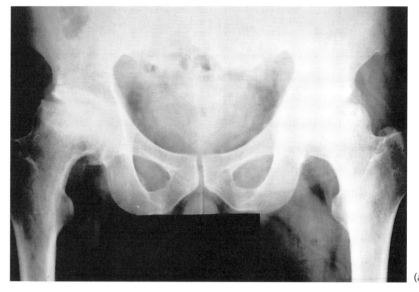

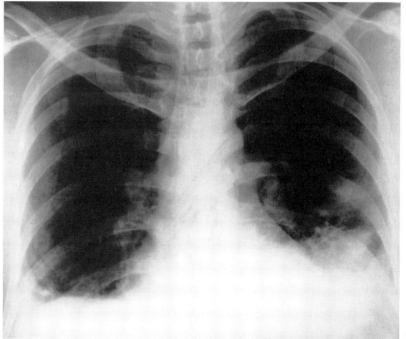

Fig. 53.1 Radiographs of patient from the Middle East who developed (a) ischaemic necrosis of the femoral heads on climbing in the Himalayas and (b) infarcted lung following operation. Sickle cell trait was responsible.

For details of the management of sickle cell disease, the reader is referred to the book by Sergeant [47]. In terms of prevention of episodes, the patient should be advised about the dangers of anaesthesia and diving and the avoidance of reduced oxygen tension during climbing and aircraft flights. The chest syndrome is managed by the use of narcotic analgesics, preferably by infusion pump, intravenous fluids, oxygen and broad-spectrum antibiotics in case of infection. Exchange transfusion is used if the patient does not improve on this regimen; blood is withdrawn in 100-mL volumes and the same amount of donor blood replaced up to about 2 L in adults every day until the proportion of haemoglobin S in the patient's blood is less

than 20% [43]. This may also be used before anaesthesia for major surgery. Increasing hypoxaemia should be treated by assisted ventilation if oronasal administration is unable to provide an adequate F_{IO_2}. In desperate cases, extracorporeal membrane oxygenation has proved life-saving [48].

There is some evidence that patients with sickle cell disease develop a restrictive pattern of lung function and pulmonary hypertension as a consequence of repeated episodes of pulmonary sickling [49]. However, the assessment of lung function may be difficult because of bodily disproportion caused by disturbance of bone growth in childhood, and specific formulae for prediction of vital capacity, total lung capacity and diffusing capacity (*D*LCO) in such patients have been published [50,51].

Immune deficiency syndromes

Many inherited abnormalities of immune defences have been described. Some, such as severe combined immunodeficiency disease, present with T-lymphocyte dysfunction and infections, including *Pneumocystis carinii* pneumonia in infancy. Others, such as Shwachman's syndrome, may present in childhood with recurrent infections and pancreatic insufficiency, mimicking cystic fibrosis [52]. The hereditary antibody deficiency syndromes may present as severe episodes of recurrent infections in infancy (such as X-linked hypogammaglobulinaemia) or as a more chronic bronchial sepsis and bronchiectasis in children and adults (such as IgA deficiency). Many of these conditions may also occur as a secondary phenomenon in adult life and may be associated with chronic bronchial sepsis or susceptibility to pneumonia. For further information on diagnosis and management, the reader is referred to relevant texts [53,54].

Niemann–Pick disease and other sphingolipidoses

These are rare hereditary diseases of sphingolipid metabolism caused by lack of specific enzymes and characterized by accumulations of abnormal lipid deposits in nervous and other tissues [55,56]. In several of them reticular radiographic shadowing on the chest film and pathological accumulations of lipid together with a fibrotic reaction have been described in the lung. Hepatosplenomegaly, mental changes, a cherry-red macula and 'sea-blue' histiocytes in the marrow are other common features. Some of these conditions occur in a mild form compatible with survival into middle age.

Acquired disorders

Connective tissue diseases

Pulmonary manifestations occur frequently in the connective tissue diseases [57,58]. There is considerable overlap between the different diseases, between the associated pulmonary manifestations and between the same pulmonary conditions in the absence of obvious collagen disease. Thus classification of the disorders is rather arbitrary and is likely to remain so until their aetiology is better understood. Those considered in this chapter are summarized in Table 53.1.

Table 53.1 Respiratory manifestations of connective tissue diseases.

Rheumatoid disease
Pleural effusion/fibrosis
Bronchopleural fistula
Pulmonary nodules and diffuse fibrosis
Caplan's syndrome
Bronchiolitis obliterans
Recurrent infections
Eosinophilic pneumonia
Pulmonary hypertension
Shrinking lung
Amyloidosis
Bronchocentric granuloma
Cricoarytenoid obstruction
Bronchiectasis

Systemic lupus erythematosus
Pleurisy/pleural effusion
Acute pneumonitis
Pulmonary haemorrhage
Interstitial fibrosis
Lymphocytic interstitial pneumonitis
Pulmonary hypertension/embolism
Segmental atelectasis
Diaphragmatic dysfunction
Infections
Drug reactions
Amyloidosis

Systemic sclerosis
Pulmonary fibrosis
Pulmonary hypertension
Aspiration pneumonia
Ventilatory failure
Relapsing pneumonitis

Sjögren's syndrome
Xerotrachea
Pulmonary fibrosis
Lymphocytic interstitial pneumonitis
Pulmonary lymphoma

Ankylosing spondylitis
Restricted chest movement
Upper lobe fibrosis

Dermatomyositis/polymyositis
Interstitial fibrosis

Polyarteritis
Pulmonary arteritis

Mixed connective tissue disease
Pleurisy/effusion
Interstitial fibrosis
Pulmonary arteritis

Giant cell arteritis
Pulmonary arteritis

Behçet's syndrome
Pulmonary arteritis/infarction

Relapsing polychondritis
Tracheal stenosis
Recurrent infection

Rheumatoid disease

Pulmonary fibrosis was first described in association with rheumatoid arthritis in the late 1940s [59,60] and Caplan [61] recognized the association of arthritis and fibrotic nodules in the chest in coal-miners in South Wales in 1953. It is now clear that the lungs and pleura may manifest many different effects of rheumatoid disease and of its treatment, although all are rare except for fibrosis and pleural effusion [62].

Pleural disease

An occasional patient with rheumatoid disease develops pleural effusion [63]. The condition is more common in men, usually in middle age, and rarely the effusion precedes evidence of joint disease. It is usually unassociated with symptoms but may cause pleurisy or, if unusually large, breathlessness. It tends to recur after aspiration. The fluid usually has a high protein and low glucose content, the latter being a useful diagnostic clue [64,65]. Another typical abnormality is a high pleural fluid/blood ratio of neurone-specific enolase, a ratio that is about unity in most conditions causing effusion but which rises to 10 or more in rheumatoid patients [66]. The effusion may appear chylous due to a high cholesterol content (Fig. 53.2). Rheumatoid factor may be present in high titre, sometimes higher than that in serum. Cytology may show large numbers of polymorphonuclear leucocytes, epithelioid cells and leucocytes containing dense granules similar to those found in joint fluid [67]. Pleural biopsy may show palisaded histiocytes characteristic of the rheumatoid nodule.

Small effusions require no treatment and may resolve spontaneously leaving pleural thickening. Larger ones should be aspirated; if they recur, chemical pleurodesis should be carried out. Persistent effusions may cause quite extensive pleural fibrosis and restriction of lung movements, and in such cases pleurectomy needs to be considered. The efficacy of corticosteroid treatment is not established for the management of rheumatoid pleural effusion. Some patients have appeared to respond and others not; a short trial is justified in patients with disease that recurs after aspiration before proceeding to pleurodesis.

Apart from effusions, patients with rheumatoid disease quite commonly show evidence of pleural thickening or adhesions at autopsy. In some cases these may be the residua of an undiagnosed effusion. Rarely, a pulmonary nodule may cavitate and rupture into the pleural space, causing pneumothorax and bronchopleural fistula [68]. Such episodes are likely to require surgical intervention to excise the nodule and to carry out pleurodesis.

Pulmonary nodules

Single or multiple nodules, usually about 1–3 cm in size though sometimes up to 10 cm, may appear on the chest film of patients, again usually male, with rheumatoid disease [69,70]. They are the least common lung manifestation of this disease. They tend to be subpleural in distribution and typically cavitate, leaving a very thin hair-line cavity that often gradually disappears (Fig. 53.3). Occasionally, nodules appear in patients without rheumatoid disease and on excision prove to be typical rheumatoid lesions; such patients may develop joint symptoms later [71].

There is no obvious relationship between the develop-

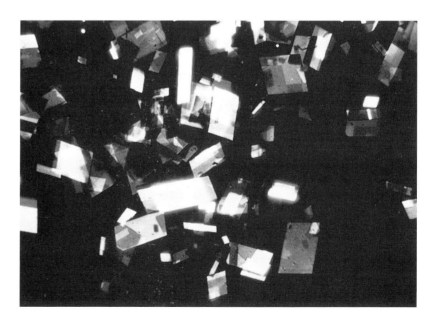

Fig. 53.2 Cholesterol crystals in pseudochylous effusion from patient with rheumatoid disease (×350).

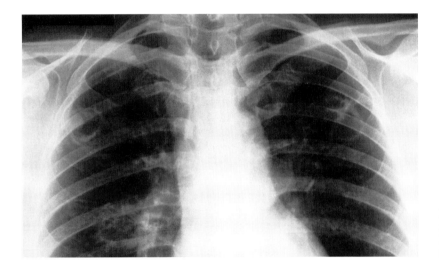

Fig. 53.3 Chest film of cavitating rheumatoid nodules in both upper lobes. Patient had long-standing seropositive rheumatoid disease.

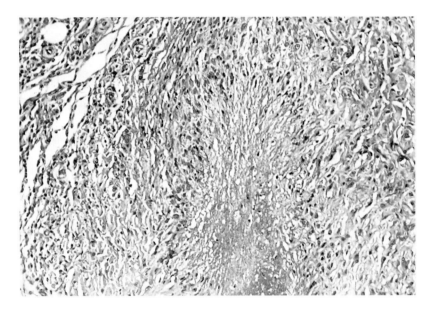

Fig. 53.4 Rheumatoid nodule showing central necrosis, a zone of palisaded histiocytes and surrounding fibrous tissue and few chronic inflammatory cells (haematoxylin & eosin ×150).

ment of nodules and the severity of the underlying rheumatoid disease, although there seems to be an association with the presence of subcutaneous nodules and with high titres of rheumatoid factor. Histologically they resemble subcutaneous nodules, with central necrosis surrounded by palisaded histiocytes and with a peripheral zone of chronic inflammatory cells (Fig. 53.4).

In general these nodules require no treatment, although excision is sometimes necessary because of anxiety that one might be neoplastic. As mentioned above, rupture into the pleura may cause bronchopleural fistula or be associated with pleural effusion, necessitating surgery.

The occurrence of such nodules in the lungs of coal-miners is called Caplan's syndrome [61]. At one time this strange immunological feature was thought to be a possible explanation of the development of progressive massive fibrosis. However, it is now apparent that

Caplan's syndrome is of rare occurrence in miners and is only very occasionally the cause of massive fibrosis.

Pulmonary fibrosis

The best-known pulmonary complication of rheumatoid disease is pulmonary fibrosis [72–74]. Most commonly this occurs as a chronic and only slowly progressive diffuse interstitial disease, maximal in the lower zones and not causing significant disability in a patient usually handicapped by joint disease. Evidence on lung function testing of some pulmonary fibrosis may be found in 30–40% of all patients with rheumatoid disease. It is more common in men. However, this description of a relatively mild condition should not blind the clinician to other possibilities since the clinical picture extends to include an aggressive and rapidly progressive arteritic type of disease, sometimes associated with digital arteritis [75]. Anything from this through desquamative interstitial pneumonitis to a burnt-out basal fibrosis may be seen.

Pulmonary fibrosis in patients with rheumatoid disease is indistinguishable either clinically or investigationally from the cryptogenic type, except for the necessary presence of evidence of the systemic disease. Up to one-third of patients with cryptogenic pulmonary fibrosis have positive rheumatoid factor in the absence of clinical evidence of rheumatoid disease, and it seems likely that the two conditions are both responses to the same cause [76]. What that is, of course, remains obscure. Finger clubbing occurs in about 50% of patients and repetitive inspiratory crackles are heard at the bases [77]. There is no clear relationship between the severity of the rheumatoid arthritis and that of the lung disease, although subcutaneous rheumatoid nodules are often present and the titre of rheumatoid factor may be high in patients with fibrosis [77,78].

Radiological appearances vary from an acute exudative pattern, through diffuse nodular and irregular, predominantly lower zone, infiltrates, to honeycombing (Figs 53.5 & 53.6). As stated above, the rate of progression is very variable. Little is known of the pathogenesis of the lung lesion, which represents a chronic inflammatory reaction with T lymphocytes and neutrophils [79]. Further discussion of the pathogenesis can be found in Chapter 31. The pathology is of interstitial fibrosis with some chronic

inflammatory cells [80], and bronchoalveolar lavage shows changes similar to those in cryptogenic pulmonary fibrosis. Immune complexes have been demonstrated in the lung in some cases but evidence of arteritis is usually absent [81,82].

Another, quite distinct, manifestation of rheumatoid lung disease is progressive upper lobe fibrosis and cavitation [83,84]. This may be unassociated with symptoms and present simply as an abnormal radiograph. However, bleeding from bronchiectatic cavities or infection of the damaged lung are not infrequent complications, while aspergilloma may also occur. The condition may mimic tuberculosis or other mycobacterial infection, chronic sarcoidosis or chronic allergic alveolitis and may cause diagnostic confusion if the clinician is not aware that it occurs. In one case it has been associated with bronchiolitis obliterans in the upper lobe airways, and the authors of this report suggested that this may play a pathogenic role; however, the presence of extensive rheumatoid disease in large airways in this patient may have been equally relevant [85]. A similar condition is well recognized in association with ankylosing spondylitis (see below). There is some evidence that the condition, when associated with rheumatoid disease, may stop progressing when the patient is treated with steroids, azathioprine or penicillamine [84,86,87].

Rheumatoid lung fibrosis is diagnosed when the above

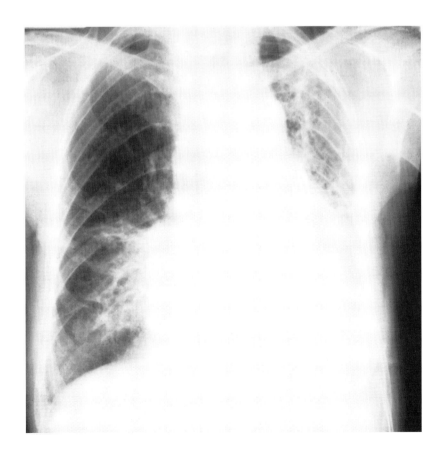

Fig. 53.5 Chest film of 60-year-old woman with mild rheumatoid disease and an acute progressive pulmonary fibrosis showing honeycombing of left lung and irregular fibrosis in right lung. There was some regression of change in the right lung after steroid therapy.

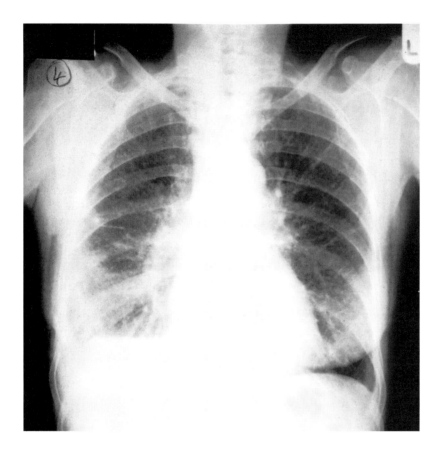

Fig. 53.6 More chronic type of rheumatoid lung showing diffuse fine fibrosis and arthritic shoulder.

clinical features occur in a patient with rheumatoid disease. The harder one looks, the more one is likely to find evidence of disease in patients with rheumatoid arthritis, although the significance of early changes in D_{LCO}, high-resolution CT or isotopic lung scans in terms of prognosis is not clear [88]. It is wise to assess the rate of progression of the lung lesion by repeating measurements of D_{LCO} over several months before embarking on treatment. If no change occurs and in view of the toxic side-effects of the drugs, it is advisable simply to reassess function at, say, 6-monthly intervals and to withhold treatment. If the patient presents with evidence of more active disease, with diffuse patchy pneumonitis radiologically, or if there appears to be deterioration in lung function, a trial of high-dose prednisolone should be given, the effect being monitored by measurements of lung volumes and D_{LCO}. If this is unsuccessful, consideration may be given to the use of azathioprine, cyclophosphamide or penicillamine, all of which have been used with apparent success in occasional cases, though none can be regarded as being of established value. In general, radiographic and CT changes of a fine irregular type, with loss of lung volume, indicate mature fibrosis and no response to therapy, whereas a more fluffy or ground-glass appearance may indicate more active inflammation and a better response.

Bronchiolitis obliterans (see also Chapter 29)

Airways obstruction appears to occur excessively frequently in patients with rheumatoid disease, even in as many as 30% of non-smokers with the disease [89,90]. However, in some patients a severe and rapidly progressive form of airways obstruction occurs, with widespread inspiratory crackles and often a mid-inspiratory squeak on auscultation [91–93]. The chest film may be normal or show only overinflation. Lung function shows severe airflow obstruction, a reduced D_{LCO} but normal K_{CO} and raised residual volume and total lung capacity measured plethysmographically; helium dilution often shows normal volumes, presumably because of inability of the gas to equilibrate with trapped air in the time available. There is a strong suspicion that in some cases the syndrome has been provoked by treatment with penicillamine [94,95] though patients have been seen who have not had this drug. The course of the condition may be progressive, with death from respiratory failure occurring within 2–3 years of onset [91]. At necropsy there is widespread fibrous obliteration of bronchioles, which are the site of an intense chronic inflammatory infiltrate. However, milder and much less rapidly progressive disease may also occur, with survival for over 10 years after the onset of symptoms [94]. There is no convincing evidence that corticosteroids are effective in preventing progression of the condition.

Other pulmonary syndromes

Pulmonary infection appears to occur relatively frequently in patients with rheumatoid arthritis [96], and the development of polyarthritis and positive rheumatoid factor has been described in patients with bronchiectasis and cystic fibrosis [97]. The significance of these observations is unclear. Conversely, bronchiectasis has been described sufficiently frequently in patients with rheumatoid disease for it to be thought that there may be a causative link or a common aetiological factor [98,99]. Chronic eosinophilic pneumonia with fever, weight loss, dyspnoea and pulmonary infiltrates has been described rarely in rheumatoid disease [100,101]; it responds to treatment with corticosteroids. Pulmonary hypertension [102,103], progressive loss of lung volume perhaps due to diaphragmatic dysfunction [104], secondary diffuse pulmonary amyloidosis [105], sclerosing mediastinitis [106] and bronchocentric granulomatosis [107–109] have all been described on rare occasions in association with rheumatoid disease. Finally, severe rheumatoid disease may affect the cricoarytenoid joints of the larynx, provoking upper airways obstruction (Fig. 53.7). One such patient treated by the author required a permanent tracheostomy.

Systemic lupus erythematosus

Systemic lupus erythematosus (SLE) is a condition occurring nine times more frequently in women than in men, with a prevalence in Californian females of 1 in 700; it is also more common in the black races, being diagnosed in 1 in 245 black women in the same state [110]. The systemic features of the disease include facial rashes, discoid skin lesions, photosensitivity, hair loss, arthropathy and renal and central nervous system lesions. Diagnosis is based on the presence of such clinical manifestations together with lupus cells in the blood, positive antinuclear antibody and antibody to double-stranded DNA. The clinical spectrum of the disease is wide, varying from acute fulminant cases with widespread arteritis and renal failure to a mild condition with transient rashes and occasional systemic involvement [111]. The known causes are few; the syndrome may follow the use of certain drugs (e.g. hydralazine, phenytoin, procainamide, chlorpromazine, penicillamine) [112] and occurs to excess in patients exposed to quartz [113,114]. It is probably influenced by both genetic and hormonal factors [115], and there is some evidence of viral transmission in animals [116]; nevertheless, in most individual patients the aetiology is obscure.

As with rheumatoid disease, SLE is also associated with a wide range of pleuropulmonary complications (see Table 53.1) [117–119]. Pleurisy or pleural effusion is the most common, occurring in about half of all patients. Pulmonary infiltrates are not infrequent and may be due to primary involvement of the lung acinus by SLE, pulmonary haemorrhage, superimposed infection or infarction, or complications such as amyloidosis or lymphocytic interstitial pneumonitis. 'Shrinking lung', originally thought to be due to progressive pulmonary disease but now usually related to bilateral elevation of myopathic diaphragms, occurs occasionally.

Pleurisy and pleural effusion

One of the most frequent clinical features of SLE, pleurisy and pleural effusion may be unilateral or bilateral and may occur just once or repeatedly [120,121]. Mild episodes may present with bilateral pain, a friction rub and no radiographic abnormality, or small bilateral effusions. More severe cases may be associated with breathlessness and persistent effusions (Fig. 53.8). Diagnosis is made from the clinical and haematological features of the disease. In the case of an effusion, the fluid is usually an exudate and has a normal glucose (though this may rarely be low) and a moderately high count of mononuclear or, sometimes, polymorphonuclear leucocytes. Immune complexes, reduced levels of complement C3 and C4, lupus cells and antinuclear factor may be present in the fluid. Pleural biopsy changes are usually non-specific, although fibrinoid deposition and haematoxylin-staining bodies may be seen. More usually the pleura is oedematous, infiltrated with mononuclear cells and covered with a fibrinous exudate [122].

The normal course is for spontaneous resolution, aided by aspiration. Pain may be relieved by non-steroidal anti-

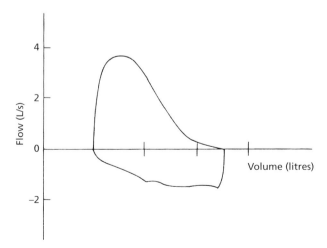

Fig. 53.7 Flow–volume loop from patient with severe rheumatoid disease and cricoarytenoid involvement showing attenuated peak flow and inspiratory flows.

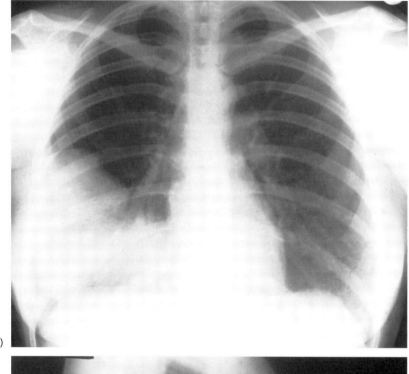

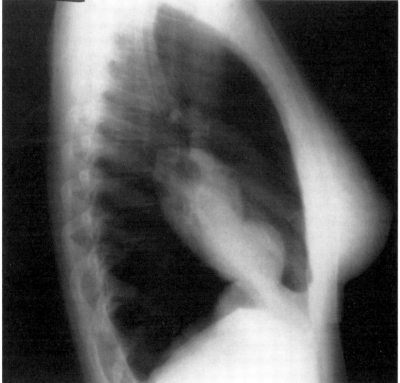

Fig. 53.8 (a) Posteroanterior radiograph of patient with systemic lupus erythematosus showing pseudotumour in right lower zone. (b) Lateral radiograph shows this to be an effusion encysted in the oblique fissure.

inflammatory drugs. In severe or persistent cases, high-dose oral steroids are usually effective. The main problem is reassuring oneself that the lesion is not due to infection or infarction, both of which occur frequently in SLE. The former may be excluded by culture of sputum, blood and pleural fluid. The latter should be suspected if the patient has the lupus anticoagulant (see below).

Lupus pneumonitis

This presentation of SLE, which occurs in some 12% of patients, usually mimics a bacterial pneumonia, the patient being ill, febrile and breathless [123–125]. Pleurisy, cough and sometimes haemoptysis may occur. Inspiratory crackles may be heard over the lung and the patient may be hypoxaemic. Pneumonic infiltrates are most frequently bilateral and basal but may be diffusely distributed and patchy. Occasionally, however, the radiograph may be apparently normal, suggesting that the episode is largely confined to the pulmonary vessels [126]. Pleural effusions may be present also.

Diagnostic difficulty arises in two respects. If the patient was not previously known to have SLE, the episode is understandably thought to be an acute infection and the diagnosis only made after antibiotics prove ineffective, bacteriology is negative and the typical haematological features are detected. On the other hand, if the patient is known to have SLE, the problem is whether the illness is acute lupoid lung or a secondary infection. Here the tendency is to assume the former, a diagnostic decision that may literally prove fatal if the patient has pyogenic or opportunist infection. Almost one-third of patients with SLE now die of infections (see below). In this situation, careful microbiological assessment should be carried out and, if necessary, both antibiotic and anti-SLE therapy used.

Lupus pneumonitis is often a severe, potentially life-threatening, disease. Pathologically, the lungs show non-specific inflammatory changes at necropsy, including mononuclear and polymorphonuclear cell alveolitis, alveolar wall oedema and sometimes an arteritis of small vessels with lymphocytes and plasma cells. Some studies have shown alveolar deposition of immunoglobulin and the presence of antinuclear antibodies in alveolar walls and capillaries [127,128], although at present lung biopsy is not helpful in making a positive diagnosis. It may of course be useful in excluding opportunist infections.

Once the diagnosis is made, the condition should be treated vigorously. There is usually a good response to high-dose (60 mg or more daily) prednisolone and this should be started immediately. If response does not occur within 2–3 days or if there is evidence of renal involvement, it would be the author's practice to add cyclophosphamide. When the patient has improved, the drugs may be slowly reduced in dosage. Lung function (volumes and D_LCO) and renal function should be monitored, stopping the cyclophosphamide first and reducing the prednisolone to as low a maintenance level as keeps the patient free of recurrence. Each patient needs to be treated as an individual, the dose of therapy being titrated against the clinical response; it is not possible to be dogmatic about treatment.

Pulmonary haemorrhage

SLE is one of the causes of acute diffuse pulmonary haemorrhage [129–132] (see Chapter 51). The patient typically presents with malaise, cough, dyspnoea and haemoptysis, which may be no more than a little streaking of the sputum or may be massive. The chest film shows bilateral, often

quite extensive consolidation, and the diagnostic clue comes from the finding of a low haemoglobin. Clinically it is indistinguishable from Goodpasture's syndrome, although antiglomerular basement membrane antibodies are not detectable.

The condition may prove fatal despite treatment and has an approximately 50% mortality rate. Appropriate oxygenation, transfusion of blood and high-dose corticosteroid and cyclophosphamide therapy are recommended when the diagnosis is suspected. If there is doubt about the diagnosis, plasmapheresis may be tried, though the evidence in the literature suggests that this does not influence survival [132].

The pathological findings, apart from extensive alveolar haemorrhage, are of non-specific alveolitis and, in some patients, an extensive neutrophil inflammatory infiltrate of small arteries, arterioles and capillaries [132,133]. Pulmonary haemorrhage may also occur in SLE secondary to uraemia or thrombocytopenia, in which case the pathological changes are simply those of haemorrhage and haemosiderosis.

Chronic interstitial fibrosis

Some evidence of chronic alveolitis is found in a majority of patients with SLE subjected to necropsy, though in some cases these may be secondary to infection or infarction, and during life abnormalities of lung function in terms of D_LCO and of the ratios of lymphocytes in alveolar lavage fluid are not infrequent [134]. Such findings do not necessarily indicate progressive lung disease and may regress [135]. Clinical evidence of chronic interstitial fibrosis, indistinguishable clinically, functionally and radiologically from the cryptogenic disease, is found rarely in SLE. Nevertheless, there are enough reports in the literature to make it clear that the association does occur occasionally and that it is associated with immune complex deposition in alveolar walls [136–138]. While it would be sensible practice to treat such patients with steroids and immunosuppressants after appropriate assessment of the severity and rate of progress of the disease, anecdotal reports suggest that it does not usually respond and has a relatively poor prognosis. Again, each case should be treated on its merits; it would be surprising if mild, non-progressive cases did not occur.

'Vanishing lung' syndrome

These patients present with increasing exertional dyspnoea and inability to take a full inspiration when they have their chest film taken. Lung function shows a restrictive pattern but usually no abnormal auscultatory signs are present in the chest. Diaphragmatic excursion is seen to be limited on screening and transdiaphragmatic pressure may be much reduced. The condition is probably due to respiratory myositis [139–142].

Some evidence of diaphragmatic weakness or elevation has been shown to be present in up to one-third of patients with SLE being studied in hospital, and is thus a relatively common feature of the disease. In symptomatic patients, a good response with improvement in diaphragmatic function has followed treatment with prednisolone.

Other pulmonary syndromes

It is quite usual to see radiological signs of linear atelectasis in SLE, often related to pleurisy, elevated diaphragms or infection [143–145]. No treatment is required except that for the primary condition. Patients with SLE are at increased risk of infection, probably largely due to the use of immunosuppressant and corticosteroid drugs; almost one-third of patients who die of SLE have evidence of serious pyogenic or opportunist infection at death [146,147]. *Pneumocystis* pneumonia, candidiasis, toxoplasmosis, aspergillosis and mycobacterial infections may be seen, as well as staphylococcal pneumonia. There is some evidence that alveolar macrophage function may be suppressed in SLE, rendering such patients more than normally liable to these infections [148].

Pulmonary embolism is a particular risk in patients with SLE with the lupus anticoagulant. This is an antiphospholipid antibody present in a small number of patients and is associated with central nervous system disease, recurrent abortions and thromboses [149,150]. It also causes a false-positive venereal disease reference laboratory (VDRL) test for syphilis. It interferes with the transformation of prothrombin to thrombin and thus causes a prolonged partial thromboplastin time. However, paradoxically, it causes an increased susceptibility to thromboses, probably as a result of its inhibition of the release of arachidonic acid metabolites from cell membranes and therefore the loss of their inhibitory effects on platelet aggregation.

Perhaps also related to the presence of the lupus anticoagulant is the development of pulmonary hypertension, which occurs in a small number of patients with SLE [151,152]; in one report, five of six patients with pulmonary hypertension had the anticoagulant. Associated vasculitis and Raynaud's disease may also be factors in the aetiology of pulmonary hypertension.

The differential diagnosis of diffuse or patchy pulmonary infiltrates in SLE should include four other possibilities: (i) some of the drugs used in its treatment (cyclophosphamide and azathioprine) may occasionally cause interstitial pneumonitis (see Chapter 55); (ii) occasionally patients with SLE develop lymphocytic interstitial pneumonia, with dense patchy infiltrates and a relatively benign course (see Chapter 40) [153]; (iii) a patient with, or even without, chronic renal involvement may rarely develop secondary amyloidosis involving the lung parenchyma (see Chapter 51) [154]; and (iv) pulmonary oedema secondary to renal failure may also occur (see Chapter 27).

Systemic sclerosis

Systemic sclerosis is a multisystem disease characterized by fibrosis of the epidermis and dermis (scleroderma), Raynaud's phenomenon and fibrosis of other organs including the kidneys, lungs, heart, gastrointestinal tract and skeletal muscles [155]. It occurs in 5–20 people per million per annum and is about three times more common in women than men. The peak incidence is between the ages of 20 and 60. There are no known geographical differences in incidence, although it does seem to be more frequent in manual workers and a number of environmental factors have been associated with an increased risk of the condition. The prognosis depends very much on which organs are involved. A relatively benign variant, scleroderma, involves only the skin, causing disfigurement and discomfort but not threatening life. However, most patients develop renal, cardiac and/or lung involvement and this reduces the 5-year survival to about 70%. One variant, known by the acronym CREST, is characterized by finger-tip *c*alcinosis, *R*aynaud's phenomenon, o*e*sophageal dysfunction, *s*clerodactyly and skin *t*elangiectasis. The skin involvement is more limited, usually being confined to the face and hands, and visceral involvement occurs later or not at all. Nevertheless, lung fibrosis or pulmonary hypertension are common accompaniments eventually.

The patient with systemic sclerosis usually presents with tight shiny skin on the hands and face, often spreading eventually all over the body. The rapidity of progression is very variable and unpredictable. Renal involvement is the main cause of death. The renal lesion appears to be a vasculitis of small arteries, with endothelial swelling, intimal thickening and a perivascular cuff of mononuclear cells, leading to intimal sclerosis and fibrinoid change and secondary kidney avascularity and infarction. These changes mimic those occurring in accelerated hypertension, which is a complication of the disease, but are not secondary to it as they may be present even if the blood pressure is normal. Similar arterial and arteriolar changes are present in the skin, where a diminution in the numbers of capillaries has also been demonstrated.

The development of renal disease is of serious import, since renal failure and malignant hypertension are likely to occur and cause death within a few years. Almost equally serious is cardiac involvement, which may present as cardiac tamponade due to pericardial effusions or fibrosis, as heart failure due to patchy myocardial fibrosis (probably also related to small vessel disease) or as syncopal attacks due to cardiac conduction disturbances

[156–159]. Lung involvement is the other important cause of death [159].

Other organs that may be involved include the oesophagus (which characteristically lacks peristaltic activity, causing dysphagia and reflux), the small intestine (leading to malabsorption), the thyroid (fibrosis) and, very occasionally, the central nervous system and cranial nerves. Systemic sclerosis may also be associated with Sjögren's syndrome, primary biliary cirrhosis and other collagen diseases.

Aetiology and pathogenesis

There is no strong evidence of genetic factors in the aetiology of systemic sclerosis [155,159]. On the other hand, there are several well-recognized environmental factors. The disease is more common in manual workers and has been associated with exposure to quartz in mining and quarrying and to vinyl chloride and other chlorinated hydrocarbons, and to ingestion of contaminated cooking oil in the notorious Spanish toxic oil syndrome [114,160–163]. A scleroderma-like syndrome has also been described during treatment with both bleomycin and L-tryptophan [164]. However, in most individual patients the aetiology is obscure.

Whatever the primary cause, the most obvious pathological lesions occur in small blood vessels and the organs they supply. It has been suggested that the initial damage caused by a number of different factors may be to the endothelial lining of those vessels, which in turn allows proteins and toxic substances access to the perivascular tissues where an inflammatory reaction leading to fibrosis occurs. A frequent feature of the disease, occurring in up to 90% of patients, is the finding of circulating antinuclear antibodies, usually of the speckled or nucleolar type; evidence suggests that the presence of anti-Scl 70 antibody is a strong predictor of lung disease in systemic sclerosis [165]. Further studies of the occurrence of such antibodies in populations exposed to quartz would be of considerable interest, since it is likely that they are produced in response to liberation of antigenic material from damaged cells.

Pulmonary fibrosis

Most patients with systemic sclerosis and the CREST variant ultimately develop lung involvement [166,167]. Pulmonary fibrosis presents as gradually increasing dyspnoea. Cough is rarely an important symptom. Bilateral inspiratory crackles are often present but their absence is not inconsistent with the diagnosis. The radiograph simply shows fine irregular, predominantly basal, fibrosis (Fig. 53.9). In some patients dyspnoea seems out of proportion to the radiological changes, and in these individuals it is likely that pulmonary vascular disease (see

below) is the predominant lesion. As in idiopathic fibrosis, CT allows estimation of the extent and to some degree the stage of the disease [168,169].

Lung function testing in the presence of radiographic and clinical abnormalities is likely to show a restrictive pattern with reduction in DLCO, although this does not usually fall below about 60% of predicted values [168,170]. Not infrequently DLCO alone is reduced, and if this reduction is severe it again suggests vascular involvement. Gallium scans may show abnormal uptake, though this is of no diagnostic value. Bronchoalveolar lavage may show further evidence of lung inflammation with increased numbers of neutrophils and eosinophils, the former being associated with a more progressive condition [171–174].

The pathological findings are of banal alveolar wall fibrosis, predominantly in the lower zones, with relatively little inflammatory cell infiltrate. Secondary bronchiolectasis may be present. Arteriolar and small arterial narrowing by intimal thickening may be present [167,175]. Recent investigations of pathogenesis have identified increased local expression of endothelin receptors in scleroderma interstitial tissue [176]; endothelins are peptide mediators involved in regulation of cell proliferation. In addition, another mediator called tissue factor, which may be involved in fibrin deposition in the lung as it is in the clotting cascade, has been found in type II pneumocytes of patients with this condition [177]. However, the mechanisms of this and other forms of lung fibrosis remain obscure.

The presence of clinical evidence of interstitial fibrosis and reduced lung function in a patient with systemic sclerosis implies a reduced life expectancy, with about a 60% 5-year survival rate [166]. However, in general the fibrosis tends to be less rapidly progressive than the idiopathic form [178] and death is due to pneumonia or other, non-respiratory, complications of the disease [159]. Cor pulmonale is rare at necropsy.

Pulmonary hypertension

In contrast to pulmonary fibrosis (but recognizing that overlap between the two conditions occurs), pulmonary hypertension is a very serious and progressive complication of systemic sclerosis, particularly in the CREST syndrome [179–181]. The patient again presents with breathlessness, but this tends to be rapidly progressive. There may be crackles in the lungs, although often there are no signs. Evidence of pulmonary hypertension, such as right ventricular heave and gallop rhythm and large jugular *a* waves, may be present. The lungs may look normal or avascular and the main pulmonary arteries may be dilated. The ECG shows evidence of right ventricular preponderance. Lung function testing shows a lowered DLCO, often of severe degree. Such patients are very likely

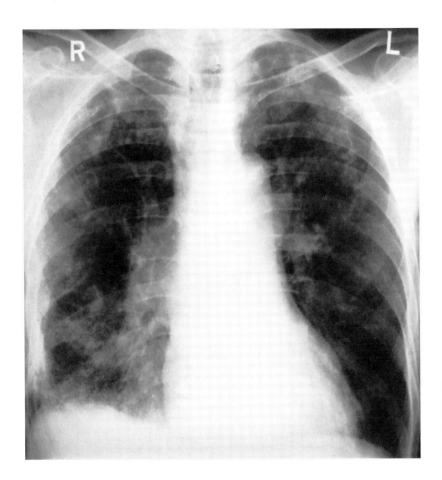

Fig. 53.9 Chest film of patient with silicosis and massive fibrosis in upper lobes who developed secondary systemic sclerosis and fine lower lobe fibrosis related to this disease. Rib fractures at right base were traumatic.

to have the antinuclear antibody anti-Scl 70, perhaps indicative of a general tendency towards vascular damage.

Pulmonary hypertension in systemic sclerosis portends a particularly bad prognosis. The patients develop cor pulmonale and most are dead within 3 years. Widespread obliterative changes are present in small arteries and arterioles and extensive arteriovenous anastamoses may be demonstrated at necropsy.

Other pulmonary syndromes

The dysphagia and gastro-oesophageal reflux associated with oesophageal disease in systemic sclerosis may be responsible for nocturnal aspiration of stomach contents and recurrent aspiration pneumonias (see Chapter 13). The rigid skin together with involvement of the muscles of respiration may cause ventilatory failure, with a restrictive pattern of lung function; in such circumstances some reversibility of the muscle weakness may occur after treatment with corticosteroids [182]. Another, very rare, syndrome responsive to corticosteroid treatment is relapsing organizing pneumonitis, which has been described in association with the CREST syndrome and primary biliary cirrhosis [183]. It presents with breathlessness and confluent areas of consolidation on the chest radiograph. Finally,

in all patients with chronic pulmonary fibrosis there appears to be an increased risk of the development of adenocarcinoma or alveolar cell carcinoma of the lung.

Treatment

With the two exceptions mentioned above, corticosteroids do not seem to be of much value in the management of systemic sclerosis unless there is evidence of overlap with other connective tissue diseases. However, there is evidence that treatment with D-penicillamine improves prognosis, may prevent development of renal and possibly lung involvement and may improve $D_{L}CO$ [184,185]. It would now be reasonable policy to treat such patients with this drug, starting with 250 mg daily and increasing the dose every fortnight to about 1.8 g daily for 2 months, then tapering it again gradually to 500 mg daily. Treatment should be continued for about 2–5 years. Side-effects include digestive disturbances, nephropathy, rashes and bone marrow suppression, some of which may require cessation of treatment. In the absence of response, little is lost by trying immunosuppressive treatment and again uncontrolled evidence suggests that cyclophosphamide may sometimes be associated with improvement in lung function [186].

There is some largely speculative evidence that patients

with pulmonary hypertension may respond to pulmonary vasodilators if treated early enough [187,188]. Hydralazine, calcium blockers and angiotensin-converting enzyme inhibitors have been tried, generally without success. Nevertheless, in view of the poor prognosis of this syndrome, carefully monitored trials of such therapy in individual patients are justified. General measures include keeping the extremities warm, lanolin for softening the skin, metoclopramide and H_2 antagonists for dysphagia and reflux and, perhaps, peripheral vasodilators.

Sjögren's syndrome

Sjögren's syndrome is characterized by a combination of dry eyes, mouth and other mucous membranes and lymphocytic infiltrates of salivary and mucous glands [189]. It is much more common in women and is often associated with rheumatoid arthritis, SLE, Raynaud's disease, scleroderma and other connective tissue disorders. In about 50% of cases, however, it is the only disease present and is called primary Sjögren's syndrome. It is of unknown aetiology, although there is a well-described association with HLA-DR3 and it may also occur in patients with either human immunodeficiency virus infection or graft-versus-host disease following marrow transplantation. Various other viral infections, including inevitably Epstein–Barr virus, have been suspected of causing the condition but no consensus has been reached.

When Sjögren's syndrome is combined with other diseases, the lungs may show any of the manifestations of those diseases. However, there is clear evidence that a proportion of patients with primary Sjögren's syndrome, ranging in different studies from 9 to 75%, develop lung involvement [190–192]. The variation in these estimates of prevalence probably reflects partly selection of the subjects and partly how thoroughly abnormalities have been sought. It seems likely that careful evaluation of symptoms, chest radiograph and lung function in patients with Sjögren's syndrome shows respiratory involvement to be present in the majority.

Pulmonary involvement

Many patients complain of a persistent dry cough with associated dry tracheobronchial mucosa [190–193]. This abnormality may be present in isolation or combined with other pulmonary lesions and has been called xerotrachea. It is associated with impaired mucociliary clearance [194]. Airways narrowing, which may be severe enough to cause reduction of forced expiratory volume in 1 s or which may only be detectable by tests of flow rates at low lung volumes, occurs in a proportion of patients. Interstitial lung disease occurs in up to one-third of patients and may present in one of two broad groups: interstitial fibrosis or diffuse lymphocytic infiltrates [195]. These conditions present no different clinical or pathological features from those occurring in the absence of Sjögren's syndrome, the patient complaining of breathlessness and radiography and CT showing diffuse irregular or patchy infiltrates respectively [196]. However, it should be noted that there is a well-recognized risk of the lymphocytic infiltrate in the lungs developing into a malignant lymphoma or reticulum cell carcinoma of highly undifferentiated type [197]. Not surprisingly, in view of the lack of airway secretions, respiratory infections and pneumonia occur relatively frequently in Sjögren's syndrome.

Treatment

No curative treatment is available for Sjögren's syndrome and local measures may be necessary for symptomatic relief. The finding of abnormal lung function in a patient with the syndrome should prompt further investigation, but it would be wise not to rush to treatment of interstitial disease with immunosuppressant drugs until follow-up makes clear whether clinically significant progression is occurring. In most cases it is not [198]. Pulmonary infiltration by lymphocytes often responds to prednisolone if thought necessary; a dose of 60 mg daily is given until improvement occurs and then tapered to a maintenance dose [197]. Azathioprine has also been used with reported initial response [195]. It is not known whether this treatment prevents progression to lymphoma; if this tumour develops, appropriate chemotherapy is necessary.

Ankylosing spondylitis

Ankylosing spondylitis is a condition in which progressive inflammation of spinal joints leads to ankylosis. It occurs predominantly in young adult males [199] and 90% of its victims carry the HLA-B27 antigen [200]. Beyond this strong genetic predisposition, the provoking cause or causes are not known. Apart from ankylosis of the spine, which may range in severity from involvement of sacroiliac joints only to development of a completely rigid bamboo spine, the joints of the chest wall, hips and knees may be involved, as may other large joints [201]. Some 20% of patients develop iritis and about 4% a proximal aortitis with aortic valve regurgitation. Amyloidosis may occasionally occur in patients with long-standing disease.

The patient usually presents with low backache, often referred down the backs of both legs, with stiffness in the mornings and on resting. The condition normally progresses only slowly and does not alter life expectancy or cause severe disability. However some patients run a more rapid course, early development of systemic signs or of limb joint involvement indicating that this is the case.

Lung involvement

The lungs are usually only involved in patients with a long history of joint disease [202–205]. Two conditions are recognized. Firstly, if there is severe involvement of the thoracic cage, a restrictive pattern of lung function may occur and rarely this may be sufficient to cause dyspnoea. Usually, however, the function of the diaphragm allows adequate ventilation [206]. Secondly, some 1% of patients with long-standing, though not necessarily severe, disease may develop upper lobe fibrosis (Fig. 53.10). Again this is rarely progressive or disabling but provides a diagnostic puzzle if the association is not known. The author has seen it occur in a patient whose only evidence of ankylosing spondylitis was sacroiliac joint fusion and HLA-B27 positivity; others have also reported this, indicating that the fibrosis is clearly not secondary to a rigid chest wall [207]. The bronchiectasis that occurs secondarily to the fibrosis may become the seat of aspergillomas and thus the cause of haemoptysis. Locally invasive aspergillosis has been reported [208]. Colonization with *Mycobacterium kansasii*, *M. avium-intracellulare* and *M. scrofulaceum* has also been reported [205,207,209], though in such cases it would be difficult to know whether the mycobacteria or the ankylosing spondylitis are the cause of the upper lobe disease.

In general, no treatment is required for the pulmonary complications of ankylosing spondylitis. The important point is to be aware of the association with upper lobe fibrosis so that the patient is spared unnecessary treatment for tuberculosis.

Other connective tissue disorders

Although respiratory muscle weakness and respiratory failure may occur in acute forms of dermatomyositis, direct lung involvement is rare in the dermatomyositis–polymyositis syndrome [210–212]. When it occurs, a subacute diffuse interstitial fibrosis with an active inflammatory component is usual. Often this is responsive to steroid treatment [213], although occasionally rapidly progressive fibrosis resistant to steroids and immunosuppressants may occur [214,215]. Bronchiolitis obliterans organizing pneumonia and diffuse alveolar damage have also been described [216]. Dermatomyositis is of course also one of the paraneoplastic syndromes associated with lung cancer. The pulmonary aspects of polyarteritis nodosa and related syndromes have been described in Chapter 38. 'Mixed connective tissue disease' is the term used to describe an illness showing features of several of the other conditions, rheumatoid, SLE, systemic sclerosis and polymyositis [217]. Not surprisingly, pulmonary fibrosis and pleurisy with effusions may be features of the syndrome, occurring in about one-quarter of the patients [218]. Management is along the lines indicated for the individual diseases above, and there is some evidence that the interstitial lung involvement may respond to corticosteroids. Giant cell arteritis may very rarely be associated with a granulomatous interstitial pneumonitis or with involvement of intrapulmonary elastic arteries [219,220].

Behçet's syndrome, a condition of unknown aetiology characterized by recurrent oral and genital ulceration, iritis, thrombophlebitis and arteritic lesions in other organs, occasionally involves the lung [221,222]. When it does, the lesions appear to be multiple recurrent infarcts with haemoptysis, caused by pulmonary arteritis and aneurysm formation. Haemoptysis may be fatal and anticoagulants are contraindicated. Recommended treatment is with high-dose prednisolone and cyclophosphamide; if haemoptysis and thrombosis persist, stanozolol or phenformin have been suggested to enhance fibrinolysis [223]. The Hughes–Stovin syndrome may be a variant of this disease; it is characterized by recurrent thrombophlebitis and pulmonary artery vasculitis and aneurysm formation [224,225].

Relapsing polychondritis is a rare condition in which recurrent episodes of inflammation, probably mediated by autoantibodies, occur in cartilage [226–230]. It is sometimes associated with rheumatoid and other collagen diseases. Inflammation and destruction of ear and nasal cartilage, episcleritis and laryngotracheobronchial damage may occur. The latter results in airway involvement by inflammatory cells, destruction of cartilage, narrowing of the lumen and increased collapsibility. The patient complains of breathlessness and stridor may be audible. The progress of the condition may be slowed by high-dose corticosteroids, but once tracheal narrowing has occurred by fibrosis the patient is likely to suffer recurrent respiratory infections and increasing breathlessness.

Some other systemic disorders with lung involvement

Rheumatic fever

Apart from the acute pulmonary effects of heart failure during rheumatic fever, a specific pulmonary infiltrative condition, rheumatic pneumonia, may occur. The patient complains of cough, dyspnoea and pleurisy and there may be haemoptysis. The radiograph may show patchy mottling or appearances suggestive of pulmonary oedema. The pathological lesions are patchy, and include alveolar wall infiltration with leucocytes, capillary endothelial necrosis and intra-alveolar haemorrhage and exudation [231]. Hyaline membranes have been described and organization with fibrosis may occur. Corticosteroids are recommended for treatment on an anecdotal basis.

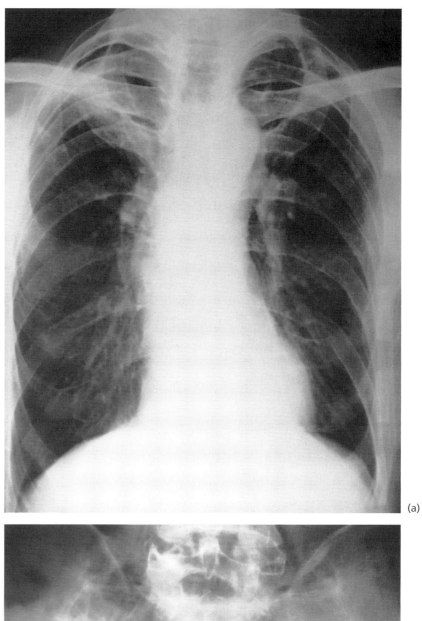

(a)

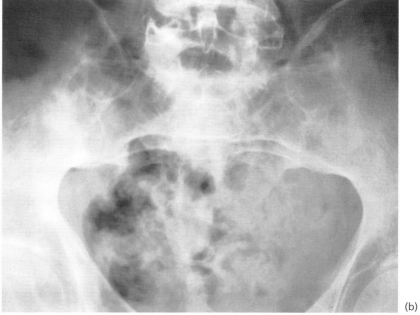

(b)

Fig. 53.10 (a) Upper lobe fibrosis with elevated hilar shadows in man with (b) sacroiliac ankylosis.

Syphilis

Diffuse consolidation of the lung may be a feature of fatal congenital or of tertiary syphilis [232–235]. Gummas may occur in trachea, bronchi or lung, where their diagnosis nowadays is a matter of considerable surprise to the pathologist examining a biopsy or specimen of lung removed under suspicion of being a carcinoma. Diffuse pulmonary fibrosis, cavitation and bronchial stricture have been described. The offending organism, *Treponema pallidum*, is sensitive to penicillin.

Ulcerative colitis

Minor abnormalities of pulmonary function, often of an obstructive type, are quite frequent in ulcerative colitis [236], although the disease may also be associated with lung disease separate from the well-known association of alveolitis with sulfasalazine (sulphasalazine) treatment (see Chapter 55). Most commonly there appears to be an inflammatory reaction affecting the airways, which may simply cause a persistent cough or may present as bronchiectasis or bronchiolitis obliterans [237–241]. In some patients the condition has presented as a progressive bronchiectasis following colectomy. It is distinct from smoking-related bronchitis and is well described in non-smokers. The pathological changes are basal cell hyperplasia, basement membrane thickening and submucosal inflammatory cell infiltration. Although the aetiology is obscure, it is likely that the disease represents a bronchial reaction to whatever environmental or immunological factor is causing the colitis. Interestingly, there is evidence of response to corticosteroids, either inhaled or systemic, unless there is a marked infective element [239]. There is also a report of an acute interstitial pneumonitis in association with ulcerative colitis and pyoderma gangrenosum, also responsive to corticosteroids [242].

Crohn's disease

Occasionally Crohn's disease, or regional enteritis, coexists with sarcoidosis, although despite the histological similarities between the two conditions this is very rare [243]. Apart from this, there are reports of interstitial lung disease, lung functional abnormalities and airway inflammation in association with Crohn's disease in both adults and children [239,244,245], though this appears to be less common than with ulcerative colitis. Amyloidosis involving the lungs may also occur [246].

Coeliac disease

There seems to be a complex relationship between coeliac disease and interstitial lung disease [247–251]. Occasionally, a syndrome of lung restriction indistinguishable from idiopathic fibrosis has been described in patients with coeliac disease. Moreover, it has been suggested that coeliac patients may be at excess risk of bird fancier's lung, although it should be noted that they often have bird antibodies in their blood derived from eggs in the diet and distinct from the true avian antibody associated with bird fancier's lung. It seems likely that there is a true but rare association of interstitial fibrosis with coeliac disease, the aetiology being obscure.

Whipple's disease

This condition of arthritis, weight loss, fever and steatorrhoea is characterized by fat-filled foamy macrophages and sarcoid-like granulomas in the intestinal wall and other affected tissues. It occurs mainly in middle-aged men and is caused by a Gram-positive bacillus also called after Whipple [252]. Some patients have been described as having patchy interstitial lung infiltrates and restrictive lung function [253].

Acute pancreatitis

Pleural effusion is a well-recognized accompaniment of acute pancreatitis (see Chapter 43). A proportion of patients acutely ill with pancreatitis may develop adult respiratory distress syndrome, and it is thought that this is due to release of inflammatory mediators in ascitic fluid that induce production of interleukin 1 and tumour necrosis factor in the lung [254,255]. Circulating pancreatic enzymes themselves may also be relevant and the author has seen one patient develop rapidly progressive lower zone emphysema after an acute attack of pancreatitis associated with very high amylase levels.

Waldenström's macroglobulinaemia

This is a condition akin to myeloma that occurs predominantly in elderly males and which is characterized by malaise, a bleeding tendency, hepatosplenomegaly and the presence of a paraprotein, usually IgM, in the blood. It generally runs a benign course. However, these patients are liable to pulmonary infections and occasionally present with pulmonary infiltrates of lymphoid or plasma cells, showing characteristic staining for the paraprotein [256,257]. In such cases, treatment with chlorambucil, melphalan or cyclophosphamide may be successful.

Renal dialysis and transplantation

Patients being treated for renal failure and those on immunosuppressants are at increased risk of pulmonary infection [258–262]. Patients on long-term dialysis may develop metastatic calcification and this has been reported to involve the lung to sufficient degree to cause respiratory failure and death. The patient presents with increasing dyspnoea, usually starting some months after the start of dialysis, and very fine pin-point shadowing may be visible on the chest film. It has also been described in patients after successful renal transplantation. CT and radiophosphate imaging provide useful methods of diagnosis when, as is often the case, the chest radiograph shows non-specific shadowing. The mechanism is usually thought to be deposition of calcium magnesium phosphate in the lungs as a result of secondary hyperparathyroidism due to low levels of 1,25-dihydroxyvitamin D_3, with reduced renal phosphate excretion. However, this seems unlikely to be the case in patients with successful renal transplants, in whom the mechanism remains obscure.

Neuromuscular disease

A wide variety of neuromuscular diseases, including muscular dystrophies, Parkinson's disease and myxoedema, may cause ventilatory insufficiency leading to recurrent infections through failure to clear secretions and to chronic respiratory failure. In selected patients, management has been much improved by domiciliary ventilatory support (see Chapter 58). These conditions are discussed in Chapter 45.

References

1 Hutchinson DCS. Natural history of alpha-1 protease deficiency. *Am J Med* 1988; 84: 3.
2 Carrell RW, Jeppsson J-O, Laurell C-B *et al.* Structure and variation of human α-1 antitrypsin. *Nature* 1982; 298: 329.
3 Fagerhol MK, Cox DW. The Pi polymorphism. Genetic, biochemical and clinical aspects of human antitrypsin. *Adv Hum Genet* 1981; 11: 1.
4 Kidd VJ, Wallace RB, Itakura K, Woo SLC. α1 Antitrypsin detection by direct analysis of the mutation in the gene. *Nature* 1983; 304: 230.
5 Crystal RG. The α1-antitrypsin gene and its deficiency states. *Trends Genet* 1989; 5: 411.
6 Lomas DA, Evans DLI, Finch JT, Carrell RW. The mechanism of Z α1-antitrypsin accumulation in the liver. *Nature* 1992; 357: 605.
7 Riccardi VM. Von Recklinghausen neurofibromatosis. *N Engl J Med* 1981; 305: 1617.
8 Upadhayaya M, Osborn MJ, Maynard J, Kim MR, Tamanoi F, Cooper DN. Mutational and functional analysis of the neurofibromatosis type 1 (NF1) gene. *Hum Genet* 1997; 99: 88.
9 Shen MH, Harper PS, Upadhayaya M. Molecular genetics of neurofibromatosis type 1 (NF1). *J Med Genet* 1996; 33: 2.
10 Ruttledge MH, Andermann AA, Phelan CM *et al.* Type of mutation in the neurofibromatosis type 2 gene (NF2) frequently determines severity of disease. *Am J Hum Genet* 1996; 59: 331.
11 Parry DM, MacCollin MM, Kaiser-Kupfer MI *et al.* Germ-line mutations in the neurofibromatosis 2 gene: correlations with disease severity and retinal abnormalities. *Am J Hum Genet* 1996; 59: 529.
12 Massaro D, Katz S, Matthews MJ, Higgins G. Von Recklinghausen's neurofibromatosis associated with cystic lung disease. *Am J Med* 1975; 38: 233.
13 Liberman BA, Chamberlain DW, Goldstein RS. Tuberous sclerosis with pulmonary involvement. *J Can Med Assoc* 1984; 130: 287.
14 Dawson J. Pulmonary tuberous sclerosis and its relationship to other forms of the disease. *Q J Med* 1954; 23: 113.
15 Van Slegtenhorst M, de Hoogt R, Hermans C *et al.* Identification of the tuberous sclerosis gene TSC1 on chromosome 9q34. *Science* 1997; 277: 805.

16 Xiao GH, Shoarinejad F, Jin F, Golemis EA, Yeung RS. The tuberous sclerosis gene product, tuberin, functions as a Rab5 GTPase activating protein (GAP) in modulating endocytosis. *J Biol Chem* 1997; 272: 6097.
17 Hams JO, Waltuck BL, Swenson EW. The pathophysiology of the lungs in tuberous sclerosis. A case report and literature review. *Am Rev Respir Dis* 1969; 100: 379.
18 Carney JA. The triad of gastric epithelioid leiomyosarcoma, functioning extra-adrenal paraganglionoma and pulmonary chondroma. *Cancer* 1979; 43: 374.
19 Broughton RBK. Primary tuberous sclerosis presenting with pleural effusion. *Br Med J* 1970; i: 477.
20 Luna CM, Gene R, Jolly EC *et al.* Pulmonary lymphangiomyomatosis associated with tuberous sclerosis. *Chest* 1985; 88: 473.
21 Westermann CJJ, Oostveen ACM, Wagenaar SS *et al.* Pulmonary tuberous sclerosis treated with tamoxifen and progesterone. *Thorax* 1986; 41: 892.
22 Wood JR, Bellamy D, Child AH, Citron KM. Pulmonary disease in patients with Marfan syndrome. *Thorax* 1984; 39: 780.
23 Hewett DR, Lynch JR, Smith R, Sykes BC. A novel fibrillin mutation in the Marfan's syndrome which could disrupt calcium binding of the epidermal growth factor-like module. *Hum Mol Genet* 1995; 2: 475.
24 McCusick VA. The defect in Marfan syndrome. *Nature* 1991; 352: 279.
25 Pyeritz RE, McKusick VA. The Marfan syndrome: diagnosis and management. *N Engl J Med* 1973; 300: 772.
26 Streeten EA, Murphy EA, Pyeritz RE. Pulmonary function in the Marfan syndrome. *Chest* 1987; 91: 408.
27 Ayres JG, Pope FM, Reidy JF, Clark TJH. Abnormalities of the lung and thoracic cage in the Ehlers–Danlos syndrome. *Thorax* 1985; 40: 300.
28 Smit J, Alberts C, Balk AG. Pneumothorax in the Ehlers–Danlos syndrome. Consequences or coincidence? *Scand J Respir Dis* 1978; 59: 239.
29 Robitaille GA. Ehlers–Danlos syndrome and recurrent haemoptysis. *Ann Intern Med* 1964; 61: 716.
30 Turner-Stokes L, Turton C, Pope FM, Green M. Emphysema and cutis laxa. *Thorax* 1983; 38: 790.

31 Beighton P. The dominant and recessive forms of cutis laxa. *J Med Genet* 1972; 9: 216.
32 Merten DF, Rooney R. Progressive pulmonary emphysema associated with congenital generalised elastolysis (cutis laxa). *Radiology* 1974; 113: 691.
33 Mehregen AH, Lee SC, Nabai H. Cutis laxa (generalised elastolysis). A report of four cases with autopsy findings. *J Cutan Pathol* 1978; 5: 116.
34 Davies BH, Tuddenham EGD. Familial pulmonary fibrosis associated with oculocutaneous albinism and platelet function defect. A new syndrome. *Q J Med* 1978; 45: 219.
35 Hermansky F, Pudlak F. Albinism associated with hemorrhagic diathesis and unusual pigmented reticular cells in the bone marrow: report of two cases with histochemical studies. *Blood* 1959; 14: 162.
36 Bednar B, Hermansky F, Lojda Z. Vascular pseudohemophilia associated with ceroid pigmentophagia in albinos. *Am J Pathol* 1964; 45: 283.
37 Fukai K, Frenk E, Almodovar C, Spritz RA. Linkage disequilibrium mapping of the gene for Hermansky–Pudlak syndrome to chromosome 10q23.1–q23.3. *Hum Mol Genet* 1995; 4: 1665.
38 Oh J, Bailin T, Fukai K *et al.* Positional cloning of a gene for Hermansky–Pudlak syndrome, a disorder of cytoplasmic organelles. *Nature Genet* 1996; 14: 300.
39 White DA, Smith GJW, Cooper JAD *et al.* Hermansky–Pudlak syndrome and interstitial lung disease: report of a case with lavage findings. *Am Rev Respir Dis* 1984; 130: 138.
40 Reynolds SP, Davies BH, Gibbs AR. Diffuse pulmonary fibrosis and the Hermansky–Pudlak syndrome: clinical course and postmortem findings. *Thorax* 1994; 49: 617.
41 Harmon KR, Witkop CJ, White JG *et al.* Pathogenesis of pulmonary fibrosis: platelet-derived growth factor precedes structural alterations in the Hermansky–Pudlak syndrome. *J Lab Clin Med* 1994; 123: 617.
42 Young RC, Castro O, Baxter RP *et al.* The lung in sickle disease: a clinical overview of common vascular, infectious and other problems. *J Natl Med Assoc* 1981; 73: 19.
43 Davies SC, Luce PJ, Win AA *et al.* Acute chest syndrome in sickle cell disease. *Lancet* 1984; i: 36.

44 Athanasou NA, Hatton C, McGee JOD, Weatherall DJ. Vascular occlusion and infarction in sickle cell crisis and the sickle chest syndrome. *J Clin Pathol* 1985; 38: 659.

45 Haupt HE, Moore BW, Bauer TW, Hutchins GM. The lung in sickle cell disease. *Chest* 1982; 81: 332.

46 Charache S, Scott JC, Charache P. Acute chest syndrome in adults with sickle cell anemia. *Arch Intern Med* 1979; 139: 67.

47 Sergeant GR. *Sickle Cell Disease*, 2nd edn. Oxford: Oxford University Press, 1992.

48 Gillett DS, Gunning KEJ, Sawicka EH *et al.* Life threatening sickle chest syndrome treated with extracorporal membrane oxygenation. *Br Med J* 1987; 294: 81.

49 Collins FS, Orringer EP. Pulmonary hypertension and cor pulmonale in the sickle hemoglobinopathies. *Am J Med* 1982; 73: 814.

50 Miller GJ, Sergeant GR. An assessment of lung volumes and transfer factor in sickle cell anaemia. *Thorax* 1971; 26: 309.

51 Miller GJ, Sergeant GR, Saunders MJ *et al.* Interpretation of lung function tests in the haemoglobinopathies. *Thorax* 1978; 33: 85.

52 Aggett PJ, Cavanagh NPC, Matthew DJ *et al.* Shwachman's syndrome. A review of 21 cases. *Arch Dis Child* 1980; 55: 331.

53 Cooper MD, Butler JL. Primary immunodeficiency diseases. In: Paul WE, ed. *Fundamental Immunology*, 2nd edn. New York: Raven Press, 1989.

54 WHO Scientific Group. Primary immunodeficiency diseases. *Clin Exp Immunol* 1995; 99 (Suppl 1).

55 Watts RWE, Gibbs DA. *Lysosomal Storage Diseases: Biochemical and Clinical Aspects.* London: Taylor & Francis, 1986.

56 Lever AML, Ryder JB. Cor pulmonale in an adult secondary to Niemann–Pick disease. *Thorax* 1983; 38: 873.

57 Eisenberg H. The interstitial lung diseases associated with the collagen-vascular disorders. *Clin Chest Med* 1982; 3: 565.

58 Hunninghake GW, Frauci AS. Pulmonary involvement in the collagen vascular diseases. *Am Rev Respir Dis* 1979; 119: 471.

59 Ellman P. The aetiology of chronic rheumatism. *Proc R Soc Med* 1947; 40: 332.

60 Ellman P, Ball RE. Rheumatoid disease, with joint and pulmonary manifestations. *Br Med J* 1948; ii: 816.

61 Caplan A. Certain unusual radiological appearances in the chest of coal-miners suffering from rheumatoid arthritis. *Thorax* 1953; 8: 29.

62 Anaya JM, Diethelm L, Ortiz LA *et al.* Pulmonary involvement in rheumatoid arthritis. *Semin Arthritis Rheum* 1995; 24: 242.

63 walker WG, Wright V. Rheumatoid pleuritis. *Ann Rheum Dis* 1967; 26: 467.

64 Carr DT, Mayne JG. Pleurisy with effusion in rheumatoid arthritis, with reference to the low concentration of glucose in pleural fluid. *Am Rev Respir Dis* 1962; 85: 345.

65 Dodson WH, Hollingsworth JW. Pleural effusion in rheumatoid arthritis. Impaired transport of glucose. *N Engl J Med* 1966; 275: 1337.

66 Nyberg P, Soderblom T, Pettersson T, Riska H, Klockars M, Linko L. Neurone-specific enolase in pleural effusions in patients with rheumatoid arthritis. *Thorax* 1996; 51: 92.

67 Boddington MM, Spriggs AI, Morton JA, Mowatt AG. Cytodiagnosis of rheumatoid pleural effusions. *J Clin Pathol* 1971; 24: 95.

68 Portner MM, Gracie WA. Rheumatoid lung disease with cavitary nodules, pneumothorax and eosinophilia. *N Engl J Med* 1966; 275: 697.

69 Panettière F, Chandler BF, Libcke JH. Pulmonary cavitation in rheumatoid disease. *Am Rev Respir Dis* 1968; 97: 89.

70 Thadani U. Rheumatoid lung disease with pulmonary fibrosis, necrobiotic nodules and pleural effusion. *Br J Dis Chest* 1973; 67: 146.

71 Eraut D, Evans J, Caplin M. Pulmonary necrobiotic nodules without rheumatoid arthritis. *Br J Dis Chest* 1978; 72: 301.

72 Stack BHR, Grant IWB. Rheumatoid interstitial lung disease. *Br J Dis Chest* 1965; 59: 202.

73 Doctor L, Snider GL. Diffuse interstitial pulmonary fibrosis associated with arthritis. *Am Rev Respir Dis* 1962; 85: 413.

74 Popper MS, Bogdonoff ML, Hughes RL. Interstitial rheumatoid lung disease: a reassessment and review of the literature. *Chest* 1972; 62: 243.

75 Hodson ME, Haslam PL, Spiro SG, Turner-Warwick M. Digital vasculitis in patients with cryptogenic fibrosing alveolitis. *Br J Dis Chest* 1984; 78: 140.

76 Scadding JG. The lungs in rheumatoid arthritis. *Proc R Soc Med* 1969; 62: 227.

77 Walker WG, Wright V. Pulmonary lesions and rheumatoid arthritis. *Medicine* 1968; 47: 501.

78 Patterson CD, Harville WE, Pierce JA. Rheumatoid lung disease. *Ann Intern Med* 1965; 62: 685.

79 Du Bois RM. Diffuse lung disease: combined clinical and laboratory studies. *J R Coll Physicians Lond* 1994; 28: 338.

80 Cruickshank B. Interstitial pneumonia and its consequences in rheumatoid disease. *Br J Dis Chest* 1959; 53: 226.

81 Turner-Warwick M. Auto-allergy and lung diseases. *J R Coll Physicians Lond* 1967; 2: 57.

82 De Horatius RJ, Albruzzo JL, Williams RC. Immunofluorescent and immunologic studies of rheumatoid lung. *Arch Intern Med* 1972; 129: 441.

83 Petrie GR, Bloomfield P, Grant IWB, Crompton GK. Upper lobe fibrosis and cavitation in rheumatoid disease. *Br J Dis Chest* 1980; 74: 263.

84 Spencer Jones J. Rheumatoid lung cavitation and response to penicillamine. *Thorax* 1987; 42: 988.

85 McGann BG, Hart GJ, Stokes TC, Harrison BDW. Obliterative bronchiolitis and upper zone consolidation in rheumatoid arthritis. *Thorax* 1983; 38: 73.

86 Locke GB. Rheumatoid lung. *Clin Radiol* 1963; 14: 43.

87 Jones JS. An account of pleural effusions, pulmonary nodules and cavities attributable to rheumatoid disease. *Br J Dis Chest* 1978; 72: 39.

88 Gabbay E, Tarala R, Will R *et al.* Interstitial lung disease in recent onset rheumatoid arthritis. *Am J Respir Crit Care Med* 1997; 156: 528.

89 Collins RL, Turner RA, Johnson AM *et al.* Obstructive pulmonary disease in rheumatoid arthritis. *Arthritis Rheum* 1976; 19: 623.

90 Geddes DM, Webley M, Emerson PA. Airways obstruction in rheumatoid arthritis. *Ann Rheum Dis* 1979; 38: 222.

91 Geddes DM, Corrin B, Brewerton DA *et al.* Progressive airway obliteration in adults and its association with rheumatoid disease. *Q J Med* 1977; 46: 427.

92 Epler GR, Snider GL, Gaensler EA *et al.* Bronchiolitis and bronchitis in connective tissue disease. A possible relationship to the use of penicillamine. *JAMA* 1979; 242: 528.

93 Schwarz MI, Lynch DA, Tuder R. Bronchiolitis obliterations: the lone manifestation of rheumatord arthritis? *Eur Respir J* 1994; 7: 817.

94 Turton CW, Williams G, Green M. Cryptogenic obliterative bronchiolitis in adults. *Thorax* 1981; 36: 805.

95 Murphy KC, Atkins CJ, Offer RC *et al.* Obliterative bronchiolitis in two rheumatoid arthritis patients treated with penicillamine. *Arthritis Rheum* 1981; 24: 557.

96 Aronoff A, Bywaters EGL, Fearnley GR. Lung lesions in rheumatoid arthritis. *Br Med J* 1955; ii: 228.

97 Mathieu J-P, Stack BHR, Dick WC, Buchanan WW. Pulmonary infection and rheumatoid arthritis. *Br J Dis Chest* 1978; 72: 57.

98 Cortet B, Flipo RM, Remy-Jardin M *et al.* Use of high resolution computed tomography of the lungs in patients with rheumatoid arthritis. *Ann Rheum Dis* 1995; 54: 815.

99 Shadick NA, Fanta CH, Weinblatt ME, O'Donnell W, Coblyn JS. Bronchiectasis: a late feature of severe rheumatoid arthritis. *Medicine* 1994; 73: 161.

100 Payne CR, Connellan SJ. Chronic eosinophilic pneumonia complicating long-standing rheumatoid arthritis. *Postgrad Med J* 1980; 56: 519.

101 Cooney TP. Interrelationship of chronic eosinophilic pneumonia, bronchiolitis obliterans, and rheumatoid disease: a hypothesis. *J Clin Pathol* 1981; 34: 129.

102 Gardner DL, Duthie JJR, McLeod J, Allan WSA. Pulmonary hypertension in rheumatoid arthritis. Report of a case with intimal sclerosis of the pulmonary and digital arteries. *Scott Med J* 1957; ii: 183.

103 Kay JM, Banik S. Unexplained pulmonary hypertension with pulmonary arteritis in rheumatoid disease. *Br J Dis Chest* 1977; 71: 53.

104 Macfarlane JD, Dieppe PA, Rigden BG, Clark TJH. Pulmonary and pleural lesions in rheumatoid disease. *Br J Dis Chest* 1978; 72: 288.

105 Tribe CR. Amyloidosis in rheumatoid arthritis. *Mod Trends Rheumatol* 1966; 1: 121.

106 Mole TM, Glover J, Sheppard MN. Sclerosing mediastinitis: a report on 18 cases. *Thorax* 1995; 50: 280.

107 Hellem SO, Kanner RE, Renzetti AD. Bronchocentric granulomatosis associated with rheumatoid arthritis. *Chest* 1983; 83: 831.

108 Berendsen HH, Hofstee N, Kapsenberg PD *et al.* Bronchocentric granulomatosis associated with seropositive polyarthritis. *Thorax* 1985; 40: 396.

109 Bonafede RP, Benatar SR. Bronchocentric granulomatosis and rheumatoid arthritis. *Br J Dis Chest* 1987; 81: 197.

110 Fessel WJ. Systemic lupus erythematosus in the community. Incidence, prevalence, outcome, and first symptoms; the high prevalence in black women. *Arch Intern Med* 1974; 134: 1027.

111 Ginzler EM, Diamond HS, Weiner M *et al.* A multicenter study of outcome in systemic lupus erythematosus. I. Entry variables as predictors of prognosis. *Arthritis Rheum* 1982; 25: 601.

112 Sim E, Gill EW, Sim RB. Drugs that induce

systemic lupus erythematosus inhibit complement component C4. *Lancet* 1984; ii: 422.

113 Ziskind M, Jones RN, Weill H. State of the art: silicosis. *Am Rev Respir Dis* 1976; 113: 643.

114 Koeger AC, Lang T, Alcaix D et al. Silica-associated connective tissue disease. *Medicine* 1995; 74: 221.

115 Shoenfeld Y, Schwartz RS. Immunologic and genetic factors in autoimmune disease. *N Engl J Med* 1984; 311: 1019.

116 Schwartz RS. Viruses and systemic lupus erythematosus. *N Engl J Med* 1975; 293: 131.

117 Segal AM, Calabrese LH, Ahmad M et al. The pulmonary manifestations of systemic lupus erythematosus. *Semin Arthritis Rheum* 1985; 14: 202.

118 Pines A, Kaplinsky N, Olchovsky D et al. Pleuropulmonary manifestations of systemic lupus erythematosus: clinical features of its subgroups. Prognostic and therapeutic implications. *Chest* 1985; 88: 129.

119 Brasington RO, Furth DE. Pulmonary disease in systemic lupus erythematosus. *Clin Exp Rheumatol* 1985; 3: 269.

120 Good JT, King TE, Antony VB, Sahn SA. Lupus pleuritis: clinical features and pleural fluid characteristics, with special reference to pleural fluid antinuclear antibodies. *Chest* 1980; 84: 714.

121 Good JT, King TE, Sahn SA. Native and drug-induced lupus pleuritis: a cause of low glucose, low pH pleural effusion. *Chest* 1980; 78: 518.

122 Miller LR, Greenberg SD, McLarty JW. Lupus lung. *Chest* 1985; 88: 265.

123 Matthay RA, Schwartz MI, Petty TL et al. Pulmonary manifestations of systemic lupus erythematosus: review of 12 cases of acute lupus pneumonitis. *Medicine* 1975; 54: 397.

124 Matthay RA, Hudson LD, Petty TL. Acute lupus pneumonitis. Response to azathioprine therapy. *Chest* 1973; 63: 117.

125 Haupt HM, Moore GW, Hutchins GM. The lung in systemic lupus erythematosus. Analysis of the pathologic changes in 120 patients. *Am J Med* 1981; 71: 791.

126 Susanto I, Peters JI. Acute lupus pneumonitis with normal chest radiograph. *Chest* 1997; 111: 1781.

127 Pertschuk LP, Moccia LF, Rosen Y et al. Acute pulmonary complications in systemic lupus erythematosus: immunofluorescence and light microscopic study. *Am J Clin Pathol* 1977; 68: 553.

128 Inoue T, Kanayama Y, Ohe A et al. Immunopathologic studies of pneumonitis in systemic lupus erythematosus. *Ann Intern Med* 1979; 91: 30.

129 Carette S, Macher AM, Nussbaum A, Plotz PH. Severe, acute pulmonary disease in patients with systemic lupus erythematosus: ten years of experience at the National Institutes of Health. *Semin Arthritis Rheum* 1984; 14: 52.

130 Eagen JW, Memoli VA, Roberts JL et al. Pulmonary hemorrhage in systemic lupus erythematosus. *Medicine* 1978; 57: 545.

131 Marino CT, Pertschuk LP. Pulmonary hemorrhage in systemic lupus erythematosus. *Arch Intern Med* 1981; 141: 201.

132 Zamora MR, Warner ML, Tuder R, Schwartz MI. Diffuse alveolar hemorrhage and systemic lupus erythematosus. Clinical presentation, histology, survival, and outcome. *Medicine* 1997; 76: 192.

133 Myers JL, Katzenstein A-LA. Microangiitis in lupus-induced pulmonary hemorrhage. *Am J Clin Pathol* 1986; 85: 552.

134 Groen H, Aslander M, van der Bootsma H, Mark TW, Kallenberg CG, Postma DS. Bronchoalveolar lavage cell analysis and lung function impairment in patients with systemic lupus erythematosus (SLE). *Clin Exp Immunol* 1993; 94: 127.

135 Cerveri I, Fanfulla F, Ravelli A et al. Pulmonary function in children with systemic lupus erythematosus. *Thorax* 1996; 51: 424.

136 Eisenberg H, Dubois EL, Sherwin RP, Balchum OJ. Diffuse interstitial lung disease in systemic lupus erythematosus. *Ann Intern Med* 1973; 79: 37.

137 Eisenberg H, Simmons DH, Barnett EV. Diffuse pulmonary interstitial disease: an immunohistologic study. *Chest* 1979; 75 (Suppl): 262.

138 Holgate ST, Glass DN, Haslam P et al. Respiratory involvement in systemic lupus erythematosus: a clinical and immunological study. *Clin Exp Immunol* 1976; 24: 385.

139 Hoffbrand BI, Beck ER. Unexplained dyspnoea and 'shrinking' lungs in systemic lupus erythematosus. *Br Med J* 1965; i: 1273.

140 Gibson GJ, Edmonds JP, Hughes GRV. Diaphragm function and lung involvement in systemic lupus erythematosus. *Am J Med* 1977; 63: 926.

141 Martens J, Demedts M, Vanmeenen MT, Dequeker J. Respiratory muscle dysfunction in systemic lupus erythematosus. *Chest* 1984; 84: 170.

142 Thompson PJ, Dhillon DP, Ledingham J, Turner-Warwick M. Shrinking lungs, diaphragmatic dysfunction, and systemic lupus erythematosus. *Am Rev Respir Dis* 1985; 132: 926.

143 Gould DM, Daves ML. A review of roentgen findings in systemic lupus erythematosus. *Am J Med Sci* 1958; 235: 596.

144 Levin DC. Proper interpretation of pulmonary roentgen changes in systemic lupus erythematosus. *Am J Radiol* 1971; 111: 510.

145 Alarcón-Segovia D, Alarcón DG. Pleuropulmonary manifestations of systemic lupus erythematosus. *Dis Chest* 1961; 39: 7.

146 Rosner S, Ginzler E, Diamond H et al. A multicenter study of outcome in systemic lupus erythematosus. II. Causes of death. *Arthritis Rheum* 1982; 25: 612.

147 Hellmann DB, Petri M, Whiting-O'Keefe Q. Fatal infections in systemic lupus erythematosus: the role of opportunistic organisms. *Medicine* 1987; 66: 341.

148 Wallaert B, Aerts C, Bart F et al. Alveolar macrophage dysfunction in systemic lupus erythematosus. *Am Rev Respir Dis* 1987; 136: 293.

149 Hughes GRV. Thrombosis, abortion, cerebral disease and the lupus anticoagulant. *Br Med J* 1983; 287: 1088.

150 Boey ML, Colaco CB, Gharavi AE et al. Thrombosis in systemic lupus erythematosus: striking association with the presence of circulating lupus anticoagulant. *Br Med J* 1983; 287: 1021.

151 Perez H, Kramer N. Pulmonary hypertension in systemic lupus erythematosus: report of four cases and review of the literature. *Semin Arthritis Rheum* 1981; 11: 177.

152 Asherson RA, Mackworth-Young CG, Boey ML et al. Pulmonary hypertension in systemic lupus erythematosus. *Br Med J* 1983; 287: 1024.

153 Yum MN, Ziegler JR, Walker PD et al. Pseudolymphoma of the lung in a patient with systemic lupus erythematosus. *Am J Med* 1979; 66: 172.

154 Nomura S, Kumagai N, Kanoh T et al. Pulmonary amyloidosis associated with systemic lupus erythematosus. *Arthritis Rheum* 1986; 29: 680.

155 Rocco VK, Hurd ER. Scleroderma and scleroderma-like syndromes. *Semin Arthritis Rheum* 1986; 16: 22.

156 Bulkley BH, Ridolfi RL, Salyer WR, Hutchins GM. Myocardial lesions of progressive systemic sclerosis: a cause of cardiac dysfunction. *Circulation* 1976; 53: 483.

157 McWhorter JE, LeRoy EC. Pericardial disease in scleroderma (systemic sclerosis). *Am J Med* 1974; 57: 566.

158 Roberts N, Cabeen W, Moss J et al. The prevalence of conduction defects and cardiac arrhythmias in progressive systemic sclerosis. *Ann Intern Med* 1981; 94: 38.

159 Owens GR, Follansbee WP. Cardiopulmonary manifestations of systemic sclerosis. *Chest* 1987; 91: 118.

160 Medsger TA, Masi AT. The epidemiology of systemic sclerosis (scleroderma) among US male veterans. *J Chron Dis* 1978; 31: 73.

161 Sluis-Cremer GK, Hessel PA, Nizolo EH et al. Silica, silicosis and progressive systemic sclerosis. *Br J Ind Med* 1985; 42: 838.

162 Veltman G, Lange C-E, Juhe S et al. Clinical manifestations and course of vinyl chloride disease. *Ann N Y Acad Sci* 1975; 246: 6.

163 Matteo IM, Izquierdo M, Fernandez-Dapica MP et al. Toxic epidemic syndrome: musculoskeletal manifestations. *J Rheumatol* 1984; 11: 333.

164 Cohen IS, Mosher MB, O'Keefe EJ et al. Cutaneous toxicity of bleomycin therapy. *Arch Dermatol* 1973; 107: 553.

165 Manoussakis MN, Constantopoulos SH, Gharavi AE, Moutsopoulos HM. Pulmonary involvement in systemic sclerosis: association with anti-Scl 70 antibody and digital pitting. *Chest* 1987; 92: 509.

166 Steen V, Owens G, Fino G et al. Pulmonary involvement in systemic sclerosis (scleroderma). *Arthritis Rheum* 1985; 28: 759.

167 D'Angelo WA, Fries JF, Masi AT, Shulman LE. Pathologic observations in systemic sclerosis (scleroderma). *Am J Med* 1969; 46: 428.

168 Wells AU, Hansell DM, Rubens MB et al. Fibrosing alveolitis in systemic sclerosis: indices of lung function in relation to extent of disease on computed tomography. *Arthritis Rheum* 1997; 40: 1229.

169 Chan TW, Hansell DM, Rubens MB, du Bois RM, Wells AU. Cryptogenic fibrosing alveolitis and fibrosing alveolitis of systemic sclerosis: morphological differences on computed tomographic scans. *Thorax* 1997; 52: 265.

170 Owens G, Fino G, Herbert D et al. Pulmonary function in progressive systemic sclerosis: comparison of CREST syndrome variant with diffuse scleroderma. *Chest* 1983; 84: 546.

171 Owens GR, Paradis IL, Gryzan S et al. The role of inflammation in the lung disease of systemic sclerosis: comparison with idiopathic pulmonary fibrosis. *J Lab Clin Med* 1986; 107: 253.

172 Rossi GA, Bitterman PB, Rennard SI *et al.* Evidence for chronic inflammation as a component of the interstitial lung disease associated with progressive systemic sclerosis. *Am Rev Respir Dis* 1985; 131: 612.

173 Wells AU, Hansell DM, Rubens MB *et al.* Fibrosing alveolitis in systemic sclerosis. Bronchoalveolar lavage findings in relation to computed tomographic appearance. *Am J Respir Crit Care Med* 1994; 150: 462.

174 Behr J, Vogelmeier C, Beinert T *et al.* Bronchoalveolar lavage for evaluation and management of scleroderma disease of the lung. *Am J Respir Crit Care Med* 1996; 154: 400.

175 Young RH, Mark GJ. Pulmonary vascular changes in scleroderma. *Am J Med* 1978; 64: 998.

176 Abraham DJ, Vancheeswaran R, Dashwood MR *et al.* Increased levels of endothelin-1 and differential endothelin type A and B receptor expression in scleroderma-associated fibrotic lung disease. *Am J Pathol* 1997; 151: 831.

177 Imokawa S, Sato A, Hayakawa H, Kotani M, Urano T, Takada A. Tissue factor expression and fibrin deposition in the lungs of patients with idiopathic pulmonary fibrosis and systemic sclerosis. *Am J Respir Crit Care Med* 1997; 156: 631.

178 Wells AU, Hansell DM, Rubens MB, Cailes JB, Black CM, du Bois RM. Functional impairment in lone cryptogenic fibrosing alveolitis and fibrosing a lveolitis associated with systemic sclerosis: a comparison. *Am J Respir Crit Care Med* 1997; 155: 1657.

179 Stupi A, Steen V, Owens G *et al.* Pulmonary hypertension in the CREST syndrome variant of systemic sclerosis. *Arthritis Rheum* 1986; 29: 515.

180 Ungerer RG, Tashkin DP, Furst D *et al.* Prevalence and clinical correlates of pulmonary arterial hypertension in progressive systemic sclerosis. *Am J Med* 1983; 75: 65.

181 Steckel RJ, Bein ME, Kelly PM. Pulmonary arterial hypertension in progressive systemic sclerosis. *Am J Roentgenol* 1975; 124: 461.

182 Chausow AM, Kane T, Levinson D, Szidon JP. Reversible hypercapnic respiratory insufficiency in scleroderma caused by muscle weakness. *Am Rev Respir Dis* 1984; 130: 142.

183 Davison AG, Epstein O. Relapsing organising pneumonitis in a man with primary biliary cirrhosis, CREST syndrome, and chronic pancreatitis. *Thorax* 1983; 38: 316.

184 Steen VD, Owens GR, Redmond C *et al.* The effect of D-penicillamine on pulmonary findings in systemic sclerosis. *Arthritis Rheum* 1985; 28: 882.

185 Steen VD, Medsger TA, Rodnan GP. D-Penicillamine therapy in progressive systemic sclerosis (scleroderma): a retrospective analysis. *Ann Intern Med* 1982; 97: 652.

186 Steen VD, Lanz JK, Conte C, Owens GR, Medsger TA. Therapy for severe interstitial lung disease in systemic sclerosis. A retrospective study. *Arthritis Rheum* 1994; 37: 1290.

187 Ocken S, Reinitz E, Strom J. Nifedine treatment for pulmonary hypertension in a patient with systemic sclerosis. *Arthritis Rheum* 1983; 26: 794.

188 Rozkovec A, Bernstein R, Asherson RA, Oakley CM. Vascular reactivity and pulmonary hypertension in systemic sclerosis. *Arthritis Rheum* 1983; 76: 1037.

189 Moutsopoulos HM, Chused TM, Mann DL

et al. Sjögren's syndrome (sicca syndrome): current issues. *Ann Intern Med* 1980; 92: 212.

190 Strimlan CV, Rosenow EC, Divertie MB, Harrison EG. Pulmonary manifestations of Sjögren's syndrome. *Chest* 1976; 70: 354.

191 Oxholm P, Bundgaard A, Madsen EB *et al.* Pulmonary function in patients with primary Sjögren's syndrome. *Rheumatol Int* 1982; 2: 179.

192 Constantopoulos SH, Papadimitriou CS, Moutsopoulos HM. Respiratory manifestations in primary Sjögren's syndrome. A clinical, functional and histologic study. *Chest* 1985; 88: 226.

193 Fairfax AJ, Haslam PL, Pavia D *et al.* Pulmonary disorders associated with Sjögren's syndrome. *Q J Med* 1981; 50: 279.

194 Matieu A, Cauli A, Pala R *et al.* Tracheobronchial mucociliary clearance in patients with primary and secondary Sjögren's syndrome. *Scand J Rheumatol* 1995; 24: 300.

195 Deheinzelin D, Capelozzi VL, Kairalla RA, Barbas Filho JV, Saldiva PH, de Carvalho CR. Interstitial lung disease in primary Sjögren's syndrome. Clinical–pathological evaluation and response to treatment. *Am J Respir Crit Care Med* 1996; 154: 794.

196 Gardiner P, Ward C, Allison A *et al.* Pleuropulmonary abnormalities in primary Sjögren's syndrome. *J Rheumatol* 1993; 20: 831.

197 Anderson LG, Talal N. The spectrum of benign to malignant lymphoproliferation in Sjögren's syndrome. *Clin Exp Immunol* 1972; 10: 199.

198 Mialon P, Barthelemy L, Sebert P *et al.* A longitudinal study of lung function with primary Sjögren's syndrome. *Clin Exp Rheumatol* 1997; 15: 349.

199 Ogryzlo MA, Rosen PS. Ankylosing (Marie–Strumpell) spondylitis. *Postgrad Med J* 1969; 45: 182.

200 Brewerton DA. HLA-B27 and the inheritance of susceptibility to rheumatic disease. *Arthritis Rheum* 1976; 19: 656.

201 Resnick DL. Patterns of peripheral joint disease in ankylosing spondylitis. *Radiology* 1974; 110: 523.

202 Zorab PA. The lungs in ankylosing spondylitis. *Q J Med* 1962; 31: 267.

203 Gacad G, Hamosh P. The lung in ankylosing spondylitis. *Am Rev Respir Dis* 1973; 107: 286.

204 Davies D. Ankylosing spondylitis and upper lobe fibrosis. *Q J Med* 1972; 41: 395.

205 Rosenow EC, Strimlan CV, Muhn JR, Ferguson RH. Pleuropulmonary manifestations of ankylosing spondylitis. *Mayo Clinic Proc* 1977; 52: 641.

206 Fisher LR, Cawley MI, Holgate ST. Relation between chest expansion, pulmonary function, and exercise tolerance in patients with ankylosing spondylitis. *Ann Rheum Dis* 1990; 49: 921.

207 Hillerdal G. Ankylosing spondylitis lung disease: an underdiagnosed entity? *Eur J Respir Dis* 1983; 64: 437.

208 Elliot JA, Milne LJ, Cumming D. Chronic necrotising aspergillosis treated with itraconazole. *Thorax* 1985; 44: 820.

209 Levy H, Hurwitz MD, Strimling M, Zwi S. Ankylosing spondylitis lung disease and *Mycobacterium scrofulaceum*. *Br J Dis Chest* 1988; 82: 84.

210 Bohan A, Peter JB, Bowman RL, Pearson CM. A computer-assisted analysis of 153

patients with polymyositis and dermatomyositis. *Medicine* 1977; 56: 255.

211 Schwarz MI, Matthay RA, Salm S *et al.* Interstitial lung disease in polymyositis and dermatomyositis: analysis of six cases and review of the literature. *Medicine* 1976; 55: 89.

212 Songcharoen S, Raju SF, Pennebaker JB. Interstitial lung disease in polymyositis and dermatomyositis. *Rheumatol* 1980; 7: 353.

213 Plotz PH, Dalakas M, Leff RL, Love LA, Miller FW, Cronin ME. Current concepts in the idiopathic inflammatory mypathies: polymyositis, dermatomyositis, and related disorders. *Ann Intern Med* 1989; 111: 143.

214 Fergusson RJ, Davidson NMcD, Nuki G, Crompton GK. Dermatomyositis and rapidly progressive fibrosing alveolitis. *Thorax* 1983; 38: 71.

215 Hashimoto Y, Natawa Y, Kurasawa K *et al.* Investigation of EB virus and cytomegalovirus in rapidly progressive interstitial pneumonitis in polymyositis/dermatomyositis by *in situ* hybridisation and polymerase chain reaction. *Clin Immunol Immunopath* 1995; 77: 298.

216 Tazelaar HD, Viggiano RW, Pickersgill J, Colby TV. Interstitial lung disease in polymyositis and dermatomyositis. Clinical features and prognosis as correlated with histologic findings. *Am Rev Respir Dis* 1990; 141: 727.

217 Sharp GC, Irvin WS, Tan EM *et al.* Mixed connective tissue disease: an apparently distinct rheumatic disease syndrome associated with a specific antibody to an extractable nuclear antigen (ENA). *Am J Med* 1972; 52: 148.

218 Prakash UBS, Luthra HS, Divertie MB. Intrathoracic manifestations in mixed connective tissue disease. *Mayo Clin Proc* 1985; 60: 813.

219 Wagenaar SS, Westermann CJJ, Corrin B. Giant cell arteritis limited to large elastic pulmonary arteries. *Thorax* 1981; 36: 876.

220 Karam GH, Fulmer JD. Giant cell arteritis presenting as interstitial lung disease. *Chest* 1982; 82: 781.

221 Chajek T, Fainaru M. Behçet's disease: report of 41 cases and a review of the literature. *Medicine* 1975; 54: 179.

222 Efthimiou J, Johnston C, Spiro SG, Turner-Warwick M. Pulmonary disease in Behçet's syndrome. *Q J Med* 1986; 58: 259.

223 Jarrett PEM, Morland M, Browse NL. Idiopathic recurrent superficial thrombophlebitis: treatment with fibrinolytic enhancement. *Br Med J* 1977; i: 933.

224 Hughes JP, Stovin PGI. Segmental pulmonary artery aneurysms with peripheral venous thrombosis. *Br J Dis Chest* 1959; 53: 19.

225 Kopp WL, Green RA. Pulmonary artery aneurysms with recurrent thrombophlebitis: the 'Hughes–Stovin syndrome'. *Ann Intern Med* 1962; 56: 105.

226 McAdam LP, O'Hanlan MA, Bluestone R, Pearson CM. Relapsing polychondritis: prospective study of 23 patients and a review of the literature. *Medicine* 1976; 55: 193.

227 Gibson GJ, Davis P. Respiratory complications of relapsing polychondritis. *Thorax* 1974; 29: 726.

228 Mohsenifar Z, Tashkin DP, Carson SA, Bellamy PE. Pulmonary function in patients

with relapsing polychondritis. *Chest* 1982; 81: 711.

229 Neilly JB, Winter JH, Stevenson RD. Progressive tracheobronchial polychondritis: need for early diagnosis. *Thorax* 1985; 40: 78.

230 Rogerson ME, Higgins EM, Godfrey RC. Tracheal stenosis due to relapsing polychondritis in rheumatoid arthritis. *Thorax* 1987; 42: 905.

231 Rich AR, Gregory JE. On the anaphylactic nature of rheumatic pneumonitis. *Bull Johns Hopkins Hosp* 1943; 73: 465.

232 McIntyre MC. Pulmonary syphilis: its frequency, pathology and roentgenologic appearance. *Arch Pathol* 1931; 11: 258.

233 Morgan AD, Lloyd WE, Price-Thomas C. Tertiary syphilis of the lung and its diagnosis. *Thorax* 1952; 7: 125.

234 Dormer BA, Friedlander J, Wiles FJ. Syphilis of the lung in Bantus. *Br J Tuberc* 1945; 39: 85.

235 Weaver RC, Branfoot AC. Gumma of the lung: a case confirmed by thoracotomy and biopsy. *Br J Dis Chest* 1970; 64: 238.

236 Godet PG, Cowie R, Woodman RC, Sutherland LR. Pulmonary function abnormalities in patients with ulcerative colitis. *Am J Gastroenterol* 1997; 92: 1154.

237 Higenbottam T, Cochrane GM, Clark TJH *et al.* Bronchial disease in ulcerative colitis. *Thorax* 1980; 35: 581.

238 Butland RJA, Cole P, Citron KM, Turner-Warwick M. Chronic bronchial suppuration and inflammatory bowel disease. *Q J Med* 1981; 50: 63.

239 Camus P, Piard F, Ashcroft T, Gal AA, Colby TV. The lung in inflammatory bowel disease. *Medicine* 1993; 72: 151.

240 Kraft SC, Earle RH, Roesler M, Esterly JR. Unexplained bronchopulmonary disease with inflammatory bowel disease. *Arch Intern Med* 1976; 136: 454.

241 Gibb WRG, Dhillon DP, Zilkha KJ, Cole PJ. Bronchiectasis with ulcerative colitis and myelopathy. *Thorax* 1987; 42: 155.

242 McCulloch AJ, McEvoy A, Jackson JD, Jarvis EH. Severe steroid-responsive pneumonitis associated with pyoderma gangrenosum and ulcerative colitis. *Thorax* 1985; 40: 314.

243 Johard U, Berlin M, Eklund A. Sarcoidosis and regional enteritis in two patients. *Sarcoid Vasculitis Diff Lung Dis* 1996; 13: 50.

244 Levine JB, Lukawski-Trubish D. Extraintestinal considerations in inflammatory bowel disease. *Gastroenterol Clin North Am* 1995; 24: 633.

245 Munck A, Murciano D, Pariente R, Cezard JP, Navarro J. Latent pulmonary function abnormalities in children with Crohn's disease. *Eur Respir J* 1995; 8: 377.

246 Beer TW, Edwards CW. Pulmonary nodules due to reactive systemic amyloidosis (AA) in Crohn's disease. *Thorax* 1993; 48: 1287.

247 Wright DH. The major complications of coeliac disease. *Clin Gastroenterol* 1995; 9: 351.

248 Lancaster Smith MJ, Benson MK, Strickland ID. Coeliac disease and diffuse interstitial lung disease. *Lancet* 1971; i: 473.

249 Hood J, Mason AMH. Diffuse pulmonary disease with transfer defect occurring with coeliac disease. *Lancet* 1970; i: 445.

250 Berrill WT, Eade OE, Fitzpatrick PF *et al.* Birdfancier's lung and jejunal villous atrophy. *Lancet* 1975; ii: 1006.

251 Hendrick DJ, Faux JA, Anand B *et al.* Is bird fancier's lung associated with coeliac disease? *Thorax* 1978; 33: 425.

252 Keren DF. 'Whipple's disease': the causative agent defined, its etiology remains obscure. *Medicine* 1993; 72: 355.

253 Symmons DPM, Shepherd AN, Boardman PL, Bacon P. Pulmonary manifestations of Whipple's disease. *Q J Med* 1985; 56: 497.

254 Denham W, Yang J, Norman J. Evidence for an unknown component of pancreatic ascites that induces adult respiratory distress syndrome through an interleukin-1 and tumor necrosis factor-dependent mechanism. *Surgery* 1997; 122: 295.

255 Montravers P, Chollet-Martin S, Marmuse JP, Gougerot-Pocidalo MA, Demonts JM. Lymphatic release of cytokines during acute lung injury complicating severe pancreatitis. *Am J Respir Crit Care Med* 1995; 152: 1527.

256 Kobayaski H, Kunio I, Hizawa K, Maeda T. Two cases of pulmonary Waldenström's macroglobulinaemia. *Chest* 1985; 88: 297.

257 Filuk RB, Warren PW. Bronchoalveolar lavage in Waldenström's macroglobulinaemia with pulmonary infiltrates. *Thorax* 1986; 41: 409.

258 Justrabo E, Genin R, Rifle G. Pulmonary metastatic calcification with respiratory insufficiency in patients on maintenance haemodialysis. *Thorax* 1979; 34: 384.

259 Evans TW, Collins M, Adams JE *et al.* Pulmonary calcification in a renal transplant recipient. *Br J Dis Chest* 1983; 77: 202.

260 Gilman M, Nissim J, Terry P, Welton A. Metastatic pulmonary calcification in the renal transplant recipient. *Am Rev Respir Dis* 1980; 121: 415.

261 McLachlan MSF, Wallace M, Seneviratne C. Pulmonary calcification in renal failure. Report of three cases. *Br J Radiol* 1968; 41: 99.

262 Breitz HB, Sirotta PS, Nelp WB *et al.* Progressive pulmonary calcification complicating successful renal transplantation. *Am Rev Respir Dis* 1987; 136: 1480.

54

OCCUPATIONAL LUNG DISEASES

ANTHONY SEATON

Most of the diseases with which this book is concerned are probably caused by the inhalation of harmful matter, be it microorganisms, tobacco smoke, allergens or other particles. While these broad classes of substances may be encountered in the general environment, many of them occur also in the workplace in greater amounts as a result of industrial processes; a broad range of lung reactions may therefore occur as a result of workplace exposure.

Historical aspects

It is likely that humans have suffered from occupational asthma since the change from hunting to agriculture as a means of providing food. However, the first recorded mention of breathlessness among handlers of grain was by Ramazzini, the father of occupational medicine, in 1713 [1]. The harmful effects of mining probably also date back to prehistory, when humans first started to dig underground for flints to make arrowheads and axes and thus exposed themselves to quartz dust. Certainly in Roman times it was recorded that mining was a dangerous trade, fit only for convicts and slaves. In 1556 Georgius Agricola [2] recorded the dangers of suffocation underground due to toxic fumes and pointed out that breathlessness due to inhalation of dust resulted in the premature death of many miners. However, these early accounts appear to have been sporadic and it was not until the Industrial Revolution in Britain that the coincidence of increasing amounts of occupational disease and adequate medical and scientific expertise allowed rapid progress to be made in their understanding. The diseases that came to attention at this time, in the eighteenth and early nineteenth centuries, were those afflicting knife grinders, pottery workers, coal-miners and stonemasons, the classical mineral pneumoconioses. By the middle of the nineteenth century, silicosis had been differentiated from tuberculosis [3] (which was of course rife in the new industrial cities at that time) and a peculiar black pigmentation of the lungs had been described in Scottish coal-miners [4]. Occupational exposure was also known to cause asthma occasionally [5].

In 1775, before the earliest descriptions of pneumoconiosis, cancer of the skin had been recognized by Pott as an occupational disease in the apprentices of chimney sweeps [6], and lung cancer was first described as an occupational disease in German metal miners in 1879 [7]. Indeed, it was as a result of the recognition that occupational factors were relevant to the genesis of cancer that scientists first started to study this disease and its mechanisms.

The twentieth century has seen an increasing recognition of the many lung diseases that can be caused by exposure to harmful substances in the workplace. Increasing use of asbestos from about 1900 until the middle of the century was clearly shown to be related to pulmonary fibrosis in 1930 [8], bronchial carcinoma in 1949 and mesothelioma in 1960 [9,10]. A range of other lung carcinogens, including radiation, arsenic, nickel, chromates and halo ethers, was described. The first of many causes of allergic alveolitis, inhalation of mouldy hay, was recorded in 1932 [11], and subsequently many other causes of this disease and of occupational asthma have been recognized. Berylliosis was described first in Germany in 1933 and in the USA in 1943 [12,13]. The public has been made dramatically aware of possible workplace hazards by a series of horrifying episodes of industrial gassings, the worst of which killed many thousands of people living around Bhopal in India in 1985, when a cloud of methyl isocyanate escaped from a factory producing pesticides [14].

Types and frequency of disease

It is now clear that many of the broad types of bronchopulmonary disease may be caused or made worse by exposure to harmful substances in the workplace. Thus pulmonary fibrosis may result from exposure to asbestos or quartz, pulmonary oedema and bronchiolitis from inhalation of toxic gas, allergic responses from exposure to organic dusts and some chemicals acting as haptens, pleurisy from inhalation of asbestos, cancer from a range of carcinogens, and infection from workplace exposure to microorganisms. The workplace may be only one factor in the causation of some of these conditions, which are discussed in more detail elsewhere in the book. A summary of lung responses to workplace hazards is given in Table 54.1.

It is difficult to know how widespread occupational lung disease is, even in advanced nations. Data obtained from workman's compensation and disability awards are likely to include only cases that fulfil quite strict criteria for diagnosis, usually from a rather selective list of conditions. Similarly, data from statutory notifications of disease are only representative of those required to be notified and again are often the tip of an iceberg. On the other hand, surveys of population samples are likely to have to rely largely on self-determination of the causes of illness and therefore probably overestimate prevalence. In the British Labour Force Survey of 1990, which questioned a random sample of the workforce in 60 000 households, some questions were added about occupational disease. The response indicated that of a workforce of about 20 million, some 30 000 people had asthma and 60 000 had other lung disease that they attributed to their work, in addition to a substantial number who thought that their lung disease was made worse by their work [15]. While these figures probably represent an overestimate, they should not be dismissed lightly, since patients often discover the relationship of their illness to work before their doctors. It might be argued that patients in general have an unsophisticated concept of disease causation, but often so do doctors. In particular, clinicians have a marked tendency to attribute disease to one cause, when epidemiology teaches that with most diseases there are multiple possible aetiological contributors. For example, it is usual

to attribute lung cancer or chronic airflow obstruction to smoking if the patient does indeed smoke. However, many epidemiological studies have shown that workers in a number of dusty industries have an increased risk of one or other of these diseases compared with non-exposed people of the same smoking status. Thus, although it can never be proved in an individual case with clinical certainty, in a population of dust-exposed workers there may be individuals who would not have developed disabling lung disease had they not been exposed to the workplace hazard. Who is to say that such people are wrong in attributing their illness to work rather than cigarettes when it is likely that both have played a part?

Perhaps the best information currently available comes from the UK SWORD survey, in which occupational and chest physicians report cases of what they think are occupationally caused lung disease on a regular and confidential basis [16,17]. Although almost certainly giving an underestimate because of failure to sample all those doctors who see such patients, this allows some estimate of incidence of such diseases to be made. Results from recent surveys have shown, as expected, that asthma and mesothelioma rank as the most commonly recognized conditions, being reported in about 950 and 650 patients each year respectively. There are good reasons to believe that the true incidences of these conditions in the UK are approximately 3000 and 1000 respectively. Two other conditions are apparently more common than was originally anticipated: acute inhalation injury, which is reported in about 300 people each year, and the syndrome of bronchial hyperreactivity following such exposures, sometimes called reactive airways dysfunction syndrome. The latter condition is responsible for a proportion, as yet undeter-

Table 54.1 Lung responses to workplace hazards.

Type of disease	Postulated mechanism	Typical exposure
Diffuse fibrosis	Macrophage-mediated Delayed hypersensitivity	Asbestos Beryllium
Nodular fibrosis	Macrophage-mediated	Quartz, coal
Emphysema	Neutrophil elastase release	Coal, cadmium
Chronic bronchitis	Airway inflammation	Dusts and fumes
Acute bronchitis	Airway inflammation	Irritant gases and fumes
Airway hyperreactivity, bronchiolitis obliterans,		
Asthma	Airway hypersensitivity	Flour, wood, isocyanates
Byssinosis	Endotoxin complement activation	Cotton dust
Allergic alveolitis	Complement activation Cytokine release	Thermophilic actinomycetes
Bronchial carcinoma	DNA damage	Asbestos, chloromethyl ether
Pleural mesothelioma	DNA damage	Asbestos

mined, of reports registered under both asthma and inhalation injury categories. It is likely that the same relative frequencies of different occupational lung diseases as reported in SWORD are present in other industrialized countries, although the actual numbers will differ in relation to the efforts made nationally to prevent them.

Deposition and clearance of particles

The details of the lung's defences are described in Chapter 4. In brief, the harmfulness of an inhaled particle depends on its inherent toxicity, its ability to penetrate to the site at which it can exert its effects and the amount retained in the lung. Penetration depends on the ability of the particle to overcome the physical forces tending to bring it into contact with the walls of the airways, namely sedimentation, impaction, interception, diffusion and electrostatic precipitation [18].

1 Sedimentation, or movement under the influence of gravity, proceeds at a rate that depends on the density and the square of the diameter of the particle; thus large dense particles fall rapidly and are deposited primarily in the nose, mouth and larger airways.

2 Impaction occurs when a particle fails to follow a change in direction of airflow and strikes the airway wall; it depends on the particle's momentum (the product of mass and velocity) so again large particles are filtered out by the larger airways.

3 Interception is a factor in the deposition of fibrous aerosols, when the ends of long thin particles strike the airway wall.

4 Diffusion occurs as a result of Brownian motion, due to bombardment of very small particles by gas molecules in the air, and is particularly important with respect to deposition on alveolar walls of particles of less than 0.5 µm. It is also the mechanism whereby inhaled toxic gases exert their effects on the airways and alveoli.

5 Electrostatic precipitation was until recently not thought to be important because of the conducting properties of mucus. However, studies in rats have shown considerably greater lung retention of highly charged compared with uncharged particles, suggesting that the effect of charge may be pathologically significant [19].

An indication of the likelihood of a particle's deposition in various parts of the respiratory tract in relation to its aerodynamic diameter, i.e. its diameter expressed in terms of it behaving as a sphere of unit density, is shown in Fig. 54.1 [20]. Another representation of lung deposition patterns is given in Fig. 54.2, which shows that the highest rate of alveolar deposition occurs with a particle size around 0.02–0.06 µm (20–60 nm). This is the size range of particles in fume and in the nucleation mode of ambient air pollution [21].

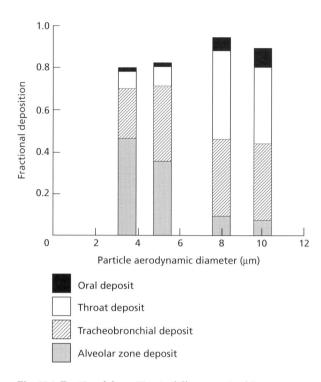

Fig. 54.1 Fractional deposition in different parts of the respiratory tract of particles of differing aerodynamic diameters. (From Emmett *et al.* [20].)

Knowledge of the physical behaviour of particles in the respiratory tract is particularly important in the design of dust-sampling instruments. These play a crucial part in monitoring the exposure of workers to aerosols in the workplace and, increasingly, in measuring exposures as part of epidemiological studies aimed at producing information about exposure–response relationships on which preventive action can be based (see Chapter 3). Such instruments are now available that can measure 'respirable' particles (<7 µm), PM_{10} (<10 µm) (Fig. 54.3) [22] and 'inspirable' particles that closely resemble in size those passing into the human nose and respiratory tract [23]; others can fractionate a mixed dust cloud into particles of different aerodynamic sizes. All these instruments allow the dusts to be weighed. However, not yet available is a simple method for measuring asbestos or other fibres in the air. These still have to be collected on a filter and then counted, a laborious and rather unreliable procedure [24].

Once deposited in the respiratory tract, the fate of a particle depends on the body's clearance mechanisms and on its ability to resist them. Larger particles, deposited on the airways, are generally cleared efficiently within 24 h by the mucociliary mechanism, though such clearance may be prolonged if the airways are damaged by cigarette smoke or fume inhalation [25,26]. Such cleared particles are either coughed up or swallowed. Particles reaching the acinus are beyond the region of cilia and production of mucus

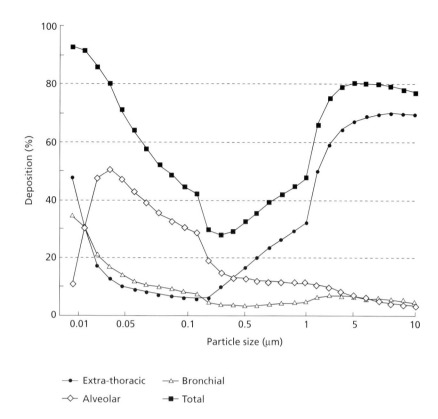

Fig. 54.2 Lung deposition and particle size: highest rate of deposition occurs with submicrometre-sized particles. (From Committee on the Medical Effects of Air Pollutants [21] with permission.)

and are cleared much more slowly [27]. Deposition occurs predominantly at bifurcations of alveolar ducts [28]. The mechanism of particle removal involves ingestion by alveolar macrophages [29] or type I alveolar epithelial cells [30]. Having ingested a particle, the type I alveolar cell either delivers it into the interstitial space of the alveolar wall, where it can be taken up by interstitial macrophages or flow with interstitial fluid into the lymphatics, or dies and passes into the alveolar lumen [31]. The macrophage also seems to have several options: it may migrate up to the mucociliary escalator, perhaps impelled by a flow of alveolar surfactant; move to the terminal airways due to a viscosity gradient [32]; or may pass between the alveolar epithelial cells, presumably temporarily unlocking the tight junctions by proteolytic enzyme action, into the interstitial space. It may then proceed into the lymphatics to pulmonary and hilar nodes, or pass back into the airways at the end of the terminal bronchiole, through lymphatic sumps [30]. It seems likely that all these mechanisms operate, though their relative importance has not been established. It is probable that alveolar clearance occurs over a prolonged period, the first particles being removed within 24 h but many remaining for months and even years [33]. The presence of dust pigment around the centre of the acinus is of course a finding familiar to all pathologists.

The harm exerted by the particle once inhaled depends on its biological, chemical and physical properties, and on the amount inhaled. Biological factors include its ability to act as a sensitizer or to overcome attack by macrophages, for example allergens such as grass pollen (up to 100 μm in diameter) provoke a primarily nasal reaction of a hypersensitivity type, while mycobacteria cause alveolar disease by being resistant to killing by macrophages. Chemical factors include the effects of gases or particle surfaces on cell or lysosomal membranes, for example the cytotoxic effects of sulphur dioxide and quartz. Physical factors apply when the particle is too large to be removed, as with asbestos fibres which are only partially ingested by macrophages. In addition, recent studies of microfine particles of less than 50 nm diameter have shown paradoxical toxicity in rats at inhaled concentrations too low to cause pathological effects when the same concentration is inhaled in the form of larger, micrometre-sized respirable particles [34]; this strongly suggests that physicochemical factors associated with particle surfaces may be responsible for toxicity in particles associated with air pollution and fumes such as those derived from welding and metal cutting [35]. Finally, the total mass of dust inhaled is clearly important, in that the lung's defences presumably evolved to enable removal of the modest amounts of particulate matter found in the ambient air (mainly bacterial, fungal and floral) and not the large amounts of inorganic matter that may be inhaled in the workplace. Nevertheless, a measure of the efficiency of these mechanisms is that a coal-miner may easily inhale 4 kg of coal dust in a lifetime but at death only about 10–30 g remain in the lungs [36].

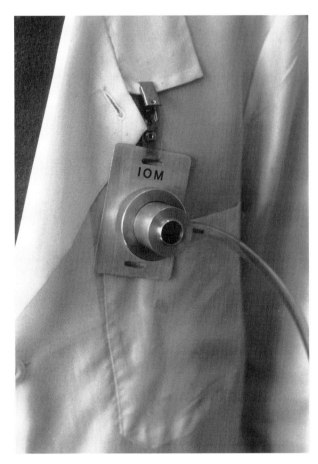

Fig. 54.3 A personal respirable dust sampler. The filter holder with size-selective orifice is close to the breathing zone and connects to a battery-operated pump on the belt.

Mineral pneumoconioses

The term 'pneumoconiosis' was coined by Zenker [37] to define a group of diseases caused by inhalation of dust. It usually implies a tissue reaction within the lung to the dust and, while strictly including diseases due to organic dusts, is generally used in relation to diseases and radiological abnormalities caused by mineral dusts. The most common pneumoconioses are coal-workers' pneumoconiosis, silicosis and asbestosis, although very many other types have been described, usually due to inhalation of mixed dusts containing silicates. They range in seriousness from asbestosis, which not only causes diffuse fibrosis but also increases substantially the patient's risk of lung carcinoma, through silicosis that causes progressive patchy nodular fibrosis, to conditions such as stannosis, siderosis and baritosis, which simply cause radiological change without physiological effects.

The inhalation of mineral dust may also have effects other than leading to pneumoconiosis, such as carcinogenesis and initiation of bronchitis or emphysema. These effects are discussed in subsequent sections.

Coal-workers' pneumoconiosis

Epidemiology

Coal-workers' pneumoconiosis is virtually confined to underground coal-miners, though it may occur in any place where a worker is exposed to high levels of coal dust in poorly ventilated conditions. Thus it has been described in coal trimmers, loading coal in the holds of ships, and in men and women sorting coal on surface screens. Coal is usually mined underground by one of two methods, long wall or room and pillar. In the former, used widely in Europe, all the coal in a seam is taken in a series of cuts by a machine across a face of up to 200 m. The roof above, usually composed of quartz-bearing rock, is supported by a row of hydraulic supports that are advanced after each cut, allowing the roof behind to fall in. The faceworkers operate the coal-cutter and roof supports in the tunnel along the face, which is ventilated by air blown down an access tunnel (roadway), across the face and out through a return roadway. The height of the face may vary from 46 cm to 2.5–3 m, depending on the height of the coal seam. Dust is generated largely by the coal-cutter but also by the movement of roof supports, by the collapse of the roof as these are moved forward, and by the transport of coal from the face. As the face progresses into the coal seam, so the roadways at either end are driven forward through coal as well as through the rocky strata. This may be done by powerful drilling machines, by placing and firing explosives or by other traditional tunnelling methods, all of which generate dust.

Room and pillar mining is used more widely in the USA. It involves driving a series of tunnels into the coal seam and linking them by cross-tunnels, leaving square pillars of coal to support the roof. Additional support is given usually by roof-bolting, where loose strata above the coal are fixed by drilling a bolt through them into firmer rock above. This form of mining is the more traditional and is used when there is sufficient coal for it to be economical to leave the pillars. It is the method widely used in mining for many other minerals.

From this brief description, it can be seen that miners may be exposed to dust not only from the coal seam but also from roof, floor and intrusions of rock (dirt bands) into the seam. Miners driving the roadway (known as hardheaders, tunnellers, rippers and brushers in different mining areas) are likely to be exposed to a mixture of mineral dusts. Other underground workers are also exposed to the same dusts, though generally more diluted, in the return roadway as well as to dust generated at points where coal is tipped from one transportation system (conveyor belt or bogie) to another. Therefore even miners working in the same colliery may show different types of pneumoconiosis depending on the work they do. It should be noted that ventilation of a mine by blowing air in one end and out the other across a long face wall does not adequately ventilate blind tunnels off the main airstream. In room and pillar mining, curtains (brattices) are hung in appropriate places to direct the flow of air away from the area where dust is being generated. In blind tunnels, forced ventilation or extraction by ducting is necessary. Again, absence of these provisions puts some men at greater risk than others.

Understanding of coal-workers' pneumoconiosis is complicated further by the fact that coal and coal dust differ dramatically from place to place. Some coals, formed under very high pressure, are particularly hard and very high in carbon content (and therefore combustibility), anthracite being the hardest of these. They are known as high-rank coals. Softer bituminous and steam coals leave more ash when burnt and are said to be of lower rank. The ash remaining in the fireplace or a coal-fired boiler is a mixture of quartz, kaolinite, mica and other silicate minerals. These are also present in the dust the miner inhales and in the lungs at postmortem, influencing the risk of pneumoconiosis and the type of pathological reaction.

Immediately after the Second World War, some 3000 men per annum were being diagnosed as having coal-workers' pneumoconiosis in the UK [38]. The realization of this epidemic led to a series of investigations by the Medical Research Council and the National Coal Board that have gone a long way to understanding the epidemiology and aetiology of the disease [39,40]. These studies have shown that the risk of pneumoconiosis varies considerably from place to place, roughly in relation to the rank of coal, high ranks being the most dangerous [41]. They have also demonstrated a relationship between a miner's exposure to respirable dust and risk of disease (Fig. 54.4); the mean of these relationships in different collieries has been used as information on which to base dust standards for protection of the workforce in coal-mines [42,43]. Other studies have shown relationships between exposure to relatively high levels of quartz in the dust and rapidly progressive pneumoconiosis or probable silicosis [44], and between dust exposure and the risks of bronchitis and emphysema [45–48]. In the UK, this information has been used by the coal industry as a basis for preventive measures and each year very few active miners are diagnosed as having pneumoconiosis; increasingly these are older men, coal-workers' pneumoconiosis in this country being a rare disease in miners under the age of 50 [49]. The disease does of course occur throughout the world, wherever coal is mined. In western Europe and the USA in general, measures of dust control have resulted in a decreased prevalence of disease, although in newly emerging industrial nations such as China and India it is likely that new cases will be seen frequently unless appropriate preventive measures are taken.

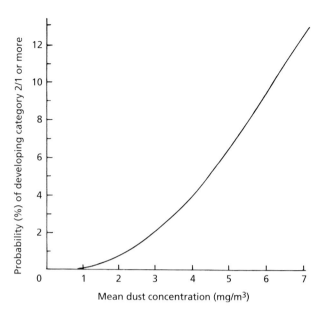

Fig. 54.4 Risk of category 2 simple coal-workers' pneumoconiosis in relation to average dust exposure over a working lifetime.

Clinical features

Chest radiography

The earliest sign of coal-workers' pneumoconiosis is nodular shadowing on the chest radiograph. These appearances are usually classified according to the International Labour Office (ILO) standard classification, which is described in Chapter 3 [50]. The nodules are most commonly of the q type (1.5–3 mm in diameter), though p (<1.5 mm) and r (>3 but <10 mm) lesions may occur, and it is quite usual to see examples of at least two of these types in any one miner's film. They are usually more profuse in the upper and middle zones. The profusion of nodules (categories 1–3) is an indirect measure of the miner's exposure to respirable dust and thus increases with increasing exposure, although progression of the p and q types does not occur after dust exposure has ceased. There is evidence that the larger nodules, which are usually relatively sparse, result from quartz exposure and represent silicotic nodules pathologically [36,51]. They may progress both in size and profusion after exposure has ceased. The very small p lesions seem to be related to the combination of pneumoconiosis and emphysema, while the q lesions represent overlapping coal macules [36]. Very rarely, the onset of severe emphysema may result in obscuration of rounded opacities, although spontaneous regresssion in the absence of emphysema does not occur in true coal-workers' pneumoconiosis. These distinctions between the radiological types of the condition are far from clear-cut since there is considerable interobserver and intraobserver variation in classifying films according to type of opacity. Typical examples are illustrated in Fig. 54.5.

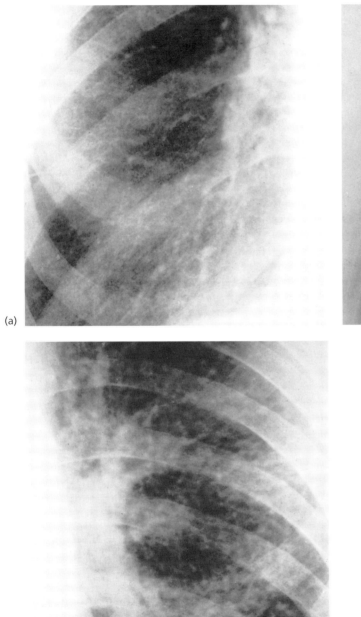

(a)

(b)

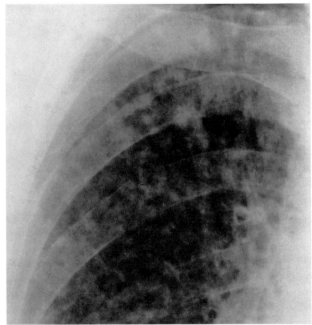

(c)

Fig. 54.5 Simple coal-workers' pneumoconiosis: (a) type p, pinpoint opacities; (b) type q, micronodular opacities; (c) type r, nodular opacities typically associated with quartz exposure.

The early nodular lesions are frequently accompanied by Kerley B lines. However, it has been recognized that coal-miners also develop other small irregular and linear shadows on their radiographs, similar to those occurring early in asbestosis [52]. These tend to occur more at the lung bases and to be of relatively low profusion, rarely more than category 1. There is evidence that their prevalence is related not only to exposure to respirable dust but also, unlike the rounded opacities, to age and cigarette smoking [53]. Pathologically and physiologically they seem to be related to the presence of emphysema

and airflow obstruction [52], and it is likely they represent paraseptal deposition of dust and the pathological reaction to it. There is no evidence that they are relevant to subsequent risks of progressive massive fibrosis (PMF).

The above description applies to simple coal-workers' pneumoconiosis, a condition in which only small opacities are present. However, a proportion of coal-miners develop so-called complicated pneumoconiosis (because originally it was thought that this was a consequence of complication of simple disease by tuberculosis) or PMF

[54,55]. This condition presents as a larger shadow, equal to or greater than 1 cm in maximum diameter, often initially in the right upper zone (Fig. 54.6). The lesion gradually grows, becomes more radiodense and causes distortion of adjacent lung and bronchi often with bullous emphysema. Frequently similar lesions appear in other parts of the lung and run a similar course. The course is very variable and often becomes arrested at a relatively early stage, although in some cases both lungs ultimately may be almost completely replaced by PMF and emphysema, with resultant cor pulmonale.

While a miner with a high category of simple pneumoconiosis is at greatest risk of developing PMF, it is now clear that simple pneumoconiosis need not be visible on a radiograph for PMF to occur [55]. Although simple pneumoconiosis does not normally progress or regress after dust exposure ceases, it has been shown that PMF commonly occurs after the miner has left the industry, sometimes as much as 20 years later [55]. This interesting fact suggests strongly that simple pneumoconiosis and PMF may be two separate diseases, both related to dust exposure. This is discussed further in the section on pathogenesis.

Massive fibrosis may present several different radiological appearances, of which at least two are relatively common and easily distinguished [56]. The most frequent appearance is as described above, initially rather indistinct and ovoid and gradually becoming more clearly demarcated and larger. This is particularly common in areas where high-rank coal is mined. The other type seems to result from aggregation of the larger r-type nodules to give a multinodular appearance initially, though ultimately this may come to resemble the other type. These appearances seem most common in miners exposed to high levels of quartz [56,57].

A few miners, especially those with rheumatoid arthritis or with rheumatoid factor in their blood, develop well-defined rounded lesions that grow to about 2–3 cm in diameter or rarely somewhat larger (Fig. 54.7). They are usually multiple and have a marked tendency to cavitate. They often occur on a background of no simple pneumoconiosis and in miners with a relatively low dust exposure. They are called Caplan's lesions and their combination with rheumatoid disease Caplan's syndrome, after the Pneumoconiosis Panel doctor who described them [58–60]. They do not have an ominous prognosis and cause no significant functional impairment, being unassociated with emphysema [61].

Symptoms and signs

The miner with simple coal-workers' pneumoconiosis has no symptoms or signs attributable to the disease. This is a particularly important fact, not always appreciated by doctors tempted to link radiological abnormality (which may be extensive) with symptoms. This is not to say that miners with simple pneumoconiosis may not become breathless; they may and often do, but this is due to some other disease such as asthma, emphysema or heart failure. Failure to appreciate this may result in the patient not

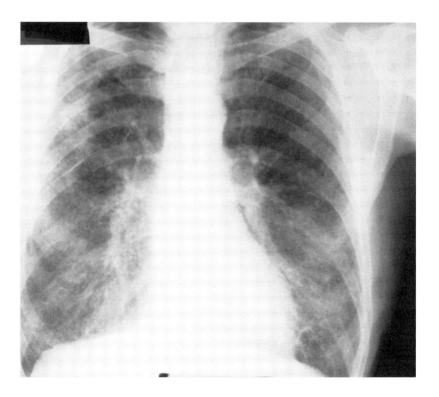

Fig. 54.6 Coal-workers' pneumoconiosis: extensive (category 3) simple pneumoconiosis with early massive fibrosis (stage A) in right upper zone.

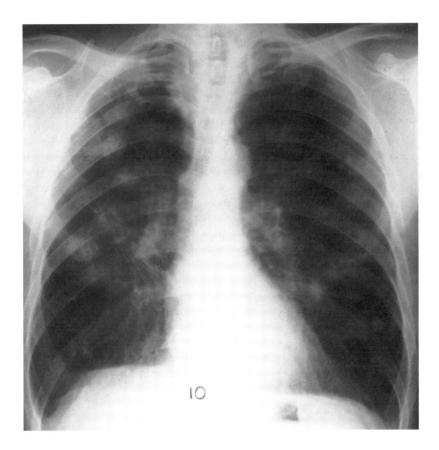

Fig. 54.7 Multiple rounded lesions of Caplan's syndrome in coal-miner with rheumatoid disease.

receiving treatment appropriate to the condition, sometimes for years. It is particularly unfortunate if this results in treatable conditions such as asthma being missed. Nevertheless, miners develop emphysema more often than other groups of workers with similar smoking habits, and this has also been shown to be related to their exposure to respirable dust [48] (see Pathogenesis).

The early stages of PMF likewise are insufficiently extensive to cause any symptoms or dysfunction. However, as the disease progresses the combination of the fibrous masses and the associated emphysema leads to increasing breathlessness. Cough is not typically a feature unless there is considerable bronchial distortion, and the breathlessness is unvarying and related to exertion. Ultimately the patient reaches the stage of hypoxic and often hypercapnic respiratory failure and cor pulmonale [62,63]. Mortality studies of coal-miners have emphasized their increased risks of dying of chronic bronchitis and emphysema, as well as pneumoconiosis [64].

There are certain other negative features of coalworkers' pneumoconiosis apart from absence of symptoms in the simple disease. These are an absence of physical signs (clubbing and crackles are not features), no increased risk of bronchial carcinoma [64,65] and no increased susceptibility to tuberculosis. However, coalminers do run an increased risk of gastric carcinoma [64], for unknown reasons (although the author is inclined to

speculate that this may be related to exposure to water underground containing *Helicobacter pylori*), and seem to be unusually susceptible to infections with opportunistic mycobacteria [66] (perhaps for the same reason).

Lung function

Several studies have indicated that coal-miners have somewhat lower forced expiratory volume in 1 s (FEV_1) than control groups but that FEV_1 does not decrease further in relation to increasing radiological category of pneumoconiosis [67,68]. This, together with the epidemiological demonstration of raised residual volume in coal-miners that increases in relation to category of pneumoconiosis [69], is consistent with the hypothesis that coal dust has an effect on airways or alveoli separate from the effect by which it causes pneumoconiosis. Studies on small numbers of miners with high categories of simple pneumoconiosis have shown changes in lung mechanics suggestive of either small airways disease or patchy emphysema [70,71]. However, in general it may be assumed clinically that a miner with simple pneumoconiosis, and without complicating chronic airways disease or emphysema, has an FEV_1 and forced vital capacity (FVC) within the normal range. Diffusing capacity is also usually normal, though slight reduction may be associated with the p type of opacities, and this has been taken to indicate that emphysema coexists with these lesions [72].

PMF may also be present without functional abnormalities. However, as the condition progresses and particularly if emphysema develops, function becomes impaired by a mixture of restriction of lung volumes and airflow obstruction [73]. Which of these is dominant depends on the size of the masses and the amount of emphysema, although severe airflow obstruction is a common feature in the late stages as a result of reduction in retractive forces across the lung, measurable as increased compliance. There is also reduction in gas transfer owing to loss of alveolar volume, and ultimately hypoxaemia and hypercapnia.

Pathology

The earliest lesion is the accumulation of coal dust in macrophages at the centre of the acinus, around the respiratory bronchioles. This lesion grows to form the typical coal macule, a stellate structure often surrounded by emphysematous changes (Fig. 54.8). Macroscopically these lesions are dispersed throughout the lung and pigmented dust is seen to have accumulated in the lymph nodes also. The macules are impalpable. In addition, in more advanced simple pneumoconiosis, palpable, somewhat larger, nodules are visible that may be stellate or rounded. They are also composed of dust, disintegrating macrophages, reticulin fibres and reticuloendothelial cells but have a firm central portion of collagen. This may be irregular or, if quartz exposure has been an important factor, arranged in concentric whorls. If the miner has had heavy quartz exposure, typical silicotic lesions may be seen.

PMF is always associated with pathological evidence of simple pneumoconiosis, though the dust foci may be so sparse as to have been invisible radiologically. The lesions are black, usually irregularly shaped and limited in number. They may be sufficiently large to destroy a whole lobe or several lobes and cavitation may be present within them (Fig. 54.9). Histologically, at least two polar types may be recognized, although most examples exhibit features somewhere between the extremes [36]. The more frequent type consists of a peripheral zone of dust, macrophages and reticuloendothelial cells surrounding a relatively acellular central area consisting of collagen around the edges and amorphous, often necrotic, tissue centrally. This material is probably largely fibronectin [74,75], which has been shown to be the major protein component of PMF. Fibronectin is produced by macrophages and fibroblasts and its normal role includes binding cells together. It is a component of reticulin on light microscopy, in that it takes up silver stains and has a fibrous form. The PMF lesion typically contains elastic laminae, the ghosts of obliterated pulmonary vessels, and is usually surrounded by quite extensive emphysema.

The other type of PMF lesion appears to be the aggregation of the fibrotic nodules described above. This is often seen clearly at the periphery of the lesion, and rings or bands of dust representing the edges of earlier lesions can be seen more centrally. Studies of the dust retained in lungs of patients with PMF suggest that the former lesion tends to be associated with exposure to large amounts of high-rank coal, while the latter type is more likely to occur in miners exposed to lower-rank coal with a high quartz and silicate content [36]. However, these relationships are not clear-cut.

A third lesion occurs less frequently than the other

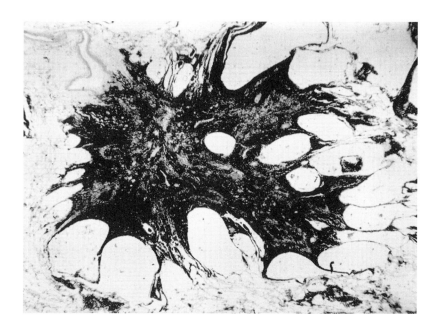

Fig. 54.8 Simple coal macule showing centriacinar accumulation of dust and cells with some surrounding emphysema.

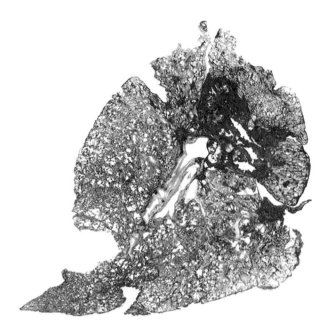

Fig. 54.9 Section of coal-miner's lung showing progressive massive fibrosis, diffuse centriacinar emphysema and relatively sparse coal macules.

two types of PMF, although at one time it was thought possible that this might be rather more common. This is the Caplan lesion, which superficially resembles a silicotic nodule in that it shows concentric pigmented and non-pigmented layers, the dust impregnation usually being relatively light [59]. There is often little background of simple pneumoconiosis and the lesions themselves are quite rounded and well demarcated. The rings consist of collagen, which often liquefies, and the whole lesion may cavitate. The periphery usually shows features constent with rheumatoid histology, with lymphocytes, plasma cells and sometimes pallisaded histiocytes. These lesions are usually muiltiple and rarely grow larger than 5 cm in diameter.

Pathogenesis

The development of simple pneumoconiosis is clearly related to two factors: the total quantity of dust inhaled and its composition [43,76]. However, these do not explain all cases and individual predisposition seems important also; this is probably related more to individual efficiency of dust clearance than to immunological differences between people, studies of which have proved unrewarding [77–79]. The composition of dust is important not only in determining the pathological type of lesion but also, almost certainly, whether pneumoconiosis occurs. Given the same levels of dust, different collieries show striking differences in prevalence of pneumoconiosis, even when factors such as migration of the workforce and differing coal and ash content have been allowed for [43]. Complex

interactions occur between different minerals in coal dust that may significantly alter their toxicity; for example, quartz may be rendered almost non-toxic when mixed with certain silicates such as illite [80]. Nevertheless, the essential mechanism of simple pneumoconiosis is likely to be dust-mediated damage to macrophages, release of cytokines accompanied by recruitment of polymorphonuclear cells, resulting in activation of fibroblasts and also local initiation of emphysema by elastolysis. This latter problem is discussed in the next section.

Equally, PMF has been shown to be related to total dust exposure and to dust composition: the more dust a miner is exposed to, the greater the risk [81]. High-rank dusts are particularly liable to provoke the amorphous type of PMF, while low-rank high-quartz dusts more commonly lead to the nodular aggregating type [43]. Why a miner's disease progresses from the simple lesion to PMF is still not clear. Sometimes it is due to progressive enlargement and aggregation of quartz-induced lesions. More commonly, however, it is a diffuse fibrosing and necrotic process with marked vasculitis and considerable accumulation of dust. Its preponderance in upper lobes and, intriguingly, its predisposition to affect taller miners speak for a mechanical cause [81]. Whether this is related to local impairment of clearance, lymphatic blockage, lymph node destruction or some other factor remains to be seen, although severe destruction of hilar nodes is almost universal in miners with PMF and progressive silicosis [82,83], and it is logical to suppose that blockage of this escape route for the dust is relevant to its accumulation in the lung and provocation of a chronic progressive inflammatory reaction there. Other theories of the aetiology of PMF now seem less likely. These include autoimmune factors, which only seem relevant to the rare cases of Caplan lesions, and tuberculosis, which is no longer relevant in the UK though it was probably important in the past. Atypical mycobacterial infection has not been investigated in detail yet. It seems unlikely but cannot be dismissed as a cause in some cases.

Coal, bronchitis and emphysema

The relationship between exposure to coal dust and chronic bronchitis and emphysema has been extremely controversial. Physicians and pathologists in mining areas have for many years believed there to be a relationship but proof has been hard to come by. In particular, in recent years the prevalence of cigarette smoking in miners has tended to hide the risks of coal dust exposure. Nevertheless, recent evidence gives strong support to the hypothesis that coal dust causes both chronic bronchitis and emphysema, adding to the effects of cigarette smoking. This evidence may be summarized as follows.

1 There is an increased prevalence of cough, sputum and reduction in FEV_1 in miners compared with controls [45,84].

2 The risk of cough and sputum increases with increasing dust exposure in smokers and non-smokers [40,85].

3 FEV$_1$ declines in relation to a miner's dust exposure [46,47,86–89].

4 There is more emphysema in the lungs of miners who have died suddenly of cardiac disease than of non-mining controls, even when matched for smoking habit [90].

5 The risk of a miner having some emphysema in the lungs at death is proportional to dust exposure during life, if there are some pathological changes of nodular pneumoconiosis in the lungs as well [48]. This relationship holds true even when the lungs of non-smokers are examined.

6 The risk of a miner dying of chronic bronchitis and emphysema increases in proportion to dust exposure [64].

The facts make a strong case for a relationship, and would fit with the hypothesis that coal dust acts as both a cause of fibrosis and an initiator of emphysema. A common pathway, via damage to macrophages and recruitment of polymorphonuclear cells, is an attractive explanation; this hypothesis has been supported by the finding that inhalation of coal-mine dust by rats at concentrations not far removed from those to which miners have been exposed causes a neutrophil alveolitis, impaired leucocyte chemotaxis and a rise in alveolar concentrations of proteolytic enzymes [91,92]. It is particularly interesting that this response occurs within weeks of the start of exposure in view of the epidemiological finding in humans of an accelerated loss of lung function in young miners over the first year or two of exposure underground, later slowing down [93]. One might speculate that it is in this period, before the lung's defences are adapted to dealing with dust, that the process leading to emphysema may be initiated in the susceptible.

Argument has centred around the relative importance of cigarettes and coal dust in causing emphysema and airflow obstruction. In practical terms this is a red herring, in that both contribute and their effects appear to be additive and dose-related epidemiologically (Fig. 54.10). Therefore, reductions of dust levels in coal-mines will reduce the numbers of workers becoming disabled, although it will not eliminate the problem. In the past, when fewer miners smoked and dust levels were exceedingly high, it is likely that coal dust was more important overall than smoking. Currently, the reverse is almost certainly true in the West. What the future holds depends on action by both industry and society.

Management and prevention

There is no treatment for coal-workers' pneumoconiosis and, as for all occupational diseases, the emphasis should be on prevention. This is achieved by reduction of dust levels in coal-mines by a combination of improved ventilation and use of water to suppress the dust at its source.

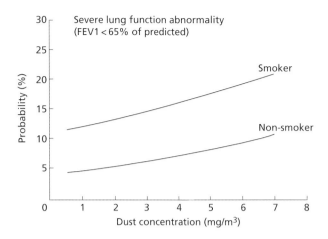

Fig. 54.10 Relationships between risk of acquiring a forced expiratory volume in 1 s (FEV$_1$) of less than 65% of predicted and dust exposure and smoking. (Derived from data in Marine *et al.* [86].)

Special attention needs to be paid to areas where ventilation may be ineffective, such as the advancing ends of roadways. On long-wall faces, the air is driven around the face down one roadway and out the other. In room and pillar mines, curtains (brattices) are used to direct the flow of air. The effectiveness of these measures is monitored by measuring the dust concentration to which miners are exposed and in many countries this is done according to statutory obligations. In the UK, the maximum allowable concentration is 7 mg/m^3, measured as respirable dust (<7 μm diameter) 70 m back from the face in the return roadway, a concentration roughly equivalent to an average of 4 mg/m^3 at the face. In the USA, dust is sampled within the breathing zone of face workers by personal monitors and a lower standard, 2 mg/m^3, is applied. Both these standards were based on epidemiological studies that predicted the average risk of category 2 simple pneumoconiosis after a lifetime's work at different dust concentrations (see Fig. 54.4). Tighter standards are generally applied for driving roadways where quartz levels may be high.

Whatever dust standard is applied, some miners will get pneumoconiosis because of variations in individual susceptibility. Therefore dust suppression should be accompanied by workforce radiographic monitoring. In the UK, chest radiographs are offered to all miners every 4 years and any worker showing signs of simple pneumoconiosis is offered work in less dusty conditions. This has the effect of reducing the risks of developing PMF. A further measure that may be taken is to offer miners personal protection by respirators, and this is the practice in the UK. However, this is not regarded as a substitute for good dust suppression.

These measures together have had a marked effect on the prevalence of pneumoconiosis in the UK and, with the dwindling numbers of men employed in a contracting industry, simple pneumoconiosis and PMF are now very rare in working miners, although the latter is still seen in retired miners [55]. National statistics in other countries are harder to find, but there is no reason to suppose that similar results would not follow similar control measures.

In the UK and some other countries, an industrial injuries insurance scheme is run by the state, miners with pneumoconiosis being entitled to benefits. This is discussed in the final section of this chapter. In practical terms, the advice given to a miner who has developed pneumoconiosis depends on his age and the coal-mine in which he works. A miner developing simple pneumoconiosis under the age of 40 is very likely to develop PMF and to have his life shortened by it. Complete cessation of further dust exposure will reduce these risks. Between 40 and 55, the risks are correspondingly smaller and PMF, when it develops, may occur too late in life to cause appreciable disablement, so the management often involves offering work in conditions where the dust level is relatively low (and in the UK this offer is a statutory obligation). A man who develops simple pneumoconiosis in his last few years underground may usually be advised that the final year or two at the face will not affect his risks of PMF and premature death appreciably. These general guidelines may be modified in individual circumstances by knowledge of the dust conditions and pneumoconiosis risks in particular mines and mining areas.

Silicosis

Epidemiology

Exposure to silica

Silicon dioxide or silica is the most abundant compound in the earth's crust, where it is mostly found in the crystalline form known as quartz, a regular tetrahedron comprising a central atom of silicon that shares four oxygen atoms with adjacent silicon atoms. Quartz may be contaminated with other elements in trace amounts that give it colour and value as ornamental gemstones, such as agate, onyx and amethyst. Different spatial arrangements of the silicon dioxide molecule are responsible for other minerals: tridymite and cristobalite are formed by heating quartz and occur naturally in some volcanic rocks. Silica may also occur in microcrystalline and amorphous forms; the former consists of tiny crystals bonded together by amorphous silica as in flint, while the latter, probably relatively non-toxic, is not crystalline and occurs as diatomite, the petrified skeletons of minute prehistoric organisms. However, calcining (heating above 1200°C) of amorphous silica converts it into a toxic crystalline form.

Since silica occurs so abundantly, exposure to its airborne dust may occur in a very wide range of circum-

Table 54.2 Some occupations in which exposure to quartz may take place.

Mining
Tunnelling
Quarrying
Stonemasonry
Sandblasting
Fettling and foundry work
Ceramics
Brick-making
Refractory kiln repair
Silica flour manufacture
Abrasive manufacture
Diatomaceous earth manufacture

stances. Some of the more important are recorded in Table 54.2. The most important numerically is cutting stone, in mining, quarrying, masonry and tunnelling. Almost all forms of mining entail a hazard of silicosis. Metal mining requires the extraction of metal-bearing ore, which is largely quartz. Even when the mineral being mined is itself a known cause of lung disease or radiological abnormalities, such as asbestos, tin or barium, the miner is usually at greater risk of silicosis. Tunnelling through granite, sandstone or other quartz-bearing rock entails an obvious hazard, although pure limestone and marble are not toxic. Stonemasonry and cleaning with abrasives are also well-known causes of silicosis. The practice of using a high-speed jet of sand for metal and stone polishing, known as sandblasting, is extremely hazardous and has been illegal in the UK since 1949. However, it continues in the USA and many other countries. Work in foundries, where molten metal is made into castings, may involve a risk of silicosis as the mould into which the metal is poured is usually made of sand bonded by resin. The sand is fused to the surface of the casting and often converted by the heat to the particularly toxic cristobalite. This is polished off the surface by a worker called a fettler, who is at potential risk of silicosis. Other foundry workers at risk are those who clean or replace the brick linings of the furnaces. These bricks (refractory bricks) are made of baked sandstone and there is also a risk of silicosis in the ceramic workers who produce them.

The production of china and earthenware involves the use of clays, usually with a low silica content, to which finely ground calcined flint may sometimes be added. The material is shaped and then fired in an oven. It is then polished, fettled and glazed, sometimes with a mixture containing powdered flint. It is clear that there are plenty of situations in this industry where silicosis may occur. Other industries with a risk of silicosis include production of silica flour, finely ground silica used as a filling in abrasives, toothpastes, polishes, paints, rubbers and plastics, production of calcined diatomaceous earths, glass-making, enamelling and production of gemstones.

Prevalence

It is not possible to know how many workers have silicosis since notification procedures differ in different countries and many workers at risk are never surveyed by radiography. However, records in some countries, notably the UK and the Scandinavian countries, allow some overall estimates to be made. In the UK, with a working population of about 20 million, the number of workers being awarded state disablement pensions each year for silicosis fluctuates between 110 and 170. However, this figure excludes an unknown but almost certainly much larger number of workers with radiological change but no disability. The workers are predominantly from foundries, mines and quarries, refractory brick-works and potteries. A Swedish case register assessed the number of workers with radiological silicosis as having fallen from about 120 to about 70 per annum between 1950 and 1975; at the same time it was apparent that the age at which the disease was first diagnosed was progressively increasing [94]. In neither the UK nor Sweden, however, is the population at risk known.

It is likely that silicosis as it occurred in the first half of this century in mining, pottery work and sandblasting is now a very rare occurrence in developed countries. The disease prevalence has been modified in these and other industries by an increased awareness of risk and by legislative action leading to better dust suppression. For example, there has been good evidence of decreasing risk in Vermont granite workers [95], Scottish granite stonemasons [96] and diatomaceous earth workers [97,98]. On the other hand, in some industries complacency about risks has allowed poor control of exposures with consequently a relatively high incidence of preventable disease. Since the last edition of this book, the author has seen severe and sometimes fatal silicosis in the UK among sandstone masons [99], 'limestone' crushers, barytes miners [100] and foundry workers, and this has also been reported in American sandblasters [101,102], bentonite miners [103] and silica flour workers [104], Indian slate pencil workers [105,106] and British slate-workers [107]. Finally, the expansion of mining and quarrying into economically poorer countries is likely to be attended by increasing numbers of victims of silicosis (Fig. 54.11), while the persistence of traditional stonemasonry in some such countries ensures that a steady number of people continue to get the disease from this occupation [108].

Relationship of exposure to risk of silicosis

While it is obvious that greater risks of silicosis attend heavier exposures, the number of studies that have attempted to relate exposure to risk in numerical terms is surprisingly small. Very heavy exposures, in industries such as sandblasting, may lead to acute silicosis and moderately heavy exposures to subacute disease. Studies of classical nodular silicosis in the Vermont granite industry have suggested that the risk of clinically important silicosis was virtually eliminated by the introduction of a dust standard of approximately $100\,\mu g/m^3$ [95]. More recent follow-up of this population has supported this conclusion [109]. Similar results have been obtained from a study of quartz-exposed workers in North Carolina [110], while a small but well-executed study of British gypsum workers has suggested an approximately 50% risk of developing small rounded opacities in workers exposed to $100\,\mu g/m^3$ for 20 years or more [111]. An important study of Canadian gold and uranium miners has estimated the risks of radiological change in relation to careful estimates of cumulative quartz exposure [112] (Fig. 54.12).

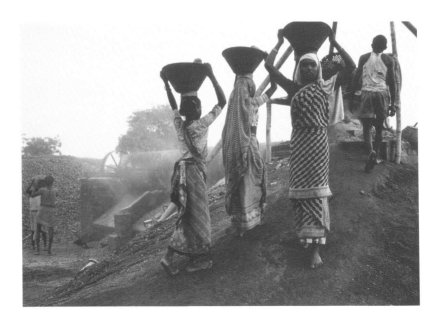

Fig 54.11 A typical roadside stonecrushing operation in India. Note the absence of any methods to prevent dust exposure.

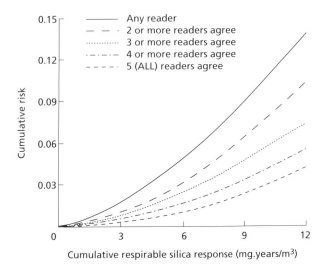

Fig 54.12 Risks of category 1 simple silicosis in Canadian hardrock miners in relation to exposure to respirable silica expressed as concentration vs. time. The different curves represent different levels of agreement between readers. (From Muir *et al.* [112] with permission.)

For category 1 pneumoconiosis to have been read by a majority of the five readers in about 3% of miners, average exposures of approximately 7 mg·year/m^3 are required, i.e. an exposure equivalent to 200 μg/m^3 for 45 years. As far as it can be interpreted, the evidence at present thus appears to show that adherence to a quartz standard of 100 μg/m^3 would prevent most serious silicosis but would not prevent the development of minor radiological opacities in a proportion of the workforce. The real challenge is to ensure adherence to such a standard. In the UK, the maximum allowable concentration for quartz is 0.3 mg/m^3, implying a maximum cumulative exposure over a 40-year working life of 20 mg·years/m^3 and therefore an approximately 6% risk of radiological change in someone exposed regularly to half that concentration, using the estimates illustrated in Fig. 54.12. Rather than regular exposures to low concentrations, in real life most workers are now probably exposed to intermittent peak concentrations, sometimes well in excess of standards, and such peaks may be more relevant to the development of serious silicosis; this was almost certainly the explanation of the outbreak described in Scottish coalminers [44].

Recent calculation of the likely exposures to quartz of two stonemasons who worked alongside each other, one of whom died from acute silicosis while the other developed PMF some years later, suggested that in the fatal case earlier prolonged exposure to low concentrations had caused fibrosis of the hilar nodes and that this was responsible for the different reactions in the two men [83]. Thus it is proposed that exposure to low concentrations over pro-

longed periods may influence the clearance of dust inhaled subsequently, and that changes for the worse in dust concentrations late in a worker's career may be particularly dangerous.

Clinical features

It is convenient for the purposes of description to categorize silicosis as chronic, accelerated and acute, though it must be borne in mind that such subdivision is not necessarily clear-cut; these terms are used in the descriptions that follow.

Chest radiography

The earliest sign of classical chronic silicosis is the appearance of small nodules, particularly in the mid and upper zones of the lungs. These are characteristically somewhat more dense than those in coal-workers' pneumoconiosis. They also have a tendency to increase in size gradually and are often of the r type (see Fig. 54.5) [44]. Calcification of small nodules sometimes occurs. There may be associated Kerley B lines at the bases and pleural thickening. Eggshell calcification of the hilar nodes is an almost pathognomonic feature, occurring only otherwise in sarcoidosis (Fig. 54.13).

Once silicosis has appeared on the chest film it tends to increase, both in profusion and in size of the nodules. This occurs even after exposure has ceased [94,113,114]. However, in this respect care should be taken to distinguish between true silicosis and mixed-dust pneumoconiosis, which may be seen in welders and some foundry workers for example and which runs a much more benign course, tending not to progress or evolve into PMF [114]. True silicosis frequently shows agglomeration of nodules to form the large masses of PMF [113] (Fig. 54.14). These typically have a multinodular appearance initially but later may consolidate into a contracted dense fibrotic mass, often surrounded by bullae. Cavitation may occur, and when it does evidence of mycobacterial infection should be sought. Pleural fibrosis is often extensive close to the PMF lesions.

Accelerated silicosis, associated with heavy exposures over a relatively short period of a few years, presents radiologically as progressive irregular upper zone fibrosis, sometimes with relatively sparse and indistinct nodularity [104]. The upper lobes may become replaced completely by PMF and the lower by emphysema (Fig. 54.15). Acute silicosis, which develops over months in response to exceedingly heavy exposures as in sandblasting or dry drilling [101,102,115–117], is characterized by appearances suggestive of pulmonary oedema (Fig. 54.16). Acute enlargement of the hilar nodes may occur with heavy exposure to quartz in individuals without prior exposure [83] (Fig. 54.17).

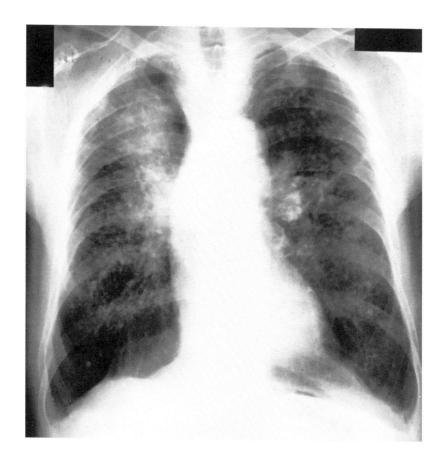

Fig. 54.13 Chest film of hardrock miner showing eggshell calcification of hilar nodes and progressive massive fibrosis in right upper zone. The nodular, r-type lesions that formed the basis of the progressive massive fibrosis are visible, particularly in the left upper zone.

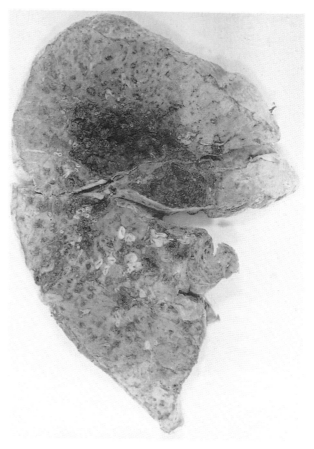

Fig. 54.14 Silicotic lung showing grey fibrotic nodules that have coalesced in the upper and middle lobes to form massive fibrosis.

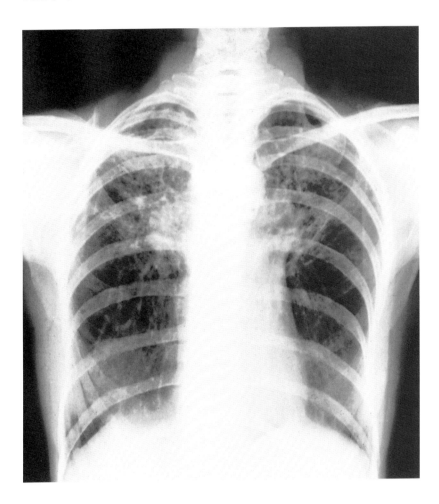

Fig. 54.15 Chest film of patient with accelerated silicosis showing irregular upper lobe fibrosis and lower zone emphysema.

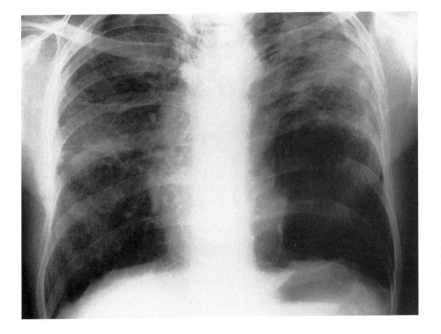

Fig 54.16 Chest film of stonemason with 6 years of exposure to 1 mg/m³ respirable quartz following 30 years of exposure to low concentrations showing diffuse finely nodular bilateral shadowing of acute silicosis shortly before his death.

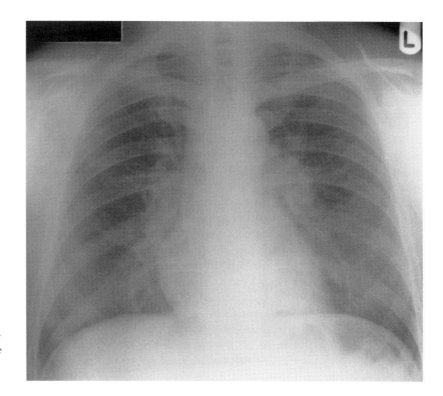

Fig. 54.17 Chest film of 25-year-old stonemason (who worked alongside the patient shown in Fig 54.16) with 6 years of exposure to respirable quartz at $1\,mg/m^3$ showing an acute enlargement of the hilar nodes. These later calcified and progressive massive fibrosis developed in the upper zones. The difference in the reactions to their recent very high exposures is likely to be due to prior fibrosis of hilar nodes in the patient in Fig. 54.16.

Symptoms and signs

In chronic silicosis the development of small nodular opacities is not associated with symptoms or signs. However, as the disease progresses to PMF, the patient may complain of shortness of breath in proportion to the size of the lesions and the extent of emphysema. A dry cough is also often present. The condition may progress with increasing disability and ultimately cor pulmonale, although this stage is now rarely reached in chronic silicosis in most of the industries classically associated with the disease. Finger clubbing and auscultatory crackles are not a feature even of late chronic silicosis. Accelerated silicosis similarly causes no abnormal signs, but differs from chronic silicosis in that breathlessness is a relatively early feature. The very rare acute silicosis presents with rapidly increasing shortness of breath and crackles may be heard in the lungs. It progresses to death in hypoxic resiratory failure within a year or two of presentation [99].

There should not be great difficulty in making the diagnosis of chronic silicosis if an occupational history is taken. However, the radiographic appearances of accelerated disease are less familiar to physicians and chronic tuberculosis, sarcoidosis or allergic alveolitis may be considered in the differential diagnosis. However, a history of a few years of heavy dust exposure should be sufficient to prevent misdiagnosis. It is important not to be misled by a patient's understanding of the nature of the dust expo-

sure. The author has seen silicosis of severe degree in workers crushing what they believed was limestone but which clearly contained high proportions of quartz. Acute silicosis may present initially mimicking bilateral bronchopneumonia or pulmonary oedema radiographically, although the history of increasing dyspnoea over a few months together with intense exposure to stone dust should make the diagnosis easy. Again, it is important not to be deterred from the diagnosis by atypical radiographic or even pathological features and to take serious account of the occupational history [99].

Lung function

Several studies have suggested that simple silicosis is not normally associated with abnormalities of lung function except in the most advanced stage (category 3) [118–121]. However, these studies have often been unable to distinguish between the effects of silicosis and possible independent effects of the dust on lung function separate from its effect in causing nodular change. Thus it may be that the functional abnormalities found are due to dust exposure, analogous to the situation in coal-miners, rather than to the development of silicosis. When abnormalities are found they are usually those of a mild mixed restrictive and obstructive pattern.

In silicotic PMF the functional changes are the same as in coal-workers' PMF, the relative amounts of obstruction and restriction depending upon the differing contributions of fibrosis and emphysema pathologically. Similar abnormalities occur in accelerated silicosis [122], while a restrictive pattern with severe hypoxaemia is to be expected in the acute disease.

Complications

Tuberculosis and other mycobacterial infections are the most important complications of silicosis, presumably largely related to reactivation of previously quiescent lesions [94,123,124]. As tuberculous infection in childhood becomes less common so the disease in silicosis will also become rarer, although it still remains a problem in societies where tuberculosis remains endemic. As tuberculosis declines, there appears to be an increase in the incidence of infections with *Mycobacterium kansasii* and *M. avium-intracellulare*, and these organisms are recognized as important pathogens of patients with silicosis in the south-eastern USA [125]. The onset of mycobacterial infection in silicosis may be insidious, but unexpected radiological change, cavitation of PMF and the development of soft patchy opacities should alert the physician to the possibility. Fever and loss of weight, though usually only occurring with advanced tuberculosis, should not be attributed to silicosis (except of the acute type). Regular sputum examination in people with silicosis is the safest method of catching the infection early.

Other complications of silicosis include pneumothorax, associated with the combination of fibrosis and bullae [123], an increased frequency of scleroderma [126], and a tendency to renal failure due to focal damage to glomeruli and proximal tubules [127–129]. Silicotic subjects have an increased prevalence of antinuclear antibodies, and it is speculated that these, and consequent tissue damage, may be related to the damage to cells and their nuclei by quartz [130].

It is possible that workers exposed to silica have an increased risk of chronic bronchitis and airflow obstruction as a consequence of non-specific effects of dust [121,131], although recent studies of the Vermont granite worker cohort suggest that this association is not universal [132]. However, this is not as clearly established as in coal-miners, and it seems that non-smokers exposed to concentrations of quartz around 0.1 mg/m^3 do not run a significant additional risk of developing emphysema [133]. There have also been suggestions that quartz may be carcinogenic, especially from a Swedish study of workers in mining, quarrying, tunnelling and iron and steel trades and from studies of North Carolina dusty trades workers, of diatomaceous earth workers and of Ontario miners [94,134–136]. This controversial subject has been investigated by the International Agency for Cancer Research in a series of specially commissioned studies intended to take account of confounding factors such as exposure to other carcinogens and cigarette smoke [137]. The results

suggest that the presence of silicosis increases the risk of a worker developing lung cancer, although the evidence associating quartz exposure without silicosis and cancer is inconsistent. Recent evidence has been reviewed with the same conclusion [138]. It seems likely to the author that any carcinogenic effect is relatively weak compared to that of asbestos for example, and that control of dust exposures sufficient to prevent silicosis is likely to prevent an excess of lung cancer also. The UK Industrial Injuries Advisory Council has included lung cancer in association with silicosis in its list of prescribed diseases.

Pathology

On macroscopic examination, the surface of silicotic lungs often shows fibrotic plaques and adhesions between visceral and parietal pleura. The lungs are pigmented and the hilar nodes are enlarged and contain fibrotic nodules that are often calcified. The cut surface of the lung is clothed with hard fibrotic nodules of varying sizes and with a characteristic whorled appearance. Emphysema is not usually as conspicuous a feature of simple silicosis as it is of coal-workers' pneumoconiosis. Where PMF has developed, it can usually be seen to have been formed by aggregation of several large simple lesions (Fig. 54.18). Cavitation of PMF may be present. Accelerated silicosis shows in addition a more irregular fibrosis in the upper zones, often with bullous emphysema in other parts of the lung. In contrast, acute silicosis looks quite different, the lungs being heavy and voluminous, without much nodular change [101].

Microscopically, the silicotic nodule arises around the respiratory bronchiole, around arterioles and in paraseptal and subpleural tissues, as well as in lymph nodes [139]. The centre of the nodule is collagen, while peripherally it shows reticulin, fibroblasts, macrophages and mononuclear cells. Dust, which may be seen to be doubly refractile using polarized light, is usually most profuse round the periphery of the nodule. However, this appearance should not be relied upon, since very fine particles of quartz may be too small to refract light and may be present in very high concentration with very little dust apparent on polarized microscopy [99]. In accelerated silicosis, in addition to nodular change, diffuse alveolar wall thickening and proliferation of type II alveolar epithelial cells may be seen [140]. In acute silicosis the alveolar walls are infiltrated by plasma cells, lymphocytes and fibroblasts, while the alveoli are filled with eosinophilic oedema fluid that is positive to periodic acid–Schiff staining [101,141]. PMF in chronic and accelerated silicosis can be seen to comprise smaller silicotic nodules at the periphery, though the centre loses this architecture and appears as a hard mass of fibrosis. Elastic ghosts of vessels may be seen within the PMF lesion and central ischaemic necrosis may occur.

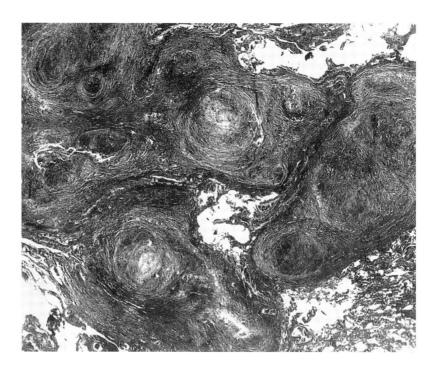

Fig. 54.18 Low-power view of silicotic nodules showing onion-skin appearance and aggregation.

Pathogenesis

The damage caused by quartz occurs at the lung acinus and in the pulmonary, hilar and mediastinal nodes. As discussed above, physical factors determine the likelihood of dust gaining access to the acinus; once there, the particles are engulfed by macrophages. It seems likely that they are then transported to the nodes where they initiate fibrosis as discussed below. With relatively low exposures, fibrosis of nodes is the only pathological consequence; however, once fibrosis has occurred the route of egress is blocked and pulmonary fibrosis starts in the acinar regions [83]. With high initial exposures, acute enlargement of hilar nodes mimicking sarcoidosis may occur, to be followed by acinar disease once the nodes have fibrosed.

It seems likely that the crystal structure and the surface properties of quartz are important in determining its toxicity. Quartz and coesite, which have tetrahedral structures, are fibrogenic experimentally whereas stishovite, which has an octohedral structure, is not [142]. Alteration of the surface of the quartz crystal by coating it with aluminium hydroxide or iron oxide reduces its toxicity, while chemical cleaning of the surface increases toxicity [143–145]. Whether the toxic effects of quartz are due to the presence of a soluble layer of silicic acid, negative ionization of its surface, piezoelectric charging or some other factor is not clear from experimental work.

Whatever the reason for the toxicity of quartz, it seems to be mediated by macrophage phagocytosis, predominantly in the interstitial space [139,146]. Large amounts of quartz ingested by macrophages cause rupture of phagosomal membranes, perhaps by peroxidation of lipids, escape of enzymes, and disruption and death of the cell [147]. However, smaller amounts of quartz do not necessarily cause rapid cell death, making it possible for macrophages to survive long enough to transport the dust within the lung, for example to hilar nodes, and to secrete bioactive materials. Among these may be reactive oxygen species and a wide range of cytokines [148–150]. One of these is probably interleukin 1, a substance that stimulates the proliferation of thymus-derived lymphocytes probably leading to transformation of B lymphocytes into plasma cells; this may also play some part in the propensity of patients with silicosis to produce autoantibodies.

Management and prevention

Once a worker has silicosis there is no treatment that affects the course of the disease. Its rate of progression varies from case to case, and the prognosis is not necessarily bad. For example, a man who develops category 1 nodular change after 30 years' work in tunnelling or quarrying is unlikely to show much progression over the next 20 years, unless his disease is due to a relatively recent high exposure. Conversely, someone who develops accelerated silicosis after a year's heavy exposure is likely to deteriorate rapidly over a few more years, and patients with acute silicosis usually die within months of presentation. Attempts to find a treatment that interferes with the toxicity of silica to phagosomal membranes, although successful to some extent *in vitro*, have not produced a drug suitable for trial in humans [151,152].

The complications of silicosis should be treated according to standard therapeutic guidelines. Evidence from the 1950s and 1960s suggests that tuberculosis responded almost as well to adequate chemotherapy in silicotics as non-silicotics [123]. The newer regimens, including rifampicin, ethambutol, isoniazid and pyrazinamide, have not been tested in a controlled manner in patients with silico-tuberculosis, although they have been shown to be successful in coal-workers' pneumoconiosis complicated by tuberculosis [153,154]. Personal experience suggests that the infection can usually be cured by modern chemotherapy but that the prognosis depends on the severity of the silicosis and the extent to which this disease is accelerated by the tuberculosis. The author's practice is to treat for 12 rather than 6 months in the belief that macrophage function in such patients may be impaired. Opportunistic mycobacterial infections should be treated along the lines suggested in Chapter 20. The patient with silicosis may be eligible for disablement benefit if symptoms and pulmonary dysfunction are present and in the UK should apply to the Department of Social Security. Civil action against a negligent employer might also be justified in individuals with disability or handicapped from pursuing their trade.

Prevention of silicosis depends on preventing exposure to respirable silica dust, which presupposes that the risk has been recognized; regrettably this is not always the case. Most countries now recognize a silica dust standard aimed at preventing exposure of the workforce to more than $100\,\mu g/m^3$ of respirable quartz. Whether this is adequate to prevent all cases is dubious, as discussed above, but, if enforced, at least prevents the most severe and rapidly developing cases [112,155]. Ideally, the use of quartz should be avoided if a safer substitute material is available. There is some evidence that inhalation of quartz mixed with other dusts leads to a less severe and progressive disease; this seems to be the case in coal-miners and foundrymen when the quartz levels, though above 100 $\mu g/m^3$, only represent a low percentage of the total dust inhaled. In such industries, a less tight standard, if based on appropriate epidemiological evidence, could be argued for. When high levels of quartz occur despite the best ventilation and water suppression that can be provided, respirators provide additional protection. In these high concentrations, the workers should be isolated from the environment by a complete helmet and suit with its own positive-pressure air supply [156].

Workers exposed to a risk of silicosis should be offered chest radiography at regular intervals, probably at least every 4 years, in order that the earliest signs of disease are detected and the worker protected from further exposure.

Asbestosis

The naturally occurring fibrous minerals known as asbestos have the common property of resistance to destruction by chemical and physical means, and have therefore acquired great usefulness to humans. There is archaeological evidence that asbestos was used in making clay pots in 2500 BC and for funeral shrouds and lamp wicks in classical times. However, widespread use of the minerals in industrial society dates back to the exploitation of the Quebec chrysotile deposits in the 1860s and the South African deposits in the 1890s. The first evidence of pulmonary fibrosis in association with asbestos use was reported at the turn of the century [157,158], and by 1930 the hazard was so well known that legislation was introduced in the UK to control the exposure of workers in asbestos factories [8]. Shortly after this, the association of asbestosis and lung cancer was reported [159], and the increased risk of this disease run by asbestos workers was confirmed epidemiologically by the 1950s [9,160]. Although it had been described as a form of lung cancer among shipyard workers in Scotland in 1947 [161], it was not until 1960 that the hitherto rare tumour, pleural mesothelioma, was shown to occur relatively frequently in South African asbestos workers [10]. Many subsequent studies have confirmed the relationship of this tumour, and of peritoneal mesothelioma, to asbestos exposure [162–165]. Thus, over the last 70 years society has been confronted with the problem of what action to take when faced with a highly dangerous but also extremely useful industrial material.

Epidemiology

Asbestos and its uses

The minerals known as asbestos, a name derived from the Greek work for unquenchable, belong to one of two mineralogical groups, the serpentines and the amphiboles. Chrysotile, or white asbestos, is the only asbestos that is a serpentine; it is a magnesium silicate with a curly configuration and is able to shear into many smaller fibrils. All the other forms of asbestos are amphiboles, straight fibres that do not shear into shorter fibrils. They include crocidolite (blue asbestos), an iron–magnesium–sodium silicate; amosite (brown asbestos) and anthophyllite, iron–magnesium silicates; and tremolite and actinolite, calcium–iron–magnesium silicates.

Chrysotile is the most widely used form of asbestos, some 4 million tonnes being produced annually by the two major producers, Russia and Quebec Province in Canada. Amosite and crocidolite are produced mainly by South Africa, about 250 000 tonnes annually reaching the world markets. Little if any tremolite, anthophyllite or actinolite is now produced commercially, although anthophyllite has been exploited in Finland in the past. Asbestos is found naturally bound into rock and is obtained largely by underground mining. The rock is crushed and the released fibres carded as in the wool industry; transport of asbestos from producer to user is now exclusively in impermeable plastic bags. The mineral has many uses, and its replacement by safer material has been a major problem for many industries. In particular, it imparts strength to cement, building materials and plastics, is an effective insulator and a durable friction material, is important in fireproofing and is useful as a filler in paints. It may be woven into fire-resistant materials. Thus people may be exposed to asbestos anywhere in the chain from the mine and crusher, the site of production of materials, to the place where the materials are used, deteriorate and are removed. Indeed, exposure to waste asbestos material at dumps is another area of concern. Of particular importance as situations where workers have been, and in some cases still are, exposed to asbestos are asbestos mills, thermal insulation, construction work and demolition, electrical repair work, railway engineering workshops, shipbuilding, ship repair and breaking, gas mask manufacture, boiler repair, and cement and friction product manufacture. Probably the most important occupation in developed countries is asbestos removal and abatement. Important exposures may also have been received by people living close to sources of heavy environmental asbestos pollution and by wives and families of asbestos workers as a result of their dusty clothes. There is little doubt also that careless disposal of asbestos waste has led to exposure of children playing on spoil heaps [166].

Prevalence

It is not possible to know how many people are suffering the harmful effects of asbestos exposure. However, some idea may be obtained from statistics published by the British Government, which indicate the number of people certified by the Pneumoconiosis Boards as having asbestosis and mesothelioma and the number of death certificates mentioning these conditions [167]. Approximately 1000 people per annum die of mesothelioma in the UK and this figure is still rising (see Fig. 43.15). About 300–400 are diagnosed as having asbestosis, most being retired from work. This figure has been static for several years. While these figures largely reflect a pathogenic response to industrial conditions in the two decades after the Second World War, amphibole forms of asbestos were imported into the UK until 1980 and chrysotile imports only started to decline about that date, so that the maximum exposures in terms of numbers of people probably occcured around 1970 [168]. The incidence of asbestos-related lung cancer is not known, since it is almost never possible in individuals to be sure whether the disease was due to asbestos, cigarettes or both. However, there is no doubt that some workers develop lung cancer who would not have done so had they not been exposed regularly to asbestos; studies of cohorts of heavily exposed asbestos workers have consistently shown lung cancer excesses as great as the numbers of mesothelioma cases. Thus in the UK although only some 50 people with asbestosis die of lung cancer each year, the numbers of patients in whom asbestos exposure may have contributed to the development of the disease may be considerably greater.

Clearly the incidence of these diseases reflects the numbers at risk of exposure and the cumulative amounts of asbestos to which they have been exposed. Incidence figures in individual countries cannot therefore be applied to other countries, where the workforce and industrial conditions may differ considerably. However, they do give some idea of the order of magnitude of the problem, for example in the UK there are 1000–2000 deaths annually from asbestos-related disease in a working population of approximately 20 million compared with about 30 000 deaths from lung cancer, largely due to cigarettes. This has been recognized as a serious public health problem, though not one that affects the general public but those members of it who work in jobs where exposure to asbestos occurs. The jobs most at risk of such exposure, as estimated from the mesothelioma statistics for England and Wales, are shown in Table 54.3.

Relationships between exposure to asbestos and disease

There are considerable difficulties in determining the relationships between exposure and response with respect to the asbestos diseases [169]. Firstly, assessment of exposure depends on reliable measurements of airborne asbestos

Table 54.3 Proportional mortality from mesothelioma in different jobs 1979–80. (from Peto *et al.* [168].)

	Proportional mortality ratio (all mean = 100) and numbers of deaths (*n*)
Metal plate work (including shipyards)	700 (110)
Vehicle body builders	619 (35)
Plumbers, gas fitters	443 (201)
Carpenters	356 (254)
Electricians	291 (161)
Upholsterers	283 (19)
Construction workers	256 (187)
Boiler operators	254 (39)
Sheet metal workers	233 (48)
Production fitters	216 (304)
Engineers	211 (105)
Plasterers	203 (27)
Welders	203 (70)
Dockers	195 (69)
Builders and handymen	164 (98)
Machine tool operators	133 (179)
Painters and decorators	131 (100)

having been made for a prolonged period of the working lives of an industrial population. The measurement of asbestos is not a simple matter, depending as it does upon counting fibres of appropriate size under the microscope, and considerable variability between different counters may occur [170]. Secondly, the response is not always easily determined. With respect to mesothelioma, the response is fairly obvious but for asbestosis it may not be; for example, early radiological change or auscultatory crackles may also be subject to considerable interobserver and intraobserver error, as well as being able to be caused by other conditions. With respect to lung cancer, the confounding factor of cigarette smoking has to be taken into account.

Despite these problems, several studies have cast light on this important matter and therefore measures to prevent the diseases are somewhat more securely based now than before. A study of Quebec miners and millers has suggested that a 1% risk of significant functional or radiological abnormalities was associated with exposures estimated to be about 200 fibre·years/mL, i.e. equivalent to 4 fibres/mL for 50 years [171]. In an American asbestos cement factory, similar results were obtained [172]; in a British asbestos textiles factory it was calculated that in order to reduce the risks so that fewer than 1% of workers would develop early signs of asbestosis (defined by the authors as 'possible asbestosis', as diagnosed by the factory doctor) over a 40-year working life the fibre concentration should be between 1.1 and 0.3 fibres/mL [173]. In the UK, regulations to cover workers in jobs with recognized exposure to asbestos were introduced in 1969 and thereafter such workers were exposed to concentrations that should not have exceeded 2 fibres/mL. One study has shown a halving of the prevalence of small radiological opacities and pleural shadows in those exposed only under the regulations [174].

These results indicate that risks are different in different industries, and it seems likely that they are indeed lower in mining, milling and cement production than in textile and insulation work. However, as shown in Table 54.3, those occupations in which mesothelioma is most likely to be found are those in which the largest numbers of people are potentially exposed to asbestos; however, these are not the industries classically recognized as being at risk during production and manufacture of asbestos products but rather those in which the risks arise from secondary exposure [168]. Thus the greatest numbers of cases occur in fitters, carpenters, plumbers and machine tool operators. It seems likely that different types of asbestos have different magnitudes of effect, crocidolite being the most dangerous, followed by amosite then chrysotile. This also becomes particularly obvious when mesothelioma is considered, although in this disease measurements of exposure have rarely been available because of the long time between exposure and development of the tumour.

Studies of workers in the Quebec industry exposed only to chrysotile have shown a very low incidence of mesothelioma [175], whereas workers exposed to amosite alone and crocidolite alone seem to have suffered higher death rates from this disease, up to 4 and 16% respectively of all deaths over about 35 years [176,177]. In particular, studies of gas mask manufacturers, who used crocidolite intensively for periods of up to 5 years during the Second World War, have shown a high mortality from mesothelioma [177,178]. While this suggests that very short exposures may be risky, there is no evidence that this is so unless the exposure is likely to have been very intense. Indeed, there is evidence that risk decreases in proportion to reduction in duration of exposure [179,180]. Careful estimates of likely rates of death among a large cohort of crocidolite workers at Wittenoom, Western Australia have predicted a likely overall mortality around 14% from mesothelioma and 10% from lung cancer, together with some 7% having asbestosis at the time of death [181].

With respect to excess risk of lung cancer, a similar gradient between asbestos types seems to exist. Prolonged exposure to chrysotile seems to increase the risk by a factor of between two and three [171,182], while exposures to amosite of more than 2 years may increase it six times [176]. In crocidolite gas mask workers, exposures of several months doubled the risk of lung cancer [177], while in the Wittenoom study it was estimated that almost half of the 10% death rate from lung cancer was attributable to the asbestos exposure [181]. With respect to lung cancer it is notable that an interaction occurs between cigarettes and asbestos such that the effects of the two probably multiply the risk [183–185]. Thus if a smoker has a risk of lung cancer 10 times that of a non-smoker and someone exposed to high levels of asbestos five times the risk of someone not exposed to asbestos, then someone who both smokes and is exposed may have up to 50 times the risk of a non-exposed non-smoker.

Several studies have suggested a relationship between asbestos exposure and other malignant diseases [186,187]. Of these, the most plausible is laryngeal carcinoma, and it seems quite likely that heavily exposed asbestos workers had an increased risk of this tumour in the past [188–190]. Some have expressed scepticism about this relationship, preferring to attribute it to failure to correct for confounding effects of smoking and alcohol [191]. However, a more likely explanation is that the risks under more recent, better regulated exposures have been much reduced. It is doubtful if the early reports of excess risk of gastrointestinal cancer were valid and it may be that they represented misdiagnosis of peritoneal mesothelioma, a condition well known to be associated with heavy asbestos exposure. There is a suspicion from a case–control study that large-cell lymphoma of the oral cavity and gastrointestinal tract, a very uncommon tumour, may be associated with asbestos [192].

Clinical features

Chest radiography

The earliest sign of asbestosis is the appearance of short linear shadows about 1–3 mm thick, predominantly in the lower lung zones. These shadows, classified as category 1s or t (see Chapter 3 for details of the ILO classification), are identical to those seen in the early stages of idiopathic pulmonary fibrosis. Moreover, they cannot be distinguished from what are probably the normal appearances of the ageing lung nor from the radiological effects associated with cigarette smoking [193]. They should not therefore be regarded as in any way diagnostic of asbestosis. As the disease progresses, these shadows become more profuse and gradually obscure the vascular pattern of the lower zones (Fig. 54.19). The individual shadows also often become thicker and take on a more irregular, sometimes stellate or blotchy, appearance. Eventually the appearance of diffuse honeycombing may become apparent. Asbestosis does not occur as a result of occasional or incidental exposure. Once the lesions have appeared they usually progress, although the rate of progression may be slow and sometimes the disease, if caught early and exposure is stopped, appears to arrest [194–196]. However, it is well

recognized that the first signs of asbestosis may occur after asbestos exposure has ceased [197,198]; in these circumstances, progression tends to be comparatively slow. When the radiological appearances of asbestosis appear for the first time after exposure to asbestos has ceased, there is almost always a prolonged history of exposure to the material, usually at relatively low concentrations.

The radiological effects of ageing and cigarette smoke do not usually extend beyond category 1 on the ILO scale of profusion, so that irregular shadows more profuse than this can be taken to indicate pulmonary fibrosis. Whether this fibrosis is due to asbestosis depends on the history of exposure, although radiological evidence may also be helpful in that the presence of pleural plaques, obliteration of costophrenic angles or diffuse pleural fibrosis is indicative of asbestos exposure. Calcified pleural plaques are indeed diagnostic of this, and if they are associated with interstitial fibrosis it is usually difficult to deny that any associated lung fibrosis is due to asbestosis. These pleural lesions are described in Chapter 43.

High-resolution CT is more sensitive than standard chest films for the detection of early interstitial fibrosis in workers exposed to asbestos and nicely demonstrates the peripheral and basal accentuation of the fibrosis. CT also shows calcified and non-calcified pleural disease and the presence of these features helps to tip the diagnostic scales in favour of an asbestos aetiology for the fibrosis in cases of clinical doubt. However, the absence of plaques on CT

Fig. 54.19 Lower part of chest film of a patient with asbestosis showing well-marked irregular fibrosis and honeycombing.

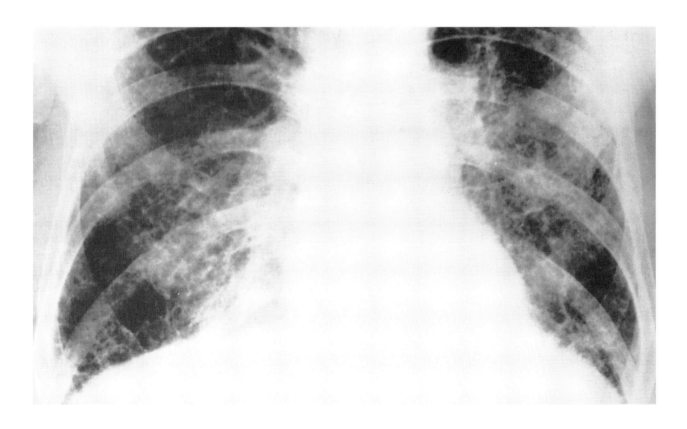

should not be taken to exclude the presence of asbestosis if there is an adequate history of exposure, since not all plaques are visible on the scan. In the author's opinion, in the absence of pleural disease it is not possible to differentiate between early asbestosis and early cryptogenic fibrosis from the CT features alone; equally pathologists are reluctant to diagnose the cause of fibrosis from macroscopic inspection of the lung! However, a few features help to increase the confidence with which a diagnosis of asbestosis can be made [199]. Pleural fibrosis with bands extending into peripheral lung are common in asbestosis (Fig. 54.20) and rare in the cryptogenic disease, while fibrosis extending into upper lobes is uncommon in asbestosis. It should be noted that reports showing clear differences between these two diseases are at serious risk of bias from selection of the relatively few 'typical' subjects studied.

Symptoms and signs

The patient always gives a history of working either directly with asbestos or adjacent to others working with the material, usually in very dusty conditions and over a prolonged period. It is most unusual nowadays in the West to see the disease in anyone who has been exposed to asbestos for less than 20 years. As mentioned above, the condition may present after exposure has ceased. The symptoms are exertional dyspnoea and, often, dry cough. The dyspnoea gradually becomes more severe and eventually may be completely disabling, the patient dying of cardiorespiratory failure. This course is uncommon, most patients developing the disease relatively late in life and their disability being moderate rather than severe. The most common presentation in the western world is a patient who has been found to have minor radiological changes (usually pleural) on a coincidental chest radiograph, has no symptoms, but has crackles audible at the bases and minimal interstitial fibrosis on CT. However death from one of the malignant complications of asbestos exposure, bronchial carcinoma or mesothelioma, is of much more frequent occurrence. Although dependent to some extent on individual susceptibility, prognosis is also related to the amount of asbestos to which the worker has been exposed; thus heavy exposures resulting in early development of disease may be expected to result in more rapid progression, whereas asbestosis developing only after 30 years of work with the material may be expected to progress very slowly and does not usually itself influence life expectancy.

The earliest sign of asbestosis is the presence of repetitive end-inspiratory crackles, heard at the lung bases posteriorly or in the axillae [200,201]. These signs are not specific to asbestosis but in the presence of a convincing history of exposure are strong evidence of the disease. As the disease progresses, the crackles become more profuse and are heard earlier in inspiration, in early expiration and further up the lung. Only at this relatively late stage in the natural history of the disease is clubbing of the digits usually present [202]. As the disease reaches its terminal stage, diminished chest wall movements, tachypnoea and evidence of cor pulmonale may be detected, with cyanosis, tall jugular *a* waves, right ventricular heave and gallop rhythm. Gross oedematous right heart failure is uncommon, the patient usually dying of hypoxic respiratory failure.

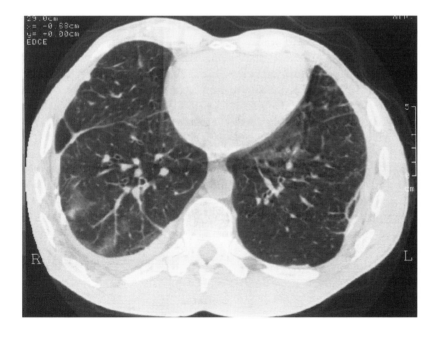

Fig. 54.20 High-resolution CT of patient with pleural fibrosis showing early interstitial fibrosis and marked pleural thickening with calcification and bands passing into the peripheral lung.

Lung function

The functional abnormalities associated with asbestosis are progressive reduction in carbon monoxide diffusing capacity, vital capacity and total lung capacity, with normal residual volume [203–205]. Compliance is decreased and lung recoil pressure increased. Hyperventilation and arterial oxygen desaturation may occur on exercise in the more advanced stages. These changes are not of course diagnostic of asbestosis but characteristic of any form of chronic pulmonary fibrosis.

Some authors, taking cognizance of the fact that the earliest pathological change involves respiratory bronchioles, have shown early changes in expiratory flow rates in subjects with relatively short but heavy exposures [206,207]. From a practical clinical point of view the most useful test for detection of significant asbestosis is the $D\text{L}CO$, and deterioration in this closely mirrors disease progression. Only as the disease reaches an advanced, and usually clinically very obvious, stage do lung volumes deviate sufficiently from the predicted range to be unequivocally abnormal. In keeping with this, the transfer coefficient ($K\text{CO}$) is usually low. However, this index of lung function may be paradoxically increased in patients with extensive pleural fibrosis [208], so the combination of pleural and pulmonary fibrosis in an asbestos worker may be associated with low $D\text{L}CO$ and alveolar volume and a relatively normal $K\text{CO}$.

Pathology

The macroscopic appearances of asbestosis are of grey-white fibrosis, most marked in the lower zones. If the disease is advanced, honeycomb changes may be apparent (Fig. 54.21). Parietal pleural plaques are usually present and diffuse fibrosis involving both layers of pleura and extending into the surface of the lung may also be seen. These pleural changes are described in Chapter 43.

Microscopically, the earliest change is an alveolitis around asbestos fibres in the respiratory bronchioles [209–211]. In experimental lesions the first response to asbestos deposition in the acinus can be seen to be an influx of macrophages, some of which disintegrate and become surrounded by fibrin and subsequently collagen [212]. The most peripheral airspaces and the interstitium are initially free of fibrosis but as the lesion develops it can be seen to spread into alveolar walls and along the respiratory bronchioles to the distal alveoli, resulting in widespread diffuse fibrosis (Fig. 54.22). The appearances of honeycombing result from a dilatation of small bronchi and bronchioles in uninvolved parts of the lung due to their retraction by surrounding fibrosis [213]. Massive areas of fibrosis have been described but are different from PMF in other pneumoconioses in that they represent confluent areas of irregular fibrosis. Caplan lesions have also been described very rarely [214].

Asbestosis may be complicated by silicosis in asbestos miners, as has been described in South Africa; when this occurs the distribution of the diffuse fibrosis may be predominantly in the upper zones of the lung. There is not thought to be an increased frequency of tuberculosis in patients with asbestosis, although workers with concomitant silicosis may develop this complication, especially if, as in South Africa, the disease is endemic in the area. As mentioned previously, the most important complication of asbestosis is bronchial carcinoma.

The feature that differentiates asbestosis from other forms of pulmonary fibrosis is the presence of asbestos in the lungs. On light microscopy, asbestos fibres are generally too fine to be seen and the clue comes from the

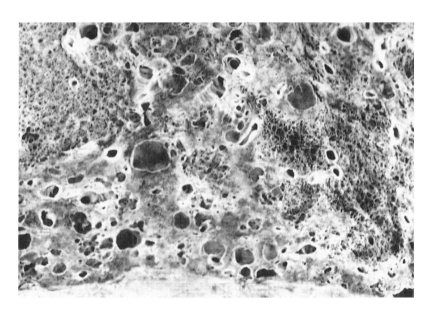

Fig. 54.21 Lung slice showing lower zone fibrosis of asbestosis. Two areas of relatively normal lung, to left and right, are separated by coarse irregular fibrosis.

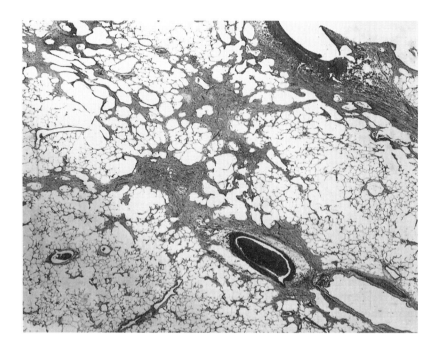

Fig. 54.22 Low-power view of early asbestosis showing peribronchiolar fibrosis.

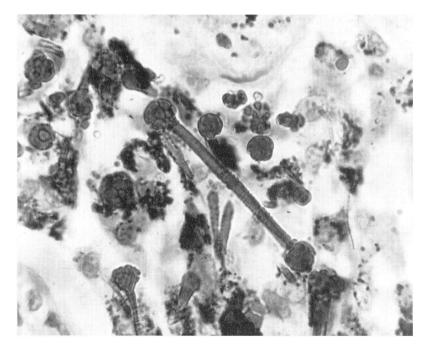

Fig. 54.23 Asbestos bodies in human lung. A few small uncoated fibres are also visible.

presence of ferruginous bodies. These are yellow-brown structures, about 2–5 μm in width and up to 150 μm in length. They have a beaded appearance and clubbed ends (Fig. 54.23) and probably derive from deposition of ferritin and protein onto the asbestos fibre within the body of macrophages. Electron microscopy shows the asbestos body to be formed around a single fibre of asbestos, usually an amphibole, though it may occasionally form around other fibrous particles [215–217]. Such structures also form around other mineral fibres, most of which do not have the same pathogenic significance of asbestos, so

care should be taken before concluding that they are indeed due to asbestos exposure. Electron microscopy with energy-dispersive X-ray spectroscopic analysis is the only sure means of identifying the minerals present in the tissue [218]. This expensive technique is not necessary for clinical purposes but is useful in research on mineral-induced lung disease and is increasingly being used in civil litigation in efforts to strengthen evidence of exposure to asbestos.

Often relatively few asbestos bodies may be seen, even in advanced asbestosis. This is because only a very small proportion of inhaled asbestos fibres are dealt with in this way by the lung's defences. Most fibres remain uncoated but are often less than 0.5 μm in diameter and therefore invisible on light microscopy. Special techniques of lung ashing and examination of residues by phase-contrast optical microscopy or electron microscopy allow an assessment to be made of the numbers of fibres that may be present in the lung. Using optical microscopy, such studies have shown up to 30 000 fibres/g of dried lung in apparently unexposed individuals, counts of 100 000 fibres/g or more in asbestos workers and over 3 million fibres/g in subjects with asbestosis [219,220]. Use of electron microscopy allows these figures to be multiplied by one or two orders of magnitude but also shows that many of the fibres in unexposed people are minerals other than asbestos [221].

Pathogenesis

In order for asbestosis to develop, sufficient numbers of fibres must penetrate to the acinar parts of the lung. The aerodynamic characteristics of fibres are such that their diameter must be less than about 3 μm in order for them to remain suspended in the inspired air to acinar level. Fibres are arbitrarily defined as structures three times as long as they are wide; thus a fibre may be of almost any length if sufficiently narrow and indeed many crocidolite fibres are only 0.1 μm in diameter. However, there is increasing evidence that in order to have a pathogenic effect fibres must be too long to be engulfed completely by macrophages and therefore fibres of less than 10 μm are probably of little

pathological significance [139,222] (Fig. 54.24). Furthermore, the shape of the fibre is probably important, such that chrysotile, with its curly configuration, is more liable to be intercepted by contact with bronchial walls than are the straight amphibole fibres [223]. Once the fibre has penetrated to acinar level, another factor of pathogenic importance is its durability [224]. This may prove to be of overriding importance in assessing the possible health effects of new fibrous substitutes for asbestos, such as glass and other synthetic fibres. A fibre that remains intact despite the attack of the lung's macrophages and the physical and chemical trauma of residence within a constantly moving organ is the one with the greatest potential harmfulness.

The mechanisms of fibrogenesis are not fully understood. *In vitro* studies show asbestos not to be very toxic to macrophages, though some studies have indicated that release of cytokines and reactive oxygen species may play a part [139]. Lavage studies in rats have shown only a moderate immediate cellular response to asbestos inhalation, in contrast to the rapid recruitment of polymorphonuclear cells that occurs with coal and quartz inhalation [225]. Nevertheless, like the human lung, the rat lung responds by production of diffuse fibrosis and bronchial carcinomas. Even more strikingly, as discussed in Chapter 43, injection of asbestos of any type into the pleura or peritoneum of a rat produces a dose-dependent incidence of mesothelioma; with appropriate doses almost 100% of rats die of this disease [226].

The epidemiological differences between the effects of chrysotile and of the amphiboles (i.e. the former seems to

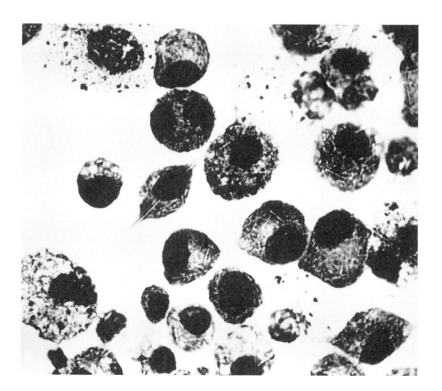

Fig. 54.24 Macrophages in culture with asbestos: several have engulfed short fibres but in two cases the fibres are too long and protrude through the cell membrane.

cause less disease dose for dose than the latter) may be explicable on the basis of two factors: (i) chrysotile is filtered out more efficiently by the airways because of its shape and its tendency to clump into groups of fibres and (ii) once inhaled, chrysotile is gradually broken up into tiny fibrils that because of their size are gradually removed by macrophages. This hypothesis explains why mesothelioma is so much less common in workers exposed to chrysotile than in those exposed to amphiboles, since in the long time period required for sufficient asbestos to migrate to the pleura chrysotile is broken up. However, it still has time to initiate the processes of fibrogenesis and bronchial carcinogenesis. In support of this hypothesis, studies of the lungs of workers exposed to a mixture of asbestos types have in general shown unexpectedly high proportions of amphiboles in relation to the amounts to which they were exposed during life [224,227].

Management

People exposed to asbestos may present to their doctors for a number of different reasons, and it is more usual to see such individuals before they develop disease than after. The usual reasons for presentation are discussed below.

1 A well person with no radiological abnormality has found that he or she has been or is currently exposed to asbestos. This is often due to the discovery of fixed asbestos materials in the house or workplace rather than to actual work with the material. Such people should be reassured that the risks of such incidental exposure are of no account. However, the physician should give general advice on future avoidance of exposure to airborne asbestos. If the workplace is the suspected source of exposure, the employer should be encouraged to seek the opinion of an occupational hygienist, and if thought necessary the regulatory authority, in the UK the Health and Safety Executive, should be contacted.

2 A fit person has been found to have pleural plaques on chest radiography. Again, the individual should be reassured once it has been established that current exposure to asbestos has ceased. Advice against smoking should be given but follow-up in clinics should not be arranged, since it serves no purpose other than to increase the subject's anxiety. There is no evidence that pleural plaques increase risks of any other disease, and any risks of lung cancer and mesothelioma relate to the history of asbestos exposure and, in the case of lung cancer, to smoking.

3 An asbestos worker presents with early irregular basal X-ray shadows and no symptoms. The diagnosis is made on the occupational history, radiological findings and presence of repetitive inspiratory crackles. Further exposure to asbestos should be discouraged, since detection at

an early stage may be associated with only very slow progression unless more asbestos is added to the load in the lungs. In the UK, if the worker has been employed, as opposed to self-employed, he or she should be encouraged to apply for pneumoconiosis benefit, which is awarded in proportion to the disability as assessed by the doctors of the Medical Board for Respiratory Diseases of the Department of Social Security. Since the risk of lung cancer is much increased, the individual should be discouraged from smoking. Such patients commonly sue their previous employers.

4 Patients presenting with late-stage, previously undiagnosed, asbestosis should be encouraged to apply for pneumoconiosis benefit. Treatment should be along routine lines for patients with respiratory failure, with provision of domestic aids, oxygen for symptomatic relief of breathlessness, diuretics for right heart failure and antibiotics for acute infections. Corticosteroids are of no value and should be avoided. In a patient of appropriate age and general health who does not smoke, transplantation would be an option (see Chapter 59).

Prevention

In taking steps to prevent asbestos-related diseases, two important points need to be borne in mind. Firstly, mesothelioma is almost always due to exposure to amphiboles and therefore avoidance of all use of these types of asbestos will eventually largely eliminate the disease. In the UK, crocidolite has effectively been excluded (by the imposition of very strict hygiene standards) since 1970 and amosite use has been restricted in the same way since 1980. Furthermore, tight regulation of asbestos removal since 1970, especially where amphiboles are concerned, should have ensured that mesothelioma would soon become a rare condition once again. However, it has now become apparent that most cases of mesothelioma occur in people working in effectively unregulated industries, with exposure to asbestos that has been *in situ* for many years, and that the epidemic of this disease is therefore likely to peak around the year 2020 and only decline to current levels some decade or two after that [168]. Secondly, asbestosis and lung cancer develop in relation to the dose of asbestos to which people are exposed. Therefore, occasional and incidental domestic or workplace exposures are likely to be of no significance. Such risks of death have been calculated to be considerably less than those associated with driving daily to work or living in a house with a smoker for example [169]. However, the risks that are run by someone working with asbestos on a regular basis are more easily imagined. While it is probable that risks of clinically significant asbestosis may be eliminated by preventing workplace exposure to more than 0.5 fibres/mL over a lifetime, these exposure levels may still entail a risk of developing lung cancer, dependent partly on the smoking habits of the workforce, rising to perhaps 6 per 1000 for men exposed to the mineral for 35 years from the age of 20. For a discussion of these risks and the assumptions made in calculating them, the reader is referred to the monograph of Doll and Peto [169].

Thus the prevention of asbestos-related disease depends on reduction or elimination of exposure to the mineral. This should be achieved by the enforcement of a strict code of practice in handling the material, by increased public awareness of its hazards (thus ensuring it is handled with respect) and by the setting of appropriate hygiene standards. Currently in the UK the maximum allowable concentration of chrysotile is 0.5 fibres/mL, while the use of crocidolite and amosite is effectively prevented by a standard of 0.2 fibres/mL. Regulations also enforce the wearing of protective clothing and full-face respirators by workers removing asbestos, effective sealing off and vacuuming of such areas and safe disposal of the waste material. Other countries have their own regulations, which range from a complete ban on the use of asbestos to none at all.

Disease due to other silicate materials

Although coal, quartz and asbestos are the three minerals containing silicon to which humans are most frequently exposed, there are other compound silicates that either occur naturally or are synthetic which may expose the lungs to hazard. In general, their toxic effects are likely to be similar to those of coal if they produce amorphous airborne dusts or similar to those of asbestos if they produce fibrous dusts. The most important such minerals are kaolin, fuller's earth, mica and cement, which are all amorphous; talc, which has a plate-like shape; and mullite, erionite, attapulgite, sepiolite and wollastonite, which are fibrous. Synthetic fibres are also considered here, as is oil-shale, which contains a complex mixture of clay minerals.

Non-fibrous silicates

Talc

Talc is a hydrated magnesium silicate with multiple uses as a lubricant and filler in cosmetics, paper and rubber manufacture, paints and building materials. It is mined in Canada, the USA, Russia, Italy and the Pyrenees, and in some of these places is associated geologically with tremolite asbestos. Cosmetic talc should be free of asbestos [228,229], but industrial grades may contain it as well as other minerals such as quartz and accordingly should be carefully handled.

The coincidence of talc and fibrous tremolite in the mineral deposits has caused some difficulty in deciding what the true effects of talc are on the lung. Talc miners have been shown to have an increased risk of pleural plaques, diffuse pulmonary fibrosis and lung cancer [230–232]. However, these effects were probably due to the tremolite (though this is of little consequence when it comes to protecting the miners and millers, who continue to be exposed to both minerals). In places where exposure has been to pure talc, the disease described is a nodular pneumoconiosis with a tendency for the small nodules to aggregate and form PMF, similar to silicosis [232]. There is no evidence that exposure to talc is carcinogenic unless associated with fibrous tremolite. A follow-up survey of people who had previously been treated for pneumothorax with insufflation of medicinal grade talc into the pleural space showed no excess mortality and no cases of mesothelioma [233].

Some rather more bizarre hazards of talc have been described. One man has been recorded as giving himself pneumoconiosis by obsessive overuse of talcum powder [234], another by enthusiastic work as a talc aerosol inspector [235] and a third by inhaling (illegally) the contents of medicinal capsules prior to performing as a punk-rock drummer [236]. Talc may also initiate bronchoconstrictive episodes when inhaled by babies [237] and is of course one of the means by which intravenous drug abusers accidentally kill themselves [238].

Kaolin and other clays

Kaolin consists mainly of the mineral kaolinite, a hydrated aluminium silicate, and is produced in south-west England, the USA, Japan, Egypt, Czechoslovakia and Germany. It is quarried by washing it out of the deposits with water and is then dried and milled for use in ceramics, paints, paper, soap and pharmaceuticals. Both simple and complicated pneumoconiosis have been described in workers in the milling and bagging plants, the pathological and radiological appearances being very similar to those of coal-workers' pneumoconiosis [239,240]. In particular, kaolin does not produce the highly collagenous lesions seen with quartz inhalation, unless the worker has been exposed to a mixed silica-containing dust. Studies of lung function in patients with kaolin pneumoconiosis have shown results similar to those described in coal-workers, with impairment associated with PMF and a possible dust-related obstructive and restrictive component in subjects with simple pneumoconiosis [241–243].

Fuller's earth is an absorbent clay that was named after its early use in fulling, the removal of grease from wool. It usually contains calcium montmorillonite, an aluminium silicate, and is obtained by quarrying in the UK, the USA and Germany. It is used as a filter, filler and binder for foundry moulds. A relatively benign simple pneumoconiosis, occasionally progressing to PMF and very similar to kaolin pneumoconiosis, has been described in production workers [244,245].

Oil-shale was mined in Scotland until 1962 for the production of mineral oil. Other deposits have been mined in France and Estonia, while enormous amounts wait to be exploited in the Rocky Mountains in the USA. The rock is crushed and heated in retorts to produce the oil which is then refined. Skin cancer is a well-known hazard of workers exposed to the oil [246], although pneumoconiosis has been described in the miners and dust-exposed surface workers [247,248]. The disease appears relatively benign, although PMF has occurred occasionally and a mixed restrictive and obstructive dysfunction has been described in the simple disease [249]. It is probably due largely to the kaolin component of the shale. Epidemiological studies have shown no associated lung cancer hazard [250].

It should be remembered that mining or quarrying and production of clays may expose workers to a risk of silicosis if the clay deposit contains substantial amounts of quartz. This may be the case with ball clays, used in earthenware and bricks, and bentonite, which is used in the same applications as fuller's earth [103,251,252]. In addition, some clay minerals such as palygorskite, attapulgite and sepiolite have a fibrous habit and are mentioned below.

Mica

There are two commercially important forms of mica: muscovite, a potassium–aluminium silicate, and phlogopite, a magnesium–aluminium silicate. The former is transparent and both are resistant to heat and electricity. They are mined in North America and India and used in furnace windows, as fillers in papers and paints, and in insulating materials in the electricity industry. There have been occasional reports of pneumoconiosis among workers exposed to ground mica, usually of a nodular type but diffuse interstitial fibrosis has been described [253–256]. However, such episodes seem to be rare.

Vermiculite is another form of mica mined mainly in the USA and South Africa and used predominantly as an insulation material. Some of the mineral deposits are contaminated with fibrous amphiboles and it is likely that the reports of radiological disease and increased cancer mortality in these workers have been largely due to this contamination [257–259].

Cement

Cement is produced by heating a crushed mixture of limestone and clay or shale in a long rotary kiln. The clinker produced is mixed with gypsum and slag, crushed, and ground in ball mills. The product consists largely of calcium silicates and aluminates. There is some evidence that cement workers may develop simple pneumoconiosis and decrement in ventilatory capacity, although adequate studies need to be carried out [260,261]. Workers handling and producing asbestos cement are at risk from exposure to the asbestos.

Fibrous silicates

Enough is now known about the nature of tissue damage from fibrous minerals to be able to generalize about risks to health from exploitation of any such new material. It is stressed that this is a generalization and that there may be exceptions; nevertheless, this information may be used as a guide to manufacturers and as a means of designing preventive measures in industry [262]. The factors that determine toxicity, in terms of both fibrogenicity and pleural carcinogenicity, are the length and diameter of the fibres to which workers are likely to be exposed and the solubility of the fibres. Fibres longer than about 10 μm are likely to be retained in the lung, while shorter fibres are likely to be removed. Thus short fibres act like amorphous dusts and are generally harmless unless inhaled in very high concentrations. Fibres wider than 3 μm are unable to reach the respiratory epithelium in sufficient numbers, and can also therefore be regarded as relatively benign. Once in the acinus, the factor that primarily determines toxicity is the solubility of the fibre and therefore its ability to remain in the tissue [263,264]. Relatively soluble fibres such as most glass fibres will dissolve quickly and cause no disease whereas insoluble fibres such as some ceramic and carbon fibres might be expected to persist much longer and ultimately lead to fibrosis and sometimes neoplasia.

Erionite

Erionite is a naturally occurring fibrous aluminium silicate found in volcanic rocks. It is not used commercially but may be the cause of disease in people who are digging through the rock. In particular, it occurs in parts of Turkey where villagers have been in the habit of cutting into the rock to make their homes and to produce building materials and stucco [265–267]. The inhabitants of these villages have been shown to have a very high rate of pleural plaques, pulmonary fibrosis, lung cancer and mesothelioma. In other words, the mineral behaves in the body like asbestos, which it resembles physically but not mineralogically. These observations have been important in supporting the hypothesis that the effects of asbestos are due to its size and shape rather than its chemical and mineralogical characteristics. They imply therefore that other minerals of similar shape and size may have similar effects and should therefore be handled with care.

Deposits of erionite occur in other parts of the world, particularly in desert areas of Nevada and Utah in the USA. There is a potential for human exposure, for example in digging missile silos, and one patient who lived and worked in such an area has been described as having pulmonary and pleural fibrosis associated with erionite in his lung [268].

Synthetic fibres

The realization that the fibrous shape of asbestos is likely to be important in the pathogenesis of disease has led to anxiety about the production and use of synthetic glass wool, rock wool, carbon and ceramic fibres, which are widely used as asbestos substitutes. Experimentally, some of these fibres have been shown to cause mesothelioma if they are introduced into the rat pleura and are sufficiently fine and long [269,270]. Studies of human workforces exposed to them have not so far shown any significant degree of hazard from mesothelioma or non-malignant respiratory disease, although there is some evidence from very large epidemiological studies in Europe and the USA of a slight increase in risk of lung cancer in workers with prolonged exposure to rock/slag wool [271,272]. Some of this risk may have been a consequence of exposure to other carcinogens in the early stages of the industry, but an open mind should be kept, especially with respect to the use of relatively insoluble fibres. Moreover, the apparently low incidence of disease may be due to the relatively low exposure of workers to fine respirable fibres and should not be taken as an indication of harmlessness if finer fibres are to be used in future applications.

Other fibrous silicates

Mullite, another aluminium silicate, occurs as a result of combustion of coal and is a component of fly ash, the ash residue from power stations. It has a fibrous shape, though the fibres tend to be short. It is commonly identified in human lungs when their mineral content is being measured by electron microscopy, although whether it is harmful has not been established. Interstitial lung disease has been described in men using it in the production of cat litter [273]. Attapulgite, palygorskite and sepiolite are fibrous clay minerals that have commercial applications as absorbents and filter materials. Again, there have been occasional reports of pulmonary fibrosis in those working with attapulgite and it seems possible that there may be a hazard with high exposures [274]. There is also a suspicion that attapulgite miners may have an excess risk of lung cancer, though this cannot be said to be firmly established [275]. In general the fibres are rather short and therefore likely to be less harmful than asbestos. Wollastonite, a fibrous calcium silicate, is used in ceramics and as an asbestos substitute. These fibres are also short but there

has been one report of possible pulmonary fibrosis and pleural plaques in exposed workers [276].

Siderosis and mixed-dust pneumoconioses

Siderosis

Pure siderosis is due to deposition of iron oxides in the lung, where they are taken up by macrophages in both the alveoli and interstitial tissue. No fibrous reaction occurs but the chest radiograph shows multiple radiodense nodules due to the presence of the iron (Fig. 54.25). The condition occurs in arc welders and oxyacetylene cutters due to the presence of iron oxides in the fume from the heated metal [277]; it should be noted that welders and cutters may also be exposed to other metals and carbon in the fume and that pneumoconiosis in such workers cannot always be assumed to be pure siderosis. Siderosis also occurs in silver polishers, who use iron oxide (jeweller's rouge) to polish the metal [278]. The radiological changes of siderosis tend to regress after exposure ceases and the condition in its pure form is not associated with abnormality of lung function [279]. There has been debate about the possible carcinogenicity of inhaled iron, based on the known increased hazard in haematite miners (see next section) and an excessive death rate from lung cancer noted by the British Registrar General. However, it seems likely that iron itself is not carcinogenic and that when cancer occurs it is probably due to concomitant exposure to other carcinogens in either cigarettes or the occupational environment.

Mixed-dust pneumoconioses

Mixed-dust pneumoconiosis is a convenient term covering pneumoconioses occurring in a variety of trades in which the inhaled dust is a mixture of silica and other substances. Strictly speaking, coal-workers' and shale-miners' pneumoconioses are mixed-dust pneumoconioses. The pathological reaction and its physiological consequences depend on the constituents of the dust though, in general, the higher the proportion of silica, the more closely the disease resembles silicosis. Haematite miners' lung is an example of this. The iron ore, haematite, was mined in Cumbria where it was noted that miners developed pneumoconiosis often after many years of exposure underground [280,281]. Both simple pneumoconiosis and PMF occurred and at postmortem the lungs were noted to be brick-red in colour [282]. Pathologically, the appearances are those of silicosis with the additional feature of accumulation of iron pigmentation. Haematite miners in the UK were shown to have an increased risk of lung cancer, although this was almost certainly related to exposure to radon daughters in the mine atmosphere [283].

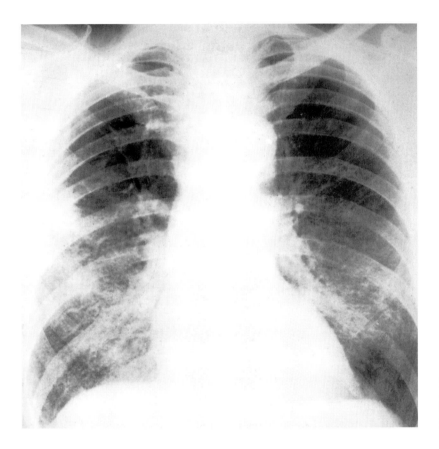

Fig 54.25 Welders' siderosis showing diffuse pin-point opacities. The peripheral lesion in the right mid zone was removed at thoracotomy and proved to be a carcinoma.

Other workers who may develop pneumoconiosis related to inhalation of a mixture of iron oxides and silica are foundry workers, especially fettlers, welders and burners, boiler scalers and ochre miners. Any worker exposed to a mixed dust containing more than about 10% quartz is liable to develop silicosis.

Berylliosis

Beryllium ore (beryl or beryllium aluminium silicate) is mined predominantly in South America. The metal is extracted from the crushed ore by heating and treatment with sulphuric acid or fluoride and is used as an alloy in the manufacture of components in X-ray equipment, atomic reactors, the aerospace industry, armaments and heat-resistant ceramics. These alloys have the properties of tensile strength, resistance to corrosion, metal fatigue and heat, as well as being non-magnetic, transparent to X-rays and of high electrical conductivity.

Effects of exposure to beryllium

Exposure to beryllium fume or salts may occur in extraction, refining or production of alloys. In the UK a few cases of berylliosis have occurred in workers producing and breaking fluorescent lights, which used to be coated with the metal, and in refinery workers [284]. The greatest experience of the harmful effects of beryllium comes from the USA, where a registry of cases has been kept at the Massachusetts General Hospital since 1952 following a postwar epidemic of the disease [285–287].

Exposure to high concentrations of beryllium fume may cause an acute toxic pneumonitis, with oedema of mucous membranes from pharynx to small airways together with pulmonary oedema [285]. The radiograph shows evidence of the pulmonary oedema and the clinical signs are tachypnoea, cyanosis and diffuse inspiratory crackles. Mild cases of the condition are usually self-limiting but severe cases may need treatment with oxygen and corticosteroids to prevent a fatal outcome. Approximately 10% of patients with acute berylliosis have progressed to the chronic form of the disease.

Chronic berylliosis was first described in 1946 [286]. It is different from other mineral pneumoconioses in that it is a systemic hypersensitivity disease, with principal effects on the lung and skin. Sensitization usually occurs by inhalation of dust or fume of the metal or its salts but may occur by introduction of beryllium into the skin through an abrasion. Only a small proportion of those exposed have developed the disease, often after a prolonged latent period and sometimes after a relatively light exposure. Cases have occurred in wives of workers, presumably from beryllium carried on clothing, and in people living close to beryllium refineries.

Clinical features

The disease may present years after exposure to beryllium has ceased [288,289]. It should be a routine in patients presenting with apparent sarcoidosis to ask about possible exposure to the metal in the past, as in ceramics, metal alloying, the nuclear industry or even dental prosthetics [290]. It has also been described in wives of such workers who have been exposed to their husbands' contaminated clothes [291]. The symptoms are cough and dyspnoea and the course of the untreated disease is usually progressive. However, an apparently self-limiting variant has been described in people exposed to beryllium in rather low concentrations [292], in whom minor radiological changes appeared and subsequently disappeared without treatment. Finger clubbing only occurs rarely and inspiratory crackles are not a feature of the early disease, although they may appear as fibrosis becomes established. Hepato-splenomegaly may occur, as may macular skin lesions, although generalized lymphadenopathy and uveitis are not features. Pneumothorax and cor pulmonale are complications of advanced disease. As in sarcoidosis, hypercalcaemia, hypercalciuria and nephrocalcinosis may also occur, but the other less common manifestations of sarcoidosis such as cardiac and neurological involvement have not been described.

The radiographic changes are initially a diffuse fine granularity that evolves into a reticulonodular pattern and finally irregular fibrosis, often of a coarse generalized type as in chronic sarcoidosis [293] (Fig. 54.26). Bilateral hilar adenopathy may occur but only when there is also evidence of interstitial lung infiltration. As would be expected, the functional changes are those associated with diffuse interstitial disease, with reduced DLCO and progressive reduction in lung volumes and compliance as fibrosis increases [294].

Pathology

The gross appearances of chronic berylliosis at an advanced stage are of irregular fibrosis with bullae and cyst formation. The important microscopic feature is the non-caseating granuloma. At an early stage, discrete follicles of epithelioid cells surrounded by lymphocytes and plasma cells are seen in the interstitial tissues and alveolar walls. Similar appearances are found in lymph nodes, skin lesions, liver and spleen. Langhans' giant cells develop by fusion of the epithelioid cells, and sarcoid-type inclusion bodies may be seen. These pathological features are indistinguishable from those of sarcoidosis (Fig. 54.27). As the disease progresses, interstitial pulmonary fibrosis occurs, which may proceed to widespread acinar destruction and dilatation of small airways, to produce honeycombing.

Pathogenesis

The characteristic immunological features of beryllium disease are cutaneous anergy to tuberculin, delayed skin reactivity to beryllium, and *in vitro* stimulation of lymphocytes by beryllium salts so that they transform into lymphoblasts and produce lymphokines such as a factor that inhibits macrophage migration [295]. In addition, the pathological features of mononuclear cells and giant cells lend weight to the concept that berylliosis is due to a delayed hypersensitivity reaction to the metal and its salts.

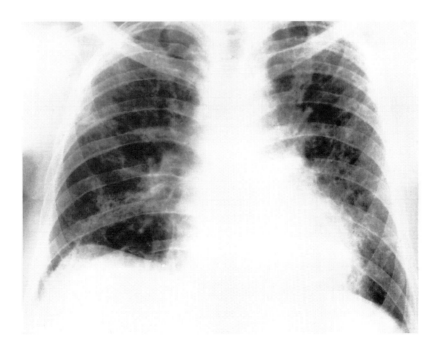

Fig. 54.26 Chronic berylliosis in ex-beryllium refiner showing diffuse irregular pulmonary fibrosis.

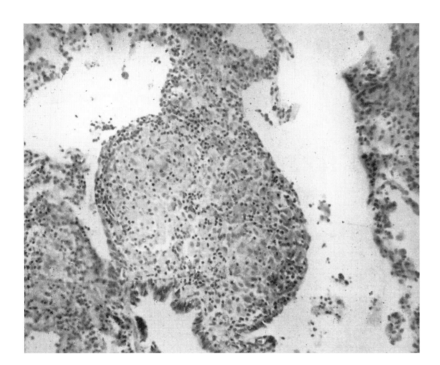

Fig. 54.27 Sarcoid-like granuloma in the lung of patient with berylliosis.

Bronchoalveolar lavage studies in patients with chronic berylliosis have shown increased cell numbers, almost 80% being lymphocytes, most of the T subtype [296]. These cells have been shown to react to beryllium more rapidly than blood lymphocytes, suggesting that a high proportion are sensitized to the metal.

It seems likely therefore that certain individuals react to inhaled or absorbed beryllium, coupled to protein as a hapten, via a cellular immune response. Perhaps ingestion of the antigen by macrophages allows persistent stimulation of the immune system, activation of T lymphocytes and production of lymphokines, which in turn stimulate further recruitment of mononuclear phagocytes leading to granuloma formation. Further discussion of the immunopathology of granulomatous disease may be found in Chapter 39.

Diagnosis and management

The disease should be suspected when someone who has worked with (or whose spouse has worked with) beryllium presents features of interstitial lung disease with histological findings suggestive of sarcoidosis [297]. There is no absolutely reliable test for berylliosis, although features that distinguish it from saroidosis include a negative Kveim test and absence of erythema nodosum, hilar adenopathy without lung changes, or uveitis. The beryllium patch test is not now recommended since it may itself lead to sensitization. The test for lymphocyte proliferation in response to beryllium sulphate using blood or bronchoalveolar lavage cells is the most reliable test of sensitization and may also reflect severity of the disease [298–301]. Studies of tissue or urine levels of beryllium have proved disappointing, since high level may be found in beryllium workers with other disease and low levels in ex-beryllium workers with berylliosis [302]. However, the use of laser microprobe mass spectrometry to analyse the content of granulomas rather than of general lung tissue has enabled the demonstration of beryllium in the granulomas and not in those of sarcoidosis [303]. Where this highly specialized chemical test is available, it is therefore possible to increase diagnostic confidence appreciably.

Since the disease usually progresses, treatment with corticosteroids is normally advised. The dose should initially be of the order of 40 mg daily and subsequent reductions guided by measurements of lung function, diffusing capacity being the most useful test. Most patients improve but few show full functional recovery and the treatment therefore needs to be continued indefinitely.

Prevention of sensitization depends on reducing the exposure of workers to as little beryllium as possible by careful occupational hygiene. A workplace hygiene standard of $2\,\mu g/m^3$ is enforced in the UK and the USA, and adherence to this may prevent most cases ocurring in future. However, its efficacy requires further study by surveillance of exposed workforces and it should be remembered that hypersensitivity diseases may not be dose-related, so that a single excursion above a relatively safe limit may produce sensitization in a susceptible worker.

Other pneumoconioses

Aluminium

Aluminium is mostly open-cast mined as bauxite ($Al_2O_5.2H_2O$), particularly in Jamaica. The ore is crushed, washed and treated with caustic soda to produce alumina, Al_2O_3, which is then reduced electrolytically after dissolution in cryolite, Na_2AlF_6. Fumes from this process, which is carried out in large vessels called pots, are responsible for pot-room asthma; this is probably due to fluoride rather than aluminium [304].

A diffuse interstitial fibrosis has been described in workers manufacturing alumina abrasives (corundum) composed of bauxite. The bauxite is ground, mixed with iron coke and melted at high temperatures, causing fumes containing both silica, mostly cristobalite, and aluminium oxide to be given off. The disease, characterized by honeycombing and a high risk of pneumothorax, has been called Shaver's disease after one of the physicians who first described it in 1947 [305]. It is possible that the condition was a variant of silicosis, probably of the accelerated type, rather than an effect of aluminium, the fumes having contained up to 30% silica. Fibrosis of the lungs has also been described in workers producing flake powder of metallic aluminium for the manufacture of fireworks, paints and armaments [306,307]. In this process, a coating of stearin was used to prevent oxide formation; when the metal was covered with either oxide or stearin it was relatively nonreactive. However, a change of process during the Second World War substituted mineral oil for stearin and this apparently allowed the reactive surface of metallic aluminium, when inhaled, to come into contact with alveolar walls and to initiate fibrosis. The doses that caused this disease were clearly very high and it seems unlikely that workers are at risk nowadays.

A report in 1962 [308] of a patient who worked in an aluminium powder-ball mill and who developed pulmonary fibrosis and progressive encephalopathy is of interest in view of the association of aluminium with the plaques in the brains of people dying with Alzheimer's disease [309]. The aluminium worker had very high levels of aluminium in his brain at death. It would seem that studies of neurological function in aluminium workers would be of interest. There has also been a report of a patient who developed alveolar proteinosis after 6 years' work as an aluminium grinder and whose lungs contained vast numbers of submicrometre-sized particles of aluminium [310], in keeping with more recent work suggesting that ultrafine particles may cause lung inflammation. The author has seen a patient who developed severe diffuse pulmonary fibrosis and died of a complicating alveolar cell carcinoma and who had a history of heavy and prolonged exposure to fume in a refinery producing aluminium from scrap. The lungs showed bronchiolitis as well as alveolitis, suggesting an inhaled cause, although aluminium was not detectable. The cause of these episodes of disease remain unclear but arouse suspicion that exposure to substances in fume generated by the processes may sometimes have toxic effects.

In contrast to the uncertainty surrounding fibrogenic effects of aluminium, there is clear evidence of an increased risk of lung cancer in workers involved in the pot room and manufacture of the anodes in aluminium refineries. The evidence strongly suggests that this relates to heavy exposure to polycyclic aromatic hydrocarbons [311].

Antimony

Antimony is mined as ores containing oxide and sulphide radicals and is used in metallic alloys, paints and pharmaceuticals. An apparently benign, non-fibrosing pneumoconiosis has been described in workers crushing the ore [312,313].

Barium

Barium is mined mostly as barytes, barium sulphate, and may be used in the production of paints, rubber and glass, and as a drilling mud in the oil industry. Miners may be exposed to quartz dust and are at risk of silicosis [100]. In contrast, workers grinding barium salts develop strikingly dense micronodular radiological shadows without any functional abnormalities (Fig. 54.28). This benign, non-fibrosing pneumoconiosis is called baritosis [314,315]. The radiographic changes tend to disappear when exposure ceases and there is no functional abnormality associated with them [316].

Carbon

Workers exposed to dust from graphite and carbon pigment may develop a form of pneumoconiosis indistinguishable from that afflicting miners of high-rank coal. Simple nodular changes and PMF have been described [317,318], and there is also evidence of some impairment of lung function in relation to exposure to carbon black [319].

Carbon fibres are now finding wide applications in industry and may be very fine and durable. While no problems have been described in workers, as with all such fibres care should be exercised in their use.

Polyvinyl chloride

The best-known hazards of polyvinyl chloride (PVC) manufacture are acro-osteolysis of the fingers and angiosarcoma of the liver due to exposure to vinyl chloride monomer [320,321]. However, a low category of

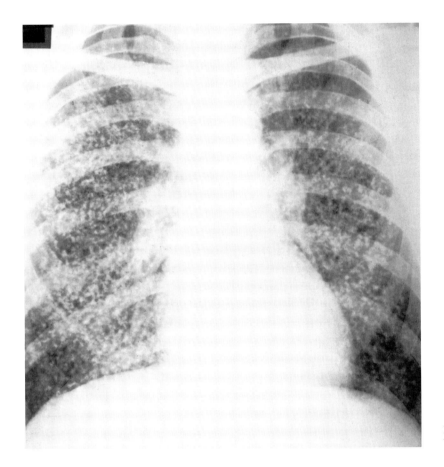

Fig. 54.28 Dense micronodular shadows of baritosis in a barium grinder.

radiological pneumoconiosis has been described in some workers and lung macules containing PVC have been demonstrated pathologically and experimentally [322–324]. It seems likely that this is a non-progressive and benign condition. Lung function changes, particularly a low $D_{L}CO$, that have been described in some workers with normal radiographs were probably due to high exposures to the monomer before controls were introduced rather than to the polymer [325].

Silicon carbide

Silicon carbide is of historical interest as Carborundum, an early US invention that saved many lives because of its use as a substitute for sandstone in knife grinding. It is widely used as an abrasive and now also used in the manufacture of synthetic fibres, known as silicon carbide whiskers. There has been a report of the development of what seems to have been a benign pneumoconiosis in two workers exposed to silicon carbide dust in refractory brick works [326]. Perhaps of more concern is the demonstration in rats injected with the fibres intrapleurally of a possible neoplastic risk [270]. A study of a cohort of silicon carbide production workers exposed *inter alia* to fibres has shown a significant increase in risk of non-malignant respiratory disease and a possible increase in risk of lung cancer [327].

Tin

Tin miners are at risk of silicosis and, if exposed to radon daughters, lung cancer [328]. Tin refiners may inhale the fume from the smelting process and develop a highly radiodense but entirely benign fine nodular pneumoconiosis. The condition has been called stannosis [329,330].

Tungsten carbide (hard metal) and cobalt

Tungsten carbide is produced, usually alloyed with cobalt and other metals, for materials requiring great hardness and resistance to heat. Pulmonary fibrosis, airways obstruction and granulomatous (giant cell) interstitial pneumonitis have been described in tungsten carbide workers [331,332]. It is probable that all these reactions are the result of inhaling the cobalt, which dissolves in coolants used in the process of grinding the hard metal [333,334]. The same syndrome has been described in diamond polishers exposed to a cobalt aerosol [335]. Ionized cobalt combines with proteins to form a hapten and has long been known as a cause of skin sensitization.

The disease presents with dry cough and breathlessness and appears to be more common in non-smokers. Inspiratory crackles may be heard and diffuse fine reticulonodular infiltrates may be seen radiographically. Detected early, the condition may remit either on cessation of exposure or following a course of corticosteroids. If exposure continues, progression to diffuse interstitial fibrosis and cor pulmonale may occur. There has been a report of a patient in whom fatal giant cell pneumonitis recurred in the transplanted lung even though exposure to hard metal had ceased [336].

In some subjects a syndrome of reversible airflow obstruction may occur. This seems to be an asthmatic response to cobalt (and sometimes also nickel) and has been reproduced by challenge testing [337,338]. Mixed patterns of asthma and interstitial disease may occur.

Occupational bronchitis

The interrelationships of occupational dust and fume exposure and clinical evidence of bronchial disease and airways obstruction have been the subject of some controversy. While it is rarely possible to recognize a distinct disease in individuals that can be called occupational bronchitis, exposures to dust and fume may increase the risk of these conditions occurring in exposed workers, whether they smoke or not. For example, an increased prevalence of chronic productive cough and of impaired expiratory flow rates has been recorded in coal-miners [40,46,47], gold-miners [121], foundry workers [339], cement workers [261], grain workers [340,341], asbestos miners [207] and coke oven workers [342]. Evidence that the reduction in lung function is related to cumulative dust exposure has been obtained from studies of South African gold-miners [121] and British coal-miners [56], while a relationship between dust exposure and prevalence of pathological emphysema in coal-miners suggests one possible mechanism [48]. There is some evidence of somewhat different patterns of response to dust inhalation in smokers and non-smokers; smokers develop classical airflow obstruction, with relatively greater reduction in FEV_1, while non-smokers tend to develop a reduction in both FEV_1 and FVC, suggesting a restrictive component [343].

Although these effects have been studied in greatest detail in coal-miners, it seems likely that the effect of dust on lung function may be a general one, possibly mediated through an alveolitic and elastolytic response of macrophages and polymorphs to the dust. It is not surprising to the author, who has visited many workplaces, that prolonged exposure to dust and fume could cause, via either bronchial irritation or alveolar inflammation, chronic sputum production and airflow obstruction, resulting in an increased prevalence of such conditions in a population. In such circumstances, as with cigarette smoking, the average effect is small but the distribution of responses in the population as a result of differences in both susceptibility and exposure may result in a few

people developing clinical disease. If, as is likely, susceptibility to the irritants inhaled from cigarettes is the same as that to other irritants, it would be expected that this effect would show mainly in smokers, especially when one considers that such effects are likely to be additive. Therefore in any dust-exposed population, one might expect to see an excess of people with disease compared with a non-dust-exposed population while in individual cases being unable to point firmly to dust as a cause. In addition, if exposures to industrial dust or fume are generally controlled, it would nowadays be unusual to see non-smoking individuals with purely dust-induced disease. This gives great opportunities for sceptics to deny that prolonged inhalation of such substances is in any way harmful, an attitude usually coloured by a need to be dogmatic in front of a judge or jury who prefer to hear that diseases have only one cause. However, a more important consideration is that such an attitude leads to a denial of the need for employers to take preventive action. Application of a precautionary principle should lead one to conclude that exposure to dust and fumes generally in industry has the potential to harm the lungs and that the exposures of workers should be minimized.

Organic dust diseases

Occupational asthma and allergic alveolitis

These conditions are considered in detail in Chapters 34 and 37 respectively.

Byssinosis

Byssinosis is a term applied to a complex of symptoms associated with the manufacture of cotton, flax and hemp [344–347]. Cotton, after picking, is cleaned and the lint separated from the seed by a process known as ginning. The lint is compressed into bales, which are then opened out by machines in a blowing room. Cleaning these machines is a very dusty job. The cotton fibres are then combed out, or carded, twisted into threads and woven. Carding and stripping the carding machine is also very dusty work. Flax is separated from the plant stems by retting (rotting, by bacterial or fungal action) followed by beating. The fibres are then carded and drawn through gills prior to spinning and weaving. Similar processes are used in the production of hemp and jute, though there is little evidence that the latter fibre is associated with byssinosis.

Acute effects of cotton exposure

Up to one-third of people exposed to cotton dust for the first time develop an acute airway reaction with often substantial fall in FEV₁ [348]. This is more likely to occur in atopic subjects and people with asthma and is associated with increased bronchial reactivity. It probably means that workers who develop this syndrome tend to leave the industry and that those who remain, some of whom later develop byssinosis, contain a relatively smaller proportion of atopic subjects [345].

The classical description of byssinosis is of a worker in a dusty area developing, usually after at least 10 years in the industry, a sensation of oppression in the chest or difficulty in breathing on the first day of the working week. A slight rise in temperature may also occur, as may cough and wheeze. The symptoms usually occur after about 2–4 h of exposure and clear some time after going home. No radiological changes occur. As the condition progresses, the symptoms may arise on subsequent working days, ultimately becoming permanent. However, longitudinal studies have shown that this progression from first day through to more persistent symptoms is not invariable, and that some workers start with symptoms on a daily basis while some even show remission despite continuing exposure [349]. For epidemiological purposes these symptoms have been used in the following classification of the disease.

Grade 0: no byssinosis.

Grade 0.5: occasional chest tightness on the first day of the working week.

Grade 1: chest tightness on the first day of every working week.

Grade 2: chest tightness on the first and following days of every working week.

Grade 3: grade 2 symptoms accompanied by evidence of permanent incapacity from diminished exercise tolerance and/or reduced ventilatory capacity.

Lung function studies have shown declines in FEV₁ both throughout a shift and throughout the week, the change over a shift being greatest on the first day [350,351]. Longitudinal decline in FEV₁ has been suggested by finding lower levels of lung function than predicted in cotton workers [352], although how far these are due to smoking and how far to cotton dust remains undecided. There is evidence that those workers who show declines in lung function over a shift are most likely to show a progressive change over several years [353]. Bronchial reactivity is increased in most workers with byssinosis and falls in indices of small airways disease have been taken to suggest that the physiological response may begin in peripheral airways and that byssinosis may be regarded as a form of occupational asthma [354,355].

In the light of newer studies of the natural history and functional effects of byssinosis, the World Health Organization has proposed a new grading system for the disease (Table 54.4).

Table 54.4 The World Health Organization grading system for byssinosis.

Grade 0	No symptoms
Byssinosis	
Grade B1	Chest tightness and/or shortness of breath on most of first day back at work
Grade B2	Chest tightness and/or shortness of breath on the first and other days of the working week
Respiratory tract irritation	
Grade RTI1	Cough associated with dust exposure
Grade RTI2	Persistent phlegm initiated or exacerbated by dust exposure
Grade RTI3	Persistent phlegm initiated or made worse by dust exposure, either with exacerbations of chest illness or persisting for 2 years or more
Lung function	
Acute changes	
No effect	A consistent decline of <5% (or an increase) in FEV₁ over a work shift
Mild effect	A consistent decline of 5–10% over the work shift
Moderate effect	A consistent decline of 10–20% over the work shift
Severe effect	A decline of 20% or more over the work shift
Chronic changes	
No effect	FEV₁ at least 80% of predicted
Mild to moderate	FEV₁ 60–79% of predicted
Severe	FEV₁ <60% of predicted

FEV₁, forced expiratory volume in 1 s.

Chronic effects of cotton exposure

This subject remains controversial. It is certainly the belief of many doctors in cotton and flax milling areas that some workers become permanently disabled by byssinosis. Cough and sputum are found more freqently among cotton workers than among controls [356] and ventilatory function tends to be impaired [357]. Several studies have shown a progressive decline in workers' FEV₁ in relation to exposure to cotton dust, in some cases of a dramatic degree [358,359]. Some of these declines are such that one would anticipate a very poor survival rate among these workers. However, mortality studies have shown either no or only small effects on mortality from chronic respiratory disease [360–362], suggesting that they may be flawed.

Necropsy studies of cotton workers with byssinosis have failed to show any distinctive pathological features [363]. There is some evidence that cotton workers have mucous gland hypertrophy and increased bronchial smooth muscle but nothing to suggest that they suffer an excess of emphysema, either pathologically or physiologically [364,365].

Pathogenesis

The prevalence of byssinosis varies from mill to mill, although the condition occurs in many different countries, including the UK, the USA, Indonesia, Sudan and India, being more prevalent in developing than developed countries [366,367]. The common factor seems to be the raw fibres, this material always being contaminated by fungi and Gram-negative bacteria. Fungal overgrowth may be responsible for weavers' cough and Gram-negative bacterial endotoxin for mill fever. Some types of cotton appear to be worse than others, while the earlier and dustier parts of the production process tend to cause more disease [368]. Washing of cotton reduces its effects in experimental studies [369].

The effects of inhalation of extract of cotton dust, namely chest tightness, cough, some fever and fall in FEV_1, have some of the features of asthma and allergic alveolitis without being typical of either. The delayed onset after challenge is similar to that of allergic alveolitis, although the functional change differs. The symptoms and reduced response on subsequent days are similar to those described in some episodes of humidifier fever [370]. It seems likely that some component of cotton bract or its fungal and bacterial contaminants is responsible, though the mechanism of this has been much debated. Early suggestions that the action is a direct one on mast cells, causing release of histamine and other mediators of smooth muscle constriction, now seem too simplistic [371]. Similarly, evidence for an antigen–antibody reaction is unconvincing, although atopic subjects do seem at slightly greater risk [372]. Inhalation of cotton dust has been shown to lead to a neutrophil response in airways, probably due to a lipid fraction of bacterial cell walls, and it may be that release of leukotrienes and platelet-activating factor by these cells plays a part in causing the disease [373]. Similar mechanisms have been invoked in the causation of asthma, pulmonary fibrosis and emphysema, diseases with very different clinical features, so this apparent explanation of the disease is really only a framework for further research. It is probable that the reaction in byssinosis is confined to the airways and is due to larger, non-respirable dust particles. Perhaps the electrostatic charge on cotton dust is also important in determining the site of action. Much more work, in both epidemiology and the study of basic mechanisms of bronchial inflammation, is necessary before byssinosis is fully understood.

Prevention and management

In the absence of knowledge of the precise cause, most attempts at control of the problem have concentrated on reducing the dust exposure of workers by enclosing machinery, ventilation and, where necessary, use of respirators. Attempts have been made to reduce the hazard by removing the soluble fraction of raw cotton by washing or steam treatment [374], although these have proved either impracticable or ineffective. In the case of steam treatment, the hazard appeared to be transferred to workers in the later stages of the process. Exclusion of very sensitive workers at an early stage is necessary and transfer of workers developing early symptoms to less dusty work is desirable. Exclusion of atopic subjects is probably of little importance, although increased susceptibility of such people to the early acute bronchoconstrictive reaction results in most leaving the industry before developing classical byssinosis. Primary prevention therefore depends on the difficult process of dust control, in accordance with national legislation on dust standards. Since byssinosis is primarily a bronchial disease, it is logical that such standards should be based on inhalable rather than respirable dust measurements and the present standard in the UK and USA takes account of this ($0.5\,mg/m^3$ measured as inhalable dust, less the coarse component known as 'fly').

Once the condition has developed, some symptomatic relief may be obtained by the use of inhaled bronchodilators and steroids if removal from the workplace proves impracticable. In the UK, industrial injuries benefits are available to victims of the disease.

Humidifier fever and related syndromes

A variety of patterns of illness has been described in people working or living in buildings with humidifiers and air conditioners. The original descriptions from the USA were of typical extrinsic allergic alveolitis, and thermophilic actinomycetes were isolated from the systems [375,376]. Since then, typical allergic alveolitis and asthma have also been described in a few individuals in British offices [377,378] and cases of allergic alveolitis due to various bacterial contaminants of nebulizers and humidifiers continue to be reported [379,380]. More characteristically, British outbreaks have consisted of episodes of malaise, fever and sometimes breathlessness, often associated with non-specific aches, occurring predominantly on the first day of the working week [381–384]. Occasionally, falls in diffusing capacity or peak flow rate have been described and the syndrome clearly has overlaps with both allergic alveolitis and occupational asthma. Usually the chest radiograph is normal and physical signs are absent from the lungs.

The common factor in all these outbreaks is the presence of profuse microbiological contamination of the humidifier system. Water and air entering the system convey microorganisms that then recirculate in the water and reproduce in sumps and on baffle plates. In such circumstances it is commonplace to find a thick jelly-like deposit on baffle plates; culture of this and of the water in the sump reveals many bacteria and fungi, together with more complex organisms such as amoebae, *Paramecium* and worms. Precipitating antibodies to the jelly and to extracts of the water are commonly present in exposed workers, whether affected or not, although recent evidence suggests that the presence of high levels of IgG antibody to humidifier water are associated with the more severe symptoms of fever, headache and chest tightness [385]. There has been much debate as to which organisms are responsible and what mechanisms are involved; amoebae, or the Gram-negative bacteria on which they feed and whose antigens they contain, have been thought to be important [386,387]. However, it seems likely that different syndromes may be related to different organisms or combinations of organisms. The mechanisms remain unresolved, though the striking similarity of humidifier fever to byssinosis has been noted [370]. It is of interest that the air conditioner was actually invented to control the temperature and humidity in cotton mills in the USA.

As far as is known, typical humidifier fever does not progress to a disabling type of lung disease and is often regarded by its victims as a 'Monday morning feeling'. Nevertheless while some of those exposed are unaffected, others may suffer more severe malaise and breathlessness. Diagnosis is made from the typical history and from the finding of a source of contaminated aerosol. Control of the problem usually requires very frequent cleaning of the systems or, preferably, change to either steam injection or the use of fresh unrecirculating water. Biocides and the use of ultraviolet light have so far proved disappointing. The efficacy of control measures may be tested by measuring antibody in the blood of exposed people or, in some outbreaks, by measurement of peak flow rates in sensitized workers.

Similar syndromes to humidifier fever have been described in cotton mills (mill fever), grain silos (grain fever) [388], piggeries (swine confinement fever) [389] and sewage works (sewage sludge fever) [390]. It is possible that Gram-negative bacterial endotoxin is responsible for these reactions. Cotton and grain workers are also at risk of the more typical features of byssinosis and occupational asthma.

Apart from the more dramatic features of humidifier fever, workers in modern offices may complain of non-specific symptoms such as headache, nasal stuffiness and general malaise. Such outbreaks have been given the rather unsatisfactory name of 'sick building syndrome' [391]. They seem to be related to a design of building intended to save energy, with little natural ventilation and much recirculation of air. Occasionally, complaints from workers have reached such a pitch that buildings have

had to be closed until their ventilation systems have been redesigned.

Finally, it should be noted that water droplets from humidifiers and cooling towers may occasionally be a source of *Legionella* infection in people working in or even visiting offices and other buildings. This disease is discussed in Chapter 13.

Toxic gases and fumes

A wide range of gases and nanometre-sized particles (fumes) may cause toxic effects on the lung and other organs if inhaled. In general their effects may be mediated by asphyxiation, local irritation, toxic absorption and allergy. All save the last are discussed here and the most common of these substances are shown in Table 54.5.

Asphyxiant gases

Asphyxiation may occur as a result of exclusion of oxygen from the air by physiologically relatively inert gases or by interference with oxygen transport within the body by inhalation of metabolic poisons. The important simple asphyxiants are carbon dioxide, nitrogen and methane, which may all be encountered in unventilated mine workings and after fires. Carbon dioxide causes hyperventilation, sweating, headache and vasodilatation, with loss of consciousness, a syndrome familar to chest physicians used to dealing with patients with chronic airways obstruction. Unconsciousness occurs rapidly and often unexpectedly when breathing nitrogen as the oxygen concentration falls to about 10%. Methane has a similar effect. It is an important problem in mines, where it may accumulate as a result of decaying vegetable matter and is released spontaneously from the coal seam. Unlike carbon dioxide, it is lighter than air and loss of consciousness may occasionally save a worker's life. Explosion is the other serious hazard associated with methane.

Management of asphyxiation depends on removal of the victim and administration of oxygen. Unfortunately, industrial accidents often produce multiple casualties, as would-be rescuers are themselves overcome by hypoxia. Self-contained breathing apparatus should be available to all workers at risk of such accidents; in most countries all miners are issued with simple oxygen-generating apparatus (self-rescuers) for use in an emergency.

The important toxic asphyxiants are carbon monoxide, phosphine, cyanides and hydrogen sulphide. Carbon monoxide is a product of incomplete combustion and is encountered classically in fires, around blast furnaces and in underground mines. It is colourless, odourless and lighter than air. It combines not only with haemoglobin (with an affinity some 200 times that of oxygen) but also with myoglobin and cytochrome oxidase, as well as shifting the oxyhaemoglobin dissociation curve to the left and

Table 54.5 Toxic fumes and gases.

Agent	Main occupations	Occupational exposure standard*
Asphyxiants		
Acrylonitrile (vinyl cyanide)	Plastics, rubber	2 ppm (MEL)
Carbon dioxide	Mining, tunnelling	5000 ppm
Carbon monoxide	Mining, foundry	50 ppm
Hydrogen cyanide	Plating, fumigation	10 ppm (MEL)
Hydrogen sulphide	Sewage, tanning, gas making	10 ppm
Methane	Mining, tunnelling	$O_2 > 17\%$
Nitrogen	Mining, tunnelling	$O_2 > 17\%$
Phosphine	Fumigation	0.3 ppm (STEL)
Irritants		
Acrolein	Plastics, rubber	0.1 ppm
Ammonia	Fertilizer, refrigeration	25 ppm
Cadmium fume	Alloying, welding	0.025 mg/m^3 (MEL)
Chlorine	Bleaching, chemicals, disinfecting	0.5 ppm
Formaldehyde	Paper, photography, preserving	2 ppm (MEL)
Hydrogen chloride	Chemicals, dyes	5 ppm (STEL)
Hydrogen fluoride	Etching, oil refinery	3 ppm (STEL)
Nitrogen dioxide	Welding, farming	3 ppm
Osmium tetroxide	Alloys	0.0002 ppm
Ozone	Welding	0.2 ppm (STEL)
Phosgene	Dyes, chemicals	0.2 ppm
Sulphur dioxide	Bleaching, smelting	2 ppm
Vanadium pentoxide	Chemicals, alloys	0.05 mg/m^3
Toxic absorption		
Arsine	Smelting, refining, scrap metal work	0.05 ppm
Copper fume	Welding	0.2 mg/m^3
Lead fume	Refining, batteries	0.05 mg/m^3
Mercury fume	Electrolysis	0.025 mg/m^3
Zinc oxide fume	Welding	5 mg/m^3

*Occupational exposure standard in UK, expressed as 8-h time-weighted average except where indicated. These values are subject to regular revision and should be taken as a general guideline only.
MEL, maximum exposure limit, measured over 10 min, that must not be exceeded.
STEL, short-term exposure limit, measured over 10 min.

impairing oxygen uptake into mitochondria [392]. The first symptom of carbon monoxide poisoning is usually headache and general malaise, which occurs with carboxyhaemoglobin concentrations around 10%. Such symptoms may persist for prolonged periods in people exposed to low concentrations of the gas from defective gas apparatus and are frequently disregarded or misdiagnosed by doctors. Higher concentrations lead to dizziness, nausea, weakness in the limbs and, at about 30%, clouding

of consciousness. Death in fit people occurs at carboxyhaemoglobin concentrations of about 50%, though lower levels may be fatal in people with coronary artery disease or if oxygen demands are higher, as during exercise. Long-term sequelae may include myocardial and cerebral infarction; in about 10% of survivors, a neuropsychiatric syndrome occurs that may include extrapyramidal signs due to damage to basal ganglia, amnesia and psychotic symptoms [393–395]. Management of carbon monoxide poisoning depends upon removal of the victim and administration of 100% oxygen. Use of a hyperbaric chamber is desirable if one is available and is advisable if the patient has been unconscious, even if recovery has occurred, in order to prevent the neurological complications.

Cyanides act by blocking the cytochrome oxidase enzyme system, preventing access of oxygen to the tricarboxylic acid cycle. They may be encountered in industry as hydrogen cyanide gas or as inorganic cyanates in metal refining, plating, laboratories and fumigation. In addition, vinyl cyanide (acrylonitrile) is a gas used in the production of synthetic rubbers. Exposure to these gases causes rapid onset of dizziness, nausea and tachypnoea; these symptoms usually serve as a warning so that the worker can escape, but if ignored unconsciousness and death ensue very rapidly. Treatment should be available in any sites where exposure may occur; the traditional kit consists of amyl nitrite for immediate inhalation and sodium nitrite with sodium thiosulphate for intravenous injection. The nitrites combine with haemoglobin to form methaemoglobin, which in turn reacts with cyanide to form cyanmethaemoglobin; this then combines with thiosulphate to form harmless thiocyanate. This reaction reduces the oxygen-carrying power of the blood because of the formation of methaemoglobin and is also less effective for treatment of vinyl cyanide poisoning. Thus the preferred treatment is usually to neutralize the cyanide by intravenous injection of dicobalt edetate, 150 mg of which contains sufficient cobalt to deal with 40% of an LD_{50} of cyanide. Up to 600 mg may be given slowly, each 300 mg being followed by 50 mL of 50% dextrose to reduce risks of the anaphylactoid side-effects of the cobalt [396]. Clearly the patients should be removed from exposure by rescuers wearing self-contained breathing apparatus and given oxygen in high concentrations.

Hydrogen sulphide is also an inhibitor of the cytochrome oxidase system and is as rapidly fatal as cyanides. It is heavier than air and has the characteristic smell of rotten eggs, although olfactory accommodation occurs rapidly so that high concentrations may not be noticed. Fatal exposures have occurred in industry, in tanning, fish processing, chemical waste disposal and natural gas production [397–399]. Survivors may develop pulmonary oedema several days after exposure. Low-level exposures are associated with conjunctivitis and keratitis and various neurological syndromes. Treatment of hydrogen sulphide poisoning requires removal from exposure, administration of oxygen and of amyl nitrite and intravenous sodium nitrite, which combine with sulphide to form sulphmethaemoglobin. Ventilatory support may be necessary for delayed pulmonary oedema and hyperbaric oxygen may help to prevent long-term neurological sequelae.

Phosphine (PH_3) is a gas used mainly in the fumigation of grain; it is introduced into cargoes in the form of tablets of aluminium phosphide, which react with water to produce the gas. Accidental poisoning of workers, particularly grain inspectors, has been described as a result of entering the holds of ships or rail freighters holding fumigated grain [400,401]. The gas poisons intracellular oxygen transport mechanisms and manifests effects particularly on heart and liver. Cardiac failure and dysrhythmias are common complications of poisoning. There is no antidote, treatment being symptomatic.

Irritant gases and fumes

Irritant gases injure the respiratory tract by causing acute inflammation when inhaled in high concentration. The main site of injury depends on the solubility of the gas, the more soluble gases exerting maximal effects more proximally. It is probable that the consequences of inhalation of irritant gases are non-specific to the particular chemical and that any one or more of a spectrum of adverse effects may follow exposure to any such gas when inhaled in sufficient concentration. Short-term reactions include cough, wheeze, acute bronchoconstriction, tracheobronchitis and laryngeal or pulmonary oedema. These may be followed by temporary or persistent bronchial hyperreactivity with a syndrome indistinguishable from bronchial asthma, often called the reactive airways dysfunction syndrome (see Chapter 36). In some subjects, airways obstruction is much less reversible and resistant to antiasthma treatment, suggesting the development of obliterative bronchiolitis.

Although this alarming array of consequences may follow acute exposure to toxic gases, fortunately in most cases complete recovery is the rule. Such episodes of gassing are not rare, and represent one of the more common causes of reports to the UK SWORD project, 1180 having been reported between 1990 and 1994 [402]. The most common agents in this series were chlorine, nitrogen oxides, phosphine, perchloroethylene, sulphur dioxide and trichloroethylene. In a further study of these data, some 70% of patients with acute exposure to irritant gases had recovered and were back at work within a week but 12% still had symptoms 1 month later, of whom about one-quarter had symptoms of asthma/reactive airways disease. It is intuitively obvious but not clearly established that the greater the exposure in terms of duration and con-

centration to a given irritant, the more likely the occurrence of longer-term sequelae. However, the nature of these episodes, which are always accidental and sporadic, means that only rarely have appropriate studies been carried out to observe the natural history of the condition. In the author's experience, which like all experience may be misleading, sometimes quite minor exposures may lead to persistent asthmatic or other respiratory symptoms [403], while in other cases major exposures with severe immediate reactions lead to full recovery. All such episodes should therefore be treated seriously and the use of corticosteroids to suppress persistent inflammation at least considered.

Ammonia

Ammonia (NH_3) is a highly irritant, soluble alkaline gas with many uses in industry. Much is used in the production of fertilizers, as well as in manufacture of synthetic fibres and plastics, explosives, nitric acid, refrigerants, pharmaceuticals and oil refining. Accidental exposure to high concentrations results in intense irritation of eyes, nose and throat with stridor due to laryngeal oedema [404]. The soluble nature of the gas results in direct damage to proximal mucous menbranes rather than to more distal parts of the lung. Death may occur through asphyxia. Management involves removal of the victim and maintenance of oxygenation for the 2–3 days until laryngeal oedema settles; this may require tracheostomy. Weakly acidic eye and mouth washes may give some symptomatic relief initially. Full recovery usually ensues, although persistent cough, bronchiolitis obliterans and bronchiectasis have been described as sequelae [405].

Chlorine

Chlorine is a heavy gas, less soluble than ammonia, used in the manufacture of alkalis, bleaches, plastics and solvents, as well as being used as a sterilizing agent. Many industrial accidents following spillages and crashes of transporters have been described [406,407]. The acute effects of inhalation are choking, chest pain and dyspnoea. Pulmonary oedma may occur immediately or after a delay of several hours, with inspiratory crackles, frothy pink sputum and radiographic changes. Management is that of non-cardiogenic pulmonary oedema; the role of corticosteroids is not established but most clinicians would probably use them. Follow-up studies of survivors of chlorine inhalation have shown equivocal results, usually confounded by ignorance of previous respiratory health and by high prevalences of smoking [408–411], but which are probably partly related to the observation made above that only a small proportion of people exposed actually develop long-term effects. Exposures to low levels of chlorine might be expected to provoke attacks of asthma in those with bronchial hyperreactivity [412].

Oxides of nitrogen

Nitrogen dioxide exists in two forms in equilibrium, NO_2 and N_2O_4, a relatively insoluble, brown, mildly irritating gas. Toxic exposures have occurred particularly in four circumstances: exposure to silo gases, arc welding, combustion of nitrogen-containing material and spills of nitric acid [413–415]. Silofillers' disease occurs when farm workers enter the top of a silo, usually shortly after ensilage has begun. Nitrogen dioxide may accumulate in this situation as a result of oxidation of nitrates in the silage; being heavier than air, the gas lies on the top and in pits. Arc welders may produce the gas by combination of nitrogen and oxygen in the heat of the arc. Exposure as a result of fires occurs when dynamite burns; this has caused accidents in mines [415]. A notorious episode occurred at the Cleveland Clinic in Ohio, when nitrocellulose X-ray film caught fire and caused over 100 deaths, many of which were thought to have been due to nitrogen dioxide [416]. Exposures in the chemical industry occur when nitric acid spills and reacts with organic material such as wood or paper.

The person exposed to nitrogen dioxide may only notice relatively mild nasal and throat irritation, though with heavy exposures cough and choking may occur. Such exposures may then lead to the progressive development of pulmonary oedema over an hour or two (Fig. 54.29), which may prove fatal. Moreover, apparent recovery may be followed 2–3 weeks later by progressive breathlessness associated with fever and diffuse lung crackles. This late reaction, which may occasionally occur after a relatively minor initial episode, is due to progressive bronchiolitis obliterans, and it also may prove fatal [417,418]. The radiograph shows diffuse punctate opacities and the lung function a predominantly restrictive pattern.

There has been much debate about the effects of prolonged low-level exposure to nitrogen dioxide, such as occur in workers exposed to diesel exhausts, people living in cities with heavy traffic pollution or in people exposed to gas cookers in their homes. Experimental chamber studies have shown that effects on airways resistance and reactivity may occur in healthy people exposed over about 2h at concentrations of up to 10 parts per million and that similar changes occur in people with asthma exposed to concentrations down to about 0.2 ppm [419]. There is some evidence that children and women living in houses with gas cookers may show increased susceptibility to pulmonary infections, increased respiratory symptoms and some reduction in ventilatory capacity [420–422].

Exposure to high levels of nitrogen dioxide should largely be prevented by appropriate education of workers. Farmers in particular should be aware of the hazards of

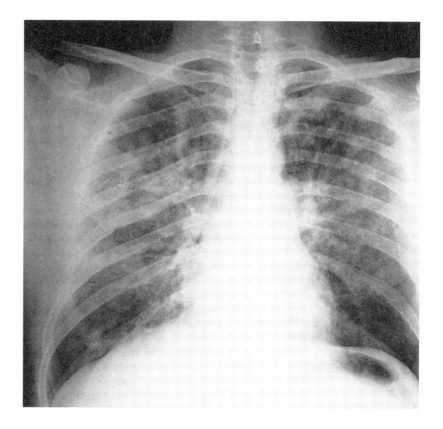

Fig. 54.29 Acute toxic pneumonitis in welder exposed to oxides of nitrogen.

silos. Management of the acute attack is as for other irritant gases, and there is anecdotal evidence that early use of corticosteroids may be of benefit both in the acute stage and in preventing bronchiolitis obliterans.

Sulphur dioxide

Sulphur dioxide (SO_2) is a heavy irritating gas. Its solubility causes it to provoke eye, throat, laryngeal and bronchial oedema, together with pulmonary oedema in severe exposures [423]. Such industrial accidents are rare but may occur in bleaching, preservation of foods, refrigeration and chemical industries. The gas is a general atmospheric pollutant, produced by combustion of fossil fuel, and is of importance in causing deterioration of limestone buildings and contributing to acid rain. Low-level exposures may contribute to the burden of chronic airflow obstruction and bronchial symptoms in exposed workers, though the evidence for this is controversial [424,425]. Experimental chamber studies of volunteers have shown subtle effects on lung function to occur at concentrations above 1–2 ppm in normal subjects and above about 0.2 ppm in those with asthma [426–428]; the role of sulphur dioxide in ambient air pollution is discussed in Chapter 11.

Ozone

Ozone (O_3) is a relatively insoluble but reactive gas that may be encountered in inert gas-shielded arc welding, the chemical industry, bleaching and industrial waste treatment. It is a respiratory irritant although severe or fatal exposures do not seem to have occurred. Occupational health interest has centred upon its long-term effects, particularly on the crews of high-flying aircraft and spacecraft, who seem to suffer an excess of symptoms attributable to respiratory irritation [429]. As discussed in Chapter 11, it is an important contributor to summer air pollution episodes and there is evidence of irritant effects in experimental studies on airways in terms of provoking changes in lung function and airway inflammation at exposures over about 0.1 ppm for several hours [427,430]. Epidemiological studies have shown relationships between rises in ambient ozone concentrations, measures of respiratory illness, and even mortality from respiratory and cardiovascular diseases [431,432].

Phosgene

Phosgene ($COCl_2$) is a heavy gas that was used as a chemical weapon in the First World War. It is now used in the production of isocyanates, pesticides, dyes and pharmaceuticals. Occasional cases of acute toxicity have been described in the chemical industry and in using carbon tetrachloride fire extinguishers. It is only mildly irritant but acts directly on the alveolar wall, causing acute pulmonary oedema [433].

Toxic fumes and vapours

Metal fumes

Metal fume fever is a condition characterized by a metallic taste followed by rigors, high fever, muscle aches and headache [434,435]. It follows a few hours after acute exposure to metal fumes, particularly zinc, copper and magnesium, and settles spontaneously, without sequelae, in 24 h. It occurs in welding, smelting and galvanizing. Episodes usually occur on first exposure to fumes after a break, tolerance then developing, and in this respect bears some resemblance to byssinosis and other causes of 'Monday fever'. It is probably due to chemotaxis within the lung of neutrophil leucocytes damaged by the very small (<1 μm) particles of metal. Recent studies of experimental zinc oxide fume inhalation have shown evidence of alveolar inflammation and release of cytokine mediators over a 24-h period following exposure [436,437], while bronchoalveolar lavage in a worker suffering from inhalation of zinc fumes has shown a lymphocytic alveolitis [438].

Metal fume may also cause direct toxic damage to the lungs and, by absorption, to other organs. A characteristic of fumes is the very small particle size, the majority being less than 0.1 μm in diameter with a high rate of alveolar deposition. Exposure to high concentrations even of relatively non-toxic substances of this size range causes an alveolitis and may lead to pulmonary oedema. This has occurred after deliberate exposure of fire-fighters and military personnel to zinc chloride fumes during training exercises [439,440]. Mercury causes a toxic pneumonitis together with neuropsychiatric symptoms [441]. Cadmium may also cause acute pulmonary oedema and renal cortical necrosis [442]. There has been debate about whether high-level or long-term low-level cadmium exposure causes fibrosis or emphysema [443,444]. There is experimental evidence that it may cause either, depending on the conditions [445], and a detailed follow-up of workers in a copper–cadmium alloy plant has shown greater physiological and radiological changes consistent with emphysema in those exposed to cadmium than in controls [446]. A mortality study has also shown a high incidence of death from chronic airways disease in such workers [447]. One unusual episode of rapidly developing emphysema after several years of exposure to cadmium at concentrations of 150–1000 μg/m³ has also been reported [448]. Vanadium exposure, encountered in cleaning oil-fired boilers and in the use of the catalyst vanadium pentoxide, is associated with an increased risk of upper respiratory and asthmatic symptoms [449,450]. A green tongue is a characteristic of acute exposure to this chemical. Manganese workers have been shown to be at increased risk of bronchitis and pneumonia [451,452] as well as extrapyramidal disorders. Osmium tetroxide is an acute respiratory irritant [453], while chromium salts may cause nasal perforation and lung cancer.

Other fumes

The exhaust gases of diesel engines contain a complex mixture of substances, including oxides of nitrogen, aldehydes and sulphur dioxide. They are undoubtedly irritant and cause cough in exposed workers, especially if the concentrations are high because the engine is labouring or working in an enclosed space such as a mine. Studies of long-term effects on lung function have proved negative [454,455] but it would be surprising if exposure to high concentrations for prolonged periods did not have some deleterious effects.

A condition similar to metal fume fever has been described in workers exposed to fumes of heated polytetrafluorethylene (Teflon) [456], while a reaction that is probably primarily an irritant bronchoconstriction may occur in workers exposed to heated PVC [457]. This condition has been called meat-wrappers' asthma. It is not clear whether it is provoked by PVC fumes or by heated adhesives from the label being affixed to the wrapping material [458]. Trimellitic anhydride, an epoxy resin hardening agent, is a known cause of occupational asthma [459]. In addition, haemorrhagic pneumonitis and haemolytic anaemia have been described in subjects exposed to its fumes [460]. Other organic substance, such as isocyanates, may be irritant in the high concentrations that occur with chemical spills and fires. While most isocyanates used in industry are diisocyanates, the notorious episode at Bhopal in Central India, in which several thousand people died of either acute asphyxiation or chemical pneumonitis, was probably caused by the highly irritant methyl isocyanate gas [14].

Smoke inhalation

Acute smoke inhalation is a not uncommon emergency in non-occupational settings, as well as being an occupational hazard of fire-fighters. Smoke may contain a wide range of chemicals, especially now that plastics and synthetic foams are so widely used in furnishings. Those exposed to smoke may asphyxiate due to lack of oxygen or carbon monoxide inhalation, or suffer acute tracheitis and pneumonitis due to irritant chemicals such as hydrogen chloride or isocyanates in the smoke. Acute falls in ventilatory capacity have been recorded in fire-fighters after smoke inhalation and the inhalation of smoke has been shown to cause an influx of neutrophils into the lung with subsequent impairment of macrophage chemotaxis [461]. While short-term effects are obvious, long-term effects of

smoke inhalation are less clear; although it is reasonable to suppose that repeated exposures would increase a person's risk of chronic airways obstruction, this has not yet been demonstrated convincingly [462]. A mortality study of fire-fighters in the USA has shown the expected 'healthy worker effect', but a somewhat increased mortality from non-malignant lung disease [463]. Long-term exposure in Nepal to wood smoke in huts also seems to lead to an increased likelihood of cough and sputum production [464].

Occupational neoplasms

Mesothelioma is discussed in Chapter 43 and asbestos carcinogenicity earlier in this chapter. Occupational lung cancer was first described in the metal miners of Schneeberg [7], and subsequently in uranium miners in Joachimstal and Colorado [465,466]. The common factor in metal mining is exposure to radon daughters, which are suspended in water droplets and inhaled by the miners. Similar increased risks of lung cancer were run by tin miners in Cornwall [328], by haematite miners in Cumbria [283] and by fluorspar miners in Newfoundland [467]. The radiomimetic, mustard gas, has been shown to have a similar effect on workers producing it [468]. Lung cancer has also been shown to occur to excess in workers exposed to arsenic [469], nickel carbonyl [470], hexavalent chromates [471], bischloromethyl ether [472,473], oils in the production of isopropyl alcohol [474], fumes in aluminium refineries and coke ovens [475,476] and printing ink [477].

In almost all patients with lung cancer, smoking is the most important aetiological factor. However, there is evidence that non-smokers exposed to these carcinogens may nevertheless develop the disease and that the two risk factors at least add up and, in the case of asbestos and cigarettes, may even multiply. It has been estimated that as many as 15% of men with lung cancer might not have developed the disease had they not also had occupational or environmental exposure to a carcinogen [478]. To the clinician, this seems an overestimate but is based on a careful review of the epidemiological literature.

Other aspects of lung cancer are discussed in Chapter 41.

Management

The diagnosis of an occupational lung disease should lead to consideration of three separate but related aspects of management: (i) the management of the patient and the condition; (ii) rehabilitation and re-employment of the patient; and (iii) prevention of the same disease in other workers [479].

The first of these involves the general principles of disease management and has been mentioned where applicable above. The acute conditions such as asthma, allergic alveolitis and inhalation injury may respond to routine therapy but are likely to recur if steps are not taken to prevent re-exposure to the causative agent. In the diseases caused by chronic exposure, such as the pneumoconioses, specific therapy is usually not available although supportive treatment may be of help. In all such patients consideration should be given to the availability of compensation (see Chapter 61). Rehabilitation of the patient if still of employable age should include consideration of return to the previous job. Since this often implies recurrence of the condition if exposures to the offending agent are not prevented, it is necessary for steps to be taken to ensure that the management of the company are aware of the hazard to their employees and have taken appropriate steps to reduce risks. In the UK, this can be achieved by an approach to the Health and Safety Executive, who will visit the workplace and ensure that the Health and Safety

at Work Act and relevant regulations are enforced. Taking this step also ensures that other workers are protected from the same hazard.

If the patient's condition is such that employment in the same job is undesirable, the management, or the company's occupational health service if one is available, may be approached to seek redeployment. In doing this it is necessary to observe the ethical principle of not revealing confidential medical information without the written consent of the patient. Only if redeployment proves impracticable or if attempted re-employment causes recurrence should retirement on the grounds of ill-health be considered. In these circumstances the patient should be advised about the benefits available, including industrial injuries benefit. In the UK, the Department of Employment runs a scheme for advising and limited retraining of disabled people. These matters are considered in more detail elsewhere [479].

References

1 Ramazzini B (1713) *De Morbis Artificum Diatriba* (translated by Wright WC). New York: Hafner Publishing, 1964.

2 Agricola G (1556) *De re metallica* (translated by Hoover HC, Hoover LH). The Mining Magazine (London) 1912.

3 Greenhow EH. Specimen of diseased lung from a case of grinder's asthma. *Trans Pathol Soc Lond* 1865; 16: 59.

4 Thomson W. On black expectoration and deposition of black matter in the lung. *Med Chir Trans* 1836; 20: 230.

5 Seaton A. Ipecachuana asthma: an old lesson. *Thorax* 1990; 45: 974.

6 Pott P. *Chirurgical Works*, Vol 3. London: Hawes, Clark & Collins, 1808: 166.

7 Harting FH, Hesse W. Der Lungenkrebs, die Bergkrankheit in der Schneeberger Gruben. *Vjschr Gericht Med* 1879; 31: 102.

8 Merewether ERA, Price CW. *Report on Effects of Asbestos Dusts on the Lungs and Dust Suppression in the Asbestos Industry.* London: HMSO, 1930.

9 Merewether ERA. Asbestosis and carcinoma of the lung. In: *Annual Report of the Chief Inspector of Factories for the Year 1947.* London: HMSO, 1949.

10 Wagner JC, Sleggs CA, Marchand P. Diffuse pleural mesothelioma and asbestos exposure in the North West Cape Province. *Br J Ind Med* 1960; 17: 260.

11 Campbell JM. Acute symptoms following work with hay. *Br Med J* 1932; 2: 1143.

12 Weber HH, Engelhardt WE. Uber eine Apparatur zur Erzeugung niedriger Staunkonzentrationen von groser Konstanz und eine Methode zur mikrogravimetrischen Staubbestimung, Andwendung bei der Untersuchung von Stauben aus Berylliumgewinnung. *Z Gesamte Hyg* 1933; 10: 41.

13 Van Orstrand HS, Hughes RC, De Nardi JM, Carmody NG. Delayed chemical pneumonitis occurring in workers exposed to beryllium compounds. *JAMA* 1945; 129: 1084.

14 Shrivastava P. *Bhopal: Anatomy of a Crisis.*

Cambridge, Massachusetts: Ballinger Publishing, 1987.

15 Davies NV, Teasdale P. *The Costs to the British Economy of Work Accidents and Work-related Ill Health.* Sudbury: HSE Books, 1994.

16 Meredith S, McDonald JC. Work-related disease in the United Kingdom 1989–1992: report on the SWORD project. *Occup Med* 1994; 44: 183.

17 Ross DJ, Sallie BA, McDonald JC. SWORD '94: surveillance of work-related and occupational disease in the UK. *Occup Med* 1995; 45: 175.

18 Brain JD, Valberg PA. Deposition of aerosol in the respiratory tract. *Am Rev Respir Dis* 1979; 120: 1325.

19 Vincent JD. On the practical significance of electrostatic lung deposition of isometric and fibrous aerosols. *J Aerosol Sci* 1985; 16: 511.

20 Emmett PC, Aitken RJ, Hannan WJ. Measurement of the total and regional deposition of inhaled particles in the human respiratory tract. *J Aerosol Sci* 1982; 13: 549.

21 Committee on the Medical Effects of Air Pollutants. *Non-biological Particles and Health.* London: HMSO, 1995: Chapter 4.

22 Hamilton RJ, Walton WH. The selective sampling of respirable dust. In: Davies CW, ed. *Inhaled Particles and Vapours.* Oxford: Pergamon Press, 1961: 465.

23 Mark D, Vincent JH, Gibson H, Lynch G. A new static sampler for airborne total dust in workplaces. *Am Ind Hyg Assoc* 1985; J 46: 127.

24 Crawford NP, Cowie AJ. Quality control of airborne asbestos fibre counts in the United Kingdom: the present position. *Ann Occup Hyg* 1984; 28: 391.

25 Pavia D, Thomson ML, Pocock SJ. Evidence for temporary slowing of mucociliary clearance in the lung caused by tobacco smoking. *Nature* 1971; 231: 325.

26 Camner P. Clearance of particles from the human tracheobronchial tree. *Clin Sci* 1980; 59: 79.

27 Bailey MR, Fry FA, James AC. The long term

clearance kinetics of insoluble particles from the human lung. *Ann Occup Hyg* 1982; 26: 273.

28 Brody AR, Roe MW. Deposition pattern of inorganic particles at the alveolar level in the lungs of rats and mice. *Am Rev Respir Dis* 1983; 126: 724.

29 Warheit BD, Chang LY, Hill LH *et al.* Pulmonary macrophage accumulation and asbestos-induced lesions at sites of fibre deposition. *Am Rev Respir Dis* 1984; 129: 301.

30 Lauweryns JM, Baert JH. Alveolar clearance and the role of the pulmonary lymphatics. *Am Rev Respir Dis* 1977; 115: 625.

31 Bowden DH. Alveolar response to injury. *Thorax* 1981; 36: 801.

32 Gross P. The mechanisms of dust clearance from the lung. *Am J Clin Pathol* 1953; 23: 116.

33 Green GM. Alveolar–bronchiolar transport mechanisms. *Arch Intern Med* 1973; 131: 109.

34 Ferin J, Oberdorster G, Penney DP. Pulmonary retention of ultra-fine and fine particles in rats. *Am J Respir Cell Mol Biol* 1992; 6: 535.

35 Seaton A, MacNee W, Donaldson K, Godden D. Particulate air pollution and acute health effects. *Lancet* 1995; 345: 176.

36 Ruckley VA, Fernie JM, Chapman JS *et al.* Comparison of radiographic appearances with associated pathology and lung dust content in a group of coalworkers. *Br J Ind Med* 1984; 41: 459.

37 Zenker FA. Uber Staubinhalationkrankheiten der Lungen. *Dtsch Arch Klin Med* 1866/7; 2: 116.

38 Fletcher CM. Pneumoconiosis of coalminers. *Br Med J* 1948; i: 1015, 1065.

39 Hart Pd'A, Aslett EA. *Chronic Pulmonary Disease in South Wales Coalminers. 1. Medical Studies.* London: HMSO, 1942.

40 Rae S, Walker DD, Attfield MD. Chronic bronchitis and dust exposure in British coalminers. In: Walton WH, ed. *Inhaled Particles III.* Old Woking, Surrey: Unwin Bros, 1971: 873.

41 Bennett JG, Dick JA, Kaplan YS *et al.* The relationship between coal rank, the preva-

lence of pneumoconiosis. *Br J Ind Med* 1979; 36: 206.

42 Jacobsen M, Rae S, Walton WH, Rogan JM. New dust standards for British coal mines. *Nature* 1970; 227: 445.

43 Hurley JF, Burns J, Copland L *et al.* Coal-workers' simple pneumoconiosis and exposure to dust at ten British collieries. *Br J Ind Med* 1982; 39: 120.

44 Seaton A, Dick JA, Dodgson J, Jacobsen M. Quartz and pneumoconiosis in coal miners. *Lancet* 1981; ii: 1272.

45 Lloyd MH, Gauld SJ, Soutar CA. Respiratory ill health among coal miners and telecommunication workers in South Wales. *Br J Ind Med* 1986; 43: 177.

46 Rogan JM, Attfield MD, Jacobsen M *et al.* Role of dust in the working environment in development of chronic bronchitis in British coal miners. *Br J Ind Med* 1973; 30: 217.

47 Love R, Miller BG. Longitudinal study of lung function in coalminers. *Thorax* 1982; 37: 193.

48 Ruckley VA, Gauld SJ, Chapman JS *et al.* Emphysema and dust exposure in a group of coal workers. *Am Rev Respir Dis* 1984; 129: 528.

49 National Coal Board Medical Service. *Annual Report 1993/94*. London: National Coal Board, 1994.

50 International Labour Office. *Guidelines for the Use of ILO International Classification of Radiographs of Pneumoconiosis*, revised edn. Geneva: International Labour Office, 1980.

51 Fernie JM, Ruckley VA. Coalworkers' pneumoconiosis: correlation between opacity profusion and number and type of dust lesions with special reference to opacity type. *Br J Ind Med* 1987; 44: 273.

52 Cockcroft AE, Wagner JC, Seal RME *et al.* Irregular opacities in coalworkers' pneumoconiosis: correlation with pulmonary function and pathology. *Ann Occup Hyg* 1982; 26: 767.

53 Dick JA, Jacobsen M, Gauld S, Pern PO. The significance of irregular opacities in the chest radiographs of British coal miners. In: *Proceedings of the VI International Pneumoconiosis Conference, Bochum, 1983*. Geneva: International Labour Office, 1984: 283.

54 Gough J. Pneumoconiosis in coal trimmers. *J Pathology* 1940; 51: 277.

55 Maclaren WM, Soutar CA. Progressive massive fibrosis and simple pneumoconiosis in ex-miners. *Br J Ind Med* 1985; 42: 734.

56 Soutar CA, Collins HPR. Classification of progressive massive fibrosis of coalminers by type of radiographic appearance. *Br J Ind Med* 1984; 41: 334.

57 Davis JMG, Chapman J, Collings P *et al.* Variations in the histological patterns of the lesions of coalworkers' pneumoconiosis in Britain and their relationship to lung dust content. *Am Rev Respir Dis* 1983; 128: 118.

58 Caplan A. Certain unusual radiological appearances in the chest of coal-miners suffering from rheumatoid arthritis. *Thorax* 1953; 8: 29.

59 Gough J, Rivers D, Seal RME. Pathological studies of modified pneumoconiosis in coal-miners with rheumatoid arthritis (Caplan's syndrome). *Thorax* 1955; 10: 9.

60 Miall WE, Caplan A, Cochrane AL *et al.* An epidemiological study of rheumatoid arthritis associated with characteristic chest X-ray appearances in coal workers. *Br Med J* 1953; ii: 1231.

61 Constantinidis K, Musk AW, Jenkins JPR, Berry G. Pulmonary function in coal-workers with Caplan's syndrome and non-rheumatoid complicated pneumoconiosis. *Thorax* 1978; 33: 764.

62 Fernie JM, Douglas AN, Lamb D, Ruckley VA. Right ventricular hypertrophy in a group of coalworkers. *Thorax* 1983; 38: 436.

63 Lapp NL, Seaton A, Kaplan KC *et al.* Pulmonary hemodynamics in symptomatic coal miners. *Am Rev Respir Dis* 1971; 104: 418.

64 Miller BG, Jacobsen M. Dust exposure, pneumoconiosis and mortality of coalminers. *Br J Ind Med* 1985; 42: 723.

65 Atuhaire LK, Campbell MJ, Cochrane AL *et al.* Mortality of men in the Rhondda Fach 1950–1980. *Br J Ind Med* 1985; 42: 741.

66 Marks J. Occupation and kansasii infection in Cardiff residents. *Tubercle* 1975; 56: 311.

67 Pemberton J. Chronic bronchitis, emphysema and bronchial spasm in bituminous coal workers. *Arch Ind Health* 1956; 13: 529.

68 Hyatt RE, Kistin AD, Mahan TK. Respiratory disease in south West Virginia coal miners. *Am Rev Respir Dis* 1964; 89: 387.

69 Morgan WKC, Burgess DB, Lapp NL, Seaton A. Hyperinflation of the lungs in coal-miners. *Thorax* 1971; 66: 585.

70 Seaton A, Lapp NL, Morgan WKC. Lung mechanics and frequency dependence of compliance in coal miners. *J Clin Invest* 1972; 51: 1203.

71 Lapp NL, Seaton A. Lung mechanics in coal workers' pneumoconiosis. *Ann N Y Acad Sci* 1972; 200: 433.

72 Seaton A, Lapp NL, Morgan WKC. The relationship of pulmonary impairment in simple coal workers' pneumoconiosis to type of radiographic opacity. *Br J Ind Med* 1972; 29: 50.

73 Lapp NL, Seaton A. Pulmonary function. In: Key MM, Kerr LE, Bundy M, eds. *Pulmonary Reactions to Coal Dust*. New York: Academic Press, 1971: 153.

74 Wagner JC, Wusteman FS, Edwards JH, Hill RJ. The composition of massive lesions in coal miners. *Thorax* 1975; 30: 382.

75 Wagner JC, Burns J, Munday DE, McGee J, O'D. Presence of fibronectin in pneumoconiotic lesions. *Thorax* 1982; 37: 54.

76 Soutar CA, Maclaren WM, Annis R, Melville AWT. Quantitative relations between exposure to respirable coalmine dust and coal-workers' simple pneumoconiosis in men who have worked as miners but who have left the coal industry. *Br J Ind Med* 1986; 43: 29.

77 Boyd J, Robertson MD, Davis JMG. Autoantibodies in coal miners: their relationship to the development of progressive massive fibrosis. *Am J Ind Med* 1982; 3: 201.

78 Dick HM, Boyd JE, Fitch M *et al.* HLA antigens in progressive massive fibrosis of coal workers. *Dis Markers* 1984; 2: 393.

79 Robertson MD, Boyd JE, Fernie JM, Davis JMG. Some immunological studies on coal-workers with and without pneumoconiosis. *Am J Ind Med* 1983; 4: 467.

80 Le Bouffant L, Daniel H, Martin JC, Bruyere S. Effect of impurities and associated minerals on quartz toxicity. *Ann Occup Hyg* 1982; 26: 625.

81 Hurley JF, Alexander WP, Hazeldine D *et al.* Exposure to respirable coalmine dust and incidence of progressive massive fibrosis. *Br J Ind Med* 1987; 44: 66.

82 Seal RME, Cockcroft A, Kung I *et al.* Central lymph node changes and progressive massive fibrosis in coalworkers. *Thorax* 1986; 41: 531.

83 Seaton A, Cherrie JW. Quartz exposures and severe silicosis: a role for the hilar nodes. *Occup Environ Med* 1998; 55: 383.

84 Leigh J, Wiles AN. Factors affecting prevalences of mucus hypersecretion and airflow obstruction in the coal industry of New South Wales, Australia. *Ann Occup Hyg* 1986; 32 (Suppl 1): 1186.

85 Leigh J, Wiles AN, Glick M. Total population study of factors affecting chronic bronchitis prevalence in the coal mining industry of New South Wales, Australia. *Br J Ind Med* 1986; 43: 263.

86 Marine WM, Gurr D, Jacobsen M. Clinically important respiratory effects of dust exposure and smoking in British coal miners. *Am Rev Respir Dis* 1988; 137: 106.

87 Soutar C, Campbell S, Gurr D *et al.* Important deficits of lung function in three modern colliery populations. *Am Rev Respir Dis* 1993; 147: 797.

88 Attfield MD, Hodous TK. Pulmonary function of US coal miners related to dust exposure estimates. *Am Rev Respir Dis* 1992; 145: 605.

89 Carta P, Aru G, Barbieri MT, Avataneo G, Casula D. Dust exposure, respiratory symptoms, and longitudinal decline in lung function in young coal miners. *Occup Environ Med* 1996; 53: 312.

90 Cockcroft A, Seal RME, Wagner JC *et al.* Post mortem study of emphysema in coal workers and non-coal workers. *Lancet* 1982; ii: 600.

91 Donaldson K, Brown GM, Brown DM *et al.* Impaired chemotactic responses of bronchoalveolar leukocytes in experimental pneumoconiosis. *J Pathol* 1990; 160: 63.

92 Brown GM, Donaldson K. Inflammatory responses in lungs of rats inhaling coalmine dust: enhanced proteolysis of fibronectin by bronchoalveolar leukocytes. *Br J Ind Med* 1989; 46: 866.

93 Seixas NS, Robins TG, Attfield MD, Moulton LH. Exposure–response relationships for coal mine dust and obstructive lung disease following enactment of the Federal Coal Mine Health and Safety Act of 1969. *Am J Ind Med* 1991; 21: 715.

94 Westerholm P. Silicosis: observations on a case register. *Scand J Work Environ Health* 1980; 6 (Suppl 2).

95 Ashe HB, Berstrom DE. Twenty-six years, experience with dust control in the Vermont granite industry. *Ind Med Surg* 1984; 33: 73.

96 Lloyd Davies TA, Doig AT, Greenberg M. A radiographic survey of monumental masonry workers in Aberdeen. *Br J Ind Med* 1973; 30: 227.

97 Cooper WC, Cralley LJ. *Pneumoconiosis in Diatomite Mining and Processing*. Washington, DC: US Department of Health, Education and Welfare, 1958.

98 Cooper WC, Jacobson G. A 21-year radiographic follow-up of workers in the diatomite industry. *J Occup Med* 1977; 19: 563.

99 Seaton A, Legge JS, Henderson J, Kerr KM. Accelerated silicosis in Scottish stonemasons. *Lancet* 1991; 337: 341.

100 Seaton A, Ruckley VA, Addison J, Brown WR. Silicosis in barium miners. *Thorax* 1986; 41: 591.

101 Buechner HA, Ansari A. Acute silico-proteinosis. A new pathologic variant of acute silicosis in sandblasters, characterised by histologic features resembling alveolar proteinosis. *Dis Chest* 1969; 55: 274.

102 Suratt PM, Winn WC, Brody AR *et al.* Acute silicosis in tombstone sandblasters. *Am Rev Respir Dis* 1977; 115: 521.

103 Phibbs BP, Sundin RE, Mitchell RS. Silicosis in Wyoming bentonite workers. *Am Rev Respir Dis* 1971; 103: 1.

104 Banks DE, Morring KL, Boehlecke BA *et al.* Silicosis in silica flour workers. *Am Rev Respir Dis* 1981; 124: 445.

105 Jain SM, Sepaha GC, Khare KC, Dubey VS. Silicosis in slate pencil workers: a clinico-radiological study. *Chest* 1977; 71: 423.

106 Saiyed HN, Parikh DJ, Ghodasara NB *et al.* Silicosis in slate pencil workers. 1. An environmental and medical study. *Am J Lnd Med* 1985; 8: 127.

107 Glover JR, Devon C, Cotes JE *et al.* Effects of exposure to slate dust in North Wales. *Br J Ind Med* 1980; 37: 152.

108 Warrell DA, Harrison BDW, Fawcett IW *et al.* Silicosis among grindstone cutters in the north of Nigeria. *Thorax* 1975; 30: 389.

109 Graham WGB, Ashikaga T, Hemenway D *et al.* Radiographic abnormalities in Vermont granite workers exposed to low levels of granite dust. *Chest* 1991; 100: 1507 1986.

110 Rice C, Harris RL, Checkoway H, Symons MJ. Dose–response relationships for silicosis from a case–control study of North Carolina dusty trades workers. In: Goldsmith DF, Winn DM, Shy CM, eds. *Silica, Silicosis and Cancer. Controversy in Occupational Medicine.* New York: Praeger, 1986: 77.

111 McDonald JC, Oakes D, Exposure–response in miners exposed to silica. In: *Proceedings of the VI International Pneumoconiosis Conference, Bochum, 1983.* Geneva: International Labour Office, 1984: 114.

112 Muir DCF, Julian JA, Shannon HS *et al.* Silica exposure and silicosis among Ontario hardrock miners. III. Analysis and risk estimates. *Am J Ind Med* 1989; 16: 29.

113 Solomon A. Massive fibrosis in gold miners: a radiological evaluation. *Environ Res* 1977; 13: 47.

114 Hughes JM, Jones RN, Gilson JC *et al.* Determinants of progression in sandblasters' silicosis. *Ann Occup Hyg* 1982; 26: 701.

115 Xipell JM, Ham KN, Price CG, Thomas DP. Acute silicoproteinosis. *Thorax* 1977; 32: 104.

116 Zimmerman PV, Sinclair RA. Rapidly fatal acute silicosis in a young man. *Med J Aust* 1977; 2: 704.

117 Banks DE, Bauer MA, Castellan RM, Lapp NL. Silicosis in surface coalmine drillers. *Thorax* 1983; 38: 275.

118 Koskinen H. Symptoms and clinical findings in patients with silicosis. *Scand J Environ Health* 1985; 11: 101.

119 Bohadana AB, Peslin R, Poncelet B, Hannhart B. Lung mechnical properties in silicosis and anthracosilicosis. *Bull Eur Physiopathol Respir* 1980; 16: 521.

120 Graham WGB, O'Grady RV, Dubuc B. Pulmonary function loss in Vermont granite workers. A long-term follow-up and critical reappraisal. *Am Rev Respir Dis* 1981; 123: 25.

121 Irwig LM, Rocks P. Lung function and respiratory symptoms in silicotic and non-silicotic gold miners. *Am Rev Respir Dis* 1978; 117: 429.

122 Jones RN, Weill H, Ziskind M. Pulmonary function in sandblasters' silicosis. *Bull Eur Physiopathol Respir* 1975; 11: 589.

123 Snider DE. The relationship between tuberculosis and silicosis. *Am Rev Respir Dis* 1978; 118: 455.

124 Sluis-Cremer GK. Active pulmonary tuberculosis discovered at post-mortem examination of the lungs of black miners. *Br J Dis Chest* 1980; 74: 374.

125 Bailley WC, Brown M, Buechner HA *et al.* Silicopathological disease in sandblasters. *Am Rev Respir Dis* 1974; 110: 115.

126 Sluis-Cremer GK, Hessel PA, Nizdo EH *et al.* Silica, silicosis, and progressive systemic sclerosis. *Br J Ind Med* 1985; 42: 838.

127 Hauglustaine D, van Damme B, Daenens P, Michielson P. Silicon nephropathy: a possible occupational hazard. *Nephron* 1980; 26: 219.

128 Bolton WK, Suratt PM, Sturgill BC. Rapidly progressive silicon nephropathy. *Am J Med* 1981; 71: 823.

129 Banks DE, Milutinovic J, Desnick RJ *et al.* Silicon nephropathy mimicking Fabry's disease. *Am J Nephrol* 1983; 3: 279.

130 Jones RN, Turner-Warwick M, Ziskind M, Weill H. High prevalence of antinuclear antibodies in sandblasters' silicosis. *Am Rev Respir Dis* 1976; 113: 393.

131 Wiles FJ, Faure MH. Chronic obstructive lung disease in gold miners. In: Walton WH, ed. *Inhaled Particles IV.* Oxford: Pergamon Press, 1977: 727.

132 Graham WG, Weaver S, Ashikaga T, O'Grady RV. Longitudinal pulmonary function losses in Vermont granite workers: a reappraisal. *Chest* 1994; 106: 125.

133 Hnizdo E, Sluis-Cremer GK, Baskind E, Murray J. Emphysema and airway obstruction in non-smoking South African gold miners with long exposure to silica dust. *Occup Environ Med* 1994; 51: 557.

134 Amandus HE, Shy C, Wing S *et al.* Silicosis and lung cancer in North Carolina dusty trades workers. *Am J Ind Med* 1991; 20: 57.

135 Checkoway H, Heyer NJ, Demers PA, Breslow NE. Mortality among workers in the diatomaceous earth industry. *Br J Ind Med* 1993; 50: 586.

136 Finkelstein MM. Radiographic abnormalities and the risk of lung cancer among workers exposed to silica dust in Ontario. *Can Med Assoc J* 1995; 152: 37.

137 Simonato A, Fletcher AC, Saracci R, Thomas TL. *Occupatioal Exposure to Silica and Cancer Risk.* IARC Scientific Publication No 97, Lyon, 1990.

138 Weill H, McDonald JC. Exposure to silica and lung cancer risk. *Thorax* 1996; 51: 97.

139 Mossman BT, Bignon J, Corn M, Seaton A, Gee JBL. Asbestos: scientific develoments and implications for public policy. *Science* 1990; 247: 294.

140 Vigliani EC, Mottura G. Diatomaceous earth silicosis. *Br J Ind Med* 1945; 5: 148.

141 Roeslin N, Lassabe-Roth C, Morand G, Batzenschlager A. La silico-proteinose aigue. *Arch Mal Prof* 1980; 41: 15.

142 Brieger H, Gross P. On the theory of silicosis. III. Stishovite. *Arch Environ Health* 1967; 15: 751.

143 Dworski M. Prophylaxis and treatment of experimental silicosis by means of aluminum. An experimental study. *Arch Ind Health* 1955; 12: 229.

144 Gross P, Westrick ML, McNerney JM.

Experimental silicosis: the inhibitory effect of iron. *Dis Chest* 1960; 37: 35.

145 Vigliani EC, Pernis B, Monaco LA. A study of the action of quartz particles on macrophages *in vitro*. In: Davis CN, ed. *Inhaled Particles and Vapours.* Oxford: Pergamon Press, 1961: 348.

146 Bowden DH, Hedgecock C, Adamson IYR. Silica-induced pulmonary fibrosis involves the reaction of particles with interstitial rather than alveolar macrophages. *J Pathol* 1989; 157: 73.

147 Gabor S, Anca Z, Zugravu E *et al. In vitro* and *in vivo* quartz-induced lipid peroxidation. In: Brown RC, Gormley IP, Chamberlain M, Davies R, eds. *The in vitro Effects of Mineral Dusts.* London: Academic Press, 1980: 131.

148 Piguet PF, Collart MA, Grau GE *et al.* Requirement of tumour necrosis factor for development of silica-induced pulmonary fibrosis. *Nature* 1990; 344: 245.

149 Lugano EM, Daubor JH, Elias JA *et al.* The regulation of lung fibroblast proliferation by alveolar macrophages in experimental silicosis. *Am Rev Respir Dis* 1984; 129: 767.

150 Schmidt JA, Oliver CH, Lepe-Zuniga JL *et al.* Silica-stimulated monocytes release fibroblast proliferation factors identical to interleukin-1. *J Clin Invest* 1984; 73: 1462.

151 Kennedy MCS. Aluminium powder inhalations in the treatment of silicosis of pottery workers and pneumoconiosis of coalminers. *Br J Ind Med* 1956; 13: 85.

152 Barhad B, Rotarn G, Lazarescu I *et al.* Our experience in polyvinylpyridin-n-oxide action on experimental lung silicosis. In: *4th International Pneumoconiosis Conference, Bucharest.* Genera: ILO, 1971: 315.

153 Dubois P, Gyselen A, Prignot J. Rifampicin combined chemotherapy in coalworkers' pneumoconio-tuberculosis. *Am Rev Respir Dis* 1977; 115: 221.

154 Jones FL. Rifampicin-containing chemotherapy for pulmonary tuberculosis associated with coal workers' pneumoconiosis. *Am Rev Respir Dis* 1982; 125: 681.

155 Hosey AD, Ashe HB, Trasko VM. *Control of Silicosis in Vermont Granite Industry. Progress Report.* Washington, DC: US Department of Health, Education and Welfare, 1957.

156 Samini B, Neilson A, Weill H, Ziskind M. The efficiency of protective hoods used by sandblasters to reduce silica dust exposure. *Am Ind Hyg Assoc J* 1975; 136: 140.

157 Lee DHK. Historical background to the asbestos problem. *Environ Res* 1979; 18: 300.

158 Murray M. Departmental committee for compensation for industrial diseases. Cmd 3495, 3496. London: HMSO, 1907.

159 Wood WB, Gloyne SR. Pulmonary asbestosis: a review of 100 cases. *Lancet* 1934; ii: 1383.

160 Doll R. Mortality from lung cancer in asbestos workers. *Br J Ind Med* 1955; 12: 81.

161 Wyers H. MD thesis, University of Glasgow, quoted by Perry KMA. Diseases of the lung resulting from occupational dusts other than silica. *Thorax* 1947; 2: 91.

162 Newhouse ML, Thompson H. Epidemiology of mesothelial tumours in the London area. *Ann N Y Acad Sci* 1965; 132: 579.

163 Elmes PC, Simpson MJC. The clinical aspects of mesothelioma. *Q J Med* 1976; 45: 427.

164 Selikoff IJ, Hammond EC, Churg J. Mortality experiences of asbestos insulation workers. In: Shappiro HA, ed. *Pneumoconio-*

sis: Proceedings of the International Conference in Johannesburg. London: Oxford University Press, 1970: 180.

165 Elmes PC, Wade OL. Relationship between exposure to asbestos and pleural malignancy in Belfast. *Ann N Y Acad Sci* 1965; 132: 549.

166 Flynn L. South Africa blacks out blue asbestos risk. *New Scientist* 1982; 94: 237.

167 Health and Safety Commission. *Health and Safety Statistics 1994–95.* Sudbury: HSE Books, 1995.

168 Peto R, Hodgson JT, Matthews FE, Jones JR. Continuing increase in mesothelioma mortality in Britain. *Lancet* 1995; 345: 535.

169 Doll R, Peto J. *Effects on Health of Exposure to Asbestos.* London: HMSO, 1985.

170 Walton WH. The nature, hazards and assessment of occupational exposure to airborne asbestos dust: a review. *Ann Occup Hyg* 1982; 25: 117.

171 McDonald JC, Liddell FDK, Gibbs GW *et al.* Dust exposure and mortality in chrysotile mining 1910–1975. *Br J Ind Med* 1980; 37: 11.

172 Weill H, Hughes J, Waggenspack C. Influence of dose and fibre type of respiratory malignancy risk in asbestos cement manufacturing. *Am Rev Respir Dis* 1979; 120: 345.

173 Berry G, Gilson JC, Holmes S *et al.* Asbestosis: a study of dose–response relationships in an asbestos textile factory. *Br J Ind Med* 1979; 36: 98.

174 Murdoch RM, Miller BG, Jacobsen M. Possible effects of the introduction of the 1969 Asbestos Regulations. *Ann Occup Hyg* 1988; 32 (Suppl 1): 505.

175 McDonald JC, Liddell FDK. Mortality in Canadian miners and millers exposed to chrysotile. *Ann N Y Acad Sci* 1979; 330: l.

176 Seidman H, Selikoff IJ, Hammond EC. Short-term asbestos work exposure and long-term observation. *Ann N Y Acad Sci* 1979; 330: 61.

177 Jones JSP, Smith PG, Pooley FD *et al.* The consequences of exposure to asbestos dust in a wartime gasmask factory. In: Wagner JC, ed. *Biological Effects of Mineral Fibres.* Lyon: International Agency for Cancer Research, 1980: 367.

178 McDonald AD. Mesothelioma after crocidolite exposure during gas mask manufacture. *Environ Res* 1978; 17: 340.

179 Newhouse ML, Berry G. Patterns of mortality in asbestos factory workers in London. *Ann N Y Acad Sci* 1979; 330: 53.

180 Hobbs MST, Woodward SD, Murphy B *et al.* The incidence of pneumoconiosis, mesothelioma and other respiratory cancer in men engaged in mining and milling crocidolite in Western Australia. In: *Biological Effects of Mineral Fibres*, Vol 2. Lyon: International Agency for Cancer Research, 1980: 615.

181 Berry G. Prediction of mesothelioma, lung cancer and asbestosis in former Wittenoom asbestos workers. *Br J Ind Med* 1991; 48: 793.

182 Peto J, Doll R, Herman C *et al.* Relationship of mortality to measures of environmental asbestos pollution in an asbestos textile factory. *Ann Occup Hyg* 1985; 29: 305.

183 Saracci R. Asbestos and lung cancer: an analysis of the epidemiological evidence on the asbestos–smoking interaction. *Int J Cancer* 1977; 20: 323.

184 Berry G, Newhouse ML, Antonis P. Combined effects of asbestos and smoking on mortality from lung cancer and mesothe-

lioma in factory workers. *Br J Ind Med* 1985; 42: 12.

185 Hammond EC, Selikoff IJ, Seidman H. Asbestos exposure, cigarette smoking and death rates. *Ann N Y Acad Sci* 1979; 330: 473.

186 Selikoff IJ, Hammond EC, Seidman H. Mortality experience of insulation workers in the United States and Canada 1943–1976. *Ann N Y Acad Sci* 1979; 330: 91.

187 Wignall BK, Fox AJ. Mortality of female gasmask assemblers. *Br J Ind Med* 1982; 39: 34.

188 Stell PM, McGill T. Asbestos and laryngeal carcinoma. *Lancet* 1973; ii: 416.

189 Morgan RW, Shettigara PT. Occupational asbestos exposure, smoking and laryngeal carcinoma. *Ann N Y Acad Sci* 1976; 271: 308.

190 Coggan D, Pannett B, Osmond C, Acheson ED. A survey of cancer and occupation in young and middle aged men. 1. Cancers of the respiratory tract. *Br J Ind Med* 1986; 43: 332.

191 Chan CK, Gee BL. Asbestos exposure and laryngeal cancer: an analysis of the epidemiologic evidence. *J Occup Med* 1988; 30: 23.

192 Ross R, Dworsky R, Nichols P *et al.* Asbestos exposure and lymphomas of the gastrointestinal tract and oral cavity. *Lancet* 1982; ii: 1118.

193 Weiss W. Cigarette smoke, asbestos and small irregular opacities. *Am Rev Respir Dis* 1984; 130: 293.

194 Sheers G. Asbestos-associated disease in employees of Devonport dockyard. *Ann N Y Acad Sci* 1979; 330: 281.

195 Coutts II, Gilson JC, Kerr IH *et al.* Progression of intrapulmonary fibrosis caused by asbestos exposure. *Thorax* 1981; 36: 232.

196 Hunt R. Routine lung function studies on 830 employees in an asbestos processing factory. *Ann N Y Acad Sci* 1965; 132: 405.

197 Becklake MR, Liddell FDK, Manfreda J, McDonald JC. Radiological changes after withdrawal from asbestos exposure. *Br J Ind Med* 1979; 36: 23.

198 Cookson W, de Clerk NH, Musk AW *et al.* The natural history of asbestosis in former crocidolite workers of Wittenoom gorge. *Am Rev Respir Dis* 1986; 133: 994.

199 Al-Jarad N, Strickland B, Pearson MC, Rubens MB, Rudd RM. High resolution computed tomography assessment of asbestosis and cryptogenic fibrosing alveolitis: a comparative study. *Thorax* 1992; 47: 645.

200 Shirai F, Kudoh S, Shibuya A *et al.* Crackles in asbestos workers: auscultation and lung sounds analysis. *Br J Dis Chest* 1981; 75: 386.

201 Murphy RLH, Sorensen K. Chest auscultation in the diagnosis of pulmonary asbestosis. *J Occup Med* 1973; 15: 272.

202 Smithers WJ. Secular changes in asbestosis in an asbestos factory. *Ann N Y Acad Sci* 1965; 132: 166.

203 Leathart GL. Pulmonary function tests in asbestos workers. *Trans Soc Occup Med* 1968; 18: 49.

204 Zedda S, Aresini G, Ghezzi I, Sartorelli E. Lung function in relation to radiographic changes in asbestos workers. *Respiration* 1973; 30: 132.

205 Williams R, Hugh-Jones P. The significance of lung function changes in asbestosis. *Thorax* 1960; 15: 109.

206 Jodoin G, Gibbs GW, Macklem PT, Becklake MR. Early effects of asbestos exposure on lung function. *Am Rev Respir Dis* 1971; 104: 525.

207 Becklake MR, Ernst P. Asbestos exposure and airway responses. In: Gee JBL, ed. *Occupational Lung Disease.* New York: Churchill Livingstone, 1984: 25.

208 Cookson WOC, Musk AW, Glancy JJ, Pleural thickening and gas transfer in asbestosis. *Thorax* 1983; 38: 657.

209 Hourihane D, O'B, McCaughey WTE. Pathological aspects of asbestosis. *Postgrad Med J* 1966; 42: 613.

210 Churg A, Wright JL, Wiggs B *et al.* Small airways disease and mineral dust exposure. *Am Rev Respir Dis* 1984; 131: 139.

211 Wright JL, Churg A. Morphology of small airways disease induced by asbestos exposure. *Hum Pathol* 1984; 15: 68.

212 Davis JMG. Electron microscope studies of asbestosis in man and animals. *Ann N Y Acad Sci* 1965; 132: 98.

213 Webster I. The pathogenesis of asbestosis. In: Shapiro HA, ed. *Pneumoconiosis: Proceedings of the International Conference in Johannesburg.* London: Oxford University Press, 1970: 117.

214 Morgan WKC. Rheumatoid pneumoconiosis in association with asbestos. *Thorax* 1964; 19: 433.

215 Churg A, Warnock ML. Analysis of the cases of ferruginous (asbestos) bodies from the general population. I. Patients with and without lung cancer. *Lab Invest* 1977; 37: 280.

216 Churg A, Warnock ML, Green N. Analysis of the cases of ferruginous (asbestos) bodies from the general population. II. True asbestos bodies and pseudo-asbestos bodies. *Lab Invest* 1979; 40: 31.

217 Churg A, Warnock ML. Analysis of the cases of ferruginous (asbestos) bodies from the general population. III. Patients with environmental exposure. *Lab Invest* 1979; 40: 622.

218 Gibbs AR, Pooley FD. Analysis and interpretation of inorganic mineral particles in 'lung' tissues. *Thorax* 1996; 51: 327.

219 Whitwell F, Scott J, Grimshaw M. Relationships between occupation and asbestos fibre content of the lungs in patients with pleural mesothielioma, lung cancer and other diseases. *Thorax* 1977; 32: 377.

220 Stovin PGI, Partridge P. Pulmonary asbestos and dust content in East Anglia. *Thorax* 1982; 37: 185.

221 Churg A, Warnock ML. Asbestos fibres in the general population. *Am Rev Respir Dis* 1980; 122: 669.

222 Davis JMG, Beckett ST, Bolton RE, Collings P. The pathological effects of asbestos clouds of different fibre dimensions on the lungs of rats. In: *V International Pneumoconiosis Conference 1978.* Bremerhaven: Wirtschaftsverlag NW, 1985: 82.

223 Timbrell V. The inhalation of fibres. In: Shapiro HA, ed. *Pneumoconiosis: Proceedings of the International Conference in Johannesburg.* London: Oxford University Press, 1970: 3.

224 Wagner JC, Pooley FD, Berry G *et al.* A pathological and mineralogical study of asbestos-related deaths in the United Kingdom in 1977. *Ann Occup Hyg* 1982; 26: 423.

225 Donaldson K, Bolton RE, Jones A *et al.* Kinetics of the bronchoalveolar leucocyte response in rats during exposure to equal airborne mass concentrations of quartz, chrysotile asbestos or titanium dioxide. *Thorax* 1988; 43: 525.

226 Bolton RE, Davis JMG, Miller B *et al.* The effect of dose of asbestos on mesothelioma

production in the laboratory rat. In: *Proceedings of the VI International Pneumoconiosis Conference, Bochum, 1983.* Geneva: International Labour Organization, 1984: 1028.

227 Rowlands N, Gibbs GW, McDonald AD. Asbestos fibres in the lungs of chrysotile miners and millers: a preliminary report. In: Walton WH, ed. *Inhaled Particles V.* Oxford: Pergamon Press, 1982: 417.

228 Cralley LJ, Key MM, Groth DH *et al.* Fibrous and mineral content of cosmetic talcum products. *Am Ind Hyg Assoc J* 1968; 29: 350.

229 Phillipson IM. Talc quality. *Lancet* 1980; i: 48.

230 Kleinfeld M, Messite J, Tabershaw IR. Talc pneumoconiosis. *Arch Ind Health* 1955; 12: 66.

231 Kleinfeld M, Messite J, Zaki MH. Mortality experiences among talc workers: a follow-up study *J Occup Med* 1974; 16: 345.

232 Gamble JF, Felner W, Dimeo MJ. An epidemiologic study of a group of talc workers. *Am Rev Respir Dis* 1979; 119: 741.

233 Research Committee of the British Thoracic Association. A survey of the long-term effects of talc and kaolin pleurodesis. *Br J Dis Chest* 1979; 73: 285.

234 Nam K, Gracy DR. Pulmonary talcosis from cosmetic talcum powder. *JAMA* 1972; 221: 492.

235 Moskowitz RL. Talc pneumoconiosis: a treated case. *Chest* 1970; 58: 37.

236 Buchanan DR, Lamb D, Seaton A. Punk rocker's lung: pulmonary fibrosis in a drug snorting fire-eater. *Br Med J* 1981; 283: 1661.

237 Gould SR, Barnardo DE. Respiratory distress after talc inhalation. *Br J Dis Chest* 1970; 66: 230.

238 Waller BE, Brownlee WJ, Roberts WC. Self-induced pulmonary granulomatosis. A consequence of intravenous injection of drugs intended for oral use. *Chest* 1980; 78: 90.

239 Lapenas D, Gale P, Kennedy T *et al.* Kaolin pneumoconiosis: radiologic, pathologic and mineralogic findings *Am Rev Respir Dis* 1984; 130: 282.

240 Wagner JC, Pooley FD, Gibbs A *et al.* Inhalation of china stone and china clay dusts: relationship between the mineralogy of dust retained in the lungs and pathological changes. *Thorax* 1986; 41: 190.

241 Kennedy T, Rawlings W, Baser M, Tockman M. Pneumoconiosis in Georgia kaolin workers. *Am Rev Respir Dis* 1983; 127: 215.

242 Altekruse EB, Chaudhary BA, Pearson MG, Morgan WKC. Kaolin dust concentrations and pneumoconiosis at a kaolin mine. *Thorax* 1984; 39: 436.

243 Ogle CG, Rundle EM, Sugar ET. China clay workers in the southwest of England: analysis of the radiographic readings, ventilatory capacity and respiratory symptoms in relation to type and duration of exposure. *Br J Ind Med* 1989; 46: 261.

244 Sakula A. Pneumoconiosis due to fuller's earth. *Thorax* 1961; 16: 176.

245 McNally WD, Trostler IS. Severe pneumoconiosis caused by inhalation of fuller's earth. *J Ind Hyg* 1941; 23: 118.

246 Scott A. On the occupational cancer of the paraffin and oil workers of the Scottish shale oil industry. *Br Med J* 1922; 2: 1108.

247 Seaton A, Lamb D, Rhind Brown W *et al.* Pneumoconiosis of shale miners. *Thorax* 1981; 36: 412.

248 Seaton A, Louw SJ, Cowie HA. Epidemiologic studies of Scottish oil shale workers. 1.

Prevalence of skin disease and pneumoconiosis. *Am J Ind Med* 1986; 9: 409.

249 Louw SJ, Cowie HA, Seaton A. Epidemiologic studies of Scottish oil shale workers. 2. Lung function in shale workers' pneumoconiosis. *Am J Ind Med* 1986; 9: 423.

250 Miller BG, Cowie HA, Middleton WG, Seaton A. Epidemiologic studies of Scottish oil shale workers. 3. Causes of death. *Am J Ind Med* 1986; 9: 433.

251 Thomas RW. Silicosis in the ball clay and china clay Indries. *Lancet* 1952; i: 133.

252 Adamis Z, Timar N. Studies on the effects of quartz, bentonite and coal dust mixtures on macrophages *in vitro*. *Br J Exp Pathol* 1978; 59: 411.

253 Pimental JC, Menezes AP. Pulmonary and hepatic granulomatous disorders due to the inhalation of cement and mica dusts. *Thorax* 1978; 33: 219.

254 Skulberg KR, Gylseth B, Skaug V, Hanoa R. Mica pneumoconiosis: a literature review. *Scand J Work Environ Health* 1985; 11: 65.

255 Davies D, Cotton R. Mica pneumoconiosis. *Br J Ind Med* 1983; 40: 22.

256 Landas SK, Schwartz DA. Mica-associated pulmonary interstitial fibrosis. *Am Rev Respir Dis* 1991; 144: 718.

257 Amandus HE, Althouse R, Morgan WKC *et al.* The morbidity and mortality of vermiculite miners and millers exposed to asbestiform tremolite/actinolite. Part III. Radiographic findings. *Am J Ind Med* 1987; 11: 21.

258 McDonald JC, Sebastien P, Armstrong B. Radiological survey of past and present vermiculite miners exposed to tremolite. *Br J Ind Med* 1986; 43: 445.

259 McDonald JC, McDonald AD, Sebastien P, Moy K. Health of vermiculite miners exposed to trace amounts of fibrous tremolite. *Br J Ind Med* 1988; 45: 630.

260 Bazas T. Effects of occupational exposure to dust on the respiratory system of cement workers. *J Soc Occup Med* 1980; 30: 31.

261 Kalacic I. Ventilatory function in cement workers. *Arch Environ Health* 1973; 26: 84.

262 Searl A. A review of the durability of inhaled fibres and options for the design of safer fibres. *Ann Occup Hyg* 1994; 38: 839.

263 Donaldson K, Brown RC, Brown G. Respirable industrial fibres: mechanisms of pathogenicity. *Thorax* 1993; 48: 390.

264 Jones AD. Respirable industrial fibres: deposition, clearance and dissolution in animal models. *Ann Occup Hyg* 1993; 37: 211.

265 Baris YI, Sahin AA, Ozesmi M *et al.* An outbreak of pleural mesothelioma and chronic fibrosing pleurisy in the village of Karain/Urgup in Anatolia. *Thorax* 1978; 33: 181.

266 Artvinli M, Baris YI. Environmental fiber induced pleuro-pulmonary diseases in an Anatolian village: an epidemiologic study. *Arch Environ Health* 1982; 37: 177.

267 Pooley FD. Evaluation of fiber samples taken from the vicinity of two villages in Turkey. In: Dement JM, Lemen R, eds. *Dusts and Disease: Occupational and Environmental Exposures to Selected Particulate and Fibrous Dusts.* Park Forest South, Illinois: Pathotox Publishers, 1979: 41.

268 Casey KR, Shigeoka JW, Rom WN, Moatamed F. Zeolite exposure and associated pneumoconiosis. *Chest* 1985; 87: 837.

269 Stanton MF, Layard M, Tegeris A *et al.* Carcinogenicity of fibrous glass: pleural

response in the rat in relation to fiber dimension. *J Natl Cancer Inst* 1977; 58: 587.

270 Donaldson K. Short term animal studies for detecting inflammation, fibrosis and preneoplastic changes induced by fibres. *IARC Sci Publ* 1996; 140: 97.

271 Simonato L, Fletcher AC, Cherrie JW *et al.* The International Agency for Research on Cancer historical cohort study of MMMF production workers in seven European countries: extension of the follow-up. *Ann Occup Hyg* 1987; 31: 603.

272 Enterline PE, Marsh GM, Henderson V, Callahan C. Mortality update of a cohort of US man-made mineral fibre workers. *Ann Occup Hyg* 1987; 31: 625.

273 Musk AW, Greville HW, Tribe AE. Pulmonary disease from occupational exposure to an artificial aluminium silicate used as cat litter. *Br J Ind Med* 1980; 37: 367.

274 Sors H, Gaudichet A, Sebastien P *et al.* Lung fibrosis after inhalation of fibrous attapulgite. *Thorax* 1979; 34: 695.

275 Waxweiler RJ, Zumwalde RD, Ness GO, Brown DP. A retrospective cohort mortality study of males mining and milling attapulgite clay. *Am J Ind Med* 1988; 13: 305.

276 Huuskonen MS, Tossavainen A, Koskinen H *et al.* Wollastonite exposure and lung fibrosis. *Environ Res* 1983; 30: 291.

277 Harding HE, McLaughlin AIG, Doig AT. Clinical, radiographic and pathological studies of the lungs of electric arc and oxyacetylene welders. *Lancet* 1958; ii: 394.

278 Barrie HF, Harding HE. Argyro-siderosis of the lungs in silver finishers. *Br J Ind Med* 1947; 4: 225.

279 Morgan WKC, Kerr HD. Pathologic and physiologic studies of welder's siderosis. *Ann Intern Med* 1963; 58: 293.

280 Cronin AJ. Dust inhalation by haematite miners. *J Ind Hyg* 1926; 8: 291.

281 Craw J. Pneumoconiosis in the haematite iron ore mines of west Cumbria. A study of 45 years of control. *J Soc Occup Med* 1982; 32: 53.

282 Stewart MJ, Faulds JS. The pulmonary fibrosis of haematite miners. *J Pathol Bacteriol* 1934; 39: 233.

283 Boyd JT, Doll R, Faulds JS, Leiper J. Cancer of the lung in iron ore (haematite) miners. *Br J Ind Med* 1970; 27: 97.

284 Jones-Williams W. A histological study of the lungs in 52 cases of chronic beryllium disease. *Br J Ind Med* 1958; 15: 84.

285 Van Ordstrand HS, Hughes R, de Nardi JM, Carmody MG. Beryllium poisoning. *JAMA* 1945; 129: l084.

286 Hardy HL, Tabershaw IR. Delayed chemical pneumonitis occurring in workers exposed to beryllium compounds. *J Ind Hyg Toxicol* 1946; 28: 197.

287 Hardy HL. Beryllium disease: a continuing diagnostic problem. *Am J Med Sci* 1961; 142: 150.

288 Hardy HL, Stoekle JD. Beryllium disease. *J Chron Dis* 1959; 9: 152.

289 Van Ordstrand HS. Diagnosis of beryllium disease. *Arch Ind Health* 1959; 19: 157.

290 Kotloff RM, Richman PS, Greenacre JK, Rossman MD. Chronic beryllium disease in a dental laboratory technician. *Am Rev Respir Dis* 1993; 147: 205.

291 Newman LS, Kreiss K. Non-occupational beryllium disease masquerading as sarcoidosis: identification by blood lymphocyte

proliferative response to beryllium. *Am Rev Respir Dis* 1992; 145: 1212.

292 Sprince NL, Kanarek DJ, Weber AL *et al.* Reversible beryllium disease in beryllium workers. *Am Rev Respir Dis* 1978; 117: 1011.

293 Weber AL, Stoeckle JD, Hardy HL. Roentgenologic patterns in longstanding beryllium disease: report of eight cases. *Am J Roentgenol* 1965; 93: 879.

294 Gaensler EA, Verstraeten JM, Weil WB. Respiratory pathophysiology in chronic beryllium disease. *Arch Ind Health* 1959; 19: 132.

295 Daniele RP. Beryllium-induced lung disease: immunologic mechanisms and diagnostic approaches. In: Gee JBL, ed. *Occupational Lung Disease.* New York: Churchill Livingstone, 1984: 183.

296 Epstein PE. Dauber lH, Rossman MD, Daniele RP. Bronchoalveolar lavage in a patient with chronic berylliosis: evidence for hypersensitivity pneumonitis. *Ann Intern Med* 1982; 97: 213.

297 Jones-Williams W. Diagnostic criteria for chronic beryllium disease (CBD) based on the UK Registry 1945–1991. *Sarcoidosis* 1993; 10: 41.

298 Williams WR, Jones-Williams W. Development of beryllium lymphocyte transformation tests in chronic beryllium disease. *Int Arch Allergy Appl Immunol* 1982; 67: 175.

299 Kreiss K, Newman LS, Mroz MM *et al.* Screening blood test identifies subclinical beryllium disease. *J Occup Med* 1989; 31: 603.

300 Newman LS, Bobka C, Schumacher B *et al.* Compartmentalized immune response reflects clinical severity of beryllium disease. *Am J Respir Crit Care Med* 1994; 150: 135.

301 Kreiss K, Wasserman S, Mroz MM, Newman LS. Beryllium disease screening in the ceramics industry. Blood lymphocyte test performance and exposure–disease relations. *J Occup Med* 1993; 35: 267.

302 Dutram FR, Cholak J, Hubbard DM. The value of beryllium determination in the diagnosis of berylliosis. *Am J Clin Pathol* 1949; 19: 229.

303 Jones-Williams W, Wallach R. Laser microprobe mass spectrometry (LAMMS) analysis of beryllium, sarcoidosis and other granulomatous diseases. *Sarcoidosis* 1989; 16: 111.

304 Kaltreider NL, Elder MJ, Cralley LU. Health survey of aluminium workers with special reference to fluoride exposure. *J Occup Med* 1972; 14: 1531.

305 Shaver CG, Riddell AR. Lung changes associated with the manufacture of alumina abrasive. *J Ind Hyg* 1947; 29: 145.

306 Mitchell J, Manning GB, Molyneux M, Lane RE. Pulmonary fibrosis in workers exposed to finely powdered aluminium. *Br J Ind Med* 1961; 18: 10.

307 Jordan JW. Pulmonary fibrosis in a worker using an aluminium powder. *Br J Ind Med* 1961; 18: 21.

308 McLaughlin AIG, Kazantzis G, King E *et al.* Pulmonary fibrosis and encephalopathy associated with the inhalation of aluminium dust. *Br J Ind Med* 1962; 19: 253.

309 Candy JM, Oakley AE, Klinowski J *et al.* Aluminium silicates and senile plaque formation in Alzheimer's disease. *Lancet* 1986; i: 345.

310 Miller RR, Churg AM, Hutcheon M, Lam S. Pulmonary alveolar proteinosis and alu-minum dust exposure. *Am Rev Respir Dis* 1984; 130: 312.

311 Armstrong B, Trembly C, Baris D, Thèriault G. Lung cancer mortality and polynuclear aromatic hydrocarbons: a case-control study of aluminium production workers in Arvida, Quebec, Canada. *Am J Epidemiol* 1994; 139: 250.

312 Cooper DA, Pendergrass EP, Vorwald AK. Pneumoconiosis in workers in an antimony industry. *Am J Roentgenol* 1968; 103: 495.

313 Kulcik I, Juck A, Gruberova J. Respiratory and pulmonary lesions caused by antimony trioxide dust. *Pracov Lek* 1962; 14: 363.

314 Arrigoni A. Le pneumoconiosis de bario. *Med Lav* 1933; 24: 461.

315 Pendergrass EP, Greening RR. Baritosis: report of a case. *Arch Ind Hyg Occup Med* 1953; 7: 44.

316 Doig AT. Baritosis: a benign pneumoconiosis. *Thorax* 1976; 31: 30.

317 Watson AK, Black J, Doig AT, Nagelschmidt G. Pneumoconiosis in carbon electrode markers. *Br J Ind Med* 1959; 16: 274.

318 Miller AA, Ramsden F. Carbon pneumoconiosis. *Br J Ind Med* 1961; 18: 103.

319 Gardiner K, Trethowan NW, Harrington JM, Rossiter CE, Calvert IA. Respiratory health effects of carbon black: a survey of European carbon black workers. *Br J Ind Med* 1993; 50: 1082.

320 Harris DK, Adams WGF. Acro-osteolysis occurring in men engaged in the polymerization of vinyl chloride. *Br Med J* 1967; 2: 712.

321 Creech JL, Johnson MN. Angiosarcoma of liver in the manufacture of polyvinyl chloride. *J Occup Med* 1974; 16: 150.

322 Soutar CA, Copland LH, Thornley PE *et al.* Epidemiological study of respiratory disease in workers exposed to polyvinyl chloride dust. *Thorax* 1980; 35: 644.

323 Arnaud A, Pommier de Santi P, Garbe L *et al.* Polyvinyl chloride pneumoconiosis. *Thorax* 1978; 33: 19.

324 Seaton A, Soutar C. Polyvinyl chloride and the lung. In: Gee JBL, Morgan WKC, Brooks SM, eds. *Occupational Lung Disease.* New York: Raven Press, 1984: 233.

325 Lloyd MH, Gauld S, Copland L, Soutar CA. Epidemiological study of the lung function of workers at a factory manufacturing polyvinyl chloride. *Br J Ind Med* 1984; 41: 328.

326 Funahashi A, Schleuter DP, Pintar K *et al.* Pneumoconiosis in workers exposed to silicon carbide. *Am Rev Respir Dis* 1983; 129: 653.

327 Infante-Rivard C, Dufresne A, Armstrong B, Bouchard P, Theriault G. Cohort study of silicon carbide production workers. *Am J Epidemiol* 1994; 140: 1009.

328 Fox AJ, Goldblatt P, Kinlen LJ. A study of the mortality of Cornish tin miners. *Br J Ind Med* 1981; 38: 378.

329 Robertson AJ, Rivers D, Nagelschmidt G, Duncumb P. Stannosis. *Lancet* 1961; i: 1089.

330 Pendergrass EP, Pryde AW. Benign pneumoconiosis due to tin oxide: a case report with experimental investigation of the radiographic density of the tin oxide dust. *J Ind Hyg* 1948; 30: 119.

331 Coates EO, Watson JHL. Diffuse interstitial lung disease in tungsten carbide workers. *Ann Intern Med* 1971; 75: 709.

332 Coates EO, Watson JHL. Pathology of the lung in tungsten carbide workers using light and electron microscopy. *J Occup Med* 1973; 15: 280.

333 Sjogren I, Hillerdal G, Andersson A, Zetterstrom O. Hard metal lung disease: importance of cobalt in coolants. *Thorax* 1980; 35: 653.

334 Davison AG, Haslam PL, Corrin B *et al.* Interstitial lung disease and asthma in hard metal workers: bronchoalveolar lavage, ultrastructural, and analytical findings and results of bronchial provocation tests. *Thorax* 1983; 38: 119.

335 Nemery B, Casier P, Roosels D, Lahaye D, Demedts M. Survey of cobalt exposure and respiratory health in diamond polishers. *Am Rev Respir Dis* 1992; 145: 610.

336 Frost AE, Keller CA, Brown RW *et al.* Giant cell interstitial pneumonitis. Disease recurrence in the transplanted lung. *Am Rev Respir Dis* 1993; 148: 1401.

337 Shirakawa T, Kusaka Y, Fujimura N *et al.* Hard metal asthma: cross immunological and respiratory reactivity between cobalt and nickel? *Thorax* 1990; 45: 267.

338 Kusaka Y, Kumagai S, Kyono H, Kohyama N, Shirakawa T. Determination of exposure to cobalt and nickel in the atmosphere of the hard metal industry. *Ann Occup Hyg* 1992; 36: 497.

339 Higgins ITT, Cochrane AL, Gilson JC, Wood CH. Population studies of chronic respiratory disease: a comparison of miners, foundry workers and others in Staveley, Derbyshire. *Br J Ind Med* 1959; 16: 255.

340 Dosman JA, Cotton DJ, Graham BL *et al.* Chronic bronchitis and decreased forced expiratory flow rates in lifetime non-smoking grain workers. *Am Rev Respir Dis* 1980; 121: 11.

341 Cotton DJ, Graham BL, Li KYR *et al.* Effects of smoking and occupational exposure on peripheral airway function in young cereal grain workers. *Am Rev Respir Dis* 1982; 126: 660.

342 Walker DD, Archibald RM, Attfield MD. Bronchitis in men employed in the coke industry. *Br J Ind Med* 1971; 28: 358.

343 Soutar CA. Occupational bronchitis. In: Harrington JM, ed. *Recent Advances in Occupational Medicine.* Edinburgh: Churchill Livingstone, 1987: 281.

344 Lee WR. Clinical diagnosis of byssinosis. *Thorax* 1979; 34: 287.

345 Niven RMcL, Pickering CAC. Byssinosis: a review. *Thorax* 1996; 51: 632.

346 Kay JP. Trades producing phthisis. *N Engl Med Surg* 1831; 1: 357.

347 Schilling RSF. Byssinosis in cotton and other textile workers. *Lancet* 1956; ii: 261.

348 Castellan RM, Olenchock SA, Hankinson JL *et al.* Acute bronchoconstriction induced by cotton dust: dose-related responses to endotoxin and othe dust factors. *Ann Intern Med* 1984; 101: 157.

349 Berry G, Molyneux MKB, Tombleson JBL. Relationship between dust level and byssinosis and bronchitis in Lancashire cotton mills. *Br J Ind Med* 1974; 31: 18.

350 Berry G, McKerrow CB, Molyneux MKB *et al.* A study of the acute and chronic changes in ventilatory capacity of workers in Lancashire cotton mills. *Br J Ind Med* 1973; 30: 25.

351 Glindmeyer HW, Lefante JJ, Jones RN *et al.* Exposure-related declines in the lung function of cotton textile workers. *Am Rev Respir Dis* 1991; 144: 675.

352 Fishwick D, Fletcher AM, Pickering CAC *et al.* Lung function, bronchial reactivity, atopic status and dust exposure in Lancashire mill operatives. *Am Rev Respir Dis* 1992; 145: 1103.

353 Christiani DC, Ye T-T, Wegman DH, Eisen EA, Dai H-E, Lu P-L. Cotton dust exposure, across shift drop in FEV_1, and five year change in lung function. *Am J Respir Crit Care Med* 1994; 150: 1250.

354 Field GB, Owen P. Respiratory function in an Australian cotton mill. *Bull Eur Physiopathol Respir* 1979; 15: 455.

355 Fishwick D, Pickering CAC. Byssinosis: a form of occupational asthma. *Thorax* 1992; 47: 401.

356 Bouhuys A, Schoenberg JBFJ, Schilling RSF. Epidemiology of chronic lung disease in a cotton mill community. *Lung* 1977; 154: 168.

357 Schacter EN, Maunder LR, Beck GJ. The pattern of lung function abnormalities in cotton textile workers. *Am Rev Respir Dis* 1984; 129: 523.

358 Beck GJ, Schacter EN, Maunder LR, Schilling RSF. A prospective study of chronic lung disease in cotton textile workers. *Ann Intern Med* 1982; 97: 645.

359 Merchant JA, Lumsden JC, Kilburn KH *et al.* Dose–response studies in cotton textile workers. *J Occup Med* 1973; 15: 222.

360 Elwood PC, Thomas HF, Sweetnam PM, Elwood JH. Mortality of flax workers. *Br J Ind Med* 1982; 39: 18.

361 Berry G, Molyneux MKB. A mortality study of workers in Lancashire cotton mills. *Chest* 1981; 79 (Suppl): 11S.

362 Hodgson JT, Jones RD. Mortality of workers in the British cotton industry in 1968–84. *Scand J Occup Environ Health* 1990; 16: 113.

363 Edwards C, McCartney J, Rooke G, Ward F. The pathology of the lung in byssinosis. *Thorax* 1975; 30: 612.

364 Pratt PC, Vollmer RT, Millar JA. Epidemiology of pulmonary lesions in nontextile and cotton textile workers: a retrospective autopsy analysis. *Arch Environ Health* 1980; 35: 133.

365 Honeybourne D, Pickering CAC. Physiological evidence that emphysema is not a feature of byssinosis. *Thorax* 1986; 41: 6.

366 Parikh JR, Bhagia LJ, Majumdar PK, Shah AR, Kashyap SK. Prevalence of byssinosis in textile mills at Ahmedabad, India. *Br J Ind Med* 1989; 46: 787.

367 El Karim MAA, Ona SH. Prevalence of byssinosis and respiratory symptoms among spinners in Sudanese cotton mills. *Am J Ind Med* 1987; 12: 281.

368 Berry G, Molyneux MKB, Tombleson JBL. Relationships between dust level and byssinosis and bronchitis in Lancashire cotton mills. *Br J Ind Med* 1974; 31: 18.

369 Petsonk EL, Olenchok SA, Castellan RM *et al.* Human ventilatory responses to washed and unwashed cottons from different growing areas. *Br J Ind Med* 1986; 43: 182.

370 Hendrick DJ. Contaminated humidifiers and the lung. *Thorax* 1983; 40: 244.

371 Antweiler H. Histamine liberation by cotton dust extract. *Br J Ind Med* 1961; 18: 130.

372 Jones RN, Butcher BT, Hammal W *et al.* Interaction of atopy and exposure to cotton dust in the bronchoconstrictor response. *Br J Ind Med* 1980; 37: 141.

373 Rylander R. Cellular and humoral mechanisms in byssinosis. In: Gee JBL, ed. *Occupational Lung Disease.* New York: Churchill Livingstone, 1985: 193.

374 Merchant JA, Lumsden JC, Kilburn KH *et al.* Preprocessing cotton to prevent byssinosis. *Br J Ind Med* 1973; 30: 237.

375 Banaszak EJ, Thiede WH, Fink JN. Hypersensitivity pneumonitis due to contamination of an air conditioner. *N Engl J Med* 1970; 283: 271.

376 Fink JN, Banaszak EJ, Thiede WH. Interstitial pneumonitis due to hypersensitivity to an organism contaminating a heating system. *Ann Intern Med* 1971; 74: 80.

377 Robertson AS, Burge PS, Weiland A. Extrinsic allergic alveolitis due to antigens from a humidifier at 15°C. *Thorax* 1985; 40: 229.

378 Burge PS, Finnegan M, Horsfield N *et al.* Occupational asthma in a factory with a contaminated humidifier. *Thorax* 1985; 40: 248.

379 Suda T, Sato A, Gemma H, Hayakawa H, Chida K. Hypersensitivity pneumonitis associated with home ultrasonic humidifiers. *Chest* 1995; 107: 711.

380 Kane GC, Marx JJ, Prince DS. Hypersensitivity pneumonitis secondary to *Klebsiella oxytoca.* A new cause of humidifier lung. *Chest* 1993; 104: 627.

381 MRC Symposium. Humidifier fever. *Thorax* 1977; 32: 653.

382 Pickering CAC, Moore WKS, Lacey J *et al.* Investigation of a respiratory disease associated with an air-conditioning system. *Clin Allergy* 1976; 6: 109.

383 Friend JAR, Gaddie J, Palmer KNV *et al.* Extrinsic allergic alveolitis and contaminated cooling water in a factory machine. *Lancet* 1977; i: 297.

384 Cockcroft A, Edwards J, Bevan C *et al.* An investigation of operating theatre staff exposed to humidifier fever antigens. *Br J Ind Med* 1981; 38: 144.

385 McSharry C, Anderson K, Speekenbrink A, Lewis C, Boyd G. Discriminant analysis of symptom pattern and serum antibody titres in humidifier-related disease. *Thorax* 1993; 48: 496.

386 Edwards JH, Griffiths AJ, Mullins J. Protozoa as sources of antigen in humidifier fever. *Nature* 1976; 264: 438.

387 Rylander R, Haglind P, Lundholm M *et al.* Humidifier fever and endotoxin exposure. *Clin Allergy* 1978; 8: 511.

388 Tse KS, Warren P, Janusz M *et al.* Respiratory abnormalities in workers exposed to grain dusts. *Arch Environ Health* 1973; 27: 74.

389 Donham KJ, Rubino M, Thedell TD, Kammermeyer J. Potential health hazards to agricultural workers in swine confinement buildings. *J Occup Med* 1977; 19: 383.

390 Rylander R, Anderson K, Belin L *et al.* Sewage workers' syndrome. *Lancet* 1976; ii: 478.

391 Finnegan MJ, Pickering CAC, Burge PS. The sick building syndrome: prevalence studies. *Br Med J* 1984; 289: 1573.

392 Committee on Medical and Biologic Effects of Environmental Pollutants. *Carbon Monoxide.* Washington, DC: National Academy of Sciences, 1977.

393 Garland H, Pierce J. Neurological complications of carbon monoxide poisoning. *Q J Med* 1967; 144: 445.

394 Smith JS, Brandon S. Morbidity from acute carbon monoxide poisoning at three year follow-up. *Br Med J* 1973; i: 318.

395 Min SK. A brain syndrome associated with delayed neuropsychiatric sequelae following acute carbon monoxide intoxication. *Acta Psychiatr Scand* 1986; 73: 80.

396 Dollery C, ed. *Therapeutic Drugs.* Edinburgh: Churchill Livingstone, 1991.

397 Donham KJ, Knapp LW, Monson R, Gustafson K. Acute toxic exposure to gases from liquid manure. *J Occup Med* 1982; 24: 142.

398 Simpson RE, Simpson GR. Fatal hydrogen sulphide poisoning in association with industrial waste exposure. *Med J Aust* 1971; i: 331.

399 Dalgaard JB, Decker F, Fallentin B *et al.* Fatal poisoning and other health hazards associated with industrial fishing. *Br J Ind Med* 1972; 29: 307.

400 Wilson R, Lovejoy FH, Rudolf J *et al.* Acute phosphine poisonong aboard a grain freighter. *JAMA* 1980; 244: 148.

401 Feldstein A, Heumann M, Barnett M. Fumigant intoxication during transport of grain by railroad. *J Occup Med* 1991; 33: 64.

402 Sallie B, McDonald JC. Inhalation accidents reported to the SWORD surveillance project 1990–1993. *Ann Occup Hyg* 1996; 40: 211.

403 Watt MM, Watt SJ, Seaton A. Episode of toxic gas exposure in sewer workers. *Occup Environ Med* 1997; 54: 277.

404 Levy DM, Divertie MB, Litzow TJ, Henderson JW. Ammonia burns of the face and respiratory tract. *JAMA* 1984; 190: 873.

405 Kass I, Zamel N, Dobry CA, Holzer M. Bronchiectasis following ammonia burns of the respiratory tract. *Chest* 1972; 62: 282.

406 Joyner RE, Durel EG. Accidental liquid chlorine spill in a rural community. *J Occup Med* 1962; 4: 152.

407 Beach FXM, Jones ES, Scarrow GD. Respiratory effects of chlorine gas. *Br J Ind Med* 1969; 26: 231.

408 Weill H, George R, Swarz M, Ziskind M. Late evaluation of pulmonary function after acute exposure to chlorine gas. *Am Rev Respir Dis* 1969; 99: 374.

409 Kowitz T, Reba RC, Parker RT, Spicer WS. Effects of chlorine gas upon respiratory function. *Arch Environ Health* 1967; 14: 545.

410 Kennedy SM, Enarson DA, Janssen RG, Chan-Yeung M. Lung health consequences of reported accidental chlorine gas exposures among pulp mill workers. *Am Rev Respir Dis* 1991; 143: 74.

411 Schwartz DA, Smith DD, Lakshminarayan S. The pulmonary sequelae associated with accidental inhalation of chlorine gas. *Chest* 1990; 97: 820.

412 Mustchin CP, Pickering CAC. 'Coughing water': bronchial hyper-reactivity induced by swimming in a chlorinated pool. *Thorax* 1979; 34: 682.

413 Hayhurst ER, Scott E. Four cases of sudden death in a silo. *JAMA* 1914; 63: 1570.

414 Moskowiz RL, Lyons HA, Cottle HR. Silo-fillers' disease: clinical, physiologic and pathologic study of a patient. *Am J Med* 1964; 36: 457.

415 Jones GR, Proudfoot AT, Hall JI. Pulmonary effects of acute exposure to nitrous fumes. *Thorax* 1973; 28: 61.

416 Gregory KL, Malinoski VF, Sharp CR. Cleveland Clinic fire survivorship study 1929–1965. *Arch Environ Health* 1969; 18: 508.

417 Becklake MR, Goldman HI, Bosman AR, Freed CC. The long term effects of exposure to nitrous fumes. *Am Rev Tuberc* 1957; 76: 398.

418 McAdams AJ. Bronchiolitis obliterans. *Am J Med* 1955; 19: 314.

419 Department of Health Advisory Group on the Medical Aspects of Air Pollution Episodes. *Third Report. Oxides of Nitrogen.* London: HMSO, 1993.

420 Shy CM, Creasan JP, Pearlman ME *et al.* The Chatanooga school children study: effects of community exposure to nitrogen dioxide. II. Incidence of acute respiratory illness. *J Air Poll Control Assoc* 1970; 20: 582.

421 Speizer FE, Ferris B, Bishop YMM, Spengler J. Respiratory disease rates and pulmonary function in children associated with NO₂ exposure. *Am Rev Respir Dis* 1980; 121: 3.

422 Jarvis D, Chinn S, Luczynska C, Burney P. Association of respiratory symptoms and lung function in young adults with use of domestic gas apparatus. *Lancet* 1996; 347: 426.

423 Charan N, Myers CG, Lakshminarayan S, Spencer TM. Pulmonary injuries associated with acute sulfur dioxide inhalation. *Am Rev Respir Dis* 1979; 119: 555.

424 Smith TJ, Peters JM, Reading JC, Castle CH. Pulmonary impairment from chronic exposure to sulfur dioxide in a smelter. *Am Rev Respir Dis* 1977; 116: 31.

425 Lebowitz MD, Burton A, Kalterborn MS. Pulmonary function in smelter workers. *J Occup Med* 1979; 21: 255.

426 Sheppard D, Wong WS, Uehara CF *et al.* Lower threshold and greater bronchomotor responsiveness of asthmatic subjects to sulfur dioxide. *Am Rev Respir Dis* 1980; 122: 873.

427 American Thoracic Society. Health effects of outdoor air pollution. *Am J Respir Crit Care Med* 1996; 153: 3.

428 Department of Health Advisory Group on the Medical Aspects of Air Pollution Episodes. *Second Report: Sulphur dioxide, Acid Aerosols and Particulates.* London: HMSO, 1992.

429 Reed D, Glaser S, Kaldor J. Ozone toxicity symptoms among flight attendants. *Am J Ind Med* 1980; 1: 43.

430 Department of Health Advisory Group on the Medical Aspects of Air Pollution Episodes. *First report. Ozone.* London: HMSO, 1991.

431 Anderson HR, Ponce de Leon A, Bland M, Bower M, Strachan DP. Air pollution, daily mortality in London: 1987–92. *Br Med J* 1996; 312: 665.

432 Buchdahl R, Parker A, Stebbings T, Babiker A. Association between air pollution and acute childhood wheezy episodes: prospective observational study. *Br Med J* 1996; 312: 661.

433 Everett ED, Overholt EL. Phosgene poisoning. *JAMA* 1968; 205: 103.

434 Doig AT, Challen PJR. Respiratory hazards in welding. *Ann Occup Hyg* 1964; 7: 223.

435 Gordon T, Fine JM. Metal fume fever. *Occup Med* 1993; 8: 504.

436 Gordon T, Chi Chen L, Fine JM *et al.* Pulmonary effects of inhaled zinc oxide in human subjects, rats and rabbits. *Int Ind Hyg J* 1994; 53: 503.

437 Blanc PD, Boushey HA, Wong H, Wintermeyer SF, Bernstein MS. Cytokines in metal fume fever. *Am Rev Respir Dis* 1993; 147: 134.

438 Ameille J, Brechot JM, Brochard P, Capron F, Dore MF. Occupational hypersensitivity pneumonitis in a smelter exposed to zinc fumes. *Chest* 1992; 101: 862.

439 Allen MB, Crisp A, Snook N, Page RL. 'Smoke bomb' pneumonitis. *Respir Med* 1992; 86: 165.

440 Evans EH. Casualties following exposure to zinc chloride smoke. *Lancet* 1945; ii: 368.

441 Seaton A, Bishop CM. Acute mercury pneumonitis. *Br J Ind Med* 1978; 35: 258.

442 Beton DC, Andrews GS, Davies HJ *et al.* Acute cadmium fume poisoning: five cases with one death from renal necrosis. *Br J Ind Med* 1966; 23: 292.

443 Bonnell JA, Kazantzis G, King E. A follow-up study of men exposed to cadmium oxide fumes. *Br J Ind Med* 1959; 16: 135.

444 Smith TJ, Petty TL, Reading JC, Lakshminarayan S. Pulmonary effects of chronic exposure to airborne cadmium. *Am Rev Respir Dis* 1976; 114: 161.

445 Niewoehner DE, Hoidal JR. Lung fibrosis and emphysema: divergent responses to a common injury. *Science* 1982; 217: 359.

446 Davison AG, Fayers PM, Newman Taylor AJ *et al.* Cadmium inhalation and emphysema. *Lancet* 1988; i: 663.

447 Armstrong BG, Kazantis G. The mortality of cadmium workers. *Lancet* 1983; i: 1424.

448 Leduc D, de Francquen P, Jacobovitz P *et al.* Association of cadmium exposure with rapidly progressive emphysema in a smoker. *Thorax* 1993; 48: 570.

449 Musk AW, Tees JG. Asthma caused by occupational exposure to vanadium compounds. *Med J Aust* 1982; i: 183.

450 Zenz C, Berg BA. Human responses to continued vanadium pentoxide exposure. *Arch Environ Health* 1967; 14: 709.

451 Bergstrom R. Acute pulmonary toxicity of manganese dioxide. *Scand J Work Environ Health* 1977; Suppl 3: 1.

452 Lloyd-Davies TA, Harding HE. Manganese pneumonitis. *Br J Ind Med* 1946; 3: 111.

453 McLaughlin AIG, Milton R, Perry KMA. Toxic manifestations of osmium tetroxide. *Br J Ind Med* 1946; 3: 183.

454 Jorgensen H, Svenson A. Studies of pulmonary function in respiratory tract syndromes of workers in an iron ore mine where diesel trucks are used underground. *J Occup Med* 1970; 12: 348.

455 Robertson A, Dodgson J, Collings P, Seaton A. Exposure to oxides of nitrogen: respiratory symptoms and lung function in British coalminers. *Br J Ind Med* 1984; 41: 214.

456 Williams N, Smith FK. Polymer fume fever: an elusive diagnosis. *JAMA* 1972; 219: 1587.

457 Sokol WN, Aelong Y, Beall GN. Meat wrapper's asthma: a new syndrome. *JAMA* 1973; 226: 639.

458 Andrasch R, Bardama EJ. Thermoactivated price label fume intolerance: a cause of meat wrappers, asthma. *JAMA* 1976; 235: 937.

459 Zeiss CR, Patterson R, Pruzanski JH *et al.* Trimellitic acid induced airway syndromes: clinical and immunologic studies. *J Allergy Clin Immunol* 1977; 60: 96.

460 Ahmad D, Morgan WKC, Patterson R *et al.* Pulmonary haemorrhage and haemolytic anaemia due to trimellitic anhydride. *Lancet* 1979; ii: 328.

461 Demarest GB, Hudson LD, Altman LC. Impaired alveolar macrophage chemotaxis in patients with acute smoke inhalation. *Am Rev Respir Dis* 1979; 119: 279.

462 Unger KM, Snow RM, Mestas JM, Miller WC. Smoke inhalation in firemen. *Thorax* 1980; 35: 838.

463 Rosenstock L, Demers P, Heyer NJ, Barnhart S. Firefighting is associated with an increased risk for mortality from non-malignant respiratory disease. *Am Rev Respir Dis* 1988; 137 (Suppl): 251.

464 Pandey MR. Domestic smoke pollution and chronic bronchitis in a rural community of the hill region of Nepal. *Thorax* 1984; 39: 337.

465 Sikl H. Uber den Lungenkrebs de Bergleuter in Joachimsthal. *Z Krebsforsch* 1930; 32: 609.

466 Lundin FE, Lloyd JW, Smith EM *et al.* Mortality of uranium miners in relation to radiation exposure, hard rock mining and cigarette smoking: 1950 through September 1967. *Health Phys* 1969; 16: 571.

467 De Villiers AJ, Windish JP. Lung cancer in a fluorspar mining community. 1. Radiation, dust and mortality experience. *Br J Ind Med* 1964; 21: 94.

468 Wada S, Miyanishi M, Nishimoto Y, Kambe S. Mustard gas as a cause of respiratory neoplasia in man. *Lancet* 1969; i: 1161.

469 Oh MG, Holder BB, Gordon HL. Respiratory cancer and occupational exposure to arsenic. *Arch Environ Health* 1974; 29: 250.

470 Doll R, Mathews ID, Morgan LG. Cancers of the lung and nasal sinuses in nickel workers: a reassessment of the period of risk. *Br J Ind Med* 1977; 34: 102.

471 Alderson MR, Ratton NS, Bidstrup L. Health of workmen in the chromate-producing industry in Britain. *Br J Ind Med* 1981; 38: 117.

472 Weiss WA, Ioser RL, Auerbach O. Lung cancer in chloromethyl ether workers. *Am Rev Respir Dis* 1979; 120: 1031.

473 McCallum RI, Wooley V, Petrie A. Lung cancer associated with chloromethyl methyl ether manufacture: an investigation at two factories in the United Kingdom. *Br J Ind Med* 1983; 40: 384.

474 Weil CS, Smyth HF, Nale TW. Quest for a suspected industrial carcinogen. *Arch Ind Hyg* 1952; 5: 535.

475 Lloyd JW. Long-term mortality of steelworkers. V. Respiratory cancer in coke in coke plant workers. *J Occup Med* 1971; 13: 53.

476 Hurley JF, Archibald RM, Collings PL *et al.* The mortality of coke workers in Britain. *Am J Ind Med* 1983; 4: 691.

477 Ask-Upmark E. Bronchial carcinoma in printing workers. *Dis Chest* 1955; 27: 427.

478 Doll R, Peto R. The causes of cancer. *J Natl Cancer Inst* 1981; 66: 1197.

479 Seaton A. Management of the patient with occupational lung disease. *Thorax* 1994; 49: 627.

DRUG-INDUCED LUNG DISEASE, OXYGEN TOXICITY AND RELATED SYNDROMES

ANTHONY SEATON

Until the widespread application of cytotoxic chemotherapy to patients with neoplastic disease, pulmonary drug reactions were relatively uncommon, usually occurring as occasional bronchospasm in response to aspirin or pulmonary infiltrates following nitrofurantoin. The introduction of cytotoxic drugs in particular has increased both the range of mechanisms and the frequency of pulmonary drug reactions, so that in some hospitals they are an important component of the differential diagnosis of pulmonary disease. The range of reactions is wide, from familiar simple pharmacological effects (e.g. opiates causing respiratory depression or β-blocking drugs causing bronchoconstriction), through less well-understood reactions (e.g. aspirin-induced asthma, eosinophilic reactions due to sulphonamides or fibrosis due to busulphan) to the infective complications of immune suppression.

Drug reactions present to the clinician as a syndrome that may be due to a number of different causes, the patient's treatment being one possibility. This chapter therefore is organized under headings denoting the main types of reaction. However, several drugs may produce different syndromes in different subjects and appear in more than one section. Table 55.1 lists the important known adverse effects on the lung of drugs grouped according to their broad therapeutic actions. For convenience, this chapter also includes some discussion of the harmful effects on the lung of oxygen and of three syndromes in which oxygen toxicity is believed to be an important component: radiation pneumonitis, paraquat poisoning and the toxic oil syndrome.

Types of reaction

Bronchoconstriction

Mechanisms

Drugs may cause bronchoconstriction in a number of different ways. The most easily understood is a direct pharmacological effect on airway smooth muscle, as when β-blockers are used for the treatment of angina or as eyedrops for glaucoma [1,2]. Similar effects have been reported following anticholinergic therapy for glaucoma [3]. The best-known pharmacological cause of asthma, aspirin, probably acts through its inhibitory action on cyclooxygenase, diverting arachidonic acid metabolism from the formation of prostaglandins to the production of leukotrienes; a genetic basis for this effect has been described that involves a leukotriene (LT)C$_4$ synthase promoter polymorphism [4,5]. Other non-steroidal anti-inflammatory drugs have a similar mechanism of action, indometacin (indomethacin) being particularly potent in this respect [6]. *In vitro* studies have shown conflicting results when considering the effects of aspirin on the cyclooxygenase of platelets [7,8] but there is some evidence of an inhibitory effect, which can be blocked by sodium salicylate and which correlates with increased respiratory burst and increased killing of *Schistosoma mansoni* [9]. Interestingly, no such effect has been found with basophils or monocytes. This raises the possibility of a role for platelets in the aetiology of aspirin-induced asthma via production of arachidonic acid metabolites.

Direct irritation of airways leading to bronchoconstriction presumably via a vagal reflex may be a mechanism in the case of asthma worsening paradoxically after inhalation of sodium cromoglicate (cromoglycate) [10] or of hypotonic nebulized solutions of ipratropium bromide [11,12]. A direct action on mast cells causing release of bronchoconstrictor substances has been suggested as a cause of wheeze following administration of morphine and codeine [13], while classical type I hypersensitivity mediated by IgE is probably the mechanism of asthma and anaphylaxis following penicillin and other antibiotics [14–16]. It should be noted that a number of drugs contain the yellow dye tartrazine, which may cause exacerbation of asthma; the mechanism of this is not known [17]. Finally, the antituberculosis drug rifampicin has important effects on the enzymatic degradation of other drugs in the liver. Of particular note is its ability to reduce the effi-

Table 55.1 Main groups of drugs having adverse effects on the lung.

Pharmacological action	Effects	Examples
Antibiotic	Bronchoconstriction Alveolitis	Penicillin Nitrofurantoin
Anti-inflammatory	Bronchoconstriction Alveolitis Bronchiolitis Pulmonary oedema	Aspirin Sulfasalazine Penicillamine Aspirin
Cardiac	Cough Bronchoconstriction Alveolitis Pulmonary oedema Pleural fibrosis Lupus syndrome	ACE inhibitors β-blockers Amiodarone Thiazides Practolol Hydralazine
Anticonvulsant	Alveolitis, lupus syndrome	Phenytoin
Psychotropic	Alveolitis Pulmonary oedema	Amitriptyline Phenothiazines
Cytotoxic	Alveolitis	Busulfan, bleomycin
	Opportunist infection	Most combinations
Analgesic	Bronchoconstriction, respiratory depression, pulmonary oedema	Opiates
Contraceptives	Pulmonary embolism	High-oestrogen pill

ACE, angiotensin-converting enzyme.

Table 55.2 Drugs causing bronchoconstriction.

Autonomic system modulators
β-Blockers
   Propranolol
   Timolol
   Oxprenolol
   Metoprolol
Anticholinesterase
   Ecothiopate

Analgesics and anti-inflammatory drugs
Opiates
   Morphine
Non-steroidal anti-inflammatory agents
   Aspirin
   Indometacin
   Naproxen
   Ibuprofen
   Mefenamic acid

Antibiotics
Penicillins
   Penicillin
   Amoxicillin
   Ampicillin
Tetracyclines
Cephalosporins
Rifampicin*

Others
Cromoglicate
Hydrocortisone sodium succinate
Tartrazine
Pancreatic extract
Iron dextran
Iodinated contrast media

*By interfering with antiasthma drugs.

cacy of corticosteroids (and the contraceptive pill) [18]. Asthmatic patients on steroids who develop tuberculosis often require their dose of steroids to be more than doubled when rifampicin therapy is introduced. Similarly, asthmatic patients on regular xanthine therapy may require a higher dose if they need treatment with rifampicin [19].

Drugs causing bronchoconstriction

The more important drugs causing bronchoconstriction are listed in Table 55.2. The most significant of these from a clinical point of view are the β-blockers and the non-steroidal anti-inflammatory drugs. Although most of the newer β-blockers have been promoted as being cardioselective, this can only be regarded as a relative advantage; subjects with asthma or airflow obstruction are quite liable to suffer exacerbations when treated with effective doses [1,20] and it is wiser to avoid the use of these drugs altogether. There is some evidence that atenolol is a less potent bronchoconstrictor than other drugs of this class.

The usual pattern of response to β-blockers is a gradual worsening of the patient's breathlessness and a failure to respond in the normal way to treatment with β-agonist drugs. The subjects usually have pre-existing asthma or airflow obstruction, although it is not uncommon for symptoms to be provoked for the first time by the use of β-blockers. Sometimes the adverse effect of the drug persists for some months after it has been discontinued [20].

Asthmatic and anaphylactic reactions to aspirin were first described not long after its introduction to therapeutics [21,22], and a syndrome comprising asthma, nasal polyps and aspirin sensitivity has been recognized since the 1920s [23,24]. Typically, the patients are middle-aged and non-atopic; the condition may be familial and occurs in 2–4% of all asthmatic subjects [25–28]. When it occurs in children, atopic features are usually absent [26]. The order in which the three features of the syndrome occur is variable, though aspirin sensitivity usually appears after the asthma and the polyps [29]. Urticaria and anaphylaxis may sometimes occur. The syndrome appears to be related to release of products of arachidonic acid metabolism via the 5-lipoxygenase pathway, notably LTE_4 [30].

Asthmatic subjects sensitive to aspirin are often found to respond similarly or to a greater degree to other non-steroidal anti-inflammatory drugs [31] and may show increased sensitivity to histamine provocation [32]. This may cause problems in the management of pain and rheumatic conditions in asthmatic subjects. As far as possible, analgesics with minimal or no anti-inflammatory action, such as paracetamol and dihydrocodeine, and local treatment should be used in these circumstances. Paradoxically, some asthmatic subjects find that their condition improves when they take aspirin or other anti-inflammatory drugs, such as indometacin and mefenamic acid [33–36]. In selected patients these drugs may therefore have a therapeutic role.

Other pharmacological causes of bronchoconstriction are rare. A number of antibiotics have occasionally provoked asthma or anaphylaxis. Several of these, notably ampicillin, cephalosporins, tetracyclines and spiramycin, have been described as causing occupational asthma in workers exposed to them during their manufacture [15,16,37,38]. Contrast media used in radiology that contain iodine and the iron dextran compound Imferon may provoke severe anaphylactic responses. A test dose should be administered before their use, though this may sometimes fail to predict a reaction following the full dose. Hydrocortisone used intravenously or intramuscularly may occasionally have the paradoxical effect of making asthma worse [39]. This appears to occur predominantly in aspirin-sensitive subjects; the mechanism is unknown, but in one case investigated by the author occurred with the sodium succinate but not the phosphate preparation. Cromoglicate may also occasionally cause bronchoconstriction. This has usually been attributed to irritation, although occasionally very severe episodes suggestive of an anaphylactic mechanism may occur; other rare side-effects of cromoglicate, including pulmonary infiltration, urticaria, eosinophilia and nasal congestion, support the idea that true allergies may occur [40,41].

Cough

Any of the drugs able to provoke asthma or bronchoconstriction may cause the symptom of cough. However, one group of drugs is notable for causing cough rarely if ever accompanied by bronchoconstriction, the angiotensin-converting enzyme (ACE) inhibitors [42,43]. These drugs are widely and successfully used in the management of hypertension and cardiac failure. The cough usually starts after several months of treatment and is of a dry irritant nature. It ceases within a few days of stopping the drug, and this is therefore an appropriate diagnostic test. The symptom, which is probably related to bradykinin release, occurs in 5–20% of patients treated with the drugs and

there is little benefit to be expected from changing to another ACE inhibitor. There is some evidence that administration of cromoglicate reduces the severity and frequency of cough in such patients, experimentally attenuating the response to inhaled capsaicin [44]. However, the patients can usually be transferred successfully to an angiotensin II antagonist, which does not have the same side-effect.

Bronchiolitis obliterans

A syndrome of progressive breathlessness associated with increasing airflow obstruction has been described in patients with rheumatoid arthritis and other collagen diseases [45,46]. A proportion, though not all, of these subjects has been treated with D-penicillamine [46,47] and it now seems possible that this drug may occasionally provoke the disease; however, it is a rare condition, in one study having occurred in only 2 of about 250 subjects with reactions to penicillamine [48]. A similar syndrome has also been described in a patient with ulcerative colitis treated with sulfasalazine (sulphasalazine) and in a patient who took an overdose of L-tryptophan [49,50]. The clinical features are difficult to distinguish from those of airflow obstruction of other causes. The breathlessness is progressive, although the rate varies from a rapid progression over weeks to a slow course over years. The airflow obstruction is irreversible and may be associated with the auscultatory signs of late inspiratory repetitive crackles and a mid-inspiratory squeak. The radiograph may show diminished peripheral markings in generalized disease or consolidation in more local disease, but is often normal.

Lung function tests show reduced forced expiratory volume in 1 s (FEV_1) and forced vital capacity (FVC) (the former to a greater extent), raised residual volume and normal total lung capacity. Diffusing capacity is typically somewhat reduced. Pathologically there is widespread obliteration by fibrous tissue of small bronchi and bronchioles, a pattern identical to that occurring occasionally after toxic gas inhalation [51] or after adenovirus infection in children [52]. Since the condition may occur in rheumatoid disease untreated by penicillamine, it may be difficult to decide on the cause. It is wiser to assume that penicillamine is responsible if this drug is being administered and to stop it, in the hope that the condition stops progressing; reversal of the airflow obstruction in these circumstances or following treatment with corticosteroids is not common but has been reported [53].

Alveolitis

Clinical features

Many drugs have been described as causing diffuse alveolitis and the spectrum of the ensuing clinical syndrome is a broad one. The patient usually presents with slowly increasing breathlessness and, sometimes, cough. Repetitive crackles may be heard in the lung and the radiograph usually shows diffuse patchy infiltration (Fig. 55.1). A raised eosinophil count may be found in the blood, and occasionally the clinical and serological features of systemic lupus erythematosus (SLE) may be present. Lung function testing reveals a reduction in diffusing capacity, sometimes associated with diminished lung volumes. In some cases this restrictive type of abnormality is associated with an obstructive pattern as well.

These features are non-specific and may give rise to diagnostic difficulty, especially if the patient is being treated for a condition that may itself cause pulmonary infiltration. It is therefore wise to consider the possibility of drug reaction in all patients presenting with diffuse lung infiltrates. In many instances, stopping the offending drug leads to an improvement in the clinical features. Further investigation is discussed in the section on diagnosis and management.

Mechanisms

It would be misleading to imply that the mechanisms of alveolitis due to drugs were clearly understood. Different drugs may cause very different reactions, and indeed the same drug may provoke different responses in different individuals. Some reactions are clearly related to the known pharmacological effects of the drug, i.e. they are direct toxic effects, while others are clearly the result of an idiosyncratic reaction. For the purposes of this section, the different reactions leading to alveolitis are divided into toxic, allergic and those related to drug-induced SLE.

Direct toxic effects of drugs may be mediated in several different ways. Some drugs, including bleomycin, cyclophosphamide and nitrofurantoin, have been shown to be able to cause the generation of toxic oxygen species or acrolein [54–56], with consequent lung damage. Others may act on the system whereby the lung matrix repairs itself, interfering with or increasing the formation of collagen. Again, bleomycin is known to cause proliferation of fibroblasts with increased formation of collagen [57], while penicillamine may impair collagen formation [58]; indeed this is partly responsible for its therapeutic efficacy.

Allergic reactions are the most frequently recognized mechanisms of drug-induced alveolitis. Their sporadic unpredictable occurrence, the common association with eosinophilia and, usually, lack of a relationship to dose are evidence in support of this hypothesis. Experimental and clinical studies have shown, for example, evidence of enhanced cell-mediated immunity or a T-lymphocyte alveolitis provoked by gold salts [59,60], nitrofurantoin [61], amiodarone [62] and methotrexate [63]. It is assumed that these drugs act as haptens, binding to plasma proteins in order to induce allergic reactions. However, the search for such antibodies has been singularly unsuccessful, leading to the hypothesis that the hapten may be a metabolic product rather than the drug itself [64]. It may be that differences between individuals in the ways in

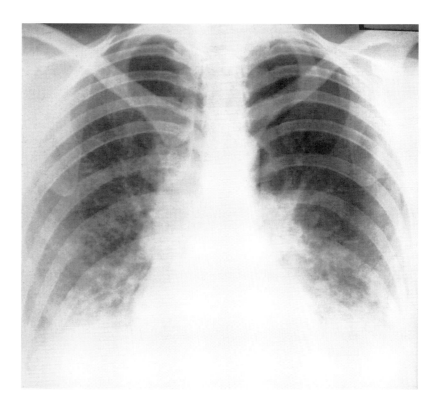

Fig. 55.1 Bilateral, predominantly lower zone, infiltrates in a patient with an acute reaction to sulphonamides.

Table 55.3 Drugs causing systemic lupus erythematosus.

Hypotensives: hydralazine, methyldopa, reserpine
Antituberculous drugs: isoniazid, para-aminosalicylic acid
Cardiac drugs: procainamide, thiazides, digoxin
Antibiotics: sulphonamides, tetracycline, penicillin
Anticonvulsants: phenytoin, primidone
Others: gold, carbamazepine, thiouracil, oral contraceptives

Table 55.4 Drugs causing alveolitis.

Antibiotics
Nitrofurantoin
Sulphonamides
Penicillins
Para-aminosalicylic acid

Anti-inflammatory
Sulfasalazine
Penicillamine
Gold

Cardiac
Antiarrhythmics
  Amiodarone
  Tocainide
  Procainamide
  Quinidine
Hypotensives
  Hydralazine
  Methyldopa
  Hexamethonium

Anticonvulsants
Phenytoin
Carbamazepine

Psychotropic
Amitriptyline
Imipramine

Cytotoxic
Antibiotics
  Bleomycin
  Mitomycin
Alkylating agents
  Busulfan
  Chlorambucil
Folic acid antagonists
  Cyclophosphamide
  Methotrexate
Nitrosourea
  Carmustine

Others
Chlorpropamide
Cromoglicate
Pituitary snuff
Cocaine

which drugs are metabolized in the liver could thus be a partial explanation for the sporadic nature of drug reactions.

Drug-induced SLE is a rare event. Originally described in patients treated with hydralazine, it has now been recorded following treatment with many other drugs [65,66], of which the most frequently used are shown in Table 55.3. Most cases are caused by hydralazine, procainamide, isoniazid and phenytoin. The condition mimics the idiopathic disease, with joint symptoms, fever, positive antinuclear factor (but less commonly anti-DNA antibodies), malaise, together with pleuropericardial disease and pulmonary infiltrates. Renal disease and malar erythema occur uncommonly and central nervous involvement and discoid lesions are very rare. The condition resolves when the drug is stopped. The drugs presumably act on the DNA of cell nuclei, and the sporadic nature of the condition suggests that allergic factors, perhaps combined with genetically determined slow metabolism, may be responsible. However the mechanisms are unknown.

Drugs causing alveolitis

Table 55.4 lists some of the more important drugs known to have caused alveolitic reactions. Of the antibiotics, the most frequent offender is nitrofurantoin, used primarily for long-term urinary antisepsis [67–70]. Two syndromes have been described. The more common, first reported in 1962, is an acute illness with cough, breathlessness and fever ensuing several weeks after the drug has been started. Crackles may be heard at the lung bases on inspiration, the radiograph usually shows bilateral diffuse micronodular or patchy infiltrates (sometimes with pleural effusion) and the diffusing capacity ($D_{L}CO$) is reduced. There is often blood eosinophilia and lung biopsy may show infiltration with inflammatory cells and eosinophils; vasculitis may also be present. The condition usually resolves rapidly when the drug is discontinued but recurs if it is restarted. Persistence with the drug may lead to fatal pulmonary fibrosis. The more chronic syndrome presents rather insidiously with cough and dyspnoea, usually after several years of treatment. The chest film shows basal infiltrates, $D_{L}CO$ is reduced, eosinophilia is inconstant and the course is progressive if the drug is not stopped. Other antibiotics seem to

cause pulmonary allergic reactions much less frequently, perhaps partly because they are rarely administered for such prolonged courses. Sulphonamides (Fig. 55.2), penicillin, ampicillin and para-aminosalicylic acid have occasionally been associated with acute eosinophilic pneumonitis [71–76].

Of the anticonvulsant drugs, phenytoin and carbamazepine have caused pulmonary reactions. The former drug causes a number of non-pulmonary toxic effects, including gum hyperplasia, hirsutism, acne and cerebellar ataxia; rarely it has been described as causing an allergic

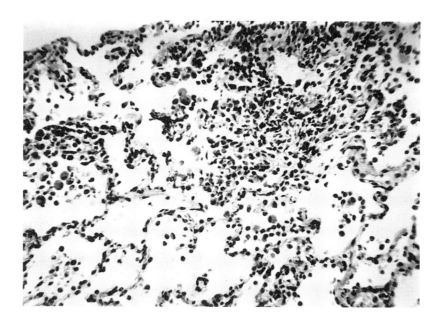

Fig. 55.2 Drill lung biopsy of patient with reaction to sulphonamides showing infiltration of alveoli with predominantly eosinophil inflammatory cells.

alveolitic reaction, with fever, cough, dyspnoea and eosinophilia [77,78]. The chest film shows diffuse interstitial shadowing sometimes with marked hilar lymphadenopathy, and occasionally generalized lymph node enlargement may cause a pseudolymphomatous syndrome [79]. Lung biopsies have shown alveolar wall and small vessel infiltration with inflammatory cells [77]. The condition resolves when the drug is stopped. A similar syndrome has been described very infrequently following the use of carbamazepine [80,81].

Several drugs used in cardiac disease may cause alveolitis. Of those used to treat dysrhythmias, amiodarone seems most frequently to have this effect [82–84]. Its action is almost certainly a direct toxic one. Radiological signs of alveolitis tend to be related to the dose, occurring in some 13% of patients on high doses and 5% of those on doses of 400 mg daily, and are often associated with other toxic manifestations such as corneal deposits [85,86]. A somewhat higher proportion of subjects develop abnormalities of lung function, and the likelihood of this is increased if a pre-existing abnormality was present. Indeed, side-effects are so frequent that amiodarone is generally only used for dysrhythmias resistant to other drugs. The clinical findings are fever, cough, dyspnoea and weight loss, usually after a few months of treatment, with interstitial shadowing on the radiograph. Subjects with pre-existing radiological abnormality seem to be at greater risk [85]. The histological features also suggest a toxic rather than allergic mechanism, with hyperplasia of type II pneumocytes and accumulation of foamy macrophages within the alveolar spaces [87,88]. The drug has a very prolonged action and its withdrawal is usually followed by slow resolution of the pulmonary abnormalities, although persistent interstitial fibrosis may remain [89,90]. Use of amiodarone should take account of this dangerous

side-effect; the dose should be the minimum required to control the dysrhythmia and the pulmonary effects should be monitored by regular measurement of the diffusing capacity.

Tocainide, a drug derived from lidocaine (lignocaine) and also used for suppression of ventricular dysrhythmias, has been reported to cause alveolitis in occasional patients [91,92]. Procainamide and quinidine may cause a syndrome resembling SLE, as may the hypotensive drugs methyldopa, hydralazine and hexamethonium [65,66,93,94]. In this syndrome, the clinical manifestations are pleurisy, sometimes associated with effusion, interstitial pneumonitis with fever, cough and dyspnoea, and positive antinuclear antibodies. The condition remits if the drug is stopped and usually also responds to corticosteroid treatment.

The most frequent of the anti-inflammatory drugs to be associated with alveolitis is sulfasalazine [95–98]. This is a drug that is broken down after ingestion to sulphapyridine and 5-aminosalicylic acid, and is used in the management of ulcerative colitis. It may cause the typical syndrome of fever, eosinophilia and pulmonary infiltration. Some patients may show evidence of airflow obstruction, probably due to involvement of the small airways. Challenge testing in one case has shown the reaction to be due to hypersensitivity to the sulphapyridine moiety [96]. As well as being associated with bronchiolitis obliterans, penicillamine may occasionally cause a diffuse type of alveolitis [99,100] or a rapidly progressive and often fatal alveolar and renal haemorrhage, mimicking Goodpasture's syndrome [101]. The alveolitis may be expected to improve on stopping the drug, although the pulmonary–renal syndrome has been reported to respond to plasmapheresis and immunosuppression [102]. Gold therapy has been occasionally associated with pneumonitis, rashes and eosinophilia in patients with rheumatoid disease [59,103–105]. There is some evidence to suggest that this is due to a cell-mediated immune response. It usually starts 1–3 months after initiation of treatment and has been shown to resolve on treatment with corticosteroids together with cessation of the gold therapy [104]. Gold may also provoke SLE.

The drugs most frequently associated with alveolitis are those used in the cytotoxic therapy of patients with neoplasms. In most cases it seems that they have a direct toxic effect on the lung cells, though occasionally allergic reactions may occur. Since they are often used in combination, it may not be possible to know which drug is responsible. Moreover, in some instances they may act with radiotherapy in a synergistic or additive manner to increase the likelihood of lung damage. In contrast to the non-cytotoxic drugs discussed above, the usual pulmonary injury with cytotoxic therapy is a progressive pulmonary fibrosis with relatively little of an inflammatory component and a tendency to cause irreversible lung damage.

Bleomycin and mitomycin are cytotoxic antibiotics, both of which cause progressive pulmonary fibrosis in 5–10% of patients (Fig. 55.3). Their effects generally seem to be related to age and dose and to be potentiated by radiotherapy. Bleomycin is used in the treatment of squamous carcinomas, lymphomas and testicular cancer. Lung toxicity presents as progressive breathlessness, cough and usually diffuse nodular radiographic infiltrates [106,107]. In a personally studied group of patients, half of those receiving more than $100 \, \text{mg/m}^2$ showed a greater than 15% fall in D_{LCO}, although some patients receiving less than $100 \, \text{mg/m}^2$ showed an appreciable fall while others receiving more than $400 \, \text{mg/m}^2$ showed none. Apart from dose, other risk factors appear to be concomitant radiation therapy or administration of high concentrations of oxygen [108]. The histological changes are of interstitial fibrosis with metaplasia of type II pneumocytes and scanty inflammatory cells [109,110]. Bleomycin toxicity usually arrests and may regress if the drug is stopped, and there is some evidence that steroid therapy may be helpful [111,112]. Occasionally, bleomycin causes a more obviously allergic type of reaction, with fever and eosinophilia [113]. This seems more likely to be responsive to steroids. Mitomycin, which is used in treating upper alimentary tract and breast cancers, has also been described as causing pulmonary fibrosis [114,115]. The features are usually indistinguishable from those caused by bleomycin, though pleural effusions have occurred [114].

Several cytotoxic drugs that act by alkylation of DNA have been shown to cause alveolitis and pulmonary fibrosis. Busulfan (busulphan) was the first cytotoxic drug reported to have this effect [116,117]. It is used in the treatment of chronic myeloid leukaemia. The symptoms of cough, breathlessness and sometimes fever may present quite rapidly and the chest film shows bilateral infiltration [118]. Lung function shows a restrictive pattern with a low D_{LCO}. About 5% of patients may develop this side-effect, usually after a prolonged course of treatment, often of several years. Many patients who develop lung fibrosis die, although cessation of therapy and treatment with steroids may allow recovery if the condition is detected sufficiently early [118]. The pathological changes are nonspecific, with damage to type I cells, proliferation and metaplasia of type II cells and interstitial fibrosis [117,119,120]. Very similar clinical features have been described, but less frequently, following treatment with the other alkylating drugs chlorambucil [121,122], cyclophosphamide [123,124] and melphalan [125,126]. Carmustine, a nitrosourea used mainly in the manage-

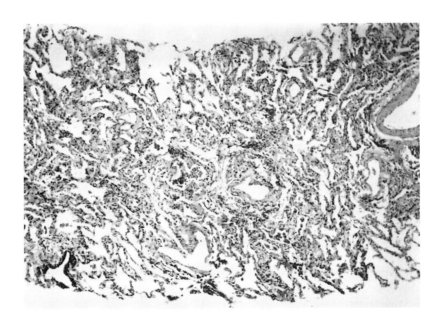

Fig. 55.3 Drill lung biopsy of patient on bleomycin therapy for end-stage lymphosarcoma showing diffuse alveolar wall fibrosis.

ment of brain tumours and lymphomas, is a more frequent cause of alveolitis and fibrosis, these effects occurring in 1–20% of patients [127,128]. The risk is related to the total dose received although, as with all these cytotoxic drugs, idiosyncratic early or acute reactions may occur [129]. In one instance, early-onset pneumonitis seems to have occurred at the site of previous lung radiotherapy, suggesting prior sensitization [130].

Pulmonary reactions leading to fibrosis have been described in association with many other cytotoxic drugs, usually when given in combination [131]. The only one of these where such reactions seem to have occurred frequently is methotrexate, a folic acid antagonist used for prolonged maintenance treatment in leukaemia and lymphomas as well as for some solid tumours. It is now used increasingly in the management of severe rheumatoid arthritis, primary biliary cirrhosis and psoriasis. The pulmonary syndrome has allergic characteristics, occurring sporadically with no obvious relation to dose. Fever, eosinophilia and pleuritis may occur in addition to the alveolitis, which usually has a granulomatous histology. Resolution usually follows cessation of therapy and institution of corticosteroid treatment [63,132–137].

Many other drugs have been described as occasional causes of a hypersensitivity type of alveolitis. Of the more commonly used, chlorpropamide, sodium cromoglicate (possibly), imipramine and amitriptyline have all caused pulmonary shadowing associated with eosinophilia [138–140]. Pituitary snuff, when produced from animal pituitaries, has been responsible for allergic alveolitis [141] and a similar syndrome has been described following recreational abuse of cocaine [142]. Aspiration of mineral oil taken as an aperient is a well-known, though uncommon, cause of patchy pulmonary fibrosis or of areas of irregular consolidation. It occurs usually in the elderly, often in association with oesophageal reflux or hiatus hernia [143]. Finally, the use of bacille Calmette–Guérin (BCG) as a tumour-suppressant drug, most notably in the treatment of bladder cancer by intravesical instillation, has resulted in disseminated disease involving lungs and other organs in a granulomatous reaction responsive to antituberculous therapy [144].

Pulmonary oedema

Acute pulmonary oedema (discussed in detail in Chapter 27) may be occasionally caused by drugs, sometimes as an idiosyncratic reaction though usually in response to an excessive dose. The mechanisms are not clear but may be a direct effect on pulmonary alveolar structures or an indirect effect mediated through the central nervous system. What evidence there is suggests that the oedema is of the high-protein increased-permeability type [145,146].

The most frequent causes of drug-induced pulmonary oedema are overdoses of aspirin and opiates. Aspirin acts to reduce prostaglandin production by inhibition of the cyclooxygenase pathway. This may have a direct effect by increasing pulmonary endothelial permeability or an indirect effect by increasing production of leukotrienes. Whatever the mechanism, patients admitted to hospital with high salicylate levels after an overdose (>40 mg/dL) are at risk of developing acute pulmonary oedema [147–149]. Fortunately the condition responds to routine management with forced alkaline diuresis, oxygen and, if necessary, assisted ventilation. Pulmonary oedema is also a frequent feature of patients admitted with an overdose of heroin or other opiates [150,151]. Again, the mechanisms are not clear and both direct and central nervous-mediated actions have been suggested. Treatment depends on the use of naloxone and assisted ventilation; recovery is to be expected in hospitalized patients.

The other drugs associated with pulmonary oedema are much less frequent causes. Sympathomimetic drugs used in high dosage for the prevention of premature labour occasionally cause the syndrome [152,153], as does hydrochlorothiazide [154,155]. The rarity of these episodes suggests an allergic mechanism. Antipsychotic drugs such as the phenothiazines and butyrophenones sometimes cause hyperpyrexia, muscle rigidity and abnormalities of the autonomic and central nervous system, the so-called neuroleptic malignant syndrome [156]; this may be associated with cardiovascular collapse and pulmonary oedema.

Pulmonary vascular disease

Oestrogen-containing oral contraceptive drugs have been shown to increase the risk of pulmonary thromboembolism in women by about six to nine times [157,158], though not the risk of subsequent recurrence [159]. They may also cause an increased risk of thrombotic stroke and myocardial infarction [160]. The effects on the clotting mechanism are probably due to the oestrogen content of the pill and the risk of thromboembolism related to its dose; there is evidence of increased activity of procoagulant factors and reduction of antithrombins [161,162]. For this reason, preparations with the lowest oestrogen content consistent with efficacy are generally prescribed. It should be remembered that the increased risk of thrombosis also applies to the use of oestrogens for other purposes, such as in the treatment of prostatic carcinoma and for the suppression of lactation. There is some evidence that some cases of pulmonary hypertension may be caused by oestrogen-containing contraceptives [163]. However, the increased frequency with which this condition was recognized in central Europe in the 1950s and 1960s was probably related to the use of an appetite-suppressant drug, aminorex [164,165]. Although the drug was not shown to cause pulmonary hypertension in animals, the epidemiological evidence in humans was strong and the drug was withdrawn. So far no other drugs have been shown to have similar effects.

Pleural and mediastinal fibrosis

Fibrosis of the pleura and underlying lung is an occasional and dose-related complication of the therapy of migraine with methysergide [166,167]. The patient usually presents after several years of treatment with shortness of breath and chest pain. The erythrocyte sedimentation rate is raised and there may be loss of weight. Chest radiography shows bilateral pleural thickening, sometimes with small effusions, and biopsy shows vascularized mature collagen. The mechanism is not known, although methysergide blocks serotonin receptors. This, together with its ability to cause fibrosis of pleura, peritoneum, and cardiac valves [168], suggests an analogy with the carcinoid syndrome in which there is overproduction of serotonin and in which cardiac valve fibrosis may also occur. Interestingly, all the other drugs that have been reported to cause pleural fibrosis are blockers of neurotransmission. Practolol blocks β-adrenergic receptors and may cause pleural, mediastinal and peritoneal fibrosis, as well as involving skin, eye and joints [169,170]. Pleuropulmonary fibrosis may present alone, in a manner identical to that following methysergide. Ergotamine blocks dopamine receptors, while bromocriptine blocks dopamine D_1 receptors and stimulates D_2 receptors. Both these drugs have been shown to cause an identical syndrome of pleural fibrosis [171,172]. Hypothetically, this observation may be explained by a balance between collagen breakdown and synthesis that is controlled by messages between involved cells, whereby receptors for these messages are blocked by the drugs [173]. In the case of carcinoid syndrome, which has also been described as a cause of pleural fibrosis [174], excess production of a neurotransmitter might cause all receptors to be blocked.

With all these drugs the course of pleural fibrosis is progressive, producing a restrictive pattern of lung function. However, the condition remits when the drug is stopped and in most instances there is reduction in symptoms and some improvement in lung function, though residual fibrosis remains on the chest film (see Figs 43.12 & 43.13).

Other pulmonary reactions to drugs

It should not be forgotten that drugs may cause lung disease in an indirect manner. Not infrequently hypoventilation and respiratory failure may be provoked by overdose or injudicious therapeutic use of narcotic or sedative drugs, particularly in the elderly or in those with previous airflow obstruction. On one occasion in the author's experience, the cause of a mysterious case of hypercapnic respiratory failure was discovered when the patient was found to have been taking large doses of a traditional Edinburgh treatment for peripheral vascular disease, prescribed by a surgeon, containing narcotic doses of barbiturates and masquerading under the name of Chief's Powder! Respiratory failure is discussed further in Chapter 24. Drugs acting on the immune system, used in the management of cancer, transplantation and vasculitic diseases, may set the scene for opportunistic pulmonary infections; these conditions are described in Chapter 52.

Diagnosis and management

The key to diagnosis of drug-induced pulmonary disease is awareness of the possibility. Most lung diseases have an external or environmental cause and it is important to exclude such possibilities in the case of alveolitis or asthma of obscure aetiology. A note should be made of all drugs taken by every patient and any drugs with unfamiliar names should be checked in reference books.

If a drug reaction seems a possibility, appropriate baseline investigations should be carried out and the drug stopped. These investigations normally include chest radiography and lung function testing, although erythrocyte sedimentation rate, temperature records and differential white cell counts may often be helpful. If several drugs are under suspicion, it is best to stop all those regarded as not essential to the patient's well-being. In the case of single drugs, cessation usually results in clinical improvement; normally this provides sufficient proof for the drug to be avoided subsequently, but if necessary when allergy is suspected a challenge test can be carried out after an interval during which the drug is not taken. This should not be performed unnecessarily as severe reactions may sometimes occur. Appropriate indications are when the drug is one of a multiple regimen and it is not clear which is responsible, or when the drug is itself a combination of two medicaments, for example Salazopyrin or Rifinah. Challenge testing should be carried out under hospital supervision and initially should use a fraction (perhaps a hundredth) of the therapeutic dose; the results should be monitored by lung function testing. It is only appropriate in suspected allergic reactions and is unlikely to be of value in diagnosing reactions due to direct toxic effects.

Lung biopsy, gallium scanning and bronchoalveolar lavage have only a small part to play in the diagnosis of these reactions, as they only show non-specific effects of a wide range of pulmonary reactions. They may of course have an important role in the differential diagnosis, by excluding other possible pathological processes. In general they are appropriately employed after drug reactions have been excluded.

Management of pulmonary drug reactions consists in stopping the offending drug and, if necessary, substituting a less harmful one. Occasionally, corticosteroid therapy may be used though its value can only be judged by anecdotal evidence in most cases. In the management of malignant disease, pulmonary side-effects are relatively frequent occurrences and cessation of the drug may result in relapse. They are therefore an important and sometimes fatal complication of therapy. Hyposensitization, or induction of tolerance, may be tried if the drug is considered essential, all alternatives are unsatisfactory and the reaction is thought to be allergic or idiosyncratic. These circumstances must be rare with respect to drug-induced lung disease, although many older chest physicians will be familiar with the techniques for management of allergic rashes to para-aminosalicylic acid and isoniazid in treating tuberculosis. The main interest in this subject currently centres on the induction of tolerance to aspirin and non-steroidal anti-inflammatory drugs [175]. There is evidence that this may be of benefit to some patients, particularly with respect to alleviation of rhinitis. However, it should be embarked upon with great care, as serious reactions can occur [176]. There is some hope that in the future leukotriene antagonists may also have a role to play in aspirin sensitivity [177].

Lipoid pneumonitis

Inhalation of oil is an occasional cause of lung disease. The reaction depends on the type of oil. Mineral oil remains in the lung, engulfed by macrophages, and may give rise to fibrosis; animal fats are hydrolysed by lung lipases and the resulting fatty acids cause acute inflammatory pneumonitis, while vegetable oils are relatively inert [178]. Animal and vegetable oils may enter the lungs by aspiration in subjects with hiatus hernia, oesophageal reflux or neuromuscular disease, and the former are an important cause of unresolved pneumonia in the elderly [179]. Mineral oil may be inhaled occasionally by shipwrecked mariners, but the important causes are the use of oily nasal drops or of liquid paraffin as an aperient [180–182]. The paraffin is usually taken daily over years and aspiration of small amounts regularly may cause a patchy diffuse granulomatosis leading to fibrosis [183]. A similar syndrome has been described in Guyana in people of Indian origin who smoked cigarettes made of tobacco to which mineral oils had been added as flavouring [184]. This blackfat tobacco-smokers' lung was an important cause of chronic pulmonary fibrosis, leading to much disablement and death in that country. Diffuse fibrosis at least partly due to inhaled paraffin has also been described in a fire-eating punk-rock drummer [185].

Oxygen toxicity and related syndromes

Mechanisms

It may seem paradoxical that oxygen, upon which animal

life depends, has the potential to harm the lung. However, oxygen became an important component of the earth's atmosphere only after the evolution of plant life and photosynthesis, and all animals may therefore be regarded as organisms that have not only turned this gas to good effect but which have also developed mechanisms for overcoming its toxic effects. These effects depend upon the relative ease with which oxygen may be reduced by cells to produce superoxide anion (O_2^-) and hydrogen peroxide (H_2O_2). These radicals are toxic to cell membranes but may also react together to form hydroxyl radical (.OH) and singlet oxygen ($^1O_2$), which are highly toxic and react with cellular chemicals leading to peroxidation of lipids, depolymerization of mucopolysaccharides, rupture of protein sulphydryl bonds and damage to nucleic acids. These reactions are utilized by phagocytic cells in the destruction of invading organisms; however, when phagocytic or other metabolizing cells are damaged they may be responsible for the destruction of adjacent cells in the tissue under attack.

Clearly, the alveolar tissues are in a vulnerable position with respect to toxic damage by oxygen, since they have to provide adequate concentrations to other tissues while resisting potential harm themselves. In common with other cells, those of the lung have developed mechanisms for defending themselves against such damage; superoxide dismutase eliminates superoxide radical, catalase and peroxidases deal with hydrogen peroxide (the green colour of infected sputum is due to the presence of myeloperoxidase from leucocytes) and substances such as glutathione, uric acid, vitamin C and vitamin E mop up free radicals. Thus the normal lung is protected by a balance between production and destruction of free radicals, a balance that may be disturbed by a number of different factors.

The inhalation of high concentrations of oxygen makes more oxygen available for conversion to free radicals and this may reach the stage of overwhelming the antioxidant defences [186,187]. However, there is evidence that gradual increase of oxygen concentration may prevent this by induction of superoxide dismutase and catalase, although experimentally there appears to a be a limit to the amount by which the catalase gene can be upregulated [188]. Overwhelming infection or recruitment of inflammatory cells to the lungs may similarly result in tissue damage by release of free radicals. Radiation therapy is particularly toxic to the lungs because of its ability to produce free radicals from cells in its path. Similarly, the herbicide paraquat acts by increasing production of superoxide radical in the lung.

Ventilator lung

Some patients requiring prolonged assisted ventilation develop a syndrome of decreasing compliance, increasing hypoxaemia and diffuse radiological shadowing. They require increasing inspired concentrations of oxygen but with decreasing effect on Pao_2. At autopsy, their lungs may present a variety of pathological appearances, including oedema, hyaline membranes, septal thickening by oedema and proliferating fibroblasts, and some interstitial fibrosis [189] (Fig. 55.4). Although in such situations it is often difficult to distinguish between the various possible causes, as there is almost always some other underlying lung disease, it is clear that hyperoxia is an important factor in the production of this damage. The condition may be reproduced in animals, where it has been shown that the sequence of pathological change consists of, firstly, an acute phase with generalized interstitial oedema, alveolar haemorrhage, capillary endothelial necrosis and damage to type I pneumocytes and, secondly, a proliferative phase in which the oedema is reabsorbed and there is hyperplasia of interstitial fibroblasts and type II pneumocytes [187]. Resolution may occur, although progressive fibrosis of the interstitial tissues is a more usual sequel in animals that survive.

Studies in humans have shown that 100% oxygen may be tolerated for up to 24h with no more than some bronchial irritation and substernal discomfort [190,191]. However, lavage studies have shown that by 18h there is early evidence of leakiness of alveoli and of liability of macrophages to release mediators of fibrogenesis [192], while physiological studies have shown falls in compliance, diffusing capacity and tracheal mucus flow rate [193–195]. It seems likely therefore that subtle changes may occur relatively early in the course of hyperoxia. However, the clinical syndrome does not usually present until after several days of exposure to high oxygen con-

centrations, the time varying inversely with the concentration. Inspired oxygen concentrations of less than 50% seem to be tolerated indefinitely [196].

The management of oxygen toxicity presents the physician with a therapeutic dilemma. Patients at risk of this problem inevitably have serious lung disease and require tissue oxygenation. Adequate inspired concentrations of oxygen must therefore be delivered to prevent hypoxic damage to other tissues. The aim should therefore be to deliver a sufficient concentration to keep the patient's blood adequately saturated but without exceeding a Pao_2 of about 13kPa (100mmHg). If this requires inspired concentrations above 50%, then this concentration has to be given, in the knowledge that far from all such patients suffer lung damage as a result and the effects of hypoxaemia are more acutely threatening. The use of appropriate methods of ventilation, such as positive end-expiratory pressure, may allow the oxygen concentration to be kept as low as possible (see Chapter 58).

Increased understanding of the mechanisms of oxygen toxicity has given rise to hope that some pharmacological therapy may eventually be helpful in the prevention of the condition [187]. Intramuscular vitamin E has been used with some success in premature infants and superoxide dismutase has been tried in paraquat poisoning [197–199]. Small doses of endotoxin have been shown to protect rats from hyperoxia, probably by increasing production of superoxide dismutase and catalase [200].

Paraquat poisoning

The herbicide paraquat kills plants by virtue of its ability to be reduced and oxidized very readily. It is thus able to

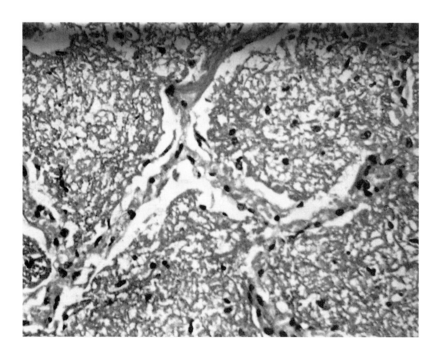

Fig. 55.4 Lung of patient who died after prolonged intensive care and ventilation for pneumonia of undetermined aetiology showing intra-alveolar fibrosis and hyaline membranes.

compete with NADP for electrons, becoming reduced to a stable free radical. In humans, it is able to react with oxygen within cells to catalyse the production of superoxide radical and hydrogen peroxide.

Most cases of paraquat poisoning occur as a result of accidental ingestion of the 20% agricultural preparation called Gramoxone, usually in the belief that it is lemonade [201,202]. It has also been taken with suicidal intent and deaths have been described following subcutaneous injection and after transcutaneous absorption in men employed to spray the poison [203]. Ingestion of the 20% solution is attended by a mortality of about 60%, the risk being related to the dose taken [204]. Deaths have also followed ingestion of the 2.5% paraquat in the Weedol granules commonly used by gardeners.

Clinical features

The patient often suffers oral and oesophageal ulceration after ingestion and may complain of abdominal pains, vomiting and diarrhoea. Toxic effects on the kidneys and liver may lead to acute renal failure and jaundice, although these conditions are self-limiting and usually resolve if the patient can be helped over them without pulmonary problems. Respiratory symptoms, with increasing breathlessness and cyanosis, commence a few days after ingestion and almost always progress remorselessly [201,205]. The chest radiograph shows diffuse opacification and there is a progressive fall in oxygen saturation. The patient usually dies of irreversible respiratory failure within 2–3 weeks of ingesting the paraquat, although occasional patients who have taken lower doses may survive despite having shown evidence of lung disease [206]. There is some evidence from studies of workers engaged in spraying paraquat, and who have absorbed it in relatively small doses through the skin, that subacute poisoning can occur which may lead to chronic interstitial fibrosis, thromboses and proliferative changes in small pulmonary arteries [203]. Similar lesions have been produced in rats by application of paraquat to the skin [203].

Pathology

The pathological appearances in humans are confused by the presence of changes that could be related to the prolonged high F_{IO_2} that has usually been given as treatment. However, identical changes occur in rats given paraquat and kept in normoxic conditions. In animal studies, the first sign of damage is oedema and ballooning of the type I and II pneumocytes [207,208]. Within a few days these cells have been destroyed, leaving the capillary endothelial cells intact. Cells that are progenitors of fibroblasts then fill the alveolar spaces, eventually developing into mature cells. The alveoli thus become organized into a mass of cellular fibrous tissue surrounded by intact capillaries. In humans, two pathological appearances have been noted [204]. In patients dying acutely after paraquat ingestion, alveolar and interstitial oedema with hyaline membranes is prominent. In those dying later, either intra-alveolar fibrosis or diffuse irregular fibrosis with dilatation of bronchioles causing a honeycomb appearance is seen. It is likely that these appearances represent progression rather than different reactions, analogous to the appearances found in animals.

Management

The essential point in management is to act early. Any unabsorbed paraquat should be removed from the gastrointestinal tract by administration of fuller's earth and by gastric or bowel lavage followed by forced diuresis, haemodialysis or charcoal haemoperfusion. Management may be guided by the plasma concentration of paraquat measured by rapid colorimetric or radioimmunoassay methods. It has been shown that if the concentration does not exceed 2.0, 0.6, 0.3, 0.16 and 0.1 mg/L at 4, 6, 10, 16 and 24 h after ingestion, survival is likely [209].

If the patient presents with evidence of jaundice, renal failure or respiratory symptoms, it is almost certainly too late for effective therapy. Unfortunately, oxygen is needed by the tissues but enhances the toxic effects of paraquat. Dialysis is unhelpful at this stage since the sequence of pulmonary damage has already begun. Corticosteroids and cyclophosphamide have their advocates [210] but are probably ineffective [211]. A logical approach would be the early use of iron chelators or superoxide dismutase to antagonize toxic oxygen radicals and D-propranolol to block paraquat receptor sites [198,212]; there is one case report of survival following vigorous treatment with desferrioxamine and acetylcysteine after bowel decontamination and haemodialysis [199]. However, almost all such patients end up on a ventilator and their chances of survival are negligible. Lung transplantation has been tried but except in one case the transplanted lung itself has succumbed to the effects of residual circulating paraquat [213,214]. The very few survivors of early pulmonary damage following paraquat ingestion or intravenous injection all probably had relatively small doses, though the fact that survival has occurred in such circumstances justifies vigorous treatment [215,216]. At present, the hopeless outlook of patients with progressive lung disease requires compassionate treatment with opiates.

Radiation pneumonitis

Irradiation of tissues causes cell death, the most actively dividing cells being those affected most readily. The effect of radiation bombardment of atoms and molecules in cells is to remove electrons. Irradiation of the water molecules in a cell first causes the generation of an unstable ion pair, H_2O^+ and an electron. These then form a hydrogen ion and a free hydroxyl radical. Further reactions result in the formation of other toxic species, including hydrogen peroxide. The presence of oxygen facilitates these reactions and high concentrations (or increased pressures) of oxygen sensitize tissues to the damaging effects of ionizing radiation [217,218]. Thus the mechanism whereby radiation may damage the lung is analogous to that of oxygen or paraquat toxicity.

As would be expected, the effects of radiation on the lung are principally on vascular endothelium and alveolar type II pneumocytes. The lung is relatively resistant to radiation up to a single dose threshold of about 6 Gy [217]. The risk of radiation damage thereafter increases sharply with increasing dose, from about 30% after a single dose of 8 Gy to 80% after 10 Gy. Higher doses may be withstood if spaced over longer intervals, with a 5% risk attending 25 Gy given over 4 weeks in 20 doses [217]. There is of course individual variability in response and other factors, such as oxygen therapy and cytotoxic drugs given simultaneously, may increase the risk [219,220].

Clinical features

Radiation pneumonitis is relatively uncommon with modern techniques of radiotherapy. It is usually seen following mediastinal treatment of lymphoma or breast carcinoma but may occur after treatment of lung cancer, pulmonary metastases or even radioiodine therapy for lung metastases from thyroid carcinoma [221–223]. The condition usually presents 1–3 months after treatment is started, though it may occur earlier or later (Fig. 55.5). If the radiotherapy was localized the only signs may be radiological, although more generalized effects may cause progressive dyspnoea associated with repetitive inspiratory crackles on auscultation. There may be a dry cough, and pleuritic pain may indicate a radiation-induced rib fracture. Skin changes, erythema, dystrophy and telangiectasia often indicate the site of radiation. Unless very extensive and severe, the pulmonary changes are usually self-limiting. The breathlessness usually subsides slowly, over weeks or months, though the patient is often left with some residual dysfunction and studies on dogs have shown restriction and reduced D_{LCO} to be likely sequels [224]. The radiological changes in the acute stage mimic pulmonary oedema, although they are normally confined to the site of treatment. Subsequent resolution in more severe cases is marked radiologically by the development of irregular fibrosis in the affected area (Fig. 55.6). Thickened pleura and dystrophic rib changes may be visible.

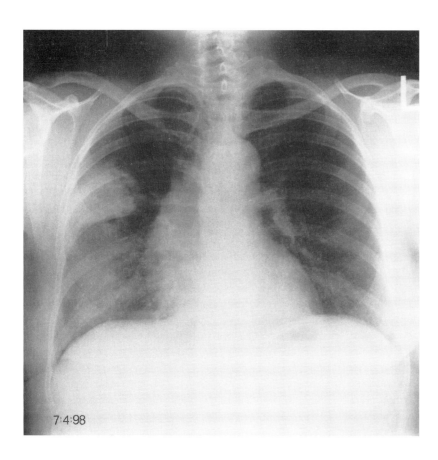

7·4·98

Fig. 55.5 Radiation pneumonitis that developed 6 weeks after therapy for carcinoma of the right breast. Note the demarcation between normal and damaged lung medially.

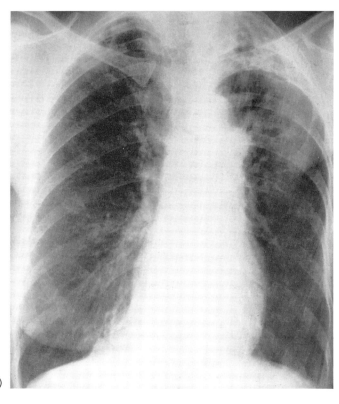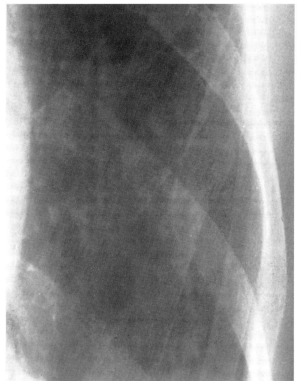

(a)

(b)

Fig. 55.6 End results of radiation therapy for breast carcinoma. Note the absent breast, left upper zone fibrosis (a) and dystrophic changes in the anterior part of the seventh rib (b).

Pathology

Since the pathological changes have been largely described in people who have died after a course complicated by oxygen therapy and infection [225], description of the earlier changes relies largely on studies of small mammals [226,227]. The appearances of classical radiation pneumonitis mimic closely those of oxygen toxicity, with initial vacuolation and necrosis of endothelial and type I cells, oedema in the alveoli and interstitial tissue and hyaline membranes. Capillary lumens become occluded by thrombi and there is proliferation of type II pneumocytes. The end stage is diffuse interstitial fibrosis, though if recovery occurs the normal alveolar epithelium may become regenerated. However, more recently a form of pneumonitis has been recognized in which hypersensitivity appears to play a part [228,229]. In these cases even local radiation to a part of the lung may cause a bilateral lymphocytic alveolitis demonstrable by bronchoalveolar lavage and sometimes by clinical symptoms and signs, these features ultimately resolving without fibrosis. This may well form the pathological basis of the transient pneumonitis often seen clinically.

Management

In most instances no special treatment is required as the condition is localized and resolves spontaneously. If it is sufficiently severe to cause breathlessness, most authorities would advise treatment with high doses (40 mg or more daily) of prednisolone, gradually reducing the dose as the condition responds [230]. Care should be taken to prevent infection and any evidence of this should result in early treatment with broad-spectrum antibiotics. If hypoxia occurs, only enough oxygen should be given to restore the Pao_2 to about 13 kPa (100 mmHg), since high alveolar tensions may aggravate the damage.

Toxic oil syndrome

An epidemic disease characterized by diffuse neurological and vascular damage occurred in Spain in 1981 and was caused by the ingestion of contaminated rapeseed oil thought to have been denatured by aniline, though the toxic component has never been identified [231,232]. In those with respiratory symptoms, the initial illness was characterized by dry cough, dyspnoea, pulmonary oedema, fever and rashes. There was usually spontaneous recovery after 2–3 weeks and then, in a proportion, vascular lesions and fatal pulmonary hypertension occurred. At a later stage scleroderma, neuropathies and joint contractures were the main problems, and long-term lung involvement was not prominent [233,234]. At necropsy, intimal proliferation and medial hypertrophy were prominent in muscular pulmonary arteries, with muscularization of pulmonary arterioles [235]. Evidence of vasculitis was also found in systemic veins and arteries. It was felt that these lesions were analogous to those occurring after radiation, suggesting that they might have been caused by the release of free oxygen radicals.

References

1 Williams IP, Millard FCJ. Severe asthma after inadvertent ingestion of oxprenolol. *Thorax* 1980; 35: 160.

2 Decalmer PBS, Chatterjee SS, Cruikshank JM *et al.* Beta-blockers and asthma. *Br Heart J* 1978; 40: 184.

3 Fratto C. Provocation of bronchospasm by eye drops. *Ann Intern Med* 1978; 88: 362.

4 Szczeklik A. Analgesics, allergy and asthma. *Br J Clin Pharmacol* 1980; 10: 401S.

5 Sanak M, Simon HU, Szczeklik A. Leukotriene C4 synthase promotor polymorphism and risk of aspirin-induced asthma. *Lancet* 1997; 350: 1599.

6 Martelli NA. Bronchial and intravenous provocation tests with indomethacin in aspirin-sensitive asthmatics. *Am Rev Respir Dis* 1979; 120: 1073.

7 Patrono C, Ciabattoni G, Venuti A *et al.* Aspirin intolerance: unaltered susceptibility of platelet cyclooxygenase to inhibition by aspirin *in vitro. J Allergy Clin Immunol* 1978; 62: 271.

8 Green A, Drzewieck G, Middleton E. Prostaglandin E$_2$ (PGE$_2$) production by platelets of asthmatic and normal subjects. *J Allergy Clin Immunol* 1980; 65: 236.

9 Ameisen JC, Capron A, Joseph M, Tonnel AB. Platelets and aspirin-induced asthma. In: Kay AB, ed. *Asthma: Clinical Pharmacology and Therapeutic Progress.* Oxford: Blackwell Scientific Publications, 1986: 226.

10 Price HV. Asthma attacks precipitated by disodium cromoglycate in a boy with α-1 antitrypsin deficiency. *Lancet* 1982; ii: 606.

11 Connolly CK. Adverse reaction to ipratropium bromide. *Br Med J* 1982; 285: 934.

12 Mann JS, Howarth PH, Holgate ST. Broncho-constriction induced by ipratropium bromide in asthma: relation to hypotonicity. *Br Med J* 1984; 289: 469.

13 Gilman AG, Goodman LS, Rall TW, Murad F. *The Pharmacological Basis of Therapeutics*, 7th edn. New York: Macmillan, 1985: 507.

14 Assem ESK, Schild HO. Detection of allergy to penicillin and other antigens by *in vitro* passive sensitisation and histamine release from human and monkey lung. *Br Med J* 1968; iii: 272.

15 Menon MPS, Das AK. Tetracycline asthma: a case report. *Clin Allergy* 1977; 7: 285.

16 Coutts II, Dally MB, Newman Taylor AJ *et al.* Asthma in workers manufacturing cyclosporins. *Br Med J* 1981; 283: 950.

17 Gerber JG, Payne NA, Oelz O *et al.* Tartrazine and the prostaglandin system. *J Allergy Clin Immunol* 1979; 63: 289.

18 Powell-Jackson PR, Gray BJ, Heaton RW *et al.* Adverse effect of rifampicin administration on steroid-dependent asthma. *Am Rev Respir Dis* 1983; 128: 307.

19 Powell-Jackson PR, Jamieson AP, Gray BJ *et al.* Effect of rifampicin administration on theophylline pharmacokinetics in humans. *Am Rev Respir Dis* 1985; 131: 939.

20 Anderson EG, Calcraft B, Jariwalla AG, Al-Zaibak M. Persistent asthma after treatment with beta-blocking drugs. *Br J Dis Chest* 1979; 73: 407.

21 Gilber GB. Unusual idiosyncracy to aspirin. *JAMA* 1911; 56: 1262.

22 Reed EN. Idiosyncracy to aspirin (acetylsalicylic acid). *JAMA* 1914; 52: 773.

23 Widal F, Abrami P, Lermoyez J. Anaphylaxie et idiosyncrasie. *Presse Med* 1922; 30: 189.

24 Prickman LE, Buchstein HF. Hypersensitivity to acetylsalicylic acid (aspirin). *JAMA* 1937; 108: 445.

25 Lockey RF, Rucknagel DL, Vanselow NA. Familial occurrence of asthma, nasal polyps and aspirin intolerance. *Ann Intern Med* 1973; 78: 57.

26 Falliers CJ. Familial coincidence of asthma, aspirin intolerance and nasal polyposis. *Ann Allergy* 1974; 32: 65.

27 Van Arsdel PP. Aspirin idiosyncracy and tolerance. *J Allergy Clin Immunol* 1984; 73: 431.

28 Giraldo B, Blumenthal MN, Spink WW. Aspirin intolerance and asthma; a clinical and immunological study. *Ann Intern Med* 1969; 71: 479.

29 Wilson JA. Nasal polypi. *Clin Otolaryngol* 1976; 1: 4.

30 Lee TH, Christie PE. Leukotrienes and aspirin-induced asthma. *Thorax* 1993; 48: 1189.

31 Szczeklik A, Gryglewski RJ, Czerniawska-Mysick G. Relationship of inhibition of prostaglandin biosynthesis by analgesics to asthma attacks in aspirin-sensitive patients. *Br Med J* 1975; i: 67.

32 Samter M, Beers RF. Intolerance to aspirin: clinical studies and consideration of its pathogenesis. *Ann Intern Med* 1968; 68: 975.

33 Szczeklik A, Gryglewski RJ, Nizankowska E. Asthma relieved by aspirin and by other cyclooxygenase inhibitors *Thorax* 1978; 33: 664.

34 Szczeklik A, Nizankowka E. Asthma improved by aspirin-like drugs. *Br J Dis Chest* 1983; 77: 153.

35 Hume M, Eddey V. Treatment of chronic airways obstruction with indomethacin. *Scand J Respir Dis* 1977; 58: 284.

36 Kordansky D, Adkinson NF, Norman PS, Rosenthal RR. Asthma improved by nonsteroidal anti-inflammatory drugs. *Ann Intern Med* 1978; 88: 508.

37 Davies RJ, Hendrick DJ, Pepys J. Asthma due to inhaled chemical agents: ampicillin, benzyl penicillin, 6 amino penicillamic acid and related substances. *Clin Allergy* 1974; 4: 227.

38 Davies RJ, Pepys J. Asthma due to inhaled chemical agents: the macrolide antibiotic spiramycin. *Clin Allergy* 1975; 5: 99.

39 Dajani BM, Sliman NA, Shubair KS, Hamzeh YS. Bronchospasm caused by intravenous hydrocortisone sodium succinate (Solu-Cortef) in aspirin sensitive subjects. *J Allergy Clin Immunol* 1984; 68: 201.

40 Sheffer AL, Rocklin RD, Goetzl EJ. Immuno-

logic components of hypersensitivity reactions to cromolyn sodium. *N Engl J Med* 1975; 293: 1220.

41 Lobel H, Machtey I, Eldror MY. Pulmonary infiltrates with eosinophilia in an asthmatic patient treated with disodium cromoglycate. *Lancet* 1972; ii: 1032.

42 Ravid D, Lishner M, Lang R, Ravid M. Angiotensin-converting enzyme inhibitors and cough: a prospective evaluation in hypertension and in congestive cardiac failure. *J Clin Pharmacol* 1994; 34: 1116.

43 Simon SR, Black HR, Moser M, Berland WE. Cough and ACE inhibitors. *Arch Intern Med* 1992; 152: 1698.

44 Hargreaves MR, Benson MK. Inhaled sodium cromoglycate in angiotensin-converting enzyme inhibitor cough. *Lancet* 1995; 345: 13.

45 Geddes DM, Corrin B, Brewerton DA *et al.* Progressive airway obliteration in adults and its association with rheumatoid disease. *Q J Med* 1977; 46: 427.

46 Epler GR, Snider GL, Gaensler EA *et al.* Bronchiolitis and bronchitis in connective tissue disease. A possible relationship to the use of penicillamine. *JAMA* 1979; 242: 528.

47 Murphy KC, Atkins CJ, Otter RC *et al.* Obliterative bronchiolitis in two rheumatoid arthritis patients treated with penicillamine. *Arthritis Rheum* 1981; 74: 557.

48 Stein HB, Patterson AC, Otter RC *et al.* Adverse effects of D-penicillamine in rheumatoid arthritis. *Ann Intern Med* 1980; 92: 24.

49 Gabazza EC, Taguchi O, Yamakami T, Machishi M, Ibata H, Suzuki S. Pulmonary infiltrates and skin pigmentation associated with sulfasalazine. *Am J Gastroenterol* 1992; 87: 1654.

50 Mar KE, Sen P, Tan K, Krishnan R, Ratkalkar K. Bronchiolitis obliterans organising pneumonia associated with massive L-tryptophan ingestion. *Chest* 1993; 104: 1924.

51 McAdams AJ. Bronchiolitis obliterans. *Am J Med* 1955; 19: 314.

52 Wohl MEB, Chernick V. Bronchiolitis. *Am Rev Respir Dis* 1978; 118: 759.

53 Ezri T, Kunichezky S, Eliraz A, Soroker D, Halperin D, Schattner A. Bronchiolitis obliterans: current concepts. *Q J Med* 1994; 87: 1.

54 Berend N. Protective effect of hypoxia on bleomycin lung toxicity in the rat. *Am Rev Respir Dis* 1984; 130: 307.

55 Gurtoo HL, Hipkens JH, Sharma SD. Role of glutathione in the metabolism-dependent toxicity and chemotherapy of cyclophosphamide. *Cancer Res* 1981; 41: 3584.

56 Martin WJ. Nitrofurantoin: evidence for the oxidant injury of lung parenchymal cells. *Am Rev Respir Dis* 1983; 127: 482.

57 Kelley J, Newman RA, Evans JN. Bleomycin-induced pulmonary fibrosis in the rat. Prevention with an inhibitor of collagen. *J Lab Clin Med* 1980; 96: 954.

58 Nimni ME, Bavetta LA. Collagen defect induced by penicillamine. *Science* 1965; 150: 905.

59 McCormick J, Cole S, Lahirir B et al. Pneumonitis caused by gold salt therapy: evidence for the role of cell-mediated immunity in its pathogenesis. *Am Rev Respir Dis* 1980; 122: 145.

60 Ettensohn DB, Roberts NJ, Condemi JJ. Broncho-alveolar lavage in gold lung. *Chest* 1984; 85: 569.

61 Back O, Linden S, Ahlstedt S. Adverse reactions to nitrofurantoin in relation to cellular and humoral immune responses. *Clin Exp Immunol* 1977; 28: 400.

62 Akoun GM, Gauthier-Rahman S, Milleron BJ et al. Amiodarone-induced hypersensitivity pneumonitis. Evidence of an immunological cell-mediated mechanism. *Chest* 1984; 85: 133.

63 Sostman HD, Matthay RA, Putman CE, Walker Smith GJ. Methotrexate-induced pneumonitis. *Medicine* 1976; 55: 371.

64 Amos HE, Lake BG, Atkinson HAC. Allergic drug reactions: an *in vitro* model using a mixed function oxidase-complex to demonstrate antibodies with specificity for a practolol metabolite. *Clin Allergy* 1977; 7: 423.

65 Demeter SL, Ahmad M, Tomashefski JF. Drug-induced pulmonary disease. Part 1. Patterns of response. *Cleve Clin Q* 1979; 46: 89.

66 Weinstein A. Drug-induced systemic lupus erythematosus. In: Schwartz R, ed. *Progress in Clinical Immunology*, Vol 4. New York: Grune & Stratton, 1980.

67 Israel HL, Diamond P. Recurrent pulmonary infiltration and pleural effusion due to nitrofurantoin therapy. *N Engl J Med* 1962; 266: 1024.

68 Hailey FJ, Glascock HW, Hewitt WF. Pleuropneumonic reactions to nitrofurantoin. *N Engl J Med* 1969; 281: 1087.

69 Holmberg L, Boman G. Pulmonary reactions to nitrofurantoin: 447 cases reported to the Swedish Adverse Drug Reaction Committee 1966–1976. *Eur J Respir Dis* 1981; 62: 180.

70 Holmberg L, Boman G, Bottiger LE et al. Adverse reactions to nitrofurantoin. Analysis of 921 reports. *Am J Med* 1980; 69: 733.

71 Fiegenberg DS, Weiss H, Kirschman H. Migratory pneumonia with eosinophilia associated with sulfonamide administration. *Arch Intern Med* 1967; 120: 85.

72 Steinfort CL, Wiggins J, Sheffield EA, Keal EE. Alveolitis associated with sulphamethoxypyridazine. *Thorax* 1989; 44: 310.

73 Daniel PT, Holzschuh J, Berg PA. Sulphadoxine specific lymphocyte transformation in a patient with eosinophilic pneumonia induced by sulphadoxine–pyrimethamine (Fansidar). *Thorax* 1989; 44: 307.

74 Reichlin S, Loveless MH, Kane EG. Loffler's syndrome following penicillin therapy. *Ann Intern Med* 1953; 38: 113.

75 Poe RH, Condemi JJ, Weinstein SS, Schuster RJ. Adult respiratory distress syndrome related to ampicillin sensitivity. *Chest* 1980; 77: 449.

76 Wold DE, Zahn DW. Allergic (Loffler's) pneumonitis occurring during antituberculous chemotherapy. *Am Rev Tuberc* 1956; 74: 445.

77 Bayer AS, Targan SR, Pitchon HE, Guze LB. Dilantin toxicity: miliary pulmonary infil-

trates and hypoxemia. *Ann Intern Med* 1976; 85: 475.

78 Michael JR, Rudin ML. Acute pulmonary disease caused by phenytoin. *Ann Intern Med* 1981; 95: 452.

79 Saltzstein SL, Ackerman LV. Lymphadenopathy induced by anticonvulsant drugs and mimicking clinically and pathologically malignant lymphomas. *Cancer* 1959; 12: 164.

80 Cullinan SA, Bower GC. Acute pulmonary hyper-sensitivity to carbamazepine. *Chest* 1975; 68: 580.

81 Stephan WC, Parks RD, Tempest B. Acute hyper-sensitivity pneumonitis associated with carbamazepine therapy. *Chest* 1978; 74: 463.

82 Rotmensch HH, Liron M, Tupilski M, Laniado S. Possible association of pneumonitis with amiodarone therapy. *Am Heart J* 1980; 100: 412.

83 Wright AJ, Brackenridge RG. Pulmonary infiltration and bone marrow depression complicating treatment with amiodarone. *Br Med J* 1982; 284: 1303.

84 Leech JA, Gallastegin J, Swiryn S. Pulmonary toxicity of amiodarone. *Chest* 1984; 85: 444.

85 Kudenchuk PJ, Pierson DJ, Greene HL et al. Prospective evaluation of amiodarone pulmonary toxicity. *Chest* 1984; 86: 541.

86 Roca J, Heras M, Rodriquez-Roisin R, Magrina J, Xaubet A, Sanz G. Pulmonary complications after long-term amiodarone treatment. *Thorax* 1992; 47: 372.

87 Marchlinski FE, Gansler TS, Waxman HL, Josephson ME. Amiodarone pulmonary toxicity. *Ann Intern Med* 1982; 97: 839.

88 Sobol SM, Rakita L. Pneumonitis and pulmonary fibrosis associated with amiodarone treatment: a possible complication of a new antiarrhythmic drug. *Circulation* 1982; 65: 819.

89 McGovern B, Garan H, Kelly E, Ruskin JN. Adverse reactions during treatment with amiodarone hydrochloride. *Br Med J* 1983; 287: 175.

90 Darmanata JI, van Zanderijk N, Duren DR et al. Amiodarone pneumonitis: three further cases with a review of published reports. *Thorax* 1984; 39: 57.

91 Perlow GM, Jain BP, Pauker SG et al. Tocainide-associated interstitial pneumonitis. *Ann Intern Med* 1981; 94: 489.

92 Braude AC, Downar E, Chamberlain DW, Rebuck AS. Tocainide-associated interstitial pneumonitis. *Thorax* 1982; 37: 309.

93 Alarcon-Segovia D. Drug-induced lupus syndromes. *Mayo Clinic Proc* 1969; 44: 664.

94 Byrd RB, Schanzer B. Pulmonary sequelae in procainamide induced lupus-like syndrome. *Dis Chest* 1969; 55: 170.

95 Jones GR, Malone DNS. Sulphasalazine induced lung disease. *Thorax* 1972; 27: 713.

96 Thomas P, Seaton A, Edwards J. Respiratory disease due to sulphasalazine. *Clin Allergy* 1974; 4: 41.

97 Williams T, Eidus L, Thomas P. Fibrosing alveolitis, bronchiolitis obliterans and sulfasalazine therapy. *Chest* 1982; 81: 766.

98 Averbuch M, Halpern Z, Hallak A et al. Sulfasalazine pneumonitis. *Am J Gastroenterol* 1985; 80: 343.

99 Camus P, Degat OR, Justrabo E, Jeannin L. D-Penicillamine-induced severe pneumonitis. *Chest* 1982; 81: 376.

100 Eastmond CJ. Diffuse alveolitis as complica-

tion of penicillamine treatment for rheumatoid arthritis. *Br Med* 1976; J i: 1506.

101 Sternlieb I, Bennett B, Scheinberg IH. D-Penicillamine induced Goodpasture's syndrome in Wilson's disease. *Ann Intern Med* 1975; 82: 673.

102 Matloff DS, Kaplan MM. D-Penicillamine-induced Goodpasture's like syndrome in primary biliary cirrhosis: successful treatment with plasmapheresis and immunosuppressives. *Gastroenterology* 1980; 78: 1046.

103 James DW, Whimster WF, Hamilton EBD. Gold lung. *Br Med J* 1978; i: 1523.

104 Winterbauer RH, Wilske KR, Wheelis RF. Diffuse pulmonary injury associated with gold treatment. *N Engl J Med* 1976; 294: 919.

105 Geddes DM, Brostoff J. Pulmonary fibrosis associated with hypersensitivity to gold salts. *Br Med J* 1976; i: 1444.

106 Yagoda A, Mukherji B, Young C et al. Bleomycin, an antitumor antibiotic. Clinical experience in 274 patients. *Ann Intern Med* 1972; 77: 861.

107 Perez-Guerra F, Harkleroad LE, Walsh RE, Costanzi JJ. Acute bleomycin lung. *Am Rev Respir Dis* 1972; 106: 909.

108 Comis RL. Bleomycin toxicity: current status and future directions. *Semin Oncol* 1992; 19 (Suppl 5): 64.

109 Luna MA, Bedrossian CWM, Lichtiger B, Salem PA. Interstitial pneumonitis associated with bleomycin therapy. *Am J Clin Pathol* 1972; 58: 501.

110 Jones AW. Bleomycin lung damage: the pathology and nature of the lesion. *Br J Dis Chest* 1978; 72: 321.

111 White DA, Stover DE. Severe bleomycin-induced pneumonitis. Clinical features and response to corticosteroids. *Chest* 1984; 86: 723.

112 Maher J, Daly PA. Severe bleomycin lung toxicity: reversal with high dose corticosteroids. *Thorax* 1993; 48: 92.

113 Holoye PY, Luna MA, MacKay B, Bedrossian CWM. Bleomycin hypersensitivity pneumonitis. *Ann Intern Med* 1978; 88: 47.

114 Orwoll ES, Kiessling PJ, Patterson JR. Interstitial pneumonia from mitomycin. *Ann Intern Med* 1978; 89: 352.

115 Andrews AT, Bowman HS, Patel SB, Anderson WM. Mitomycin and interstitial pneumonitis. *Ann Intern Med* 1979; 90: 127.

116 Oliner H, Schwartz R, Rubio F, Dameshek W. Interstitial pulmonary fibrosis following busulphan therapy. *Am J Med* 1961; 31: 134.

117 Heard BE, Cooke RA. Busulphan lung. *Thorax* 1968; 23: 187.

118 Burns WA, McFarland W, Matthews MJ. Busulphan-induced pulmonary disease. Report of a case and review of the literature. *Am Rev Respir Dis* 1970; 101: 408.

119 Littler WA, Kay JM, Hasleton PS, Heath D. Busulphan lung. *Thorax* 1969; 24: 639.

120 Koss LG, Melamed MR, Mayer K. The effect of busulphan on human epithelia. *Am J Clin Pathol* 1965; 44: 385.

121 Rose MS. Busulphan toxicity syndrome caused by chlorambucil. *Br Med J* 1975; ii: 123.

122 Godard P, Marty JP, Michel FB. Interstitial pneumonia and chlorambucil. *Chest* 1979; 76: 471.

123 Topilow AA, Rothenberg SP, Cottrell TS. Interstitial pneumonia after prolonged treatment with cyclophosphamide. *Am Rev Respir Dis* 1973; 108: 114.

124 Mark GJ, Lehimgar-Zadeh A, Ragsdale BD.

Cyclophosphamide pneumonitis. *Thorax* 1978; 33: 89.

125 Goucher G, Rowland V, Hawkins J. Melphalan-induced pulmonary interstitial fibrosis. *Chest* 1980; 77: 805.

126 Westerfield BT, Michalski JP, McCombs C, Light RW. Reversible melphalan-induced lung damage. *Am J Med* 1980; 68: 767.

127 Aronin PA, Mahaley MS, Rudnick SA *et al.* Prediction of BCNU pulmonary toxicity in patients with malignant gliomas. *N Engl J Med* 1980; 303: 183.

128 Durant JR, Norgard MJ, Murad TM *et al.* Pulmonary toxicity associated with bischloroethylnitrosourea (BCNU). *Ann Intern Med* 1979; 90: 191.

129 Patten GA, Billi JE, Rotman HH. Rapidly progressive, fatal pulmonary fibrosis induced by carmustine. *JAMA* 1980; 244: 687.

130 Thomas PS, Agrawal S, Gore M, Geddes DM. Recall lung pneumonitis due to carmustine after radiotherapy. *Thorax* 1995; 50: 1116.

131 Allen J, Cooper D, White DA, Matthay RA. Drug-induced pulmonary disease. Part 1. Cytotoxic drugs. *Am Rev Respir Dis* 1986; 133: 321.

132 Schwartz IR, Kajani MK. Methotrexate therapy and pulmonary disease. *JAMA* 1969; 210: 1924.

133 Robbins KM, Gribetz I, Strauss L *et al.* Pneumonitis in acute lymphatic leukaemia during methotrexate therapy. *J Pediatr* 1973; 82: 84.

134 Walden PAM, Mitchell-Heggs PF, Coppin C *et al.* Pleurisy and methotrexate treatment. *Br Med J* 1977; ii: 867.

135 Hargreaves MR, Mowat AG, Benson MK. Acute pneumonitis associated with low dose methotrexate treatment for rheumatoid arthritis. Report of five cases and review of published reports. *Thorax* 1992; 47: 628.

136 Carroll GJ, Thomas R, Phatouros CC *et al.* Incidence, prevalence and possible risk factors for pneumonitis in patients with rheumatoid arthritis receiving methotrexate. *J Rheumatol* 1994; 21: 51.

137 Sharma A, Provenzale D, McKusick A, Kaplan MM. Interstitial pneumonitis after low-dose methotrexate treatment in primary biliary cirrhosis. *Gastroenterology* 1994; 107: 266.

138 Bell RJM. Pulmonary infiltration with eosinophils caused by chlorpropamide. *Lancet* 1964; i: 1249.

139 Burgher LW, Kass I, Schenken JR. Pulmonary allergic granulomatosis: a possible drug reaction in a patient receiving cromolyn sodium. *Chest* 1974; 66: 84.

140 Wilson IC, Gambill JM, Sandifer MG. Loeffler syndrome occurring during imipramine therapy. *Am J Psychiatry* 1963; 119: 892.

141 Harper LO, Burrell RG, Lapp NL, Morgan WKC. Allergic alveolitis due to pituitary snuff. *Ann Intern Med* 1970; 73: 581.

142 Oh PI, Balter MS. Cocaine induced eosinophilic lung disease. *Thorax* 1992; 47: 478.

143 Kennedy JD, Costello F, Balikian JP, Herman PG. Exogenous lipoid pneumonia. *Am J Roentgenol* 1981; 136: 1145.

144 Kesten S, Title L, Mullen B, Grossman R. Pulmonary disease following intravesical BCG. *Thorax* 1990; 45: 709.

145 Hormaechea E, Carlson RW, Rogove H *et al.* Hypovolemia, pulmonary edema and

146 Katz S, Aberman A, Frand UI *et al.* Heroin pulmonary edema. Evidence for increased pulmonary capillary permeability. *Am Rev Respir Dis* 1972; 106: 472.

147 Granville-Grossman KL, Sargeant HGS. Pulmonary oedema due to salicylate intoxication. *Lancet* 1960; i: 575.

148 Heffner JE, Sahn SA. Salicylate-induced pulmonary edema. *Ann Intern Med* 1981; 95: 405.

149 Bowers RE, Brigham KL, Owen PJ. Salicylate pulmonary edema: the mechanism in sheep and review of the clinical literature. *Am Rev Respir Dis* 1977; 115: 261.

150 Steinberg AD, Karliner JS. The clinical spectrum of heroin pulmonary edema. *Arch Intern Med* 1968; 122: 122.

151 Frand UI, Shim CS, Willams MH. Methadone-induced pulmonary edema. *Ann Intern Med* 1972; 76: 975.

152 Tinga DJ, Aarnondse JG. Post-partum pulmonary oedema associated with preventive therapy for premature labour. *Lancet* 1979; i: 1026.

153 Elliott HR, Abdulla U, Hayes PJ. Pulmonary oedema associated with ritodrine infusion and betamethasone administration in premature labour. *Br Med J* 1978; ii: 799.

154 Steinberg AD. Pulmonary edema following ingestion of hydrochlorothiazide. *JAMA* 1968; 204: 825.

155 Dom MR, Walker BK. Non-cardiogenic pulmonary edema associated with hydrochlorothiazide therapy. *Chest* 1981; 79: 482.

156 Smego RA, Durack DT. The neuroleptic malignant syndrome. *Arch Intern Med* 1982; 142: 1183.

157 Vessey MP, Weatherall JAC. Venous thromboembolic disease and the use of oral contraceptives. A review of mortality statistics in England and Wales. *Lancet* 1968; ii: 94.

158 Vessey MP, Doll R. Investigation of relation between use of oral contraceptives and thromboembolic disease. *Br Med J* 1968; ii: 199.

159 Badaracco MA, Vessey MP. Recurrence of venous thromboembolic disease and use of oral contraceptives. *Br Med J* 1974; i: 215.

160 Inman WHW, Vessey MP. Investigation of deaths from pulmonary, coronary and cerebral thrombosis and embolism in women of child-bearing age. *Br Med J* 1968; ii: 193.

161 Carvalho ACA, Vaillancourt RA, Cabral RS *et al.* Coagulation abnormalities in women taking oral contraceptives. *JAMA* 1977; 237: 875.

162 Potter L. Oral contraceptives, blood clotting and thrombosis. *Br Med Bull* 1978; 34: 151.

163 Kleiger RE, Boxer M, Ingham RE, Harrison DC. Pulmonary hypertension in patients using oral contraceptives: a report of six cases. *Chest* 1976; 69: 143.

164 Gurtner HP, Gertsch M, Salzmann C *et al.* Haufen sich die primar vascularen Formen des chronischen Cor pulmonales? *Schweiz Med Wochenschr* 1968; 98: 1579, 1695.

165 Gurtner HP. Pulmonary hypertension produced by ingestion of substances. *Bull Eur Physiopathol Respir* 1969; 5: 435.

166 Graham JR. Cardiac and pulmonary fibrosis during methysergide therapy for headache. *Am J Med Sci* 1967; 254: 1.

167 Hindle W, Posner E, Sweetnam MT, Tan RSH. Pleural effusion and fibrosis during

treatment with methysergide. *Br Med J* 1970; i: 605.

168 Graham JR, Suby HI, LeCompte PR, Sadowsky NL. Fibrotic disorders associated with methysergide therapy for headache. *N Engl J Med* 1966; 274: 359.

169 Marshall AJ, Eltringham WK, Barritt DW *et al.* Respiratory disease associated with practolol therapy. *Lancet* 1977; ii: 1254.

170 Hall DR, Morrison JB, Edwards FR. Pleural fibrosis after practolol therapy. *Thorax* 1978; 33: 822.

171 Taal BG, Spierings ELH, Hilvering C. Pleuropulmonary fibrosis associated with chronic and excessive intake of ergotamine. *Thorax* 1983; 38: 396.

172 Wiggins J, Skinner C. Bromocriptine induced pleuropulmonary fibrosis. *Thorax* 1986; 41: 328.

173 Seaton A. Pleural fibrosis in carcinoid syndrome. *Q J Med* 1993; 86: 350.

174 Moss SF, Lehner PJ, Gilbey SG *et al.* Pleural involvement in the carcinoid syndrome. *Q J Med* 1993; 86: 49.

175 Nasser SM, Patel M, Bell GS, Lee TH. The effect of aspirin desensitisation on urinary leukotriene E_4 concentrations in aspirin-sensitive subjects. *Am J Respir Crit Care Med* 1995; 151: 1326.

176 Stevenson DD, Pleskow WU, Simon RA *et al.* Aspirin-sensitive rhinosinusitis asthma: a double-blind crossover study of treatment with aspirin. *J Allergy Clin Immunol* 1984; 73: 500.

177 Dahlen B, Margolskee DJ, Zetterstrom O, Dahlen SE. Effect of the leukotriene receptor antagonist MK-0679 on baseline pulmonary function in aspirin sensitive asthmatic subjects. *Thorax* 1993; 48: 1205.

178 Pinkerton H. The reaction to oils and fats in the lung. *Arch Pathol* 1928; 5: 380.

179 Volk BW, Nathanson L, Losner S *et al.* Incidence of lipoid pneumonia in a survey of 389 chronically ill patients. *Am J Med* 1951; 10: 316.

180 Wagner JC, Adler DI, Fuller DN. Foreign body granulomata of the lungs due to liquid paraffin. *Thorax* 1955; 10: 157.

181 Salm R, Hughes EW. A case of chronic paraffin pneumonitis. *Thorax* 1970; 25: 762.

182 Spickard A, Hirschmann JV. Exogenous lipoid pneumonia. *Arch Intern Med* 1994; 154: 686.

183 Brown AC, Slocum PC, Putthoff SL, Wallace WE, Foresman BH. Exogenous lipoid pneumonia due to nasal application of petroleum jelly. *Chest* 1994; 105: 968.

184 Miller GJ, Ashcroft MT, Beadnell HMSG *et al.* The lipoid pneumonia of blackfat tobacco smokers in Guyana. *Q J Med* 1971; 40: 457.

185 Buchanan DR, Lamb D, Seaton A. Punk rocker's lung: pulmonary fibrosis in a drug snorting fire-eater. *Br Med J* 1981; 283: 1661.

186 Deneke SM, Fanburg BL. Normobaric oxygen toxicity of the lung. *N Engl J Med* 1980; 303: 76.

187 Frank L, Massaro D. Oxygen toxicity. *Am J Med* 1980; 69: 117.

188 Yoo JH, Erzurum SC, Hay JG, Lemarchand P, Crystal RG. Vulnerability of the human airway epithelium to hyperoxia. Constitutive expression of the catalase gene in human bronchial epithelial cells despite oxidative stress. *J Clin Invest* 1994; 93: 297.

189 Nash G, Biennerhasset JB, Pontoppidan H. Pulmonary lesions associated with oxygen

therapy and artificial ventilation. *N Engl J Med* 1967; 276: 368.

190 Comroe JH, Dripps RD, Dumke PR, Dening M. Oxygen toxicity. *JAMA* 1945; 128: 710.

191 Van der Water JM, Kagey KS, Miller IT *et al*. Response of the lung to six to 12 hours of 100 per cent oxygen inhalation in normal man. *N Engl J Med* 1970; 283: 621.

192 Davis WB, Rennard SI, Bitterman PB, Crystal RG. Early reversible changes in human alveolar structures induced by hyperoxia. *N Engl J Med* 1983; 309: 878.

193 Burger EJ, Mead J. Static properties of the lungs after oxygen exposure. *J Appl Physiol* 1969; 27: 191.

194 Caldwell PRB, Lee WL, Schildkraut HS, Archibald ER. Changes in lung volume, diffusing capacity and blood gases in men breathing oxygen. *J Appl Physiol* 1966; 21: 1477.

195 Sackner MA, Landa J, Hirsch J, Zapata A. Pulmonary effects of oxygen breathing. A 6-hour study in normal men. *Ann Intern Med* 1975; 82: 40.

196 Clark JM, Lambertson CJ. Pulmonary oxygen toxicity: a review. *Pharmacol Rev* 1971; 23: 37.

197 Ehrenkranz RA, Bonta BW, Ablow RC, Warshaw JB. Amelioration of bronchopulmonary dysplasia after vitamin E administration. *N Engl J Med* 1978; 299: 546.

198 Fairshter RD, Rosen SM, Smith WR *et al*. Paraquat poisoning: new aspects of therapy. *Q J Med* 1976; 45: 551.

199 Llheureux P, Leduc D, Vanbinst R, Askenasi R. Survival in a case of massive paraquat ingestion. *Chest* 1995; 107: 285.

200 Frank L, Yam J, Roberts RJ. The role of endotoxin in protection of adult rats from oxygen-induced lung toxicity. *J Clin Invest* 1978; 61: 269.

201 Anon. Poisoning from paraquat. *Br Med J* 1967; iii: 690.

202 Bullivant CM. Accidental poisoning by paraquat: report of two cases in man. *Br Med J* 1966; i: 1272.

203 Levin PJ, Klaff LJ, Ross AG, Ferguson AD. Pulmonary effects of contact exposure to paraquat: a clinical and experimental study. *Thorax* 1979; 34: 150.

204 Higenbottam T, Crome P, Parkinson C, Nunn J. Further clinical observations on the pulmonary effects of paraquat ingestion. *Thorax* 1979; 34: 161.

205 Smith P, Heath D. Paraquat lung: a reappraisal. *Thorax* 1974; 29: 643.

206 Hudson M, Patel SB, Ewan SW, Smith CC, Friend JA. Paraquat-induced pulmonary fibrosis in three survivors. *Thorax* 1991; 46: 201.

207 Smith P, Heath D. The ultrastructure and time sequence of the early stages of paraquat lung in rats. *J Pathol* 1974; 114: 177.

208 Smith P, Heath D, Kay JM. The pathogenesis and structure of paraquat-induced pulmonary fibrosis in rats. *J Pathol* 1974; 114: 57.

209 Proudfoot AT, Stewart MS, Levitt T, Widdop B. Paraquat poisoning: significance of plasma paraquat levels. *Lancet* 1979; ii: 330.

210 Addo E, Poon-King T. Leucocyte suppression in treatment of 72 patients with paraquat poisoning. *Lancet* 1986; i: 1117.

211 Vale JA, Meredith TJ, Buckley BM. Paraquat poisoning. *Lancet* 1986; i: 1439.

212 Van der Wal NA, Smith LL, van Oirschot JF, van Asbeck BS. Effect of iron chelators on paraquat toxicity in rats and alveolar type II cells. *Am Rev Respir Dis* 1992; 145: 180.

213 Matthew H, Logan A, Woodruff MFA, Heard B. Paraquat poisoning: lung transplantation. *Br Med J* 1968; iii: 759.

214 Licker M, Schweizer A, Hohn L, Morel DR, Spiliopoulos A. Single lung transplant for adult respiratory distress syndrome after paraquat poisoning. *Thorax* 1998; 53: 620.

215 Gardiner AJS. Pulmonary oedema in paraquat poisoning. *Thorax* 1972; 27: 132.

216 Hendry MS, Williams PS, Ackrill P. Recovery from severe pulmonary damage due to paraquat administered intravenously and orally. *Thorax* 1984; 39: 874.

217 Duncan W, Nias AHW. *Clinical Radiobiology*. Edinburgh: Churchill Livingstone, 1977.

218 Nonn RA, Gross NJ. Effects of radiation on the lung. *Curr Opin Pulm Med* 1996; 2: 390.

219 Einhorn L, Krause M, Hornback N, Furnas B. Enhanced pulmonary toxicity with bleomycin and radiotherapy in oat cell lung cancer. *Cancer* 1976; 37: 2414.

220 Mah K, Keane TJ, Van Dyk J, Braban LE, Poon PY, Hao Y. Quantitative effect of combined chemotherapy and fractionated radiotherapy on the incidence of radiation-induced lung damage: a prospective clinical study. *Int J Radiat Oncol Biol Phys* 1994; 28: 563.

221 Gross N. Pulmonary effects of radiation therapy. *Ann Intern Med* 1977; 86: 81.

222 Rall JE, Alpers JB, Lewallen CG *et al*. Radiation pneumonitis and fibrosis: a complication of radioiodine treatment for carcinoma of the thyroid. *J Clin Endocrinol* 1957; 17: 1263.

223 Whitfield AGW, Bond WH, Kunkler PB. Radiation damage to thoracic tissues. *Thorax* 1963; 18: 371.

224 Teates CD. Effects of unilateral thoracic irradiation on lung function. *J Appl Physiol* 1963; 20: 628.

225 Jennings FL, Arden A. Development of radiation pneumonitis. *Arch Pathol* 1962; 74: 351.

226 Adamson IYR, Bowden DH, Wyatt JP. A pathway to pulmonary fibrosis: an ultrastructural study of mouse and rat following radiation to the whole body and hemithorax. *Am J Pathol* 1970; 58: 481.

227 Jennings FL, Arden A. Development of experimental radiation pneumonitis. *Arch Pathol* 1961; 71: 437.

228 Roberts CM, Foulcher E, Zaunders JJ *et al*. Radiation pneumonitis: a possible lymphocyte-mediated hypersensitivity reaction. *Ann Intern Med* 1993; 118: 696.

229 Morgan GW, Breit SN. Radiation and the lung: a re-evaluation of the mechanisms mediating pulmonary injury. *Int J Radiat Oncol Biol Phys* 1995; 31: 361.

230 Douglas AC. Treatment of radiation pneumonitis with prednisolone. *Br J Dis Chest* 1959; 53: 346.

231 Toxic Epidemic Study Group. Toxic epidemic syndrome, Spain, 1981. *Lancet* 1982; ii: 697.

232 Tabuenca JM. Toxic allergic syndrome caused by ingestion of rape-seed oil denatured by aniline. *Lancet* 1981; ii: 567.

233 Alonso-Ruiz A, Calabozo M, Perez-Ruiz F, Mancebo L. Toxic oil syndrome. A long-term follow-up of a cohort of 332 patients. *Medicine* 1993; 72: 285.

234 Kaufman LD, Izquierd-Martinez M, Serrano JM, Gomez-Rieno JJ. 12-year follow-up study of epidemic Spanish toxic oil syndrome. *J Rheumatol* 1995; 22: 282.

235 Fernandez-Segoviano P, Esteban A, Martinez-Cabruja R. Pulmonary vascular lesions in the toxic oil syndrome in Spain. *Thorax* 1983; 38: 724.

SOME PAEDIATRIC INFLUENCES ON ADULT LUNG DISEASE

GEORGE RUSSELL

This chapter focuses on developments in our understanding and management of a few relatively common paediatric disorders that have implications for adult physicians. In the last two decades there have been major changes in the ability of paediatricians to ensure the survival of infants and children afflicted by illnesses that in the past would have proved fatal. These changes have led to the survival of many children with chronic respiratory ailments who are now entering adult life with impaired respiratory reserve. With the physiological decline in lung function that is an inevitable part of ageing, even such adults who are initially symptom-free are likely eventually to experience premature respiratory insufficiency and to have a considerable impact on adult respiratory services.

This impact has already been felt for cystic fibrosis, which enjoys the dubious distinction of being the most common recessively inherited fatal condition in populations of northern European stock, a gene frequency of 1 in 25 resulting in a disease prevalence of 1 in 2500. The prognosis for cystic fibrosis diagnosed during childhood is constantly improving, the current odds for a child born in 1983–85 entering his or her teens being just under 90% for girls and just over 90% for boys [1]. This means that the great majority of children with cystic fibrosis survive into adulthood, supporting previous estimates [2] that prolonged survival would soon be the norm. Not unexpectedly, prolonged survival has brought additional complications in its wake. In particular, diabetes mellitus and liver disease are seen with increasing frequency, with the result that the long-term care of affected individuals becomes ever more complex, posing major logistic and financial problems for adult respiratory services.

The identification of the gene responsible for cystic fibrosis has enabled accurate prenatal diagnosis following determination of the carrier status of the parents, either by initial examination of the mother's genotype followed by that of the father (sequential screening) or by examining DNA obtained from both parents simultaneously (couple screening). Whichever technique is adopted, the applicability of this approach is limited by the impossibility of testing for more than a handful of the known pathological mutations in the cystic fibrosis gene and by the need to obtain genetic material from the father as well as the mother. Although prenatal diagnosis initially using amniotic fluid levels of microvillar enzymes and later specific gene testing has been available for more than a decade, there is no evidence that it has had any effect on the overall numbers of children born with cystic fibrosis in the UK [1], though the effect in individual centres has been dramatic [3]. It is therefore possible that if funding were made available for antenatal diagnosis, the numbers of affected infants might eventually fall.

Universal antenatal screening leading to termination of pregnancy raises important ethical issues. Although cystic fibrosis remains a fatal disorder, the constantly improving survival mentioned above, with further improvements such as gene therapy on the therapeutic horizon, make the case for termination much less clear-cut than was the case only a few years ago.

The other form of screening still under debate is neonatal screening, most efficiently performed by examining a blood spot for immunoreactive trypsin, followed by gene mutation analysis to eliminate the large numbers of false positives identified when immunoreactive trypsin is used alone [4]. This approach reduces the number of inappropriate treatments and investigations to which affected children are usually subjected before a diagnosis is made, and allows the family to make informed decisions regarding further procreation. Several studies have now shown that in the long term patients diagnosed by screening fare better in terms of nutrition and decline in lung function than those diagnosed clinically [5,6]. There is therefore considerable pressure to introduce universal neonatal screening, which may produce further improvements in the prognosis for affected children.

Another result of modern paediatric treatment has been the dramatic fall in neonatal mortality resulting from intensive care, which has led to the survival of increasing numbers of extremely premature infants who at one time would have been considered previable. Unfortunately, the impressively good mortality statistics found in most neonatal units have been bought at a heavy price in neuro-developmental disability and, of interest to adult respiratory physicians, bronchopulmonary dysplasia [7], more commonly known simply as chronic lung disease.

The aetiology of chronic lung disease remains obscure, although its incidence is related to low birthweight and gestational age, the barotrauma of artificial ventilation, and oxygen administration in the neonatal period. Immature antioxidant defences may play a part; during fetal life the infant exists in a hypoxic environment and has no need of such defences, so that antioxidant enzyme systems do not appear until late in gestation [8]. The prematurely born infant is therefore ill prepared for the much higher oxygen tensions prevailing in the extrauterine world, particularly if surfactant deficiency necessitates the administration of high concentrations of oxygen.

Pathologically, bronchopulmonary dysplasia is characterized by diffuse alveolar damage with increased capillary permeability, with an infiltrate of inflammatory cells, principally neutrophils, and the release of inflammatory mediators including neutrophil elastase [9] and leukotrienes [10], which are presumably responsible for the bronchial hyperreactivity that characterizes the disorder in its later stages.

In the neonatal period, the diagnosis of bronchopulmonary dysplasia is based on respiratory distress lasting for longer than 4 weeks, oxygen dependency persisting beyond 36 weeks' postconceptual age [11] and a wide variety of radiographic abnormalities. In later infancy, laboratory assessment shows hypoxaemia and sometimes hypercarbia, associated with abnormalities of pulmonary function including increased airways resistance, air trapping with increased functional residual capacity (FRC), decreased lung compliance with increased work of breathing, bronchial hyperreactivity and, in some, pulmonary hypertension. These changes may be associated with growth failure, and it is commonly observed that the lung changes seldom improve until the child begins to thrive.

Management has tended to focus on anti-inflammatory agents such as dexamethasone [12], diuretics and the avoidance of barotrauma and hyperoxia by meticulous attention to ventilator technique. The condition tends to improve over time, and oxygen dependency seldom persists beyond the first year of life. However, functional abnormalities persist throughout childhood, with slightly impaired lung function at rest but substantial impairment of the ventilatory response to exercise and reduced aerobic capacity [13]. Few studies have been performed on adult survivors [14] but currently available information suggests that these children are entering adult life with considerably impaired lung function and exercise tolerance.

Recent improvements in the respiratory management of premature babies, such as high-frequency oscillatory ventilation and surfactant therapy, may have led to some reduction in the proportion of survivors of neonatal intensive care who have chronic lung disease [15], a benefit that may be offset by an overall increase in survival. The continuing increase in the prevalence of chronic lung disease now poses substantial financial and social burdens for society in general and affected families in particular. Zimmerman [16] cites a newspaper report estimating that in 1988 the annual cost of this condition was $2.4 billion throughout the USA, a figure that has undoubtedly increased since then. As they appear in ever greater numbers over the next few years, the adult survivors of chronic neonatal lung disease will contribute significantly to the burden of adult lung disease.

The survival of sufferers from paediatric respiratory disease represents an obvious contribution to adult respiratory disease. More subtle are the long-term effects of environmental influences on the lungs of the unborn baby, of which the most obvious, and certainly the most extensively investigated, is maternal smoking. This is associated with a wide variety of adverse effects on the fetus, ranging from increased fetal loss by way of spontaneous abortion, stillbirth and neonatal death to growth retardation and an increased prevalence of respiratory symptoms during childhood. Data from the British Birth Survey showed that the adverse effects of smoking during pregnancy could be separated from those of passive smoking postnatally, and strongly suggested that intrauterine exposure was more important than postnatal exposure [17]. These epidemiological observations are supported by abnormalities of lung function; in two separate studies, Tager and colleagues [18] and Hanrahan and colleagues [19] have shown a decrease in maximum expiratory flow at FRC of about 50% in the offspring of mothers who smoked during pregnancy, pointing to the presence of significant airways disease. In an era when, contrary to the general trend in the UK, the prevalence of smoking is increasing in young females, the effects of maternal smoking are particularly worrying. Although the case for discouraging maternal smoking during pregnancy is overwhelming, in practice these mothers tend to stick tenaciously to their habit.

The role of intrauterine nutrition has attracted considerable interest since Barker's observations on the relationship between birthweight and the subsequent development of chronic obstructive pulmonary disease [20]. Although this study did not take account of prematurity or smoking, both of which are likely to have effects independently of birthweight, decreased lung function between the ages of 59 and 70 years and death from chronic obstructive pulmonary disease were related to low birthweight. Barker speculated that intrauterine influences which retard fetal weight gain may permanently constrain the growth of the airways. The association of congenitally small airways with postnatal lung disease is supported by the observation of Martinez and colleagues [21] that children with evidence of impaired airway function in infancy are prone to develop wheeze in association with viral infection. Against a background of ever-increasing survival rates for premature and low birth-weight infants, these findings are a source of anxiety to neonatologists and chest physicians alike.

Interference with intrauterine lung growth also occurs in association with a variety of conditions that result in intrauterine compression or interfere with fetal breathing movements. These include the more obvious space-occupying lesions, such as diaphragmatic hernia and pleural effusion, as well as congenital lung abnormalities, such as cystic adenomatoid malformation, external compression from asphyxiating thoracic dystrophy, interference with respiratory muscle activity in spinal muscular atrophy, muscular dystrophy and anterior abdominal wall defects, and pulmonary constriction due to reduced amniotic fluid volume following prolonged rupture of membranes and renal agenesis. Studies on children who survived in previous generations suggest a relatively benign prognosis, with little interference with daily activities, although modest impairment of lung function is common [22,23] as is bronchial hyperreactivity [24]. Whether the prognosis for the current generation of children surviving more severe abnormalities with the help of high-frequency ventilation and extracorporeal membrane oxygenation will be equally benign remains to be seen, but it seems more than likely that survivors will enter adult life with more severely impaired lung function.

Even after delivery at a normal birthweight, the child's lungs are anatomically small, functionally immature and are still growing and developing. It is no great surprise therefore that they should be exquisitely sensitive to the effects of inhaled toxins and that passively inhaled tobacco smoke should have a marked effect on respiratory morbidity. The effects of passive smoking have been assessed in many studies over the years, with wide variations in the methods used to both assess exposure to smoke and define respiratory morbidity. Associations have long been established between passive smoking and pneumonia and bronchiolitis in infancy [25] and with wheeze, cough and other respiratory symptoms in older children [26,27]. Although the effects of passive smoking on lung function are less dramatic than those of intrauterine exposure to tobacco smoke, several studies [28,29] have shown significant adverse effects on lung function and growth. The overall effect amounts to a reduction in forced expiratory volume in 1 s (FEV_1) of the order of 5–10%. Passive smoking during childhood has also been associated with a variety of other effects during childhood, including bronchial hyperreactivity [30], glue ear and sudden infant death syndrome [31], and is said to

account for 17% of cases of lung cancer in adult non-smokers [32]. Smoking is strongly related to social deprivation, and in a recent study of Aberdeen schoolchildren we were unable to detect any effect of deprivation on respiratory morbidity that could not be explained by parental smoking.

Childhood infections also have important long-term effects on the lungs. In the past, measles and whooping cough were responsible for many cases of bronchiectasis, although this problem has now all but disappeared with the advent of successful vaccines for these conditions. These days, acute bronchiolitis is the most important lower respiratory tract infection presenting to paediatricians. It is an acute viral infection of the lower respiratory tract that affects large numbers of infants each winter, being by far the most common single cause of admission to hospital in this age group. It is usually, but by no means invariably, associated with infection by the respiratory syncytial virus (RSV), which can be identified in lower respiratory tract secretions by rapid immunofluorescent techniques. The infection usually begins in the upper respiratory tract, nasal obstruction frequently resulting in feeding problems. Over the next day or two, cough, wheeze and dyspnoea become progressively more severe. On examination, the findings include tachypnoea, inspiratory chest wall recession, evidence of hyperexpansion, and various combinations of fine and coarse crackles with wheezes. The illness runs a variable course, although most patients admitted to hospital require nasal suction, oxygen and nasogastric tube feeding. A few run a more severe course and require ventilatory support. The use of nebulized ribavirin in the management of these infants remains controversial [33]. However, there are hopes that an effective vaccine against RSV will be available soon, although paediatricians with long memories will recall that previous attempts to develop a vaccine were bedevilled by the development of vaccine-enhanced illness, reflecting the complex immunology of the disease.

It is unclear why some children develop bronchiolitis in response to RSV infection, while others develop nothing worse than a bad cold. A number of environmental factors have been implicated, particularly maternal smoking [34–36]. Although the evidence of a clinical association between bronchiolitis and atopy is conflicting, bronchiolitis is associated with increased numbers of airway mast cells [37] and the immunological response to RSV includes the production of IgE antibodies [38], which in turn is related to the frequency of subsequent wheeze.

Following the acute infection, there is considerable respiratory morbidity over the next few years, at least half the affected infants going on to develop recurrent wheeze. In many children these symptoms are transient and have disappeared by school age, but in others they persist into later childhood [36]. It is notable that most follow-up studies of infants who have had bronchiolitis have shown that abnormalities of pulmonary function are much more common than symptomatic disability, so that yet a further group of children are entering adult life with reduced respiratory reserve, predisposed to chronic obstructive pulmonary disease in later life [39]. Bronchitis and pneumonia in early childhood have also been associated with chronic obstructive pulmonary disease in late adult life [40]; it is likely that many of these individuals actually suffered from bronchiolitis that had not been identified as a separate disorder during their infancy.

The most common chronic respiratory disease in childhood is asthma, the prevalence of which appears to be increasing for reasons that are unclear. In common with other atopic disorders, asthma has a strong genetic component [41]. A recent twin study from Norway suggested that about 75% of the variation in the liability to asthma was genetic, the remaining 25% being accounted for by environmental influences not shared by the twins [42]; given the extent to which twins normally share identical environments, these influences must indeed be subtle. Postulated environmental influences include maternal smoking (as discussed above), low birthweight, low maternal age [43], early exposure to allergens (including exposure *in utero*), exposure to viral infection [37], lack of exposure to infection, excessive vaccination, lack of bacille Calmette–Guérin (BCG) vaccination and reduced antioxidant reserves [44].

Although atmospheric pollution is popularly believed to be responsible for the recent increase in the prevalence of asthma, studies in children living in the Highlands of Scotland [45] have shown a high prevalence of wheeze and asthma in a notably unpolluted area, studies in the north of England have shown no difference between the prevalence of respiratory symptoms between young men living in urban and rural areas [46], and studies in Surrey actually showed a significantly lower prevalence of asthma-like symptoms in children living near motorways [47].

Nevertheless, whatever the reason, it does appear that the prevalence of childhood asthma has increased [48] and is continuing to increase [49]; in a recent review, Sears [50] states that of more than 20 sequential studies, none has shown a decrease in asthma prevalence with time. Clearly the genetic constitution of the population has not changed in a single generation, and environmental influences must be responsible. The increase in asthma-like symptoms has been accompanied by a similar increase in eczema and hay fever [48,49], whereas the prevalence of wheeze triggered only by upper respiratory tract infection has remained relatively static at around 7%. Wheeze is roughly twice as common following atopy-related asthma in childhood as following infection-related wheeze [51,52] so unless a correctable cause is found for the increase in childhood asthma, adult respiratory physicians can anticipate a continuing increase in asthma-related activity over the coming decades. Based on data from the papers cited above, it can be estimated that we are on course for an adult asthma prevalence of 25%.

This brief review has tried to demonstrate that the prognosis and prevalence of many childhood respiratory diseases are changing, and that these changes are likely to be translated into important changes in the spectrum of disease seen in adult respiratory practice. As far as chest disease is concerned, the child is truly father of the man.

References

1 Dodge JA, Morison S, Lewis PA *et al*. Incidence, population and survival of cystic fibrosis in the UK, 1968–95: UK Cystic Fibrosis Survey Management Committee. *Arch Dis Child* 1997; 77: 493.

2 Elborn JS, Shale DJ, Britton JR. Cystic fibrosis: current survival and population estimates to year 2,000. *Thorax* 1991; 46: 881.

3 Brock DJ. Prenatal screening for cystic fibrosis: 5 years' experience reviewed. *Lancet* 1996; 347: 148.

4 Wilcken B, Wiley V, Sherry G, Bayliss U. Neonatal screening for cystic fibrosis: a comparison of two strategies for case detection in 1.2 million babies. *J Pediatr* 1995; 127: 965.

5 Dankert-Roelse JE, te Meerman GJ. Long term prognosis of patients with cystic fibrosis in relation to early detection by neonatal screening and treatment in a cystic fibrosis centre. *Thorax* 1995; 50: 712.

6 Weaver LT, Green MR, Nicholson K *et al*. Prognosis in cystic fibrosis treated with continuous flucloxacillin from the neonatal period. *Arch Dis Child* 1994; 70: 84.

7 Northway WH, Rosan RC, Porter DY. Pulmonary disease following respiratory therapy of hyaline membrane disease: bronchopulmonary dysplasia. *N Engl J Med* 1967; 267: 357.

8 Autor AP, Frank L, Roberts RJ. Developmental characteristics of pulmonary superoxide dismutase: relationship to idiopathic respiratory distress syndrome. *Pediatr Res* 1976; 10: 154.

9 Ogden BE, Murphy SA, Saunders GC *et al*. Neonatal lung neutrophils and elastase/proteinase inhibitor balance. *Am Rev Respir Dis* 1984; 130: 817.

10 Mirro R, Armstead W, Leffler C. Increased airway leukotriene levels in infants with severe bronchopulmonary dysplasia. *Am J Dis Child* 1990; 144: 160.

11 Shennan AT, Dunn MS, Ohlsson A *et al*. Abnormal pulmonary outcomes in premature infants: prediction from oxygen requirement in the neonatal period. *Pediatrics* 1988; 82: 527.

12 Ng PC. The effectiveness and side effects of dexamethasone in preterm infants with bronchopulmonary dysplasia. *Arch Dis Child* 1994; 68: 330.

13 Santuz P, Baraldi E, Zaramella P *et al*. Factors limiting exercise performance in long-term survivors of bronchopulmonary dysplasia. *Am J Respir Crit Care Med* 1995; 152: 1284.

14 Northway WH, Moss RB, Carlisle KB *et al*. Late pulmonary sequelae of bronchopulmonary dysplasia. *N Engl J Med* 1990; 323: 1793.

15 Jackson IC, Truog WE, Standaert TA *et al*. Reduction in lung injury after combined surfactant and high-frequency ventilation. *Am J Respir Crit Care Med* 1994; 150: 534.

16 Zimmerman JJ. Bronchoalveolar inflammatory pathophysiology of bronchopulmonary dysplasia. *Clin Perinatol* 1995; 22: 429.

17 Taylor B, Wadsworth J. Maternal smoking during pregnancy and lower respiratory tract illness in early life. *Arch Dis Child* 1987; 62: 766.

18 Tager IB, Hanrahan JP, Toseson TD *et al*. Lung function, pre- and post-natal smoke exposure and wheezing in the first year of life. *Am Rev Respir Dis* 1993; 147: 811.

19 Hanrahan JP, Tager IB, Segal MR *et al*. The effect of maternal smoking during pregnancy on early infant lung function. *Am Rev Respir Dis* 1992; 145; 1129.

20 Barker DJP, Godfrey KM, Fall C *et al*. Relation of birth weight and childhood respiratory

infection to adult lung function and death from chronic obstructive airways disease. *Br Med J* 1991; 303: 671.

21 Martinez FD, Wright AL, Taussig LM *et al.* Asthma and wheezing in the first six years of life. *N Engl J Med* 1995; 332: 133.

22 Chatrath RR, el-Shafie M, Jones RS. Fate of hypoplastic lungs after repair of congenital diaphragmatic hernia. *Arch Dis Child* 1971; 46: 633.

23 Helms P, Stocks J. Lung function in infants with congenital pulmonary hypoplasia. *J Pediatr* 1982; 101: 918.

24 Ijsselstijn H, Tibboel D, Hop WJ *et al.* Long-term pulmonary sequelae in children with congenital diaphragmatic hernia. *Am J Respir Crit Care Med* 1997; 155: 174.

25 Fergusson DM, Horwood LJ, Shannon FT. Parental smoking and parental illness in infancy. *Arch Dis Child* 1980; 55: 358.

26 Ware JH, Dockery DW, Spiro A *et al.* Passive smoking, gas cooking and respiratory health of children living in six cities. *Am Rev Respir Dis* 1984; 129: 366.

27 Somerville SM, Rona RJ, Chinn S. Passive smoking and respiratory conditions in primary school children. *J Epidemiol Community Health* 1988; 42: 105.

28 Tager IB, Weiss ST, Muno A *et al.* Longitudinal study of maternal smoking and pulmonary smoking in children. *N Engl J Med* 1983; 309: 699.

29 Cook DG, Whincup PH, Papacosta O *et al.* Relation of passive smoking as assessed by salivary conitine concentrations and questionnaire to spirometric indices in children. *Thorax* 1993; 48: 14.

30 Frischer T, Kuehr J, Meinert R *et al.* Maternal smoking in early childhood: a risk factor for bronchial responsiveness to exercise in primary-school children. *J Pediatr* 1992; 121: 17.

31 Haglund B, Cnattinguis S. Cigarette smoking as a risk factor for sudden infant death syndrome: a population based study. *Am J Public Health* 1990; 80: 29.

32 Janerich DT, Thompson WD, Varela LR *et al.* Lung cancer and exposure to tobacco smoke in the household. *N Engl J Med* 1990; 323: 632.

33 Prober CG, Wang EE. Reducing the morbidity of lower respiratory tract infections caused by respiratory syncytial virus: still no answer. *Pediatrics* 1997; 99: 472.

34 Murray M, Webb MSC, O'Callaghan C *et al.* Respiratory status and allergy after bronchiolitis. *Arch Dis Child* 1992; 60: 1064.

35 McConnochie KM, Roughman KJ. Wheezing at 8 and 13 years: changing importance of bronchiolitis and passive smoking. *Pediatr Pulmonol* 1989; 6: 138.

36 Pullan CR, Hey EN. Wheezing, asthma and pulmonary dysfunction 10 years after infection with respiratory syncytial virus in infancy. *Br Med J* 1982; 284: 1665.

37 Castleman WL, Sorkness RL, Lemanske RF, McAllister PK. Viral bronchiolitis during early life induces increased numbers of bronchiolar mast cells and airway hyperresponsiveness. *Am J Pathol* 1990; 137: 821.

38 Welliver RC, Wong DT, Sun M *et al.* The development of respiratory syncytial virus-specific IgE and the release of histamine in nasopharyngeal secretions after infection. *N Engl J Med* 1981; 305: 841.

39 Kattan M, Keens TG, Lapierre JG *et al.* Pulmonary function abnormalities in symptom free children after bronchiolitis. *Pediatrics* 1977; 58: 683.

40 Shaheen SO, Barker DJ, Holgate ST. Do lower respiratory tract infections in early childhood cause chronic obstructive pulmonary disease? *Am J Respir Crit Care Med* 1995; 151: 1649.

41 Sandford A, Weir T, Pare P. The genetics of asthma. *Am J Respir Crit Care Med* 1996; 153: 1749.

42 Harris JR, Magnus P, Samuelsen SO, Tambs K. No evidence for effects of family environment on asthma. *Am J Respir Crit Care Med* 1997; 156: 43.

43 Infante-Rivard C. Young maternal age: a risk factor for childhood asthma? *Epidemiology* 1995; 6: 178.

44 Seaton A, Godden DJ, Brown K. Increase in asthma: a more toxic environment or a more susceptible population? *Thorax* 1994; 49: 171.

45 Austin JB, Russell G, Adam MG *et al.* Prevalence of asthma and wheeze in the Highlands of Scotland. *Arch Dis Child* 1994; 71: 211.

46 Devereux G, Ayatollahe T, Ward R *et al.* Asthma, airways responsiveness and air pollution in two contrasting districts of Northern England. *Thorax* 1996; 51: 169.

47 Waldron G, Pottle B, Dod J. Asthma and the motorways: one district's experience. *J Public Health Med* 1995; 17: 85.

48 Ninan TK, Russell G. Respiratory symptoms and atopy in Aberdeen schoolchildren: evidence from two surveys 25 years apart. *Br Med J* 1992; 304: 873.

49 Omran M, Russell G. Continuing increase in the prevalence of respiratory symptoms and diagnosed atopy in Aberdeen schoolchildren. *Br Med J* 1996; 312: 34.

50 Sears MR. Epidemiology of childhood asthma. *Lancet* 1997; 350: 1015.

51 Ross S, Godden DJ, Abdalla M *et al.* Outcome of wheeze in childhood: the influence of atopy. *Eur Respir J* 1995; 8: 2081.

52 Godden DJ, Ross S, Abdaiia M *et al.* Outcome of wheeze in childhood. Symptoms and pulmonary function 25 years later. *Am J Respir Crit Care Med* 1996; 149: 106.

57

DIVING AND THE LUNG

STEPHEN J. WATT

The term 'diving' refers to activities carried out underwater that necessitate either a breath-hold or the use of breathing apparatus. It includes recreational snorkelling and scuba diving, deep breath-hold record attempts and a range of commercial activities using various types of breathing apparatus. It also includes specialized techniques such as closed-circuit breathing apparatus with oxygen for covert military operations and deep commercial diving using saturation techniques and the use of helium or other alternative inert gases. All these activities have important implications for respiratory physiology and pathology. What makes the underwater environment dramatically different from other toxic environments is the density of water and its impact on the ambient environmental pressure.

The lung is of critical importance in diving for several reasons. Apart from the necessity to maintain adequate gas exchange, the lung is the largest gas-containing space in the body and hence plays an important role in the maintenance of buoyancy. At the same time there is a risk of rupture due to overpressurization, which may lead to fatal consequences such as tension pneumothorax or air embolism. Furthermore, the lung has a crucial role in protecting the body from the pathological effects of gas bubbles formed during the ascent phase or decompression from a dive. Without this benefit, activities underwater would be much more restricted by decompression sickness.

This chapter describes the major effects of the underwater environment on lung physiology, potential pathological outcomes and the importance of assessment of lung function in determining an individual's fitness to dive.

Physics and physiology

Diving physics

On land at sea level, humans are exposed to an ambient pressure of 100 kPa (760 mmHg), this pressure resulting from the mass of gas in the earth's atmosphere above sea level. Since gas is compressible, as altitude increases the pressure falls in a non-linear relationship with height. However, water is effectively non-compressible and is much denser than air. Therefore, underwater the pressure increases rapidly and linearly with depth; for every 10 m of seawater (msw) depth the pressure increases by 100 kPa. This substantial pressure change has important implications.

The gas laws are particularly important to the understanding of diving physiology. Boyle's law states that for a given mass of gas, the volume is proportional to the absolute pressure. Thus a balloon holding 10 L of air at sea level (100 kPa) reduces in volume to 5 L on descent to 10 msw (200 kPa) and to 1 L at 90 msw (1000 kPa). This is of direct relevance to the breath-hold diver who may take a large inspiration to total lung capacity (TLC) on the surface but at only 10 msw finds the lung volume close to functional residual capacity (FRC). The world record for breath-hold diving is in excess of 120 msw [1], which takes the diver's intrathoracic gas volume well below normal residual volume (RV). A diver using breathing apparatus underwater maintains relatively normal lung volumes, but a much greater mass of gas is required. The implications of the increase in gas density are described below.

Dalton's law states that in a mixture of gases, the total pressure exerted by the gas mixture is the sum of the partial pressures of each of the constituent gases in the mixture. Hence in air at 100 kPa, the pressure results from a P_{N_2} of 79 kPa, a P_{O_2} of 20.9 kPa plus small contributions from carbon dioxide and noble gases. If air is breathed at 10 msw, where the total pressure is 200 kPa, the resultant partial pressures are doubled, i.e. a P_{N_2} of 158 kPa and a P_{O_2} of 41.8 kPa. While gas concentrations are frequently used in medicine, the body's physiological response is to partial pressure; thus breathing air at 10 msw produces the same oxygen tension and physiological effect as breathing 40% oxygen at sea level.

Henry's law deals with the solution of gases and states

that the amount of gas dissolving in a fluid depends upon the partial pressure of the gas to which the fluid is exposed. This means that as the partial pressure increases, the amount of gas that can dissolve in body tissues increases. At sea level the average human has the equivalent of 1 L of nitrogen dissolved in body tissues. At 10 msw, after adequate time for complete equilibration, double that mass of gas has dissolved. This additional gas dissolved in tissues while the diver is exposed to increased pressure must come out of solution on or after return to the surface and is the source of the gas bubbles that cause decompression illness.

Immersion

Immersion in water has a number of important consequences for the lung. The pressure differential from the feet to the chest when standing upright is almost 1.5 m of water. This is sufficient to have important circulatory effects. The additional hydrostatic pressure on the dependent limbs tends to force blood from the legs up into the chest. This has been measured and amounts to about 700 mL additional intrathoracic blood volume within the large vessels and the pulmonary circulation [2]. The increase in intrathoracic blood volume has secondary effects. Right heart pressures rise [2] and may result in a diuresis and hence a loss of total plasma volume [3]. The increase of blood volume in the pulmonary capillary vasculature may affect ventilation–perfusion balance mechanisms [3,4]. However, the most striking impact is a direct mechanical reduction in lung volumes, with a reduction in vital capacity (VC) of about 300 mL [5] that results mainly from the blood volume shift [2], though direct hydrostatic compression contributes. These measurements have been made in subjects standing erect in water with the head above the surface and are made after a period of stabilization [3,6]. In diving, posture is variable and so the available VC may change. The additional blood within the pulmonary circulation also appears to increase closing volume [7] and reduce flow rates at low lung volume [6]; hence it is associated with earlier closure of airways on expiration. This may be of considerable importance during rapid ascent as a possible cause of gas trapping [5,7].

The large pressure differential across the height of the body also imposes problems associated with the work of breathing. Normally, in the absence of airflow, there is no significant pressure differential between the mouth and the alveolar spaces of the lung. When submerged, there may be 30 cmH$_2$O pressure differential between the mouth and the centre of the lung in the erect posture. This results in an additional workload to be overcome in order to inhale gas and imposes a further limitation on VC. The pressure differential is reduced when the diver is in a horizontal position and reversed when head down. In practice divers usually find that a slight head-down posture is most comfortable during heavy exertion (finning). This reduces the workload of inspiration but imposes a small expiratory resistance.

Breath-hold diving

Although breath-hold diving represents the simplest form of underwater activity, it generates some interesting physiological consequences. The breath-hold diver encounters all the problems of pressure change, immersion and buoyancy; in addition, gas exchange during a breath-hold dive is complex [8]. As the diver descends commencing with the lung at TLC, all the alveolar gas tensions rise in proportion to the increase in ambient pressure. Thus at 10 msw both alveolar Po$_2$ and Pco$_2$ have doubled. At depth, Po$_2$ falls with consumption, while Pco$_2$ is altered by production and solution. On ascent all gas tensions fall. If the alveolar Pco$_2$ has been reduced by hyperventilation before the dive, there is a delay in stimulation of ventilation by carbon dioxide and no hypoxic stimulus as a result of the elevated Po$_2$. In this circumstance, Po$_2$ may reduce sufficiently on ascent to result in an acute hypoxic episode known as shallow water blackout.

Although the importance of the diving reflex is uncertain in humans, it can readily be demonstrated and results in a significant bradycardia [9,10] and disturbance of left ventricular function [11]. At the same time, the efficiency of gas exchange is influenced by alterations in the distribution of pulmonary blood flow [12].

Breathing apparatus

Diving means using underwater breathing apparatus. Although very good, most breathing apparatus systems produce an impact on ventilation. This is because there is an inevitable dead space, and a resistance to breathing during both inspiration (mainly until the demand valve opens) and expiration (breathing out through the exhaust valve). Though small, the combined effect of resistance and dead space causes a significant increase in the work of breathing associated with any given workload [13]. These effects are in addition to the reduction in VC and increase in the work of breathing associated with immersion.

The effect of immersion and breathing apparatus is well demonstrated in a study by Dressendorfer and colleagues [14] in which volunteers exercised in air and immersed in water to the neck with and without breathing apparatus. For similar levels of workload (oxygen consumption), minute ventilation was reduced from a control value of 146 L/min to 130 L/min when immersed and to 108 L/min when immersed and using breathing apparatus. A degree of carbon dioxide retention is inevitable.

Gas density

With increasing pressure the diver's air or breathing gas becomes more dense. This imposes significant limitations on ventilation [15] that can be assessed by measurement of maximum voluntary ventilation (MVV). At 100 kPa, MVV is approximately 180–200 L/min. When breathing air, the effect of gas density is readily detected at quite shallow depths, for example at 30 msw (400 kPa) MVV is reduced to 100 L/min and at 50 msw (600 kPa) to 65 L/min [15,16]. On the surface, MVV is only sustainable for 20–30 s and the maximum sustainable ventilation over a period of several minutes is 70–80% MVV [17].

Underwater, for the same workload (oxygen consumption and carbon dioxide production) approximately the same minute ventilation is required to maintain a similar alveolar $P\text{co}_2$. Lung volume remains relatively unchanged. The mass of carbon dioxide produced remains the same, although it occupies a smaller volume within the alveoli. As a result the alveolar concentration of carbon dioxide is reduced but the partial pressure exerted is unchanged. The net effect of this is that if high levels of exertion are achieved underwater, it may be physiologically impossible to maintain adequate alveolar ventilation and carbon dioxide retention occurs. This is a well-recognized cause of loss of consciousness underwater. Various studies have demonstrated that divers tend to retain carbon dioxide [18–20] and that carbon dioxide retention underwater may reach dangerous levels without the diver recognizing the problem [21].

Decompression illness

Pulmonary barotrauma

Barotrauma is the term given to tissue damage that results from a change in pressure within a gas-containing space in or around the body. It can therefore affect the middle ear, sinuses, bowel, spaces between the body and the mask or suit and the lung. Pulmonary barotrauma is potentially the most serious pressure-related illness because of the severity of the outcome of arterial gas embolism.

Barotrauma may affect the lung in two ways. The lung may be compressed due to a rise in ambient pressure when the diver cannot breathe in (lung squeeze). This may occur either during a deep breath-hold dive or where breathing gas supply is lost during a rapid descent. The first scenario has been described above. The breath-hold diver takes a large breath, closes the glottis and descends. As pressure rises, the lung volume decreases. Around or below RV, there is increasing likelihood that the thorax and lung tissue are not adequately compliant to reduce in volume and hence the relative vacuum in the alveoli leads to rupture of alveolar walls and results in alveolar exudate and haemorrhage [22]. During the subsequent ascent, gas

within the lung re-expands and the diver surfaces with symptoms of cough, haemoptysis and sometimes breathlessness [20]; disturbance of blood gas tensions may result from the alveolar haemorrhage.

This event is rare in circumstances where the diver has a breathing gas unless there is a failure of gas supply. In the absence of a non-return valve, a surface supplied diver's lungs are effectively compressed by the hydrostatic pressure. Alternatively it may affect a scuba diver attempting to descend quickly. To do this he or she maintains a low lung volume in order to reduce buoyancy. If at this point the diver is unable to breathe in due to loss of gas supply, there is increasing loss of buoyancy and acceleration downwards with progressive reduction of lung volume.

Barotrauma of the lung on ascent (burst lung) is of much greater importance both numerically and in terms of morbidity and mortality. It occurs when the diver is breathing compressed gas underwater. The diver breathes with normal lung volumes at depth. On ascent the volume of gas in the chest expands and the diver must therefore breathe out to enable the expanding gas to escape. During a controlled ascent this is achieved by breathing normally. During a rapid ascent the diver may need to breathe out continuously or at least keep the mouth and glottis open. If the expanding gas is unable to escape from the lung, the transpulmonary pressure increases and the lung may rupture. It seems that rupture most likely occurs at alveolar level and that gas then expands and spreads throughout the interstitial tissues of the lung. This may result in alveolar haemorrhage [23]. The gas makes its way following the line of least resistance to the hilum [24] and from there may spread up into the mediastinum (Fig. 57.1), down into the retroperitoneal space [25,26] or through the parietal pleura into the pleural space (Fig. 57.2). Alternatively, gas may rupture through the visceral pleura into the pleural space. Finally, the tissue damage within the lung may allow the gas access to the pulmonary venous system and expanding gas then passes to the left heart and into the systemic circulation resulting in severe neurological injury or death [27].

Theoretically, any pathological lesion that interferes with gas escaping from the lungs in an evenly distributed fashion may result in shear stress forces between parts of the lung and lead to rupture. In addition, a lung that has previously ruptured spontaneously is likely to be at increased risk. Lesions which might do this are localized bullae, areas of fibrosis or scarring or major obstructions to the bronchial tree. The importance of generalized airflow limitation is difficult to assess. On normal expiration the airways tend to close and trap gas in the alveolar space. However, on ascent, gas escape is only partly by normal expiration because expanding gas tends to splint the airways open and hence vents itself. Forceful attempts to expire might themselves be harmful by prevention of gas

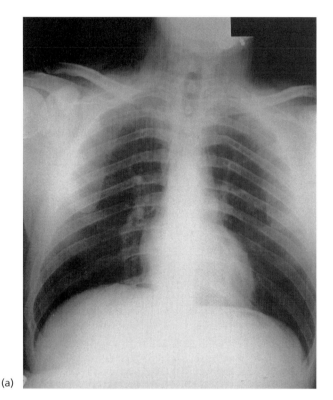

(a)

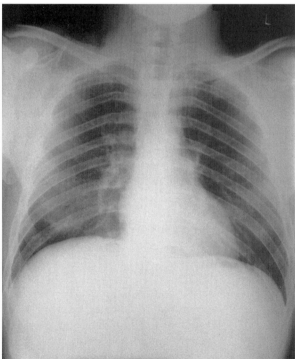

(b)

Fig. 57.1 (a,b) Two chest radiographs of a diver taken during decompression in a chamber after pulmonary barotrauma showing pneumomediastinum. Expansion of the mediastinal gas resulted in prolonged decompression.

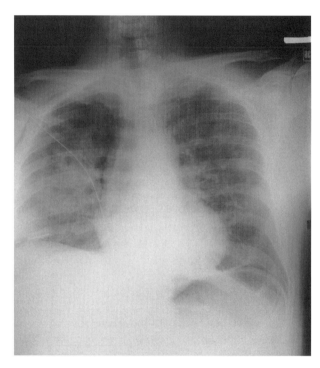

Fig. 57.2 Chest radiograph of a diver following pulmonary barotrauma of ascent showing extensive peripheral shadowing. Diver surfaced with tension pneumothorax.

escape because of airway closure. Such airway closure occurs at an earlier phase of expiration than normal because of the additional fluid in the pulmonary circulation.

A recent study of submarine escape trainees has demonstrated that the risk of pulmonary barotrauma appears to relate better to the lung volume, i.e. forced vital capacity (FVC), than to forced expiratory volume in 1s (FEV_1), though the association is weak [28]. This is a logical finding and is consistent with the other medical evidence available. In the water, VC is restricted by fluid shift to the lung but tidal volume remains unchanged. Inspiratory reserve volume (IRV) is, therefore, reduced. If during normal ticlal breathing, a diver commences ascent but fails to breathe out, IRV represents the volume by which the lung can expand before reaching normal maximal volume. Hence if IRV is small as it may be in a diver with a Cow VC, the lung may be at greater risk of rupture.

In most cases pulmonary barotrauma occurs as a result of an uncontrolled ascent. Two common scenarios are recognized. Exhaustion of the scuba diver's compressed gas supply leaves the diver struggling to obtain a last breath of air from the empty cylinder. The diver has to make a potentially strenuous ascent and, despite knowing that there is no further breathing gas available, must remember to breathe out continuously. Although considerable effort is placed on diver training to cope with this event, it is difficult to breathe out adequately and it remains a high-risk situation. An alternative but increasingly common scenario is loss of buoyancy control. As the diver commences ascent, air within the diver's dry suit or buoyancy compensator expands and provides increased buoyancy and an accelerating ascent. This gas must be dumped (exhausted from the suit) through valves in order to maintain neutral buoyancy and control. Valve failure or inversion into the feet-up position may make it impossible to dump gas and hence an explosive ascent to the surface with a grossly overinflated suit occurs.

As gas expands within the lungs and is unable to escape, the transpulmonary pressure increases and the lung may rupture when the pressure exceeds 60 cmH$_2$O [29]. It appears that it is distension of the lung rather than simply the pressure that is important, since in animal experiments the transpulmonary pressure that can be tolerated can be substantially increased by supporting the chest with binders [29]. In the diver a certain amount of chest movement restriction may be imposed by suit and harness. Nevertheless, pulmonary barotrauma has been reported after dives from very shallow depths of less than 2 msw and has also been reported after breath-hold dives [30,31].

Pulmonary barotrauma should be suspected whenever respiratory symptoms occur after a dive, particularly if there is a history of rapid or uncontrolled ascent. In most cases the presentation is immediately after the dive but delay in onset of symptoms is reported [32] and may be common when pneumomediastinum is the only manifestation. Pneumothorax may present with typical symptoms following surfacing from a dive. However, if the lung ruptures during the ascent phase of the dive more than a few metres from the surface and produces pneumothorax, the continued expansion of the gas within the pleural cavity results in tension that may have fatal results. The symptoms and signs of pneumothorax are no different from pneumothorax in any other situation and treatment is also the same, with one exception. If pneumothorax occurs to a diver who is in, or retrieved to, a closed diving bell or decompression chamber, the opportunity exists to relieve symptoms by compression. This results in reduction of the volume of the gas in the pleural space and relief of tension. This offers an emergency therapy or means of controlling symptoms while arrangements for pleural drainage are made.

Pneumomediastinum usually results in central chest discomfort, hoarse voice and sometimes breathlessness. Symptoms are rarely sufficient to require active treatment, but again recompression does offer an emergency treatment if large volumes of mediastinal gas are causing circulatory disturbance. Pneumomediastinum has caused considerable difficulty when it has occurred during deep saturation diving, since the gas expands so much during decompression and must be absorbed during this period. The decompression may therefore have to be considerably prolonged to allow time for gas absorption. Pneumomediastinum may present with some delay after surfacing from a dive with symptoms of neck discomfort and voice change associated with subcutaneous emphysema. Pneumoperitoneum is a relatively rare occurrence but causes diagnostic difficulty since the patient may present with abdominal pain and have radiological evidence of free gas in the peritoneum.

Pneumothorax, pneumomediastinum and pneumoperitoneum are all helped by breathing 100% oxygen since this speeds up the elimination of the inert gas from the gas space [33]. This technique depends on the concentration of oxygen rather than the partial pressure and hence is of very limited application in saturation diving since 100% oxygen can only be given on the surface or at relatively shallow depths (to 18 msw).

Arterial gas embolism usually presents with symptoms very soon after reaching the surface. The diver may give a shriek on arrival at the surface, probably due to the release of gas under pressure from the chest. It seems possible that it is at this time, when the intrathoracic pressure falls, that gas is best able to pass through the pulmonary venous system. Thus in at least some cases the arrival of gas in the cerebral circulation probably occurs within seconds of arrival on the surface. The presentation is with acute onset of major cerebral disturbance, loss of consciousness, blindness, hemiplegia, convulsion, etc. [27,34]. Sudden death may result from embolization of the coronary circulation. The natural history of this condition is variable, some patients making a rapid and complete recovery without treatment, others having permanent neurological injury despite rapid treatment [19,27]. Recompression rapidly reduces the volume of gas within the circulation and if achieved at an early stage may produce complete resolution of all symptoms [27]. Recompression is usually followed by hyperbaric oxygen treatment [35], which has three aims: (i) it reduces the inert gas load within the vascular space and other tissues, (ii) it may provide oxygenation to tissues that remain hypoxic as a result of the injury and (iii) it may help to prevent reperfusion injury in those tissues which had lost their blood supply.

Because of the severity of the outcome of pulmonary barotrauma, considerable efforts are made to prevent its occurrence. These efforts follow two avenues. The most important depends upon diver training, primarily to ensure that the circumstances leading to an emergency or uncontrolled ascent do not occur and, secondarily, to reduce the risks should an emergency ascent become essential. Considerable argument exists about whether practical emergency ascent training causes more harm than it prevents [36]. The second area is to identify individuals who may be at increased risk of pulmonary barotrauma. This is considered to be a crucial component of a diver's medical assessment for fitness. A variety of conditions have been considered potential risk factors, including the presence of lung bullae or cysts [37], previous spontaneous pneumothorax, localized airways obstruction and generalized airways obstruction [38]. Theoretically any condition that impairs lung compliance may also represent a risk, particularly if this is patchy since this may result in shear stress within the lung as it expands. Impairment of lung compliance has been demonstrated in a number of survivors of pulmonary barotrauma [39] but it is not clear whether this represents a pre-existing risk factor or a result of the injury.

Barotrauma may also occur to the thorax rather than to the lung. A number of incidents have occurred where a diver has experienced an uncontrolled ascent that has resulted in overpressurization of the lung but without any evidence of its rupture. Nevertheless, these divers have suffered from considerable and prolonged chest discomfort which appears to arise from the chest wall. In some the symptoms settle over a few months but in others the discomfort has persisted for years.

Mild degrees of pulmonary overpressurization occurring on ascent but insufficient to cause barotrauma may result in restriction of venous return to the heart and syncope [40].

Decompression sickness (the lung as a bubble filter)

The lung, or rather the pulmonary circulation, plays a critical role in the prevention of decompression illness. Decompression illness results from the formation of gas bubbles within body tissues from inert gas previously dissolved in tissues. As the ambient pressure falls, tissues become supersaturated with inert gas that may then come out of solution. Gas in tissues results in limb pain (the bends), constitutional symptoms of fatigue and malaise and diverse neurological manifestations. More severe episodes may cause respiratory symptoms, circulatory collapse and even death. Bubbles form in many tissues but a considerable proportion find their way into peripheral capillaries and travel through the venous circulation to the lung [41–43]. A gas bubble acts as a foreign surface, thus provoking a response from the coagulation system and being rapidly transformed into a small protein–platelet embolus with a gas nucleus [44]. These microbubbles pass into the pulmonary circulation and are trapped within the pulmonary capillary bed [45]. The quantity of gas bubbles formed during or after a decompression can be monitored using ultrasound imaging or Doppler techniques [46,47]. Neurological manifestations of decompression illness appear to be associated with the appearance of bubbles within the arterial circulation [47]. Bubbles may gain access to the arterial circulation in the presence of a right-to-left cardiac shunt, for example atrial septal defect [48] or patent foramen ovale [49,50], in the presence of intra-

pulmonary shunting or when the volume of bubbles is sufficient to cause a rise in pulmonary arterial pressure above a threshold, as has been demonstrated in an animal model [51,52]. There is growing evidence that pulmonary abnormalities that may be associated with a disturbance of pulmonary circulation are risk factors for neurological decompression illness [53].

Pulmonary decompression sickness presents with severe symptoms of chest tightness, breathlessness and cough and is due to massive bubble embolization of the pulmonary capillary bed, usually as result of severe decompression stress (omitted decompression). Fortunately, such presentations are rare but are often fatal and almost inevitably associated with severe neurological manifestations. However, mild respiratory symptoms of transient chest tightness and cough are commonly reported in divers shortly before the onset of neurological symptoms and may represent a lesser degree of pulmonary bubble embolization.

Obstructive airways disease has been identified as an independent risk factor [53] and there are anecdotal case reports of decompression sickness in association with unilateral absent pulmonary artery [50].

The process of bubble capture within the pulmonary capillary bed is also a cause of concern with regard to possible long-term effects. A fall in diffusing capacity (D_{LCO}) occurs after deep saturation dives [54], where the potential for bubble formation is present over several days, but has also been reported after short air dives to 50 msw [55].

Other diving-related pulmonary illness

Oxygen toxicity

While oxygen is essential for life, it is unfortunately also toxic when breathed at increased pressure. Oxygen causes two major varieties of acute toxic effect. At partial pressures above about 130 kPa, neurological effects may occur that can include muscular twitching, jerks and convulsions. The risks increase with partial pressure and are also increased with exertion and carbon dioxide retention. Hence partial pressures of up to 300 kPa may be used therapeutically with a resting patient but pressures above 150 kPa are a significant risk to a diver in the water. A convulsion may have a fatal outcome for a diver using a simple scuba demand valve held in the mouth by the teeth, and hence a band mask or helmet that enables the diver to use an oronasal mask is a crucial safety precaution when oxygen-enriched breathing mixtures are used. Divers who use oxygen-enriched breathing gas mixtures to obtain a decompression advantage are at risk of cerebral oxygen toxicity [53].

Oxygen also exerts a direct toxic effect on the lung.

Minor abnormalities of lung function have been demonstrated after breathing oxygen at partial pressures of less than 50 kPa [56] and animal experiments have demonstrated histological abnormalities after exposure to oxygen at partial pressures of 60 kPa [57]. In practice, divers tolerate partial pressures of up to 50 kPa for prolonged periods without any obvious symptoms [58]. Above a partial pressure of 50 kPa the onset of symptoms is dose dependent in terms of both partial pressure and duration [59,60]. Acute symptoms of chest soreness on inspiration and cough may occur after 2–3 h at 300 kPa or after longer exposure at lower partial pressure [61]. If exposure is continued, the symptoms progress to include severe discomfort on inspiration, breathlessness and ultimately pulmonary oedema and respiratory failure with the development of diffuse alveolar damage. There have been a number of attempts to characterize the physiological abnormality. The earliest abnormality on investigation is a reduction of VC [61], although it is not clear whether this is a direct result of early development of oedema or simply a result of discomfort on inspiration. At a later stage a more obvious restrictive defect develops and is associated with impairment of diffusing capacity (D_{LCO}) [61]. This is a reversible effect and symptoms usually subside over a period of 24–48 h after the end of exposure. The mechanism of oxygen toxicity appears to be the result of local tissue P_{O_2} increasing the concentration of oxygen free radicals and overcoming the body's normal defence mechanisms. This results in a primary endothelial lesion [62,63]. Evidence for the vascular nature of the lesion is supported by animal studies demonstrating abnormal endothelial cell biochemistry [64–66] as well as by human studies [67,68].

In practice, the development of pulmonary oxygen toxicity presents a problem in the management of decompression illness where divers are treated with quite prolonged periods of hyperbaric oxygenation. This is particularly true when the provocative dive involved the use of oxygen during the decompression or when treatment needs to be repeated. However, tolerance to oxygen can be increased by brief interruptions to the exposure [69,70] and hence most treatment regimens [58] use intermittent oxygen rather than continuous treatment. The use of relatively hyperoxic breathing gas mixtures during saturation diving has also raised concerns about possible long-term effects [71]. It has been standard practice during saturation diving for the breathing gas in chambers to be maintained with a partial pressure of oxygen of about 40 kPa [58]. While divers are working in the water this is increased to about 80 kPa and in the decompression phase to about 50 kPa. Hence divers may be exposed to partial pressures above 40 kPa for periods of up to a month at a time. Small decrements in diffusing capacity (D_{LCO}) have been observed after deep saturation dives [54,72] and there is

some evidence to suggest that oxygen exposure may be at least partially responsible [73].

Near drowning

Many emergency situations in diving may lead to inhalation of water and partial or near drowning. Lesser degrees of water inhalation are probably very common due to leaky demand valves and may be the cause for the so-called saltwater aspiration syndrome [74]. It appears that humans who drown may inhale only very small quantities of water [75]; animal models have shown that very small amounts of inhaled water produce substantial disturbance of lung function, with reduction in lung volume and fall in both compliance and Sa_{O_2} [76]. Hence patients who have suffered a near-drowning incident are inevitably hypoxaemic with a substantial shunt [77]. Clinical examination may reveal little or no abnormality. A chest radiograph may also be normal but may show the development of diffuse alveolar damage (adult respiratory distress syndrome) during the first 12–24 h (Figs 57.3 & 57.4). Hence such patients should always be assessed in hospital and remain under observation during the first 24 h. Management is supportive and may require administration of oxygen, ventilation, antibiotic therapy for secondary infection and other intensive care support. Most patients recover fully, although complete recovery of lung function may take months. A few patients show evidence of permanent lung injury [78] but of more significance is the substantial proportion who survive with permanent neurological injury following the period of hypoxaemia [79].

Most near-drowning accidents in divers occur when the diver is on or close to the surface. However, inhalation of water can occur as a result of various situations at depth, including buddy breathing exercises, failure of demand valve or exhaustion of gas supply. In these situations the immediate effect of water inhalation is partially masked by the increased partial pressure of oxygen in the breathing gas. For example, at 20 msw the diver breathing air has a partial pressure of oxygen equivalent to breathing 60% oxygen on the surface. This may be sufficient to maintain a normal Sa_{O_2}. However, the exertion required to ascend, while at the same time the partial pressure of oxygen in the alveoli is falling, may result in loss of consciousness on arrival at the surface due to acute hypoxia [80,81].

Many diving fatalities are recorded as drowning and while this may be the final pathological insult, other events may have led to incapacitation in the water. The postmortem examination of divers is complex since the presence of gas in tissues may be of considerable importance. Radiological examination [82] and other specialized techniques may be valuable [83,84].

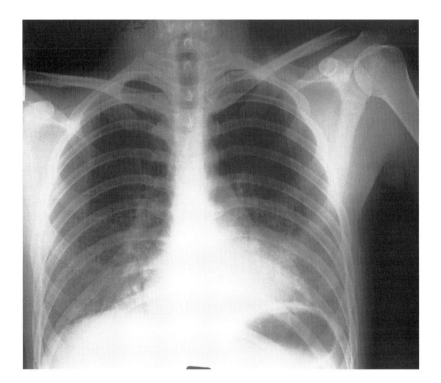

Fig. 57.3 Chest radiograph of a diver after a near-drowning incident showing bilateral lower zone interstitial shadowing. Diver recovered with administration of supplementary oxygen only.

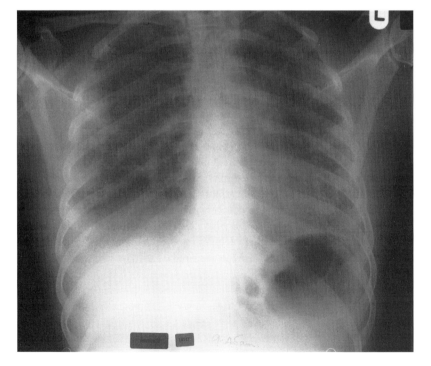

Fig. 57.4 Chest radiograph of a diver following a severe near-drowning incident showing widespread interstitial shadowing. Diver developed adult respiratory distress syndrome and was left with permanent impairment of lung function.

Trauma

Commercial divers are exposed to a number of underwater hazards that arise from the use of special tools. The use of oxygen cutting equipment has become widespread. This technique involves production of an electric arc using a welding rod. However, the rod is hollow and oxygen is fed under pressure through the rod into the arc in order to accelerate the rate at which the metal is burned. A number of major injuries have occurred as a result of this technique in which either oxygen or steam has collected in the pocket in close vicinity to the cut in progress and then exploded. The effects of the underwater blast have included direct chest trauma, pneumothorax and damage to the diver's helmet resulting in near drowning. Underwater blast may result in extensive tissue injury, particularly where there is a tissue–gas interface such as at the lung surface [85,86] (Fig. 57.5). Characteristically divers sustaining this injury suffer considerable widespread chest pain suggestive of multiple rib fractures. The management is largely dictated by the depth of the incident and whether the diver is recovered to the surface or to a diving bell and pressure chamber.

Although diving illness and environmental problems have been the major contributors to diving fatalities in the past [87], these problems have become progressively better controlled and trauma is becoming increasingly important as a cause of both morbidity [88] and mortality.

Hypoxia

In most circumstances the diver breathes a gas that has a partial pressure of oxygen higher than that in air on the surface. However, hypoxia may occur in a number of specific circumstances. The diver may be supplied with a breathing gas mixture containing too little or no oxygen. For example a mixture containing only 2% oxygen provides an adequate partial pressure at 100 msw but results in severe hypoxaemia at 10 or 20 msw. The breathing gas

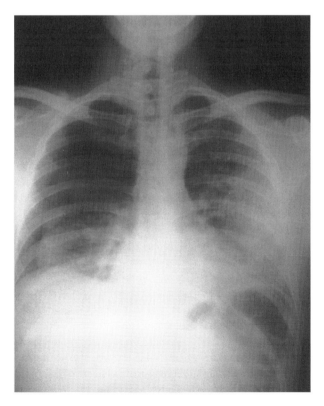

Fig. 57.5 Chest radiograph of a diver taken in a saturation chamber following an underwater explosion showing a pneumothorax on the right and extensive peripheral shadowing more marked on the left.

may be contaminated, for example the intake for an air compressor may include exhaust gas from the compressor's petrol engine resulting in carbon monoxide toxicity. The diver may lose breathing gas supply, and during the exertion of returning to the surface oxygen consumption may exceed the total available in the lung [80,81].

Rebreathing apparatus, which is extensively used for covert operations, also carries a risk of hypoxaemia. This is essentially a closed-circuit breathing system dependent on absorption of carbon dioxide and an adequate supply of oxygen. The supply of oxygen to the circuit needs to be adequate to meet the oxygen consumption of a diver, which may be high when the diver is shallow and not impeded by gas density, yet controlled such that at deeper depths when the diver is resting the oxygen partial pressure does not reach potentially toxic levels. These requirements demand complex equipment and training of the divers.

Cold gas

Diver's breathing gas is always cold since, with the exception of closed-circuit apparatus, it is almost inevitably supplied from a compressed gas source. The implications of breathing cold dry gas may be important for individuals with cold-induced wheeze. There are also considerable difficulties when helium is used as the inert gas because of its thermal characteristics. Helium has very high thermal conductivity and as a result respiratory heat loss is greatly increased, since the breathing gas acts as a heat conductor from the body core [89]. As the depth and gas density increases, the heat capacity of the breathing gas increases to the extent that respiratory heat loss exceeds the body's total heat production and hypothermia becomes inevitable unless the breathing gas is heated. In practice, this becomes essential below depths of 180 msw. Attempting to breathe cold helium–oxygen mixtures at great depth is difficult to tolerate and induces bronchorrhoea.

Cold exposure also has a significant impact on the circulation, with peripheral vasoconstriction, shift of fluid volume to the core and a resulting increase in pulmonary blood volume and rise in right heart pressures [90]. These effects are additive to those of immersion and may contribute to the phenomenon of immersion-induced pulmonary oedema [91], a condition that appears to be more likely in individuals with established or labile hypertension.

Long-term effects of diving on the lung

Considerable concern exists about the possibility that diving may have some adverse effect on the lung. There is no doubt that divers have larger lung volumes than standard reference populations [92–95]. This may be partly the result of selection but there is evidence from submarine escape tank instructors that a significant increase in lung volume can occur during a term of duty [96], presumably as a result of repetitive breath-hold diving acting as respiratory muscle training. However, in populations of commercial and military divers a consistent finding is a greater increase in FVC than FEV_1 [94,97]. Further investigation of the resulting reduction in the FEV_1/FVC ratio has indicated reduced flow at low lung volumes, which may represent a pathological injury to small airways [98–100]. Few longitudinal studies are available but do suggest a reduction in lung volume at a faster rate than anticipated from standard prediction equations [71,101]. These data are difficult to interpret since the change in lung volume during early adult life may not follow a progressive decline even though lung growth may continue until the late twenties [102]. If correct, a more rapid decline than predicted equations suggest may not be abnormal. After deep saturation dives, small but significant reductions in diffusing capacity (DLCO) have observed [54,93]. In some cases there has not been complete recovery. The two factors that may contribute to this are an effect due to long-term exposure to an elevated partial pressure of oxygen, insufficient to induce acute symptoms [73,103], and an inflammatory response to repetitive delivery of gas bubbles to the pulmonary vasculature during prolonged decompressions. Bubbles certainly result in an acute effect on the pulmonary vascular bed [104–106] and the extent of recovery is unclear. However, this effect would also be anticipated in air divers, who do not appear to be subject to the same effect on lung function [107].

Assessment of fitness to dive

Rationale

For the reasons obvious from the foregoing discussion, assessment of pulmonary fitness is of considerable importance to the diver. In the UK, commercial divers must undergo a statutory medical examination on an annual basis according to guidelines issued by the Health and Safety Executive [108]. Similar but less extensive medical examination systems are operated by the sport diving organizations and there is a considerable literature concerning this subject [109,110]. Although it is often argued that recreational diving does not require the same medical standards as commercial diving, the safety issues are the same and in practice the risks associated with recreational diving are often greater. It is more important to consider fitness in relation to the type of diving the individual will undertake.

In the UK, the medical examination of commercial divers must be carried out by a doctor approved by the Health and Safety Executive. Although the medical examination of sport divers may be performed by any doctor, there is a strong argument for seeking advice from a doctor with appropriate knowledge of diving and the medical issues involved.

The objectives of assessment of fitness are to ensure that the potential diver is not suffering from a pre-existing condition that represents an increased risk to the health of the diver and his/her buddies and to ensure an adequate exercise capacity in order to cope with the physical exertion of diving. These two objectives are closely related since involvement in a rescue of an injured or incapacitated diver may be the most strenuous activity a diver has to undertake. It is important to recognize that all diving activities rely upon the divers providing mutual support in the event of emergency. In recreational diving this is known as the buddy system; in most commercial operations, a standby diver is a legal requirement. The diver's ability to respond to assist another diver forms the most important baseline for standards of fitness in terms of exercise capacity. It is reasonable for any diver to expect that other divers who may be required to assist in an emergency are not inefficient in this respect as a result of poor fitness.

Medical history

The medical history should be free from symptoms of undue exertional breathlessness, cough, chest pain or other limitations to exercise. A history of significant lung disease that may have resulted in a permanent impairment of lung function or structure should be investigated further. Significant kyphosis or other restriction of thoracic movement, diaphragmatic paralysis, etc. represent contraindications. Previous spontaneous pneumothorax is a contraindication as this indicates the presence of an anatomical defect that has ruptured under normal environmental conditions. Although the risk of recurrence falls with time, such defects are more likely to rupture under conditions of increased transpulmonary pressure and the occurrence of a pneumothorax underwater is likely to be fatal due to the tension associated with increasing pleural gas volume on ascent. Conversely, following an uncomplicated traumatic pneumothorax the individual may be able to return to diving, provided that complete recovery occurs. In this situation it is presumed that the lung was normal initially and that complete recovery can occur. Hence provided that lung function and chest radiography returns to normal, the individual can return to diving; high-resolution CT provides greater confidence of the absence of any structural lesion after such trauma. Thoracic surgery is generally considered to represent a contraindication since there is a high risk of pleural adhesion following thoracotomy. For this reason surgical prevention of recurrent pneumothorax by pleurectomy does not change the situation regarding unfitness to dive.

Exercise underwater

Unfortunately, there is very little information available that provides an accurate measure of the workload in terms of oxygen consumption associated with a diver rescue. Similarly, the relationship between aerobic performance on the surface and work capacity in the water is uncertain. Exercise tests underwater using fin swimming as the exercise have demonstrated that oxygen consumptions of up to 2.5 mL/kg/min can be achieved [18]. This is substantially less than levels achieved on the surface during treadmill walking, which may reflect the different types of muscles involved and the fact that the diver is weightless.

Despite these limitations some assessment of exercise capacity is valuable. In the absence of contrary evidence, it can be assumed that there is a relationship between performance on the surface and underwater ability. A reasonable fitness standard is to require divers to achieve an aerobic performance level that is not below the 50th percentile for individuals in that age group. However, since exercise tolerance falls with age, it would be prudent to use age 40 as the reference age group for all divers over 40. In practice this standard presents little difficulty for the vast majority of divers both recreational and commercial.

Lung function

The diver's lung function should be normal or, if there is any impairment, this should not be sufficient to affect the diver's ability to exercise underwater. The diver's lungs should not have any anatomical or physiological abnormality that increases the risk of pulmonary barotrauma and the diver should not have any condition that might impair the function of the lung as a bubble filter.

From considerations of pulmonary physiology during exercise and diving, the symptomatic effect of a significant deviation from normal lung function is likely to be magnified in the underwater environment. Hence anyone with abnormal breathlessness on the surface should be considered unfit to dive. The possible exception to this is asthma where the symptoms and functional abnormality is transient (see below).

Investigations

A chest radiograph is considered essential before commencing diving and is an absolute requirement for commercial divers, although some sport diving associations permit diving without a previous chest film. The purpose of the chest radiograph is to exclude major anatomical defects such as bullae, areas of fibrosis or scarring that may contribute to air trapping or be associated with impaired compliance and hence represent a risk factor for lung rupture [37,38]. Small old scars due to previous pulmonary tuberculosis do not appear to represent a risk.

Lung function is usually assessed by simple spirometric indices of FEV_1, FVC and peak expiratory flow rate or flow–volume loop analysis. The purpose is to exclude individuals with diminished lung volume or evidence of airways obstruction. Airways obstruction and the associated air trapping may represent a risk factor for pulmonary barotrauma, although the evidence to support this theoretical risk is limited. However, given that medical examiners have tended to exclude those with obvious abnormalities from diving, the absence of epidemiological evidence to support a risk is not all that surprising. Fortunately, pulmonary barotrauma is a very rare problem and in most cases there is an obvious dive-related provocative factor. This makes assessment of the risk associated with a pre-existing medical problem very difficult. A recent study of submarine escape trainees has demonstrated that the risk of pulmonary barotrauma appears to relate better to the lung volume, i.e. FVC, than to FEV_1, although the association is weak [28].

The results of lung function tests should be considered in association with the exercise test result. An individual with poor exercise performance and impaired or marginally reduced lung function resulting in poor exercise tolerance is very likely to have substantial difficulty underwater and is unfit. Conversely, if lung function is good, the individual with poor exercise tolerance should be able to demonstrate an improvement with training. A repeat FEV_1 after an exercise test also provides a simple screen for the presence of exercise-induced wheeze.

The lung as a bubble filter

This is a more controversial area but one likely to become of much greater importance in the future. It is established that the lung acts as a filter to remove bubbles from the circulation and that appearance of bubbles in the arterial circulation is associated with decompression sickness. The Divers Alert Network (DAN) study [111], which set out to look for an association between asthma and pulmonary barotrauma, found an association with diving incidents but not with barotrauma, suggestive of a possible increased risk of decompression illness. This may be related to intrapulmonary shunting since cardiac shunt is a well-recognized risk factor [48–50]. A study by Wilmshurst and colleagues [53] also provides evidence for a relationship between decompression illness and lung disease.

Returning to dive after a diving accident

There is little published information about the risk of returning to dive following a diving injury. A critical issue is whether lung function returns to normality after an episode of pulmonary barotrauma. There is some published evidence of individuals having repeated episodes [20], although not all these cases had objective evidence of lung rupture. Colebatch and colleagues [39] found evidence of impairment of lung compliance in survivors of pulmonary barotrauma but it is unclear whether this abnormality existed before, or resulted from, the incidents. It is generally agreed that a diver who experiences an episode of pulmonary barotrauma during normal diving practice should be regarded as having a pre-existing risk factor and be advised not to dive. The diver in whom pulmonary barotrauma occurs as a result of an explosive ascent may be assumed to have had normal lungs before the incident. Hence if a complete recovery is made with a return to normal lung function and no anatomical abnormality can be demonstrated by high-resolution or spiral CT, a return to diving may be possible.

Asthma

Asthma represents a special situation because it is increasingly common, a growing number of asthmatic subjects wish to dive and because symptoms are transient. The issue has been extensively considered [112,113]. There is no doubt that some asthmatics can and do dive regularly [114] but they may be at increased risk. The DAN study in the USA found that although there was no over-representation of people with asthma among individuals with episodes of pulmonary barotrauma, there was an over-representation of asthmatics when all categories of diving accident were considered together. This is probably a significant finding since many asthmatic patients have received and taken medical advice not to dive. Similarly in an Australian study of diving fatalities, 9% of cases had a diagnosis of asthma [115]. There are various anecdotal reports of both barotrauma in patients with asthma [116] and acute breathlessness occurring in the water [117]. It seems reasonable that there is an increased risk but it may not apply to all patients with asthma.

Potential problems for the diver with asthma would include impairment of exercise capacity, inability to tolerate breathing apparatus, effect of medication on cardiac function, incapacitation due to an episode of wheezing while underwater (which may be provoked by breathing cold gas), breathing dense gas and the possible increased risk of decompression sickness.

Bronchodilator agents, particularly β_2 stimulants, all have a cardiac effect that may result in unexpected interaction with the cardiac stimuli associated with diving such as immersion, cold and the diving reflex. On the other hand, their potential protective effect against episodes in the water is used as an argument to support their regular use before diving by some. The diver should be able to go into the water without significant risk of an episode occurring, and the need or desire to take a dose before a dive suggests that symptom control is inadequate. Other agents used prophylactically, such as salmeterol or eformoterol, also indicate more severe symptoms or greater difficulty in control. Theophyllines are a contraindication because of cardiac and gastric side-effects and because (at least in the UK) their use indicates poor control [118]. Intensive bronchodilator therapy and theophylline therapy may represent a risk for decompression illness as a result of intrapulmonary shunt.

At present, some patients with asthma may be certified fit to dive provided that they can meet the following criteria.

1 When well they are free of symptoms, with normal lung function and no impairment of exercise capacity.

2 They should not dive if they have current symptoms.

3 They should not have exercise- or cold-induced symptoms.

4 Their asthma should be stable, predictable and well controlled and they should not have a regular need for use of relief bronchodilator.

5 Patients whose asthma is well controlled on inhaled steroids may meet these criteria even if they use inhaled bronchodilator regularly before each inhaled steroid.

To establish compliance with these criteria an accurate record of previous health from a general practitioner is essential. Asthmatics should be able to demonstrate normal exercise tolerance and the absence of exercise-induced symptoms. Patients whose asthma is brittle, who have had a recent history of severe episodes or who have a regular requirement for relief inhaler therapy or other additional support therapy should be advised not to dive. Above all, patients with asthma need to be informed of the possible increase in risk for asthmatics who dive and that diving when their asthma is troublesome may substantially increase the risk. They should be aware of how to control these risks by modifying their diving practice. Unfortunately, it is very difficult to predict how a patient with asthma will respond to their first diving experience [117].

References

1 *Diver* 1993; 38: 40.

2 Arborelius M, Balldin UI, Lilja B, Lundgren CEG. Hemodynamic changes in man during immersion with the head above water. *Aerospace Med* 1972; 43: 592.

3 Flynn ET, Saltzman HA, Summitt JK. Effects of head-out immersion at 19.18 Ata on pulmonary gas exchange in man. *J Appl Physiol* 1972; 33: 113.

4 Lollgren H, Von Neiding G, Krekeler H,

Smidt U, Koppenhagen K, Frank H. Respiratory gas exchange and lung perfusion in man during and after head-out water immersion. *Undersea Biomed Res* 1976; 3: 49.

5 Robertson CH, Engle CM, Bradley ME. Lung volumes in man immersed to the neck: dilution and plethysmographic techniques. *J Appl Physiol* 1978; 44: 679.

6 Prefaut C, Lupich E, Anthonisen NR. Human lung mechanics during water immersion. *J Appl Physiol* 1976; 40: 320.

7 Dahlback GO, Lundgren CEG. Pulmonary air-trapping induced by water immersion. *Aerospace Med* 1972; 43: 768.

8 Lanphier EH, Rahn H. Alveolar gas exchange during breath-hold diving. *J Appl Physiol* 1963; 18: 471.

9 Song SH, Lee WK, Chung YA, Hong SK. Mechanism of apneic bradycardia in man. *J Appl Physiol* 1969; 27: 323.

10 Sterba JA, Lundgren CEG. Diving bradycardia and breath-holding time in man. *Undersea Biomed Res* 1985; 12: 139.

11 Frey MAB, Kenney RA. Changes in left ventricular activity during apnoea and face immersion. *Undersea Biomed Res* 1977; 4: 27.

12 Lopez-Majano V, Data PG, Martignoni R, Lossredo B, Arborelius M. Pulmonary blood flow distribution in erect man in air and during breath-hold diving. *Aviat Space Environ Med* 1990; 61: 1107.

13 Morrison JB, Butt WS, Florio JT, Mayo IC. Effects of increased O_2–N_2 pressure and breathing apparatus on respiratory function. *Undersea Biomed Res* 1976; 3: 217.

14 Dressendorfer RH, Morlock JF, Baker DG, Hong SK. Effects of head-out water immersion on cardiorespiratory responses to maximal cycling exercise. *Undersea Biomed Res* 1976; 3: 177.

15 Wood LDH, Bryan AC. Effect of increased ambient pressure on flow–volume curve of the lung. *J Appl Physiol* 1969; 27: 4.

16 Maio DA, Farhi LE. Effect of gas density on mechanics of breathing. *J Appl Physiol* 1967; 23: 687.

17 Shepherd RJ. The maximum sustained voluntary ventilation in exercise. *Clin Sci* 1967; 32: 167.

18 Lanphier EH, Camporesi EM. Respiration and exercise. In: Bennett PB, Elliott DH, eds. *The Physiology and Medicine of Diving*, 3rd edn. London: Baillière Tindall, 1982: 99.

19 Elliott DH, Harrison JAB, Barnard EEP. Clinical and radiological features of 88 cases of decompression barotrauma. In: Shilling CW, Beckett MW, eds. *Underwater Physiology VI*. Bethesda, Maryland: FASEB, 1978: 527.

20 Leitch DR, Green RD. Recurrent pulmonary barotrauma. *Aviat Space Environ Med* 1986; 57: 1039.

21 Warkander DE, Norfleet WT, Nagasawa GK, Lundgren CEG. CO_2 retention with minimal symptoms but severe dysfunction during wet simulated dives to 6.8 atm abs. *Undersea Biomed Res* 1990; 17: 515.

22 Strauss MB, Wright PW. Thoracic squeeze diving casualty. *Aerospace Med* 1971; 42: 673.

23 Balk M, Goldman JM. Alveolar haemorrhage as a manifestation of pulmonary barotrauma after scuba diving. *Ann Emerg Med* 1990; 19: 930.

24 Macklin MT, Macklin CC. Malignant interstitial emphysema of the lungs and mediastinum as an important occult complication in many respiratory diseases and other conditions: an interpretetion of the clinical literature in the light of laboratory experiment. *Medicine* 1944; 23: 281.

25 Schriger DL, Rosenberg G, Wilder RJ. Shoulder pain and pneumoperitoneum following a diving accident. *Ann Emerg Med* 1996; 16: 1281.

26 Rashleigh-Belcher C, Ballham A. Pneumoperitoneum in a sport diver. *Br J Accid Surg* 1996; 16: 47.

27 Leitch DR, Green RD. Pulmonary barotrauma in divers and the treatment of cerebral arterial gas embolism. *Aviat Space Environ Med* 1986; 57: 931.

28 Benton PJ, Woodfine JD, Francis TJR. A review of spirometry and UK submarine escape training tank incidents (1987–1993) using objective diagnostic criteria. In: *Are Asthmatics Fit to Dive?* Kensington, Maryland: Undersea and Hyperbaric Medical Society, 1996: 17.

29 Schaeffer KE, McNulty WP, Carey C, Liebow A. Mechanisms in development of interstitial emphysema and air embolism on decompression from depth. *J Appl Physiol* 1958; 13: 15.

30 Kol S, Weisz G, Melamed Y. Pulmonary barotrauma after a free dive: a possible mechanism. *Aviat Space Environ Med* 1993; 64: 236.

31 Bayne CG, Wurzbacher T. Can pulmonary barotrauma cause cerebral air embolism in a non-diver? *Chest* 1982; 81: 648.

32 Krzyzak J. A case of delayed onset pulmonary barotrauma in a scuba diver. *Undersea Biomed Res* 1987; 14: 553.

33 Daugherty CG. Inherent unsaturation in the treatment of pneumothorax at depth. *Undersea Biomed Res* 1990; 17: 171.

34 Gillen HW. Symptomatology of cerebral gas embolism. *Neurology* 1968; 18: 507.

35 Dutka AJ. A review of the pathophysiology and potential application of experimental therapies for cerebral ischaemia to the treatment of cerebral arterial gas embolism. *Undersea Biomed Res* 1985; 12: 403.

36 Gorman D, Richardson D. The SPUMS workshop on emergency ascent training. *SPUMS J* 1993; 23: 236.

37 Maklem H, Emhjellen S, Horgen O. Pulmonary barotrauma and arterial gas embolism caused by an emphysematous bulla in a scuba diver. *Aviat Space Environ Med* 1990; 61: 559.

38 Calder IM. Autopsy and experimental observations on factors leading to barotrauma in man. *Undersea Biomed Res* 1985; 12: 165.

39 Colebatch HJH, Smith MM, Ng CKY. Increased elastic recoil as a determinant of pulmonary barotrauma in divers. *Respir Physiol* 1976; 26: 55.

40 Thorsen E, Segedal K, Kambestad BK. Mechanisms of reduced pulmonary function after a saturation dive. *Eur Resp J* 1994; 7: 4.

41 Smith KH, Spencer MP. Doppler indices of decompression sickness: their evaluation and use. *Aerospace Med* 41: 1970; 1396.

42 Masurel G, Gardette B, Comet M, Kisman K, Guillerm R. Ultrasonic detection of circulating bubbles during Janus IV excursion dives at sea to 460 and 501 MSW. *Undersea Biomed Res* 1978; 5 (Suppl): 29.

43 Brubakk AO, Petersen R, Grip A *et al*. Gas bubbles in the circulation of divers after ascending excursions from 300 to 250 MSW. *J Appl Physiol* 1986; 60: 45.

44 Philp RB, Inwood MJ, Warren BA. Interactions between gas bubbles and components of the blood: implications in decompression sickness. *Aerospace Med* 1997; 43: 946.

45 Butler BD, Hills BA. The lung as a filter for microbubbles. *J Appl Physiol* 1979; 47: 537.

46 Spencer MP, Clarke HF. Precordial monitoring of pulmonary gas embolism and decompression bubbles. *Aerospace Med* 1972; 43: 762.

47 Nishi RY. Doppler and ultrasonic bubble detection. In: Bennett PB, Elliott DH, eds. *The Physiology and Medicine of Diving*, 4th edn. London: WB Saunders, 1993: 433.

48 Wilmshurst PT, Ellis BG, Jenkins BS. Paradoxical gas embolism in a scuba diver with an atrial septal defect. *Br Med J* 1986; 293: 1277.

49 Moon RE, Camporesi EM, Kisslo JA. Patent foramen ovale and decompression sickness in divers. *Lancet* 1989; i: 513.

50 Wilmshurst PT, Byrne JC, Webb-Peploe MM. Relation between interatrial shunts and decompression sickness in divers. *Lancet* 1989; ii: 1302.

51 Butler. BD, Hills BA. Transpulmonary passage of venous air emboli. *J Appl Physiol* 1985; 59: 543.

52 Butler BD, Katz J. Vascular pressures and passage of gas emboli through the pulmonary circulation. *Undersea Biomed Res* 1988; 15: 203.

53 Wilmshurst PT, Davidson C, O'Connell G, Byrne C. Role of cardiorespiratory abnormalities, smoking and dive characteristics in the manifestations of neurologicical decompression illness. *Clin Sci* 1994; 86: 297.

54 Thorsen E, Segadal K, Myrseth E, Pasche A, Gulsvik A. Pulmonary mechanical function and diffusion capacity after deep saturation dives. *Br J Ind Med* 1990; 47: 242.

55 Dujic Z, Eterovic D, Denoble P, Krstacic G, Tocili J, Gosovic S. Effect of a single air dive on pulmonary diffusing capacity in professional divers. *J Appl Physiol* 1993; 74: 55.

56 Griffith DE, Holden WE, Morris JF, Min LK, Krishnamurthy GT. Effects of common therapeutic concentrations of oxygen on lung clearance of ^{99m}Tc DTPA and broncho alveolar lavage albumin concentration. *Am Rev Respir Dis* 1986; 134: 233.

57 Dobuler KJ, Catravas JD, Gillis NC. Early detection of oxygen-induced lung injury in conscious rabbits. *Am Rev Respir Dis* 1982; 126: 534.

58 Saturation Diving. In: *United States Navy Diving Manual*, Revision 3. Flagstaff, Arizona: Best Publishing Company, 1991; 2: 53.

59 Fisher AB, Hyde RW, Puy RJM, Clark JM, Lambertson CJ. Effect of oxygen at 2 atmospheres on the pulmonary mechanics of normal man. *J Appl Physiol* 1968; 24: 529.

60 Clark JM, Jackson RM, Lambertson CJ, Gelfand R, Hiller WDB, Unger M. Pulmonary function in men after oxygen breathing at 3.0 ata for 3.5 hours. *J Appl Physiol* 1991; 71: 878.

61 Clark JM. Oxygen toxicity. In: Bennett PB, Elliott DH, eds. *The Physiology and Medicine of Diving*, 3rd edn. London: Baillière Tindall, 1982: 200.

62 Bruce Davis W, Rennard SI, Bitterman PB, Crystal RG. Pulmonary oxygen toxicity: early reversible changes in human alveolar structures induced by hyperoxia. *N Engl J Med* 1983; 309: 878.

63 Crapo JD, Barry BE, Foscue HA, Shelburne J. Structural and biochemical changes in rat lungs occurring during exposures to lethal

and adaptive doses of oxygen. *Am Rev Respir Dis* 1980; 122: 123.

64 Block ER, Fisher AB. Depression of sero-tonin clearance by rat lungs during oxygen exposure. *J Appl Physiol* 1977; 42: 33.

65 Allen MC, Watt SJ. Effect of hyperbaric and normobaric oxygen on pulmonary endothelial cell function. *Undersea Hyperbaric Med* 1993; 20: 39.

66 Kistler GS, Caldwell PRB, Weibel ER. Development of fine ultra-structural damage to alveolar and capillary ling cells in oxygen poisoned rats. *J Cell Biol* 1967; 33: 605.

67 Puy RJM, Hyde RW, Fisher AB, Clark JM, Dickson J, Lambertson CJ. Alterations in the pulmonary capillary bed during early oxygen toxicity in man. *J Appl Physiol* 1968; 24: 537.

68 Nash G, Blennerhasset JB, Pontoppidan H. Pulmonary lesions associated with oxygen therapy and artificial ventilation. *N Engl J Med* 1967; 279: 368.

69 Penrod KE. Effect of intermittent nitrogen exposures on tolerance to oxygen at high pressures. *Am J Phys* 1956; 186: 149.

70 Hendricks PL, Hall DA, Hunter WI, Haley PJ. Extension of pulmonary O_2 tolerance in man at 2 ata by intermittent O_2 exposure. *J Appl Physiol* 1977; 42: 593.

71 Radermacher P, Muth CM, Santak B, Wenzel J. A case of breath holding and ascent-induced circulatory hypotension. *Undersea Hyperbaric Med* 1993; 20: 159.

72 Thorsen E, Hjelle J, Segedal K, Gulsvik A. Exercise tolerance and pulmonary gas exchange after deep saturation dives. *J Appl Physiol* 1990; 68: 1809.

73 Thorsen E, Segedal K, Reed JW, Elliott C, Gulsvik A, Hjelle J. Contribution of hyperoxia to reduced pulmonary function after deep saturation dives. *J Appl Physiol* 1993; 75: 657.

74 Edmonds C. A salt water aspiration syndrome. *Milit Med* 1970; 135: 779.

75 Harries MG. Drowning in man. *Crit Care Med* 1981; 9: 407.

76 Modell JH. *The Pathophysiology and Treatment of Drowning and Near Drowning.* Springfield, Illinois: CC Thomas, 1996.

77 Colebatch HJH, Halmagyi DFJ. Lung mechanics and resuscitation after fluid aspiration. *J Appl Physiol* 1961; 16: 684.

78 Laughlin JJ, Eigen HE. Pulmonary function abnormalities in survivors of near drowning. *J Pediatr* 1982; 100: 26.

79 Modell JH, Graves SA, Kluck EJ. Near-drowning: correlation of level of consciousness and survival. *Can Anaesth Soc J* 1980; 27: 211.

80 Harpur GD. Hypoxia in out of air ascents: a preliminary report. *SPUMS J* 1984; 14: 24.

81 Watt SJ, Ross JAS, Stephenson RN. Hypoxia of ascent: an underestimated cause of impaired consciousness on surfacing. *Undersea Biomed Res* 1994; 21 (Suppl): 58.

82 Nelson EE. Internal carotid artery dissection associated with scuba diving. *Ann Emerg Med* 1995; 25: 103.

83 Calder IM. A method for investigating specialised accidents with special reference to diving. *Forensic Sci Int* 1997; 27: 119.

84 Calder IM. Use of post mortem radiographs for the investigation of underwater and hyperbaric deaths. *Undersea Biomed Res* 1987; 14: 113.

85 Williams ERP. Blast effects in warfare. *Br J Surg* 1942; 30: 38.

86 Wakely PG. Effect of underwater explosions on the human body. *Lancet* 1945; i: 715.

87 Bradley ME. Commercial diving fatalities. *Aviat Space Environ Med* 1984; 55: 721.

88 Gunnyeon WJ, McLeod TNN, Rhodes PM, Ross JAS, Watt SJ. A diving medical emergency service experience of 211 cases arising during commercial diving in the North Sea. *Undersea Biomed Res* 1992; 19 (Suppl): 21.

89 Sterba JA. Thermal problems: prevention and treatment. In: Bennett PB, Elliott DH, eds. *The Physiology and Medicine of Diving,* 4th edn. London: WB Saunders, 1993: 301.

90 Glasser EM, Berridge FR. Effects of heat and cold on the distribution of blood within the human body. *Clin Sci* 1950; 9: 181.

91 Wilmshurst PT, Crowther A, Nuri M, Webb-Peploe MM. Cold-induced pulmonary oedema in scuba divers and swimmers and subsequent development of hypertension. *Lancet* 1989; i: 62.

92 Hong SK, Rahn H, Kang DH, Song SH, Kang BS. Diving pattern, lung volumes and alveolar gas of the Korean diving woman (ama). *J Appl Physiol* 1963; 18: 457.

93 Cotes JE, Davey IS, Reed JW, Rooks M. Respiratory effects of a single saturation dive to 300 meters. *Br J Ind Med* 1987; 44: 76.

94 Crosbie WA, Clarke MB, Cox RAF *et al.* Physical characteristics and ventilatory function of 404 commercial divers working in the North Sea. *Br J Ind Med* 1977; 34: 19.

95 Cimsit M, Flook V. Pulmonary function in divers. In: Bachrach AJ, Matzen MM, eds. *Underwater Physiology VIII.* Bethesda, Maryland: Undersea Medical Society, 1981: 245.

96 Carey CR, Schaefer KE, Alvis HJ. Effect of skin diving on lung volumes. *J Appl Physiol* 1956; 8: 519.

97 Clifford GM, Smith DJ, Searing CSM. A comparison of lung volumes between divers and submariners in the Royal Navy. *J R Nav Med Serv* 1984; 70: 143.

98 Crosbie WA, Reed JW, Clarke MC. Functional characteristics of the large lungs found in divers. *J Appl Physiol* 1979; 46: 639.

99 Davey IS, Cotes JE, Reed JW. Does diving exposure induce airflow obstruction? *Clin Sci* 1983; 65: 48p.

100 Thorsen E, Segedal K, Kambestad B, Gulsvik A. Divers' lung function: small airways disease. *Br J Ind Med* 1990; 47: 519.

101 Watt SJ. Effect of commercial diving on ventilatory function. *Br J Ind Med* 1985; 42: 59.

102 Burrows B, Knudson RJ, Taussig LM, Lebowitz MD. A descriptive analysis of the growth and decline of the FVC and FEV_1. *Chest* 1983; 83: 717.

103 Thorsen E, Segedal K, Reed J *et al. Effects of raised partial pressure of oxygen on pulmonary function in saturation diving.* Bergen: Norwegian Underwater Technology Centre, 1992.

104 Perkett EA, Brigham KL, Meyrick B. Continuous air embolisation into sheep causes sustained pulmonary hypertension and increased pulmonary vasoactivity. *Am J Pathol* 1988; 132: 444.

105 Albertine KH, Weiner-Kronish JP, Koike K, Staub N. Quantification of damage by air emboli to lung microvessels in anaesthetized sheep. *J Appl Physiol* 1984; 57: 1360.

106 Flick MR, Milligan SA, Hoeffel JM, Goldstein IM. Catalase prevents increased lung vascular permeability during air emboli in unanesthetized sheep. *J Appl Physiol* 1988; 64: 929.

107 Watt SJ. Lung function in commercial air and saturation divers. *Undersea Biomed Res* 1994; 21 (Suppl): 25.

108 Health and Safety Executive. *MA1: the Medical Examination and Assessment of Divers.* London: HMSO, 1998.

109 Davis JC. *Medical Examination of Sport Scuba Divers,* 2nd edn. San Antonio: Medical Seminars, 1986.

110 Elliott DH. *Medical Assessment of Fitness to Dive.* London: Biomedical Seminars, 1995.

111 Corson KS, Dovenbarger JA, Moon RE, Hodder S, Bennett PB. Risk assessment of asthma for decompression illness. *Undersea Biomed Res* 1991; 18 (Suppl): 16.

112 Neuman TS, Bove AA, O'Connor RD, Kelsen SG. Asthma and diving. *Ann Allergy* 1994; 73: 344.

113 Elliott DH. *Are Asthmatics Fit to Dive?* Kensington, Maryland: Undersea and Hyperbaric Medical Society, 1996.

114 Farrell PJS, Glanvill P. Diving practices of scuba divers with asthma. *Br Med J* 1990; 300: 166.

115 Edmonds C, Walker D. Scuba diving fatalities in Australia and New Zealand. *SPUMS J* 1989; 19: 94.

116 Weiss LD, Van Meter KW. Cerebral air embolism in asthmatic scuba divers in a swimming pool. *Chest* 1995; 107: 1653.

117 Martindale JJ. Scuba divers with asthma. *Br Med J* 1990; 300: 609.

118 British Thoracic Society, National Asthma Campaign and Royal College of Physicians of London. The British guidelines on asthma management: 1995 review and position statement. *Thorax* 1997; 52: S1.

58

ASSISTED VENTILATION

JOHN M. SHNEERSON

Principles of ventilation

Mechanical ventilators transfer gas into and out of the lungs with the aim of optimizing oxygen transport and carbon dioxide elimination from the body. To achieve this they have to not only ventilate the lungs but also ensure that the mixing of gases within the lungs is efficient, that ventilation and perfusion are well matched and that the ventilator itself does not impair cardiac output. The ventilator therefore acts as an external pump that supplies energy to supplement or replace the activity of the normal respiratory pump. In addition, the ventilator has to fulfil at least some of the roles of the respiratory control system by determining the pattern of respiration. None of the currently available ventilators approaches the complexity and adaptability of the normal respiratory control system, although the microprocessors of modern ventilators are becoming increasingly sophisticated. There is an increasing number of methods of respiratory support that vary in the degree of assistance they provide and which almost merge with spontaneous respiration.

All the positive-pressure ventilators that are applied to the airway work on the principle that if the pressure in the ventilator exceeds that in the patient's alveoli, gas will enter the lungs. This contrasts with spontaneous and negative-pressure ventilation, in which the alveolar pressure is less than atmospheric pressure during inspiration. Positive-pressure ventilators require a source of pressurized gas to be delivered at a controllable flow or pressure to the patient without dilution with ambient air. The flow of inspired gas is intermittent in true mechanical ventilation but may be continuous in for instance continuous positive airway pressure (CPAP) support. The expired gas is conducted away from the patient without contaminating the inspired gas except in the dead space of the circuit close to the patient. Expiration is usually passive and due to the elastic recoil of the lungs and chest wall, but can be modified in various ways by the ventilator as well as by the patient's effort.

Negative-pressure ventilators differ from positive-pressure systems in that a subatmospheric pressure is applied intermittently around the chest and abdomen within a rigid and impervious enclosure so that air is drawn in through the mouth and nose. No appliance is required around or inside the airway and a source of pressurized gas is not needed since the energy of the ventilator is applied to the chest wall rather than to the airway. Negative-pressure systems are therefore a method of external ventilation in contrast to internal ventilation as typified by positive-pressure systems using a tracheostomy or endotracheal tube.

Control of inspiration

There are a number of ways in which inspiration can be influenced by the ventilator controls, the most important of which are discussed below.

Initiation of inspiration and termination of expiration

This is often called ventilatory triggering or cycling, although the latter term is confusing because it is also used to designate the changeover from inspiration to the start of expiration. Inspiration can be initiated by one or more of the following methods.

Time

The expiratory time can be preset so that inspiration follows after a predetermined interval or, on some ventilators, the total time for the inspiratory cycle can be set and the inspiratory–expiratory (I/E) ratio fixed.

Pressure

The development of a negative pressure by the patient's inspiratory effort can be sensed by the ventilator controls and used to trigger the inspiratory phase of the machine. The usual trigger threshold is 0.5–2 cmH$_2$O. Lower thresholds may lead to triggering of the ventilator by, for instance, cardiac impulses, small leaks or non-respiratory movements. Conversely, if the threshold is too high the patient's inspiratory work may be excessive and failure to trigger the ventilator may lead to incoordination between the patient and the ventilator.

Flow

Inspiration can be triggered when the flow generated by the patient increases above a threshold value set by the ventilator. This is used with some pressure-preset ventilators.

Volume

Inspiration can be initiated when a preset volume has been expired.

Termination of inspiration and initiation of expiration

Inspiration can be terminated by time, pressure, flow or volume criteria. In general the termination of inspiration by pressure is unsatisfactory and leads to incoordination between the patient and the ventilator. Flow cycling promotes coordination but is only suitable for pressure-preset ventilators. Time or volume cycling are appropriate for constant-flow generators.

Inspiratory pressure and flow waveforms

Flow generators

Ventilators that generate a predetermined flow rate and which have a fixed inspiratory time deliver a predictable tidal volume. The inspiratory flow may be constant, a half sine, ramp or a reverse ramp waveform, although there is remarkably little difference between these in most clinical situations. The adequacy of the mixing of inspired gas with air already in the lungs probably depends more on the inspiratory time than on the pattern of flow. The tidal volume is hardly altered by changes in the elastance or resistance of the ventilator circuit or patient, but in the presence of a leak the flow remains unchanged and the volume delivered to the patient falls. The airway pressure is determined by the elastance and resistance of the upper airways, lungs and chest wall and of the ventilator and circuit.

Pressure generators

This type of ventilator generates a predetermined pressure waveform that is often but not always a square wave. The inspiratory flow rate and tidal volume is determined by the transpulmonary pressure, which in turn is determined by the elastance and resistance of the lungs and the

patient's effort. The transpulmonary pressure is greatest initially when the pleural pressure is least and the inspiratory flow rate then decreases towards zero as the pressures in the airways equilibrate. Pressure generators do not provide a fixed tidal volume since this varies with the elastance and resistance of the patient, ventilator and circuit, although they can compensate for leaks by increasing their flow rate in order to maintain the preset pressure waveform.

Inspiratory limitation

Inspiratory limitation is a technique used to protect the patient against an excessive pressure or volume delivered by the ventilator. The unwanted gases are vented through a relief valve. Protection against high pressure is needed particularly with flow generators when the elastance and resistance are increased, and against increased volume delivery with pressure generators when they are reduced or if the patient's inspiratory effort increases.

End-inspiratory pause

An end-inspiratory pause is the period after the delivery of the inspired gas but before expiration starts. The airway pressure falls to a plateau level which, since there is no airflow, reflects the elastance of the respiratory system and is independent of the airflow resistance. During the pause, air enters alveoli which have prolonged time constants and their recruitment is thought to improve ventilation–perfusion matching, particularly in patients with diffuse lung diseases.

Sigh

A sigh can be mimicked by positive-pressure ventilators by the introduction of a periodic large inspiration. The depth of the mechanical sigh is usually 1.5–2 times the usual tidal volume and the frequency is often between 1 in 60 and 1 in 100 breaths. Sighs can reverse small airway closure and improve ventilation–perfusion matching but are not as effective as positive end-expiratory pressure (PEEP) or other manipulations of the ventilator controls, such as increasing the tidal volume.

Inspiratory–expiratory ratio, frequency and inspiratory–expiratory times

These various indices of ventilation are interrelated and alteration of one influences the others. Shortening the inspiratory time increases the flow rate in volume-preset generators and, particularly if it falls to less than about 1 s, the distribution of the inspired gas to the alveoli is impaired. Conversely, a prolonged inspiratory time may be uncomfortable and although it promotes gas mixing it also increases the mean airway pressure. A reduction in the expiratory time may lead to air trapping and increased end-expiratory pressure (auto-PEEP).

An increase in the respiratory frequency at any fixed I/E ratio reduces both the inspiratory and expiratory time. An I/E ratio of 1:2–2.5 is satisfactory for subjects with normal respiratory mechanics. A lower ratio reduces the mean airway pressure and increases the cardiac output but at the cost of a deterioration in ventilation–perfusion matching. Increasing the I/E ratio has the opposite effect. The extreme is inverse ratio ventilation, where the inspiratory time exceeds the expiratory time. This assists oxygenation through prolonging the inspiratory time and increasing the end-expiratory volume but may significantly reduce cardiac output.

Control of expiration

The most important methods of influencing expiration include the following.

Expiratory retard

This is a method of prolonging expiration by increasing the resistance of the expiration valve, usually by narrowing its diameter. It is equivalent to pursed-lip breathing in emphysema. Like this, it moves the equal pressure point proximally and so reduces air trapping. It differs from PEEP or CPAP in that the resistance does not have a threshold value above which it is brought into action. Expiratory retard has the disadvantage of raising the mean intrathoracic pressure and reducing cardiac output.

Negative end-expiratory pressure

Negative end-expiratory pressure can be achieved by entraining air in the expiratory limb of the ventilator circuit by the Venturi effect. This reduces the expiratory pressure and thereby increases the venous return to the right ventricle. However, it may cause narrowing or closure of small airways and distal lung collapse.

Positive end-expiratory pressure

PEEP is the maintenance of pressure above atmospheric at the end of expiration but is in practice applied throughout the expiratory phase. The term is restricted to a positive pressure applied during ventilation, in contrast to expiratory positive airway pressure (EPAP) or CPAP, which refer to manipulations during spontaneous breathing. PEEP is maintained by introducing a threshold resistor in the expiratory circuit. It tends to prevent airway closure during expiration with the result that the end-expiratory volume increases. This improves ventilation–perfusion matching

and raises Pa_{O_2}, particularly in restrictive disorders such as diffuse lung fibrosis and neuromuscular diseases [1]. The elastance of the lungs falls unless they become hyperinflated, in which case it increases. The increased lung volume and intrathoracic pressures may also lead to pneumothorax and other pulmonary barotrauma. Cardiac output and venous return are reduced as a result of the increased mean intrathoracic pressure. This may be clinically important especially if the cardiac output is already low, if the blood volume is reduced or if autonomic reflexes are impaired.

Modes of ventilation

There is a spectrum of respiratory assistance between the extremes of spontaneous independent respiration and completely controlled mechanical ventilation (Figs 58.1 & 58.2). In the centre of this spectrum are the partial ventilatory support techniques which, if they can maintain ventilation adequately, are usually preferable to controlled ventilation since ventilation–perfusion matching is better and respiratory muscle strength and coordination are preserved. Partial support techniques can be adjusted according to the patient's requirements. For instance, the frequency, tidal volume, level of pressure support and method of triggering can all be individually adjusted so that the patient has some degree of control over the respiratory pattern. The nomenclature of the modes of ventilation is complex and inconsistent [2], but in general they are distinguished by the methods by which inspiration is assisted or triggered. The most important techniques are discussed below.

Controlled mechanical ventilation

Controlled mechanical ventilation delivers inspired gas at a preselected pressure (pressure controlled) or volume (volume controlled) with a fixed inspiratory and expiratory time. These techniques are suitable if the patient is unable to trigger additional breaths but not when respiratory drive and muscle strength remain. Controlled mechanical ventilation is indicated if the patient is sedated and given muscle paralysing agents, is unconscious, or has no respiratory muscle effort due to complete paralysis of the respiratory muscles as in high cervical tetraplegia.

Assist and assist control ventilation

In these techniques a preset tidal volume is delivered by the ventilator with a preselected inspiratory time. The ventilator can be cycled into inspiration by time or this can be triggered by a reduction in pressure caused by the patient's inspiratory effort. However, in assist ventilation a back-up rate provided by time-cycling into inspiration is

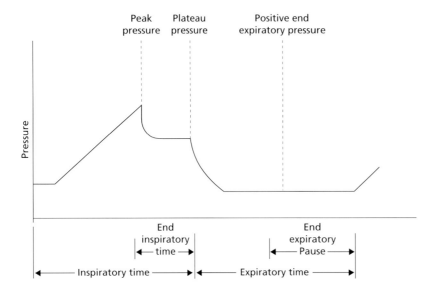

Fig. 58.1 Pressure–time relationships during controlled mechanical ventilation with positive end-expiratory pressure.

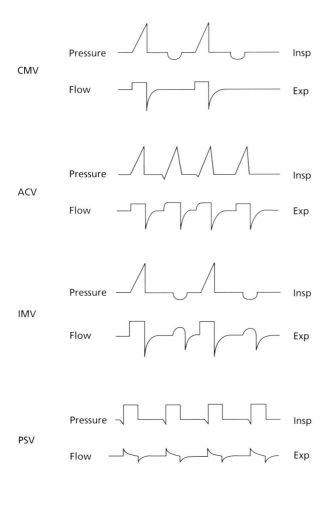

Fig. 58.2 Flow and pressure changes with different modes of ventilation. During controlled mechanical ventilation (CMV), patient effort does not result in airflow in contrast to assist control ventilation (ACV). The flow rate is determined by the patient when using pressure support ventilation (PSV), continuous positive airway pressure (CPAP) and spontaneous breath with intermittent mandatory ventilation (IMV).

absent. The degree of patient effort can be modified by altering the pressure threshold for triggering into inspiration and the back-up rate. Assist control is a safer technique than assist if there is any doubt about the respiratory drive or respiratory muscle strength or endurance.

Intermittent mandatory ventilation and synchronized intermittent mandatory ventilation

In intermittent mandatory ventilation (IMV) and synchronized intermittent mandatory ventilation (SIMV), the ventilator delivers breaths of a preset volume with a preset inspiratory time. Additional spontaneous breaths can be taken through the ventilator, which therefore should have a low resistance and an adequate supply of fresh gas available, usually from a reservoir, between the controlled breaths. In IMV the machine breaths are delivered at regular intervals independent of the timing of the patient's spontaneous breaths, but in SIMV they are synchronized within limits with the patient's spontaneous breaths. This avoids breath stacking, which is common with IMV. The patient's work of breathing can be regulated by changing the IMV or SIMV rate and by the addition of inspiratory pressure support to the spontaneous breaths. IMV and SIMV therefore provide a combination of assisted and spontaneous inspirations that differ in their pressure and flow characteristics.

Inspiratory pressure support ventilation

With this technique the ventilator delivers an inspiration with a preset pressure waveform that usually results in a decelerating or reversed ramp pattern of airflow (Fig. 58.3). Inspiration is terminated either by a fall in the flow rate or by time; the expiratory time is determined either by the patient pressure- or flow-triggering the next inspiration or by time. The patient therefore has more control over the respiratory pattern than with the previous modes but a preselected tidal volume is not guaranteed. This depends on the elastance and resistance of the patient's respiratory system and the ventilator circuit, as well as on the patient's inspiratory effort. Pressure support ventilation does not provide a reliable tidal volume if the patient's mechanics change. However, it is able to compensate for air leaks. The ventilator is usually flow-cycled, which gives a shorter response time than with pressure cycling. Pressure support enables the work of breathing to be graduated by altering the applied inspiratory pressure.

High-frequency ventilation

High-frequency ventilation is the term used to describe ventilatory techniques in which the respiratory frequency is greater than 60/min. Air can be delivered using conventional positive-pressure ventilators at a high frequency, with jet ventilators and high-frequency oscillators. Oscillation can be applied directly to the column of gas in the airway or externally to the chest wall. This method can be used without intubation, although mechanical coupling to the patient is often difficult. With each of these techniques both inspiration and expiration are usually active and although the tidal volume is smaller than with conventional frequency ventilation, alveolar ventilation can be maintained. The pressure swings are much less than with conventional techniques and this minimizes the risk of pulmonary barotrauma and the reduction of cardiac output. However, high-frequency ventilation may increase the end-expiratory volume, particularly if the

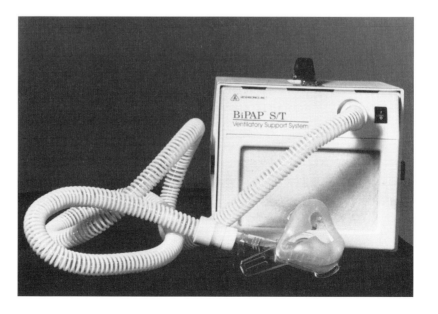

Fig. 58.3 Bilevel pressure-support ventilator.

expiratory time is excessively reduced. It has not found wide application but can be of value with laryngeal surgery and in the management of bronchopleural fistulae, since the inspired gas is not preferentially directed through the low-impedance fistula as it is in conventional ventilation.

Other modes

A wide range of other modes of ventilation has been introduced over the last few years, including proportional assist ventilation, mandatory minute ventilation and airway pressure release ventilation. The current indications for these are limited [3].

Aims of ventilation

Mechanical ventilation is only one component of the overall management of patients with ventilatory failure, and it is important to have clearly defined aims whenever a patient is ventilated. These vary between individuals but the most important are described below.

Control of arterial blood gases

In general, the Po_2 should be kept between 8 and 12 kPa (60–90 mmHg), at which levels the oxygen saturation is usually over 90%. This may require supplemental oxygen as well as ventilation if the gas-exchange function of the lungs is severely impaired. Wherever possible, the Pco_2 should be brought within the normal range in order to improve the hypercapnic drive and to make withdrawal of ventilatory support easier. Occasionally, patients with very abnormal respiratory mechanics cannot be ventilated without the peak inspiratory pressure rising to levels where barotrauma is a significant risk (40–50 cmH$_2$O) and in these situations controlled hypoventilation (permissive hypercapnia) may be the best policy [4,5]. Conversely, hyperventilation to reduce the Pco_2 to around 4 kPa (30 mmHg) is indicated if ventilation is used to reduce intracranial pressure.

Substitution for a failed or inactivated respiratory pump

In certain circumstances, for example anaesthesia, the patient carries out no respiratory work and the ventilator substitutes for this. The controlled mode in which the patient's tidal volume, respiratory frequency and inspiratory and expiratory times are preset is usually used.

Supplementation of the patient's respiratory activity

In these circumstances the patient contributes to respira-

tion but the ventilator acts as an additional external energy source. It is important to try to synchronize the patient's and the ventilator's respiratory cycles. For instance, if the patient exhales during an inspiration with a volume-preset ventilator, the pressure limit would be reached early and air vented from the system. Conversely, with a pressure-preset ventilator, synchronization of the patient's inspiration with the ventilator's inspiration increases the tidal volume.

Modification of the patient's respiratory activity

The ventilator not only provides respiratory support for the patient but also interacts with the patient's respiratory control system and modifies the respiratory pattern. This may occur as a result of an improvement in the blood gases, which alters the biochemical respiratory drive, and also by relieving anxiety and discomfort by providing adequate respiratory support. More complex interaction is also possible involving breath-to-breath and intra-breath reflex changes to the respiratory drive, which are determined by the type of ventilatory support [6].

Treatment of the underlying condition

Mechanical ventilation can to a limited degree treat as well as support ventilatory failure. Most of its effects are transient, but with long-term nocturnal ventilation some must persist long enough to explain the clinical and physiological improvement seen during the day. The possible mechanisms of these improvements are changes in the following parameters.

Respiratory drive

Mechanical ventilation can improve respiratory drive by lowering $Paco_2$ and relieving hypoxic depression of the respiratory centres and sleep deprivation. It also has more subtle and dynamic interactions with the patient's respiratory drive through reflexes, as mentioned earlier.

Respiratory muscle function

Respiratory muscle fatigue has been postulated as a cause of ventilatory failure and of difficulty in weaning, although this has only been demonstrated in a few circumstances. It is more likely that the respiratory control mechanisms adapt to prevent fatigue developing. Nevertheless, the practice of resting the respiratory muscles, particularly during acute illnesses or when the patient is systemically unwell, is probably advisable in order to avoid near-fatiguing work. In other circumstances, increasing the patient's work of breathing using partial respiratory support techniques may increase respiratory muscle strength and endurance and improve their coordination.

Respiratory mechanics

Ventilation can improve both lung and chest wall compliance though these effects persist for only a short period after ventilation has been discontinued [7].

Ventilation–perfusion matching

Gas exchange in the lungs depends on the degree of matching of ventilation and perfusion, and this is hard to optimize during ventilation. Regional perfusion is affected by factors such as gravitational forces, lung disease, vascular tone and lung volume as well as cardiac output. The increase in intrathoracic pressure with positive-pressure ventilation reduces intrathoracic blood volume, right ventricular inflow and left ventricular outflow. These problems are most marked if the inspiratory pressure is high and the inspiratory time prolonged or if the mean expiratory pressure is raised as with PEEP and CPAP.

The distribution of inspired gas is very heterogeneous in lung disease. Overdistention of alveoli is thought to be the cause of pulmonary barotrauma. This may be manifested as pneumothorax, pneumomediastinum, sub-cutaneous emphysema, interstitial emphysema or pneumopericardium. These complications appear to be most closely related to the peak inspiratory pressure and the tidal volume.

In general, ventilation–perfusion matching usually improves if the inspiratory time can be prolonged, with or without an end-inspiratory pause to assist equilibration of gases within the alveoli, and if the tidal volume is increased, with or without PEEP or sighs to prevent airway closure.

Control of upper airway function

An impaired cough, swallowing or speech is common in neuromuscular disorders. Airway protection and access to tracheobronchial secretions with a cuffed tracheostomy or endotracheal tube may be as important as ventilatory support. The same considerations apply to patients who are unconscious, for instance after a drug overdose.

Complete or partial weaning

Ventilation is usually only a temporary phase, although occasionally long-term nocturnal non-invasive ventilatory support is required. It is particularly effective in neuromuscular and skeletal disorders but also in selected patients with chronic airflow obstruction [8]. In effect, these patients are only partially weaned although they may return to an active life during the day.

Gas exchange during ventilation

The main aim of ventilation is to sustain adequate alveolar gas exchange for the patient's metabolic requirements. However, not all the gas leaving the ventilator reaches the alveoli and it has three distinct destinations, as discussed below.

Leaks

The gas leaving the ventilator follows the path of lowest impedance, which may be into the lungs or through leaks in the system. These may occur within the ventilator or its circuit, at the interface with the patient or within the patient. For instance, gas may leak around a cuffed endotracheal or tracheostomy tube or around a face or nasal mask; with the latter, leaks through the mouth are commonly a problem as well. Leaks within the patient may occur through a bronchopleural fistula or by air passing through the cricopharyngeal sphincter into the oesophagus rather than the trachea.

Dead space ventilation

There are two main parts of the dead space: the volume of the ventilator circuit and the anatomical and physiological dead space. The volume within the ventilator and its circuit depends on the length and diameter of the connecting tubing plus the pressure under which the gas enters the circuit. The tubing is distensible and accommodates 2–3 mL of gas for every 1 cmH$_2$O inspiratory pressure (the compressible volume). The volume of the interface of the system with the patient, such as a face or nasal mask, also contributes to the dead space. The dead space of a nasotracheal or orotracheal tube is greater than that of a tracheostomy tube, and with a face mask the dead space exceeds that of a nasal mask or mouthpiece.

Within the patient, the anatomical dead space may be partially bypassed by a tracheostomy but not by non-invasive techniques. The physiological dead space usually increases during ventilation, especially if this causes hyperinflation.

Alveolar ventilation

The rest of the inspired gas is distributed to the alveoli according to factors such as the inspiratory time, the inspiratory pressure and flow waveform and the elastance and resistance of the patient's respiratory system. In most lung diseases the mechanical properties of the lungs are heterogeneous and inspired gas is distributed irregularly. An increase in tidal volume or inspired pressure may simply distend those alveoli with the shortest time constants without improving gas exchange. Recruitment of alveoli with longer time constants may be achieved by adding an end-inspiratory pause or by prolonging the inspiratory time.

Tracheostomy and endotracheal tube ventilation

Composition of tubes

Rubber tubes were used for many years but they tend to perish and are irritant, probably because of the sulphides they contain. As a result most modern tubes are made of silver or synthetic materials. Silver tubes are light and inert and their thinness increases the ratio of internal to external diameter. They also have efficient low-resistance speaking valves. They are expensive but durable. Most modern endotracheal and tracheostomy tubes are synthetic, usually plastic, acrylic, silicone or PVC. They are virtually non-antigenic and most are thermoplastic so that they adapt to the shape of the patient's airway once they are in place. This pliability reduces the risk of tracheal injury. Polyurethane armoured tubes contain a coiled steel spring that prevents them kinking at sites of pressure such as close to the teeth.

Length and diameter of tubes

An endotracheal or tracheostomy tube should be no longer than anatomically required so that its dead space is reduced to a minimum. A tube that is too long may enter one or other main bronchus, usually the right, so that only this lung is inflated and the other collapses. Conversely, if the tube is too short the cuff may damage the vocal cords and the tube may become displaced. Translaryngeal and tracheostomy tubes have a significant resistance which, if airflow is laminar, increases in inverse proportion to the fourth power of the radius. A slightly narrower tube therefore has a disproportionately large effect on airflow resistance. With narrow tubes it may be difficult to obtain an adequate seal with the tracheal wall when the cuff is inflated. However, larger tubes are more likely to traumatize the trachea and larynx and make it more difficult to speak. In general, the diameter of an endotracheal or tracheostomy tube should not exceed two-thirds the diameter of the trachea.

Special tube features

Some tracheostomy tubes have a fenestration or hole in the outer tube that is designed to lie in the tracheal lumen to assist expiration of air through the vocal cords and upper airway during speech and weaning (Fig. 58.4).

Inner tubes are not a feature of translaryngeal tubes but are useful for tracheostomy tubes when these are likely to be required for prolonged periods. The inner tube is slightly longer than the outer tube and as a result secretions accumulate on it rather than on the outer tube. The inner tube can be removed and cleaned, usually twice daily, so that the outer tubing needs to be changed less frequently than would otherwise be the case. The inner tube occludes any fenestration and attaches to the ventilator connections and speaking valves.

Cuffed and cuffless tubes

Cuffless tubes were used almost exclusively before the

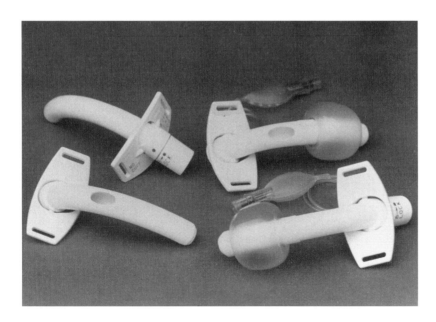

Fig. 58.4 Synthetic tracheostomy tubes. Clockwise from bottom left: uncuffed fenestrated, non-fenestrated, cuffed fenestrated, non-fenestrated.

Copenhagen poliomyelitis epidemic of 1952 [9], but since that time they have been largely superseded by cuffed tubes. Nevertheless, cuffless tubes have the advantages that pressure necrosis of the tracheal wall due to the cuff does not occur. It is easier to speak with a cuffless tube since it occupies less of the tracheal lumen than a cuffed tube.

Cuffless tubes are used in particular in neonates and young children, in whom tracheal damage can easily occur with a cuffed tube, and in adults when there is upper airway obstruction and no risk of aspiration. The most common situation is after laryngectomy, but they are also used during weaning from positive-pressure ventilation and in some patients for long-term tracheostomy ventilation when speech is required and aspiration is not a problem [10].

Cuffless tubes do not protect the airway and the leak of air during inspiration through the upper respiratory tract can be uncomfortable and poorly tolerated. For these reasons, cuffed tubes are more commonly used. The new low-pressure high-volume cuffs have superseded the older high-pressure low-volume cuffs and have greatly reduced the risk of tracheal damage. The pressure required within the cuff depends on the airway pressure during ventilation and on the pressure required to prevent aspiration of material into the tracheobronchial tree. This is determined by the relative diameters of the trachea and tube, the elastance of the cuff, and on the height of the column of secretions lying above the cuff and their density. The factor limiting cuff pressure is the circulation of blood through the tracheal capillaries, and therefore it should be kept below $25\,cmH_2O$ wherever possible. The pressure on the anterior wall of the trachea is usually greater than on the posterior wall because the latter is more distensible, and cuff damage is therefore usually greatest anteriorly.

Early complications (see ref. 11)

Pneumothorax, pneumomediastinum and mediastinal emphysema

These complications occur in up to 5% tracheostomies.

Incisional haemorrhage

Troublesome postoperative bleeding occurs in about 5% of tracheostomies. The wound should be packed and if the bleeding persists surgical exploration may be required.

Tube displacement

This can be a serious complication if it occurs during the first 4–5 days postoperatively. It is usually the result of inadequate securing of the tube and may be precipitated by a bout of coughing. A false channel anterior to the trachea can easily be created during attempts to reinsert the tube. This is best attempted using a fibreoptic laryngoscope or bronchoscope as a guide.

Tube blockage

This may be due to accumulation of mucus or blood within the tracheostomy tube and can usually be prevented by frequent suctioning.

Tracheostome wound infection and tracheobronchial aspiration

Aspiration is usually due to an inadequately inflated cuff.

Late complications

Tracheal stenosis and related complications

These are most common in infants and elderly patients and if the cuff pressure is excessive, particularly if the tube is of wide diameter or moves excessively. Damage may occur at the site of the tracheostome itself, at the level of the cuff or at the tip of the tracheostomy tube, especially if the tube is too large or if it is positioned at an incorrect angle. The initial changes are loss of the ciliated epithelium and mucous glands and development of squamous metaplasia. Following this, the mucosa may ulcerate and the cartilage can be damaged. This leads to dilatation, the formation of a flaccid segment of trachea, or to fibrous stenosis. These complications may require resection of the affected segment, repeated dilatations or stenting.

Tracheo-oesophageal fistula

This occurs in less than 1% of tracheostomies and is due to necrosis of the posterior wall of the trachea. It is often associated with the presence of a nasogastric tube in the oesophagus. It should be suspected if food or other gastric contents can be aspirated from the trachea, if there is an air leak around the cuff associated with abdominal distension, or if an increasing amount of air is required to fill the cuff. Surgery is required to repair the defect.

Tracheo-innominate artery fistula

This is due to erosion through the tracheostomy anteriorly at the level of the clavicle. It may present with obvious pulsation of the tracheostomy tube or small (sentinel) haemoptyses. Repositioning of the tube or use of a tube of a different length may be required. Urgent surgical treatment is needed, although only about 25% of patients survive.

Tube obstruction

This is usually due to secretions and should be prevented by adequate humidification and frequent suctioning.

Tracheobronchial aspiration

This is usually due to use of an inadequate cuff pressure or inappropriate deflation of the cuff.

Swallowing difficulty

The presence of a tracheostomy tube may impair elevation of the larynx, which is required to open the cricopharyngeal sphincter and to enable swallowing to proceed normally [12].

Tracheostome infection

This is a common problem in intensive care units but is infrequent when long-term tracheostomies are cared for in the home.

Mask and mouthpiece ventilation

Nasal intermittent positive-pressure ventilation was introduced in the early 1980s and since then has become widely used [13]. The ventilators that are suitable are similar to those used with tracheostomies and endotracheal tubes, although humidification of the inspired air is usually not required since the air passes through the upper respiratory tract.

Nasal and face masks

Nasal ventilation is possible with cannulae that fit within the nose and which distend during inspiration to seal on to the mucosa. They may cause pressure areas and soreness and an alternative is a design that seals on to the external nares. However, this type of interface can become displaced and in general a mask is preferred [14]. The standard nasal masks are made of silicone and fit snugly around the nose (Fig. 58.5). It is important to select a mask of the correct width and length in order to minimize air leaks and the risk of pressure areas, particularly over the bridge of the nose. Some models have a foam nasal support that reduces the pressure in this area. The masks are secured by straps which are tightened gently. The tension should be equal all around the mask so that it fits closely. Some designs of headgear have soft cotton caps to increase the stability of the mask (Fig. 58.6).

Face masks surround the mouth as well as the nose, but otherwise they work on similar principles to nasal masks. However, the standard designs are less comfortable and less well fitting than the standard nasal masks. Face masks also have a greater dead space, with a risk of rebreathing, and tend to be more claustrophobic than nasal masks.

Individually made masks are an alternative to the standard models. They may be more comfortable and reduce the air leaks and the dead space. There are a variety of methods of constructing individually made masks, but most involve making a mould of the nose.

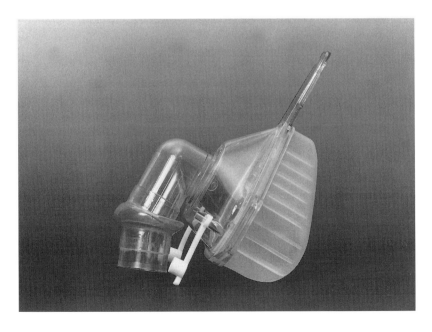

Fig. 58.5 Silicone nasal ventilation mask.

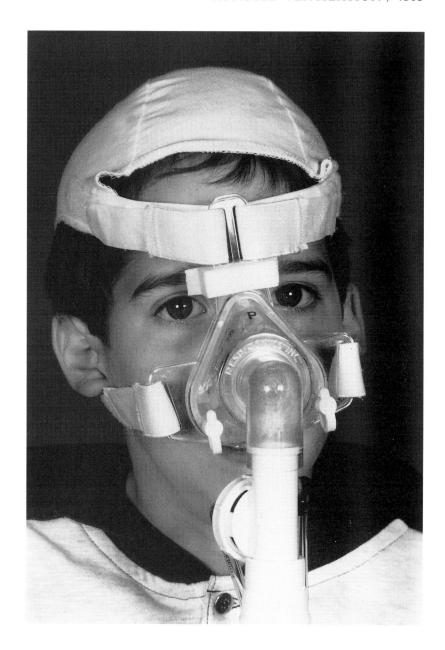

Fig. 58.6 Nasal mask and headgear in position on patient.

Complications

Nasal ulcers

Ulceration of the skin over the bridge of the nose is a common problem [15]. It is usually due to the mask being fitted too tightly or to prolonged initial use of mask ventilation before the skin has hardened (Fig. 58.7). The use of high airway pressures that require the mask to be tighter than usual in order to minimize air leaks may contribute to skin ulceration. Occasionally the ulcer becomes infected, usually with *Staphylococcus aureus*, and it may be difficult to continue with mask ventilation until the ulcer heals. It is important to try to prevent ulceration of the skin, although once this is established it may be necessary to either protect the skin with Granuflex or change to an alternative method of ventilation such as nasal seals, at least temporarily.

Displacement of the mask

This is usually the result of a poorly fitting or inadequately secured mask; some patients regularly remove the mask, particularly during sleep.

Air leaks around the mask

These are usually due to poorly fitting or inadequately

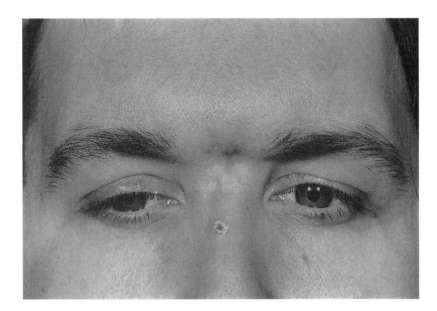

Fig. 58.7 Scar on bridge of nose and crusting inferiorly from use of two different nasal masks.

secured masks but may be difficult to avoid, especially with face masks. Air leaks may lead to conjunctivitis if they are directed into the eyes.

Air leaks through the mouth

These are a problem particularly if the pressure within the mouth is high or if the oral muscles are weak or inactivated, for instance during rapid eye movement (REM) sleep. A chin strap or collar may be required to help close the mouth, and attention to the head and neck position and ventilator settings is required. If these methods fail, a face mask rather than a nasal mask should be used.

Upper airway and head symptoms

These are related to the high flow or pressure of dry air entering the upper airway. A dry or blocked nose may develop but are less common than with CPAP. A dry mouth occurs particularly if there is a large mouth leak. Nasal symptoms often respond to a steroid inhaler and adjustment of the ventilator settings may be of help.

Abdominal distension

This is caused by air entering the oesophagus rather than the trachea. It is most common in patients with neuromuscular disorders in whom the pharyngeal pressure during inspiration exceeds that which the cricopharyngeal sphincter can withstand. The airway pressure is raised if the elastance or resistance of the lungs and chest wall is increased or if there is poor coordination between the patient and the ventilator. Frequent belching, nausea,

vomiting, abdominal distension and the passing of flatus may develop. Reduction of the peak airway pressure is usually indicated, although this may reduce the alveolar ventilation unless other adjustments are made to the ventilator settings. Better coordination between the patient and ventilator lowers the pharyngeal pressure and may relieve the patient's symptoms.

Upper airway obstruction

This may occur at any level in the upper airway between the base of the tongue and the larynx. The mechanisms are uncertain but probably include passive airway closure possibly related to the flow or pressure waveform in the upper airway and active contraction of the upper airway muscles [16]. It can be detected by ballooning of the cheeks or neck and by failure of the chest and abdomen to expand during the ventilator's inspiratory phase. It often causes an increased mouth leak and occasionally abdominal distension, particularly if the obstruction is at laryngeal level. Attention to the head and neck position, provision of a collar and improved coordination of the patient and ventilator's respiratory cycles may all be of help.

Initiation of mask ventilation

Patients who have never tried nasal or face mask ventilation often find it difficult to adjust to the mask and to the high flow of air required. After an initial explanation it is best to place the mask over the patient's nose or face in a comfortable position with a low inspiratory flow rate or pressure. The mask position is checked to make sure that there is little air leak around it. The tidal volume or pressure support level is gradually increased while the trigger threshold is kept at a low level. Attention is paid to the patient's comfort and with reassurance the ventilator settings are adjusted in order to ensure adequate alveolar ventilation, that the patient feels enough air is being delivered and that the timing of inspiration and expiration is appropriate. The expiratory time is adjusted so that it is slightly longer than the patient's usual expiratory time in order to encourage triggering of the next inspiration. The headgear is then secured and further fine adjustments to the ventilator settings carried out, ideally in the light of continuous monitoring of oxygen saturation and transcutaneous P_{CO_2}.

Mouthpieces

Positive-pressure ventilation through the mouth has never been widely used, possibly because of difficulties in developing a satisfactory mouthpiece [17]. The types of ventilator used are similar to those for nasal, face mask, tracheostomy and endotracheal tube ventilation. The inspired gas requires humidification since it bypasses the nose, which is the physiological air conditioner. The ventilator circuit usually needs careful mounting so that the mouthpiece is stable and does not become displaced.

A variety of mouthpieces have been developed but none are very satisfactory. Most include a flange that lies between the lips and the teeth. Plaster moulds of the upper and lower teeth can be taken so that mouthpieces can be fashioned to fit precisely, but in general those that contact the tongue or palate are poorly tolerated and lead to the production of excessive saliva. Mouthpieces are held in place by straps which operate on a similar principle to those of nasal and face masks; in some designs these form an external seal over the lips as well as stabilizing the mouthpiece.

Complications

The main complications of mouth positive-pressure ventilation include the following.

Nasal leaks

These are significant in around 50% of subjects but are determined by palatal function at least as much as by nasal patency. Leaks are also determined by mouth pressure, which varies with the elastance and airflow resistance of the lungs and chest wall. Nasal leaks can be reduced by nasal plugs or nasal clips.

Dental complications

Mouthpieces may loosen teeth and change their position. This often results in an open bite or a gap where the mouthpiece is positioned. This can be avoided by individually moulded dental acrylic bite plates, although a lip seal is needed with these as well to prevent any air leaks from the mouth. Dental development is particularly impaired in children below the age of 4 years.

Mouth leaks

These are a problem particularly if there is weakness of the lips or cheek muscles, as in many neuromuscular disorders.

Abdominal distension

The factors causing this are similar to those described for nasal and face mask ventilation.

Advantages and disadvantages of mask and mouthpiece ventilation

A tracheostomy is indicated in order to bypass upper airway obstruction, to gain access to tracheobronchial secretions and, if the tube is cuffed, to attempt to reduce aspiration as well as to provide ventilatory support. The non-invasive techniques only achieve the latter but all have the advantage of not requiring an artificial airway, which impairs coughing, swallowing and speech, and they can be used intermittently. This makes them suitable for patients who are being weaned from ventilation or who require intermittent long-term use. However, they are unsuitable if the patient is unconscious, uncooperative or requires continuous ventilation for more than 2 or 3 days, or has a weak cough with profuse tracheobronchial secretions. Masks and mouthpieces do not protect the airway and a significant risk of aspiration is generally considered to be a contraindication to their use. Nasal ventilation is usually the method of choice, although a face mask may be required if air leaks through the mouth are a problem. Mouthpiece ventilation is an alternative and is also indicated for intermittent use during the day if the patient is almost completely dependent on the ventilator. The subject can take occasional ventilator breaths between spontaneous respirations. At night there is an increased risk of displacement of the mouthpiece relative to nasal and face masks unless the mouthpiece is carefully constructed.

Negative-pressure ventilation

With all the negative-pressure techniques, the chest and abdomen are enclosed in an airtight rigid chamber; in most of the earlier designs the rest of the body up to the neck was also enclosed in the chamber [18]. The advantages of this are that chest wall expansion is not limited by contact with the sides of the negative-pressure device and only one airtight seal around the neck is required. The first of these ventilators to be effective clinically was the 'iron lung' or tank ventilator developed by Drinker in 1928 [19]. This and subsequent modifications were widely used during poliomyelitis epidemics until the 1950s [9] but since then have been largely superseded by positive-pressure techniques. Negative-pressure systems comprise both the chamber, which interfaces with the patient, and a ventilator or pump that provides the source of energy to support respiration.

Types of ventilator

Negative-pressure ventilators or pumps are pressure generators that work in the controlled mode. Most are servo-controlled and their speed of response determines how completely they adapt to changing air leaks. The extent to which the preset pressure is maintained in the presence of a constant leak also varies between ventilators [20]. The negative pressure required to ventilate each patient is determined by the elastance and resistance of the patient's respiratory system and the ventilator circuit. The peak negative pressure is in practice usually 30–40 cmH$_2$O [21] but depends in part on the pressure waveform generated by the ventilator. The peak pressure required is least when a square pressure wave rather than a half sine wave is produced. Upper airway obstruction is a complication [22,23], probably related most closely to the peak negative pressure and therefore should be less of a problem with ventilators producing a square pressure wave. The frequency and I/E ratio should be adjusted to be comfortable for each patient and to facilitate coordination with the ventilator.

Types of chamber

Tank ventilation

Most of the modern tank ventilators are constructed of aluminium although some are plastic. The patient's body rests on a mattress within the chamber and a headrest supports the head and neck and prevents kinking of the upper airway. In some tank ventilators the head or feet can be elevated and in others the whole tank can rotate 180° in order to facilitate postural drainage [24]. Some observation of the patient is possible through portholes, which also enable catheters and monitor leads to be passed and physiotherapy to be carried out (Fig. 58.8). This type of ventilator has the disadvantage that access to the patient is limited and it is large, heavy and expensive. There are few centres in the UK with experience in their use. An airtight, comfortable neck seal is difficult to achieve and patients often find it awkward to lie in one position for long periods.

Jacket ventilation

With jacket (wrap or poncho) ventilators the functions of rigidity and imperviousness to air are separated into two structures. An inner framework of metal or plastic provides the rigidity and this is covered by an airtight garment. This seals around the arms, neck and usually the waist. Some designs have a back plate and some include the legs as well as the trunk. The air within the jacket is intermittently evacuated by a pump similar to that used for tank and cuirass ventilation.

Jackets, like tank ventilators, do not restrain the

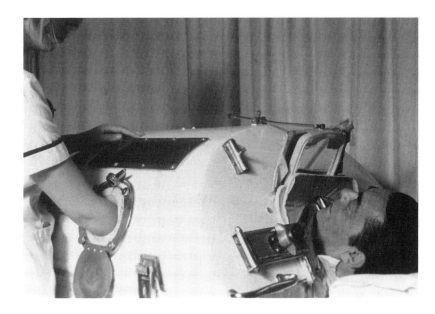

Fig. 58.8 Tank ventilator: patient receiving physiotherapy while being treated.

expansion of the rib cage or the abdomen but can be awkward to put on and cold because of air leaks. They are slightly more efficient than cuirasses, although their greater size and cumbersome nature has restricted their use.

Cuirass ventilation

The earlier cuirass models were often ineffective because they fitted poorly and were inadequately designed. Individually constructed cuirasses are much more comfortable and effective in reducing leaks and are less likely to cause pressure sores (Fig. 58.9). They should enclose the anterior abdominal wall, which is then able to expand during inspiration. Movement of the lateral aspect of the chest should also be unrestricted. Individually constructed cuirasses can be made to fit patients even if there is a severe thoracic deformity such as scoliosis [25] (Fig. 58.10), although the cuirass may need to be modified if the patient grows or changes in weight. They are light and durable and unlike nasal and face masks do not cause claustrophobia. They rarely cause abdominal distension via aerophagy but can induce upper airway obstruction,

particularly during REM sleep. This may be due to loss of tone of the upper airway dilator muscles or to loss of the normal sequence of activation of the upper airway muscles during inspiration. Obstruction can be minimized by lowering the peak airway pressure and by selecting a negative-pressure pump producing a square pressure wave.

Acute respiratory failure

Indications for ventilation

The most common indications for ventilatory support in acute respiratory failure are severe pneumonia, asthma, adult respiratory distress syndrome (ARDS) and acute infective exacerbations of chronic bronchitis and emphysema. There are no fixed criteria for initiating ventilatory support but in general this is required if the arterial blood gases are deteriorating, particularly if $P\text{CO}_2$ is rising, and if the patient is becoming confused, distressed or hypotensive. In acute as opposed to acute-on-chronic respiratory failure, intubation is almost invariably required together with sedation with or without muscle paralysis.

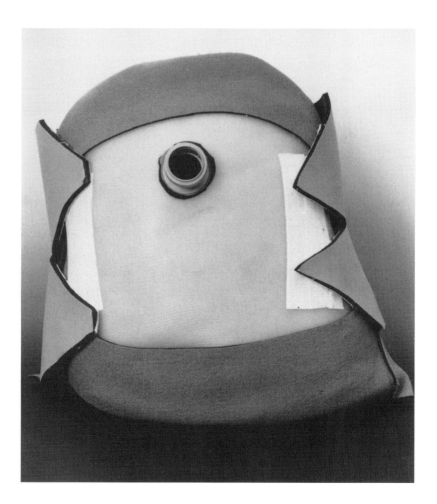

Fig. 58.9 Cuirass ventilator showing velcro attachment for back strap and connector for ventilator circuit.

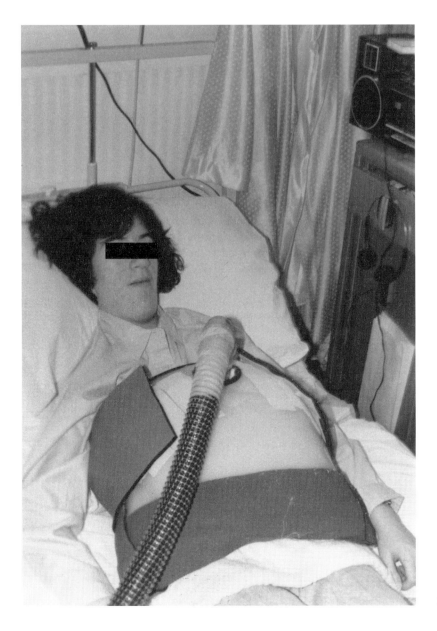

Fig. 58.10 Cuirass in position on patient.

Patients with asthma have expiratory flow limitation that leads to an increase in the end-expiratory volume and pressure (auto-PEEP) unless the expiratory time is sufficiently prolonged for the tidal volume to be completely expired. In order to preserve an adequate expiratory time, the inspiratory time is shortened and the respiratory frequency reduced. A small tidal volume is required to minimize the risk of barotrauma, which correlates with the peak inspiratory pressure. PEEP may be required to overcome auto-PEEP.

Patients with pneumonia have an increased pulmonary elastance that may lead to high peak inspiratory pressures with a volume-preset ventilator unless this is pressure-limited. Pressure-controlled ventilation with a rapid respiratory rate may be preferable. Similar considerations apply to patients with ARDS, although if this is severe the

inspiratory time may need to be prolonged so that it is longer than the expiratory time (inverse ratio ventilation) in order to improve oxygenation and to recruit alveoli with long time constants. The disadvantage of this is that the mean intrathoracic pressure increases and this reduces cardiac output and may cause auto-PEEP to develop. At a low level this may be beneficial in holding open small airways but at higher levels can be associated with excessive hyperinflation.

The optimal management of acute infective exacerbations of chronic bronchitis and emphysema has not been established. In some studies approximately 25% of patients admitted to hospital required intubation and the survival to discharge from hospital was 60–75% [26,27]. Recently, non-invasive ventilation has been recommended as an alternative to intubation, but none of the studies has shown any survival benefit [28–30]. However, non-invasive ventilation may allow intubation to be avoided in some patients, particularly those whose respiratory failure is not very severe and who do not have profuse secretions [28–30]. Ventilation with a face mask is usually preferably to a nasal mask because most of these patients have large air leaks through the mouth. It is important that the cause of the acute infective exacerbation is promptly and effectively treated while ventilation is being supported.

Weaning

Weaning implies two separate but closely related processes: the termination of mechanical ventilation and the removal of any artificial airway. In general the indications for weaning are the opposite of those for initiation of mechanical ventilatory support, and the factors that prevent weaning are similar to those that cause respiratory failure and require ventilatory support. The most important of these factors are listed below.

1 *Respiratory drive.* This may be reduced if the level of consciousness is impaired by sedatives for instance, or if the patient is deprived of sleep. It is also reduced if there is a metabolic alkalosis or chronic hypercapnia.

2 *Respiratory pump.* Respiratory muscle function can be impaired by malnutrition, hypoxia, hypercapnia, acidosis, hypercalcaemia, hypophosphataemia and hypomagnesaemia.

3 *Airflow obstruction.* Hyperinflation increases lung elastance and places the inspiratory muscles at a mechanical disadvantage, as well as rendering them too short to generate their maximum force. Airflow obstruction also increases the resistive work of the respiratory pump.

4 *Alveolar disorders.* Pulmonary oedema, pneumonia and other alveolar disorders increase lung elastance and the work of breathing as well as impairing gas exchange.

5 *Metabolic demand.* This is increased if the patient is febrile or anxious.

6 *Cardiovascular effects.* Oxygen transport is reduced by factors such as anaemia, low cardiac output or hypoxia, which may lead to pulmonary vasoconstriction.

Most of these factors are amenable to treatment, which should be carried out before trying to wean the patient from the ventilator. In general, weaning should be attempted when the capacity of the respiratory pump exceeds the load on it. A variety of predictors of successful weaning have been suggested [31,32] but are of limited value; these include tidal volume greater than 5 mL/kg, forced expiratory volume in 1s (FEV_1) greater than 10 mL/kg, vital capacity greater than 10–15 mL/kg, maximum inspiratory pressure greater than 20–30 cmH_2O, minute ventilation less than 10 L/min and maximum voluntary ventilation twice the resting minute ventilation. In practice an overall clinical assessment is usually more accurate and it is particularly important to bear in mind the patient's level of consciousness and ability to cough and swallow before weaning is attempted.

Many patients can be weaned rapidly with a short trial of T-piece spontaneous breathing followed by extubation. This principle can be extended so that patients breathe spontaneously for gradually lengthening intervals over a period of days or sometimes weeks but receive ventilatory support in between. Alternatively, gradual weaning can be achieved not by intermittent spontaneous ventilation but by steadily reducing the degree of support that the ventilator supplies. Partial respiratory support techniques are suitable for this method of weaning [33,34]. With assist control, for instance, the trigger threshold can be gradually increased and with IMV and SIMV the frequency of the machine breaths is reduced. With pressure support ventilation the pressure level is gradually lowered. In these ways the patient's work of breathing can be graduated and steadily increased. If weaning is delayed, non-invasive techniques, including nasal and face mask ventilation and tank ventilation, may be required, although in practice many patients undergo a tracheostomy before these techniques are used [35,36]. Non-invasive ventilation should not be used for weaning unless the patient's swallowing and coughing have been assessed or if there is upper airways obstruction.

Long-term ventilatory support

Indications

Long-term ventilatory support is usually indicated if respiratory failure causes troublesome symptoms, potentially serious complications such as polycythaemia or pulmonary hypertension or is likely to lead to these problems or to premature death. Symptoms may include frequent wakening from sleep at night, feeling unrefreshed on waking in the morning, early morning headaches, daytime sleepiness and personality change, physical fatigue, breathlessness or ankle swelling. These symptoms can be effectively relieved by both positive-pressure and negative-pressure ventilation [37]. Long-term ventilation has also been attempted prophylactically in patients with Duchenne's muscular dystrophy before ventilatory failure has developed but this has not proved to be of any benefit [38].

Effects on prognosis

The effect of ventilation on prognosis has not been definitely established as there have been no long-term controlled studies. However, survival in neuromuscular and skeletal disorders with home ventilation is good, especially in scoliosis and non-progressive neuromuscular dis-

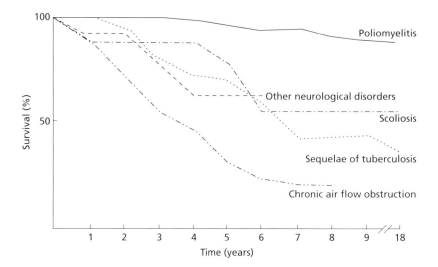

Fig. 58.11 Actuarial survival during treatment with ventilatory assistance. (From Shneerson [49] with permission.)

orders [39–42] (Fig. 58.11). In rapidly deteriorating conditions the prognosis is determined not only by the ventilatory failure but also by other complications, such as bulbar dysfunction which may lead to aspiration pneumonia [43]. In chronic bronchitis, emphysema and bronchiectasis, the prognosis is worse than in neuromuscular and skeletal disorders [42,44–46]. The survival with tracheostomy or nasal mask ventilation is similar to that observed with long-term oxygen therapy using oxygen for 12 h or more daily [47,48]. However, comparisons between these studies are difficult, since it is uncertain whether patients started on oxygen and mechanical ventilation at similar stages in their natural history and none has controlled for smoking, which may have been more important than either of the treatments in influencing survival.

The prognosis for patients with the sequelae of tuberculosis, including those who underwent a thoracoplasty, lies between these two groups, presumably because these subjects have both a chest wall defect due to surgery and extensive lung disease as a result of the tuberculous infection [50]. Non-invasive ventilation has also been used successfully in selected patients with cystic fibrosis [51], particularly as a bridge to transplantation.

Effects on quality of life

There are few studies of the effects of long-term ventilation on quality of life but the published reports suggest that this can be good [52–54], even in progressive neuromuscular disorders [55–57]. The quality of life is related less to the physical limitations than to the mental state of the patient. All the techniques for supporting ventilation do nevertheless interfere to some extent with the activities of normal life, and in some cases with the patient's self-esteem. Nocturnal support is less intru-

sive than continuous treatment and in general patients prefer non-invasive systems to tracheostomy ventilation [58].

Physiological effects of treatment

The arterial blood gases can be improved both during the day and at night. This improvement is apparent within a few days, complete within around 1 month and, in the absence of progression of the underlying disorder, these values are usually maintained for several years [39,41,59,60]. The mechanisms by which the blood gases are improved are not clear, but the most important effects probably include the following.

Improvement of the respiratory drive

Ventilation can influence respiratory drive by lowering $Paco_2$, which reduces the cerebrospinal fluid bicarbonate level and thereby increases the response to hypercapnia. Hypoxic depression of the respiratory centres can also be reversed and restoration of a more normal sleep architecture relieves sleep deprivation and increases the respiratory drive through mechanisms that are largely unknown at present.

Relief of respiratory muscle fatigue

Muscle fatigue has been postulated as a cause of respiratory failure but it is more likely that the central respiratory control mechanisms adapt their output to prevent fatigue from developing. None the less, it is possible that ventilatory support provided in the long term, even if only at night, improves respiratory muscle strength, endurance or coordination so that spontaneous ventilation is more effective during the day.

Other mechanisms

An improvement in chest wall compliance, caused by a reduction in the stiffness of the soft tissues of the chest wall (due to the restricted range of tidal movements) and also by a decrease in lung elastance via reopening of small airways, may contribute to the blood gas changes. Other effects of ventilation, such as improvement in ventilation–perfusion matching and relief of upper airway obstruction, are transient.

Selection of method of ventilatory support

Patients with poor bulbar function impairing swallowing and coughing are at risk of aspiration and usually require a cuffed tracheostomy tube. A tracheostomy is also needed if there is upper airway obstruction that prevents the non-invasive techniques from being effective. However, these are preferable for patients without these complications and in whom support is required only intermittently. This is usually confined to the night-time but some subjects require some additional support during the day. If ventilation is required for more than about 16 h per day, tracheostomy ventilation may be more convenient than non-invasive techniques, particularly in young children. Patients who are totally dependent on the ventilator are usually best treated with tracheostomy ventilation.

The choice between a nasal or face mask positive-pressure system and negative-pressure ventilation can be difficult. Many patients with neuromuscular and skeletal disorders can be adequately ventilated by either method, and whichever is preferred by the patient should be provided. For patients with severe hypoxia and hypercapnia and with markedly abnormal respiratory mechanics, mask ventilation appears to be more effective than negative-pressure ventilation. If mask ventilation is selected, the question arises as to whether to choose a volume- or pressure-preset system. The former compensates better for abnormal respiratory mechanics since it delivers a fixed tidal volume but is less able to cope with leaks either around the mask or through the mouth. A pressure-preset ventilator should be preferred if leaks are a problem and usually if the patient has a strong respiratory drive or an erratic respiratory pattern. These instruments not only have better flow-triggering systems than volume-preset ventilators but also generate a higher tidal volume in response to continuing inspiratory effort during the machine's inspiratory cycle. However, pressure-preset ventilators are unreliable if the patient's respiratory mechanics change, for instance due to retained secretions, bronchoconstriction or changes in sleep stage or, in the longer term, with changes in weight or during infections. The addition of PEEP may be of use in patients with upper airway obstruction causing sleep apnoeas in addition to ventilatory failure and if auto-PEEP is present and is significantly increasing the initial inspiratory work of breathing.

Home or hospital care

Ventilatory support is almost invariably initiated in hospital, often in intensive care units, although long-term hospital care is rarely preferable once the medical condition is stable. Whether treatment in the home is successful depends on the ability of the patient, the family and other attendants or carers being physically able to manage the equipment and also on their understanding of how to use it and cope with any problems that may develop. It is important to assess the psychological state of the patient and the type and extent of support from his or her family before discharge.

Patients who require home ventilation often have other disabilities such as limb weakness that may prevent them from becoming independent in managing their equipment. The patient's previous ability to cope with stress and acceptance of the respiratory support equipment are two factors that predict whether the patient will be able to continue with ventilatory support. These issues are particularly important with the more invasive forms of treatment, especially those requiring a tracheostomy. It is important to try to motivate the patient and family by realizing not only what the outcome might be if treatment is discontinued but also the benefits likely to be obtained if treatment is successful.

Ventilatory support should be as safe in the home as in hospital if care is taken in stabilizing the patient's condition before discharge. Occasionally, deaths occur in the first few days after discharge but these are remarkably few in large centres [61].

An important aspect of home care is the degree of independence that it enables the patient to maintain. This should be encouraged while the patient is still in hospital by gradually transferring responsibility for the patient's care from the health professionals to the patient and family and other carers [62]. Before discharge it is important to assess all the practical aspects of care in the home and to make any necessary modifications and to anticipate any difficulties which might arise.

Care is usually cheaper if the patient is cared for in the home rather than in hospital. This is particularly so if non-invasive forms of ventilatory support are provided, but for patients with multiple disabilities, usually due to chronic neuromuscular disorders, home care can be more expensive [63]. The cost is mainly determined by the number and grade of carers required. There may be as many as 10 for a patient with a high cervical spinal cord lesion.

Once the patient has returned home, it is important that he or she knows how to cope with any problems that may arise. Ideally a hospital telephone helpline number should be available continuously. It is usually not necessary to monitor any physiological indices such as oxygen satura-tion in the home, although regular clinical reassessment is essential since the patient's condition may alter and the ventilatory requirements change. All ventilators need regular servicing, and accessories such as nasal masks need replacing.

References

1 Corbridge TC, Hall JB. The assessment and management of adults with status asthmaticus. *Am J Respir Crit Care Med* 1995; 151: 1296.

2 Blanch PB, Jones M, Layton AJ, Camner N. Pressure preset ventilation. Part 1. Physiologic and mechanical considerations. *Chest* 1993; 104: 590.

3 Sassoon CSH. Positive pressure ventilation: alternate modes. *Chest* 1991; 100: 1421.

4 Tuxen DV. Permissive hypercapnic ventilation. *Am J Respir Crit Care Med* 1994; 150: 870.

5 Feihl F, Perret C. Permissive hypercapnia: how permissive should we be? *Am J Respir Crit Care Med* 1994; 150: 1722.

6 Fabry B, Guttmann J, Eberhard L, Bauer T, Haberthur C, Wolff G. An analysis of desynchronization between the spontaneously breathing patient and ventilator during inspiratory pressure support. *Chest* 1995; 107: 1387.

7 McCool FD, Mayewski RF, Shayne DS, Gibson CJ, Griggs RC, Hyde RW. Intermittent positive pressure breathing in patients with respiratory muscle weakness: alterations in total respiratory compliance. *Chest* 1986; 90: 546.

8 Shneerson J. The changing role of mechanical ventilation in COPD. *Eur Respir J* 1996; 9: 393.

9 Lassen HCA. A preliminary report on the 1952 epidemic of poliomyelitis in Copenhagen with special reference to the treatment of acute respiratory insufficiency. *Lancet* 1953; i: 37.

10 Bach JR, Alba AS. Tracheostomy ventilation: a study of efficacy with deflated cuffs and cuffless tubes. *Chest* 1990; 97: 679.

11 Stauffer JL, Olson DE, Petty TL. Complications and consequences of endotracheal intubation and tracheotomy: a prospective study of 150 critically ill adult patients. *Am J Med* 1981; 70: 65.

12 Bonanno PC. Swallowing dysfunction after tracheostomy. *Ann Surg* 1971; 174: 29.

13 Bach JR. Update and perspectives on non-invasive respiratory muscle aids. Part 1. The inspiratory aids. *Chest* 1994; 105: 1230.

14 Bach JR, Sortor SM, Saporito LR. Interfaces for non-invasive intermittent positive pressure ventilatory support in North America. *Eur Respir Rev* 1993; 3: 254.

15 Meecham Jones DJ, Braid GM, Wedzicha JA. Nasal masks for domiciliary positive pressure ventilation: patient usage and complications. *Thorax* 1994; 49: 811.

16 Delguste P, Aubert-Tulkens G, Rodenstein DO. Upper airway obstruction during nasal intermittent positive pressure hyperventilation in sleep. *Lancet* 1991; 338: 1295.

17 Bach JR, Alba AS. Sleep and nocturnal mouthpiece IPPV. Efficiency in post-poliomyelitis ventilator users. *Chest* 1994; 106: 1705.

18 Shneerson JM. Non-invasive and domiciliary ventilation: negative pressure techniques. *Thorax* 1991; 46: 131.

19 Drinker PA, McKhann CF. The iron lung, first practical means of respiratory support. *JAMA* 1985; 225: 1476.

20 Smith IE, King MA, Shneerson JM. Choosing a negative pressure ventilation pump: are there any important differences? *Eur Respir J* 1995; 8: 1792.

21 Kinnear W, Petch M, Taylor G, Shneerson J. Assisted ventilation using cuirass respirators. *Eur Respir J* 1998; 1: 198.

22 Levy RD, Bradley TD, Newman ST, Macklem PT, Martin JG. Negative pressure ventilation: effects on ventilation during sleep in normal subjects. *Chest* 1989; 95: 95.

23 Bach JR, Penek J. Obstructive sleep apnea complicating negative-pressure ventilatory support in patients with chronic paralytic/restrictive ventilatory dysfunction. *Chest* 1991; 99: 1386.

24 Kelleher WH. A new pattern of 'iron lung' for the prevention and treatment of airway complications in paralytic disease. *Lancet* 1961; ii: 1113.

25 Brown L, Kinnear W, Sergeant K-A, Shneerson JM. Artificial ventilation by external negative pressure: a method for manufacturing cuirass shells. *Physiotherapy* 1985; 71: 181.

26 Kettel LJ, Diener CF, Morse JO, Stein HF, Burrows B. Treatment of acute respiratory acidosis in chronic obstructive lung disease. *JAMA* 1971; 217: 1503.

27 Bone RC, Pierce AK, Johnson RL. Controlled oxygen administration in acute respiratory failure in chronic obstructive pulmonary disease: a re-appraisal. *Am J Med* 1978; 65: 896.

28 Brochard L, Mancebo J, Wysocki M *et al.* Non-invasive ventilation for acute exacerbations of chronic obstructive pulmonary disease. *N Engl J Med* 1995; 333: 817.

29 Kramer N, Meyer TJ, Meharg J, Cece RD, Hill NS. Randomized, prospective trial of noninvasive positive pressure ventilation in acute respiratory failure. *Am J Respir Crit Care Med* 1995; 151: 1799.

30 Bott J, Carroll MP, Conway JH *et al.* Randomised controlled trial of nasal ventilation in acute ventilatory failure due to chronic obstructive airways disease. *Lancet* 1993; 341: 1555.

31 Tobin MJ, Yang K. Weaning from mechanical ventilation. *Crit Care Clin* 1990; 6: 725.

32 Goldstone J, Moxham J. Weaning from mechanical ventilation. *Thorax* 1991; 46: 56.

33 Esteban A, Alia I, Ibanez J, Benito S, Tobin MJ. Modes of mechanical ventilation and weaning. A national survey of Spanish hospitals. *Chest* 1994; 106: 1188.

34 Brochard L, Rauss A, Benito S. Comparison of three methods of gradual withdrawal from ventilatory support during weaning from mechanical ventilation. *Am J Respir Crit Care Med* 1994; 150: 896.

35 Smith IE, Shneerson JM. A progressive care programme for prolonged ventilatory failure: analysis of outcome. *Br J Anaesth* 1995; 75: 399.

36 Shneerson JM. Are there new solutions to old problems with weaning? *Br J Anaesth* 1997; 78: 238.

37 Fragoso CAV, Kacmarek RM, Systrom DM. Improvement in exercise capacity after nocturnal positive pressure ventilation and tracheostomy in a post-poliomyelitis patient. *Chest* 1992; 101: 254.

38 Raphael J-C, Chevret S, Chastang C, Bouvet F. Randomised trial of preventive nasal ventilation in Duchenne muscular dystrophy. *Lancet* 1994; 343: 1600.

39 Leger P, Jennequin J, Gerard M, Lassonnery S, Robert D. Home positive pressure ventilation via nasal mask for patients with neuromuscu-loskeletal disorders. *Eur Respir J* 1989; 2 (Suppl 7): 640S.

40 Splaingard ML, Frates RC, Jefferson LS, Rosen CL, Harrison GM. Home negative pressure ventilation: report of 20 years of experience in patients with neuromuscular disease. *Arch Phys Med Rehabil* 1985; 66: 239.

41 Bach JR, Alba AS. Management of chronic alveolar hypoventilation by nasal ventilation. *Chest* 1990; 97: 52.

42 Robert D, Gerard M, Leger P *et al.* La ventilation mécanique à domicile définitive par tracheotomie: de l'insuffisance respiratoire chronique. *Rev Fr Mal Respir* 1983; 11: 923.

43 Curran FJ, Colbert AP. Ventilator management in Duchenne muscular dystrophy and post-poliomyelitis syndrome: twelve years' experience. *Arch Phys Med Rehabil* 1989; 70: 180.

44 Simonds AK, Elliott MW. Outcome of domiciliary nasal intermittent positive pressure ventilation in restrictive and obstructive disorders. *Thorax* 1993; 50: 604.

45 Leger P, Bedicam JM, Cornette A *et al.* Nasal intermittent positive pressure ventilation: long-term follow-up in patients with severe chronic respiratory insufficiency. *Chest* 1994; 105: 100.

46 Muir J-F, Girault C, Cardinaud J-P, Polu J-M. Survival and long-term follow-up of tracheostomized patients with COPD treated by home mechanical ventilation. A multicenter French study in 259 patients. *Chest* 1994; 106: 201.

47 Nocturnal Oxygen Therapy Trial Group. Continuous or nocturnal oxygen therapy in hypoxemic chronic obstructive lung disease. *Ann Intern Med* 1980; 93: 391.

48 Report of the Medical Research Council Working Party. Long term domiciliary oxygen therapy in chronic hypoxic cor pulmonale complicating chronic bronchitis and emphysema. *Lancet* 1981; i: 681.

49 Shneerson JM. *Disorders of Ventilation*. Oxford: Blackwell Scientific Publications, 1988.

50 Jackson M, Smith I, King M, Shneerson JM.

Long term non-invasive domiciliary assisted ventilation for respiratory failure following thoracoplasty. *Thorax* 1994; 49: 915.

51 Piper AJ, Parker S, Torzillo PJ, Sullivan CE, Bye PTP. Nocturnal nasal IPPV stabilizes patients with cystic fibrosis and hypercapnic respiratory failure. *Chest* 1992; 102: 846.

52 Kinnear W, Hockley S, Harvey J, Shneerson J. The effects of one year of nocturnal cuirass-assisted ventilation in chest wall disease. *Eur Respir J* 1988; 1: 204.

53 Goldstein RS, Psek JA, Gort EH. Home mechanical ventilation: demographics and user perspectives. *Chest* 1995; 108: 1581.

54 Pehrsson K, Olofson J, Larsson S, Sullivan M. Quality of life of patients treated by home mechanical ventilation due to restrictive ventilatory disorders. *Respir Med* 1994; 88: 21.

55 Oppenheimer EA. Decision-making in the respiratory care of amyotrophic lateral sclerosis: should home mechanical ventilation be used? *Palliat Med* 7 (Suppl 2): 49.

56 Bach JR. Amyotrophic lateral sclerosis: communication status and survival with ventilatory support. *Am J Phys Med Rehabil* 1993; 72: 343.

57 Oppenheimer EA. Amyotrophic lateral sclerosis: care, survival and quality of life on home mechanical ventilation. In: Robert D, Make BJ, Leger P, Goldberg AI, Paulus J, Willig T-N, eds. *Proceedings of 4th International Conference on Home Mechanical Ventilation.* Lyon, Paris: Arnette-Blackwell, 1995: 249.

58 Bach JR. A comparison of long-term ventilatory support alternatives from the perspec-

tive of the patient and care giver. *Chest* 1993; 104: 1702.

59 Sawicka EH, Loh L, Branthwaite MA. Domiciliary ventilatory support: an analysis of outcome. *Thorax* 1988; 43: 31.

60 Heckmatt JZ, Loh L, Dubowitz V. Night-time nasal ventilation in neuromuscular disease. *Lancet* 1990; 335: 579.

61 Bach JR, Alba AS. Intermittent abdominal pressure ventilator in a regimen of non-invasive ventilatory support. *Chest* 1991; 99: 630.

62 Fischer DA. Long-term management of the ventilator-dependent patient: levels of disability and resocialization. *Eur Respir J* 1989; (Suppl 7): 651S.

63 Goldberg AI, Frownfelter D. The ventilator-assisted individuals study: *Chest* 1990; 98: 428.

59
LUNG TRANSPLANTATION

TIMOTHY W. HIGGENBOTTAM

Clinical lung transplantation, which developed during the 1980s [1], has awakened interest in many hitherto neglected chronic lung diseases. Its emergence not as an experimental but as a clinical treatment has not only spurred our understanding of the new diseases associated with the transplant lung, but has also seen the introduction of new alternative medical and surgical treatments of chronic lung disease.

Philosophy of lung transplantation and its consequent limitations

The replacement of diseased organs with healthy engrafted ones offers a number of therapeutic opportunities for the patient with chronic lung disease.

1 It enables replacement with lungs able to provide adequate ventilation and gas exchange in patients with respiratory failure [2].

2 Where there is advanced pulmonary hypertension, a normal pulmonary vascular resistance can be restored [3].

3 Extensive lung sepsis, as in cystic fibrosis, can be treated by removal and replacement with relatively clean and uninfected bilateral lung grafts [4].

It is important to understand that a transplant patient has traded the old diseased lungs for engrafted organs that to varying degrees are involved in an alternative chronic disease, namely lung rejection. Depending on the adequacy of control of rejection with immunosuppressive treatment, the normal function of the graft will decline over time and most transplant patients are ultimately likely to die of a transplant-related disease [5].

Donation of organs, except in the case of living related donors (see below), requires that a person has to die. An obligation of the transplant doctor is to make the most effective use of this precious gift. Presently, the need in lung disease is to extend the life of a fatally ill patient. Selection of patients involves the most careful assessment of their untreated chances of survival, and this is then compared with the chances of survival after the lung transplant. Study of the natural history of many chronic lung diseases has been stimulated by this need [6].

Human donation of organs for transplantation can clearly never offer sufficient transplants to treat a significant number of patients with chronic lung disease, and thus only a selected few can benefit. This realization has spurred the quest for xenograft or animal organ transplantation and, more recently, has encouraged thought of cloning organs from single stem cells.

History

Few of the early lung transplant recipients treated during the 1960s survived more than a few days. Technical problems with the surgery, acute lung injury of the engrafted lung and poorly effective immunosuppressive treatments all contributed to these failures [7].

In 1979 the first reports appeared of the use of cyclosporin as an immunosuppressive drug in patients with liver and renal transplants. This fungal-derived antibiotic was significantly better than the earlier immunosuppressives, azathioprine and steroids. Cyclosporin was tried first in cardiac transplants and in 1981 its use was reported in lung transplantation [1].

The initial operation of choice was heart–lung transplantation, where the graft is made up of the heart and lungs harvested *en bloc* in a single exercise. This operation provides an immediately functioning heart even when the underlying disease is advanced. Pulmonary hypertension secondary to uncorrectable congenital heart disease is the main indication for this form of surgery. Few centres worldwide are still using this method, as the alternative, double lung transplantation, allows the donor heart to be used separately in another cardiac recipient.

In the 1980s, Cooper developed the single lung transplant [8]. Initially used in patients with cryptogenic fibrosing alveolitis, this was soon extended for use in emphysema. *En bloc* double lung and, more recently, sequential bilateral lung transplantation are used in patients with lung sepsis and in patients with primary pulmonary hypertension. The initial immunosuppressive treatment was with cyclosporin and steroids, azathioprine being added later. New therapies are coming into clinical practice each year offering fewer side-effects and better immunosuppression. A major contribution to the advance of this form of surgery was the development of techniques in medical management that allowed early diagnosis of complications, rejection and infection and simplified the patient's home care. These are described later.

Indications

All forms of life-threatening chronic lung disease can be treated with this form of treatment.

Emphysema and chronic obstructive lung diseases

These cause respiratory failure, and patients often die of intercurrent pneumonia or hypercapnic respiratory failure. Over the last decade there have been several studies of the natural history of these diseases. An adult with a forced expiratory volume in 1 s (FEV_1) of less than 1 L or under 25% of the predicted value has only a 30% chance of surviving untreated for 3 years. However, medical treatments, specifically long-term oxygen therapy, can double the survival chance in those patients with an FEV_1 of less than 1.5 L, Pao_2 less than 6.5 kPa (50 mmHg) and $Paco_2$ greater than 6.5 kPa (50 mmHg).

Patients are now selected according to their FEV_1 values and when long-term oxygen therapy is no longer effective or cannot be considered because of the risk of hypoventilation causing significant hypercapnia. An alternative surgical treatment that should now be considered is lung volume reduction surgery for patients without respiratory failure where diffuse disease is observed on high-resolution CT (HRCT) [9] (see Chapter 23). HRCT is used prior to consideration of lung transplantation, not only to confirm the diagnosis of emphysema but also to detect evidence of bronchiectasis. This renders single lung transplantation unsatisfactory, as infection can spread from the native to the engrafted lung. Therefore the finding of bronchiectasis requires bilateral lung transplantation.

Pulmonary fibroses

To the specific condition of cryptogenic fibrosing alveolitis one can add other forms of diffuse lung fibrosis, including sarcoidosis and diffuse fibrosis associated with the connective tissue diseases including scleroderma, as suitable for consideration for transplant surgery.

The characteristic feature of advanced lung fibrosis found in these conditions is the poor prognosis. In cryptogenic fibrosing alveolitis only a few patients make any sig-

nificant response to medical treatment. When decline in lung volumes or diffusing capacity for carbon monoxide ($DLco$) occurs in an otherwise suitable patient despite appropriate corticosteroid and immunosuppressive therapy, it is wise to refer early in the progression of disease for consideration for surgery [10]. As noted in Chapter 31, a number of patients with cryptogenic fibrosing alveolitis show rapid progression and if such patients are not controlled with limited doses of corticosteroids they also should be referred early for consideration for transplantation.

Ideally there should be histological proof of diagnosis in patients with diffuse lung fibrosis, as a number of diseases can be difficult to differentiate from cryptogenic fibrosing alveolitis (see Chapter 31). In explant lungs the author has observed *Mycobacterium tuberculosis*, plexogenic pulmonary hypertension and carcinoma in clinically diagnosed patients.

Primary pulmonary hypertension

The natural history of this disease is now well described and the effectiveness of medical treatments known (see Chapter 26). This has allowed a straightforward approach to selection of patients for surgery [10]. The prognosis can be determined by the haemodynamic measurements obtained at a diagnostic right heart catheter study and from this analysis treatment can be determined [11].

1 Medical treatment in the form of anticoagulation is offered to all patients. This improves survival, presumably by reducing intravascular pulmonary thrombosis.

2 In those patients with a right atrial pressure below 2 kPa (15 mmHg), a cardiac index above 2.1 L/min/m² and an $S\bar{v}o_2$ of more than 63% and in whom there is a capacity to vasodilate when given prostacyclin, a potential treatment is an oral calcium channel blocker such as diltiazem. Given in a dose to maintain a systemic arterial pressure of 100/70 mmHg, this often improves symptoms and survival.

3 When the patient has developed right heart failure, i.e. right atrial pressure greater than 2 kPa (15 mmHg), cardiac index less than 2.1 L/min/m² and $S\bar{v}o_2$ less than 63%, a continuous intravenous infusion of either prostacyclin or iloprost (a stable analogue) improves survival and quality of life.

Lung transplantation is considered when this sequence of medical treatment fails to control symptoms and where there is evidence that the disease is progressing. It has been suggested that prostacyclin and iloprost can achieve 5-year survival rates of 80%, which exceed the rates seen with transplantation [11,12].

Cystic fibrosis

Lung transplantation has contributed to the unravelling of

the genetics of this common inherited disease (see Chapter 30). It was demonstrated early in the 1980s that when patients with cystic fibrosis underwent heart–lung transplantation the typical mucosal abnormality of ion transport did not recur in the engrafted lung [13]. This excluded notions of a contributing humoral factor and placed the pathogenic emphasis on the mucosa.

The main prognostic measures in advanced cystic fibrosis are FEV_1 values below 25% of those predicted, arterial hypoxia with Pao_2 values below 6.5 kPa (50 mmHg) and, most importantly, an elevated $Paco_2$, which provides evidence of hypoventilation. Hypoventilation carries a poor prognosis [14].

Patients can be considered for transplantation before the development of respiratory failure when there is a history of life-threatening haemoptysis or uncontrolled pulmonary sepsis. In these circumstances a careful appraisal of the patient is required, weighing up the relative risks of the underlying pulmonary problem and the risks from lung transplantation.

Tumours

There is only limited information on the outcome of lung transplantation on patients with cancers. However in other forms of solid organ transplantation it is recommended that 5 years' freedom from the original cancer should elapse before transplant surgery is considered [10]. This advice precludes the use of lung transplantation as a treatment for all forms of lung cancer. Certainly case reports indicate a high recurrence rate for even tumours of low malignancy such as alveolar cell carcinoma [10].

One special indication for lung transplantation is the development of diffuse lung fibrosis as a result of chemotherapy for lymphomas. Again the empirical advice is to wait for a 5-year period of freedom from relapse before surgery is considered.

Lung transplantation in children

The results of lung transplantation have been poorer in children, considered as a group, than in adults. This has been the result of higher incidence rates of pulmonary infections and greater difficulty in the diagnosis and treatment of acute lung rejection [15]. However, in the child with advanced lung disease transplantation offers an effective treatment. The main indication is pulmonary hypertension, either primary or secondary to congenital heart disease or pulmonary dysplasia. A number of children with cystic fibrosis require transplant surgery, although the usual age range for transplantation in this condition is 18–25 years.

Assessment of the patient's untreated survival chances is undertaken in the same way as in the adult. The recommendation is that this is performed in a unit specializing in childhood lung transplantation.

Surgical techniques

Heart–lung transplantation

The era of lung transplantation began in 1981 with the successful use of heart–lung transplantation (HLT) for pulmonary hypertension [1]. After excision of the heart and lungs of the donor *en bloc*, the trachea is anastomosed in the recipient just above the carina. The integrity of the anastomosis is maintained as a result of extensive collateral arterial blood supply to the lower trachea from the coronary arteries. Airway complications had been a major limiting factor in earlier attempts at lung transplantation. The advantages of HLT include the benefits from simultaneous engraftment of the heart, allowing immediate restoration of normal cardiac output, an important factor in patients with severe pulmonary hypertension.

The operation requires cardiopulmonary bypass. As a result, there is an age limit for patients of 55 years. There is also a significantly higher risk of perioperative bleeding despite the introduction of aprotinin to limit this complication. Further disadvantages are that the heart can also be involved in chronic rejection, although this is not isolated from the same process in the lungs. The use of both lungs and heart limits the number of potential recipients who can benefit from the donation. The 'domino' operation, where the recipient's heart is used and donated to a second recipient, is one way of maximizing effective use of the organs [16].

As a result of the limited number of donors, most centres have confined HLT to the treatment of pulmonary hypertension secondary to uncorrectable congenital heart disease. However, certain centres have retained HLT for cystic fibrosis and primary pulmonary hypertension. Internationally the results are poorer from HLT than from other forms of lung transplantation [15].

Single lung transplantation

Single lung transplantation was first used to treat cryptogenic fibrosing alveolitis but quickly gained a place also for emphysema [9]. Its advantages are that potentially two lung recipients and one cardiac recipient can be treated with organs from one donor. No cardiopulmonary bypass is needed and so patients up to the age of 65 years are being considered for this form of transplantation. Perioperative bleeding is limited.

A number of technical innovations to achieve good healing of the bronchial anastomosis have been tried. These include wrapping the omentum around the suture line or telescoping the donor bronchus into that of the recipient. Each approach has its advocates but careful harvesting of the graft appears equally important in determining successful outcome. It is essential to exclude bronchiectasis in patients with either cryptogenic fibrosing alveolitis or emphysema, as the remaining native lung infects the transplant and compromises the chances of success. HRCT is the test of choice.

Operations for single lung transplantation in patients with emphysema involve selection of donor lungs that have a total lung capacity (TLC) to match that predicted by the height and age of the recipient. After surgery the lungs adopt the size determined by the thoracic vertebral height; as a result a patient with emphysema has a reduction in TLC, while in cryptogenic fibrosing alveolitis the TLC increases [17]. This nicely demonstrates an important physiological point, namely that the volume of the lung is determined by the size of the thoracic cavity.

Double lung transplantation

This operation is now performed as two sequential lung transplants, one side followed by the other. There usually is no need for cardiopulmonary bypass. Again the risk of bleeding is less than in HLT. This is the operation of choice for cystic fibrosis and bronchiectasis, and is also now advocated for patients with primary pulmonary hypertension [18]. Single lung transplants are used in some centres for this disease, although acute pulmonary oedema in the postoperative period and disabling breathlessness if obliterative bronchiolitis develops in the graft limit the efficacy of this operation. Again the opportunity to use the donor heart for another cardiac recipient is retained.

Living-related donation of lungs

The delays in obtaining donor organs and the rapid decline in the clinical state of children with cystic fibrosis awaiting a lung transplant led to the development in California of the procedure of living-related donation [19]. Both parents of a cystic fibrosis child donate a lobe of lung, which are then tailored to fit into the thorax on each side. The risks to the donor have been determined to be small and the engraftment is no worse than with cadaveric transplant. The need for close matching between the donor and recipient is not necessarily a limiting factor, as more distant relatives than parents have been used as donors. This procedure has been mainly restricted to children with cystic fibrosis.

Selection criteria

Patients evaluated for lung transplantation should have received maximal or optimal medical treatment for the disease but nevertheless have declining lung function. Lung transplantation is rarely an option for the acutely ill patient requiring intensive care. Concurrent illness should be adequately treated and preventative care instituted for common illnesses [10].

Older patients survive less well than the younger transplant patient. Currently the maximum ages advised for surgery on the basis of survival chances are 55 years for HLT, 65 years for single lung transplantation and 60 years for double lung transplantation. Certain medical conditions that affect the results of lung transplantation can be considered to be contraindications if untreated, and some of these remain absolute contraindications. Current corticosteroid therapy is not a contraindication, but the dose should be reduced to 20 mg or less per day.

For every patient an individual assessment is needed and careful counselling is required. Most centres admit the potential recipient for a period of time to engage all the specialists involved and to undertake appropriate tests.

Relative contraindications

1 Symptomatic and asymptomatic osteoporosis require treatment before transplantation of the lungs. This requires full investigation and appropriate objective measurements of improvement by bone densitometry.
2 Severe musculoskeletal disease of the thorax.
3 Obesity or cachexia; weight needs to be between 70 and 130% of the ideal.
4 Substance abuse, including nicotine, alcohol and narcotics. Freedom from abuse for 6 months is needed.
5 Psychosocial problems must be resolved before surgery.
6 Requirement for invasive ventilation is a relative contraindication but this is not applied to patients on non-invasive ventilatory support.
7 Colonization with fungi and mycobacteria are not absolute contraindications but special care needs to be observed where single lung transplantation is considered.

Absolute contraindications

1 Major dysfunction of another organ, such as liver or kidneys, precludes lung transplantation, unless combined multiorgan transplantation is considered.
2 Progressive neuromuscular disease.
3 Infection with human immunodeficiency virus (HIV).
4 Infection with hepatitis B (antigen positivity) and hepatitis C with liver disease.

Donor selection and lung preservation

Selection of donors has become a critical part of the lung transplant programme. Less than 30% of potential donors can contribute lungs, a situation quite unlike that with other solid organ transplants. This reflects the frequency with which the lungs are infected or oedematous in patients who have died from brain injury or stroke. Patients cannot become donors if positive for HIV or hepatitis B or C nor if they have evidence of malignant disease.

Lung donors are confined to people who have been non-smokers under the age of 45 years. The ideal lung donor should have a clear chest radiograph, normal gas exchange and no evidence of pneumonia. Most centres send out teams to manage potential donors in order to reduce the risks of fluid overload and to check for pneumonia prior to death. Assisted ventilation is optimized before the harvesting operation.

The donor operation involves cannulation of the pulmonary artery and infusion of either prostacyclin or prostaglandin E_2 [20]. This causes vasodilatation of the pulmonary circulation in order to allow the cold preservation fluid to be subsequently distributed through the lungs. It may also have some cytoprotective effects. The lungs and heart or heart–lung block are preserved inflated at 4°C. A number of different types of preservation fluid are used but all are limited to total ischaemic times below 4 h. If this time is exceeded, the engrafted lungs develop significant reperfusion injury.

Donors and recipient are matched according to ABO blood group. Usually cytomegalovirus-positive donors are matched with positive recipients.

Perioperative care

Intravenous immunosuppressive treatment is given before surgery in the form of cyclosporin, azathioprine and steroids, which are continued postoperatively until food is taken by the patient. Early extubation, allowing the patient to breathe spontaneously soon after surgery, is the ideal. Mobilization and oral feeds are started as soon as possible. The main limitation to this is acute lung injury after surgery and this usually occurs as a result of surgical complications. Patients are given broad-spectrum antibiotics and fluid is restricted to avoid pulmonary oedema. Nursing takes place in a separate intensive care area, although isolation is no longer practised. Once mobilized, the patients can return to general wards.

Management of complications

There are two main acute complications: infection and rejection of the lung. These occur most frequently in the first postoperative months but can occur at any stage of the transplant. Many of the early developments in lung transplantation focused on the diagnostic techniques and methods of monitoring graft function.

Daily spirometry

For adults, both acute rejection and infection of the trans-

planted lungs cause a fall in FEV_1. Using daily measurement with a pocket spirometer it is possible to detect the complication before chest radiographic abnormalities develop [21]. The fall in FEV_1 is an indication, along with the respiratory symptoms of breathlessness and cough, for undertaking a transbronchial lung biopsy and bronchial lavage.

Transbronchial lung biopsy

It was early realized that histology of small lung biopsies of the lung transplant is able to differentiate lung infections from acute lung rejection [22]. Characteristically the histology in rejection shows a perivascular infiltrate of activated lymphocytes. Occasionally the bronchioles are also involved in a similar infiltration. Treatment is with daily intravenous methylprednisolone (0.5–1 g) for 3 days followed by oral prednisolone in reducing dosage over 3 weeks. The lymphocytic infiltration clears with this treatment.

Common oppportunistic infections can also be recognized from the histology of the biopsies. In cytomegalovirus pneumonia there are characteristic inclusion bodies in the epithelial cells. A foamy intra-alveolar exudate is seen in *Pneumocystis carinii* pneumonia. Herpes simplex infections also have characteristic inclusions. Bronchial lavage allows further cytological examination and culture for bacterial infections.

Immunosuppressive treatment

The principal immunosuppressive treatments are cyclosporin [8] (or the equivalent tacrolimus [23]), azathioprine (or mycophenolate [24]) and oral prednisolone. The doses of cyclosporin or tacrolimus are monitored by means of blood levels of the drug. Renal function is carefully monitored as both cyclosporin and tacrolimus injure the kidneys. The white cell count is maintained at $6 \times 10^9/L$ if azathioprine is used. There are a large number of new immunosuppressive treatment regimens under investigation [25] and the pattern of treatment will certainly change over the next few years.

Prophylactic antibiotic and antiviral treatment

All patients receive immediate prophylactic postoperative antibiotics. After 2 days, guided by the cultures of the bronchial aspirate from the donor lungs, further antibiotics are given. Patients receiving organs from a donor with positive serology to *Toxocara* spp. receive pyrimethamine postoperatively [1].

During periods when augmented immunosuppression is used to treat acute rejection, it is useful to cover patients who received organs from a cytomegalovirus-positive donor with intravenous ganciclovir. Oral co-trimoxazole is used in the same way to avoid *P. carinii* pneumonia during augmentation of immunosuppression.

Results

Heart–lung transplantation

The outcome of HLT is that most patients attain their predicted normal values for FEV_1, vital capacity and TLC within 3 months of the surgery [26]. Their exercise tolerance is not as good as predicted for their height and age, probably as a result of the denervated heart being unable to increase cardiac output equivalently to normal [27]. In contrast, denervation of the lung affects neither control of breathing nor the perception of breathlessness. Indeed bronchoconstriction can be demonstrated in the transplanted lung, particularly at times of acute rejection when bronchial hyperresponsiveness as seen in asthma is well described. In all these functions, vagal innervation of the lungs appears unimportant [28].

Single lung transplantation

As one native lung remains, the improvement in lung function is less impressive than with double transplantation or HLT. However the FEV_1 and TLC return towards normal and the exercise tolerance often exceeds that seen after HLT [9].

Double lung transplantation

These patients benefit from two lungs and retain a normally innervated heart. Lung function is normal and exercise capacity exceeds that seen after HLT.

Later complications

A number of chronic complications limit the success of lung transplantation and contribute to early deaths.

Airway anastomosis

Tracheal and bronchial dehiscence are recognized complications of poor vascularization of the anastomoses. While uncommon in HLT, errors in surgical technique in single and bilateral lung transplantation are punished by this problem. Diagnosis is by a combination of bronchoscopy and HRCT. Conservative management is the only successful approach, but fatalities are common.

More common in single and bilateral lung transplantation are the complications of either bronchial stenosis or bronchomalacia. The diagnosis is made by bronchoscopy and treatment is with expandable Gianturco stents. These complications are both the result of ischaemia of the anastomosis.

Obliterative bronchiolitis

This is the most common cause of late death from lung transplantation and contributes significantly to morbidity after surgery. It is estimated that in 5 years one-third of patients die from this complication, one-third are disabled by it, while the remainder remain free of the problem [5]. The principal risk factor appears to be the frequency of acute rejection in the first 3 months after surgery [29]. Some have also implicated infection, as with cytomegalovirus. The abnormality is a proliferative obliteration of the bronchioles by a fibromuscular process [30]. It is often associated with bronchiectasis and suppurative airway disease [31].

The functional consequence of obliterative bronchiolitis is irreversible airways obstruction, characterized by a progressive fall in FEV_1. Augmentation of immunosuppression can limit the rate of loss of function but seldom restores lost FEV_1. A simple descriptive scheme of the disorder depends on the degree of fall in FEV_1 and is called the bronchiolitis obliterans syndrome grading [26]. It has predictive value for survival. Presently the only preventive treatment that has been shown to work is the use of nebulized budesonide, an inhaled corticosteroid, usually effective in asthma. When this is given for a year in daily doses of $500\mu g$ to patients experiencing more than three rejection episodes in the first 3 months, it not only prevents obliterative bronchiolitis but also reduces the patient's requirements for oral prednisolone [32].

Effectiveness and costs

There has been sufficient time to observe the long-term effectiveness of lung transplantation in extending life and improving the quality of life. However there have been no randomized controlled trials of transplantation nor any direct comparisons with medical treatments. The few studies of the quality of life after transplantation have in the main been descriptive rather than analytic. Studies of cost are now being undertaken and some preliminary work has been reported.

Survival

There are differences in the ability of HLT and single and bilateral lung transplantation to extend life. These reflect frequency of use and the number of centres undertaking sufficient transplants to maintain skills. International registries report annually on outcome data [15]. There are ranges of values that should help the clinician decide on the merits of the operations.

1 HLT: 5-year actuarial survival 30–60%.
2 Single lung transplantation: 5-year survival 60–80%.
3 Bilateral lung transplantation: 5-year survival 50–70%.

The original disease also influences outcome. Emphysema provides the best survival figures for single lung transplantation. Primary pulmonary hypertension has the poorest survival figures from any type of lung transplant surgery in adults. Children also have poorer survival figures.

Quality of life

Observational studies comparing patients before and after lung transplantation indicate substantial improvements for all three transplant operations [33]. Many of the measurements relate to activity and these correlate well with the enhanced exercise tolerance. Clearly all these studies focus on those patients who are well and do not systematically study those who have complications such as obliterative bronchiolitis.

Costs

A few studies have addressed the costs of lung transplantation. Ramsey and colleagues [34] considered cost in relation to the improvement in quality of life. In particular, the cost per quality-adjusted life-year (QALY) was estimated. A figure for single lung transplantation in the USA was $176 000 per QALY. Most of the costs concern the initial hospital costs, although a significant cost is incurred by complications such as bronchiolitis and infections. No such figure has been calculated in Europe. For comparison, in the UK the usual limit for cost-effectiveness of a new treatment is regarded as £25 000 per QALY [35].

One alternative approach to costs has been to consider the comparative costs of medical care, and this has been used to study cystic fibrosis [36]. Of interest, overall there was no cost reduction after lung transplantation surgery. Furthermore, there was no overall reduction in the number of admissions to hospital. These observations are of importance when a clinician advises the patient in making choices of types of care.

The future

The prospects for lung transplantation are not limited by the costs but more by the availability of potential donors. It has been estimated that in the UK some 900 patients would benefit from lung transplantation each year. The total number of deaths from head injuries and strokes where transplant organs could be donated is about 2000 per year [37]. Even with a perfect donation scheme there remains a large difference between the resource and the need. This has led to a number of strategies to increase the availability of transplantable organs.

Xenograft transplants

The use of organs from another animal species has been prevented by an acute haemorrhagic injury, understanding of which has recently rapidly expanded [38]. It appears that there is an acute activation of complement, the process being facilitated by two receptors expressed on human endothelial cells, decay accelerating factor (DAF) and membrane cofactor protein (MCP). Research workers have overcome this by using transgenic animals, where the human receptors DAF and MCP are expressed on the endothelium of the pig [39]. Such animals can be used to donate hearts and kidneys, and it is possible that the lungs might also be used. Routine immunosuppressive therapy is still required to prevent the cellular and humoral rejection.

Sadly, however, this form of transplantation probably will not become a reality. There is evidence that the porcine genome contains retroviruses that are expressed in human cells when exposed to pig cells, and currently there is a moratorium on this form of transplant surgery.

Cloning of organs

This has all the elements of science fiction. However the notion is that from a single cell it should be possible to develop a complete organ. Limited success has been reported experimentally with limbs and if achieved this would clearly offer the opportunity of using the patient's own tissue to develop a new organ such as a lung.

Conclusion

We are entering the third decade of lung transplantation. New issues of cost and effectiveness need to be studied. Immunosuppressive therapies are improving, both in effectiveness and avoidance of toxic effects. Potentially new sources of organs may become available. After a prolonged stage of evaluation and experiment, lung transplantation is now established as an effective treatment for specific types of disease.

References

1 Wallwork J. In: *Heart and Heart–Lung Transplantation.* Philadelphia: WB Saunders, 1989.
2 Penketh A, Higenbottam T, Hakim M, Wallwork J. Heart–lung transplantation in patients with end-stage lung disease. *Br Med J* 1987; 295: 311.
3 Dawkins K, Jamieson SW, Hunt SA *et al.* Long-term results, haemodynamic and complications after combined heart and lung transplantation. *Circulation* 1985; 71: 919.
4 Scott J, Higenbottam TW, Hutter J *et al.* Heart–lung transplantation in cystic fibrosis. *Lancet* 1988; ii: 192.

5 Sharples LD, Scott JP, Higenbottam TW *et al.* Risk factors for survival following combined heart–lung transplantation. *Transplantation* 1994; 57: 218.

6 D'Alonzo GE, Barst RJ, Ayres SM *et al.* Survival in patients with primary pulmonary hypertension. *Ann Intern Med* 1991; 115: 343.

7 Higenbottam TW, Otulana BA, Wallwork J. Transplantation of the lung. *Eur Respir J* 1990; 3: 594.

8 Toronto Lung Transplant Group. Unilateral lung transplantation for pulmonary fibrosis. *N Engl J Med* 1986; 314: 1140.

9 Cooper JD, Patterson GA, Sundarsan RS *et al.* Results of 150 consecutive bilateral lung volume reduction procedures in patients with severe emphysema. *J Thorac Cardiovasc Surg* 1996; 112: 1319.

10 Maurer J, Frost A, Glanville AR, Estenne M, Higenbottam TW. International guidelines for the selection of lung transplant candidates. *J Heart Lung Transplant* 1998; 17(7): 703.

11 Higenbottam TW, Butt Y, McMahon A, Westerbeck R, Sharples L. Long-term intravenous prostaglandin treatment of severe pulmonary hypertension. *Heart* 1998; 80(2): 151.

12 Barst R, Rubin L, Long W *et al.* A comparison of continuous intranvenous epoprostenol with conventional therapy for primary pulmonary hypertension. *N Engl J Med* 1996; 334: 296.

13 Wood A, Higenbottam TW, Jackson M *et al.* Airway mucosal bioelectric potential differences in cystic fibrosis after lung transplantation. *Am Rev Respir Dis* 1990; 140: 1645.

14 Kerem E, Reisman J, Corey M *et al.* Prediction of mortality in patients with cystic fibrosis. *N Engl J Med* 1992; 326: 1187.

15 Hosenpud JD, Bennet LE, Keck BM *et al.* The registry of the international society for heart and lung transplantation: fourteenth official report 1997. *J Heart Lung Transplant* 1997; 16: 691.

16 Scott JP, Aravot DJ, Mullins PA *et al.* The ethics of domino heart transplantation. In: Land W, Dossetor JB, eds. *Organ Replacement Therapy: Ethics, Justice and Commerce.* Berlin: Springer-Verlag, 1991.

17 Otulana BA, Mist BA, Scott JP, Higenbottam TW. The effect of recipient lung size on lung physiology after heart–lung transplantation. *Transplantation* 1989; 48: 625.

18 Bando K, Paradis IL, Keenan RJ *et al.* Comparison of outcomes after single and bilateral lung transplantation for obstructive lung disease. *J Heart Lung Transplant* 1995; 14: 692.

19 Armitage JM, Kurland G, Michaelis M *et al.* Critical issues in pediatric lung transplantation. *J Thorac Cardiovasc Surg* 1995; 109: 60.

20 Hakim M, Higenbottam TW, Bethune D *et al.* Selection and procurement of combined heart and lung grafts for transplantation. *J Thorac Cardiovasc Surg* 1988; 95: 474.

21 Otulana B, Higenbottam TW, Ferrari L *et al.* The use of home spirometry in detecting acute lung rejection and infection after heart lung transplantation. *Chest* 1990; 97: 353.

22 Clelland C, Higenbottam TW, Scott JP *et al.* Histological changes in the transbronchial biopsy after acute lung rejection in heart lung transplants. *J Pathol* 1990; 161: 105.

23 European FK506 Multicentre Liver Study Group. Randomised trial comparing tacrolimus (FK506) and cyclosporin in prevention of liver allograft rejection. *Lancet* 1994; 344: 423.

24 European Mycophenolate Mofetil Cooperative Study Group. Placebo-controlled study of mycophenolate mofetil combined with cyclosporin and corticosteroids for prevention of acute rejection. *Lancet* 1995; 345: 1321.

25 Akamine S, Katayama Y, Higenbottam T, Lock T. Developments in inhaled immunosuppressive therapy for the prevention of pulmonary graft rejection. *Bio Drugs* 1998; 9: 49.

26 Cooper JD, Billingham M, Egan T *et al.* A working formulation for the standardisation of nomenclature and for staging chronic dysfunction of lung allografts. *J Heart Lung Transplant* 1993; 12: 713.

27 Otulana BA, Higenbottam TW, Scott JP, Wallwork J. A possible role for mixed venous blood changes in the hyperventilation of exercise in heart–lung recipients. *Chest* 1990; 97: 88S.

28 Higenbottam TW, Otulana BA, Wallwork J. The physiology of heart–lung transplantation in man. *News Physiol Sci* 1991; 70: 2287.

29 Sharples L, Dennis C, Higenbottam TW *et al.* Risk factors for survival following heart–lung transplantation. *J Heart Lung Transplant* 1994; 57: 218.

30 Yousem SA, Dauber JA, Keenan RD *et al.* Efficacy of the transbronchial biopsy in the diagnosis of bronchiolitis obliterans in heart–lung transplant recipients. *Transplantation* 1989; 47: 893.

31 Theodore J, Starnes V, Lewiston NJ. Obliterative bronchiolitis. *Clin Chest Med* 1990; 11: 309.

32 Takao M, Higenbottam TW, Audley T *et al.* Effects of inhaled nebulised steroids on acute and chronic lung fuction in heart–lung transplant patients. *Transplant Proc* 1995; 27: 1284.

33 Caine N, Sharples LD, Dennis C, Higenbottam TW, Wallwork J. Measurement of health-related quality-of-life before and after heart–lung transplantation. *J Heart Lung Transplant* 1996; 15: 1047.

34 Ramsey SD, Patrick DL, Albert RK *et al.* The cost effectiveness of lung transplantation: a pilot study. *Chest* 1995; 108: 1594.

35 Higenbottam TW, Ward SE, Brennan A *et al.* Prostacyclin and iloprost in the treatment of primary pulmonary hypertension. Guidance note for purchasers 97/02. Trent Institute for Health Services Research, 1998.

36 Dennis C, Caine N, Sharples L *et al.* Heart lung transplantation for end-stage respiratory disease in patients with cystic fibrosis at Papworth Hospital. *J Heart Lung Transplant* 1993; 12: 893.

37 Cooper D. Xenografting: how great is the need? *Xenograft* 1993; 1: 25.

38 Nowak R. Xenotransplants set to resume. *Science* 1996; 266: 1148.

39 White DJG. hDAF transgenic pig organs: are they concordant for human transplantation? *Xenograft* 1996; 4: 50.

60

TERMINAL CARE IN RESPIRATORY DISEASE

DOUGLAS SEATON

I have often thought upon death, and I find it the least of all evils.

Francis Bacon (1561–1626)

Death must be distinguished from dying, with which it is often confused.

Sydney Smith (1771–1845)

The inevitability of death, its unpredictability, the surprising perception that it can be regarded as a benign event and the important distinction between death itself and the process of dying are all germane to any consideration of medical care in its broadest sense; for no matter how hard we strive to educate ourselves about the prevention of disease and the provision of 'healthcare', all clinicians are, in the natural course of events, also responsible for the provision of 'dying care', and can do much good to patients and their relatives by a kindly and sensible approach to these matters. The opportunities for such care begin with the realization that the coming of death as a consequence of a firmly diagnosed disease is certain and not far removed in time and that increasing attention should be paid to the relief of suffering, both physical and psychological. It is at this point of realization that efforts may be turned away from the trials of investigative procedures or attempts at cure that rather than prolonging life may in reality be simply making the process of dying more protracted.

Truthful explanation

The possession of the knowledge that a patient is dying gives the physician an opportunity to offer appropriate support to all concerned. Imparting this knowledge can be distressing for the patient and the family as well as the doctor, and how this is done is a delicate matter for which no simple formula exists. Events unfold according to circumstances so that sometimes the patient learns before close relatives, sometimes the reverse occurs and sometimes the truth is told to both together. It is common for the spouse or relatives to seek to protect the patient from the knowledge that their disease is incurable and fatal. Such reactions are natural enough, particularly when voiced in response to the sudden realization of the true state of affairs. They may sometimes be right, at least for a time, but more often than not their judgement in this situation is inevitably clouded by emotion, for the deliberate concealment of the truth from the patient is an act of denial that increases the stresses between individual members of the family, the patient and the doctor, creating a world of make-believe in which interpersonal relationships become strained and in which suspicion, fear and mistrust are fostered. Family members who take this view may be reassured that in the doctor's experience patients who are denied the truth are likely to suffer more than those who have a greater awareness of their situation so that they can come to terms with it.

How patients are told that their illness is fatal is a matter of individual judgement. It is most difficult when the patient is outwardly in reasonable health, in which case the concept may be introduced gradually in terms of what can and cannot be done in the way of management. This often allows the patient to ask the relevant questions and to be supplied with answers that lead as far towards the truth as he or she wishes to go at that particular time. These disclosures should be made gently and by degree. A 'screening question' may be asked at the outset to try to establish the patient's perception of the position. The whole truth need not come out at first but a line of communication is set up so that the patient can establish trust in the doctor and in the authenticity of the information supplied, but can also be given time to adjust to the new situation that has arisen. This stepwise approach seems entirely reasonable and care should be taken not to 'assault the patient with truth' that he or she is not yet ready to handle [1]. Not infrequently the patient has realized the seriousness of the position and that recovery is not taking place. In this situation fairly frank explanations of the true state of affairs may bring a sense of relief, being received with openly expressed gratitude.

When the truth is told it should be accompanied by a

positive statement of the physician's intention to continue to offer supportive treatment and to deal with symptoms effectively whenever they should happen to arise. A failure to provide such assurances may produce a sense of abandonment and isolation stemming from the belief that 'nothing more can be done'. The provision of a firm statement of support may help to provide the patient with a much-needed sense of security and comfort despite the fact that life is drawing to its conclusion.

Relief of symptoms

Although much can be done to relieve the physical and psychological symptoms of patients who are dying, there is evidence that our hospitals have fallen short of meeting basic needs [2,3]. The first step is to question the patient carefully about those symptoms that are most troubling. Where there is doubt in the presence of multiple symptoms, the principal symptom is usually easily sought out by asking the question: 'If there was one symptom that you could get rid of, which one would you choose first?' The answer frequently helps the physician to direct therapeutic efforts more usefully, while still taking account of secondary symptoms. A more formal symptomatic enquiry, system by system, may unearth other information of value in general management.

Whereas the event of death itself may be regarded as a merciful release, the process of dying can hardly be regarded as pleasurable, and the prospect of physical discomfort may produce a good deal of trepidation. Firm reassurance that uncomfortable symptoms will be effectively combatted may ease the mind of the worried patient. It is up to the individual physician to be sufficiently informed about the various therapeutic options available in order to fulfil such a promise. Clearly therapeutic intervention cannot abolish discomfort totally but it can nevertheless provide a considerable measure of relief.

Pain

The perception of pain is entirely subjective and may well be influenced by mood, so that if individuals are depressed, anxious or lonely, painful sensations are likely to be more problematical than if their mood has been elevated by any of a number of circumstances, among which is included the provision of kind and courteous general care.

Having established that pain is present, some effort must be made to assess its significance. Patients may sometimes behave in a more reticent and stoical manner towards their medical practitioner than to other members of their family, and a clearer picture of the degree of incapacity caused by pain may be obtained from the spouse, partner or the nursing staff.

Once it has been established that pain is a problem, attention should be turned towards the likely cause. This can usually be inferred from the site and nature of the discomfort, which may be due to involvement of the chest wall, bones, nerves, nerve roots or brain. Patients with cancer more often than not have more than one pain and how far to investigate the source depends upon their general condition. In appropriate circumstances, plain radiographs, isotope bone scans or CT may be required. This is only the case if the result of the investigation is likely to influence mangement; for example, if it is suspected that there is localized involvement of bone or other structures that may respond to palliative radiotherapy. The instigation of adequate analgesia need not await the results of such tests. Patients are likely to benefit from a frank explanation of the cause of the pain, and if this is not forthcoming will only be worried all the more by doubt and uncertainty, whereas if they are clear about the mechanism then they will be better be able to adjust and come to terms with it.

Although it is possible to grade pain according to a visual analogue scale and to record the degree of incapacity by devices such as the Karnovsky scale [4], from a practical standpoint, in patients with cancer, pain may be regarded as mild if it responds adequately to a simple non-narcotic analgesic such as paracetamol or aspirin, and moderate if it requires a weak narcotic analgesic such as codeine or dextropropoxyphene (commonly prescribed with paracetamol as co-proxamol). Any pain that is uncontrolled by the foregoing or is partly controlled but still significantly limits activity should be regarded as being severe and should be treated with a potent opioid (narcotic) analgesic such as morphine [5]. There is a plethora of analgesic preparations available and rather than wander randomly through a jungle of unfamiliar or less well-known preparations, it behoves the physician to develop a simple therapeutic 'three-rung ladder' (Table 60.1) and stick to it [6].

Table 60.1 Vertical progression of oral analgesia in cancer-associated pain (see text).

Morphine sulphate (controlled-release preparations)	Same daily dose	Once or twice daily
Morphine sulphate (immediate-release preparations)	5–10 mg titrated upwards	Every 4 h
Co-codamol 30/500	Two tablets	Every 4–6 h
Codeine phosphate	30–60 mg	Every 4–6 h
Paracetamol	1 g	Every 4–6 h

Lower rung

Paracetamol is a suitable lower-rung preparation often used for mild pain relief. Aspirin, which has both analgesic and anti-inflammatory properties, may be taken as an alternative at a dose of 600 mg every 4–6 h, although one of the many other non-steroidal anti-inflammatory drugs may be used instead. Aspirin intolerance may be reduced if it is taken after meals.

Middle rung

Drugs belonging to the family of weak opioid analgesics, such as codeine or dextropropoxyphene, occupy the middle rung. Dihydrocodeine is a semisynthetic analogue that has no particular advantage over the standard weak opioid codeine. In the UK, dextropropoxyphene 32.5 mg is commonly prescribed in combined form with paracetamol 325 mg as co-proxamol. Combinations of codeine with paracetamol also exist and when these are used it makes sense to prescribe a formulation that contains a therapeutic 30-mg dose of codeine (co-codamol 30/500) rather than one of those containing only 8 mg (co-codamol 8/500), unless the patient is very elderly in which case increased sensitivity to codeine and other narcotics may occur. These middle-rung analgesics are likely to be more acceptable than morphine to patients earlier in their disease, and when taken in combined form with paracetamol are probably as effective as low-dose morphine.

Upper rung

Strong opioid analgesics like morphine and diamorphine are on the upper rung of the analgesic ladder. Some physicians may feel a reluctance to prescribe regular opioids unless they regard the patient as 'terminal'. Any such fears are misplaced and morphine may be continued safely for many months if need be. Stepping sideways on a ladder has never been a very wise course of action and if a non-opioid or a weak opioid analgesic proves ineffective at standard dosage, there is no point in using another similar drug; one should rather go directly to a strong opioid such as morphine (referred to by Sir William Osler as GOM or 'God's own medicine').

The principles are that this drug is prescribed orally by preference, that it should be taken regularly to prevent pain from recurring, that the dose should be tailored upwards according to the patient's needs and that there is no upper dose limit; thus the patient's pain may require anything between 2.5 mg and 2500 mg every 4 h to control it, good control being commonly achieved with 250 mg daily or less.

Morphine may be dispensed as an oral solution (mor-phine elixir), the prescription having to be written in full in order to comply with the law [7] and to avoid embarrassing delays and telephone calls from the outpatient pharmacist, for example 'morphine hydrochloride 5 mg, chloroform water to 5 mL'.

Alternatively there are now prepared proprietary formulations of morphine sulphate solution such as Oramorph oral solution in strengths of 10 mg per 5 mL and 100 mg per 5 mL. The amount to be dispensed must be written *in figures and words*, for example 'supply 200 mL (two hundred millilitres)', followed by the amount to be taken, for example '10 mL every 4 hours'.

The same applies to morphine sulphate 10 and 20 mg immediate-release tablets (Sevredol). There is no particular advantage in prescribing oral diamorphine rather than morphine itself, as the former is itself biotransformed to morphine and other metabolites. The advantages of parenteral diamorphine are outlined below.

Morphine 5 or 10 mg every 4 h is a reasonable starting dose for pain that is continuous, as is frequently the case with malignancy, although 2.5 mg may be preferred in an elderly or frail patient or one with renal insufficiency. This continuous type of pain should not be treated with as-required or prn prescriptions, unless these are used to augment a regular strong opioid analgesic should breakthrough pain occur between doses. Such top-up or rescue supplementation can be given as often as necessary (e.g. hourly) but is an indication that pain control is incomplete and that the regular 4-hourly doses need to be increased. Doses of morphine sulphate oral solution or tablets are therefore increased gradually according to response, the usual dose for control being 5–30 mg every 4 h, although as mentioned above sometimes very much larger amounts are required. A steady pharmacokinetic state is reached in about 24 h and the dose can therefore be adjusted daily. It is usual to increase the dose by 30–50% at each step and a double dose at bedtime helps to ensure sleep. An example of morphine dose titration is given in Table 60.2.

As frequent dosage can be tiresome for the patient and awkward for the ward, modified-release morphine sulphate tablets (5, 10, 15, 30, 60, 100 and 200 mg) provide a convenient alternative for maintainance treatment, once the patient's total daily dose requirements (including rescue doses for breakthrough pain) have been determined using the 4-hourly regimen, being prescribed *at the same total daily dose* but using a 12-hourly regimen (e.g. MST Continus) [9]. The top-up or rescue dose of immediate-release morphine should be one-third of the 12-hourly dose of MST Continus, this being equivalent to an extra 4-hourly dose (Table 60.2). Modified-release morphine sulphate capsules (30, 60, 90, 120, 150 and 200 mg) for once-daily dosing have become available more recently (MXL). The modified-release preparations tend to

Table 60.2 Morphine dose titration: an example of initial treatment with a standard formulation leading to maintenance treatment with a twice-daily controlled-release formulation. (After O'Neill [8] with permission.)

Day	Doses given	Total on that day	Starting dose on next day
Day 1	10 mg 4-hourly, plus three 10-mg prn doses	90 mg	15 mg 4-hourly (90/6)
Day 2	15 mg 4-hourly, plus two 15-mg prn doses	120 mg	20 mg 4-hourly (120/6)
Day 3	20 mg 4-hourly	120 mg	
	Pain is controlled, no breakthrough dosage required		
Day 4 and on	60 mg twice daily (*controlled release*) plus 20-mg prn doses (standard formulation) should breakthrough pain occur		

achieve an attenuated peak plasma level in about 2–4 h compared with about 1 h for the immediate-release preparations.

It is clear from the foregoing that 'normal' doses of narcotic analgesics, such as might be used for the short-term relief of postoperative pain, do not apply in the management of chronic pain associated with incurable cancer. Respiratory tolerance to these high doses develops [10].

Route of administration

When analgesics are required, the oral route should be used wherever possible as injections are inconvenient for patients and increase their sense of dependence on those who are taking care of them.

If the patient cannot swallow, then strong opioid analgesics should be given either as morphine suppositories (morphine sulphate or hydrochloride suppositories 10, 15, 20 or 30 mg) or by injection. In the lower dose range of morphine, buprenorphine 200–400 µg sublingually every 6–8 h is an alternative. Buprenorphine binds partially to opioid receptors and may block the access of full agonists, such as morphine, to the same receptors, thereby partially antagonizing its effect if taken concurrently. A transdermal formulation of the potent opioid analgesic fentanyl has been developed, being applied in the form of a cutaneous patch. These are changed every 72 h and are available in different strengths designed to deliver 25, 50, 75 and 100 µg of fentanyl per hour. The system appears to be effective but as with other controlled-release formulations, immediate-release preparations may still be required for breakthrough pain [11,12].

Diamorphine (heroin) tends to be preferred for injection in the UK as it is more soluble than morphine; 20 mL of water is required to dissolve 1 g of morphine, whereas only 1.6 mL is needed to dissolve 1 g of diamorphine. It is an advantage to be able to give the same dose in a smaller volume in patients who need large doses of subcutaneous opioid [13]. There is no point in giving diamorphine orally as it is a prodrug of morphine. Diamorphine is only legally prescribable in the UK and Canada. Hydromorphone, which has now become available in the UK (so far only in oral form, 1 mg dose equivalent to 7.5 mg morphine), has similar properties and is used in place of diamorphine in the USA and elsewhere (where a parenteral form is available). When used subcutaneously, diamorphine should be given at one-third of the oral dose of morphine that had previously controlled pain satisfactorily, in order to achieve the same effect, whereas if subcutaneous morphine is used it should be given at half the oral dose. If intravenous morphine is used (e.g. in patients with peripheral venous shutdown or in those who already have intravenous access established for some other reason), the equivalent dose is one-third of that given orally [14]. It is not usual practice to give morphine intramuscularly in a palliative setting as subcutaneous injections are less painful. A fine 'butterfly' needle may be used for regular subcutaneous injections.

A syringe driver (such as a portable, pocket-sized Graseby type MS16A pump) is a very useful method for delivering diamorphine in the terminal phase when the patient is disinclined or unable to swallow, being less disturbing than repeated injections. It may also allay fears on the part of the relations that the last dose of a 4-hourly subcutaneous morphine regimen 'carried off' the patient should death happen to come shortly after such an injection. However, it is a mistake to use this form of treatment while the patient is still able to swallow comfortably. Diamorphine is available in 5, 10, 30, 100 and 500 mg ampoules. Water for injection rather than 0.9% saline should be used for strengths greater than 40 mg/mL in order to avoid precipitation. The pumps run at a preset rate measured in millimetres of syringe plunger movement per hour. Thus the diamorphine (and any other compatible medication that needs to be infused as well) may be made up with water or saline to 8.5 mL total volume, which when drawn up in a 10-mL disposable plastic syringe occupies 50 mm of barrel length. The driver can then be set to run at 2 mm/h, emptying its contents over 25 h. The syringe is connected to the patient by a disposable butterfly cannula with integral 60 or 100 cm tubing, the butterfly needle being being bent to about 45° and secured on the upper arm, thigh, abdomen or chest with a light proprietary dressing such as OpSite or Tegaderm. The conversion from oral morphine to 24-h or, in this case, 25-h subcutaneous diamorphine is achieved by dividing the previous day's dose of oral morphine by three (Table 60.3). A list of drugs compatible with diamorphine is contained in the British National Formulary [14].

Table 60.3 Approximate dose equivalence of some opioid analgesics to oral morphine.

	Ratio
Diamorphine orally	2:3
Diamorphine subcutaneous	1:3
Morphine intravenous	1:3
Morphine subcutaneous	1:2
Morphine per rectum	1:1
Hydromorphone orally	1:7.5

For the oral route morphine is preferable to diamorphine; for the parenteral routes diamorphine is preferable to morphine (see text).

Bony pain and sequelae

Bone pain, like visceral and neuropathic pain, tends to be somewhat less responsive to narcotic analgesics. When pain is localized and caused by direct involvement of the chest wall by tumour or by bony metastases, palliative radiotherapy may be very helpful and can often be delivered as a single treatment to a painful area. Indometacin (indomethacin) or other non-steroidal anti-inflammatory drugs may be useful in controlling bony pain, presumably as a result of their inhibition of prostaglandins, which are released during osteolysis [15]. They may also be used to supplement a regular strong opioid in the same situation [16]. In the same manner these drugs are very effective in relieving the pain of hypertrophic pulmonary osteoarthropathy (see Chapter 41). Preliminary data exist to suggest that bisphosphonates, such as oral clodronate or parenteral pamidronate, might be helpful in reducing bone pain from metastatic disease [15,17].

Pathological fractures of long bones are fortunately an infrequent occurrence in lung cancer. When they do occur they are almost always situated in the femur or the humerus. An orthopaedic opinion should be sought unless the patient is very close to death, as otherwise internal fixation and postoperative radiotherapy need to be considered. Sometimes prophylactic internal fixation is carried out when a large lytic metastasis is found in a weight-bearing long bone, this again being followed by radiotherapy. Patients with spinal instability secondary to destructive metastatic bony involvement may require orthopaedic stabilization followed by radiotherapy.

Those with spinal cord compression may be treated by surgical decompression and stabilization or by radiotherapy or both. Surgery is more likely to be undertaken in those with paraplegia or urinary retention of less than 24 h duration, when the block on magnetic resonance imaging or CT involves less than three contiguous vertebral segments and when the patient's life expectancy is likely to be more than a few weeks [18].

Intractable pain

Pain in lung cancer that persists despite treatment with large doses of narcotic analgesics is unusual, 80% of patients responding to the measures outlined above. Occasionally, pain is difficult to control and alternative methods may be required to achieve adequate relief. Morphine is usually effective in controlling 'tissue-damage' (or nociceptive) pain, in which the pain is produced by the stimulation of nerve endings in non-neural tissue, whereas it tends to be ineffective in neurogenic pain (e.g. trigeminal neuralgia, postherpetic neuralgia, thalamic pain and pain from brachial plexus involvement by tumour), in which impulses are produced as a result of neural dysfunction and do not follow classic pain pathways. The reasons for the occasional resistance of tissue-damage pain to the action of morphine may be related to the ratio of one of its opiate receptor-binding metabolites (morphine 3-glucuronide) to another (morphine 6-glucuronide) in different patients, the former tending to antagonize analgesic activity whereas the latter is itself a potent analgesic. Thus those with a high ratio of 3-glucuronide/6-glucuronide may be relatively resistant to the analgesic effect of morphine on nociceptive pain and may experience so-called paradoxical pain [19]. It has been suggested that these patients may be more responsive to methadone, which follows different metabolic pathways to morphine [20]. Patients with neurogenic pain may sometimes respond to a tricyclic antidepressant such as amitriptyline (for 'burning' discomfort) or to an anticonvulsant such as sodium valproate or carbamazepine (for 'shooting' pains). The analgesic effect of the tricyclic group appears to be unrelated to any antidepressant effect and these drugs (mixed reuptake inhibitors) seem to be more effective in this regard than the newer selective serotonin reuptake inhibitors such as paroxetine. The dose of amitriptyline should be started as low as 10 mg at night in order to improve patient acceptability, and should be titrated up at weekly intervals with proper explanation of its minor but tiresome adverse effects. Low doses in the range 25–75 mg nocte are usually settled for and an added benefit is a degree of nocturnal sedation. Failure of amitriptyline to control opioid-resistant neurogenic pain may then lead to the substitution of sodium valproate, titrating up from 200 mg twice daily to a maximum of 1600 mg daily or, alternatively, carbamazepine starting with 200 mg at night increasing to 400 mg twice daily according to tolerance and response [21]. Dexamethasone 8 mg daily may reduce oedema around tumours that are compressing nerves.

One non-invasive technique that can be beneficial in chest wall pain is transcutaneous electrical nerve stimulation (TENS), in which patients must be taught properly how to deliver an electical stimulus from a small battery-operated device by cutaneous surface electrodes either to the painful area itself or to the nerve roots subtending that area. The stimulus, which the patient must feel, is transmitted by myelinated fibres to the spinal cord, thereby blocking the transmission of pain signals according to the gate control theory of pain [22]. It is not easy to know which patients are likely to respond and any beneficial effect may gradually decline over some weeks.

Nerve blocks are a matter for the specialist in pain relief and are carried out in appropriate circumstances as a last resort; these procedures should be planned after due discussion with the patient and the close relatives. They involve the injection of a neurolytic substance such as phenol or alcohol into the immediate proximity of the appropriate nerve trunk or root, with permanent alteration of nerve function [23]. The likely effects, which may be motor as well as sensory, may be simulated if a local anaesthetic block is used first. Intractable thoracic pain may respond to paravertebral or intercostal nerve block. Another technique for nerve block involves the use of a cryotherapy probe. Clearly, the source of the pain needs to be accurately determined and the destruction of nervous tissue selective in order to relieve pain successfully and to avoid motor damage. Dorsal sensory nerve roots may be interrupted by radiofrequency thermocoagulation, a technique that can also be used to carry out a percutaneous spinothalamic tractotomy. The application of these specialized procedures depends upon local interest and expertise but are seldom required in the management of lung cancer.

Side-effects of narcotic analgesics

Patients frequently react badly to the prospect of being prescribed strong opioid analgesics, fearing that such treatment will 'drug them up' and render them incapable of all normal activity. They can be reassured on this count but should be warned that they may feel some drowsiness for the first 3 days or so. Effects on cognition are minimal once patients have been established on a stable dose and such patients should be permitted to drive should they so wish [24]. However, they should not drive when morphine is being started or increased in response to worsening pain [25].

Nausea or vomiting should be anticipated and may occur at the onset of treatment in up to two-thirds of patients. This can be prevented by the use of cyclizine 50 mg or metaclopramide 10 mg, each taken three times a day before meals. Haloperidol 1.5 mg at night or twice daily may also be effective. These symptoms often subside spontaneously so that it is possible to withdraw the antiemetic within a few days.

Constipation is an inevitable consequence and the main nuisance of opioid analgesics. It should always be anticipated, whenever these are used, by the use of regular laxatives and patients should be forewarned. This aspect of management is important and is dealt with below in more detail.

Cough

A cough causing distress in terminal lung disease requires symptomatic treatment and, in addition, an explanation of the cause of the cough, coupled with reassurance that it is not going to cause choking or suffocation; a description of how it can be dealt with does much to help the patient's flagging morale. Assuming that the patient is not already taking morphine, codeine linctus 30 mg three or four times daily can be tried initially. Patients in whom this is ineffective may be started on morphine, which can be titrated against response in the manner described above for pain. Methadone may be effective for night-time cough as it has a relatively long half-life.

There are a number of other symptomatic remedies that may be tried for additional relief. These include inhalations of benzoin tincture, one teaspoonful of which is put in a pint of hot water and the vapour breathed in by the patient from a Nelson's inhaler. The sensation of warm moist aromatic air is comfortable and may assist difficult expectoration. Sometimes the patient may feel the presence of viscid sputum that has great trouble in breaking free and, if a moist inhalation is ineffective, carbocisteine or another mucolytic agent sometimes produces symptomatic relief, although the cost of such preparations may outweigh their benefit. Simple change of posture and physiotherapy may also help these patients, who may be advised to try lying with the affected lung uppermost in order to facilitate the drainage of obstinate bronchial secretions. Advanced bronchioloalveolar cell carinoma may unusually produce extremely copious and salty-tasting sputum, the sheer volume of which provides the patient with an exhausting and unbearable problem that is best dealt with by regular and increasing doses of morphine.

Inhalations of nebulized solutions of local anaesthetic may prove effective in intractable cough where other measures have failed. They suffer from the disadvantage of anaesthetizing the mouth and pharynx so that fluids or food may be inadvertently aspirated if taken within 1 h of the dose. Lidocaine (lignocaine) up to 5 mL of 2% solution every 6 h may be used; alternatively, bupivicaine 0.25% solution has been recommended at a dose of up to 5 mL every 8 h [26,27].

Dyspnoea and associated symptoms

As with other respiratory symptoms in the terminally ill, the advice that treatment for shortness of breath is available and effective and that support is at hand may provide reassuring comfort. Relaxation techniques and simple measures such as the provision of a fan may increase comfort. Sometimes breathlessness in advanced malignancy may be treated by attention to the cause, such as those listed below.

1 Obstruction of a large central airway by tumour that may be responsive to radiotherapy, laser treatment or stenting (see Chapter 41). Stridor in this situation may also be temporarily relieved by breathing a commercially available mixture of helium and oxygen (4:1). Dexamethasone 16 mg daily may also help.

2 Restriction of the movement of the affected hemithorax by the presence of a pleural effusion, in which case relief may be obtained by thoracentesis (see Chapter 43). In both these cases the clinician has to make a judgement on whether active intervention will improve the patient's comfort. If the end is seemingly very close, then invasive measures are probably unwarranted. Sometimes surprisingly large effusions may occur in the absence of symptoms, in which case they should be left alone. At other times simply changing the posture of a recumbent patient with unilateral lung disease so that the 'good lung' is dependent improves oxygenation [28].

When reaccumulation of a symptomatic effusion occurs, further aspiration is merited; if the reaccumulation has been rapid, some form of sclerosant such as 500 mg tetracycline added to 50 mL of normal saline and 10 mL 1% lidocaine in a 60-mL syringe can be introduced intrapleurally after drainage, left overnight and any residual fluid removed the next day [29,30]. A slurry of talc in saline may be similarly used. Even with lidocaine and other analgesia, this procedure is often painful and a useful outcome not always forthcoming.

Sometimes dyspnoea may result from associated disease such as pneumonia or an exacerbation of chronic bronchitis; symptomatic relief using nebulized bronchodilators may be achieved in the latter case. The giving or withholding of antibiotics depends on the physician's assessment of whether the symptoms of infection are causing distress and whether further prolongation of life is likely to be wished for by either the patient or close relatives. It may sometimes be important to gain some extra time if, for example, a close relation is travelling from afar or if legal or other affairs need settling. At other times pneumonia may provide a welcome release to all concerned.

Frequently in terminal respiratory malignancy, treatment cannot usefully be addressed to the cause of breathlessness, which may be diffuse neoplastic spread, and remedies are directed to the symptom of dyspnoea itself. Once again a strong opioid analgesic such as morphine is required and can be used in similar doses to those already described for the relief of pain. This has the advantage of suppressing respiratory drive centrally and of decreasing anxiety and distress. It also relieves any associated chest pain, which may itself be making breathing difficult and uncomfortable. The association of chronic obstructive airways disease with advanced malignancy is not a contraindication to the use of morphine in a patient whose life is drawing to its close and who is experiencing significant dyspnoea.

Nebulized morphine or diamorphine has been used in attempts to control dyspnoea. Reports of its efficacy in cancer have been based on uncontrolled observations and are therefore open to question [13,31,32]. As might be expected, doses used vary widely, from 5 mg morphine added to 5 mL of normal saline to as much as 50 mg diamorphine. Conflicting results have been reported when this form of treatment has been used in other patient groups, including those with dyspnoea due to severe chronic lung and heart disease [33–35]. Benzodiazepines such as diazepam starting with a small dose such as 2 mg three times daily may also help to alleviate the anxiety associated with breathlessness and are worth trying. Sublingual lorazepam 2.5–5 mg has a rapid onset of action and a short half-life, lending itself to self-administration for the management of more acute dyspnoea that may be associated with panic.

Although the provision of oxygen may have little to offer in a physiological sense, the availability of an oxygen cylinder to a person who feels the need for 'more air' may be a source of some comfort to both the patient and family. This having been said, the proper provision of morphine is likely to reduce such feelings of need for what is often a psychological crutch.

As a dying patient weakens to the extent that coughing is no longer easy, loose secretions may be heard to rattle in the larger airways during respiration. By this time the patient's conscious level may be sufficiently depressed for the sensation to go unnoticed and it may be a greater source of distress to those about the bed who have to listen to it. Repositioning of the patient may help in this respect. The traditional remedy is the atropine-like substance hyoscine hydrobromide, given at a dose of 400–600 μg every 4 h subcutaneously as necessary or infused subcutaneously at a dose of 1.2–2.4 mg over 24 h. The rationale for this is that it dries bronchial secretions and that it is less likely than atropine to cause central nervous system stimulation. The extent to which it is effective is somewhat doubtful.

Dehydration

Whereas it is good practice to keep patients who still have a chance of recovery well hydrated and nourished when they are too ill to swallow, this line of action makes little sense in a patient who is dying; indeed there is a strong body of opinion among hospice workers that dehydration is symptomatically beneficial in terminal patients, reducing the problems of urinary incontinence and also those of loose bronchial secretions referred to in the previous section [36]. It is sensible to avoid intravenous or nasogastric tube rehydration in such circumstances. Attention can instead be paid to mouth care [37], keeping the patient's mouth moistened with 2-mL aliquots of cool water by syringe or with chips of ice.

Haemoptysis

The small haemoptyses that occur commonly in association with lung cancer are a source of anxiety to the patient and firm reassurance that they do not presage a major bleed may be all that is required. If the haemoptysis persists and is of sufficient volume to continue to cause the concern, palliative radiotherapy may very well be helpful and should be requested (see Chapter 41). In the mean time, an oral haemostatic agent such as tranexamic acid or etamsylate (ethamsylate) that tends to reduce capillary bleeding can be tried, although there are no published controlled trials to support the clinical impression that they may help in this situation. A major haemorrhage is rare, but should one occur and if the patient survives and remains conscious, an immediate intravenous injection of 5–10 mg morphine is advisable and may if necessary be followed by a similar dose of diazepam by the same route in order to reduce fear and awareness. The patient should not be left alone and blood stains on the bed linen should be covered with red or green towelling to reduce further alarm [31].

Constipation

Constipation is an inevitable consequence of any terminal illness that is protracted and is a cause of considerable anxiety to patients unless dealt with adequately. It is best to anticipate it and treat from an early stage with laxatives, particularly in patients taking narcotics or other constipating drugs. Opioids are one of the major causes of constipation in terminal illness, tending to increase smooth muscle tone with suppression of peristalsis while also increasing sphincter tone and reducing the awareness of rectal distension. Other factors contributing to constipation are anorexia, leading to a poor intake, dehydration, inactivity and general debility. Hypercalcaemia or the use of tricyclic antidepressants may also be contributory and the possibility of spinal cord compression should not be forgotten.

It is routine to combine a stool-softening laxative with a bowel stimulant, since a single agent of either class may produce an inadequate effect. There are numerous laxatives available, the liquid preparations being referred to by some patients as 'engine oil'. It is best to become familiar with a few but to be prepared to make some adjustments according to patient preference.

Although liquid paraffin is avoided in other longer-term situations because of its propensity to cause lipoid pneumonia, it is a suitable stool softener for use in patients with terminal conditions, a dose of 10–30 mL being taken on retiring (as combined with magnesium hydroxide in Milpar). Other agents that have stool-softening effects include the bulking agents methylcellulose, which may produce bloatedness, and lactulose, which draws water into the bowel osmotically and which has a sickly taste. Examples of bowel stimulants include senna taken in tablets or as granules 15–30 mg or bisacodyl tablets 10 mg, both taken on retiring. These preparations have effect within the following 10–12 h [38]. Another very useful alternative is the stimulant dantron (danthron), combined with a stool softener such as poloxamer (i.e. co-danthramer) or the surfactant docusate (i.e. co-danthrusate), both being available as capsules (two at night or up to three four times daily) or as a suspension usually to be taken at night.

If the patient remains constipated for more than 2 days and examination reveals formed stools in the rectum, then two glycerol suppositories may be used for their stimulant effect, an alternative stimulant suppository being bisacodyl 10 mg which may produce rapid results. Both of these should act within an hour or so. If examination shows the rectum to be empty then a high phosphate enema, delivered via a soft catheter inserted 20 cm into the rectum to prevent immediate expulsion, may be used. Unusually an impacted rectum requires manual evacuation combined with some form of sedation. High soap and warm water enemas are sometimes required for gross constipation that has been neglected but this is also unusual.

Miscellaneous symptoms

Anorexia

Anorexia and weight loss are frequent accompaniments of advanced malignant disease. The mechanism is obscure but is likely to be multifactorial, apparently being related to the production of cytokines and to tumour type rather than size. Some predisposing factors are readily identifiable and can be dealt with appropriately.

Nausea

Nausea resulting from opiates may be controlled with an antiemetic such as cyclizine (50 mg) or metoclopramide (10 mg), each to be taken three times a day before meals. Haloperidol 1.5 mg at night or twice daily may also be effective. Mouth care should be meticulous. Nausea and vomiting occurring as a result of chemotherapy may be effectively prevented by a selective serotonin receptor antagonist such as ondansetron [39]. This drug, as well as granisetron and tropisetron, acts by antagonizing 5-HT_3 receptor-mediated activation of afferent gastrointestinal neurones before they can trigger the brainstem centres that initiate vomiting. Prednisolone 15–30 mg daily frequently improves the appetite as well as having a mild euphoriant effect but does not result in lost weight being regained [40]. An alcoholic drink before meals may also be helpful. Dexamethasone reduces vomiting due to raised intracranial pressure from brain metastases (see below).

Dysphagia

Dysphagia may be caused by a sore or dry mouth and may be managed with regular mouth rinses. If the patient is too weak to drink, 2 mL of water can be placed in the dependent side of the mouth with a syringe every 30 min or small pieces of ice may be used for the same purpose. Nystatin suspension 200 000 units four or five times daily may be used if oral thrush is present; alternatively amphotericin lozenges may be sucked. Ketoconazole 200 mg daily for 5 days is effective in difficult cases and fluconazole 50 mg daily for 1–2 weeks may be taken if oeophageal candidiasis is suspected or confirmed by barium swallow. The latter drug may be taken long term in patients with recurrent candidiasis associated with AIDS. Oesophagitis occurring following irradiation of the mediastinum may be treated with the proprietary antacid Mucaine, which contains a local anaesthetic oxetacaine (oxethazaine), and patients can be reassured that the discomfort will resolve completely in a week or two. Extrinsic oesophageal compression may result from mediastinal lymph node metastases or direct extension of a tumour into the mediastinum, the diagnosis being confirmed by a radiographic contrast swallow examination. How this is managed depends not only on the general fitness of patients but also on their views about what they would like to be done. When symptoms are mild, a blender may produce food of the right consistency to pass the obstruction, but eventually dysphagia and regurgitation for liquids including saliva will occur and aspiration pneumonia will supervene. If the patient wishes for nothing further to be done, then heavy sedation with morphine is appropriate in order to relieve their inevitable distress. However, if the patient is sufficiently fit, a thoracic surgical opinion can be obtained concerning the insertion of a palliative oesophageal tube, or palliative radiotherapy may be considered.

Hiccups

Hiccuping is occasionally very persistent and troublesome in a small minority of patients with thoracic cancer. There are a large number of both central and peripheral causes, including gastric distension and mediastinal invasion by tumour. Physical stimulation of the back of the pharynx with a nasal catheter, iced water or the like may stop it and is worth trying [41]. Gastric

distension may be caused by gross hepatomegaly ('squashed stomach syndrome') and patients may be helped by practical advice to take small meals followed by 10 mg metoclopramide, which promotes normal gastric emptying. Activated dimeticone (dimethicone), an antifoaming agent, may also be used as a deflatulent in such cases, 10 mL being taken after meals. Chlorpromazine may be necessary for a severe episode of hiccups but is sedating and may cause postural hypotension, particularly in the elderly. It can be tried orally at first at a dose of 10–25 mg three times daily followed by a single slow intravenous dose of 25 mg if necessary. Other treatments sometimes used include carbamazepine, nifedipine, baclofen, haloperidol, ketamine, phenytoin and, in extreme cases, intravenous lidocaine [42,43].

Sleeplessness

Sleeplessness may be due to a readily identifiable cause such as pain, in which case appropriate analgesia can be given. Where no such cause is evident, a benzodiazepine such a temazepam 10 mg may be given. Alternatively, nitrazepam 5 mg at night may provide some anxiolytic effect the next day as this has a longer half-life. Benzodiazepines may produce confusion in elderly patients in whom clomethiazole (chlormethiazole) two capsules at night is a useful alternative.

Symptoms due to cerebral metastases

Nausea, vomiting and pain are dealt with as outlined in earlier sections of this chapter. The decision about whether to treat more actively using steroids and/or radiotherapy must take account of the patient's general situation as well as the attitude of any close family. No particular benefit may be seen in achieving a temporary respite in a patient who is clearly in the terminal phase of the disease. In other circumstances, more active management might be considered to be in their best interests. Dexamethasone 16 mg daily for 1–2 weeks is given in order to reduce oedema around metastases. If there is no response, the drug can be rapidly tailed off. If response does occur, the dose may be reduced by 2 mg per week to a 'maintenance' dose of about 4 mg daily. Recurrent symptoms sometimes respond to an increase in the dose to its original level. A response to dexamethasone may encourage the radiotherapist to treat with palliative cranial irradiation. The opposite usually deters them from intervening.

Epileptic seizures

Epileptic seizures are treated in conventional manner with an oral anticonvulsant such as phenytoin 150–600 mg daily. If the parenteral route is required, diazepam 10 mg may be given intravenously over 2 min to control a persistent fit and may be repeated if necessary. An emulsified form, Diazemuls, is best used to avoid thrombophlebitis. Another option if intravenous access is difficult is to give diazepam as a rectal solution, also at a dose of 10 mg. Phenobarbital (phenobarbitone) may then be given twice daily intramuscularly if the oral route remains unavailable. When the patient is in the terminal phase, fits may be controlled by subcutaneous midazolam, given by syringe driver at a dose of 20–40 mg per 24 h. This is also suitable for very restless patients (see below) and is compatible with diamorphine.

Confusion, restlessness and delirium

Confusion in elderly ill patients is often attributed to their inability to adapt to changed circumstances or an altered environment. Whether or not this is true, it is worth spending some time thinking through possible physical causes of confusion that might be amenable to treatment. Psychotropic drugs, including narcotic analgesics, benzodiazepines and corticosteroids, should all be suspected. Metabolic disturbances, such as uraemia, hypercalcaemia or a low blood glucose due to regular oral hypoglycaemic therapy, may be responsible for disturbances of consciousness. Confusion or agitation may also arise as a result of systemic infection, hypoxaemia or urinary retention. Sedative drugs are required if confusion cannot be settled by identification and treatment of any such cause (provided that there is no response to simple reassurance) and if it is causing distress or if it is likely to result in physical injury to the patient or anyone else. In mild cases of confusion and restlessness, haloperidol 1.5–5 mg at bedtime may be sufficient. For severe delirium, haloperidol 5–10 mg may be given subcutaneously or intravenously, being repeated hourly until the patient is settled, after which it may be continued orally if necessary. Alternatives are thioridazine 25 mg three times daily, which has to be taken orally, and chlorpromazine 50 mg intramuscularly or orally followed by 25–50 mg three times daily, the latter drug being useful if more sedation is required. Levomepromazine (methotrimeprazine) is a more heavily sedating alternative for restlessness and confusion in the terminal stage, being infused subcutaneously at a dose of 20–100 mg per 24 h. When necessary this can be combined with diamorphine in the same syringe driver. A good nursing technique is invaluable in dealing with such patients and every attempt should be made to understand and calm them. It should never be assumed that patients cannot understand what is being said in their presence and the relatives feel better if they can be given a physical explanation for the disturbance rather than be left with the impression that the doctors and nurses do not know what is going on.

Psychological aspects

Attempts to unravel the psychology of dying are beyond the scope of this chapter. Suffice to say that the journey may be charged with many strong emotions and that appropriate action on the part of those in a position of care may work strongly to diminish the unpleasantness and to provide comfort and support in the face of suffering [44]. It is dangerous to generalize about the nature of an individual's response to the revelation that life will shortly end, but nevertheless such generalizations have been made and are widely quoted.

Kübler-Ross [45] describes five stages: first denial and isolation, then anger followed by bargaining, then depression and finally acceptance, the passage through these stages respresenting a gradual process of realization. In reality many reactions are encountered and they do not necessarily occur in any particular sequence. Initial incomprehension is almost invariably followed by apprehension and various mental acrobatics that are apparently performed to avoid the perception of unpleasant reality. Bargaining is said to occur if patients 'do deals' with their own conscience to behave in a certain manner in order to improve the chances of a more successful outcome. Denial may be tested by asking patients whether they have times when they feel that they may not 'beat' the illness after all. Patients are likely to experience sadness, depression or despair but may also display hopefulness and optimism and may slip in and out of these different emotions from day to day as they seek to cope with their illness. It is to be hoped that the inevitability of new circumstances is eventually accepted and that this acceptance brings with it an inner tranquillity. Certainly this peace of mind is the major objective of terminal care, as it brings comfort to the patient and is a source of strength to the family, whereas anger and resentment does the reverse. As has been previously emphasized in this chapter, it is generally thought that kindly, open and supportive discussion helps the patient to achieve acceptance.

Organization

Most patients with terminal cancer die in hospital in the UK, and the type of terminal care that they receive is influenced not only by the training and attitudes of those who look after them but also by the other demands inevitably placed upon the staff of busy acute wards. One of the achievements of the hospice movement has been to promote discussion and to disseminate a greater understanding of the needs of the dying [46]. Whereas the acute hospital ward cannot produce the same physical environment, nevertheless it should be possible to transpose some of the organizational practices and the general ethos of the hospice or 'continuing care' unit to the management of terminal patients in any hospital. Such care depends upon good liaison between the senior nurse on the ward, the medical team and the social worker, and time spent talking not only to the patient but also to the family and the general practitioner is in itself therapeutic. Physiotherapists and occupational therapists also play an important role in helping the patient to remain as independent as practicable. The family should be allowed to come and go as they please and should be made to feel welcome on the ward, rather than being restricted to predetermined visiting hours. Their anxieties should be listened to and an attempt should be made to deal with them in a well thought out manner. When practicable, home visits or excursions with the relations should be allowed and whenever possible the patient should be discharged with the provision of adequate social support and district nursing care. Specialized care such as that given by Macmillan nurses may be made available and provision should be made for readmission if the need arises.

The anxieties of patients should be appreciated; many fear separation from their family and home and are happier in their own surroundings if this can be arranged. A fear of dependence on others is also common and this may be alleviated by avoiding an impatient or patronizing attitude, so that care is delivered as though it was a privilege rather than a chore. Concerns about how the surviving relatives will cope may be prominent and if voiced are best dealt with in a practical manner, sometimes with the help of a sympathetic social worker, hospital chaplain or other minister of religion. A study that asked patients from whom they most wanted emotional support and from whom they most got it indicated that their first choice was their doctor and that senior doctors were perceived as providing more emotional support than junior colleagues, leading to the conclusion that this form of comfort stemmed from what was thought to be the provision of accurate and authoritative information [47,48].

References

1 Saunders C. Appropriate treatment, appropriate death. In: Saunders C, ed. *The Management of Terminal Malignant Disease*. London: Edward Arnold, 1984.
2 Mills M, Davies HTO, Macrae WA. Care of dying patients in hospital. *Br Med J* 1994; 309: 583.
3 Cleeland CS, Gonin R, Hatfield AK *et al.* Pain and its treatment in outpatients with metastatic cancer. *N Engl J Med* 1994; 330: 592.
4 Karnofsky DA, Burchenal JH. The clinical evaluation of chemotherapeutic agents in cancer. In: *Evaluation of Chemotherapeutic Agents*. New York: Columbia University Press, 1949.
5 Twycross RG. Relief of pain. In: Saunders C, ed. *The Management of Terminal Malignant Disease*. London: Edward Arnold, 1984.
6 World Health Organisation. *Cancer Pain Relief and Palliative Care*. Geneva: WHO, 1990.
7 *British National Formulary*, Vol 37. London: British Medical Association and the Royal Pharmaceutical Society of Great Britain, 1999: 6.
8 O'Neill WM. Pain in malignant disease. *Prescribers' J* 1993; 33: 250.
9 Hanks GW, Trueman T. Controlled-release tablets are effective in twice daily dosage in chronic cancer pain. *R Soc Med Int Congr Series* 1984; 64: 103.
10 Walsh TD. Opiates and respiratory function in advanced cancer. *Recent Results Cancer Res* 1984; 89: 115.
11 Cherny NI. Opioid analgesics, comparative features and prescribing guidelines. *Drugs* 1996; 51: 713.
12 Hanks GWC, de Conno F, Ripamonti C. Morphine in cancer pain: modes of administration. *Br Med J* 1996; 312: 823.
13 Regnard CFB, Davies A. *A Guide to Symptom Relief in Advanced Cancer*. Manchester: Haigh and Hochland, 1986.
14 *British National Formulary*, Vol 36. London: British Medical Association and the Royal

Pharmaceutical Society of Great Britain, 1998: 14.
15 Davis CD, Hardy JR. Palliative care. *Br Med J* 1994; 308: 1359.
16 Ventafridda V, Fochi C, De Conno D, Sganzerla E. Use of non-steroidal anti-inflammatory drugs in the treatment of pain in cancer. *Br J Clin Pharmacol* 1980; 10 (Suppl 2): 343S.
17 Levy MH. Pharmacologic treatment of cancer pain. *N Engl J Med* 1996; 335: 1124.
18 Galasko CSB. Orthopaedic principles and management. In: Doyle D, Hanks GWC, Macdonald N, eds. *Oxford Textbook of Palliative Medicine*. Oxford: Oxford Medical Publications, 1993.
19 Bowsher D. Paradoxical pain when the metabolites of morphine are in the wrong ratio. *Br Med J* 1993; 306: 473.
20 Morley JS, Miles JB, Wells JC *et al.* Paradoxical pain. *Lancet* 1993; 340: 1045.
21 Sykes J, Johnson R, Hanks GW. Difficult pain problems. *Br Med J* 1997; 315: 867.
22 Melzack R, Wall PD. Pain mechanisms: a new theory. *Science* 1965; 150: 971.
23 Arner S. The role of nerve blocks in the treatment of cancer pain. *Acta Anaesthesiol Scand* 1982; Suppl 74: 104.
24 Vainio A, Ollila J, Matikainan E *et al.* Driving ability in cancer patients receiving long-term morphine analgesia. *Lancet* 1995; 346: 667.
25 Smith AM. Patients taking stable doses of morphine may drive. *Br Med J* 1996; 312: 56.
26 Heyse-Moore L. Respiratory symptoms. In: Saunders C, ed. *The Management of Terminal Malignant Disease*. London: Edward Arnold, 1984.
27 Davis CL. Breathlessness, cough and other respiratory problems. *Br Med J* 1997; 315: 931.
28 Seaton D, Morgan WKC, Lapp NL. Effect of body position on gas exchange after thoracotomy. *Thorax* 1978; 34: 518.
29 Wallach HW. Intrapleural tetracycline for

malignant pleural effusions. *Chest* 1975; 68: 510.
30 Dhillon DP, Spiro SG. Malignant pleural effusions. *Br J Hosp Med* 1983; 29: 506.
31 Ahmedzai S. Palliation of respiratory symptoms. In: Doyle D, Hanks GWC, Macdonald N, eds. *Oxford Textbook of Palliative Medicine*. Oxford: Oxford Medical Publications, 1993.
32 Tooms A, McKenzie A, Grey H. Nebulised morphine. *Lancet* 1993; 342: 1123.
33 Masood AR, Reed JW, Thomas SHL. Lack of effect of inhaled morphine on exercise-induced breathlessness in chronic obstructive pulmonary disease. *Thorax* 1995; 50: 629.
34 Farncombe M, Chater S. Case studies outlining use of nebulized morphine for patients with end-stage chronic lung and cardiac disease. *J Pain Symptom Manage* 1993; 8: 221.
35 Young JH, Daviskas E, Keena VA. Effect of low dose nebulised morphine on exercise endurance in patients with chronic lung disease. *Thorax* 1989; 44: 387.
36 Twycross RG, Lichter I. The terminal phase. In: Doyle D, Hanks GWC, Macdonald N, eds. *Oxford Textbook of Palliative Medicine*. Oxford: Oxford Medical Publications, 1993.
37 Regnard C, Allport S, Stephenson L. Mouth care, skin care and lymphoedema. *Br Med J* 1997; 315: 1002.
38 Godding EW. Therapeutic agents. In: Avery Jones F, Godding EW, eds. *Management of Constipation*. Oxford: Blackwell Scientific Publications, 1972.
39 Markham A, Sorkin EM. Ondansetron. *Drugs* 1993; 45: 931.
40 Loprinzi CL, Goldberg RM, Burnham NL. Cancer associated anorexia and cachexia. *Drugs* 1992; 43: 499.
41 Salem MR, Baraka A, Rattenborg CC *et al.* Treatment of hiccups by pharyngeal stimulation in anaesthetized and concious subjects. *JAMA* 1967; 202: 126.
42 Howard RS. Persistent hiccups. *Br Med J* 1992; 305: 1237.

43 Dunst MN, Margolin K, Horak D. Lidocaine for severe hiccups. *N Engl J Med* 1992; 329: 890.

44 Fallowfield L. Psychosocial interventions in cancer. *Br Med J* 1995; 311: 1316.

45 Ross EK. *On Death and Dying.* London: Tavistock, 1970.

46 Bulkin W, Lukashok H. Rx for dying: the case for hospice. *N Engl J Med* 1988; 318: 376.

47 Slevin ML, Downer S, Cody M *et al.* The evaluation of emotional support by patients with cancer. *Br J Cancer* 1990; 63: 11.

48 Slevin ML. Quality of life: philosophical question or clinical reality. *Br Med J* 1992; 305: 466.

61

MEDICOLEGAL ASPECTS OF LUNG DISEASE

ANTHONY SEATON

At its simplest, the law exists to protect citizens, their property and the environment within which they exist from harm due to the actions or omissions of others. Doctors may become involved in legal processes in their role as citizen, as when they are sued by an aggrieved patient or, fortunately rarely, accused of a criminal offence such as unlawful killing, or in their role as medical expert when asked to give evidence about the causation and consequences of disease. This chapter is concerned with the latter role, relating particularly to lung disease.

The great majority of cases in which a medical expert is likely to be involved occur under the civil, as opposed to the criminal, law. The difference is important with respect to the legal definition of proof, a matter not always appreciated by doctors. In criminal law, in which a crime is alleged to have been committed, it is necessary for the prosecution to prove a case 'beyond reasonable doubt'. This form of proof is similar to that with which we are familiar in our clinical role, in which we pursue the investigation of a patient until fairly certain that we know the diagnosis. In contrast, in civil proceedings it is only necessary for the litigant (sometimes referred to as the plaintiff or pursuer) to prove the case 'on the balance of probabilities', i.e. greater than 50% likelihood or more likely than not. This test applies to all matters in contention, such as the presence of a particular disease, the likelihood of something having caused it and whether appropriate measures were taken to prevent it. In most jurisdictions, civil cases are argued before a judge, both parties being represented by lawyers who examine their own witnesses and cross-examine those called on behalf of the other side. The judge arrives at a verdict and decides the amount of the award in damages. In contrast, in the USA all cases are argued before a jury, which is responsible not only for the verdict but also for assessing the amount of the award. In general the award of damages takes account of all financial losses, both actual and likely future ones, in terms of earnings, expenses and so on, and of pain and suffering. Again, in the USA an additional sum is often added by the

jury, so-called punitive damages, often adding considerably to the award.

A further difference between the USA and most other jurisdictions is the method of obtaining the services of a lawyer. In most countries, the transaction involves a fee for service, usually calculated on the basis of guidelines issued by the relevant professional body. This means that the costs of litigation are considerable and, as has been found by many who have sued unsuccessfully for libel, ruinous. The costs may be recovered if the action is successful, at the discretion of the judge, but if the litigation is unsuccessful they fall upon the litigant. Thus only the very wealthy can usually afford to embark on legal action unsupported by some other agency. In the USA this problem has been overcome by the introduction of a system of contingency fees, lawyers agreeing to act for a client on a speculative basis with an agreement that they will pay the costs if unsuccessful but will take a percentage of the damages if successful. The introduction of a similar system is likely in the UK, and has already been introduced by some law firms. From the experience in the USA it seems to be associated with inflationary pressures on court settlements and acts as a stimulus to an ambulance-chasing form of legal behaviour. However, it does ensure that anyone with a reasonable case can obtain legal representation. In the UK, most injured workers manage at present to obtain support from their trade union, a powerful reason for being a member of one, or from the state through legal aid. Legal aid is means-tested and is likely to be available to fewer people in future as part of an effort to control government expenditure.

Compensation

No-fault benefits

It is not uncommon for a doctor to be asked by a patient if he or she is entitled to compensation for some work-related lung disease. In these circumstances, it is wise to advise the patient to consult a lawyer, preferably through the trade union. If the patient is not a member, limited advice may be obtained from the Citizens' Advice Bureaux or similar organizations. However, there is some useful advice that a doctor can give. Most importantly, doctors should be aware of the system of no-fault benefits available in their country or state. In the UK there is a state-funded system of industrial injuries benefits available to all employed people (but not self-employed, who have to make their own insurance arrangements) who suffer an injury or illness as a result of their work, funded from the social security budget. While any work-caused injury is potentially eligible for compensation, benefits for illnesses are only available if the illness is prescribed, i.e. on a list agreed by Parliament. This list is updated regularly as a result of the recommendations of an independent committee of experts, the Industrial Injuries Advisory Council, who base their advice on the medical, mainly epidemiological, evidence relating diseases to work. The lung diseases currently prescribed on this list are shown in Table 61.1.

Before advising a patient to seek industrial injuries benefit, the doctor should ensure first that the patient is or was employed as opposed to self-employed. It is also the case that this system of compensation is not available to

Table 61.1 Prescribed occupational lung diseases in the UK.

Disease	Prescribed occupation
Anthrax	Contact with animals or their products
Tuberculosis	Medical or laboratory contact
Extrinsic allergic alveolitis	Agriculture, malt work, mushroom growing, bird handling, bagasse handling
Asthma	Exposure to a sensitizing agent
Byssinosis	Contact with cotton or flax dust
Various poisonings	Exposure to mercury, cadmium, nickel carbonyl, beryllium, nitrogen oxides
Pneumoconiosis	Mining, quarrying, ceramics, foundary work, asbestos handling, etc.
Mesothelioma	Asbestos handling
Lung cancer	Nickel refining, asbestos handling (if asbestosis or diffuse pleural fibrosis is also present), and in the presence of silicosis
Nasal cancer	Nickel refining, woodwork, shoe manufacture
Bilateral pleural fibrosis	Asbestos handling

For full details, see *Notes on the Diagnosis of Occupational Disease* (1979) HMSO, London; and leaflets published by the Department of Social Security: NI 3 (pneumoconiosis) and NI 238 (asthma).

members of the armed services, who may however be able to obtain war pensions instead. Secondly, it is necessary to be reasonably sure that the disease was caused, and not simply made worse, by work. Thirdly, the illness must be one that is on the list of prescribed diseases and the patient must have been working in a trade in which a relevant exposure is likely to have occurred. Alternatively, if the illness occurred as a consequence of an accidental exposure, say to a toxic gas or fume, benefits may be claimable for an industrial injury rather than for a prescribed disease. If these conditions are fulfilled, the patient should be told that it is worth applying for benefits and an explanation of the process given. Application must be made by the patient to the local branch of the Department of Social Security (DSS), where a form needs to be completed, indicating the disease being claimed for and the work that the patient has been doing. There then follows an interview with an insurance officer, whose job is simply to ensure that the applicant has indeed been employed and is eligible for benefits if the prescribed disease is present. The papers are then sent to the regional panel of DSS doctors specializing in respiratory diseases, whose role is to determine, on the balance of probabilities, whether the patient has the prescribed disease and to determine the extent of disablement ascribable to it. This determination is expressed in terms of loss of faculty, i.e. loss of the functional abilities of a healthy person of the same age and sex, account being taken of the employability of the individual as a result of the illness. A percentage figure for loss of faculty is arrived at and this is usually applied by the insurance officer to calculate the benefit payments. A sum for 100% disability is agreed by Parliament each year. In some circumstances, a lump sum payment may be made to the claimant, but more usually an annual pension is awarded and this may be adjusted after further medical assessments in the light of improvement or deterioration in the patient's condition. Such reviews usually take place every 2 years. If a patient is unsuccessful in claiming benefit, there is a mechanism for appeal to a Medical Appeals Tribunal, chaired by a lawyer and including doctors with special experience of lung disease.

This system of state benefits was introduced at a time when injured workers were effectively unable, because of the costs of litigation and lack of a system of social security, to obtain any compensation and were often rendered indigent. It remains in force now despite a comprehensive system of sickness benefits available to those unable to work for whatever cause, and therefore provides people injured at work with benefits additional to those available to someone injured, say, in a domestic accident or suffering from some illness as a result of ill-fortune. It may therefore be regarded as something of an anomaly, and in recent years there has been a progressive erosion of the value of the benefits payable. At one time it served to limit the numbers of people seeking redress through the courts, but more recently an award of benefits is often taken as an indication that a claim in civil law is likely to be successful; this is far from always the case, since in civil litigation it is necessary not only to show that the disease is present and was caused by the work but also to prove that it occurred as a consequence of the employer's negligence. If a patient is successful in obtaining damages in a civil case, any state benefits paid in respect of the illness are repayable.

Civil litigation

When patients wish to sue their employer, the main role of the doctor is in advising them whether they have a work-related disease or not, and it is then up to patients to seek advice from a lawyer. The date at which this advice is given should be recorded, since in most jurisdictions there is a limited time available from the moment the patient became aware that the illness was caused by work for the lawyer to lodge a claim against the employer(s). This so-called time bar sometimes becomes an issue when a patient only decides to see a lawyer after hearing of a successful claim by a colleague, most commonly for a relatively trivial condition such as pleural plaques.

The process of civil litigation involves the issue of a writ, or a statement that the litigant is suing the employer for a stated sum in compensation for suffering and loss incurred as a result of illness caused by the negligence of the person sued. The negligence is defined in terms of the defender's failure to comply with the law as it obtained at the time the injury occurred. This is then answered by the lawyers acting for the defender, who generally enter a robust denial of any negligence or of any knowledge that the litigant has indeed suffered any injury. These documents appear to represent irreconcilable views but can be taken to be opening moves in a prolonged game in which evidence is obtained and challenged, leading in most cases to an agreement between the parties prior to appearing in court. Occasionally, however, the case actually reaches the courts and is argued before a judge, witnesses being examined and cross-examined by advocates. This outcome should always be anticipated by any doctor writing a report for a lawyer.

Lawyers, like doctors, specialize and some firms are particularly effective in the area of work-related illness. The good lawyer seeks the opinion of a doctor recognized as an expert in the field of lung disease as to what the illness is, what is likely to have been the cause, to what extent the patient is disabled and the likely prognosis. In general, advice is not sought from a chest physician as to whether or not the person being sued was negligent, since this is a legal matter. However, the lawyer may require advice about the state of medical knowledge at the time the injury is alleged to have occurred in order to determine whether the defender could reasonably have foreseen the consequences of the alleged negligence. Both parties to the litigation seek advice independently from experts, both in respect of diagnosis and disability and often also in relation to conditions in the workplace. Having obtained such evidence as they require, they usually consult with a trial lawyer (barrister in England, advocate in Scotland) and decide how to proceed. The costs of a court hearing are considerable, and in most cases settlement can be arrived at by a process of discussion (or a game of cat-and-mouse) between opposing lawyers, the decision often being reached shortly before the hearing and indeed sometimes on the first day. This settlement is usually reached on the basis of a payment, including costs, by the defender to the litigant without accepting responsibility for the injury. If after such an offer is made and refused the case proceeds to trial and the litigant is subsequently awarded a smaller sum in damages than that offered, the responsibility for costs of the action may fall on the litigant. There is thus a good incentive to accept a reasonable offer.

If the case proceeds to trial, the lawyers state their positions before the judge and call witnesses. All witnesses, whether giving evidence about conditions in the workplace at the relevant time or an expert opinion, are led through their evidence by the lawyer for whom they are acting and then cross-examined by the lawyer for the other side, whose job it is to discredit them. At this point, every word and opinion written in a report may be subject to the most detailed inquisition. Any papers quoted in support of statements by an expert may be dissected, and the opinions put forward by one doctor are likely to be challenged by those of another. The whole process requires not just a cool head but also an unshakeable ability to justify all one says and all one has already committed to paper. It is never an enjoyable experience and can be likened to an anatomy viva prolonged, sometimes, for a day or two! This possible outcome should be borne in mind by anyone writing a report for a lawyer. With the agreement of the judge, witnesses may be recalled to deal with matters brought up in subsequent evidence and some trial lawyers may ask experts to assist them through the course of the trial with informal medical advice. Once the evidence has been heard, the lawyers summarize their cases and the judge eventually delivers a decision and, if finding for the plaintiff, decides on an appropriate sum in damages and costs.

The system in the USA differs in several ways. The trial lawyer may often conduct both the investigative and trial parts of the action, and is likely to wish to maximize the chances of success by giving advice to the expert on such matters as how to address a jury, how best to present a case and so on. Witnesses are often required to make a deposition before the case comes to court; lawyers call this 'being deposed' and it involves being questioned for a prolonged period by the lawyer from the other side in order to find out what evidence will be given and just how knowledgeable the witness really is. If the case comes to trial it is argued before a jury and all sorts of stratagems are used to convince the jurors of a witness's veracity and expertise. The process is undoubtedly less gentlemanly than the British version, and clearly the lawyers for the litigant, being on a contingency fee, have a lot more at stake than just professional pride. In both systems, however, when a case comes to court the arguments are usually finely balanced and the most important factors in determining the outcome are the expertise and skill of the advocate and the competence of the expert witnesses.

Role of the doctor as expert

From what has been said above, a doctor should not agree to write an expert medical opinion unless he or she has a particular knowledge of the subject and should confine any opinions to those pertaining to these areas of expertise. There may be a temptation to overstep these limits in support, perhaps, of one's patient but this should be resisted for fear of having to justify them in the witness box in the face of conflicting evidence from a real expert and from the literature. A doctor is approached by lawyers from one or other side, and here again there is a temptation to slant one's evidence in favour of that side. While this is understandable and may indeed be encouraged by some lawyers, it is unwise since it leads to difficulties in justifying the opinion under cross-examination and possible loss of credibility as an expert. An expert should give as honest and impartial advice as possible and it is for the lawyers to act as advocates. It can be argued that good lawyers want to know the truth, even if it does not support their case, since this helps to decide on settlement and thus minimize costs. This does not mean that an expert should not point out possible defences or weaknesses in the other side's case, where such matters fall within his or her field of expertise. In an ideal world, the opinions of experts about an individual patient should differ little, and this in fact is frequently the case with respect to disease and its causation. There is often greater scope for disagreement with respect to prognosis, though even here agreement is usually possible by compromise. Exchange of medical reports prior to trial, in the expectation of being able to resolve relatively small differences, is becoming more common in British actions and is a desirable tendency.

Expert medical report

A report is written in response to a letter requesting advice from a lawyer, and that letter should ask the questions that the lawyer wishes answered. In general there are four: what disease does the client suffer from, is it likely that the illness was caused by the client's work, how disabled is the client and what is the prognosis? If the doctor is an expert in occupational medicine, the lawyer may in addition wish to know whether the precautions taken to prevent disease were reasonable in the light of knowledge at the time in question. The letter may ask the expert to examine the patient or it may simply request an opinion on various records, statements by others and radiographs.

The format of the report is of course a matter for the individual doctor, although it is sensible to have one's personal style and stick to it in order to avoid neglecting any important matters. It is usual to head it with a note of the case and a statement of what was done and when. If the doctor has not previously worked for the lawyer requesting advice, it may be helpful to state one's qualifications, both formal and in respect of one's expertise in the case at hand, and it is usual to provide the lawyer with a short curriculum vitae. Clinical and research experience with respect to the alleged condition are relevant, as are any personal publications on the subject. However, it is worth noting that any such publications can appear in court at a later stage if they appear to contradict any part of the evidence given in the report or orally in court, and may result in dramatic loss of credibility! The author has come across a report written by an expert denying the existence of a condition that he himself had described some two decades previously, an act of carelessness that destroyed his case.

The report should then detail the findings from the history and examination of the litigant, from careful reading of any written material provided or from both. It is usually sensible to seek corroboration of the clinical history, which may be imperfect on account of forgetfulness or deliberate deceit, from hospital and general practice notes. The lawyer should be asked to obtain these prior to seeing the client if at all possible and they should normally be reviewed prior to writing a definitive report. Particular care should be taken over the occupational history, since this is crucial to determining if work was likely to have been responsible for the condition. If the illness is thought to have been caused by an acute exposure to toxic gas, full details of the episode are necessary together with their temporal relationship to the onset of symptoms. All available evidence as to what gases or fumes were involved, where the exposure took place and for how long, and what were the likely concentrations should be considered. Lawyers are often able to provide data sheets and witness statements in such circumstances and should be asked to obtain them if they are not available. It is of course essential to form an opinion on the health of the client prior to the accident and how it has changed as a result. In the case of illness thought to be due to longer exposure, as in the case of mineral dust diseases, a lifetime occupational history is essential, again making particular note of possible levels and duration of exposure to harmful substances. This information on likely exposures is often disputed in actions that reach the court, and it is crucial to convince oneself that the individual's history is consistent with the disease that is present.

It is usual as part of the process of examination to include certain tests, depending on what has been done before. A chest radiograph is clearly essential in many cases, as are lung function tests. However, in the case of occupational asthma it is useful to remember that the legal test of proof is on the balance of probabilities, and such tests as serial peak flow rates and challenge with suspected antigen are rarely necessary. Indeed, challenge testing has potential hazards and should only be considered as part of a clinical rather than medicolegal investigation.

Having recorded the findings, it is usual to provide a commentary written in non-technical language. This is conveniently set out under headings corresponding to the questions asked by the lawyer. Thus, the first section might be headed 'What does the client suffer from?', the next 'What are the likely causes?', then 'How disabled is the client?' and finally 'What is the prognosis?'

In assessing disablement, a particular problem commonly arises when the litigant has two or more conditions. A sensible balanced judgement should be made as to which are the main contributors to disability. For example, is is not uncommon to see people whose disability has been attributed to pleural fibrosis when they have normal lung function but clear evidence of ischaemic heart disease. The author has seen patients with breathlessness due not only to this condition but also undiagnosed atrial septal defect and motoneurone disease, in all of whom an expert had confidently attributed the symptom to pleural disease. The patient with atrial septal defect was actually cured of his symptom as a result of entering the process of litigation, having missed this benefit from the normal medical process.

In discussing disablement, it is important to differentiate between impairment, disability and handicap. An abnormality of lung function is a measure of *impairment*, and is convincing evidence of lung disease if the tests have been done carefully and reliably. In this respect it is always wise to check the original traces if the tests were not done personally. However, it does not of itself provide a measure of *disability*, which takes account of the expected activity levels of a person of the same age and sex. A person with abnormal lung function may be free of disability because the impairment does not interfere with normal activities, while someone with normal lung function may be disabled because of psychological breathlessness due to anxiety about, for example, a spurious diagnosis. The level of disability is assessed from the history and its likely cause is judged by considering the results of the lung function tests. *Handicap* is a measure of the amount to which individuals are prevented from pursuing their normal lives and therefore takes account of their work. Thus someone with occupational asthma due

to spraying isocyanate paints may no longer show any impairment of function or disability but may be severely handicapped in the job market because of an inability to work in the paint-spraying trades. All these points and the subtle distinctions between them need to be considered in writing that part of the report that answers questions about level of disability.

The question of prognosis is often critical if the disease is proved, since it is an important factor in determining the level of damages. If available, serial lung function tests and radiographs from the client's records are invaluable in determining prognosis and should never be ignored. It is common for doctors to take unduly optimistic or pessimistic views, depending on which side they are appearing for. This is unwise, since cases often take years to come to court and it can be embarrassing to see someone hale and hearty whom one confidently predicted would be on his last legs, or vice versa. If possible, one's prognosis should be based on epidemiological and clinical studies in the literature as well as one's own experience. The prognosis should cover not only the disease or diseases in question but also any other disease that may follow in the future as a complication of the present illness or its causes. This is particularly relevant with respect to asbestos, where damages paid to people with benign pleural plaques takes account of the future possibilities of developing mesothelioma.

This section discussing the findings and their implications should then be followed by a succinctly expressed opinion that the writer would have no difficulty defending under cross-examination. There is the likelihood of challenge in all these parts of the report; the diagnosis and the cause are usually contested and there is plenty of scope for debate on level of disability and prognosis. This opinion should state in simple terms the views arrived at on each of these points. If there is insufficient evidence on which to arrive at a conclusion, even on the balance of probabilities, this should be stated and a recommendation for further medical or legal investigation should be made. In these circumstances it is usual to offer to write a supplementary report when the further information has been produced.

Appearing in court

Receipt of a carefully argued report should assist a lawyer to decide whether the case is worth pursuing, abandoning or settling out of court. Whichever side the report is written for, a clear, honest and straightforward opinion is of much greater value than an equivocal one, even if it does not support the side who have requested it. If it is decided to pursue the case, nothing is likely to be heard for a year or two as various legal procedures are followed and further evidence obtained. The most likely outcome is agreement to settle, usually just before the hearing. Before this, it is usual for the lawyer to have a conference, and if the medical evidence is in dispute the doctors who have written reports are usually asked to attend. This helps the trial lawyer to prepare the case and courtroom tactics and is an opportunity to test the strength of the expert evidence. Thereafter the expert is summoned to court, and it is usually possible to negotiate a time within fairly tight limits. Evidence is given under oath and commences with a benign examination by the lawyer on the same side. It is usual to be asked to describe one's qualifications and position and the lawyer also asks some questions designed to demonstrate to the judge one's unique and unrivalled expertise, in comparison to the experts on the other side. The written report is likely to be discussed and the opinions expressed therein reiterated. The fun then begins with the cross-examination, when the other side's lawyer tries to show, albeit politely at first, that one's expertise is insubstantial and that the report was written on the basis of a poor appreciation of the facts of the case; in short, that one's opinion is of no value compared to that of the other experts. In the course of this there may be detailed discussion of papers from the literature that have been included as evidence and which have to be interpreted for the judge. It is as well to have read these papers carefully beforehand. After the cross-examination, the original lawyer has a chance to re-examine the expert in order to correct any false impression that may have been given and to direct the judge's attention back to the essentials of one's evidence.

All one's evidence in British civil courts is addressed to the judge, who should be spoken to with due deference and addressed by the proper title, usually 'my lord/lady'. The judge often intervenes with questions and requests for clarification or explanation. In courts in the USA, one gives one's evidence to the jurors, and this should be given at an appropriate level of comprehensibility. Again, the judge also intervenes from time to time for clarification. It is unusual to be asked to attend court throughout a hearing, although occasionally a lawyer might value an expert's comments on the evidence of other witnesses, and wish to hold conferences during the course of the trial. Generally, however, it is possible to arrange to attend simply to give evidence and then disappear.

Trends in litigation

The respiratory disease medicolegal industry in the USA has been built on asbestos, though there is substantial activity also with respect to coal, quartz and chronic airflow obstruction. In the UK, there has been and continues to be much asbestos litigation, most concerned with benign pleural disease and mesothelioma. However, occupational asthma and acute lung disease due to inhalation of toxic substances are common conditions, as

discussed in Chapters 34, 36 and 54, and there is a rising trend of litigation in these areas. Chronic airflow obstruction in groups of workers where epidemiological evidence suggests an increased risk, such as coal-miners and welders, has also been an increasing cause of litigation. Changes in the value of, and access to, disability benefits and reduction in regulation of industry as part of British government policy is likely to lead to a rising trend both of litigation and of the diseases that provoke it.

Postscript

Books such as this are not written overnight and, since this chapter was originally drafted, new Civil Procedure Rules have been introduced for actions in the English and Welsh (but not Scottish) courts. These respond to a report by Lord Justice Woolf which took a refreshing look at the waste of public money on much of this litigation. The Rules are happily consistent with the advice given above and should eliminate much of the unsatisfactory behaviour of doctors and other self-styled 'experts' taking on the role of advocate. They should also reduce the likelihood of busy and expensive doctors having to appear in court. With repect to experts, the Rules indicate that:

1 Evidence should be confined to that which is reasonably required to resolve the proceedings.

2 It is the duty of an expert to *help the court*.

3 This duty overrides any obligation to the person from whom the expert has received instruction.

The court will approve the appointment of experts and may direct that only one such be appointed, to be agreed by the two parties. The Rules set down the form and content of the report, as follows. It must:

1 be addressed to the court;

2 give details of the qualifications of the expert;

3 give details of the literature relied upon;

4 state who carried out any tests and give that person's qualifications;

5 where there is a range of opinion, summarize that range and give reasons for the expert's own opinion;

6 contain a summary of the conclusions reached;

7 contain a statement that the expert understands his/her duty to the court;

8 contain a statement setting out the written and oral instructions received; and

9 state as follows: 'I believe the facts I have stated in this report are true and that the opinions I have expressed are correct'.

This last statement may form an appropriate note on which to end this book. It is our hope that the facts stated herein mostly turn out to be true and that the opinions which we have expressed are sensible and ultimately benefit our patients.

INDEX

Note:
  Abbreviations:
    ARDS Adult respiratory distress syndrome
    BAL Bronchoalveolar lavage
    COPD Chronic obstructive pulmonary disease
    SLE Systemic lupus erythematosus
  Page numbers in **bold** refer to pages on which tables are located. Page numbers in *italics* refer to pages on which illustrations are found.
  This index is in letter-by-letter order whereby hyphens and spaces in index headings are ignored in the alphabetization.
  vs denotes differential diagnosis or comparisons.
  Volume 1 pp. 1–828; Volume 2 pp. 829–1542.

alveolar microlithiasis 1339–40
alveolar proteinosis *see* pulmonary alveolar
     proteinosis
alveolar sacs 15
alveolar ventilation 15, 27–8, 28
     mechanical ventilation 1501–2
alveolar wall 15–16
     cells *see* pneumocytes
     thickening
          cryptogenic fibrosing alveolitis 878,
               879
          silicosis 1422
alveoli 15
     anatomy and physiology 766–7
     collapse
          neonatal respiratory distress
               syndrome 712
          pulmonary embolism 722
     destruction in COPD 642
     development 3
     exudate, radiation pneumonitis 427
     number 3, 9
     rupture 1205
     structure 9, 15
     total surface area 15
alveolitis
     asbestosis 1429
     cryptogenic fibrosing *see* cryptogenic
          fibrosing alveolitis
     drug-induced 1460–5
          clinical features 1460–1
          drugs causing 1462, 1462–5
          mechanisms 1461–2
     fibrosing *see* fibrosing alveolitis
     hypersensitivity type 1465
     lymphocytic, radiation pneumonitis
          1471
Alzheimer's disease 1439
amantadine 242–3
     influenza 242, 243, 349
          prophylaxis 243
     structure *242*
ambroxol 1337
amenorrhoea 516, 862
American Thoracic Society
     antimycobacterial drugs susceptibility
          testing 567
     COPD definition 617
     lung sounds 116
     opportunistic mycobacterial disease 567
     pneumonia treatment guidelines 369,
          370–1
     questionnaires 75, 76
     severe pneumonia definition 373
     theophylline doses 254
     tuberculosis chemoprophylaxis
          499–500, *500*
amfebutamone 317
amikacin 213, 216
     tuberculosis 551, *551*
aminoglycosides 212–16
     administration, distribution and
          excretion 213
     adverse effects 213–14, *214*
          ototoxicity 864
     choice and uses 214
     in cystic fibrosis 864
     drug interactions 214
     nebulized 216
     spectrum of activity 212–13
     see also gentamicin
aminopenicillins 196–8
     pneumonia 368

aminophylline 252, 253, 255
     acute severe asthma treatment 987
     administration 254
     diaphragmatic fatigue 1236
     rectal administration 255
     uses/indications 256
aminorex, primary pulmonary
          hypertension after 755
amiodarone, side-effects 1463
amitriptyline 1528
ammonia fumes 1446
amniotic fluid embolism 722
amniotic membranes, premature rupture
          1315
amoebiasis 604–6
     empyema 449
     hepatic 1160
     thoracic 604–6
amoebic liver abscess 605, 1160
amoebic lung abscess 605, *606*
amosite 1174, 1424
amoxicillin 196–7
     administration and dose 197
     adverse effects 197
     bronchiectasis 817
     epiglottitis 340
     pneumonia 365
     prophylactic, pneumonia prevention
          383
     resistance/susceptibility 196–7
     sinusitis 344
amoxicillin–clavulanate (co-amoxiclav)
          197–8
amphiboles 1424, 1431, 1432
amphotericin 228–30
     administration, distribution and
          excretion 228–9
     adverse effects 229, 1350
     blastomycosis 578
     coccidioidomycosis 580
     dosage 229
     lipid formulations 229
     spectrum of activity 228
     structure *228*
     uses/indications 229–30, 1350
ampicillin 196–7
     administration and dose 197
     adverse effects 197
     bronchiectasis 817
     Moraxella catarrhalis pneumonia 411
     pneumococcal pneumonia 380
     resistance/susceptibility 196–7
ampicillin–sulbactam (sultamicillin) 197
amylases 1164
amyloidosis 1291, 1337–9, *1338*
     bronchiectasis complication 823
     classification 1337, *1337*
     generalized and localized types 1337,
          1337
     mediastinal 1291
     primary 1337
     secondary 1337
     tuberculosis complication 523
anaemia
     aplastic 228
     iron deficiency 1331, 1333
     megaloblastic 210
     zidovudine causing 237
anaerobes
     antibiotic sensitivity 468, 472
     culture and specimens for 468
     in saliva 460
     sputum culture 413

anaerobic infections
     acute sinusitis 342
     bronchiectasis and 809
     empyema 447, 448
     hospital-acquired pneumonia 372
     management 453–4
          clindamycin 219
          metronidazole 217–18
anaerobic threshold 55
anaesthesia
     percutaneous fine-needle biopsy 173
     topical
          complications 168–9
          fibreoptic bronchoscopy 153–4
anaesthetic agents, local, cough reflex
          inhibition 84, 1529
analeptic drugs 280
analgesia/analgesics *see* pain relief
anaphylactic reactions
     amphotericin 229
     cephalosporins 200
     early asthmatic response 908
anaphylaxis
     immunotherapy for asthma and 991
     management 195, 249
     penicillin reaction 195
anatomical dead space 13–14, 26–7, *27*,
          1501
     measurement 27, *27*
     type II respiratory failure 698–9
anatomy
     airways 11–14
     alveoli 766–7
     bronchi 9, *11*
     bronchioles 829
     endothelial cells 20, *21*
     left recurrent laryngeal nerve 19
     lung *10*, 10–11
     lymphatic ducts 1165–6
     mediastinum 1269
     nose *342*
     paranasal sinuses 341, *342*
     pleura 23, 1152, 1182
     pulmonary artery and arterioles 19, *20*
     in pulmonary oedema 766–8
     thoracic duct 1165–6
     thymus gland 1278–9
     turbinates *342*
Ancylostoma braziliense 1022
Ancylostoma duodenale 608
aneurysm
     aortic *see* aortic aneurysm
     carotid arteries 1298
     pulmonary arteriovenous 1322–6
angiitis, pulmonary lymphocytic *see*
          pulmonary lymphocytic angiitis
angina pectoris 248, 992
angiofollicular hyperplasia 1342
angiogenesis, asthma 918
angiography *see* pulmonary angiography
angioma, pulmonary and pulmonary
          cavernous *see* arteriovenous
          malformations
angioneurotic oedema 709
angioplasty, superior vena cava
          obstruction 1114
angiosarcoma (Kaposi's sarcoma) *see*
          Kaposi's sarcoma
angiotensin-converting enzyme (ACE)
     inhibitors, cough 104, 1460
     serum levels in sarcoidosis 1055–6
angiotensin I 20
angiotensin II 20